Current Techniques
in Small Animal Surgery

Current Techniques in Small Animal Surgery

Edited by
M. JOSEPH BOJRAB, DVM, MS, PhD
Diplomate, American College of Veterinary Surgeons
Professor and Head of Small Animal Surgery
Department of Veterinary Medicine and Surgery
University of Missouri
Columbia, Missouri

Consulting Soft Tissue Editor
STEPHEN W. CRANE, DVM
Diplomate, American College of Veterinary Surgeons
Professor of Surgery, Head of Companion Animal and Special Species
  Medicine
School of Veterinary Medicine, North Carolina State University
Raleigh, North Carolina

Consulting Bone and Joint Editor
STEVEN P. ARNOCZKY, DVM
Diplomate, American College of Veterinary Surgeons
Director, Laboratory of Comparative Orthopaedics
Hospital for Special Surgery
New York, New York

LEA & FEBIGER PHILADELPHIA

LEA & FEBIGER
600 Washington Square
Philadelphia, Pennsylvania 19106
U.S.A.

Library of Congress Cataloging in Publication Data

Main entry under title:
Current techniques in small animal surgery.

Bibliography: p.
Includes index.
1. Veterinary   surgery.   2. Dogs—Surgery.   3. Cats—Surgery.
I. Bojrab, M. Joseph.
SF911.C87 1983   636.089'7   82-24929
ISBN 0–8121–0862–0

PRINTED IN THE UNITED STATES OF AMERICA

Print No. 4 3 2

Preface

The second edition of *Current Techniques of Small Animal Surgery* continues to provide veterinary surgeons with a concise, up-to-date collection of current surgical techniques. This edition has been expanded and made more complete than the first edition, based on suggestions and comments from readers of the first edition. We have concentrated on improving and upgrading the line drawings for accuracy, clarity, and uniformity because they play an important role in the message of this text. Whenever a multiauthor text of this magnitude is assembled, some differences among authors will exist, but such differences do not detract from the major mission of this text, to provide a working, practical surgical reference.

Included in the expansion of this second edition is a section on surgical techniques for exotic species. This section describes the surgical procedures a practitioner is most often requested to perform on exotic animals. Other new subjects included in this edition are traumatic wounds and burns, suture materials, electrosurgical techniques, and restraint techniques.

Again, it must be emphasized that this text was not meant to replace more basic surgical texts. It mainly represents current accepted technique and not basic pathophysiology. For this reason, this text is complemented by *Pathophysiology in Small Animal Surgery*.

Doctors Arnoczky and Crane, Consulting Co-Editors, deserve my deepest gratitude for their tremendous help and advice. Above all, the more than one hundred contributors deserve thanks not only for their superior contributions, but also for their prompt and enthusiastic response.

I want to take this opportunity to thank the consulting artists, Mr. Don Conner and Dr. Kay Schwink, for their competent and dedicated work.

Columbia, Missouri   M. JOSEPH BOJRAB

Contributors

JOSEPH W. ALEXANDER, DVM, MS

Diplomate, American College of Veterinary Surgeons
Associate Professor of Surgery
Coordinator of Surgical Services
Virginia-Maryland Regional College of Veterinary
* Medicine*
Virginia Polytechnic Institute
Blacksburg, Virginia

WESLEY D. ANDERSON, DVM, PhD

Professor and Chairman of Veterinary Anatomy
College of Veterinary Medicine
The Ohio State University
Columbus, Ohio

STEVEN P. ARNOCZKY, DVM

Diplomate, American College of Veterinary Surgeons
Director, Laboratory of Comparative Orthopaedics
Associate Research Scientist
Head, Division of Laboratory Animal Resources
Hospital for Special Surgery
Associate Professor of Surgery
Cornell University Medical College
New York, New York
Adjunct Associate Professor of Surgery
New York State College of Veterinary Medicine
Cornell University
Ithaca, New York

DENNIS N. ARON, DVM

Diplomate, American College of Veterinary Surgeons
Assistant Professor of Small Animal Surgery
College of Veterinary Medicine
University of Georgia
Athens, Georgia

KATHLEEN P. BARRIE, DVM, MS

Diplomate, American College of Veterinary
* Ophthalmologists*
Adjunct Assistant Professor of Comparative
* Ophthalmology*
College of Veterinary Medicine
University of Florida
Gainesville, Florida
Ophthalmologist
Animal Eye Clinic
Tampa, Florida

C. W. BETTS, DVM

Diplomate, American College of Veterinary Surgeons
Professor and Section Chief of Small Animal Surgery
School of Veterinary Medicine
North Carolina State University
Raleigh, North Carolina

ANTHONY P. BLACK, BVSc

Fellow, Australian College of Veterinary Scientists
* (Surgery)*
Consultant Small Animal Surgeon
Sydney, Australia

MARK S. BLOOMBERG, DVM, MS

Diplomate, American College of Veterinary Surgeons
Assistant Professor and Chief of Small Animal
* Surgery*
College of Veterinary Medicine
University of Florida
Gainesville, Florida

RICHARD H. BÖHNING, JR., DVM

Director and Surgeon
Post Road Veterinary Hospital
New Rochelle, New York

M. JOSEPH BOJRAB, DVM, MS, PhD

Diplomate, American College of Veterinary Surgeons
Professor and Head of Small Animal Surgery
School of Veterinary Medicine
University of Missouri
Columbia, Missouri

EUGENE M. BREZNOCK, DVM, PhD

Diplomate, American College of Veterinary Surgeons
Associate Professor of Surgery
School of Veterinary Medicine
Chief of Small Animal Surgery
Veterinary Medical Teaching Hospital
University of California
Davis, California

RONALD M. BRIGHT, DVM, MS

Diplomate, American College of Veterinary Surgeons
Associate Professor of Small Animal Surgery
College of Veterinary Medicine
University of Florida
Gainesville, Florida

NANCY M. BROMBERG, VMD, MS

Director
Eye Clinic for Animals
Washington, D.C.

H. EDWARD CABAUD, MD

Research Orthopaedist
Letterman Army Institute of Research
Assistant Clinical Professor of Orthopaedics
School of Medicine
University of California
San Francisco, California

DENNIS D. CAYWOOD, DVM, MS

Diplomate, American College of Veterinary Surgeons
Head of Small Animal Surgery
Associate Professor of General and Orthopedic
*   Surgery*
College of Veterinary Medicine
University of Minnesota
St. Paul, Minnesota

VINCENT W. CHAFFEE, DVM, MS, PhD

Diplomate, American College of Veterinary Surgeons
Director of Veterinary Sciences
Whittaker-Toxigenics
Decatur, Illinois

THOMAS R. CHRISTIE, DVM

Diplomate, American College of Veterinary Surgeons
Staff Surgeon
Burleigh Road Animal Hospital
Brookfield, Wisconsin

ROGER M. CLEMMONS, DVM, PhD

Assistant Professor of Medical Science
College of Veterinary Medicine
University of Florida
Gainesville, Florida

BEN H. COLMERY, III, DVM

Assistant Adjunct Professor of Small Animal Surgery
*   and Medicine*
College of Veterinary Medicine
Michigan State University
East Lansing, Michigan
Director
Westarbor Animal Hospital
Ann Arbor, Michigan

ELLIOTT CRAIG, DVM

Staff Surgeon
Houston Veterinary Referral Hospital
Houston, Texas

STEPHEN W. CRANE, DVM

Diplomate, American College of Veterinary Surgeons
Professor of Surgery
Head of Companion Animal and Special Species
*   Medicine*
School of Veterinary Medicine
North Carolina State University
Raleigh, North Carolina

JAMES E. CREED, DVM

Diplomate, American College of Veterinary Surgeons
Professor of Veterinary Medicine and Surgery
Veterinary Teaching Hospital
Oklahoma State University
Stillwater, Oklahoma

DENNIS T. CROWE, DVM

Diplomate, American College of Veterinary Surgeons
Assistant Professor of Small Animal Surgery
College of Veterinary Medicine
Director of Shock-Trauma Team
Small Animal Teaching Hospital
University of Georgia
Athens, Georgia

MARK J. DALLMAN, DVM, MS, PhD

Assistant Professor of Veterinary Medicine and
*   Surgery*
Veterinary Teaching Hospital
University of Missouri
Columbia, Missouri

WILLIAM R. DALY, DVM

Diplomate, American College of Veterinary Surgeons
Staff Surgeon
Houston Veterinary Referral Hospital
Houston, Texas

MARY L. DULISCH, DVM, MS

Diplomate, American College of Veterinary Surgeons
Staff Surgeon
Angell Memorial Animal Hospital
Boston, Massachusetts

THOMAS D. EARLEY, DVM, MS

Director
Greater Atlanta Veterinary Referral Surgical Practice
Marietta, Georgia

MAX G. EASOM, DVM

Surgical Practitioner
Lakeland, Florida

DAVID F. EDWARDS, DVM

Diplomate, American College of Veterinary Internal
*   Medicine*
Assistant Professor of Pathobiology
College of Veterinary Medicine
University of Tennessee
Knoxville, Tennessee

ERICK L. EGGER, DVM

Diplomate, American College of Veterinary Surgeons
Assistant Professor of Veterinary Medicine
College of Veterinary Medicine and Biomedical
*   Sciences*
Colorado State University
Fort Collins, Colorado

MARK H. ENGEN, DVM

Diplomate, American College of Veterinary Surgeons
Practitioner

Puget Sound Animal Hospital for Surgery
Kirkland, Washington

GEORGE E. EYSTER, VMD

Diplomate, American College of Veterinary Surgeons
Professor of Cardiology
College of Veterinary Medicine
Michigan State University
East Lansing, Michigan

EDWARD C. FELDMAN, DVM

Diplomate, American College of Veterinary Internal
*   Medicine*
Assistant Professor of Reproduction
School of Veterinary Medicine
University of California
Davis, California

GRETCHEN L. FLO, DVM, MS

Professor of Surgery
College of Veterinary Medicine
Michigan State University
East Lansing, Michigan

DEAN R. GAHRING, DVM

Diplomate, American College of Veterinary Surgeons
Chief of Surgical Services
San Carlos Veterinary Hospital
San Diego, California

PAUL C. GAMBARDELLA, VMD, MS

Diplomate, American College of Veterinary Surgeons
Assistant Professor and Head of Small Animal
*   Surgery*
School of Veterinary Medicine
Tufts University
Boston, Massachusetts

KIRK N. GELATT, VMD

Diplomate, American College of Veterinary
*   Ophthalmologists*
Dean and Professor of Comparative Ophthalmology
College of Veterinary Medicine
University of Florida
Gainesville, Florida

JERRY A. GREENE, DVM, MS

Director
Academe Animal Hospital
Tampa, Florida

KENNETH M. GREENWOOD, DVM

Diplomate, American College of Veterinary Surgeons
Surgical Practitioner
Atlanta, Georgia

ROBERT M. GWIN, DVM, MS

Diplomate, American College of Veterinary
*   Ophthalmologists*
Director of Animal Research Facility
Dean A. McGee Eye Institute
Oklahoma City, Oklahoma
Adjunct Associate Professor
University of Oklahoma
Norman, Oklahoma

COLIN E. HARVEY, BVSc, MRCVS

Diplomate, American College of Veterinary Surgeons
Professor of Surgery
School of Veterinary Medicine
University of Pennsylvania
Philadelphia, Pennsylvania

H. JAY HARVEY, DVM

Diplomate, American College of Veterinary Surgeons
Assistant Professor of Surgery
New York State College of Veterinary Medicine
Cornell University
Ithaca, New York

HOWARD M. HAYES, JR., DVM

Staff Veterinarian
Environmental Epidemiology Branch
National Cancer Institute
National Institutes of Health
Bethesda, Maryland

MELVIN L. HELPHREY, DVM

Diplomate, American College of Veterinary Surgeons
Practitioner
Gulf Coast Veterinary Surgical Referral Service
Seminole, Florida

RALPH A. HENDERSON, JR., DVM

Diplomate, American College of Veterinary Surgeons
Associate Professor and Chief of Small Animal
*   Surgery*
Department of Small Animal Surgery and Medicine
Auburn University
Auburn, Alabama

WILLIAM B. HENRY, JR., DVM

Diplomate, American College of Veterinary Surgeons
Director of Surgical Services
South Shore Veterinary Associates
South Weymouth, Massachusetts
Clinical Professor of Surgery
School of Veterinary Medicine
Tufts University
Associate Orthopedist
Harvard Medical School
Associate Orthopedist
Massachusetts General Hospital
Boston, Massachusetts

MICHAEL R. HERRON, DVM

Diplomate, American College of Veterinary Surgeons
Professor of Small Animal Surgery
College of Veterinary Medicine
Texas A & M University
College Station, Texas

H. PHIL HOBSON, DVM

Diplomate, American College of Veterinary Surgeons
Professor and Chief of Small Animal Surgery
College of Veterinary Medicine
Texas A & M University
College Station, Texas

R. BRUCE HOHN, DVM, MS

Diplomate, American College of Veterinary Surgeons
Professor of Orthopedic Surgery
Head of Small Animal Surgery
College of Veterinary Medicine
Professor of Surgery
College of Medicine
The Ohio State University
Columbus, Ohio

DONALD R. HOWARD, DVM, PhD

Diplomate, American College of Veterinary Surgeons
Associate Dean of Academic Affairs
Professor of Surgery
School of Veterinary Medicine
North Carolina State University
Raleigh, North Carolina

DONALD A. HULSE, DVM

Diplomate, American College of Veterinary Surgeons
Professor of Surgery
School of Veterinary Medicine
Louisiana State University
Baton Rouge, Louisiana

DENNIS A. JACKSON, DVM, MS

Diplomate, American College of Veterinary Surgeons
Staff Surgeon
Animal Hospital for Referral Surgery
Vancouver, British Columbia, Canada

WILLIAM F. JACKSON, DVM, DSc (HON), MSc

Diplomate, American College of Veterinary Surgeons
and American College of Veterinary
Ophthalmologists
Practitioner
Animal Medical Clinic
Lakeland, Florida
Adjunct Clinical Professor of Comparative
Ophthalomology
College of Veterinary Medicine
University of Florida
Gainesville, Florida

PAUL B. JENNINGS, JR., VMD, MMEDSc(SURG)

Diplomate, American College of Veterinary Surgeons
Lieutenant-Colonel
Veterinary Corps
Commander
167th Medical Detachment
United States Army
Stuttgart, West Germany

DUDLEY E. JOHNSTON, BVSc, MVSc

Diplomate, American College of Veterinary Surgeons
Professor of Small Animal Surgery
School of Veterinary Medicine
University of Pennsylvania
Philadelphia, Pennsylvania

GARY R. JOHNSTON, DVM, MS

Diplomate, American College of Veterinary Radiology
Assistant Professor of Small Animal Clinical
Sciences
College of Veterinary Medicine
University of Minnesota
St. Paul, Minnesota

KENNETH G. KAGAN, VMD

Diplomate, American College of Veterinary Surgeons
Assistant Professor of Surgical Sciences
College of Veterinary Medicine
University of Florida
Gainesville, Florida

RONALD J. KOLATA, DVM

Diplomate, American College of Veterinary Surgeons
Associate Research Professor of Comparative
* Medicine*
School of Medicine
St. Louis University
St. Louis, Missouri

D. J. KRAHWINKEL, JR, DVM

Diplomate, American College of Veterinary Surgeons
Professor and Director of Surgery
College of Veterinary Medicine
University of Tennessee
Knoxville, Tennessee

JILL K. KUSBA, DVM

Practitioner
Milwaukee, Wisconsin

JOHN J. LAMMERDING, VMD

Diplomate, American College of Veterinary Surgeons
Director of Surgery
West Los Angeles Veterinary Medical Group
Los Angeles, California

GEORGE E. LEES, DVM, MS

Diplomate, American College of Veterinary Internal
* Medicine*
Associate Professor of Small Animal Medicine and
* Surgery*
College of Veterinary Medicine
Texas A & M University
College Station, Texas

ROBERT L. LEIGHTON, VMD

Diplomate, American College of Veterinary Surgeons
Professor of Surgery
School of Veterinary Medicine
University of California
Davis, California

NANCY A. LEITING, DVM

Associate Veterinarian
Niles Animal Hospital
Niles, Illinois

ARNOLD S. LESSER, VMD

Diplomate, American College of Veterinary Surgeons
Director and Surgeon
Flushing Veterinary Hospital
Flushing, New York

ALAN J. LIPOWITZ, DVM, MS

Diplomate, American College of Veterinary Surgeons
Associate Professor of Small Animal Surgery
College of Veterinary Medicine
University of Minnesota
St. Paul, Minnesota

CHARLES G. McLEOD, JR., DVM

Diplomate, American College of Veterinary
Pathologists
Chief of Comparative Pathology Branch
United States Army Medical Research Institute of
Chemical Defense
Aberdeen Proving Ground
Edgewood, Maryland

REUBEN MERIDETH, DVM

Practitioner
Eye Clinic for Animals
Tucson, Arizona

DENNIS J. MEYER, DVM

Diplomate, American College of Veterinary Internal
Medicine
Assistant Professor of Medical Sciences
College of Veterinary Medicine
University of Florida
Gainesville, Florida

JAMES L. MILTON, DVM

Diplomate, American College of Veterinary Surgeons
Associate Professor of Surgery
Department of Small Animal Surgery and Medicine
Auburn University
Auburn, Alabama

CECIL P. MOORE, DVM

Diplomate, American College of Veterinary
Ophthalmology
Assistant Professor of Surgical Sciences
School of Veterinary Medicine
University of Wisconsin
Madison, Wisconsin

WILLIAM W. MUIR, DVM

Diplomate, American College of Veterinary
Anesthesiologists
Professor and Chairman of Veterinary Clinical
Sciences
Professor of Physiology and Pharmacology
College of Veterinary Medicine
The Ohio State University
Columbus, Ohio

A. WENDELL NELSON, DVM, PhD

Diplomate, American College of Veterinary Surgeons
Head of Small Animal Surgery
Veterinary Teaching Hospital
Professor of Clinical Sciences
College of Veterinary Medicine and Biomedical
Sciences
Colorado State University
Fort Collins, Colorado

CARL A. OSBORNE, DVM, PhD

Diplomate, American College of Veterinary Internal
Medicine
Professor and Chairman of Small Animal Clinical
Sciences
College of Veterinary Medicine
Professor of Pediatrics
College of Medicine
University of Minnesota
St. Paul, Minnesota

ROBERT B. PARKER, DVM

Diplomate, American College of Veterinary Surgeons
Assistant Professor of Surgery
College of Veterinary Medicine
University of Florida
Gainesville, Florida

JOHN L. PARKS, DVM

Diplomate, American College of Veterinary Surgeons
Referral Surgeon
Eastchester Animal Clinic
Scarsdale, New York

MICHAEL M. PAVLETIC, DVM

Diplomate, American College of Veterinary Surgeons
Assistant Professor of Small Animal Surgery
School of Veterinary Medicine
Tufts University
Boston, Massachusetts

JAMES F. PEDDIE, DVM

Staff Surgeon
Conejo Valley Veterinary Clinic
Thousand Oaks, California

ROBERT L. PEIFFER, JR., DVM, PhD

Diplomate, American College of Veterinary
Ophthalmologists
Adjunct Associate Professor and Section Chief of
Ophthalmology
School of Veterinary Medicine
North Carolina State University
Raleigh, North Carolina
Associate Professor of Ophthalmology and Pathology
School of Medicine
University of North Carolina
Chapel Hill, North Carolina

MARK E. PETERSON, DVM

Staff Endocrinologist
Animal Medical Center
Director of Clinical Medicine
Cornell University Center for Research Animal
Resources
Cornell University Medical College
New York, New York
Assistant Professor of Medicine
New York State College of Veterinary Medicine
Cornell University
Ithaca, New York

GHERY D. PETTIT, DVM

Diplomate, American College of Veterinary Surgeons
Professor of Veterinary Clinical Medicine and
Surgery

Head of Small Animal Surgery
College of Veterinary Medicine
Washington State University
Pullman, Washington

LLEWELLYN C. PEYTON, DVM, MS

Assistant Professor of Large Animal Surgery
College of Veterinary Medicine
University of Florida
Gainesville, Florida

N. GAIL POWELL, DVM

Director
Atlanta Veterinary Eye Clinic
Avondale Estates, Georgia

RAYMOND G. PRATA, DVM

Diplomate, American College of Veterinary Surgeons
Director of Surgery
Animal Medical Center
New York, New York

CURTIS W. PROBST, DVM

Assistant Professor of Small Animal Surgery
College of Veterinary Medicine
Michigan State University
East Lansing, Michigan

CLARENCE A. RAWLINGS, DVM, PhD

Diplomate, American College of Veterinary
* Surgeons*
Professor of Small Animal Medicine, Physiology, and
* Pharmacology*
Chief of Staff of Small Animal Surgery
Veterinary Teaching Hospital
College of Veterinary Medicine
University of Georgia
Athens, Georgia

WAYNE R. RENEGAR, DVM

Surgical Consultant
Veterinary Surgery of New England
Hanson, Massachusetts
Surgical Consultant
Whitman Animal Hospital
Whitman, Massachusetts

DANIEL C. RICHARDSON, DVM

Diplomate, American College of Veterinary Surgeons
Assistant Professor of Small Animal Surgery
School of Veterinary Medicine
Purdue University
West Lafayette, Indiana

JOHN J. ROBERTSON, DVM

Clinical Instructor in Surgery
School of Veterinary Medicine
University of Missouri
Columbia, Missouri

WILLIAM G. RODKEY, DVM

Chief of Operative Services Group
Letterman Army Institute of Research
San Francisco, California

EBERHARD ROSIN, DVM, PhD

Diplomate, American College of Veterinary Surgeons
Associate Professor of Surgical Sciences
School of Veterinary Medicine
University of Wisconsin
Madison, Wisconsin

DONALD L. ROSS, DVM

Assistant Director of the Vivarium
School of Dentistry
University of Texas
Director
Houston Veterinary Dental Clinic
Houston, Texas

WILLIAM W. RYAN, DVM

Diplomate, American College of Veterinary Surgeons
Staff Surgeon
Oradell Animal Hospital
Oradell, New Jersey

ALFRED G. SCHILLER, DVM, MS

Diplomate, American College of Veterinary Surgeons
Assistant Head of Veterinary Clinical Medicine
College of Veterinary Medicine
University of Illinois
Urbana, Illinois

ANTHONY SCHWARTZ, DVM, PhD

Diplomate, American College of Veterinary Surgeons
Associate Professor and Chairman of Surgery
School of Veterinary Medicine
Tufts University
Staff Surgeon
Angell Memorial Animal Hospital
Boston, Massachusetts

HOWARD B. SEIM, III, DVM

Diplomate, American College of Veterinary Surgeons
Assistant Professor of Surgery
College of Veterinary Medicine and Biomedical
* Sciences*
Colorado State University
Fort Collins, Colorado

ROBERT R. SELCER, DVM

Diplomate, American College of Veterinary Internal
* Medicine*
Associate Professor of Neurology and Neurosurgery
College of Veterinary Medicine
University of Tennessee
Knoxville, Tennessee

VICTOR M. SHILLE, DVM, PhD

Diplomate, American College of Theriogenology
Associate Professor of Reproduction
College of Veterinary Medicine
University of Florida
Gainesville, Florida

PETER K. SHIRES, BVSc, MS, MRCVS

Diplomate, American College of Veterinary Surgeons
Assistant Professor of Surgery
School of Veterinary Medicine

Louisiana State University
Baton Rouge, Louisiana

KENNETH R. SINIBALDI, DVM

Diplomate, American College of Veterinary Surgeons
Staff Surgeon
Seattle Veterinary Hospital for Surgery
Seattle, Washington

JAMES E. SMALLWOOD, DVM, MS

Professor of Anatomy
School of Veterinary Medicine
North Carolina State University
Raleigh, North Carolina

KENNETH W. SMITH, DVM, MS

Diplomate, American College of Veterinary Surgeons
Professor Emeritus of Clinical Science
College of Veterinary Medicine and Biomedical
* Sciences*
Colorado State University
Fort Collins, Colorado

SHARON STEVENSON, DVM, MS

Diplomate, American College of Veterinary Surgeons
Postgraduate Research Pathologist
School of Veterinary Medicine
University of California
Davis, California

STEVEN G. STOLL, DVM

Diplomate, American College of Veterinary Surgeons
Practitioner
North Park Animal Clinic
Spokane, Washington

DAVID R. STOLOFF, DVM, MS

Diplomate, American College of Veterinary Surgeons
Staff Surgeon
Rowley Memorial Hospital
Springfield, Massachusetts

ELIZABETH A. STONE, DVM, MS

Diplomate, American College of Veterinary Surgeons
Assistant Professor of Surgery
School of Veterinary Medicine
University of Pennsylvania
Philadelphia, Pennsylvania

JOSEPH M. STOYAK, VMD

Lecturer in Surgery
School of Veterinary Medicine
Tufts University
Boston, Massachusetts
Chief of Staff and Director of Surgical Service
Rowley Memorial Hospital
Springfield, Massachusetts

GUY B. TARVIN, DVM

Diplomate, American College of Veterinary Surgeons
Surgical Practitioner
San Diego Veterinary Referral Service
San Diego, California

WILLIAM J. TAYLOR, DVM

Practitioner
Mountain Vista Animal Clinic
Las Vegas, Nevada

JERRY A. THORNHILL, DVM

Diplomate, American College of Veterinary Internal
* Medicine*
Assistant Professor of Small Animal Medicine
School of Veterinary Medicine
Purdue University
West Lafayette, Indiana

AMELIA A. TOOMEY, DVM

Practitioner
West Allis, Wisconsin

ERIC J. TROTTER, DVM, MS

Diplomate, American College of Veterinary Surgeons
Associate Professor of Surgery
New York State College of Veterinary Medicine
Cornell University
Ithaca, New York

THOMAS M. TURNER, DVM

Staff Surgeon
Berwyn Veterinary Associates
Berwyn, Illinois
Associate in Orthopedics
Rush Medical School
Chicago, Illinois

PHILIP B. VASSEUR, DVM

Diplomate, American College of Veterinary Surgeons
Assistant Professor of Surgery
School of Veterinary Medicine
University of California
Davis, California

STANLEY D. WAGNER, DVM

Assistant Professor of Small Animal Surgery
Veterinary Medical Teaching Hospital
Kansas State University
Manhattan, Kansas

DON R. WALDRON, DVM

Assistant Professor of Surgery
School of Veterinary Medicine
Louisiana State University
Baton Rouge, Louisiana

TOMMY L. WALKER, DVM, MS

Diplomate, American College of Veterinary Surgeons
Associate Professor of Surgery
College of Veterinary Medicine
University of Tennessee
Knoxville, Tennessee

LARRY J. WALLACE, DVM, MS

Diplomate, American College of Veterinary Surgeons
Professor of Small Animal Orthopedic Surgery
College of Veterinary Medicine
University of Minnesota
St. Paul, Minnesota

RICHARD WALSHAW, BVMS, MRCVS

Diplomate, American College of Veterinary Surgeons
Associate Professor of Small Animal Surgery
College of Veterinary Medicine
Michigan State University
East Lansing, Michigan

A. I. WEBB, BVSc, PhD, MRCVS

Diplomate, American College of Veterinary
* Anesthesiologists*
Assistant Professor and Chief of Anesthesia
College of Veterinary Medicine
University of Florida
Gainesville, Florida

WALTER E. WEIRICH, DVM

Diplomate, American College of Veterinary Surgeons
Professor and Head of Small Animal Clinics
School of Veterinary Medicine
Purdue University
West Lafayette, Indiana

CORNELIS J. G. WENSING, DVM, PhD

Professor of Anatomy and Embryology
School of Veterinary Medicine
State University of the Netherlands
Utrecht, Netherlands

GEORGE P. WILSON, VMD, MSc

Diplomate, American College of Veterinary Surgeons
Professor of Surgery
College of Veterinary Medicine
The Ohio State University
Columbus, Ohio

JAMES W. WILSON, DVM, MS

Diplomate, American College of Veterinary Surgeons
Assistant Professor of Surgical Sciences
School of Veterinary Medicine
University of Wisconsin
Madison, Wisconsin

WAYNE E. WINGFIELD, DVM, MS

Diplomate, American College of Veterinary Surgeons
Professor of Medicine
Chief of Emergency Medicine and Intensive Care
Veterinary Teaching Hospital
College of Veterinary Medicine and Biomedical
* Sciences*
Colorado State University
Fort Collins, Colorado

STEPHEN J. WITHROW, DVM

Diplomate, American College of Veterinary Surgeons
Associate Professor of Surgery
Chief of Clinical Oncology Service
College of Veterinary Medicine and Biomedical
* Sciences*
Colorado State University
Fort Collins, Colorado

E. DAN WOLF, DVM

Diplomate, American College of Veterinary
* Ophthalmologists*
Assistant Professor of Comparative Ophthalmology
College of Veterinary Medicine
University of Florida
Gainesville, Florida

DANIEL J. YTURRASPE, DVM, PhD

Diplomate, American College of Veterinary Surgeons
Staff Surgeon
White-Ivie Small Animal Hospital
San Bruno, California

ROBERT D. ZENOBLE, DVM, MS

Diplomate, American College of Veterinary Internal
* Medicine*
Associate Professor of Small Animal Surgery and
* Medicine*
School of Veterinary Medicine
Auburn University
Auburn, Alabama

Contents

Section C: Miscellaneous Orthopedic Techniques and Disorders

Part 1

Soft Tissue

Section A: Introductory Considerations

1 * Suture Materials

Characteristics and Selection of Currently Available Suture Materials

by STEPHEN W. CRANE

Suture technology has advanced significantly in the past decade. The current definitive trend is toward abandoning some of the suture products that have been used for almost a century in favor of newly developed synthetic materials. These sutures have improved physical and chemical characteristics that allow many of them to approximate closely the criteria for an "ideal" suture material. The purpose of this chapter is to review principles of suture selection as they relate to currently available suture products in veterinary surgical practice.

Ideal Suture Materials

The properties of an ideal suture material have been frequently described, but have yet to be obtained in any single product. Among ideal features are high initial tensile strength coupled with ultimate and total biodegradability at a predictable rate. This feature is desirable because the breaking, bursting, and tensile strengths of the wound are initially zero, but rapidly increase over a period of days and weeks. The wound slowly increases in strength as the scar matures over months and years.

Another important feature of the ideal suture material is total bioinertness. The suture material should not predispose the patient to pain, swelling, loss of function or motion, febrile response, allergy, delay in wound healing, carcinogenesis, or infection. In its physical properties, the ideal suture material should be fine in caliber, yet strong and supple, and it should not retain "memory" of its packaging configuration. The material should pass through tissues without friction, grabbing, cutting, or vibrating. The suture should handle as well, or better, when wet as when dry and should tie into the commonly used surgical knots with precision and ease. Once tied, the loss of strength at the knot should be minimal. The security of the knot should be absolute, with no tendency for slipping or hygroscopic swelling and loosening. The ideal material should also be totally sterile, packaged for the convenient maintenance of sterility, readily available, and inexpensive. It would be ideal if the material could be resterilized by pressurized steam or ethylene oxide without altering its physical or chemical characteristics. Polydioxanone, a monofilament synthetic absorbable material, fulfills many of the requirements of an ideal suture material.

Effect on Wound Healing

Suture material, being placed within and across the wound, exerts an influence on healing. Historically, this influence has been negative, and concerted efforts have been made to identify more biologically compatible and less-reactive suture materials. Another approach has been the development of metal clips and staples, wound tapes, and a variety of tissue adhesives, in an attempt to obviate sutures. Some of these products, staples in particular, offer technical and biologic advantages and are currently accepted alternatives.

Importantly, how any suture material is used—the judgment and manual craft used in suture technique—is often equally or even more significant than the type of suture material selected. For example, it is considered proper surgical technique to implant the minimum-needed quantity of suture material within the wound. This teaching results from common clinical experiences and controlled research, which indicated that a wound is more susceptible to infection when a suture is present. This observation causes one to appreciate that any suture material is a toxic, foreign-body prosthesis that inhibits normal tissue defenses and the local events in primary wound healing. The burden imposed by excessive numbers of sutures, overly large sutures, sutures that are tied too loosely or too tightly, bulky knots, and suture ends that are too long can contribute greatly to the production of an inflamed wound, excessive dead space, and predisposition to fluid accumulation, delayed healing, infection, and dehiscence.

Despite the critical importance of suture technique to uncomplicated primary wound healing, the selection of suture material itself is also extremely important to the success of the surgical procedure and the postoper-

Table 1-1. *Available Suture Materials*

Suture's Generic Description	*Trade Name*	*Origin*	*Size-to-Strength Ratio* *Knot-pull Tensile Strength*	*Relative Knot Security*	*Handling Ease*
"Plain catgut" spun and bonded collagen filaments	—	Mammalian collagen, usually derived from intestinal submucosa	Relatively low	Knots may loosen when wet	Very good
"Chromacized catgut"	—	As above, but "tanned" in solutions of chromium salts	Relatively low	Knots may loosen when wet	Very good
Braided polyglycolic acid	Dexon-S	Glycolic acid polymer	High	Good	Fair
Coated, braided polyglycolic acid	Dexon-Plus	Glycolic acid, polymer coated with surfactant	High	Good	Very good
Coated braided polyglactin 910	Coated Vicryl	Glycolic-lactic acid copolymer, coated with calcium stearate	High	Good	Fair
Monofilament Polydioxanone	PDS	Paradioxanone polymer	Very high	Good	Very good
Braided or twisted silk	—	Silkworm cocoon fibers	Moderate	Good	Excellent
Braided polyester fiber	Dacron Mersilene Polydek	Extruded synthetic resin polymers	Very high	Fair	Fair
Coated, braided polyester fiber	Ethibond Tevdek Ticron	As above, but coated or impregnated with Teflon polybutilate or silicone	Very high	Fair to poor, requires proper technique	Fair
Silicone treated, braided nylon	Surgilon	Polyamide polymer	High	Fair to good	Very good
Monofilament nylon	Dermalon Ethilon	Extruded polyamide filament	High	Fair (poor in large sizes)	Fair to poor (stiff)
Monofilament polypropylene	Prolene Surgilene	Polymerized polyolefin hydrocarbons	Very high	Fair (poor in large sizes)	Fair to good
Monofilament polyethylene	Dermalene	Linearly polymerized ethylene	High	Good	Good
Monofilament stainless steel wire	—	Ductile surgical-grade stainless steel alloy	Very high	Excellent	Poor
Twisted multifilament stainless steel wire	Flexon	As above	Very high	Excellent	Fair to good
Polyfilament polyamide polymer encased in outer tubular sheath	Suprylon Vetafil Braunamid	Polyamide polymer	High	Good	Very good
Surgical linen	—	Vegetable fibers (flax)	Low	Good	Poor
Surgical cotton	—	Vegetable fibers (long-staple cotton)	Low (higher when wet)	Good	Poor
Stainless steel and tantalum clips	Hemoclip Versa-Clip	Malleable surgical-grade steel or tantalum	N.A.	N.A.	Excellent

Tissue Reactivity	Duration and Mode of Degradation	Comments
Very high	U.S.P. does not classify absorption in terms of days; many factors influence rate of absorption, including chromatization; degradation is by proteolytic enzymes and phagocytic cells; loss of tensile strength is unpredictable, but one-third of strength is usually lost in first week	A material useful for inciting local inflammation and subsequent fibrosis
High		A traditional nonabsorbable that is being replaced by synthetic absorbable products in many practices
Initially moderate, but low during absorption	Absorbed by hydrolysis; main by-products of degradation are CO_2 and water	More controlled physical characteristics, rate of absorption, less tissue reaction, and improved performance in contaminated or infected tissues are advantages to these suture materials over chromacized catgut; Dexon-Plus handles best
Initially moderate, but low during absorption		
Initially moderate, but low during absorption		
Initially modest, but low during absorption	Hydrolytic degradation of polymer is slower than for braided synthetic absorbable sutures. 58% strength remains at 4 weeks. Complete absorption at 180 days.	Advantages include monofilament configuration, and extreme strength. Retention of suture strength and absorption is 2 to 3 times that of braided absorbable products.
Moderately high	Mechanical fragmentation and breakage often occur within one year	Contraindicated in urinary system, biliary system, or in presence of infection and contamination
Low	Permanent and relatively nonreactive; excellent retention of tensile strength	Extremely strong material with good flex durability; useful for prosthetic implantation
Low	Coatings fragment with time and increase tissue reaction	Passes through tissue with ease and handles better than uncoated polyester suture
Very low	Nylon possesses a slow loss of tensile strength with release of polyamide radicals; these have bacteriostatic properties that inhibit infection	40% stronger than silk with better permanence and less tissue reactivity; handles much better than monofilament nylon
Very low		An excellent general-purpose material; care is required making knots
Extremely low	Permanent and nonreactive	Suture of choice for many nonabsorbable applications; care is required in making knots
Low	Slow loss of tensile strength	A useful, general-purpose nonabsorbable suture; preferred over nylon, steel, and polyfilament sutures for skin closure
Low	Permanent; poor flex durability	Many buried steel sutures eventually break
Low	Permanent; better flex durability than monofilament wire	Handles better than monofilament wire; may be suture of choice in some ligament-bone and tendon repair
Low (if outer envelope breaks, reaction increases)	Outer envelope subject to breakage	Loses strength when autoclaved, yet must be sterilized prior to use; good skin closure material, but should not be buried in tissue
High	Loss of mechanical strength within months	Not recommended; substitute a stronger and less-reactive nonabsorbable suture
High	Loss of mechanical strength and fragmentation is present within one year	Not recommended; substitute a stronger and less-reactive nonabsorbable suture
Very low	Permanent	Clips allow rapid and convenient vessel and small-pedicle ligation

ative responses of local tissues. Because of the differences in suture materials, it is convenient to classify suture materials by category, based on their physical and chemical configurations and their fate in biologic tissue.

Physical Characteristics

Physical features that affect the suitability of a suture material for a particular task are size, direct-pull tensile strength, knot-pull tensile strength, characteristics of spinning, twisting, or braiding, surface smoothness and coefficient of friction, surface coating or fiber impregnation with lubricants, and uniformity of manufacture. These and other features influence the "stiffness" of the suture, the handling characteristics, the strength available per unit of cross-sectional area, and the knot security.

The volume of interstitial space available between filaments to harbor fluid, cellular debris, and bacteria are other important characteristics of braided materials, as opposed to monofilament suture materials. Knot security is an important feature of a suture material for obvious reasons. The weakest point in the individual suture or in a continuously placed suture is at the knot because tension forces are converted into shearing forces at crossing points within the tied knot loops. The magnitude of pull force necessary to break the knot varies with the size of the suture loop, the type of material, and the suture diameter. The relative knot security is described as knot slippage divided by knot breaking strength. Knot security is influenced by the quality of the knot tied (does it interlock or slip?), by the surface coefficient of friction, and by the size of the suture material. The larger the material, the stiffer the material, and the more "slippery" the suture, the more careful the surgeon must be to create properly interlocking, flat, and "snugged-down" square knots.

It is stated that braided sutures usually handle better than monofilaments. Another generalization is that the interstices between fibers of a braided suture material enhance the chances for clinical infection through the consequences of surface fluid capillary action. Broken braided or polyfilament sutures may also fistulate. The chemical nature of the suture material, any by-products of suture degradation, the duration of the suture's existence within the tissue, and the surgeon's technique also influence the predisposition to infection and fistulization.

Chemical Characteristics

The origins of suture-material filaments are plants or animals or a variety of man-made products. The generic chemical composition is, of course, elemental in determining the characteristics and biologic reactions of the material. As mentioned, the chemical by-products of degradation of some materials, nylon in particular, may be important inhibitors of bacterial colonization and infection.

Absorbable Versus Nonabsorbable Suture

Traditionally, the rate of loss of tensile strength of a suture material after implantation determines whether it is classified as absorbable or nonabsorbable. Absorbable materials are considered to have little if any tensile strength remaining after 60 days in an in vivo environment, and should eventually be completely removed from the body. These sutures are derived from both nature and man-made sources. Their applications, of course, are when only short-term holding power is needed. Body-wall closure, subcutaneous tissue closure, mucosal approximations of tubular viscera, corneal-scleral suturing, and joint capsule closures are examples of tissue coaptations in which absorbable materials are frequently used.

Nonabsorbable sutures are also derived from both natural and synthetic sources. Long-term stabilizations of any type require nonabsorbable materials, including those situations in which sutures are employed as a prosthesis, or when a prosthesis is implanted. Such nonabsorbable material is also indicated whenever clinical judgment predicts delayed wound healing for any reason. For example, nonabsorbable materials, such as polypropylene, are frequently selected for body-wall closures in debilitated patients undergoing emergency celiotomy. Some veterinarians prefer to approximate the mucosa of tubular viscera with absorbable sutures and then to close the nonluminal layers with a nonabsorbable product. Obviously, nonabsorbable materials should be used in tissues that are subject to movement and are normally slow to heal, such as tendons, ligaments, and bone. Importantly, certain nonabsorbable suture materials are the strongest, most flexible, and least reactive of the materials and, therefore, offer significant advantages in many applications.

Recommendations for Selection

Table 1-1 reviews several aspects of commonly used materials in veterinary surgical practice. Although most of this material is summarized from current literature, the "comments" should be considered as my own opinion.

References and Suggested Readings

Edlich, R. F., et al.: Physical and chemical configuration of sutures in the development of surgical infection. Ann. Surg., *177*:679, 1973.

Postlethwait, R. W.: Five year study of reaction to synthetic sutures. Ann. Surg., *196*:54, 1979.

Ray, J. A., et al.: Polydioxanone (PDS), a novel monofilament synthetic absorbable suture. Surg. Gynecol. Obstet., *153*:497, 1981.

Thacker, J. G., et al.: Mechanical performance of sutures in surgery. Am. J. Surg., *133*:713, 1977.

2 * Electrosurgical Techniques

Electrosurgical Techniques in Small Animal Practice

by ROBERT B. PARKER

Electrosurgical units are probably among the most frequently used and least understood surgical instruments. Little information is available in the veterinary literature concerning basic electronics, proper surgical techniques, and potential hazards. Judicious use of electrosurgery can be of great benefit to the veterinarian in maintaining a bloodless field, but indiscriminate use can create serious complications. The following discussion describes available electrosurgical methods and apparatus and provides a guideline for their proper use.

Electrolysis

Electrolysis implies a unidirectional, direct-current flow that produces strong polarity in the anode and cathode (Fig. 2-1). The system is of low voltage and amperage. When the electrodes are inserted into the body, hydroxides are produced at the treatment cathode by the following formula:

$$2\,NaCl + 4\,H_2O \rightarrow 2\,NaOH + 2\,H_2 \text{ (cathode)}$$
$$\searrow 2\,HCl + O_2 \text{ (anode)}$$

The hydroxides liquify tissue, yet produce minimal discomfort.

Electroepilation has been used in ophthalmic surgery for treatment of ectopic cilia or distichiasis. The fine-cathode electrode is passed to the base of the cilia, where the current and hydroxides liquify and destroy the ciliary root.

Electrocautery

The use of cautery to control hemorrhage dates back to ancient times, when a hot iron was used to cauterize wounds. More sophisticated microcautery is now available, but the technique of direct heat application is the same.

Low-voltage current is used to heat the treatment electrode, and therefore, electrical energy does not pass through the body (Fig. 2-2). The destructive effect is heat coagulation, and the temperature is proportional to the intensity of the current flowing through the resistance of the tip.

Advantages of this technique are (1) the degree of tissue damage is apparent, (2) it coagulates well in a bloody field, and (3) it is inexpensive and simple. The disadvantages are (1) tissue destruction can be extensive and (2) large lesions are slowly destroyed.

Electrocautery units are generally reserved for minor surgical procedures, such as dewclaw or tail

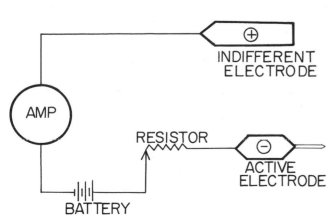

Fig. 2-1. *Basic circuit diagram for an electrolysis unit.*

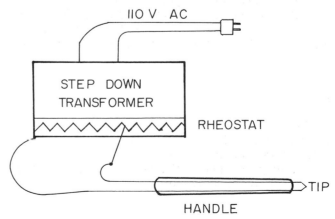

Fig. 2-2. *Basic circuit diagram for a thermal electrocautery unit.*

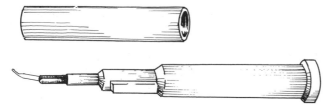

Fig. 2-3. *Disposable electrocautery unit.*

removal in puppies. Disposable electrocautery units, frequently used in ophthalmic surgery, provide fine hemostasis by pinpoint heat application (Fig. 2-3).

High-Frequency Electrosurgery

Most electrosurgical units available today fall into this category. The unit is essentially a radio transmitter that produces an oscillating high-frequency electrical field of 500,000 to 100,000,000 hertz (cycles per second). Above 10,000 hertz, current can be passed through the body without pain or muscle contraction. In contrast to electrocautery, the treatment electrode is not hot, but serves to deliver electrical energy at a concentrated area. The electrosurgical effect is determined by (1) the tissue resistance, (2) the mode of application, and (3) the amount and type of current. These factors can be modified to produce the desired surgical response.

Body tissue and fluids have a definite electrical impedence or resistance. Heat is produced by the resistance to current flow as electrical energy is absorbed and converted to thermal energy. Because resistance is inversely proportional to surface area, resistance decreases as the current spreads over the body.

The mode of application can be either uni- or biterminal. Biterminal application, used most frequently with cutting or coagulation, implies the use of an indifferent electrode or "ground plate" (Fig. 2-4). The indifferent electrode collects the current when it has passed through the body and dissipates it over a large surface area to produce a low-current density. Because heat production is inversely proportional to the contact area, the large size of the indifferent electrode evenly distributes the heat to prevent burning. The active electrode concentrates the same energy at a small point and produces the surgical effect (Fig. 2-5).

With the uniterminal technique, the patient is not incorporated into the electrical circuit. An indifferent

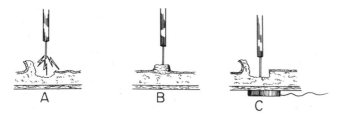

Fig. 2-4. *Uniterminal techniques, electrofulguration (A) and electrodesiccation (B). Biterminal techniques, electrotomy and electrocoagulation (C).*

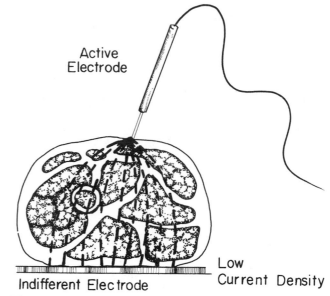

Fig. 2-5. *High current density at the active electrode and low current density with a properly placed indifferent electrode.*

electrode is not used, and the electrical energy is absorbed by the patient and is radiated into the air. Thus, sparking is produced at the tip and is directly applied to the lesion to cause either fulguration or desiccation (see Fig. 2-4).

Most modern electrosurgical units provide different wave forms to bring about either cutting or coagulation. An undamped, continuous sine wave makes the most effective cutting current (Fig. 2-6). Little hemostasis is achieved with a pure sine wave. In older units, a triode vacuum tube was used to produce the sine wave, but newer solid-state units use electronic circuitry to yield a more refined current. A series of damped or interrupted waves achieve coagulation with limited

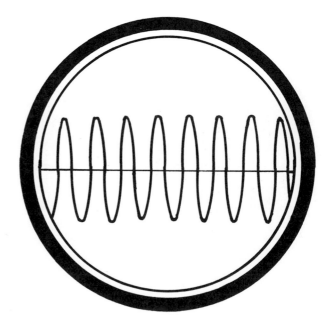

Fig. 2-6. *Undamped, continuous sine waves.*

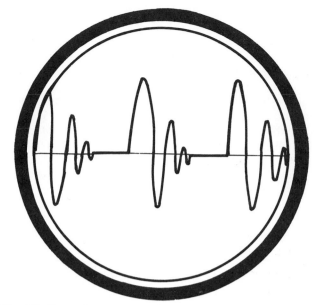

Fig. 2-7. *Damped waves.*

cutting capability (Fig. 2-7). Blended currents are possible, to produce a combined cutting and coagulation mode (Fig. 2-8). The more expensive units are capable of varying the "on-to-off" time to accomplish degrees of cutting versus coagulation.

Surgical Techniques

These include electrotomy, electrocoagulation, and electrofulguration and electrodesiccation.

ELECTROTOMY

Electroincision of any tissue causes greater tissue damage than sharp incision; therefore, the veterinarian must weigh the advantages of reduced blood loss and

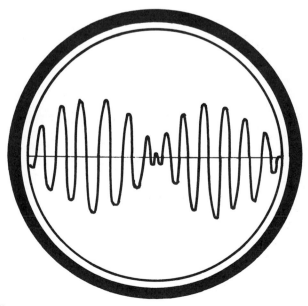

Fig. 2-8. *Blended waves.*

operating time against the disadvantages of increased tissue destruction and healing time. Electroincision of the skin heals primarily, but a definite lag is seen in the ultimate healing of the wound. Healing does occur, however, and maximal breaking strength is achieved.

The primary indications for electroincision of the skin are in patients with clotting disorders or when anticoagulant treatment is anticipated, such as with cardiopulmonary bypass procedures. Because of the initial delay in wound healing, it is recommended that skin sutures remain approximately 2 to 3 days longer with a skin incision made with an electrosurgical unit. The amount of coagulation and necrosis is proportional to the amount of heat produced and its duration of contact. Therefore, it is best to use a smooth, swift stroke when using an electrosurgical scalpel.

An electrosurgical scalpel has been used to cut virtually every type of tissue; its use in division of muscle or other highly vascular tissue is generally accepted procedure. By using blended currents, muscular tissue can be divided with less blood loss and in less operating time. The small blood vessels traversing muscular tissue can be effectively coagulated without the necessity of using ligatures that are difficult to place unless one includes significant amounts of normal tissue. With electrotomy of muscular tissues, particular attention should be made to large vessels; they can be incompletely coagulated, may retract, and may form a hematoma. If muscle twitching is a problem, one should tense the muscle between one's fingers to facilitate transection.

Although I do not routinely use them, electrosurgical scalpels and loops have been advocated for performing tonsillectomies, uvulectomies, ventriculocordectomies, anal sacculectomies, and skin tumor resections.

ELECTROCOAGULATION

The electrosurgical apparatus is extremely useful for coagulation of small bleeding vessels. A damped wave pattern provides the ultimate current for coagulation. Proper technique is required, and the technique of "frying tissue until it pops" is to be avoided. This practice is comparable to mass ligation of a bleeding point, and both lead to unnecessary tissue necrosis.

Vessels less than 1.5 mm in diameter can be sealed by pinpoint electrocoagulation. If larger vessels are coagulated by this method, delayed breakdown and hemorrhage may occur. Because fluids are current conductors, the field must be dry in the area surrounding the bleeding vessel. There are two ways to coagulate a bleeding vessel properly. The first is to apply the activated tip directly onto the vessel. The end point of coagulation is determined by tissue contraction and color change. A more precise method is to occlude the vessel initially with a hemostat or plain tissue thumb forceps. The active electrode is applied directly to the surgical instrument, which carries the current directly to the vessel. Care should be taken to prevent unwanted coagulation by not allowing the instrument to rest on normal tissue when the current is applied.

ELECTROFULGURATION AND ELECTRODESICCATION

These electrosurgical techniques cause dehydration and superficial destruction by a high-voltage, high-frequency current. These techniques are uniterminal, an indifferent electrode is not used. Electrofulguration damages tissue by electrical energy transmitted through an electrical arc or spark. Electrodesiccation is similar, although the electrode directly touches the lesion (see Fig. 2-4). Tissue damage is deeper than with fulguration and may be difficult to control. Electrofulguration of perianal fistulas following a sharp "deroofing" procedure has produced encouraging results. Electrodesiccation has been used for removal of superficial skin lesions.

Precautions

Accidental burns are probably the most frequently observed complication of electrosurgery. It is imperative that an adequate indifferent electrode ("ground plate") be incorporated in the system. Because of its large surface area, the indifferent electrode normally provides a low-current density to complete the electrosurgical circuit. If contact between the patient and plate is inadequate, however, high-density electrical current can easily cause a burn (Fig. 2-9). Although the indifferent electrode is designed to be the preferential pathway for the current, a faulty connection between the plate and the unit can result in a burn where the patient touches the metal operating table or the attachment sites of electrical monitoring equipment. More expensive units have a 60-cycle monitoring current flowing through the "ground-plate" system. A break in the ground wire or in its ground-plate connection interrupts the monitoring current and sounds an alarm. Electrolyte jellies and a large area of contact with the patient are recommended to lower skin resistance and to provide a more intimate contact between the skin and the indifferent electrode.

Explosions and fire are potential hazards when inflammable anesthetics, such as ether, chloroform, and cyclopropane, and inflammable skin preparations, such as alcohol, are used.

Electrical channeling occurs when the treatment electrode is used on tissue that has a thin connection to the body. An example is the testicle mobilized out of the scrotum. If electrocoagulation is used, electric energy will be channeled or funneled along the spermatic cord and will cause heat damage.

Cardiac pacemakers are being implanted with increasing frequency in veterinary medicine, and the veterinary surgeon should be aware that high-frequency electric energy may cause a cardiac arrest by interfering with the operation of the pacemaker.

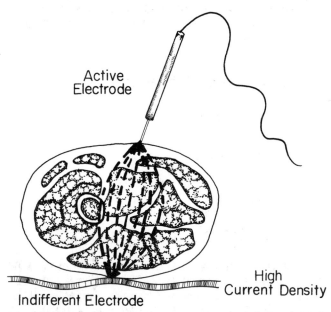

Fig. 2-9. *High current density produced at the indifferent electrode with improper technique.*

References and Suggested Readings

Battig, C. G.: Electrosurgical burn injuries and their prevention. JAMA, *204*:91, 1968.

Giddard, D. W., Jones, W. R., and Wescott, J. W.: Electrosurgical units: particular attention to tube, spark gap and solid state generated currents—their differences and similarities. J. Urol., *107*:1051, 1972.

Glover, J. L., Bendick, P. J., and Link, W. J.: The use of thermal knives in surgery: electrosurgery, lasers, plasma scalpel. Curr. Probl. Surg., *15*:7, 1978.

Greene, J. A., and Knecht, C. D.: Electrosurgery: a review. Vet. Surg., *9*:27, 1980.

Greene, J. A., and Knecht, C. D.: Healing of sharp incisions and electroincisions in dogs: a comparative study. Vet. Surg., *9*:42, 1980.

Ormrod, A. N.: Electrosurgery: its usefulness and limitations for the small animal surgeon. Vet. Rec., *75*:1095, 1963.

Swerdlow, D. B., et al.: Electrosurgery: principles and use. Dis. Colon Rectum, *17*:482, 1974.

Wald, A. S., Mazzia, V. D. B., and Spencer, F. C.: Accidental burns associated with electrocautery. JAMA, *217*:916, 1971.

3 * Restraint Techniques

Restraint Techniques for Prevention of Self-Trauma

by Howard B. Seim, III, James E. Creed, *and* Kenneth W. Smith

Numerous techniques to prevent self-trauma have been described, and even more have been used by practicing veterinarians. This chapter deals with an assortment of devices that we have learned about or have created for the prevention of self-trauma. We describe methods of assembly, materials necessary, specific indications, contraindications, and complications of each device.

Self-trauma prevention techniques can be divided into two groups: chemical agents and mechanical devices. Those included are as follows:

Chemical Restraint Agents
  Tranquilizers
  Noxious-tasting agents
    Variton*
    Bitter apple
    Obtundia†
    Tabasco
    Stoma-nil‡
    Thumb-sucking preparations§

Mechanical Restraint Devices
  Elizabethan collar
  Body brace
  Side bar
  Stockinette body bandage
  Emergency ear laceration protector
  Ear laceration protector
  Taping ears to the head
  Cast
  Schroeder-Thomas splint with sheet aluminum
  Soft padded bandage
  Hobbles
    Hock, carpal, stifle-to-tail
  Tail-tip protector

*Schering Corp., Kenilworth, NJ 07033
†Otis Clapp & Sons, Inc., 143 Albany Street, Cambridge, MA 02139
‡Dow B. Hickam, Inc., P.O. Box 35413, Houston, TX 77035
§Thum, Num Specialty, Inc., P.O. Box 326, Murrysville, PA 15668

Chemical Restraint Agents

Tranquilizers have been advocated to restrain patients from inflicting self-trauma. These drugs must be used with some caution, as they are often insufficient when used alone. In combination with other devices, however, these agents are often efficacious.

Noxious-tasting agents should also be used with discretion. Some patients endure the taste of a particular one, so these substances are not always dependable. Many such agents are available; alternating them helps to prevent the patient from becoming accustomed to one. The combined use of mechanical restraint devices and chemical agents has been helpful in controlling intractable patients.

Mechanical Restraint Devices

ELIZABETHAN COLLAR

Materials
  Commercial
    Plastic collars‖
    Cardboard collars#
  Handmade
    Cardboard
    X-ray film
    Plastic bucket or waste basket

Method of Assembly. Cardboard collars are best suited for dogs weighing 15 to 30 lb. X-ray film can be used to construct collars for cats and small dogs (under 15 lb). Regardless of material selected, the method of assembly is the same. An appropriately sized circle is cut from material used. The collar's size is dependent on the size of dog and the purpose for which the collar is to be used. When completed, the collar should extend 1 to 2 inches beyond the patient's nose. A cut is then made from the edge of the circle to the center. A small circle, slightly larger than the patient's neck, is then cut from the center. Adhesive tape

‖ Buster collar, Dr. Jorgensen Laboratories, P.O. Box 872, Loveland, CO 80537
#Medicollar, Evsco Pharmaceutical Corp., P.O. Box 29, Harding Highway, Buena, NJ 08310

may be applied to the edge of the circular cut to protect the neck from any sharp edges. The collar is then placed around the patient's neck, and the edges are overlapped until the collar fits snugly. It should be tight enough to allow no more than one finger between the edge of the collar and the patient's neck. The collar is then secured by taping the overlapping edges (Fig. 3-1). The inside and outside edges should be taped to prevent trauma to the patient's face and to keep the edges from catching on objects. After application, rostral traction should be applied on the collar to make sure it will not slip off.

An alternate method for construction of an effective cardboard collar is to cut the center just large enough to permit forcing it over the head and ears. The result is a flat collar instead of a cone shape. The advantages of this type collar are comfort, acceptance, and better peripheral vision; disadvantages are ease with which the collar can slip off and greater width. The patient's personality largely determines which technique one should employ.

Cardboard and x-ray film collars should not be used on large dogs (over 30 lb). Cardboard is not durable

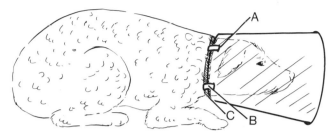

Fig. 3-2. *Waste basket extending well beyond dog's nose. A, hole cut in bottom of basket 1 to 2 cm from cut edge; B, gauze tied to form loop; C, leather collar or gauze tied around neck.*

enough and x-ray film is not large enough to be effective. Instead, plastic buckets, waste baskets, or commercially available Elizabethan collars should be used.

Commercially available collars are similar in function to those previously described. The major difference is in their attachment to the patient. Plastic loops located around the inner edge of the Elizabethan collar are used to attach it to a leather or gauze collar placed around the patient's neck. The collar should be tight enough so as not to slip over the head. Such collars are durable and come in several sizes.

Plastic buckets or waste baskets of medium size can also be used for large dogs. They protect the front legs more effectively than regular Elizabethan collars. A circle is cut out of the bottom of the bucket just large enough to slip over the patient's head. Cloth tape or elastic adhesive tape* bandage is placed over the resulting sharp plastic edge to protect the patient's neck. Four or more holes are punched around the bottom of the bucket about 1 cm away from the cut edge. Gauze bandage is then placed through each hole and is tied to itself to form a loop. A leather or gauze collar is threaded through these loops and is secured around the dog's neck (Fig. 3-2). The only disadvantage of this variation of an Elizabethan collar is that the amount of material extending beyond the patient's muzzle can make eating and drinking difficult. Feeding and watering the patient on a slightly elevated surface help to eliminate this problem, or it may be necessary to remove the plastic bucket for feeding and watering.

INDICATIONS. Elizabethan collars are versatile, widely accepted, and have few contraindications or complications. These collars prevent self-trauma if they are large enough to prevent the animal from licking, scratching, or chewing the affected area. These collars are especially useful for preventing self-trauma following surgical procedures and can also be used in conjunction with other mechanical restraint devices.

CONTRAINDICATIONS. Elizabethan collars are not effective in restraining patients from fore and hind extremity mutilation, unless long plastic waste baskets or large plastic cone-shaped collars are used.

COMPLICATIONS. The most devastating potential complication is from applying the collar too tightly, which

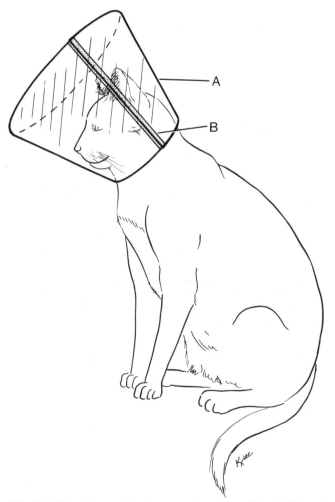

Fig. 3-1. *Elizabethan collar. A, x-ray film (14 × 17 inch); B, taped overlapped edge of film.*

*Elasticon Elastic Tape, Johnson & Johnson Products, Inc., New Brunswick, NJ 08903

may result in death of the patient by suffocation. This complication can be prevented by following these rules: (1) never place an Elizabethan collar on an anesthetized patient, (2) always secure the collar or roll gauze so that one finger can be easily placed between the patient's neck and the collar, and (3) watch the patient for the first few minutes after application to assess respiratory function.

BODY BRACE

MATERIALS

> Aluminum rod* (3/16-, 1/4-, 5/16-, and 3/8-inch width; 6- and 12-foot length)
> One-inch cloth tape
> Splint bender*

METHOD OF ASSEMBLY. The circumference of the base of the neck is measured or is estimated by using the thumb and forefinger of both hands; either method must allow for padding. With the aid of a splint bender, or a round object, the rod is bent into a circle and a half. Each protruding rod is cut to a length equal to the distance from the base of the neck to the flank. Both rods are then bent at approximately 60° to the circle, so that the ring will rest comfortably on the shoulders of the dog with the ends protruding caudally toward the flanks. The circle and tips of the rods are then padded with cotton and tape for greater comfort.

The apparatus is placed with the padded ring resting against the shoulders and the rods along both sides of the thorax and abdomen (Fig. 3-3). Lateral rods are taped around the cranial abdomen with cloth tape, to secure the rods to the patient's side and to help prevent dorsoventral movement. This device is comfortable for the patient and can be used for extended periods of time.

With a few simple additions, the body brace also can be constructed to act as a tail lifter. An aluminum rod is

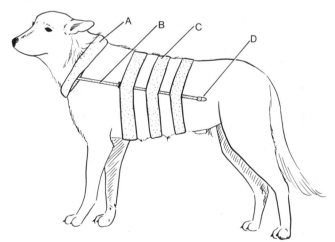

Fig. 3-3. *Body brace: aluminum rod adjacent to each side of trunk. A, padded ring; B, lateral rod; C, tape encircling trunk; D, padded end of rod.*

*Kirschner, P.O. Box 459, Aberdeen, MD 21001

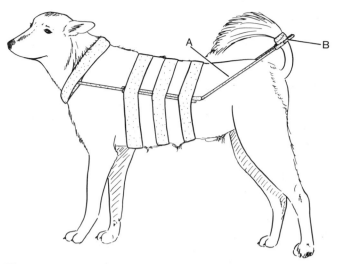

Fig. 3-4. *Body brace with angled aluminum rod added to keep tail elevated. A, angled rod taped to lateral rod of body brace; B, tail taped to apex of tail lifter rod.*

bent back on itself to form a 30- to 45°-angled apex. Sufficient tail lifter rod is allowed to secure it with tape to each lateral rod of the body brace (Fig. 3-4). The triangular portion, located caudally, is bent upward about 45° at the flank, so that the apex is situated 10 to 15 cm above the base of the tail. Once situated comfortably, the tail lifter rod is securely taped to the body brace; then the base of the tail is taped to the apex of the tail brace (Fig. 3-4).

INDICATIONS. The body brace is indicated to protect the body caudal to the base of the neck, including the thorax, abdomen, anal region, and hind legs above the hocks. It is especially useful for patient's that will not tolerate an Elizabethan collar.

With the tail lifter added, this device has been useful following surgical procedures for perianal fistulas and perianal neoplasms. Elevation of the tail facilitates ventilation, drainage, and local medication of the anal region.

CONTRAINDICATIONS. The head, neck, and forelegs are not adequately protected with this device, nor is it effective on the cat.

COMPLICATIONS. Lateral rods that are improperly padded or are too tightly taped may cause discomfort, skin irritation, and areas of necrosis. These problems are easily prevented by regular examination of the lateral rods, by application of padding as needed, and by not taping the trunk too tightly. The neck ring should be snug, but not compromising. If the patient exhibits respiratory dyspnea, the rods should be loosened.

SIDE BAR

MATERIALS

> Aluminum rod
> One-inch cloth tape
> Leather collar

METHOD OF ASSEMBLY. Another useful device is a side bar. A leather collar is fixed around the patient's neck,

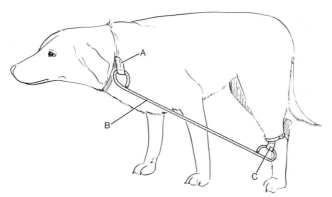

Fig. 3-5. *Side bar.* A, *end of bar taped to collar (collar can also be run through ring);* B, *aluminum bar (additional rods can be added for increased strength);* C, *end of bar taped to collar.*

and a smaller collar is placed around the hind leg just above the hock. A ring is formed in each end of a suitable length of adequately sized aluminum rod. The bar is attached to the collars by adhesive tape; one should leave about 5 cm of slack at each attachment (Fig. 3-5). In giant breeds of dogs, 2 or 3 ⅜-inch aluminum rods should be taped together to provide sufficient strength. The advantages of this method are the ease of application and the minimal amount of materials necessary for construction. The disadvantages are the awkward gait created by the device, and the possibility of the animal's tangling its legs in the bar. The patient must be confined to a kennel or a small room to avoid excessive trauma where the strap encircles the leg. This device is infrequently used, but it is helpful in selected cases.

INDICATIONS. A side bar prevents licking and chewing of the ipsilateral hind foot and hock.

CONTRAINDICATIONS. A side bar does not protect the contralateral side. It is not usually tolerated by cats.

COMPLICATIONS. Some dogs may not tolerate a side bar because their feet may become tangled around the bar.

STOCKINETTE BODY BANDAGE

MATERIALS
Stockinette (2, 3, 4, and 6 inch*)

METHOD OF ASSEMBLY. An appropriate size of stockinette is selected. A 3-inch size is used for cats and small dogs (under 15 lb), and a 4- to 6-inch size is used for larger dogs. The length of stockinette is measured from the patient's head to the rump. Four small holes are cut in the stockinette to accommodate the legs. The stockinette is placed on the patient, with the legs protruding through the holes. In male dogs, a hole must also be cut for the prepuce. If added bulkiness is desired, several layers of stockinette can be comfortably applied.

INDICATIONS. A stockinette body bandage can be used to protect surgical wounds, and lacerations of the thorax or abdomen. The bandage is comfortable, inexpensive, and does not slip off.

*Distributed by Whittaker General Medical, Richmond, VA 23228

CONTRAINDICATIONS. This bandage cannot be used for protection of the head, neck, legs, tail, or anal area.

COMPLICATIONS. Aggressive scratching, especially in cats, may cause a nail to be caught in the stockinette. This problem can be prevented by clipping the patient's nails when the bandage has been applied.

EMERGENCY EAR LACERATION PROTECTOR

MATERIALS
Stockinette
Old sock

METHOD OF ASSEMBLY AND APPLICATION. A stockinette or a sock is cut so as to create an opening at both ends. The patient's ears are folded over the top of the head. The sock or stockinette is then slipped over the patient's head to hold the ears in place. The edges of the sock or stockinette are then taped to the hair over the back of the neck and forehead to secure it to the head.

INDICATIONS. This quick, temporary immobilizing device prevents further trauma and bleeding of a lacerated ear. It can also be used as a final bandage cover for ears previously taped to the head.

CONTRAINDICATIONS. It is not intended to be the only treatment for pinna lacerations.

COMPLICATIONS. The bandage is tolerated by most patients, but it is important to include enough hair in the tape to prevent slipping forward or backward. Patients not tolerating the bandage may require concurrent use of an Elizabethan collar.

EAR LACERATION PROTECTOR

MATERIALS
One- and 2-inch cloth tape

METHOD OF ASSEMBLY AND APPLICATION. Once an ear laceration has been sutured, a gauze sponge is placed over the laceration to protect the suture line. The ear is then thoroughly dried. A strip of 2-inch cloth tape is placed on the lateral side of the pinna, over the gauze covered laceration, and extended 4 to 6 cm beyond the tip of the ear. The tape is then doubled over on itself and is taped back to the medial side of the pinna. One-inch cloth tape is then used to encircle the ear gently, and the tape should extend beyond the pinna. Excessive tape distally is trimmed to be parallel to the ear tip (Fig. 3-6). It is important that a large area of adhesive tape be in contact with the ear. Subsequent shaking of the head will result in whiplash of the tape instead of the tip of the ear.

INDICATIONS. This protector is used for lacerations of the ear involving the tip of the pinna.

CONTRAINDICATIONS. In patients with marginal auricular dermatitis, the adhesive may act as an irritant and may perpetuate the condition.

COMPLICATIONS. Some patients may find the device annoying and may try to scratch it off. If this occurs, an Elizabethan collar can be used in conjunction with the device.

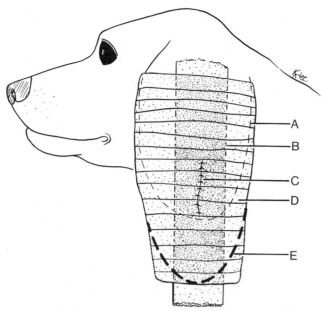

Fig. 3-6. *Ear laceration protector. A, edge of pinna; B, two-inch tape on both sides of pinna; C, sutured laceration; D, one-inch tape encircling ear; E, line for trimming off extra tape.*

TAPING EARS TO HEAD

MATERIALS

    Two-inch cloth tape
    Stockinette
    Elastic adhesive tape
    Sponge-rubber doughnuts

METHOD OF APPLICATION. The traumatized area or lesion is protected with a gauze sponge or nonadherent*† pad. A strip of 2-inch cloth tape is applied to the medial and lateral aspects of the pinna of both ears, so that it extends 15 cm from the tip of the ear to form tape stirrups. The tape stirrups are then passed over the opposite side of the dog's head and around the neck. Care must be taken not to apply excessive tension. The stirrups are then extended by taping 3 or 4 added revolutions around the head. The external ear canal should remain exposed. A doughnut 7 to 10 cm in diameter cut from a soft rubber material can be placed over each ear canal. A stockinette is then placed over the head and is taped to the bandage.

INDICATIONS. This is a good method of protecting the ears from continued shaking. Because the ear canals remain exposed to air, this apparatus can be used as an adjunct to medical or surgical management of otitis externa.

CONTRAINDICATIONS. The bandage should not be used in patients with severe dermatitis of the pinna because adhesive tape increases the irritation.

COMPLICATIONS. It is still possible for the patient to scratch the bandage and ear canal with a rear paw. This

*Telfa Surgical Dressing, Kendall Co. Hospital Products, Boston, MA 02101
†Micropad Dressing, Medical Products Division, 3M Co., 3M Center, St. Paul, MN 55101

problem can be solved by concurrent use of an Elizabethan collar.

The bandage is removed by cutting the tape under the chin; the tips of the ears can inadvertently be cut if the bandage is removed by cutting tape on top of the head.

CAST

MATERIALS

    Hexalite orthopedic tape‡
    Cutter Cast 7 casting tape§
    Plaster‖
    Light Cast II WB (weight-bearing) casting tape#

METHOD OF ASSEMBLY. Routine application of a cast has been described.[1,2]

INDICATIONS. Casts protect a limb below the elbow and stifle and are especially useful for the initial protection of carpal and tarsal lick granulomas.

CONTRAINDICATIONS. This technique should not be used if draining wounds will be covered by the cast.

COMPLICATIONS. Improper application compromise the circulation to the toes, and dry gangrene may result. Some patients chew excessively on a cast.

SCHROEDER-THOMAS SPLINT WITH SHEET ALUMINUM

MATERIALS

    Aluminum rod
    Cotton
    Cloth tape
    Splint bender
    Sheet aluminum

METHOD OF ASSEMBLY. Construction of a Schroeder-Thomas splint has been described.[2,3] Once the splint has been secured to the patient's extremity, the area to be protected is covered with a light sheet of durable aluminum or tin (Fig. 3-7). The aluminum is taped securely in place to the vertical rods over the area requiring protection. Immediately distal to the aluminum sheet, the aluminum bars are not wrapped with tape, to ensure that the protected area will be well ventilated (Fig. 3-7).

INDICATIONS. A regular Schroeder-Thomas splint is especially useful in hygroma of the elbow, where it is applied postoperatively to prevent trauma from lying on the elbow. It is also used to protect wounds and skin lesions of the legs from licking and chewing. When all else fails, tin or aluminum may be applied around the splint. Aluminum can be used to protect adequately any part of the fore or hind extremity that is included in the

‡ Hexcel Medical Products, 11711 Dublin Boulevard, Dublin, CA 94566
§ Cutter Biological, Division of Cutter Laboratories, Inc., 2200 Powell Street, Emeryville, CA 94608
‖ Zoroc, Johnson & Johnson Products, Inc., New Brunswick, NJ 08903
Orthopedics Co., Inc., 2990 Red Hill Avenue, Costa Mesa, CA 92626

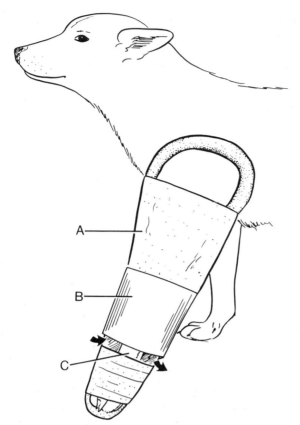

Fig. 3-7. *Schroeder-Thomas splint with sheet aluminum secured to splint. A, tape covering Schroeder-Thomas splint; B, sheet aluminum; C, leg left uncovered to provide ventilation.*

Schroeder-Thomas splint. Generally speaking, this is below the elbow and stifle.

CONTRAINDICATIONS. Protection is not offered above the distal humerus or femur.

COMPLICATIONS. The only complication of this device is from inappropriate application or construction of the splint, which may result in decubital sores, swollen toes, necrosis of toes, and stiff joints from prolonged immobilization.

SOFT PADDED BANDAGE

MATERIALS

> Cloth tape
> Cast padding* or cotton
> Conforming gauze†
> Elastic adhesive tape or conforming adhesive bandage‡

METHOD OF ASSEMBLY. Tape stirrups are placed on the medial and lateral aspects of the extremity, to extend 10 to 12 cm beyond the end of the limb. Cast padding or cotton is then wrapped up the limb starting at the toes.

*Specialist cast padding, Johnson & Johnson Products, Inc., New Brunswick, NJ 08903
†Kling elastic gauze bandage, Johnson & Johnson Products, Inc., New Brunswick, NJ 08903
‡Vet Wrap, Animal Care Products, 3M Co., 3M Center, St. Paul, MN 55101

Enough padding is used to cover the desired area adequately and to create the bulkiness necessary for protection. Conforming gauze is then applied up the extremity; one should apply enough pressure to conform the cotton snugly to the limb. The ends of the tape stirrups are then folded back and are taped to the outside of the bandage. An elastic tape or bandage is used to cover the gauze. This layer of material adds strength to the bandage, as well as additional protection to the area being covered.

INDICATIONS. This device is indicated for protection of extremities below the elbow and stifle.

CONTRAINDICATIONS. Protection is not offered above the elbow or stifle. Extremely aggressive patients may need a combination of a soft padded bandage and a chemical restraint or an Elizabethan collar.

COMPLICATIONS. Complications arise from improperly applied bandages. If a bandage is too tight, the patient's circulation may be compromised; if it is too loose, pressure sores, decubital ulcers, or slippage will result. Experience helps to dictate the appropriate method of application.

HOBBLES

MATERIALS
> One-inch cloth tape

METHOD OF ASSEMBLY. When applying stifle-to-tail hobbles, encircling tape should be applied just distal to the stifle joint of either leg, and to the midportion of the tail (Fig. 3-8). It is important that adequate hair-to-tape contact be made to preclude slipping of tape down the leg or tail. The hobble should be long enough

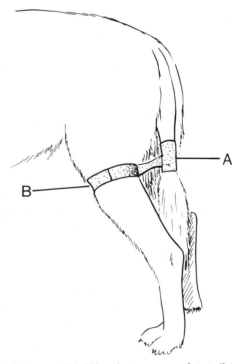

Fig. 3-8. *Stifle-to-tail hobbles. A, tape secured to tail; B, tape secured just distal to stifle.*

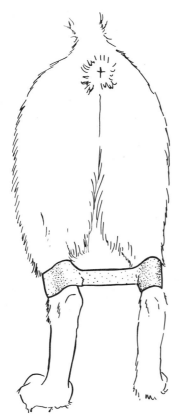

Fig. 3-9. *Hock hobbles.*

to allow normal defecation, but short enough to stop the damaging effect of continued tail-wagging.

Tape hobbles can also be applied just proximal to each hock or carpus. The hobbles must be long enough to permit the dog to walk and short enough to be restrictive (Fig. 3-9).

INDICATIONS. Stifle-to-tail hobbles are used exclusively to prevent trauma to the tip of the tail resulting from constant wagging of the tail in a confined area.

Hock hobbles are used to prevent patients from scratching the head and fore quarters. Such hobbles are also useful when a patient persists in scratching an Elizabethan collar, or when such a collar allows the patient to lick or chew the perineal region. Carpal hobbles prevent a patient from removing an Elizabethan collar with the front feet.

CONTRAINDICATIONS. Hock or carpal hobbles should not be used on patients that cannot be confined to a cage or kennel. If allowed free run, a patient may continually stumble and fall.

COMPLICATIONS. The tape should be checked daily for evidence of skin irritation, slipping, or breaking. Ex-

tremities should be examined for swelling, redness, and temperature. If problems develop, the device should be removed. If the patient chews at hobbles, an Elizabethan collar or a body brace should be applied.

TAIL-TIP PROTECTORS

MATERIALS

    Gauze sponges
    Roll or conforming gauze
    Conforming adhesive bandage or elastic adhesive tape
    Hexalite, Light Cast, Cutter Cast 7, or Orthoplast

METHOD OF ASSEMBLY. The tip of the tail is wrapped with a gauze sponge and conforming gauze for initial padding. Cloth or elastic tape can be used to hold the padding in place. It is imperative to include 7 to 10 cm of hair in the tape cover to keep the apparatus from slipping off. Hexalite, Light Cast, Cutter Cast 7, or Orthoplast is molded to form a guard over the tip of the tail. A final cloth tape or elastic wrap is used to hold the cast in place.

INDICATIONS. Tail protectors are especially useful in large, long-tailed, short-haired breeds that have had recent tail amputations or trauma to the tip of the tail. Other indications are lacerations, abrasions, or crushing trauma requiring coaptation and prevention of further trauma.

CONTRAINDICATIONS. Patients with paresthesia from neurologic disorders, such as cauda equina syndrome, must have the underlying cause corrected for such a device to be helpful.

COMPLICATIONS. This coaptation device is not designed to protect the tail from constant licking or chewing. If that is a problem, concurrent use of an Elizabethan collar is indicated.

In conclusion, judicious use of devices and agents to prevent self-trauma often reduces morbidity from a surgical procedure or prevents a small lesion from becoming a major problem. The most frequent mistake is waiting too long to apply such a device or agent.

References and Suggested Readings

1. Hohn, R. B.: Principles and application of plaster cast. Vet. Clin. North Am., 5, 1975.
2. Knecht, C. D., et al.: Fundamental Techniques in Veterinary Surgery. Philadelphia, W. B. Saunders, 1975.
3. Leonard, E. P.: Orthopedic Surgery of the Dog and Cat. Philadelphia, W. B. Saunders, 1960.

4 * Central Nervous System

Ventriculoperitoneal Shunt for Hydrocephalus

by ROGER M. CLEMMONS

Hydrocephalus is defined as an abnormal accumulation of cerebrospinal fluid (CSF) within the ventricular system of the brain accompanied by a concomitant loss of cerebral white matter or gray matter. This condition is a common neurologic disorder of miniature breed dogs and offers a unique challenge to the clinician for diagnosis and treatment. My purpose is to discuss a simple and inexpensive surgical treatment for hydrocephalus.

Pathophysiology of Hydrocephalus

Hydrocephalus develops as a sequel to excessive formation of CSF, to decreased absorption of CSF, or to a loss of cerebral tissue volume. The pathophysiology of the former two conditions is important because these causes of hydrocephalus are likely to respond to CSF shunting procedures. The third condition is not likely to respond to either surgical or medical management.

As a result of excessive fluid accumulation in the ventricular system from increased formation or decreased absorption of CSF, a disequilibrium of forces exists at the ventricular-cerebral interface.[3] Because the ventricular surface is semipermeable, there is a net flux of CSF into the periventricular extracellular fluid compartment. A concomitant decrease must occur in other cranial structures because no "dead space" exists within the cranial cavity. Cerebral vascular structures are most easily compressed, and with increased production of extracellular fluid from the ventricles, the periventricular white matter's reabsorptive capacity is overloaded. The vasculature of the white matter thereby collapses and leads to the development of periventricular white matter ischemia. Because oligodendroglia are sensitive to ischemic insult, demyelination and ventricular enlargement result. Therefore, early treatment must be given for maximal benefit to the patient.

Some authors[2] have not seen elevated intracranial pressure in dogs with hydrocephalus. In human patients likely to benefit from CSF shunting, however, transient or constantly increased ventricular pressure is common.[7] Although the CSF pressure may be within normal levels in most dogs, increased intracranial pressure does occur in hydrocephalus and may play a significant role in the progression of this disorder. Hydrocephalus in the dog is associated with a higher initial resistance to CSF absorption, but an increased absorptive capacity.[9] The mean rate of CSF formation is also found to be reduced. These findings suggest that canine hydrocephalus would be expected to exhibit low or normal ventricular pressures, but that minor changes in CSF volume would result in pressure increases that could not be normally transmitted or dispersed. Fluctuations in intraventricular pressure, as seen in man, would lead to periods of abnormally high pressures.

Diagnosis

The variability of signs of canine hydrocephalus often makes the diagnosis by clinical criteria alone difficult. In young animals in which a dome-shaped calvarium, open fontanelles, and a downcast gaze are also associated with neurologic dysfunction, however, the diagnosis may be easier. Confirmatory laboratory examinations include electroencephalography and radiology.

The electroencephalogram of hydrocephalic dogs is characterized by high-amplitude, slow wave activity. This pattern is accentuated during sleep, but remains abnormal even during the alerting response. Although a correlation does appear to exist between the electroencephalographic changes and the degree of ventricular enlargement, these findings do not correlate with the clinical signs.

Noncontrast radiographs may show some flattening of the gyral impressions upon the calvarium, but such changes are not pathognomonic. Contrast ventriculography with air on a positive-contrast agent adequately outlines an enlarged ventricular system. Metrizamide* ventriculography may also provide useful information about CSF circulation patterns and may indicate sites

---

*Amipaque, Winthrop Laboratories, 90 Park Avenue, New York, NY 10016

of obstruction to CSF flow.[5] In addition, this technique may be useful in demonstrating shunt patentcy.

Laboratory evaluation of ventricular fluid pressure, volume, and chemical and cellular characteristics may furnish helpful information about the underlying cause of hydrocephalus.

Surgical Technique

The decision to place a ventriculoperitoneal shunt should be based upon the progression of clinical signs. The triad of dementia, gait abnormalities, and incontinence is an accurate predictor of responsiveness to shunting procedures in humans[4] and can be used in the dog.

The choice of anesthesia should be considered carefully because agents that increase the intracranial pressure may have disastrous consequences. Although halothane increases intracranial pressure, this effect can be minimized by hyperventilating the animal for several minutes with oxygen-rich gases prior to the addition of halothane to the breathing mixture. Owing to the rapidity with which anesthetic depth can be altered with halothane, it is currently the agent of choice.

The animal is positioned in ventral recumbancy, and the calvarium, the neck, and the right, dorsolateral body surface to the paralumbar fossa are surgically prepared. The area is draped, preferably with a barrier drape material.

A slightly paramedian incision is made over the surface of the calvarium. The subcutaneous tissue and musculature overlying the bony calvarium is dissected free at approximately half the distance from the lateral canthus of the eye to the occipital protuberance and 1 to 1½ cm from the midline. At this point, a bur hole sufficient to pass the shunt tubing is made through the skull. In small dogs and cats with a thin calvarium, the skull may be carefully cut away with a sharp scalpel blade. The dura is incised, and a shortened, sharpened mare's catheter* is inserted into the ventricular cavity. The ventricular end of the shunt tubing is then introduced through the mare's catheter or through the hole made by the catheter in the cerebral tissue. The length of shunt tubing to be inserted into the ventricle should be determined by the depth required to enter the ventricle with the catheter. The shunt tubing is fixed in place with nonabsorbable suture material passed through a hole in the outer cortical lamina of the calvarium. The muscular layers are apposed around the tubing. Once CSF is noted flowing distally in the shunt tubing, the tubing is clamped to prevent excessive CSF loss.

Alligator forceps are passed subcutaneously through a small skin incision every 9 to 12 cm and are used to pull the distal end of the shunt tubing to the paralumbar fossa. At this point, the peritoneal end of the shunt tubing is bluntly thrust through the body wall and into the peritoneal cavity by grasping it with hemostatic forceps. An additional 15 to 25 cm of shunt tub-

*Jensen-Salsbury Laboratories, 520 West 21st Street, Kansas City, MO 64141

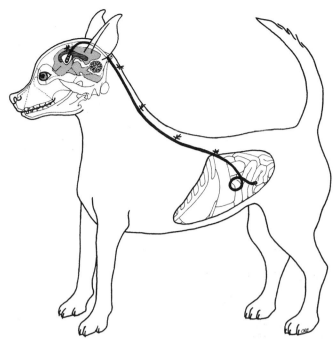

Fig. 4-1. *Ventriculoperitoneal shunt in place. A silicone shunt tube connects the lateral ventricle with the peritoneal cavity and runs subcutaneously from the head down the side of the body to the paralumbar fossa. An excess of shunt tubing in the peritoneal cavity allows for some growth of the animal.*

ing should be allowed to lie freely in the peritoneal cavity. The flow of CSF from the tube should be monitored for a few minutes to ensure shunt patency. The skin incisions are closed in a routine manner (Fig. 4-1).

The advent of silicone† materials for shunt tubing has greatly improved the success rate for these procedures.[1] Several shunt systems have been described for ventriculoperitoneal shunting employing special valves, pumping devices, and catheter tips. That these devices are expensive often mitigates against the decision to use the technique in veterinary practice. The technique previously described is compatible with the use of these materials. This technique uses silicone rubber tubing that does not incorporate a valve device. The tubing is cut to an appropriate length, the ventricular end is perforated on the sides, and the sharp edges are rounded over a flame (Fig. 4-2). This material is readily sterilized by ethylene oxide or autoclave. The peritoneal end may be cut to length at the time of operation.

Any increase in intraventricular pressure is dissipated through the shunt by the passage of CSF into the

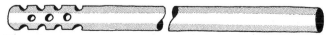

Fig. 4-2. *The shunt is made of inexpensive silicone material. The ventricular end of the shunt has perforated sides for maximal passage of CSF. The peritoneal end may be cut to length during the surgical procedure.*

†Silastic Medical Products Division, Dow Corning Corp., P.O. Box 1767, Midland, MI 48640

peritoneal cavity. Although the absence of valves potentially allows the passage of material in either direction, this possibility has not led to complications in clinical applications. This method has been successful in canine and feline patients with hydrocephalus in which shunting was performed. Its major advantages have been low cost, simplicity of application, and ease of correction.

Postoperative Management and Complications

Aseptic surgical technique is essential to ensure postoperative success. The routine use of antibiotics is not indicated. If their use is indicated, however, the veterinarian must consider the lack of a normal blood-brain barrier in the choice of an agent. For example, penicillins are known to be epileptogenic and should be used with caution.

The complications associated with the procedure and shunt tubing described should be comparable to those with other systems. In general, these complications can be broken into certain categories: shunt failure due to device failure[8] and infections secondary to the shunt.[6,10] The simplicity of the selected design of the system described may, in fact, reduce the complication rate. In patients with hydrocephalus, the practicality of this system may allow considerable salvage of neurologic tissue.

References and Suggested Readings

1. Ames, R. H.: Ventriculo-peritoneal shunts in the management of hydrocephalus. J. Neurosurg., 25:525, 1967.
2. Averill, D. R.: Diagnosis and treatment of hydrocephalus in the dog. Proc. Kal Kan Symp., September 28 to 30, 1978.
3. Berger, M. P., and Brumback, R. A.: Pathophysiologic mechanisms of hydrocephalus. J. Clin. Psychiatry, 39:143; 148, 1978.
4. Black, P. McL.: Idiopathic normal-pressure hydrocephalus: results of shunting in 62 patients. J. Neurosurg., 52:371, 1980.
5. Drayer, B. P., and Rosenbaum, A. E.: Studies of the third circulation: Amipaque CT cisternography and ventriculography. J. Neurosurg., 48:946, 1978.
6. Finney, H. L., and Roberts, T. S.: Nephritis secondary to chronic cerebrospinal fluid-vascular shunt infection: "shunt nephritis." Childs Brain, 6:189, 1980.
7. Lamas, E., and Lobato, R. D.: Intraventricular pressure and CSF dynamics in chronic adult hydrocephalus. Surg. Neurol., 12:287, 1979.
8. Little, J. R., Rhoton, A. L., and Mellinger, J. F.: Comparison of ventriculoperitoneal and ventriculoatrial shunts for hydrocephalus in children. Mayo Clin. Proc., 47:396, 1972.
9. Sahar, A., Hochwald, G. M., Kay, W. J., and Ransohoff, J.: Spontaneous canine hydrocephalus: cerebrospinal fluid dynamics. J. Neurol. Neurosurg. Psychiatry, 34:308, 1971.
10. Sugarman, B., and Massanari, R. M.: *Candida* meningitis in patients with CSF shunts. Arch. Neurol., 37:180, 1980.
11. Vastola, E. F.: CSF formation and absorption estimates by constant flow infusion method. Arch. Neurol., 37:150, 1980.

5 * Peripheral Nervous System

Tendon Transfer for Treatment of Sciatic Paralysis

by ARNOLD LESSER

Damage to the sciatic nerve is a common sequel to certain pelvic or proximal femoral fractures. Reports on the treatment for peripheral nerve palsy in veterinary medicine have been scant, as compared to human medicine in which the transfer of muscles and their tendons in such diseases as spina bifida, neuromuscular atrophies, cerebral palsy, and especially poliomyelitis has been practiced frequently and successfully. A tendon transfer is defined as the relocation of the tendon of insertion to another location to substitute its muscle for a paralyzed muscle in the same region. A tendon transplant is the relocation of a whole segment of tendon, or tendon and muscle, whereas a tendon transfer is the relocation of the tendinous insertion only. Tendon transfers have been used for the treatment of both radial and sciatic nerve paralysis in the dog and cat. The alternative usually consists of arthrodeses of the carpus or hock or amputation of the leg.

Sciatic paralysis may include both the tibial and peroneal branches as they course together; or in some cases, only the peroneal nerve is affected, and the tibial nerve is spared. Therefore, the extent of the paralysis may vary. In either instance, the animal is able to bear some weight on the leg owing to the function of the quadriceps (femoral nerve), which extends the stifle and can swing the leg because of the function of the extensors and flexors of the hip (obturator, cranial, and caudal gluteal nerves). The animal cannot push off the ground, however, because of the flaccid paralysis of the hock and digits. If only the peroneal nerve is damaged, then the animal can extend and maintain the hock off the ground. With a total sciatic paralysis, the hock is flaccid, and the animal supports weight with the plantar surface of the calcaneous and tarsus bones in contact with the ground. A muscular branch leaving the sciatic nerve at the level of the greater trochanter innervates the biceps femoris and the semitendinosus muscles. These two muscles participate in the calcaneal (Achilles) tendon and, if spared, allow the animal to hold its hock off the ground. Therefore, an animal's

ability to extend his hock joint does not exclude a damaged tibial nerve. In either case, unless the foot is swung forward sufficiently with the limb, the toes remain flexed. On contact with the ground, the dorsal aspect of the paw is traumatized, leading to chronic ulceration and flexion contracture.

The object in restoring function is to regain extension (dorsiflexion) of the digits as the foot lands and fixation of the hock to provide push-off strength when the stifle is fixed and the hip is extended. Arthrodesis

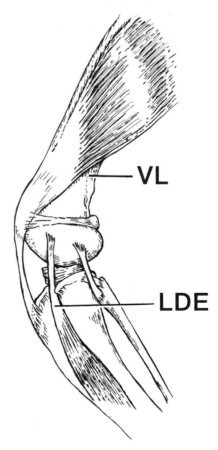

Fig. 5-1. *The anatomic location of the structures involved. VL, vastus lateralis muscle; LDE, long digital extensor muscle. (From Lesser, A. S.: The use of a tendon transfer for the treatment of a traumatic sciatic nerve paralysis in the dog. Vet. Surg., 7:85, 1978.)*

of the talocrural, intratarsal, and tarsal metatarsal joints accomplishes this end, but requires extensive surgical procedures and deprives the animal of the original shock-absorbing mechanisms of all these now fused and rigid joints. A transfer of the origin of the long digital extensor muscle to the vastus lateralis muscle, combined with arthrodesis of only the talocrural joint, can be used to bring about a more functional repair (Fig. 5-1).

Criteria for Surgical Management

Before a plan can be made to substitute one muscle for another, certain criteria must be met: (1) the muscle and tendon chosen for transfer must be sufficient in size and strength for their new function; (2) the unit should be transferred in as straight a line as possible for efficiency of action and should be attached as close to the insertion of the paralyzed tendon as possible; (3) the tendon must be placed under sufficient tension (slightly greater than normal) with the joint in the desired position; (4) the transferred tendon's sheath should be retained, or at least the tendon should be passed through tissue that will allow it to glide; tunnels through bone, fascia, or an interosseous membrane may lead to adhesions; (5) all contractions must be released prior to transfer, so that the joint to be activated is in its proper position; a transfer cannot be expected to overcome a deformity; (6) the loss of function of the transferred tendon must be accounted for either by synergists or arthrodesis; (7) if possible, one should use an agonist rather than an antagonist; (8) the transferred muscle and tendon should have had sufficient range of excursion in their normal position to allow adequate range of motion in their new role; (9) the neurovascular bundle must not be excessively stretched or kinked; and (10) the muscle picked for transfer must not be affected by the same disorder; this last can be ascertained by the nature of the disease, the function of the limb, electromyography, or nerve and muscle stimulation.

The long digital extensor muscle is used because it provides the major extensor tendons of the digits and has an easily mobilized tendon of origin. With a sciatic paralysis, no muscles are viable distal to the stifle, so the vastus lateralis is the closest muscle to fit most of the criteria. If only the peroneal nerve is affected, then the tibialis caudalis or the flexor digitorum longus muscles can be transferred to the insertion of the long digital extensor. The transfer of the long digital extensor to the vastus lateralis muscle is described here.

Sufficient time should be allowed for function to return or for the nerve to regenerate. This process could take up to 6 months, but the clinical status of the patient in terms of ulceration of the paw, flexion contractures, and disuse atrophy of the leg (especially the VL) must be taken into consideration when planning the timing of the operation. If the animal refuses to use the leg at all and is having problems with chronic ulceration, it is better to perform the transfer early than to wait and end up with a useless limb.

Surgical Technique

A lateral parapatellar incision through the skin and lateral retinaculum is made from the proximal tibia to the distal third of the vastus lateralis muscle. The retinaculum must be retracted cranially off the vastus lateralis to expose the muscle's insertion on the patella. The insertion is then incised close to the patella; one must be careful to preserve sufficient tendon with the muscle to be available for the anastomosis to the long digital extensor (Fig. 5-2A). The vastus lateralis muscle is freed by bluntly dissecting its attachment to the joint capsule caudomedially and to the rectus femoris cranially. The cranial edge of the vastus lateralis muscle and the lateral edge of the rectus femoris muscle blend together, but can be separated. This dissection should allow the distal fourth of the vastus lateralis muscle and tendon to be mobilized caudally. An incision is then made in the lateral joint capsule over the origin of the long digital extensor muscle; one must be careful not to incise the underlying tendon (Fig. 5-2A). The long digital extensor tendon is excised from the lateral condyle, is exteriorized superficially to the joint capsule, and is anastomosed to the prepared vastus lateralis tendon. The long digital extensor muscle is moved caudally from where it lies in the extensor notch of the tibia when it is anastomosed to the vastus lateralis muscle (Fig. 5-2B). It is necessary to incise the fascia over the tibialis cranialis muscle to allow the

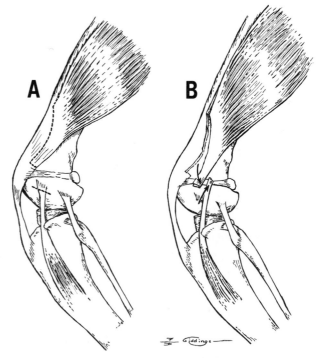

Fig. 5-2. A and B, The origin of the long digital extensor muscle is detached from the lateral femoral condyle, and the vastus lateralis and its tendon of insertion is separated from the patella and for 3 cm from the quadriceps mass. (From Lesser, A. S.: The use of a tendon transfer for the treatment of a traumatic sciatic nerve paralysis in the dog. Vet. Surg., 7:85, 1978.)

long digital extensor this movement. This procedure allows the anastomosed unit to lie in a straight line.

The anastomosis is completed by drawing the origin of the long digital extensor through two stab incisions made with a No. 11 blade in the vastus lateralis insertion (Fig. 5-3). This end is accomplished by passing mosquito forceps through the incision in the vastus lateralis tendon, grasping a stay suture placed in the long digital extensor origin, and pulling it through. This process is repeated for the second stab incision, and then the two tendons are sutured with interrupted nonabsorbable 4-0 sutures (Fig. 5-3, inset). Before suturing, traction is placed on the origin of the long digital extensor muscle; this traction should cause the toes to dorsiflex. In delayed cases, the body of the long digital extensor muscle may have to be freed from adhesions by applying traction on its insertion through a second distal incision at the hock. Care must be taken to ensure enough tension on the muscle when the anastomosis is complete. Some tension is always lost postoperatively, and therefore, the anastomosis should be under as much tension as possible during the operation. The digits should be in dorsiflexion when the long digital extensor and vastus lateralis muscles are sutured, and strong resistance to flexion of the digits

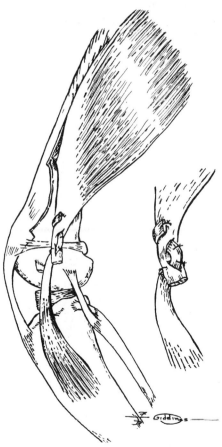

Fig. 5-3. *The origin of the long digital extensor muscle is drawn through two stab incisions in the vastus lateralis tendon of insertion and is sutured with 4-0 nylon. (From Lesser, A. S.: The use of a tendon transfer for the treatment of a traumatic sciatic nerve paralysis in the dog. Vet. Surg., 7:85, 1978.)*

should be met when the anastomosis is complete. The veterinary surgeon should test this at the operating table.

The ultimate aim of this procedure is the extension of the digits as the stifle is extended by the quadriceps muscle just prior to weight bearing, during the forward-swing phase of gait. In this procedure the entire LDE is used as the tendon of insertion. Because a long distance is spanned between the transferred muscle and the point of action (the digits), the correct tension is vital. This is also the reason that arthrodesis of the talocrural joint is included. Without the arthrodesis, some of the contractile force of the vastus lateralis muscle is expended in flexing the talocrural joint instead of dorsiflexing the digits. The arthrodesis also provides resistance for a flaccid hock during the weight-bearing and push-off phases of gait. The talocrural arthrodesis can be performed at the same time or prior to the tendon transfer.

It is important for the animal to use the transfer as early as possible. If the arthrodesis is painful, or if it is not completely stable, it can prevent use of the leg for a number of weeks; this situation can lead to restrictive adhesions at the anastomotic site. For that reason, it is recommended that the arthrodesis be performed first and that the tendon transfer be delayed until the animal is willing to bear weight on the leg. Moreover, any contracture of the superficial or deep flexor muscles of the digits should be released by transection prior to the muscle transfer.

In smaller dogs and cats, the transfer has been performed successfully without the use of a talocrural arthrodesis. It is not certain at this time whether this finding represents a function of the weight and size of these patients or the nature of their deficits. Beagles with experimentally induced sciatic paralysis did not function with tendon transfers alone, but did bear weight properly after the addition of talocrural arthrodesis. Conversely, talocrural arthrodesis alone has not proved sufficient in clinical cases.

The foot should be maintained in dorsiflexion, and the anastomosis should be protected with a molded splint covering the crus and paw. The splint should remain for 10 days and then ideally should be used daily for short periods for another 2 weeks. The problem is to protect the anastomosis while still allowing the animal to use the leg to prevent adhesions from restricting the tendon at the site of the anastomosis. A normal gait without knuckling is usually seen 3 weeks postoperatively. At this time, the splint can be removed permanently.

References and Suggested Readings

Crenshaw, A. H.: Campbell's Operative Orthopaedics. Vol. 2. 5th Ed. St. Louis, C.V. Mosby, 1971.

Lesser, A. L.: The use of a tendon transfer for the treatment of a traumatic sciatic nerve paralysis in the dog. Vet. Surg., 7:85, 1978.

Lesser, A. L.: Experimental evaluation of tendon transfer for the treatment of sciatic nerve paralysis in the dog. Vet. Surg., 9:72, 1980.

Peripheral Nerve Injury and Repair

by WILLIAM G. RODKEY *and* H. EDWARD CABAUD

Peripheral nerve injuries may result from simple compression, crushing, stretching, laceration, or complete transection.[4,10] Such injuries occur commonly in animals because the anatomic location of many nerves leaves them vulnerable to trauma.[7] Causes of peripheral nerve injuries include vehicle accidents, fractures, gunshot wounds, bite wounds, lacerations, and iatrogenic causes such as malplaced injections or surgical accidents. Although peripheral nerve injuries are rarely life-threatening, the consequences may be devastating if these injuries are not treated appropriately.

Morphology and Pathophysiology

The anatomy and physiology of peripheral nerves are complex and are intimately related.[10] Through a broad knowledge of nerve morphology (Fig. 5-4), the veterinary surgeon first must set the stage mechanically for a repaired nerve to heal. Then, because nerve healing and regeneration are basic physiologic and biochemical processes, a maximum return of function can be expected only when one bases the management of nerve injuries on a thorough understanding of the appropriate biologic features.

Each peripheral nerve has as its basic unit many axons that are extensions of nerve cell bodies in or near the spinal cord. The axons, which consist of fluid axoplasm within a cell membrane, may be myelinated or unmyelinated. The myelin sheath for each myelinated axon is formed by a series of Schwann cells, but many unmyelinated axons may be ensheathed by one Schwann cell.[2,10] Nodes of Ranvier are the junctional areas between Schwann cells, and they are found at discrete intervals over the entire length of a myelinated axon. Nerve conduction velocity is much more rapid in myelinated fibers where the action potential appears to jump from one node of Ranvier to the next. Conduction is slower in unmyelinated axons because the action potential is continuous over the entire length of each nerve fiber.[4,10]

The axon and Schwann cell units are surrounded by and are separated from each other by loose interstitial tissue, the endoneurium, which is of connective tissue origin and is composed of collagen fibrils, fibroblasts, and a capillary system that provides nourishment to the nerve fibers.[4,7,10] The perineurium, the next connective tissue layer, is a tubule that encases bundles of nerve fibers. The nerve bundles are called fascicles or funiculi, and each one may contain from only a few to several thousand nerve fibers.[1,8,10] The perineurium provides support, and it acts as a diffusion barrier to keep out various substances and to maintain a controlled environment similar to that of the central nervous system.[4]

The epineurium is the outer layer, which surrounds the entire nerve. It is composed of areolar connective tissue and contains collagen fibrils that are thicker than those found in the endoneurium and perineurium.[9] The fibroblasts of the epineurium produce the collagen that provides strength to a repaired nerve, but overproduction as a result of an inflammatory response may lead to detrimental fibrosis and scarring following nerve injury.[4,6,9,10]

The extent of derangement of the described neural anatomic features that results from trauma determines the severity of nerve injury. As more structures are injured, spontaneous recovery is decreased and less chance exists for a full return of function of the traumatized nerve. The mildest degree of trauma results only in transient loss of nerve function and is called neurapraxia. Actual anatomic disruption does not take place, but nerve conduction is blocked.[7] No degenerative changes occur, and full functional recovery is the usual outcome. An example of neurapraxia is contusion of the peripheral nerve as a result of blunt trauma.

The next nerve injury in degree of severity is called axonotmesis. In this condition, a portion of the axons are disrupted, but all endoneurial tubules and connective tissue elements remain intact.[7] Examples of this type of intrafascicular trauma include crush injury and severe stretching of the nerve. Following such injury, wallerian degeneration occurs.[10] The axons and their myelin sheaths distal to the point of injury undergo degeneration and are phagocytized. This same degenerative process, called axonal degeneration, occurs for a distance proximal to the injury, usually involving only one to three nodes of Ranvier. Following axonotmesis, axons regrow spontaneously. The time required for functional recovery, however, is dependent on extent of injury and the distance from the denervated end organs.

The most severe injury is a complete separation of the nerve trunk, with a gap between the severed ends. This type of injury is called neurotmesis, and it is exemplified by a complete nerve laceration.[7] The distal segment of the nerve undergoes wallerian degeneration, and axonal degeneration occurs in the proximal segment. Because the severed ends frequently are malaligned or are widely separated, spontaneous recovery of normal function is not likely. Such injuries require surgical realignment to provide regenerating axons the opportunity to reach and to reinnervate their appropriate end organs.

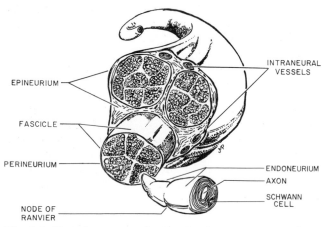

EPINEURIUM

FASCICLE

PERINEURIUM

NODE OF
RANVIER

INTRANEURAL
VESSELS

ENDONEURIUM
AXON

SCHWANN
CELL

Fig. 5-4. *Normal anatomy of a peripheral nerve.*

Nerve Healing and Regeneration

Many factors influence healing, regeneration, and ultimate return of function of injured peripheral nerves. Some of the adverse circumstances can be minimized with proper clinical management, but certain other factors continue to plague all efforts to completely regenerate nerve tissue.

The mechanism of the injury determines the initial degree of anatomic disruption. A complete, sharp laceration of a nerve usually is much more amenable to repair and regeneration than is a complete avulsion injury. The avulsion likely would have retrograde effects because of the severe stretching of the nerve,[9] and thus multiple axonal injury sites might have to be overcome by individual regenerating axons before the nerves could reinnervate their end organs.

The condition of the end organ also must be considered. Extensive trauma to the denervated area may preclude return of function, regardless of the success of nerve regeneration.

Prolonged delays in reinnervation often decrease the chances of an ultimate return of function. Such delays might occur because of the level, that is, distance from the end organ, of the nerve injury or because of a protracted period between injury and surgical repair. In either case, the distal nerve segment may fibrose and may thereby hinder the advancing axons, or the end organ may undergo irreversible atrophy and fibrosis. The age and the nutritional status of the patient also influence nerve healing. Nerves in young patients heal more rapidly and completely than those of older patients. Properly nourished patients have a faster rate of nerve regeneration than those with nutritional deficiencies.[10]

The veterinary surgeon performing the neurorrhaphy also has a great influence on the final result. A meticulous neurorrhaphy performed with atraumatic technique is much more likely to succeed than one performed in a less-refined manner. Improper handling can be expected to produce greater inflammation and fibroplasia, both deterrents to axon regeneration. Axons start to regrow soon after injury. In fact, recent work by us[2] has confirmed that axon regeneration is well advanced long before wallerian degeneration is complete. New endoneurial tubules are formed for the regenerating axons, and the old tubules may be of little importance to the reinnervation process. Therefore, concerted efforts should be made to counteract those adverse factors, previously described, that delay or prevent the early and rapid regrowth of axons to the appropriate end organs.

Surgical Considerations and Techniques

Peripheral nerve repairs should be undertaken only after life-threatening problems have been resolved and vital functions have been stabilized. Although we prefer immediate primary repair of severed nerves whenever possible, delayed or secondary repair at times may be necessary. Gross wound contamination, existing local infection, and extensive associated soft-tissue trauma are reasons for delay.[6,10] Definitive repair, however, should not be delayed any longer than necessary.

At the time of exploration and neurorrhaphy, the entire involved limb should be prepared and draped for the surgical procedure. Skin incisions must be of sufficient length to permit adequate exposure of proximal and distal segments, and the limb may have to be manipulated into various positions during the nerve repair. As an additional consideration, if the use of nerve grafts (discussed later) is anticipated, the donor sites must also be prepared and draped before the surgical procedure is started.

Knowledge of the surgical anatomy of the involved area is essential. A long or extensile skin incision should be made over the course of the nerve to be repaired, extending proximally and distally equal distances from the site of injury. The deep incision should be continued through fascial planes if possible, or muscles should be divided parallel to their fibers.

Both the proximal and distal segments usually retract after nerve severance, and the ends may be several centimeters apart. If a delayed secondary repair is being performed, the nerve ends may be imbedded in scar tissue, or they may be adherent to other vital structures. For these reasons, we prefer initially to identify and isolate the nerve segments several centimeters proximal and distal to the original point of injury, and then to continue surgical dissection until the nerve ends can be located and freed from the surrounding tissue. The segments then are more accessible for debridement, mobilization, and repair.

If it is decided to delay definitive repair, the nerve ends should be identified to simplify finding them later. We prefer to place a bright-blue monofilament 5-0 or 6-0 suture through the epineurium of each end and tie it, thus loosely approximating the nerve ends. The bright-blue suture and the nerve segments usually are found readily during the subsequent procedure.

NERVE DEBRIDEMENT

In nearly all cases, the ends of the nerve segments require some debridement prior to surgical anastomosis. In acute cases involving a clean, sharp laceration of the nerve, minimal debridement is indicated in order to preserve the nerve's length. Uneven tags of nerve tissue should be trimmed, so that the two nerve ends have flush contact. In cases of more extensive trauma, each nerve end must undergo careful debridement transection until the veterinary surgeon is satisfied that healthy neural tissue has been reached. In more chronic cases, bulbous neuromas and gliomas may be found on the respective proximal and distal ends, and they must be removed by progressive serial transection until normal nerve tissue can be identified.[11] If a nerve has received only a partial laceration, care must be taken to debride only the injured fascicles while leaving intact fascicles undisturbed.

Several methods of nerve debridement transection are used, but we prefer the following technique. The

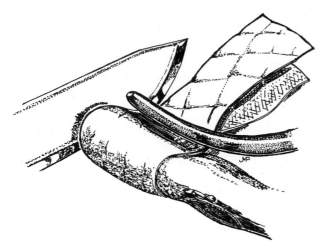

Fig. 5-5. *Debridement transection of a nerve end. The end has been wrapped circumferentially so a flush cut may be made. (Drawing based on photograph from Braun, R. M.: Epineurial nerve repair. In Management of peripheral nerve problems. Edited by G. E. Omer and M. Spinner. Philadelphia, W. B. Saunders, 1980.)*

nerve segment to be debrided is wrapped circumferentially with a soft material such as a Penrose drain, wide umbilical tape, or even moistened paper. This circumferential wrap must gently compress the nerve without crushing it. As a result of the circumferential compression, the portion of nerve undergoing debridement transection is changed from being soft and deformable to one that is firm and easy to stabilize. Consequently, the debridement transections can be made evenly and accurately by placing the nerve on a wooden tongue blade and by cutting it with a new scalpel or razor blade. Each transection must be made with a sharp blade, preferably a new one, to produce an even cut and to avoid any crushing action resulting from a dull blade. The debridement transections should be made perpendicular to the long axis of the nerve, so that each end will have a flush face (Fig. 5-5).

INSTRUMENTATION

Peripheral nerve surgery requires certain special instruments, and an appropriately trained assistant is also necessary for many procedures. Some form of optical magnification is needed to see adequately the anatomic structures of the nerve, and thus to minimize inadvertent surgical trauma. Variable-power operating microscopes are ideal because they are versatile and provide excellent optical acuity. More practical, however, are optical loupes, which provide from 2- to 6-fold magnification. These loupes may be obtained with adjustable or fixed intraocular space and working distance. They are adequate for most procedures, but certain situations involving small nerves may require 8- to 16-fold magnification.

Most of the surgical exposure of the nerve can be accomplished with standard instruments; however, to manipulate and suture the nerve appropriately one needs, at a minimum, microsurgical scissors, a micro-

needle holder, fine-tip jeweler's forceps, and tissue forceps with microfine teeth. Many other microsurgical instruments are available for use in various situations, but they are not required for routine neurorrhaphy. Suture material preferences are discussed later.

PRINCIPLES OF NEURORRHAPHY

Many techniques for repairing injured peripheral nerves have been reported in the surgical literature, yet no single technique has proved to be conclusively superior. The methods presented in this discussion are those that we have found practical and have given consistently good results. Regardless of the method used, the veterinary surgeon must adhere to certain principles to achieve the ultimate goal of return of nerve function.

Ideally, the nerve repair should be done as soon after injury as possible. Prolonged delays result in fibrosis of the distal nerve segment and degeneration of the end organ.

Atraumatic surgical technique must be used to minimize local inflammation and subsequent scar-tissue formation. Excessive scar tissue at or around the nerve repair site only serves to inhibit axon regrowth.

One goal of proper debridement of the nerve ends is to remove all nonviable ischemic tissue. Although an adequate blood supply is essential, hemorrhage must be avoided. Excessive blood clots at the repair site may promote scar formation; however, some remaining clot stabilizes the repair. Continued bleeding usually can be controlled by applying direct pressure with moistened lint-free sponges.

Proper anatomic alignment of the nerve ends is extremely important. Although it is not possible, nor is it necessary, to align individual endoneurial tubules, every effort should be made to match the fascicles of the two nerve ends. Failure to do so might prevent a significant number of the regenerated axons from reaching appropriate end organs. At times, however, accurate matching simply is not possible, owing to the normal variation of fascicular patterns between the proximal and distal nerve stumps.[8,9,10]

Tension at the repair site may stimulate detrimental scar-tissue formation.[9,10] Efforts must be made to minimize both longitudinal and circumferential tension. Longitudinal tension often can be decreased by extensive mobilization of both nerve segments, but care must be taken to avoid compromising the blood supply to the nerve. Longitudinal tension also can be lessened by flexing surrounding joints. Circumferential tension can be avoided by careful suture placement, so that the nerve ends are made flush without impaction or overlap.

The suture material used for the neurorrhaphy should be as nonreactive as possible to preclude foreign-body scar formation. A minimal number of the smallest-size sutures practical should be used to appose the nerve ends. We prefer size 8-0 to 10-0 monofilament nylon because it produces minimal suture granuloma formation when properly used.[3,8]

EPINEURIAL NERVE REPAIR

A large percentage of nerve injuries are suitable for epineurial suture techniques. Acute cases in which nerve loss is minimal are especially amenable to this type of repair. Epineurial neurorrhaphy is our preference whenever appropriate. Less magnification is required, and technically it is the least difficult and most rapid to perform.

The nerve ends are exposed and debrided as described. A light-colored soft material, such as a piece of a latex rubber balloon, is placed in the surgical field to act as a background against which the surgeon can more easily distinguish anatomic details. The light background also facilitates finding and handling the fine suture material when looking through magnification loupes or an operating microscope.

The nerve ends should be examined in detail, so that the fascicles of the 2 segments can be matched as closely as possible. Longitudinal blood vessels in the epineurium also should be matched to assure rotational alignment. When proper alignment has been determined, the first 2 sutures are placed 180° apart. Size 8-0 monofilament nylon* on a BV-2 or BV-3 needle† is preferred. These sutures must pass only through the epineurium and not through the underlying neural elements. When the first 2 sutures are tied, long tags are left so that the nerve may be manipulated without handling. The nerve then may be rotated with the suture tags in order that the back side of the nerve may be sutured more easily. At no time should any portion of the nerve other than the epineurium be grasped with forceps. Next, 2 sutures are placed opposite each other and 90° from the first 2 sutures (Fig. 5-6).

At this point, the neurorrhaphy should be examined carefully for alignment and distraction or impaction. Additional sutures may not be required, but this decision must be based on the appearance of the repair. If more sutures are deemed necessary to assure a stable neurorrhaphy, only the minimum number actually needed should be placed. In only a few cases have we found it necessary to place more than 6 or 7 sutures in an epineurial neurorrhaphy without tension, and usually 4 or 5 sutures are adequate. Prior to closing the surgical wound, any long suture tags should be cut short. Hemostasis must be attained, and excessive blood clots should be removed.

PERINEURIAL NERVE REPAIR

Perineurial, or fascicular, nerve repairs require more magnification and are more tedious to perform than epineurial repairs, but they have gained popularity with the improvement in microsurgical techniques. More accurate fascicular coaptation can be achieved with perineurial repairs, and this type of repair may be indicated when a few distinct fascicles can be identified clearly in both nerve segments (Fig. 5-7). We do not recommend this neurorrhaphy technique, however, when many small fascicles are present.

The injured nerve is exposed and is debrided as described, and a light-colored background is placed in the surgical site. With the aid of an operating microscope and working with an 8- to 16-fold magnification, the epineurium is dissected away from the nerve ends. The length of epineurium removed should equal one to two times the nerve diameter. The fascicles from each segment should be matched by size and location in preparation for anastomosis.

Size 9-0 or 10-0 Ethilon on a BV-5 or BV-6 needle is used to repair one fascicle at a time. Extreme care must be used to pass the suture through only the peri-

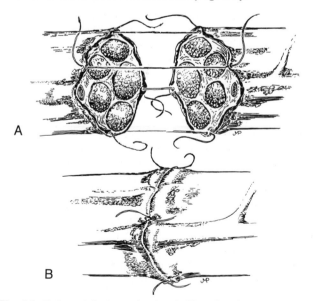

A

B

Fig. 5-6. *Epineurial neurorrhaphy. A, Note that the suture passes through only the epineurium and does not touch any neural elements. B, The two segments have flush contact. Rotational alignment has been maintained by using a surface blood vessel as a landmark.*

*Ethilon, Ethicon, Inc., Somerville, NJ 08876
†Ethicon, Inc., Somerville, NJ 08876

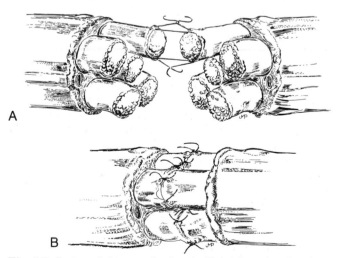

A

B

Fig. 5-7. *Perineurial neurorrhaphy. A, The epineurium has been dissected from the nerve ends and individual fascicles have been exposed. The suture penetrates the perineurium only and does not touch the nerve fibers. B, Precise fascicular coaptation has been achieved in the completed perineurial neurorrhaphy.*

neurium while avoiding the underlying nerve fibers. Two sutures placed 180° apart are used to repair each fascicle. They must be positioned and tied with great finesse to avoid distraction or impaction at the neurorrhaphy site. As previously discussed, hemostasis must be attained prior to closing the surgical wound.

NERVE GRAFTS

Management of peripheral nerve injuries in which a gap exists between the nerve ends because of an actual loss of nerve tissue is a difficult clinical problem. Such loss of nerve tissue may be due to extensive original trauma, or it might result from resection of terminal neuromas and gliomas at the time of secondary repairs. Two methods of gaining usable nerve length and overcoming such gaps have been mentioned previously, that is, positioning of joints and nerve mobilization. These and other techniques, however, are not adequate when an irreducible gap exists between the nerve segments.

The use and value of autogenous interfascicular nerve grafts to bridge large gaps have been described.[5,8] The problems of repairing a nerve under some degree of tension, however, where joints must be flexed, nerves must be mobilized, and vascularity is diminished, are not overcome completely by the use of interfascicular nerve grafts. Interfascicular grafting involves interposition of an avascular nerve segment that loses all endoneurial elements and also requires two separate neurorrhaphies that regenerating axons must cross. Regardless of these limitations, no other practical option may exist, and nerve grafting offers an excellent chance for recovery of function.

Interfascicular grafts consist of one or more free, autogenous donor nerve segments placed from each fascicle in the proximal nerve segment to the corresponding fascicle in the distal segment. Because fascicular patterns vary greatly and frequently are different in the two ends because of a loss of nerve tissue, the original fascicular pattern cannot be restored. The total number of grafts needed is not definite, but the total cross-sectional area of all grafts should approximate that of the nerve to be grafted.

Numerous small nerve segments are used rather than one large nerve trunk, in an attempt to increase surface-area contact and to gain maximum survival of the nerve graft. A whole nerve trunk used as a free graft frequently undergoes central fibrotic changes due to delayed revascularization. Several small cutaneous nerve segments, on the other hand, are more likely to survive because the reduced diameter across which vascular ingrowth must occur restores circulation quickly throughout the entire nerve segment. Therefore, a healthy vascular wound bed without scar tissue is essential for optimal graft survival.

Donor nerves for autogenous grafts should be easily accessible, and their removal must not leave the patient with any significant nerve deficit. The caudal cutaneous sural nerve is ideal for grafting, and it is our choice in more than 90% of cases. Several centimeters of suitable graft can be obtained from the sural nerve even in small patients. Similarly, no complications yet have been observed following removal of one or both sural nerves from several species of animals. The lateral antebrachial cutaneous nerve is the only other donor nerve that we have used for autogenous grafts. It is more difficult and time-consuming to harvest than is the sural nerve, but its removal also is well tolerated by the patient.

The technique of nerve grafting is similar to that of perineurial fascicular repairs, as described. The injured nerve segments are exposed, debrided, and undergo dissection to isolate and identify the individual nerve fascicles. At this point, the injured nerve and the size of the gap are assessed carefully to estimate the quantity of donor nerve needed for grafts. The donor nerve(s) then are harvested, and they must be protected with moist sponges until they are used. One graft at a time is cut from the donor nerve. Its length should be about 10% greater than the actual nerve gap. This extra length helps ensure that there will be no tension at either the proximal or distal suture line. It also allows for some shrinkage of the graft during the avascular period. Excessive graft length and redundancy must be avoided, however, because axon regrowth is prolonged by the extra distance.

The first graft of appropriate size is laid across the nerve gap. With the aid of an operating microscope using 8- to 16-fold magnification, the graft is sutured to a fascicle of the proximal segment. Using the perineurial suture technique described, the anastomosis requires 2 sutures of size 10-0 Ethilon (BV-5 or BV-6 needle) placed 180° apart. The distal end of the graft is left free at this time. Next, the second graft is cut from the donor nerve at the appropriate length, and then it is sutured to a fascicle of the proximal segment in the same fashion. The procedure is repeated until all proximal neurorrhaphies have been completed. Finally, the distal neurorrhaphies are done one graft at a time, making sure that each graft connects the corresponding proximal and distal fascicles. All suture lines must be without tension (Fig. 5-8).

Prior to wound closure, the grafts should be manipulated gently in an attempt to increase surface-area contact with the wound bed. If the nerve segments are left as a tightly packed cable, revascularization of the inner segments will be delayed. They may become fibrotic, and such fibrosis will slow axon regrowth.

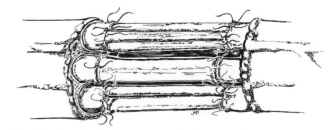

Fig. 5-8. *Interfascicular nerve grafts. Corresponding proximal and distal fascicles are bridged by the grafts. Note that two or more graft segments may be required for the larger fascicles.*

Postoperative Care

The extent of postoperative limb protection and immobilization required will vary with the severity of injury and the type of neurorrhaphy performed. A padded bandage for 7 to 10 days is adequate for an epineurial or perineurial neurorrhaphy performed without tension. If moderate tension exists, the limb should be immobilized rigidly for 3 weeks.[10] If joints have been positioned and the repair is under tension, the limb should be fixed rigidly in its operative position for 3 weeks, then at weekly intervals for the next 2 to 4 weeks, the limb should be returned gradually to a neutral position. After nerve grafting, the limb should be protected with semirigid fixation, such as a plaster splint, for 7 to 10 days before full mobilization is permitted.

Insensitive or anesthetic portions of the limb must be protected during the reinnervation process to prevent self-mutilation. Good general nursing and wound-care principles should be followed to expedite functional recovery of the limb. Physical therapy, to include active and passive exercise, is started as early as possible to help maintain joint motion and muscle tone.

Note

The opinions or assertions contained herein are our private views and are not to be construed as reflecting the views of the Department of the Army or the Department of Defense.

References

1. Cabaud, H. E., Rodkey, W. G., and McCarroll, H. R.: Peripheral nerve injuries: studies in higher nonhuman primates. J. Hand Surg., 5:201, 1980.
2. Cabaud, H. E., Rodkey, W. G., and Nemeth, T. J.: Progressive ultrastructural changes following peripheral nerve transection and repair. J. Hand Surg. 7:353, 1982.
3. Cabaud, H. E., et al.: Epineurial and perineurial fascicular nerve repairs: a critical comparison. J. Hand Surg., 1:131, 1976.
4. Ketchum, L. D.: Peripheral nerve repair. In Fundamentals of Wound Management. Edited by T. K. Hunt and J. E. Dunphy. New York, Appleton-Century-Crofts, 1979.
5. Millesi, H., Meissel, G., and Berger, A.: The interfascicular nerve grafting of the median and ulnar nerves. J. Bone Joint Surg. [Am.], 54:727, 1972.
6. Peacock, E. E., and VanWinkle, W.: Wound Repair. Philadelphia, W. B. Saunders, 1976.
7. Raffe, M. R.: Peripheral nerve injuries in the dog (Part I). Compend. Contin. Ed. Small Anim. Pract., 1:207, 1979.
8. Rodkey, W. G., Cabaud, H. E., and McCarroll, H. R.: Neurorrhaphy after loss of a nerve segment: comparison of epineurial suture under tension versus multiple nerve grafts. J. Hand Surg., 5:366, 1980.
9. Sunderland, S.: The anatomical basis of nerve repair. In Nerve Repair and Regeneration: Its Clinical and Experimental Basis. Edited by D. L. Jewett and H. R. McCarroll, Jr. St. Louis, C. V. Mosby, 1980.
10. Sunderland, S.: Nerves and Nerve Injuries. Edinburgh, Churchill-Livingstone, 1978.
11. Swaim, S. F.: Peripheral nerve surgery. In Canine Neurology: Diagnosis and Treatment. Edited by B. F. Hoerlein. Philadelphia, W. B. Saunders, 1978.

6 * Eye

Lids

Surgery of the Eyelids

by KATHLEEN P. BARRIE

Morphology

The eyelids can be separated surgically into two layers: the skin and orbicularis oculi muscle, and the tarsus and palpebral conjunctiva (Fig. 6-1). In dogs, cilia (eyelashes) are present only on the upper eyelid. The cat does not possess true eyelashes. Eyelid skin is pliable and can be easily stretched for sliding grafts. The

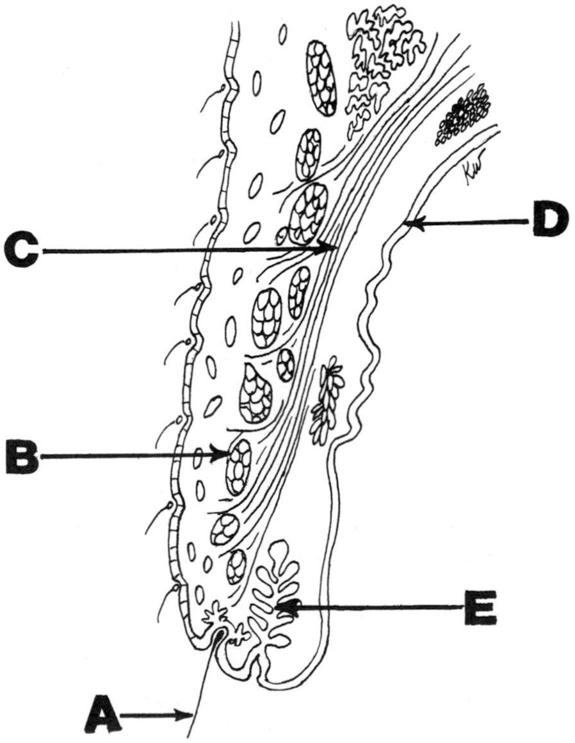

Fig. 6-1. *Sagittal section of the upper eyelid.* A, *cilia;* B, *orbicularis oculi muscle;* C, *tarsus;* D, *palpebral conjunctiva;* E, *meibomian gland.*

orbicularis oculi muscle, as a sphincter muscle, closes the palpebral fissure. The superior portion has the greatest strength for eyelid closure. Sensory innervation is by the trigeminal nerve; motor innervation is by the facial nerve.

The levator palpebrae superioris muscle is responsible for opening the upper eyelid and is innervated by the oculomotor nerve. The Müller muscle, a smooth muscle, complements the activity of the levator palpebrae superioris. The levator anguli oculi medialis is a small muscle that also elevates the medial portion of the upper lid and is innervated by the facial nerve.

The tarsal plate, a fibrous sheet, is not well defined in animals. It continues with the septum orbitale to attach to the periosteum of the orbital rim. The thin, pliable palpebral conjunctiva contains goblet cells, accessory lacrimal glands, and lymphoid follicles.

The meibomian glands are situated within the tarsus. There are 20 to 40 glands per eyelid; their ducts are distributed along a furrow within the lid margin forming the "gray line." Other eyelid glands include the glands of Zeis (modified sebaceous glands associated with the eyelashes), the glands of Moll (sweat glands associated with the eyelashes), and the glands of Krause and Wolfring (accessory lacrimal glands).

The almond-shaped palpebral fissure is maintained by the medial and lateral canthal ligaments (condensations of the tarsus) and the lateral retractor anguli oculi muscle (Fig. 6-2).

Entropion

Entropion is the inversion of the eyelid and its margin that causes eyelashes and lid hairs to irritate the cornea and conjunctiva. Entropion can be divided into three types: (1) anatomic (congenital), (2) spastic, and (3) cicatricial.

Anatomic entropion is the most common type in companion animals. Breed dispositions include chow-chow, Kerry blue terrier, St. Bernard, English bulldog, toy and miniature poodle, Irish setter, Doberman

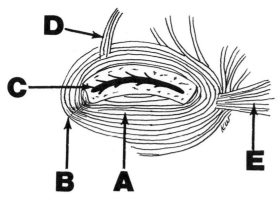

Fig. 6-2. *Muscles of the canine eyelid.* A, *orbicularis oculi muscle;* B, *medial canthus;* C, *palpebral fissure;* D, *levator anguli oculi muscle;* E, *lateral retractor anguli oculi muscle*

pinscher, Great Dane, Norwegian elkhound, and many of the sporting breeds. The defect may be due to a lateral canthal defect in the giant breeds, or it may be related to micropalpebral fissure in the chow-chow and Kerry blue terrier. Entropion also occasionally affects the lower eyelid of the Persian cat. The relationships of the globe, the tarsus, and the muscles of the eyelids are the determining factors in the development of anatomic entropion.

Spastic entropion is usually associated with contractions of the orbicularis oculi muscle because of ocular irritation, as in ulcerative keratitis. The entropion is usually unilateral, although it may be bilateral when associated with anatomic entropion or with corneal and conjunctival diseases. Therefore, the extent of spasm must be evaluated before a surgical procedure is performed. Topical anesthesia helps to define the blepharospastic component of entropion.

Cicatricial entropion is caused by the fibrosis and contracture of the eyelids due to trauma, chronic inflammation, neoplasia, or surgery. This condition is usually unilateral and should be distinguished from spastic entropion.

Several surgical procedures are used to repair entropion. The choice of procedure and the extent of correction is dependent on the underlying cause of the disease. Correction of the corneal or conjunctival disease by medical therapy may resolve spastic entropion. Anatomic and cicatricial entropion are usually treated surgically. Unless the cornea is irritated, anatomic entropion should not be corrected until the animal is approximately 6 to 9 months of age or has reached mature body size. Early correction may result in ectropion in the adult or may only partially correct the entropion. The use of ocular lubricants is indicated to help protect the cornea in the young animal. Temporary everting sutures may also be indicated.

The procedure selected to correct entropion is determined by the location, the severity, and the cause of

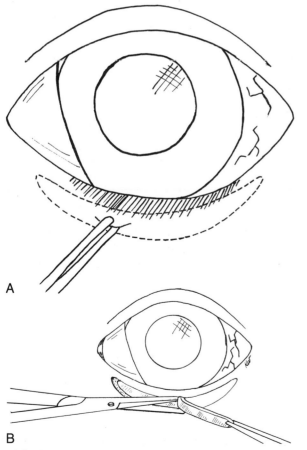

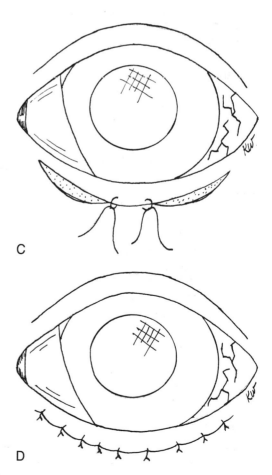

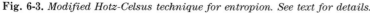

Fig. 6-3. *Modified Hotz-Celsus technique for entropion. See text for details.*

the condition. The modified Hotz-Celsus procedure is the most basic and can be adapted to most types of entropion. The amount of skin to be removed is ascertained, prior to anesthetizing the patient, by (1) digitally pulling the lids away; (2) noting depigmented, moistened skin; and (3) relieving the blepharospastic component by applying a topical anesthetic. An incision is made in the skin parallel to and 2 to 4 mm from the eyelid margin. The length of the incision should extend 1 to 2 mm beyond the affected portion of the eyelid; the depth should include the orbicularis oculi muscle. The ends of the first incision are joined by a ventral elliptical incision (Fig. 6-3*A*). The excised area is removed with scissors or scalpel (Fig. 6-3*B*). The central 2 sutures are placed first to provide maximum eversion (Fig. 6-3*C*). The sutures pass through the skin and subcutaneous tissue and, in severe cases, incorporate the orbicularis oculi muscle to enhance correction. The remaining sutures are placed at an angle about 3 mm apart from the center outward . The final result is a normal contour to the eyelid margin (Fig. 6-3*D*).

Postoperative antibiotic and corticosteroid ointment is applied tid to the eyelid to prevent secondary infection and to decrease pruritis. Complications of entropion repair are undercorrection (entropion) or overcorrection (ectropion). Subsequent entropion is easier to correct than postoperative ectropion.

MEDIAL CANTHOPLASTY

Medial entropion occurs frequently in the toy and miniature poodle, Pekingese, pug, and English bulldog. Clinical signs of epiphora, pannus, and keratitis of the medial quadrant of the cornea are often related to an inversion of the medial canthus, especially that of the lower eyelid.

A minor defect can be corrected by removing a triangular section of skin and orbicularis oculi muscle from the medial lower eyelid. The apex of the triangle should be below the lower lacrimal punctum (Fig. 6-4*A*). The triangular section of skin and orbicularis oculi muscle is excised with a scalpel (Fig. 6-4*B*). The incision is closed with 4-0 to 6-0 nonabsorbable simple interrupted sutures (Fig. 6-4*C*). The completed incision produces a normal contour to the eyelid margin (Fig. 6-4*D*). A more complex procedure is needed for lower and upper eyelid entropion, lagophthalmos, or exposure keratitis. This procedure combines entropion repair with a permanent medial tarsorrhaphy. Care must be taken to avoid the lacrimal drainage system. Cannulation of both puncta with 4-0 nylon is occasionally necessary to visualize and define these structures.

To evert the medial canthus, mosquito forceps are placed 5 mm lateral to the puncta in the conjunctiva (Fig. 6-5*A*). Fine scissors are used to remove a section of eyelid margin 1 to 2 mm from the puncta on both the

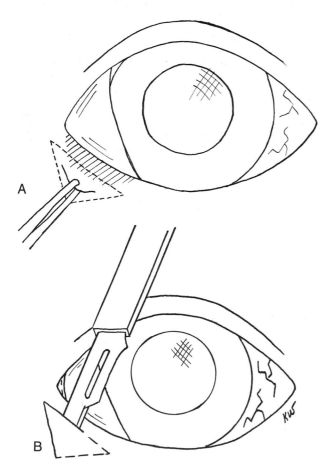

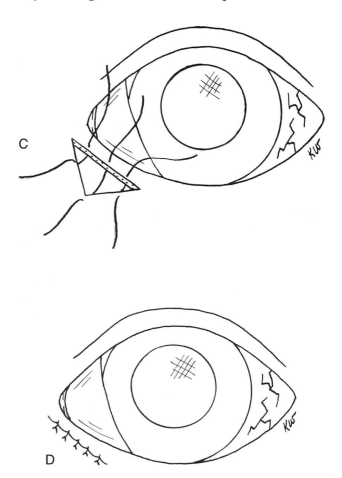

Fig. 6-4. *Medial entropion repair. See text for details.*

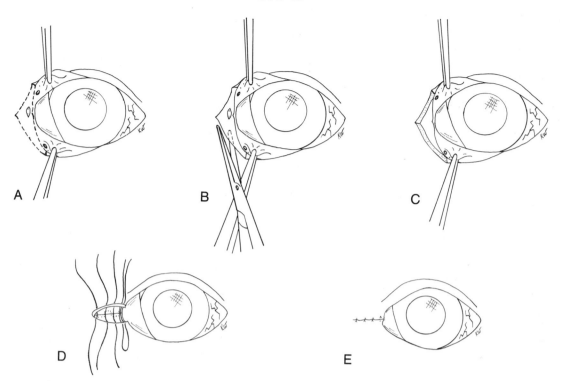

Fig. 6-5. *Medial canthoplasty. See text for details.*

upper and lower lid (Fig. 6-5*B*). The incision is continued into the medial canthus. The amount of canthal tissue removed depends on the extent of entropion. Completion of this incision includes the caruncle (Fig. 6-5*C*). The defect is closed by apposing the conjunctiva with a continuous 6-0 or 7-0 absorbable suture. The skin is apposed with simple interrupted 4-0 to 6-0 nonabsorbable sutures. Care must be taken in reforming the medial canthus. A 5-0 mattress nonabsorbable suture is meticulously placed at the wound's edge. The final result is a smaller palpebral fissure and a normal lid contour (Fig. 6-5*D* and *E*).

Postoperative care consists of topical antibiotic and corticosteroid ointment applied tid. Some type of protective collar can be used to prevent self-mutilation. Complications include possible injury to the lacrimal puncta with resultant epiphora, undercorrection, and overcorrection. If undercorrection occurs, skin sutures may contact the cornea and may produce keratitis.

LATERAL CANTHOPLASTY

Some breeds, such as the Norwegian elkhound, have an almond-shaped palpebral fissure with lateral entropion of the lower eyelids. To correct the lateral entropion, a modified Hotz-Celsus technique can be used. An elliptical incision made around the lateral canthus extends 2 mm beyond the affected lid (Fig. 6-6*A*). The orbicularis oculi muscle and skin are excised with a scalpel (Fig. 6-6*B*). The incision is closed by placing the first suture in the center of the wound to provide maximum eversion (Fig. 6-6*C*). The remaining incision is closed with simple interrupted 4-0 to 6-0 nonabsorbable sutures (Fig. 6-6*D* and *E*).

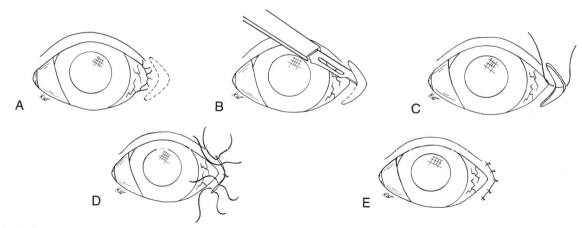

Fig. 6-6. *Modified Hotz-Celsus technique for lateral entropion. See text for details.*

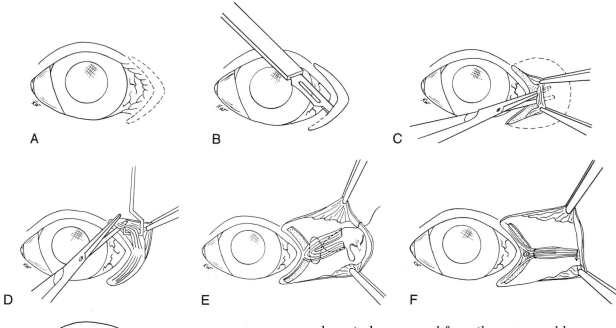

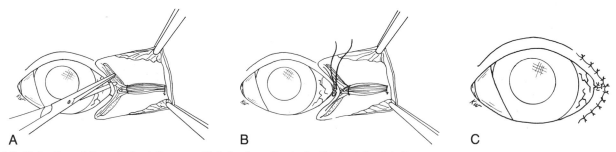

Fig. 6-7. *Lateral canthoplasty. See text for details.*

Large and giant breeds of dogs often have lateral entropion and a poorly functional or absent lateral retractor anguli oculi muscle, resulting in a round palpebral fissure. The surgical procedure to correct this defect uses a pedicle section of the orbicularis oculi muscle to serve as a lateral canthal ligament.

An elliptical skin incision is made around the lateral canthus about 3 to 4 mm from the eyelid margin (Fig. 6-7A). The skin is reflected to expose the orbicularis oculi muscle (Fig. 6-7B). Dissection is continued laterally for 2 to 3 cm; 2 strips of orbicularis oculi muscle are constructed and dissected free, leaving the muscle attached at the lateral canthus (Fig. 6-7C and D). The size of the muscle strips is approximately 2 by 6 mm. They are sutured to the periosteum of the temporal process of the zygomatic bone with a 1-0 to 2-0 absorbable figure-8 suture (Fig. 6-7E and F). Skin may

have to be removed from the upper and lower eyelids to correct additional entropion. The subcutaneous tissue is closed with simple interrupted 4-0 to 6-0 nonabsorbable sutures, and normal eyelid contour results (Fig. 6-7G).

In severe cases, shortening of the palpebral fissure is also indicated.* Shortening of the palpebral fissure involves removing equal amounts of lid margin from the upper and lower eyelids (Fig. 6-8A). The first suture is placed carefully at the eyelid margin with a 5-0 to 6-0 nonabsorbable mattress suture (Fig. 6-8B). The remaining incision is closed with simple interrupted 4-0 to 6-0 nonabsorbable sutures (Fig. 6-8C). Simply shortening the palpebral fissure is also useful for lagophthalmos, exophthalmos, and chronic exposure keratitis of the brachycephalic breeds.

Topical antibiotic and corticosteroid ointment is applied to the eye and incisions tid for 5 to 7 days. Postoperative complications can result from breakdown of the suture in the periosteum or removal of insufficient tissue. Overcorrection with resultant chronic conjunctivitis may also occur.

---

*Editor's note: An alternate procedure is the pocket-flap cantho-plasty closure, which may be used medially or laterally. See the following section of this chapter.

Fig. 6-8. *Reduction of the palpebral fissure with lateral canthoplasty. See text for details.*

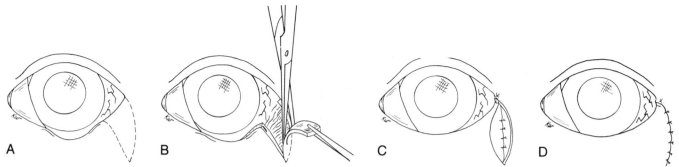

Fig. 6-9. *Ectropion repair. See text for details.*

Ectropion

Ectropion is an eversion of the lower eyelid and its margin that exposes the conjunctival and corneal surfaces. Its causes can be divided into five groups: (1) congenital, (2) physiologic due to fatigue, (3) paralytic, (4) cicatricial, and (5) iatrogenic. Congenital ectropion occurs frequently in the St. Bernard, American cocker spaniel, Newfoundland, and bloodhound. The condition may result in ocular disease. In general, affected eyes are subject to environmental irritation producing chronic conjunctivitis; if the lower lacrimal punctum is everted, epiphora results. Ectropion can also be associated with an abnormal lateral retractor anguli oculi muscle and macropalpebral fissure.

Surgical correction is indicated if ectropion results in persistent ocular disease. Removal of a large triangular piece of eyelid tissue laterally is one of the less-complicated ectropion repair procedures (Fig. 6-9A). The size of the triangle removed is dependent on the degree of ectropion. The appropriate portion of eyelid skin is removed with fine scissors (Fig. 6-9B). The conjunctiva is closed with 6-0 absorbable simple interrupted sutures (Fig. 6-9C). Care is taken not to penetrate the palpebral surface of the conjunctiva. The lateral canthus is reestablished with a 5-0 nonabsorbable mattress suture. The remaining incision is closed with 4-0 to 6-0 nonabsorbable simple interrupted sutures (Fig. 6-9D).

The Kuhnt-Helmbold technique is used for moderate ectropion (Fig. 6-10A). The eyelid is split into 2 layers—skin and orbicularis oculi muscle, and tarsoconjunctiva—with a No. 15 Bard-Parker blade or No. 64 Beaver blade to a depth of 10 mm (Fig. 6-10B). A "V"-shaped wedge of tarsoconjunctiva is removed from the medial aspect of the incision (Fig. 6-10C). The amount removed is dependent on the extent of ectropion. The tarsoconjunctiva is reapposed with simple interrupted 6-0 absorbable sutures, with the knots on the tarsal side to prevent corneal ulceration. Lateral to this incision, a similar "V" is removed from the skin and orbicularis oculi muscle layer (Fig. 6-10D and E). The 2 skin incisions are closed with 4-0 to 6-0 nonabsorbable simple interrupted sutures (Fig. 6-10F).

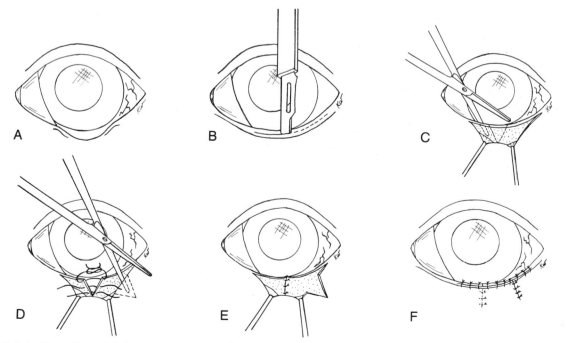

Fig. 6-10. *Kuhnt-Helmbold method for ectropion repair. See text for details.*

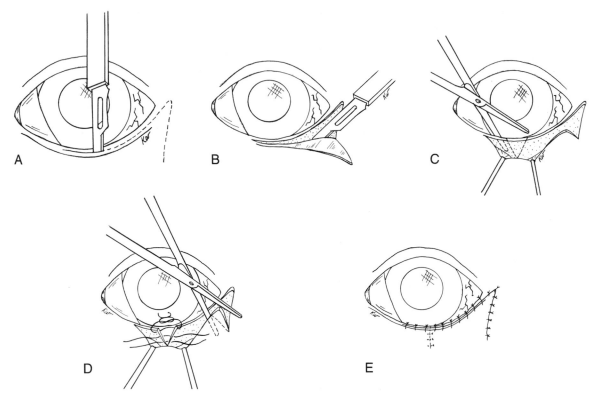

Fig. 6-11. *Kuhnt-Szymanowski procedure for ectropion repair. See text for details.*

Another technique for large ectropion defects is the Kuhnt-Szymanowski procedure, which tightens and lifts the eyelid. The lateral half of the eyelid is split into skin and orbicularis oculi muscle and tarsoconjunctiva layers to a depth of 10 to 15 mm. The incision is continued to the lateral canthus following the natural curve of the eyelid; the length of the incision is dependent on the extent of ectropion (Fig. 6-11A). At the end of the incision, another incision is followed downward and inward to meet the lower cut (Fig. 6-11B). A "V"-shaped wedge is removed from the conjunctiva and skin and is closed as described by the Kuhnt-Helmbold technique (Fig. 6-11C and D). The procedure is completed by apposing the skin and eyelid margin with several 4-0 to 6-0 nonabsorbable simple interrupted sutures (Fig. 6-11E).

Cicatricial ectropion results from scarring and con-traction of the eyelid. The "V-to-Y" method is the most fundamental correction. A "V" incision is made through the skin and orbicularis oculi muscle, with the base of the "V" at the eyelid margin (Fig. 6-12A). The skin is freed from the underlying scar with tenotomy scissors by blunt dissection, and the scar tissue is excised (Fig. 6-12B). The skin is undermined at the apex of the "V" to establish a sliding graft (Fig. 6-12C). The incision is closed in a "Y" shape with several 4-0 to 6-0 nonabsorbable simple interrupted sutures (Fig. 6-12D).

Postoperatively, topical antibiotic and corticosteroid ointment is applied to the eye and eyelid tid for 5 to 7 days. A protective collar may be needed to prevent self-mutilation. A complication of ectropion repair may be undercorrection with continued sagging of the lower eyelid. If too much eyelid is removed, entropion may result. Full-thickness resections can result in

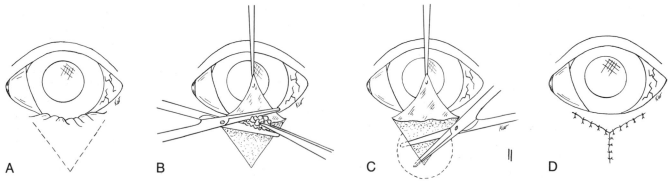

Fig. 6-12. *"V-Y" procedure for correction of cicatricial entropion. See text for details.*

micropalpebral fissure. In general, one-quarter of the eyelid is the maximum amount of tissue that can be excised without a relief lateral canthotomy.

Blepharoplasty

Many different blepharoplastic techniques are available, including skin grafts, full-thickness eyelid grafts, and pedicle grafts. Such procedures are indicated in eyelid tumors and in extensive lacerations. The goal of any procedure is to restore the physiologic function and the normal appearance of the eyelids as closely as possible.

General surgical principles, including atraumatic technique, are imperative in eyelid reconstruction. The specific procedure used depends both on the extent and location of the defect and on the patient. In relation to the size of the lesion, to replace one-quarter of the eyelid's length, a simple closure can be used; for defects up to half the eyelid's length and mediolateral canthal defects, sliding skin grafts or "Z" plasty can be used; for medial canthal defects, a pedicle graft can be used; for defects greater than half the eyelid's length, sliding grafts or "bucket handle" procedures are applicable.

Because blepharoplastic procedures usually require more surgical time, tissue handling, and larger wounds, systemic antibiotics are administered 5 to 7 days postoperatively. Topical antibiotic and corticosteroid ointment is applied to the eye and eyelid incision tid for 5 to 7 days. If much postoperative swelling and pruritus are present, low doses of corticosteroid may be administered parenterally. Some type of protective collar prevents self-mutilation. Tranquilizing the patient may also be helpful.

SIMPLE EYELID LACERATION

Eyelid lacerations usually heal readily, owing to a plentiful local blood supply. A contaminated wound requires pretreatment with topical and systemic antibiotics, minimal debridement, and proper closure (Fig. 6-13A and B). The tarsoconjunctiva is closed with 6-0 absorbable suture. The sutures are placed in the tarsal layer without penetrating the palpebral conjunctival mucosa. The skin and eyelid margin are then apposed with 4-0 to 6-0 nonabsorbable sutures. The first suture is placed meticulously at the eyelid margin in a horizontal mattress pattern to maintain the eyelid's contour, followed by simple interrupted sutures (Fig. 6-13C).

"V" PLASTY

"V" plasty is applicable in any full-thickness eyelid defect. This procedure can be used in defects involving less than one-third of the eyelid. The apex of the "V" is distal to the eyelid margin. The eyelid is cut with tenotomy scissors to remove the triangular piece of tissue. The defect is closed in a manner similar to a laceration repair, using a two-layer closure apposing initially the conjunctiva and then the skin (see Fig. 6-13).

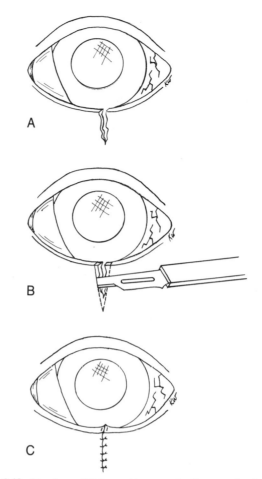

Fig. 6-13. *Simple eyelid laceration repair. See text for details.*

"Y-TO-V" PLASTY

The "Y-to-V" plasty is used to increase tension on the eyelid margin, as indicated with entropion. The first incision is made so that the arms of the "Y" incorporate the defect (Fig. 6-14A). The flap is undermined in order that the apex of the arms of the "Y" can be pulled down to the bottom of the stem of the "Y" to form a "V" (Fig. 6-14B). The skin is apposed with 4-0 nonabsorbable simple interrupted sutures (Fig. 6-14C).

FOUR-SIDED EXCISION

The four-sided excision ("upside-down" or "rightside-up" house) is used in larger full-thickness eyelid resections. The defect is removed with fine scissors en bloc in the shape of an upside-down house (Fig. 6-15A and B). Adjacent conjunctiva is closed with 6-0 absorbable suture placed in the tarsal layer without penetrating the conjunctiva (Fig. 6-15C). The eyelid margin is re-established with a 4-0 to 6-0 mattress suture. The skin is closed with simple interrupted 4-0 to 6-0 nonabsorbable sutures (Fig. 6-15D). This method distributes suture tension along the incision line and minimizes the possibility of a "notch" or defect at the eyelid margin.

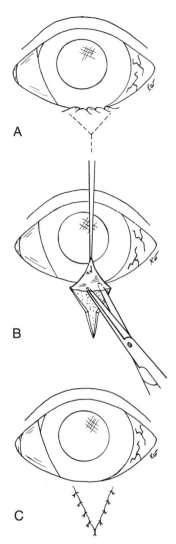

Fig. 6-14. *"Y-V" plasty. See text for details.*

SLIDING SKIN GRAFT

The sliding skin graft is used to close large defects in the eyelid associated with lacerations and excision of neoplasms. A full-thickness resection of the mass is performed, removing some adjacent normal eyelid (Fig. 6-16A). Once the tissue is excised, the palpebral conjunctiva is undermined extensively to fill the inner aspects of the defect. The palpebral conjunctiva must be adequately mobile to relieve tension at the suture line, to prevent contracture of the graft. The vertical incisions are extended to twice the length (height) of the original incision through the skin and orbicularis oculi muscle. The sliding skin graft is prepared by removing equilateral-triangular wedges of skin (Fig. 6-16B). The base of the flap is wider to decrease lateral tension, to provide maximum vascularity, and to compensate for limited contracture. The sliding skin graft is undermined by blunt dissection and is moved into the defect (Fig. 6-16C). The mobilized palpebral conjunctiva is first sutured to the eyelid margin on each side of the defect with 6-0 absorbable full-thickness suture. The skin graft is positioned slightly above the existing eyelid margin. The skin margins are apposed with 6-0 simple interrupted nonabsorbable sutures. The first sutures are placed at the eyelid margin and base in a mattress pattern. The remaining skin incisions are closed with 4-0 to 6-0 nonabsorbable simple interrupted sutures (Fig. 6-16D). The sliding skin flaps may be lined with tissues other than conjunctiva such as autogenous buccal mucosa.

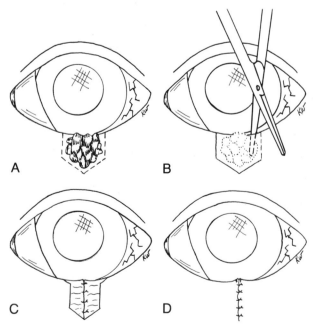

Fig. 6-15. *Four-sided excision. See text for details.*

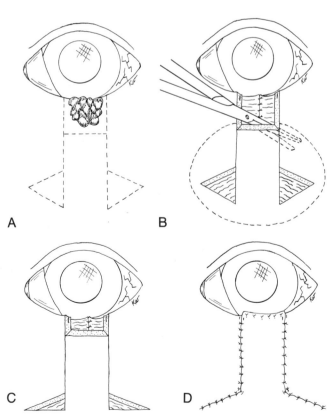

Fig. 6-16. *Sliding skin flap. See text for details.*

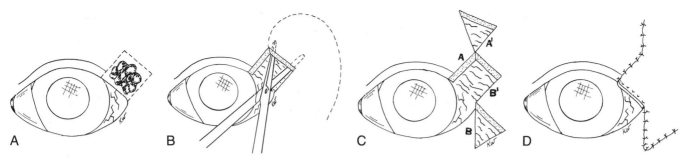

Fig. 6-17. *Sliding "Z" plasty. See text for details.*

SLIDING "Z" PLASTY

The sliding "Z" plasty is used to repair lateral eyelid defects. The defect is removed en bloc (Fig. 6-17*A*). Adjacent palpebral conjunctiva is pulled together with 6-0 absorbable suture to appose the inner defect. The adjacent skin is extensively undermined from the subcutaneous tissues (Fig. 6-17*B*). Equivalent triangular pieces of skin are removed dorsally and ventrally. The sides of the triangles are the same width as the defect. The free margin of the flap is advanced forward, thereby closing the triangular defects (A' to A and B' to B) (Fig. 6-17*C*). The skin and palpebral conjunctiva are apposed at the new eyelid margin with simple interrupted 6-0 nonabsorbable suture. The skin is closed with simple interrupted 4-0 to 6-0 nonabsorbable suture (Fig. 6-17*D*).

"BUCKET HANDLE" (FULL-THICKNESS) EYELID GRAFT

The "bucket handle" technique is used for eyelid defects involving at least half the entire eyelid. A full-thickness incision is made in the lower eyelid, and the neoplasm is excised (Fig. 6-18*A*). A full-thickness advancement flap is made in the upper eyelid 5 mm from the eyelid margin (Fig. 6-18*B*). A lower eyelid advancement flap is also prepared. Both upper and lower flaps are separated into layers comprising the tarsoconjunctiva and the skin and orbicularis oculi muscle (Fig. 6-18*C*). The tarsoconjunctiva from the upper eyelid is advanced and is apposed to the lower tarsoconjunctiva with simple interrupted 6-0 absorbable sutures (Fig. 6-18*D*). The skin and orbicularis oculi muscle of the upper eyelid are manipulated under the bridge and are sutured to the lower eyelid with 4-0 to

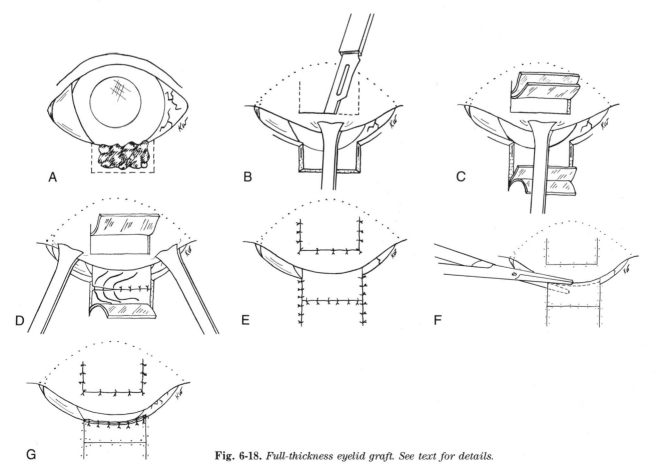

Fig. 6-18. *Full-thickness eyelid graft. See text for details.*

6-0 nonabsorbable suture. The raw edge of the bridge is sutured to skin to help prevent retraction (Fig. 6-18*E*). A temporary tarsorrhaphy may also be performed to take tension off the suture lines.

Two weeks postoperatively, the eyelids are incised at the palpebral fissure (Fig. 6-18*F*). The new eyelid margin is sutured in place with 6-0 nonabsorbable suture (Fig. 6-18*G*). The upper eyelid is also resutured to its normal state. It may be necessary to freshen the dorsal surface of the bridge before resuturing. A similar procedure can be used when only tarsoconjunctiva from the upper eyelid is used to fill a defect in the lower eyelid. If the same technique as the "bucket handle" is used, only the tarsoconjunctiva is mobilized. The tarsoconjunctiva is separated from the skin by blunt dissection. Two parallel incisions are made perpendicular to and 2 to 3 mm from lid margin through the palpebral conjunctiva. The tarsoconjunctiva is protracted and is apposed to the lower lid conjunctiva at the edge of the defect. A sliding skin flap is performed in the lower eyelid as described previously (see Fig. 6-17). A temporary tarsorrhaphy is used to relieve tension on the tarsoconjunctival flap. Two weeks postoperatively, the tarsoconjunctiva is cut in the palpebral fissure. The conjunctiva is then sutured at both eyelid margins.

PEDICLE GRAFT FOR EYELID AGENESIS

Eyelid agenesis of the lateral upper eyelid is not uncommon in cats, but is rare in dogs. The defect usually involves the eyelid margin and is of full thickness (Fig. 6-19*A*). Extensive lesions usually cause ocular irritation and disease necessitating surgical correction.

The upper eyelid defect is prepared to receive the new graft by splitting the defect into 2 layers, comprising the skin and orbicularis oculi muscle and the tarsoconjunctiva (Fig. 6-19*B* and *C*). The nasal aspect is trimmed. The horizontal pedicle graft is prepared by making 2 incisions through the skin of the lower eyelid. The first incision is parallel to the eyelid margin approximately 2 mm from the margin. The second incision is parallel to the first, making a 3-mm strip (Fig. 6-19*D*). The pedicle flap is rotated to the upper eyelid defect (Fig. 6-19*E*) and is sutured in place with 4-0 to 6-0 nonabsorbable simple interrupted sutures (Fig. 6-19*F*).

Lid Splitting for Distichiasis

Lid splitting is used to remove aberrant cilia from the eyelid margin. Distichia are abnormally located cilia usually emerging from or just medial to the openings of the meibomian glands in both upper and lower eyelids. Distichiasis can also result from chronic meibomianitis caused by metaplasia of these glands. It occurs most commonly in spaniels and poodles, although all breeds can be affected. The long, silky, aberrant cilia rarely cause problems, whereas those that are coarse and stiff can produce corneal ulceration. Persistent corneal ulceration that does not respond to treatment may be due to extra eyelashes. Therefore, magnification is recommended in examination of the eyelids. Other signs associated with cilia disease are epiphora, blepharospasm, and keratitis.

Several modes of treatment are possible. Lid splitting is the most drastic of the surgical treatments and is

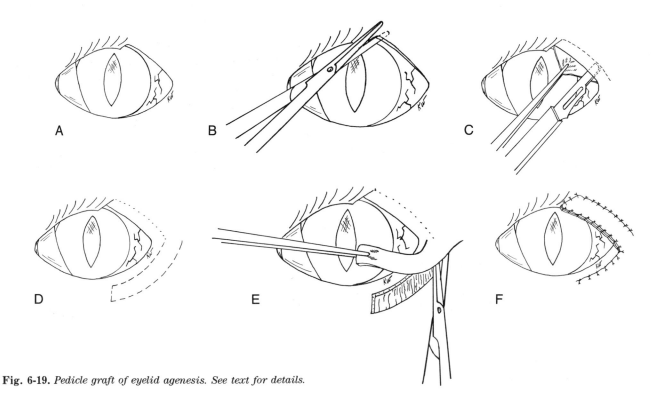

Fig. 6-19. *Pedicle graft of eyelid agenesis. See text for details.*

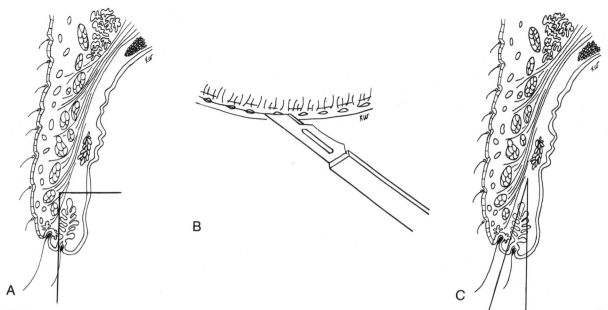

Fig. 6-20. *Lid splitting procedure for aberrant cilia. See text for details.*

seldom necessary. Resection of the tarsoconjunctiva requires magnification. The eyelid is split into the skin and orbicularis oculi muscle layer and the tarsoconjunctiva layer. The free eyelid margin is tensed with a tongue depressor or chalazion clamp. Once adequate tension is achieved, an incision is made along the meibomian gland openings (gray line) with a No. 15 Bard-Parker or a No. 64 Beaver blade (Fig. 6-20A and B). The incision is deep enough to include the meibomian gland and cilia follicle (perpendicular lines in Fig. 6-20A). The base of the incised tissue is cut and removed. A more difficult but precise procedure is the removal of the meibomian gland and cilia follicle with a "V" incision. An incision is made 2 mm across the gland and 4 mm deep (Fig. 6-20C). The "V" incision minimizes tissue loss, but requires eyelid stability, magnification, and delicate instrumentation. Postoperative therapy after lid splitting consists of topical antibiotic and corticosteroid preparations tid for 5 to 7 days to help decrease postoperative inflammation, pruritus,

and cicatration. Complications can be cicatricial entropion, fibrosis, and most commonly, recurrence of cilia.

Lateral Canthotomy

Temporary lateral canthotomy is used to increase exposure of the globe or conjunctival fornices during surgery and to facilitate replacement of the globe for proptosis. Permanent lateral canthotomy can be used to correct micropalpebral fissure.

The full-thickness lateral canthus is incised from the commissure to the conjunctival cul-de-sac. A hemostat may be preplaced on the canthus before cutting to minimize hemorrhage. The canthus is incised with sharp scissors on a line parallel to the palpebral fissure (Fig. 6-21A). Improved exposure of the globe is achieved with the lateral canthotomy (Fig. 6-21B). Closure of the permanent lateral canthotomy consists of apposing the conjunctiva to skin with nonabsorbable

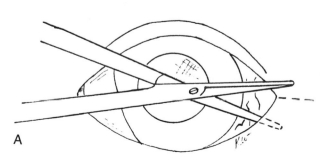

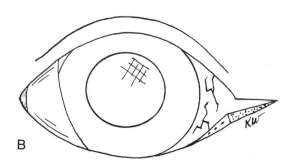

Fig. 6-21. *Lateral canthotomy. See text for details.*

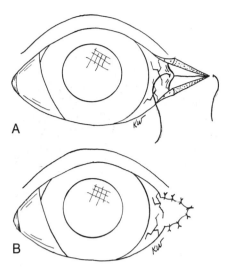

Fig. 6-22. *Permanent lateral canthotomy for correction of micropalpebral fissure. See text for details.*

6-0 silk simple interrupted sutures (Fig. 6-22*A*). An enlarged palpebral fissure results (Fig. 6-22*B*). A 2-layer closure strengthens the canthotomy, that is, (1) 6-0 absorbable tarsoconjunctival sutures in a continuous pattern and (2) 6-0 nonabsorbable simple interrupted skin sutures.

References and Suggested Readings

Fox, S. A.: Ophthalmic Plastic Surgery, 4th Ed. New York, Grune & Stratton, 1970.

Gelatt, K. N.: Veterinary Ophthalmology. Philadelphia, Lea & Febiger, 1981.

Magrane, W. G.: Canine Ophthalmology. 3rd Ed. Philadelphia, Lea & Febiger, 1977.

Prince, J. H., Diesem, C. D., Eglitis, I., and Ruskell, G. L.: Anatomy and Histology of the Eye and Orbit in Domestic Animals. Springfield, IL, Charles C Thomas, 1960.

Pocket-Flap Canthoplasty

by Cecil P. Moore

Permanent partial tarsorrhaphy or canthus closure has many applications in the treatment of canine eye disease. Indications for medial canthus closure include exophthalmos with lagophthalmos and exposure keratitis, ventral medial entropion with medial canthal trichiasis, or post-traumatic proptosis with lateral deviation of the globe. Lateral canthal closure may be indicated in cases of buphthalmos with corneal insensitivity, inversion of the lateral canthus (lateral canthal entropion) with blepharospasm, or macropalpebral fissure (with entropion, ectropion, or blepharospasm). I favor a two-layer pocket-flap technique because it is simple to perform, the results are cosmetic, it stabilizes the lid margins and results in a strong permanent closure, it may be combined with other techniques, and it may be used at either the lateral or medial canthus.

Instruments and materials necessary to perform this procedure include a No. 3 Bard-Parker handle with a No. 15 blade, small 1 by 2 rat-tooth forceps, small sharp-blunt tissue scissors, Allis tissue forceps, 4-inch Mayo-Hager needle holders, mosquito forceps, 4-0 silk with swaged-on cutting needle, and 5-0 monofilament nylon with swaged-on cutting needle. Prior to the operation, the desired amount of closure is determined. This amount varies from one-fifth to one-third the length of the lid fissure, depending upon the patient and the reason for performing the canthoplasty.

Surgical Procedure

The procedure is started by splitting the thickness of both upper and lower lids for the predetermined length of the closure. The lid may be stabilized by grasping the midportion of the eyelid with atraumatic forceps. The lid margin is incised on the meibomian gland line (Fig. 6-23) with a No. 15 Bard-Parker blade. The tip of the scalpel blade is firmly directed into the substance of the lid, where it splits the thickness and forms a pocket. This step is facilitated by a to-and-fro sweeping motion, followed by a reversal of the blade's direction. The pocket is of adequate depth when the distal snap-on hub of the scalpel handle contacts the lid margin (Fig. 6-24). Identical pockets are made in the upper and lower eyelids.

Marginal splitting incisions of the upper and lower lids should meet at the canthus to form a continuous incision. With small 1 by 2 rat-tooth forceps, the skin margin of the split lid farthest from the canthus is grasped. Using blunt-sharp tissue scissors, the skin margins of the upper and lower split eyelids are removed (Figs. 6-25 and 6-26). This technique facilitates a primary skin closure at the conclusion of the operation. Again, starting away from the canthus, the blunt blade of the tissue scissors is inserted into the dorsal lid pocket, and a right-angle cut is made in the conjunctival side of the pocket (Fig. 6-27). This cut creates a triangular flap that will be anchored in the ventral pocket (Fig. 6-28), which is left intact.

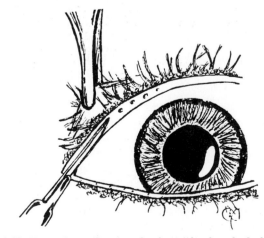

Fig. 6-23. *Using the meibomian glands as a landmark, the lid margins are incised for the predetermined length.*

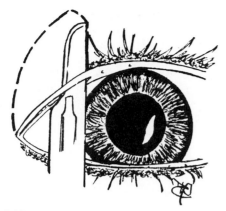

Fig. 6-24. *When the lid has been split, the blade is moved to and fro and forms a pocket the depth of the blade tip.*

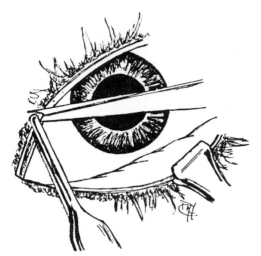

Fig. 6-25. *The skin side of the split lid is grasped with forceps and incised with tissue scissors.*

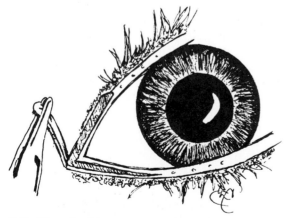

Fig. 6-26. *When the skin margins have been incised, they are reflected to the canthus. Corresponding strips of upper and lower eyelid margins are joined at the canthus and removed.*

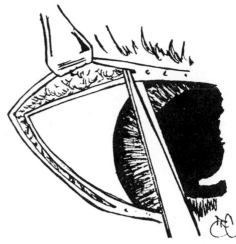

Fig. 6-27. *A right-angle cut of the conjunctival side of the upper lid pocket is made farthest from the canthus with tissue scissors.*

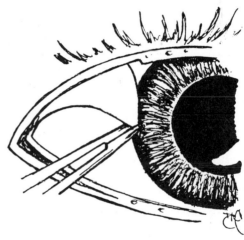

Fig. 6-28. *A triangular flap is created to be secured into the ventral pocket.*

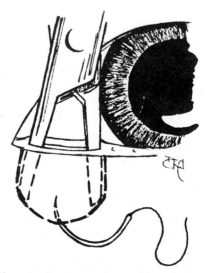

Fig. 6-29. *Mosquito forceps are inserted into the lower lid pocket, and the jaws are spread. See text for details.*

Mosquito forceps are inserted into the ventral pocket, and the jaws are opened (Fig. 6-29). From the skin side of the pocket, 4-0 silk suture with a swaged-on cutting needle is passed into the pocket ventrally and is grasped with the mosquito forceps. The needle is carried into the pocket, out the lid margin, and up to the point of the upper conjunctival flap, where it is inserted through the tip of the triangular flap (Figs. 6-29 and 6-30). Mosquito forceps are reinserted into the ventral pocket to allow the needle to pass through the lower incision. The needle is then passed from the pocket externally through the skin near its original entrance (Fig. 6-31). By tightening the suture, the upper lid flap is pulled into the lower lid pocket (Fig. 6-32). Once the flap is secured, the silk suture is tied, and the ends are left long for easy retrieval when the suture is later removed.

Final steps are the formation of a new canthus and the closing of the skin margins. Starting away from the original canthus, nonabsorbable 5-0 monofilament nylon with a swaged-on cutting needle is used to oppose the skin edges carefully. Proper placement of this first suture is essential to achieve proper function and cosmetic results (Fig. 6-33). At least 5 throws are made

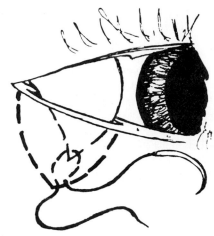

Fig. 6-32. *The upper lid flap is pulled into the lower lid pocket and tied.*

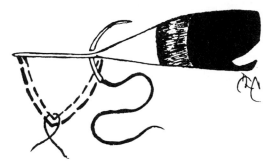

Fig. 6-33. *Placement of the first skin suture is critical to cosmesis and to function of the canthoplasty.*

in tying the nylon suture. The ends of the first suture may be left long, so that they can be tied back away from the globe by incorporating them into the adjacent skin suture. The remainder of the skin portion of the lids is sutured, using a simple interrupted pattern with 5-0 monofilament nylon (Fig. 6-34). Antibiotic ophthalmic ointment is placed in the eyes t.i.d., and sutures are removed 14 days postoperatively.

Advantages of the pocket-flap canthal closure include correction of both inversions and eversions of the lid; this correction thus stabilizes the lid margins. Pulling the conjunctival portion of the upper eyelid into the pocket of the lower eyelid has a straightening effect that is particularly helpful in cases of lateral canthal laxity. In exophthalmic states, distribution of the tear is facilitated by improved blink response.

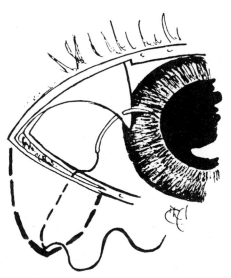

Fig. 6-30. *The needle is carried up and is inserted through the point of the triangular flap.*

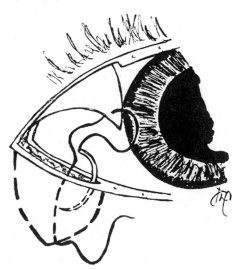

Fig. 6-31. *When the triangular flap has been engaged by the 4-0 silk suture, the needle is inserted back down through the lower lid incision and is placed through the skin.*

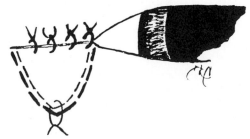

Fig. 6-34. *The procedure is completed by suturing the remainder of the skin portion of the eyelids.*

Tears are also conserved because of the reduced surface area of the exposed globe. Strong, permanent, fibrous adhesions that form between the dorsal flap and the ventral pocket thereby stabilize the closure and prevent stretching. If overcorrection occurs with this technique, a portion of the closure may be reopened surgically by cutting with tissue scissors. Following canthoplasty, the animal's appearance is frequently improved, and little scarring is apparent. In some cases, additional lid procedures, such as entropion, ectropion, or anchoring canthoplasties, may be performed either concurrently or later.

In medial canthal closure using the pocket-flap technique, the function of the lower lacrimal punctum is preserved, whereas the drainage of the upper punctum is questionable. Epiphora has not clinically been a problem postoperatively because the lower punctum apparently provides adequate drainage. The secretory potential of the conjunctival mucosa on the caudal side of the dorsal conjunctival flap placed in the ventral pocket has been questioned, but it has not been a problem. Similarly, splitting of the lids at the level of the meibomian glands has produced no complications.

References and Suggested Readings

Jensen, H. E.: Canthus closure. Compend. Contin. Ed. Small Anim. Pract., 1:735, 1979.

Wyman, M.: Ophthalmic surgery for the practitioner: permanent medial tarsorrhaphy. Vet. Clin. North Am., 9:322, 1979.

Surgical Procedures of the Conjunctiva

by NANCY BROMBERG

Symblepharon

Symblepharon is an adhesion between the bulbar and palpebral conjunctiva. Symblepharon may result from physical or chemical trauma, surgical procedures, inflammatory processes, or infectious diseases. Corneal burns due to hot liquids, lye, chemicals, and soap or detergents can cause extensive damage. The raw, granulating surfaces of conjunctiva adhere to each other and may heal by cicatrization. Neonatal or juvenile herpes keratoconjunctivitis in felines can cause conjunctival adhesions onto the surface of the cornea that may be significant enough to inhibit movement of the eyelids, to obstruct nasolacrimal drainage, or to compromise a significant portion of the visual axis of the cornea.

Symblepharon may limit the size of the cul-de-sac and may interfere with globe mobility. Partial or incomplete symblepharon involves only part of the cul-de-sac. In partial posterior symblepharon, attachment between the two conjunctival surfaces obliterates part of the posterior fornix (Fig. 6-35, B), whereas in partial anterior symblepharon, the adhesions do not extend to the fornix (Fig. 6-35, A). In total symblepharon, the entire fornix is obliterated. In all types, the cornea is fre-

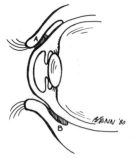

Fig. 6-35. *Partial anterior* (A) *and partial posterior* (B) *symblepharon.*

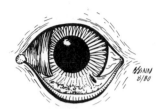

Fig. 6-36. *Corneal involvement in symblepharon.*

quently involved, causing it to be partially obstructed by an opaque and vascularized surface epithelium that replaces normal transparent epithelium (Fig. 6-36).

In cases of partial symblepharon that cause little or no visual impairment and mild cosmetic disturbance, treatment is not usually necessary. Repair is indicated, however, in patients in which the fornix is obliterated, causing marked restriction of ocular mobility or severe visual or cosmetic disturbance.

Problems in freeing the globe and reattachment postoperatively are frequently encountered, particularly if both surfaces are left without epithelium. When symblepharon affects a small area, it is possible to sever the adhesions and to repair the defect by undermining the adjacent conjunctiva, by protracting it over the nonepithelialized surfaces, and by apposition with 7-0 or 8-0 absorbable ophthalmic polyglactin 910* or polyglycolic acid† suture. The operative site should be checked daily and should be manipulated to prevent new adhesions. Several authors recommend the use of doughnut-shaped scleral implants or soft contact lenses to maintain the cul-de-sac.

When the conjunctival adhesions are larger and the cornea is involved, resection should begin in clear cornea just beyond the symblepharon. The conjunctiva attached to the cornea is grasped with forceps and is removed by laminar keratectomy. The veterinary surgeon should be careful to avoid perforating the corneal attachment, which may be thin. Peripheral to the cornea, dissection is continued under the surface of the conjunctiva until all adhesions are severed and the globe rotates freely. The edges of the normal bulbar and palpebral conjunctiva are undermined and are united with a small absorbable suture (Figs. 6-37 and 6-38). If the wound is large, or the undermining excessive, a buccal mucosa graft is performed. The graft is

*Vicryl, Ethicon, Inc., Somerville, NJ, 08876
†Dexon, Davis & Geck, Inc., Manati, PR 00701

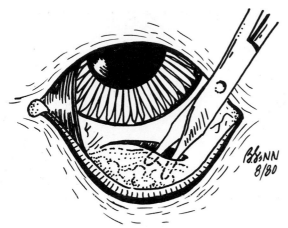

Fig. 6-37. *Dissection under the conjunctional surface severs adhesions.*

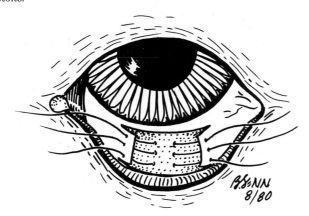

Fig. 6-38. *The conjunctival edges are undermined and then sutured.*

obtained from the inside lip or gum and consists only of epithelium and a minimal amount of supporting tissue. The graft is apposed to adjacent conjunctiva with 7-0 or 8-0 absorbable sutures, which are anchored to the sclera to prevent graft contraction.

Symblepharon can be repaired without mucous membrane or conjunctival grafts when only one nonepithelialized surface is present or when two such surfaces can be separated until epithelialization occurs (Fig. 6-39). This aim can be accomplished by lining the

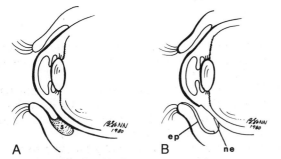

Fig. 6-39. A *and* B, *Symblepharon repair without mucous membrane or conjunctival grafts.* s, *symblepharon;* ne, *nonepithelialized surface;* ep, *epithelialized surface.*

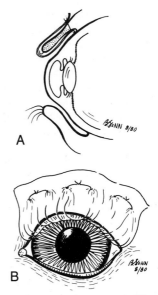

Fig. 6-40. A *and* B, *Placement of sutures holding plastic lining in place.*

eyelid with gas-sterilized household plastic wrap or other clear plastic. A piece of plastic is cut long enough to extend from canthus to canthus and from the upper part of the outer eyelid, around the lid margin, up into the fornix, turning down partially onto the bulbar surface. Three equidistant mattress sutures are placed through the plastic before insertion into the fornix. The sutures are passed through the fornix and appear on the front of the eyelid, where they penetrate the plastic. This procedure allows insertion of the plastic into the fornix and holds it in place (Fig. 6-40). The plastic material can be removed in 2 to 3 weeks. The aim of such an operation is to maintain separation of the nonepithelialized surfaces until the existing conjunctiva can proliferate and can extend along the surface to cover the more nearly normal cul-de-sac.

The use of ophthalmic ointment postoperatively may also reduce the likelihood of readhesion. Pyogranuloma resulting from inclusion of ointment within the wound is a consideration, but has not been a clinical problem.

Conjunctival Flaps

Conjunctival flaps are used to treat corneal ulcers unresponsive to medical therapy or those in danger of perforation, as well as corneal lacerations and, occasionally, keratopathies. The choice of surgical treatment of corneal ulcers is based on several criteria: (1) the severity, size, and depth of the ulcer; an epithelial defect may not be large, but if stromal loss is significant, the ulcer may be best treated surgically; (2) condition of the stroma; (3) rate of progression of the ulcer; a rapidly progressing ulcer may respond more favorably to surgical treatment; (4) if Descemet's membrane is exposed, surgical treatment is generally the best; and (5) initial or recurrent corneal ulcer.

The conjunctival flap has several advantages over the nictitating membrane flap or medical treatment alone: (1) the conjunctiva provides a vascularized tissue in intimate contact with the corneal defect; (2) the conjunctiva also provides tissue to fill in stromal defects, as well as support for the cornea; (3) a partial conjunctival flap allows observation of the defect and direct application of medication on the cornea; and (4) the conjunctival flap, if small and thin, permits vision.

Manipulation of the eyelids or globe should be avoided if one suspects a weak cornea. Anesthesia induction and surgical preparation should be carried out gently, to avoid corneal rupture. All manipulations of the globe must be made under anesthesia to avoid increasing intraocular pressure, which may rupture the defect.

The flap should consist of conjunctiva only. The conjunctiva is thin, elastic, and nearly transparent. If deeper tissues such as Tenon's capsule are incorporated in the flap, the flap loses elasticity and is more difficult to position. The flap should be transparent enough to permit some vision. Thicker flaps lose transparency and cannot be left in place permanently. It is essential to undermine the conjunctiva adequately to eliminate tension on the flap. Adequate undermining and proper suturing of the flap avoid dehiscence and premature contraction. After transposition, the deep conjunctival surface adheres to the area of the corneal epithelial defect.

The versatile conjunctival flap may be used in the treatment of corneal ulcers in several ways.

PARTIAL (HOOD) FLAP

A partial conjunctival flap is used for corneal ulcers with stromal loss near the limbus. The technique is as follows:

1. The conjunctiva is incised near to and concentric with the limbus using blunt scissors such as Steven's tenotomy scissors. A lateral canthotomy or a lid speculum may be used to increase exposure (Fig. 6-41).
2. The conjunctiva is undermined and is dissected from the underlying Tenon's capsule sufficiently

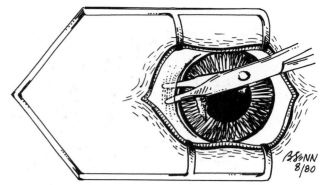

Fig. 6-42. *Undermining and dissection for partial conjunctival flap.*

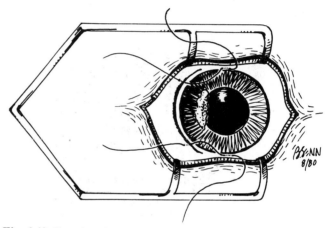

Fig. 6-43. *Securing the partial conjunctival flap in position.*

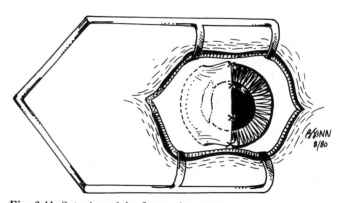

Fig. 6-44. *Suturing of the flap to the cornea.*

to provide a flap that can be extended over the corneal defect. Undue tension on the flap is to be avoided (Fig. 6-42).
3. The flap is anchored into position by suturing the conjunctiva to the sclera at the limbus with 6-0 or 7-0 absorbable ophthalmic polyglactin 910 or polyglycolic acid suture (Fig. 6-43).
4. The flap may be additionally sutured to the cornea with 7-0 to 9-0 absorbable ophthalmic suture. Sutures are placed in the stroma at half-depth or slightly deeper (Fig. 6-44).

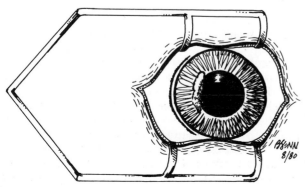

Fig. 6-41. *Incision for partial conjunctival flap.*

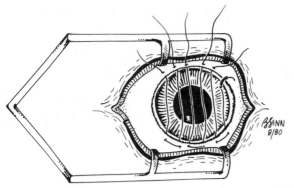

Fig. 6-45. *Suturing of the free edges for total conjunctival flap.*

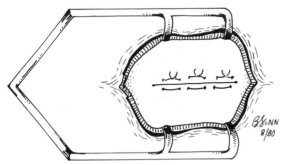

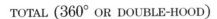

Fig. 6-46. *Mattress sutures in place (see Fig. 6-45).*

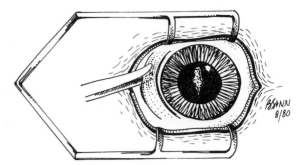

Fig. 6-47. *Incision for conjunctival bridge flap.*

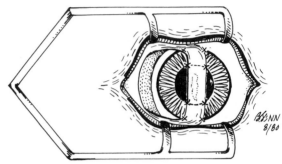

Fig. 6-48. *Anchoring the conjunctival bridge flap in position.*

TOTAL (360° OR DOUBLE-HOOD)

Total conjunctival flaps provide full corneal coverage circumferentially. They can be applied to large corneal ulcers and provide a contiguous vascular supply, protection, and support to the cornea. The technique follows:

1. The conjunctiva is incised at the limbus and is undermined as illustrated in Figures 6-41 and 6-42 for partial conjunctival flaps.
2. Undermining is continued for 360°, dissecting the entire perimeter of conjunctiva back from the limbus. Dissection behind the nictitating membrane may be difficult. The conjunctival flap should be kept thin and mobile enough to allow the dorsal and ventral aspects of the flap to be sutured together without tension.
3. The free edges of the conjunctiva are sutured using an interrupted mattress pattern with 5-0 or 6-0 polyglycolic acid suture. The mattress suture avoids irritation to the underlying cornea. A pursestring suture can also be used (Figs. 6-45 and 6-46).

BRIDGE FLAP

The conjunctival bridge flap is used primarily for central corneal ulcers. It provides a controlled, non-corneal blood supply to the cornea, as opposed to circumferential corneal neovascularization, which would

occur if the ulcer were to heal naturally. The technique is as follows:

1. The conjunctiva is incised at the limbus and is undermined as previously illustrated in Figures 6-41 and 6-42 for partial flaps.
2. A second concentric incision in the conjunctiva is made. The distance between incisions is determined by the size of the corneal defect (Fig. 6-47).
3. This strip of conjunctiva is dissected free and, attached at both ends, is moved to lie over the corneal defect. The flap should cross the cornea vertically, to avoid displacement during blinking.
4. The flap is anchored into position by suturing the conjunctiva to the sclera at the limbus with 6-0 or 7-0 absorbable ophthalmic suture. It is additionally sutured to the cornea over the defect with 7-0 to 9-0 absorbable ophthalmic suture. From 6 to 8 sutures may be needed around the defect (Fig. 6-48).

Postoperative Considerations

Conjunctival flaps are left in place 2 to 3 weeks. Medical therapy is continued during this period. While use of ointments is preferred with both partial and complete flaps, solutions can be used with a bridge flap. When the conjunctival flap is released, a portion of the flap will adhere to the corneal lesion. The conjunctiva is trimmed around this area. The remaining conjunctiva atrophies in time. When releasing a bridge flap, the dorsal and ventral aspects of the flap are transected close to the lesion. After release, they retract to the limbus. If healing of the cornea is complete, topical corticosteroids may be used with caution to decrease scarring.

References and Suggested Readings

Bistner, S., Aguirre, G., and Batik, G.: Atlas of Veterinary Ophthalmic Surgery. Philadelphia, W. B. Saunders, 1977.

Blogg, J. R.: The Eye in Veterinary Practice. Philadelphia, W. B. Saunders, 1980.

Choy, A. E., Asbell, R. L., and Taterka, H. B.: Symblepharon repair using a silicone sheet implant. Ann. Ophthalmol. 9:197, 1977.

Fox, S. A.: Ophthalmic Plastic Surgery. 4th Ed. New York, Grune and Stratton, 1970.

Gelatt, K. N.: Veterinary Ophthalmology. Philadelphia, Lea & Febiger, 1981.

Kaufman, H. E., and Thomas, E. L.: Prevention and treatment of symblepharon. Am. J. Ophthalmol. 88:419, 1979.

Magrane, W. G.: Canine Ophthalmology. 3rd Ed. Philadelphia, Lea & Febiger, 1977.

Severin, G. A.: Veterinary Ophthalmology Notes. 2nd Ed. Fort Collins, CO, Colorado State University Press, 1976.

Stallard, H. B.: Eye Surgery. 5th Ed. Baltimore, Williams & Wilkins, 1973.

Lacrimal Apparatus and Nictitating Membrane

Surgical Procedures of the Nictitating Membrane

by NANCY BROMBERG

Partial Excision of Cartilage

Eversion of the cartilage of the nictitating membrane occurs spontaneously in several breeds of dogs. Inheritance may be a factor in the development of the defect in the German short-haired pointer and other breeds. The eversion may be related to an unequal growth rate of the cartilage or the adherent conjunctival surfaces during development. Iatrogenic eversion can be caused by improper nictitating membrane suturing. It occasionally occurs in hunting dogs secondary to trauma to the nictitating membrane. Eversion of the cartilage occurs more frequently than inversion. In some dogs with a unilateral defect, eversion of the cartilage in the unaffected nictitating membrane can be elicited by protracting the membrane. The T-junction appears to be the weakest site of the cartilage (Fig. 6-49).

Eversion of the cartilage, characterized by the scroll-like appearance of the nictitating membrane's free border, may be unnoticed by the owner if the disorder is unaccompanied by clinical signs (Fig. 6-50). It may be either unilateral or bilateral. Presenting signs include slight epiphora and seromucoid discharge. Eversion of the cartilage reduces the effectiveness of the nictitating membrane in distribution of the preocular tear film and, consequently, may cause irritation or exposure keratitis. Examination of the nictitating membrane reveals the deformity.

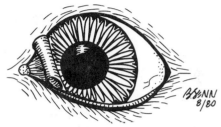

Fig. 6-50. *Characteristic scroll-like appearance of eversion of the cartilage.*

Surgical correction of the cartilage deformity requires careful dissection and excision of the abnormal portion of cartilage (Figs. 6-51, 6-52, and 6-53). Incision through the conjunctiva on the bulbar surface of the nictitating membrane and removal of the affected section permit the margin of the membrane to return to normal position and conform to the surface curvature of the cornea. The veterinary surgeon should avoid removing lacrimal tissue at the base of the third eyelid.

Because the everted area is usually at the junction of the T-stem and extensions, local excision of the affected cartilage can be accomplished. Occasionally, eversion of the T-junction is accompanied by deformity of the tips of the T at the medial and lateral extents of

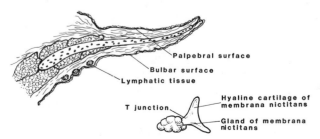

Fig. 6-49. *Schematic diagram illustrating the regional anatomy of the nictitating membrane.*

Palpebral surface
Bulbar surface
Lymphatic tissue
T junction
Hyaline cartilage of membrana nictitans
Gland of membrana nictitans

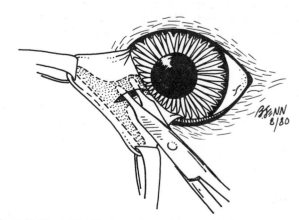

Fig. 6-51. *The nictitating membrane is everted, exposing the bulbar surface with thumb forceps. A No. 15 Bard-Parker or a No. 64 Beaver blade, or Steven's tenotomy scissors, is used to incise the bulbar conjunctiva overlying the everted portion of the cartilage.*

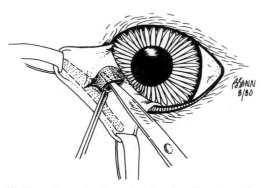

Fig. 6-52. *Blunt dissection is used to free the affected cartilage from the underlying and overlying conjunctiva. Caution must be used not to perforate the conjunctiva.*

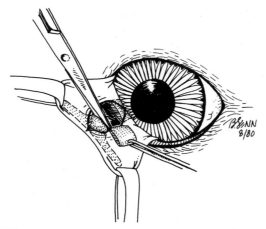

Fig. 6-53. *The affected portion of cartilage is excised once it has been dissected free of its conjunctival attachments. Any hemorrhage, usually minimal, is controlled by pressure or electrocautery. No suturing is necessary to close the conjunctival defect.*

the nictitating membrane margin. When only the tips of the cartilage are involved, these portions alone should be excised. The conjunctiva is closely adhered to the cartilage, and it is therefore difficult to remove portions of the cartilage without damaging overlying or underlying conjunctiva.

Topical antibiotic or antibiotic and corticosteroid ointment is used for one week postoperatively.

Partial Excision of the Gland

Protrusion of the gland of the nictitating membrane over the free edge is usually the result of gland hypertrophy (Fig. 6-54). This condition is commonly called "cherry eye." Although not considered a congenital anomaly, it usually occurs early in life. The breeds predisposed to this condition are the American cocker spaniel, Pekingese, beagle, and Boston terrier. A hereditary weakness of the connective tissue between the cartilage and the gland has been implicated. When seen unilaterally, the unaffected eye should also be evaluated for the potential to prolapse. Inflammation and hypertrophy of the gland, causing epiphora and conjunctivitis, occurs secondary to the exposure of the conjunctival surface of the nictitating membrane.

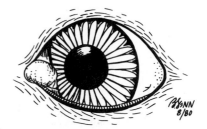

Fig. 6-54. *Protrusion of the gland of the nictitating membrane from its bulbar surface.*

Use of an antibiotic and corticosteroid preparation after repositioning of the gland often reduces the inflammation and edema associated with gland protrusion. Surgical excision may be the only permanent correction, however. The roles of the lacrimal gland and the gland of the nictitating membrane in tear production vary from dog to dog; that is, in a given patient, either the orbital gland or the third eyelid gland may be the predominant source of tears. Removal of the gland of the nictitating membrane may reduce tear production by 30 to 50%. Because of the possibility of resultant keratoconjunctivitis sicca, the surgical excision of the entire gland is discouraged. Only the exposed portion of the gland should be removed, leaving as much glandular tissue as possible (Figs. 6-55 and 6-56). An alternate method is to replace the glandular tissue by means of an inverting suture technique, thus preserving the tissue and the gland's function. (See the following contribution to this chapter.)

The excised tissue should be examined histologically because malignant adenocarcinomas of this gland are not uncommon.

Nictitating Membrane Flap

Nictitating membrane flaps are useful for certain types of exposure keratitis and for specific cases of corneal ulceration in which protection from drying and exposure would benefit medical therapy. These flaps act as a "bandage" for covering the globe in cases such as (1) facial nerve compromise, with decreased orbicularis oculi muscular function and lagophthalmus; (2) lid

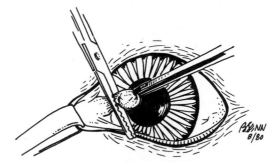

Fig. 6-55. *Straight mosquito forceps are used across the base of the prolapsed portion of the glandular tissue. Alternatively, the conjunctiva may be incised and the prolapsed portion of the gland clamped. Short-acting general anesthesia is usually adequate.*

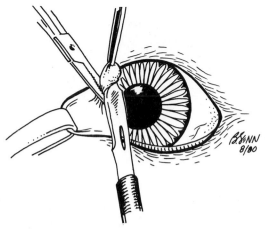

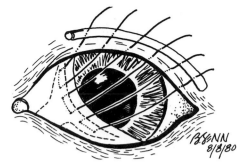

Fig. 6-57. *Nictitating membrane flap.*

Fig. 6-56. *The glandular tissue is excised with a small scalpel blade, such as a No. 15 Bard-Parker, or with scissors. The hemostat is left in place a minute or so to control hemorrhage. No suturing is necessary.*

lacerations; (3) severe palpebral conjunctival chemosis; and (4) globe subluxations secondary to retrobulbar swellings.

A nictitating membrane flap is easy to perform, often without the use of general anesthesia. It can be used to cover the globe temporarily in cases of multiple trauma when other, lifethreatening injuries have a higher priority of treatment.

In cases of corneal ulceration, the nictitating membrane flap has limited application. It is used only for protection of the cornea and support, not to replace stromal tissue or to provide increased vascularity. Disadvantages are that the flap decreases the amount of medication reaching the cornea. It also renders the eye temporarily blind and prevents evaluation of the healing process of the corneal lesion. In severe corneal disease, the use of a thin conjunctival flap may be preferred, as described in the previous contribution to this chapter. Use of a nictitating membrane flap should be avoided in cases of corneal ulceration or keratitis because of the risk of keratoconjunctivitis sicca. In superficial corneal lesions, in which friction between the cornea and the third eyelid is detrimental, an alternate method may be used; that is, one should suture the third eyelid directly to the globe. Mattress sutures are used to anchor the third eyelid to Tenon's layer of the dorsal globe.

In many dogs, the procedure can be performed with local anesthesia to desensitize the upper eyelid and topical anesthesia of the cornea and nictitating membrane. Some systemic sedation is usually necessary, and the use of a short-acting anesthetic agent better allows corneal culture, biopsy, and debridement. The upper lid should be clipped and surgically prepared.

The nictitating membrane is handled gently. It is grasped with serrated forceps (nontoothed) and is pulled across the cornea in its natural direction. This maneuver determines the location of the sutures in the eyelid, so as to draw the nictitating membrane across the cornea in a normal, nonwrinkled position. Mattress

sutures are placed through the eyelid near the fornix, using a stent such as a rubber band, a piece of plastic intravenous tubing, or gauze. A nonabsorbable ophthalmic suture material such as 4-0 silk with a swaged-on cutting needle should be used. The suture is then passed through the nictitating membrane from the palpebral surface without penetrating the bulbar surface. This technique allows a thick bite of tissue without exposing suture material to the cornea. The stitches should either pass behind or go through the cartilage of the nictitating membrane for extra support; this is especially important with the central stitch. Three sutures are generally used to distribute tension evenly across the nictitating membrane margin. These sutures are preplaced, and tension is adjusted so that all are under equal tension, in order to hold the flap in place but not strangulate tissue (Fig. 6-57).

The nictitating membrane flap should be checked frequently. Sutures placed under too much tension or placed too closely to the free margin may undergo pressure necrosis and dehiscense. Loose sutures may cause corneal abrasion. Because the nictitating membrane flap obscures visualization of the cornea, complications may go unobserved. The flap should be released and the globe inspected if evidence of a degeneration, such as copious discharge, or pain is present.

Depending on the underlying condition, the nictitating membrane flap is left in place for 2 to 3 weeks. When medicating an eye with a nictitating membrane flap, it is important to keep the eye free of discharge and to use ointments rather than solutions. Ointments are retained longer; thus, medication is more likely to reach the cornea and to maintain contact.

References and Suggested Readings

Bistner, S., Aguirre, G., and Batik, G.: Atlas of Veterinary Ophthalmic Surgery. Philadelphia, W. B. Saunders, 1977.

Bromberg, N. M.: The nictitating membrane. Compend. Contin. Ed. Small Anim. Pract., 11:627, 1980.

Gelatt, K. N.: Veterinary Ophthalmology. Philadelphia, Lea & Febiger, 1981.

Helper, L. C., Magrane, W. G., Koehm, J., and Johnson, R.: Surgical induction of keratoconjunctivitis sicca in the dog. J. Am. Vet. Med. Assoc., 165:1185, 1978.

Severin, G. A.: Veterinary Ophthalmology Notes. 2nd Ed. Fort Collins, CO, Colorado State University Press, 1976.

Alternate Technique for Prolapsed Gland of the Third Eyelid (Replacement Technique)

by CECIL P. MOORE

The function of the gland of the third eyelid in production of aqueous tear is discussed in the previous section of this chapter. Because of its important contribution to total tear volume, retention of this tissue is desirable in cases of gland prolapse (Fig. 6-58). The technique described here is a replacement procedure that offers an alternative to partial or total resection of the gland.

Preservation of the gland involves the placement of subconjunctival retention sutures to retract and to anchor it. Instruments necessary for the procedure include 2 mosquito forceps, Bard-Parker handle with No. 15 blade or a Beaver handle with No. 64 blade, fine 1 by 2 rat-tooth forceps, small, blunt tissue scissors, 7-0 absorbable suture with swaged-on microcutting needle, and Castroveijo ophthalmic needle holders.

Surgical Procedure

The third eyelid is grasped and suspended by mosquito forceps on nasal and temporal sides. An elliptical incision is made through the conjunctiva over the prolapsed gland (Fig. 6-59). A horizontal ellipse of conjunctiva, approximately 3 to 4 mm at its widest point, is dissected free with small blunt tissue scissors and is removed, exposing the glandular tissue. Later, as the procedure is completed, this maneuver will facilitate more exact apposition of the conjunctiva. The conjunctival margins are freed from the gland by blunt dissection, so that connective tissue is exposed deep (bulbar) to the gland as well as distally near the edge of the nictitating membrane. Hemorrhage is controlled by applying gentle pressure with a cotton-tipped applicator.

Following separation of the conjunctiva from the glandular tissue, a 7-0 absorbable suture (polyglycolic acid*, polyglactin 910†, or chromic catgut) with swaged-on microcutting needle is passed deep to the gland and is anchored under the conjunctiva to the epibulbar connective tissue (Fig. 6-60). This suture is carried to the opposite side of the gland, and the needle is passed into subconjunctival connective tissue near the margin of the third eyelid (Fig. 6-61). The first suture is preplaced, so that approximately one-third of the gland is demarcated. The suture is left untied. Similarly, a second suture is placed deep on the opposite side of the gland, then is passed over the exposed gland and anchored under the conjunctiva near the edge of the nictitating membrane (Fig. 6-62). If properly placed, these sutures will overlie the gland, dividing it into thirds. Once the sutures are in place, each suture is drawn together with a surgeon's throw while gentle downward pressure is applied to the gland (Fig. 6-63).

*Dexon, Davis & Geck, Inc., Manati, PR 00701
†Vicryl, Ethicon, Inc., Somerville, NJ 08876

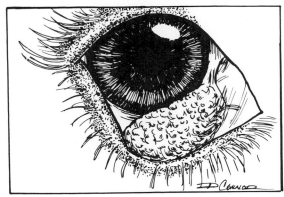

Fig. 6-58. *Typical appearance of prolapsed third eyelid gland.*

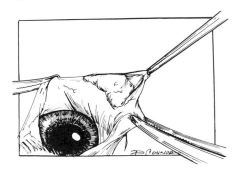

Fig. 6-59. *Elliptical incision.*

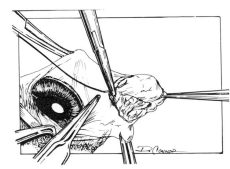

Fig. 6-60. *Initial anchor suture.*

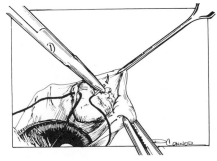

Fig. 6-61. *Initial suture carried to the opposite side of the gland.*

This technique inverts the prolapsed tissue (Fig. 6-64). The procedure is completed by tying the knots and by trimming the sutures close to the knots, thus minimizing corneal irritation from frictional rubbing of long suture ends. Correctly placed knots will lie under the conjunctiva. No sutures are placed in the conjunctiva because inversion of the gland results in apposition of

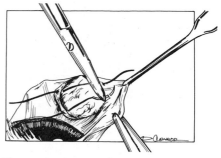

Fig. 6-62. *Placement of a second suture.*

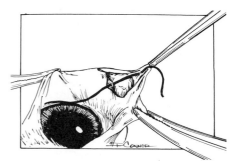

Fig. 6-63. *Initial suture is drawn together and tied.*

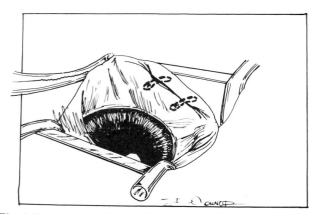

Fig. 6-64. *Inversion of the prolapsed tissue. The dotted lines indicate that suture and knots lie under the conjunctiva.*

the conjunctival margins. Buckling and redundancy of the conjunctiva are minimized by the initial removal of the conjunctival strip.

This inverting technique immediately corrects the prolapse (Fig. 6-65). Postoperatively, antibiotic ophthalmic ointment is applied to the eye tid for 7 days

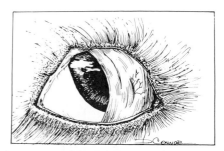

Fig. 6-65. *Appearance of third eyelid immediately after operation.*

when re-evaluation is recommended. At that time, fluorescein dye is applied to assess the cornea for possible frictional irritation. Sutures do not need to be removed with this procedure.

Reference and Suggested Reading

Blogg, J. R.: Surgical replacement of a prolapsed gland of the third eyelid ('cherry eye')—a new technique. Aust. Vet. Pract., *9*:75, 1979.

Lacrimal System

by Reuben Merideth

The lacrimal system consists of a tear-secreting mechanism coupled with a tear-drainage apparatus. The preocular tear film (POTF), a composite secretion, maintains the health and the optical clarity of the cornea. The drainage apparatus channels tears from the lacrimal lake at the medial canthus to the nasal cavity. In healthy subjects, this system provides for continuous turnover of the POTF with minimal ocular discharge.

Dysfunction of the lacrimal system results from either an inappropriate tear production or an ineffective drainage. Lacrimation, an excessive production of aqueous tears, is generally the consequence of corneal and conjunctival irritation or uveitis. Epiphora is the overflow of tears due to inadequate drainage of tears through the nasolacrimal apparatus. The most frequent problem in small animal ophthalmology is the insufficient production of one or more components of the POTF.

Keratoconjunctivitis Sicca

The clinical signs of inadequate tear production, keratoconjunctivitis sicca (KCS), are a dull lackluster cornea with a thick, ropy mucous discharge and a hyperemic conjunctiva. If the onset is acute, corneal ulceration usually complicates the disease.

Acute KCS may result from lacrimal gland infection, trauma, or drug toxicities.[4] The sudden absence of the aqueous secretion should be considered an ophthalmic emergency. The cornea acutely deprived of POTF soon desiccates, and corneal malacia and rapidly progressive ulcers may develop. Clinically, the patient exhibits intense ocular pain with blepharospasm and frequent corneal ulceration. If unchecked, corneal perforation and staphyloma often result.

Acute KCS may necessitate both medical and surgical management. Medical treatment includes the administration of lacrimomimetics and lacrimogenics, in addition to broad-spectrum topical antibiotics. Conjunctival grafts and nictitating membrane flaps may be considered for the rapidly deteriorating cornea. These biologic bandages provide support and nutrition to aid in the healing process. Both procedures are discussed previously in this chapter.

The more common, chronic form of KCS is characterized by the previously mentioned signs, pigment infiltration and neovascularization of the cornea. Both processes contribute to corneal opacification and decrease in vision. Signs are similar in the cat, but with much less corneal pigmentation.

KCS must be differentiated from other types of conjunctivitis. In addition to a complete ophthalmic examination, the Schirmer tear test is used to measure aqueous tear production. The test involves placing a commercially available strip of filter paper, 5 by 35 mm,* in the cul-de-sac of the lower lid. The length of test-strip wetting in 60 seconds is correlated to tear production. The test is conducted by measuring basal and reflex production without topical anesthetic (Schirmer I), by measuring basal tear production with topical anesthetic (Schirmer II). Normal Schirmer I values are 21.0 mm (S.D. ± 4.2 mm) per 60 seconds in the dog[4] and 16.9 mm (S.D. ± 5.7 mm) per 60 seconds in the cat.[11] Values of less than 5 mm of wetting in 60 seconds are diagnostic for KCS, whereas values between 6 and 14 mm of wetting in 60 seconds are suggestive of aqueous tear-film deficiency. This test should be performed before excessive manipulations of the eyelids or adnexa and prior to the instillation of solutions that may alter the results, such as topical anesthetic agents or artificial tears.

Another test of tear-film integrity, tear-film breakup time, has had limited application in veterinary ophthalmology. The mucin layer of the POTF enhances maintenance of a confluent tear film. A mucin deficiency accelerates the tear-film breakup. Visualization of tear-film breakup is improved by the instillation of one drop of fluorescein solution and slit-lamp biomicroscopic magnification. The eyelids are retracted, and the time is recorded from the last blink to the appearance of islands devoid of tears. The average time in man is normally 25 seconds or longer.[8] Times under 15 seconds are indicative of a mucin-layer deficiency of the POTF.

Conjunctival cytologic examination aids in the diagnosis of KCS. Cytologic specimens should be obtained from the palpebral conjunctiva at a point midway between the lid margin and the fornix. The specimen is gently spread on a glass slide. A variety of special stains are available, although the Wright-Giemsa and the Gram stains are sufficient. A normal specimen consists of nonkeratinized epithelial cells with an occasional goblet cell. Few neutrophils and bacteria may be noted. Keratinized epithelial cells typically predominate in chronic KCS, along with increased numbers of goblet cells. Abundant neutrophils and bacteria suggest bacterial conjunctivitis, a frequent secondary complication. Ideally, biopsy of the lacrimal or accessory lacrimal gland may also aid in the determination of an etiologic diagnosis.

*Schirmer Tear Test Strips, Alcon Laboratories, 6201 South Freeway, Fort Worth, TX 76134

MEDICAL MANAGEMENT

All patients with chronic KCS should be managed medically for 6 to 8 weeks. Transient decreases in tear production frequently respond to medical therapy, thereby obviating the need for long-term treatment or an operation. Surgical procedures should be reserved for those patients that cannot be effectively controlled by medical management or in which the treatment procedure proves unacceptable to the owners.

The aim of medical management is to replace tear volume and to stimulate tear production. Effective tear volume can be increased by the instillations of lacrimomimetic or mucomimetic agents to supplement existing tears, and by the stimulation of endogenous aqueous secretion with lacrimogenic agents.

Lacrimomimetic agents must simulate several properties of natural tears. First, they must be hydrophilic, to aid in cleansing the cornea. Additionally, they should lubricate the corneal surface sufficiently to permit normal lid function. Drug-to-cornea contact times must be long enough to make the use of these agents acceptable. Lacrimogenic agents are parasympathomimetics and therefore stimulate the production of the aqueous tears. For these agents to be effective, functional glandular tissue must be present, although intact innervation is not necessary. Pilocarpine is widely used for this purpose, at divided daily doses of 2 to 4 mg, and may be instilled topically or administered systemically in the food. Side effects may arise irrespective of route of administration. Side effects include ptyalism 30 minutes after treatment. More severe toxic effects include vomiting, heart block, and pulmonary edema.[10] The lacrimogenic effects usually persist for 6 to 8 hours.[3] These agents should be considered only for those patients without cardiovascular and respiratory diseases.

Antibiotics are indicated when secondary bacterial conjunctivitis is present. Topical corticosteroids may provide some symptomatic relief and may aid in the dispersion of the pigmentary keratopathy.

INDICATIONS FOR SURGICAL TREATMENT

Surgical treatment should be limited to those patients in which medical management is ineffective or compliance is a problem. Obviously, not all cases of KCS are amenable to surgical correction. Mucin-deficient KCS does not benefit from an increase in an already adequate aqueous phase of tears. Similarly, exposure keratitis secondary to lagophthalmia shows little improvement with a parotid duct transposition, but benefits from a permanent partial tarsorrhaphy to reduce exposure. Neurogenic deficits to the salivary glands may be concomitant and may negate the benefit of parotid duct transposition.

Transposition of the duct of the parotid salivary gland was first described in 1950 in human surgery. The application to veterinary surgery was in 1966, by Lavignette.[7] The technique is based on the similarity of parotid salivary and lacrimal gland secretions.

SURGICAL ANATOMY

The parotid salivary gland is a V-shaped structure located at the base of the auricular cartilage. Its rostral border is the masseter muscle and the temporomandibular joint. The main duct is formed by the convergence of 2 to 3 smaller ductules just proximal to the gland. The duct, about 1.5 mm in diameter, extends approximately 6 cm rostrally in the mesocephalic dog and transcends the superficial aspect of the masseter muscle. Its secretions enter the buccal cavity by a papilla located lateral to the caudal aspect of the fourth upper premolar (carnassial) tooth.[2]

The papilla of the zygomatic salivary duct is located adjacent to the molar teeth. The zygomatic duct is shorter than the parotid duct, and the catheter can be passed only 2 cm or less.

PRESURGICAL CONSIDERATIONS

Before the operation, the functional capability of the parotid salivary gland should be assessed.[5] Topical application of a bitter agent to the tongue should stimulate a profuse salivation if the gland is neurologically intact. Paradoxically, 1% atropine sulfate can provide the necessary taste stimulus (the pharmacologic effect of atropine is to decrease parotid salivary secretions). Following stimulation, the openings of the parotid ducts should be viewed directly by the veterinary surgeon for evidence of salivary flow.

SURGICAL PROCEDURES

Two approaches have been developed for transposition of the parotid duct. The open technique, involving isolation and dissection of the duct through a skin inci-sion, has been employed successfully in cats and dogs.[4] An alternate, closed approach, described by Jensen, involves dissection through an oral incision.[5]

OPEN APPROACH. The open approach provides optimum surgical exposure facilitating dissection, reduces the potential for duct transection and rotation and allows identification of the buccal nerves and facial vein.

General anesthesia is induced in the patient. Preoperative atropinization is not recommended because it decreases salivary secretions. The parotid salivary duct is catheterized with a darkly colored suture (Fig. 6-66); the tip of a 1-0 to 2-0 monofilament nylon suture is blunted by lightly flaming. The initial passage of suture is difficult because of the tortuous path of the distal duct beneath the submucosa. This distal curvature can be straightened and passage can be facilitated by grasping the mucosa rostral to the papilla and pulling the mucosa and duct forward. The suture is passed until it reaches the gland. The exposed suture is left in situ with at least 1 to 2 cm external to the papilla.

A pledget of cotton soaked with antiseptic solution is placed over the papilla when the area has been treated with surgical scrub solution. The lip is returned to its normal position.

The lateral aspect of the face is prepared for aseptic surgery and is draped appropriately. The nylon suture can usually be palpated through the skin and serves to mark the incision site. The incision over the catheterized duct is made through the skin and superficial facial muscles. The duct is isolated and is dissected with Steven's tenotomy scissors (Fig. 6-67). Mobilization and elevation of the duct are facilitated by retraction with one-eighth-inch sterile umbilical tape.

Dissection is continued proximally to the base of the gland where the ductules converge, and distally to the

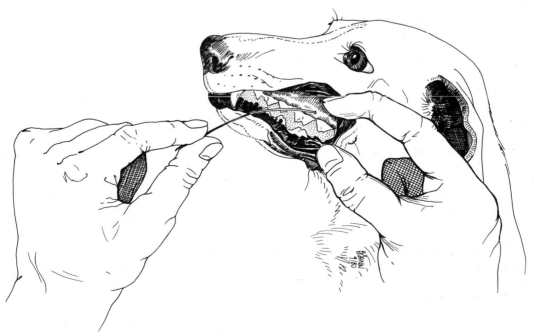

Fig. 6-66. *Catheterization of parotid salivary duct with a monofilament nylon suture. The parotid duct papilla is located above the carnassial tooth cranial to the zygomatic papilla.*

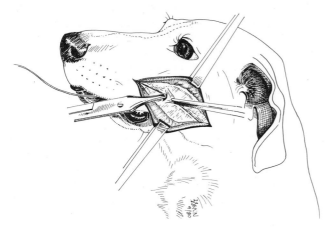

Fig. 6-67. *The catheterized duct is dissected beneath the buccal nerves and facial vein at the cranial aspect of the incision.*

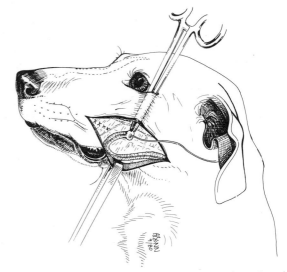

Fig. 6-68. *The freed duct is transposed to the ventrolateral conjunctival fornix through a subcutaneous tunnel.*

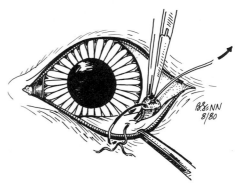

Fig. 6-69. *The mucosa collarette is anchored to the conjunctiva by four to six absorbable sutures.*

papilla below the buccal nerves and their communicating branch and the facial vein. Both these structures are superficial to the duct and left intact.

The lateral surgical site is protected and covered. The papilla and a surrounding 3-mm collar of buccal mucosa are incised from the buccal mucosa by an oral approach. The papilla and duct are dissected, totally freeing the parotid duct. The mucosal incision should not penetrate deeper than the submucosa. The oral incision is closed with an inverting suture pattern to avoid exposure of the sutures within the mouth. The instruments used orally are set aside because of contamination; the veterinary surgeon regloves.

A subcutaneous tunnel is fashioned from the parotid gland toward the ventrolateral fornix of the eye using straight mosquito forceps. The tunnel is extended until it can be appreciated subconjunctivally. The conjunctiva is incised, and a second mosquito forceps is grasped between the jaws of the first. The path is reversed until the second forceps appears in the primary skin incision. With the second forceps, the mucosa collar surrounding the papilla is grasped and is elevated to the conjunctival fornix (Fig. 6-68). Great care is exercised in the handling of duct and papilla. Twisting is avoided because it compromises the ability of the duct to serve as an effective conduit for salivary fluid. Excessive mucosa is trimmed, and the papilla is apposed to conjunctiva with four to six simple interrupted sutures of polyglycolic acid placed circumferentially (Fig. 6-69).

Subcutaneous tissue is apposed using a 4-0 absorbable suture. The skin is apposed by a simple interrupted pattern of nonabsorbable suture.

CLOSED TECHNIQUE. The closed approach involves dissection of the parotid salivary duct entirely through the oral cavity. Advantages include decreased postoperative edema and dissection of the duct without manipulation of the facial vein and branches of the buccal nerve.[5] Disadvantages include greater risk of contamination from the oral cavity and "blind" dissection.

Preoperative evaluation and preparation are the same as for the open technique, including catheterization of the duct. A 3- to 4-mm peripapillary section of mucosa is excised with the parotid duct papilla. The

duct and papilla are manipulated by traction on the collarette. The duct is freed from adjacent mucosa and the submucosal connective tissues with tenotomy scissors. Once the papilla is free, the buccal incision is extended caudally to permit continued dissection of the duct. A sufficient length of duct is isolated to permit redirection to the lateral canthus without stretching the duct. A subcutaneous tunnel is fashioned to the lateral canthus, as in the open technique.

The conjunctival incision creates an opening in the ventrolateral fornix. The duct and papilla with surrounding mucosa are directed into place; one must take care to avoid twisting or stressing the duct. Excess mucosa is trimmed, and the peripapillary mucosa is apposed to the conjunctiva with single interrupted 6-0 polyglycolic sutures. The buccal incision is closed in an inverting pattern of absorbable 5-0 sutures.

POSTOPERATIVE MANAGEMENT

Postoperative management usually consists of 5 to 7 days of systemic broad-spectrum antibiotics. Frequent applications of hot packs to the operative site facilitate resolution of the local swelling. Topical instillations of antibiotics and corticosteroid ophthalmic preparations are administered at least qid.

Patency and function of the transposed duct are evaluated on the first postoperative day. Epiphora is usually detectable with the first meal. Atropine placed on the tongue can also be used to stimulate salivation. The duct should function immediately postoperatively; however, postsurgical edema may decrease initial secretion. Topical lacrimomimetics should be continued for 4 to 5 days. Several small meals daily can be used to stimulate salivation. Skin sutures are removed in 7 to 10 days. All medications are usually discontinued 2 to 3 weeks postoperatively.

COMPLICATIONS

Complications are usually related to surgically induced trauma and to deposits of crystal-like precipitates on the cornea. Excessive manipulations, torsion, and transection may compromise the function of gland and duct. Periductular fibrosis can occur slowly over several weeks. Fibrotic constriction can be localized by dilation of the duct proximal to the stricture. Careful excision of the surrounding fibrous tissues can relieve the constriction and may permit function to return.

Deposits of crystal-like precipitates may occur on cornea and lid margins. Their microscopic form and physical properties suggest calcium carbonates, phosphates, or oxalates.[4] These precipitates are solubilized by 0.25 to 1.0% Na_2 EDTA ointment.

In a few patients, some owners have complained of epiphora of sufficient severity to necessitate relocating the parotid duct to its original site.[12] Successful ligation of the transposed duct without complications has also been reported.[6]

Nasolacrimal Drainage Apparatus

The nasolacrimal drainage apparatus is the conduit through which tears flow from the medial canthus for a variable distance into the nasopharynx of the nasal cavity. The lacrimal puncta receive the tears and are located on the inner surface of lid margins 3 to 4 mm from the medial canthus. The puncta in the dog are two slit-like openings located on the dorsal and ventral lid margins. They are connected by canaliculi to a diverticulum analogous to the lacrimal sac in man and continue as the nasolacrimal duct to the nasal cavity.

Congenital absence, trauma, inflammation, neoplasia, infections, and foreign bodies can compromise the system at several points. The inability to drain tears results in epiphora; the location of the site of blockage presents a diagnostic challenge to the clinician.

DIAGNOSTIC TECHNIQUES

Any patient with epiphora should be evaluated systematically to arrive at an etiologic diagnosis. Initial diagnostic procedures include the Schirmer tear test (to rule out lacrimation) and examination by magnification for anatomic variation and presence of the puncta.

The primary nasolacrimal drainage test is conducted before manipulation of the lids and consists of topical instillation of fluorescein and a few drops of artificial tears in each eye. Appearance of fluorescence in the nasal cavity or pharynx can be enhanced with an ultraviolet (Wood's) lamp or cobalt blue light. Normal transit time may be as long as 7 minutes in small animals. Longer times or absence of flow suggest blockage of the drainage apparatus. This passive drainage test evaluates the functional integrity of the system; structural integrity can be evaluated by the positive-pressure nasolacrimal flush.

Most patients permit flushing of the nasolacrimal system under topical anesthesia; some may require tranquilization. A 22- to 23-gauge gold-tipped lacrimal cannula is attached to a flush bottle or a syringe.

The upper lacrimal punctum is usually cannulated, and steady ejection pressure is applied. An imperforate lower punctum balloons initially under positive pressure. Mucopurulent debris and foreign bodies, such as plant awns, may be expelled. Any resistance at this level is indicative of obstruction in the canaliculi or lacrimal diverticulum.

Once the patency of the upper portion of the apparatus is established, the lower lacrimal punctum is occluded by digital pressure, and the flush is continued. The solution should normally appear at the external nares. If the patient's head is elevated, and in most brachycephalic dogs, a gagging reaction may signal nasopharyneal passage.

Other diagnostic techniques include catheterization and radiographic studies. Both these procedures require general anesthesia of short duration.

Dacryocystorhinography involves the injection of radiopaque dye to outline the nasolacrimal system. This technique is well documented and requires a minimum of two views to analyze the pathway of the system properly.[4]

Catheterization of the nasolacrimal system has both diagnostic and therapeutic implications.[9] Catheterization can be accomplished antegrade in most dogs and retrograde in approximately 50% of all dogs. Initial catheterization is performed using 2-0 monofilament nylon through the superior lacrimal punctum (Fig. 6-70). Longer-term catheterization with large-diameter

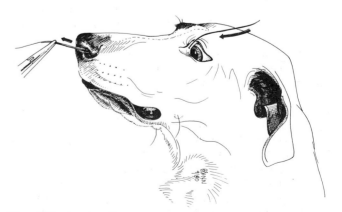

Fig. 6-70. *A monofilament nylon suture is passed antegrade through the dorsal lacrimal punctum to the nasal punctum.*

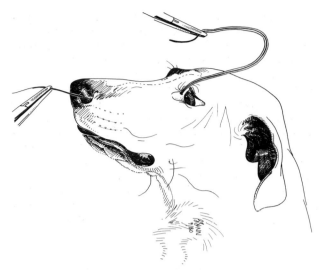

Fig. 6-71. *Polyethylene or Silastic tubing is threaded through the duct over the preplaced monofilament suture.*

catheters aids in maintaining patency during periods of medication and support during healing.

Once the nylon suture has been passed, a length of polyethylene 50 to 90 tubing or Silastic tubing is passed over the suture. A hemostat is applied to the suture at the end of the tubing. Steady traction from the nasal end of the suture and gentle manipulation direct the tubing through the nasolacrimal duct (Fig. 6-71). Once in place, the tubing is transfixed to adjacent skin by sutures. In general, most catheters are maintained 2 to 8 weeks. Topical antibiotics and corticosteroid or antibiotic solutions are generally administered while the tube is in place.

Imperforate lacrimal puncta are a congenital anomaly; breeds of dogs predisposed are the toy and miniature poodle, American cocker spaniel, and Bedlington terrier.[4] Clinical signs occur only when the lower lacrimal punctum is involved, and the condition can be unilateral or bilateral. The lacrimal punctum is usually occluded by a redundant flap of mucosa; however, absence of the connecting canaliculus may occur concurrently. Accurate evaluation is important to define the extent of the abnormality.

SURGICAL PROCEDURE FOR IMPERFORATE LACRIMAL PUNCTUM

An imperforate lacrimal punctum can be opened with a canaliculus knife or a No. 11 Bard-Parker blade or scissors. Positive pressure created by retrograde flushing of the opposite normal lacrimal punctum creates a bleb at the site of the incision (Fig. 6-72). A 2- to 3-mm slit (Figs. 6-73 and 6-74) orifice is created. In similar fashion, a small lacrimal punctum can be surgically enlarged to facilitate drainage. Postoperative management includes frequent topical instillations of antibiotic and corticosteroid solutions for 7 to 10 days to prevent fibrous adhesions and to maintain patency.

In some instances, restoration of normal structural and functional integrity of the nasolacrimal drainage

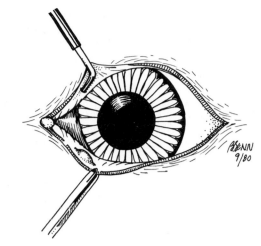

Fig. 6-72. *An imperforate lacrimal punctum, under a positive-pressure flush, will bulge and create a bleb.*

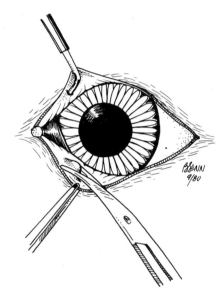

Fig. 6-73. *Scissors can be used to fashion a lacrimal orifice while maintaining positive pressure.*

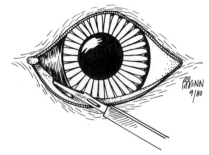

Fig. 6-74. *A No. 11 Bard-Parker blade can be used to enlarge a small lacrimal punctum.*

apparatus is impossible. Trauma, chronic inflammation, and cicatrization are common causes of irreparable damage. For those rare cases in which epiphora is unacceptable, an artificial or alternate drainage route can be fashioned. One technique, conjunctivorhinostomy, involves the creation of mucosa-lined fistula from the ventromedial conjunctival fornix to the nasopharynx.[1] Another technique, conjunctivoralostomy, creates a similar fistula to the oral cavity.[4]

CONJUNCTIVORHINOSTOMY

In addition to the standard ophthalmic surgical instruments including an eyelid speculum, tenotomy scissors, and toothed forceps, Steinmann's pins, a hand-held manual drill chuck, and a malleable probe are needed.

Preoperative measures include a periorbital scrub and aseptic preparation of the conjunctival fornix by topical instillations of broad-spectrum antibiotics tid. General anesthesia is induced, and an endotracheal tube with inflatable cuff is positioned. Intraoperative hemorrhage into the nasopharynx must be anticipated.

The eyelid speculum is positioned so that the surgical site in the ventromedial orbital rim can be visualized. Overlying soft tissue is dissected to the orbital periosteum of the lacrimal bone or maxillary bone, depending on breed and orbital conformation.

Starting with a small Steinmann's pin, the overlying bone is trephined manually. The direction of the pin is from the nasal canthus to the ipsilateral external narcs. The shaft of the pin retropulses the globe, which must be protected during the drilling process. Entry into the nasal cavity is noted by a sudden decrease of resistance. Larger pins are then progressively passed until the width of the bony canal equals the diameter of the catheter.

The catheter, constructed before the operation, should measure approximately 40 mm in length, with a collar or flange at one end. The diameter of catheters ranges from 2 mm outside diameter for small dogs to 4 mm for large dogs. Polyethylene tubing can be heat-flanged, and its rigid nature facilitates placement.

Once proper size of the tract is established, it is flushed repeatedly with physiologic saline solution. The catheter, supported by the malleable probe, is threaded through the tract (see Fig. 6-70). An inability to position the catheter suggests that conjunctival mucosa or fibrous tissues have not been completely removed. On achieving an adequate placement, the catheter is sutured to adjacent conjunctiva with several 5-0 nylon sutures. The patency of the tube is tested by flushing with physiologic saline solution.

Postoperative management involves the frequent daily applications of antibiotic and corticosteroid solutions. The catheter should remain in situ for 2 months; however, the sutures may be removed 2 to 3 weeks postoperatively. From 4 to 8 weeks are necessary for the surgical tract to become lined with mucosa.[1]

An alternate technique is to establish a permanent fistula between the ventral conjunctival fornix and oral cavity using a subcutaneous route. A tunnel is fashioned from the middle aspect of the ventral conjunctival fornix between the nictitating membrane and the lower lid. The tunnel is extended into the oral cavity in an area dorsal to the fourth premolar tooth. A large catheter of proper size is positioned and is stabilized by nonabsorbable sutures. The catheter is left in situ for 6 to 8 weeks.

References and Suggested Readings

1. Covitz, D., Hunziker, J., and Koch, S. A.: Conjunctivorhinostomy: a surgical method for the control of epiphora in the dog and cat. J. Am. Vet. Med. Assoc., *171*:251, 1977.
2. Evans, H. E., and Christensen, G. C.: Miller's Anatomy of the Dog. 2nd ed. Philadelphia, W. B. Saunders, 1979.
3. Gelatt, K. N.: Veterinary Ophthalmic Pharmacology and Therapeutics. 2nd Ed. Bonner Spring, KS, VM Publishing, 1978.
4. Gelatt, K. N., and Gwin, R. M.: Canine lacrimal and nasolacrimal systems. *In* Veterinary Ophthalmology. Edited by K. N. Gelatt. Philadelphia, Lea & Febiger, 1981.
5. Jensen, H. E.: Keratitis sicca and parotid duct transposition. Compend. Contin. Ed. Small Anim. Pract., *109*:721, 1979.
6. Kuhns, E. L., and Keller, W. I.: Effects of postsurgical ligation of a transposed parotid duct. VM SAC *74*:515, 1979.
7. Lavingnette, A. M.: Keratoconjunctivitis sicca in a dog treated by transposition of the parotid salivary duct. J. Am. Vet. Med. Assoc., *148*:778, 1966.
8. Lemp, M. A., et al.: Dry eye secondary to mucus deficiency. Trans. Am. Acad. Ophthalmol. Otolaryngol., *75*:1223, 1971.
9. Severin, G. A.: Nasolacrimal duct catheterization in the dog. J. Am. Anim. Hosp. Assoc., *8*:13, 1972.
10. Taylor, P.: Cholinergic agonists. *In* Goodman and Gilman's The Pharmacologic Basis of Therapeutics. 6th Ed. Edited by A. G. Gilman, L. S. Goodman, and A. Gilman. New York, Macmillan Publishing, 1980.
11. Veith, L. A., Cure, T. H., and Gelatt, K. N.: The Schirmer tear test in cats. Mod. Vet. Pract., *5*:48, 1970.
12. Vierheller, R.: Personal communication.

Cornea

Surgery of the Cornea

by N. Gail Powell

Corneal surgery requires a general understanding of the pathophysiologic and anatomic dynamics of corneal diseases. Many corneal diseases can be managed medically. Surgery is sometimes the primary treatment, however.

The most superficial layer of the cornea is the epithelium, which is several cell layers thick. The underlying basement membrane is important in the healing of superficial ulcers. Newly regenerated epithelial cells adhere to the anterior stromal face by an intact basement membrane; this adhesion requires several weeks. The high regenerative power facilitates rapid healing of superficial corneal wounds. The healing process involves both cell migration and mitosis.[16] The epithelial cells normally produce a minimal amount of collagenase. Upon injury, however, the rapidly dividing epithelial cells produce more collagenase; this process predisposes the collagen fibers of the stroma to destruction.

The corneal stroma (substantia propria corneae) comprising the majority of the corneal thickness undergoes slow regeneration. This layer is arranged in a lamellar pattern that makes the stroma an ideal surgical tissue to separate for excisional procedures such as superficial keratectomy and keratoplasty.

The posterior limit of the stroma is Descemet's membrane, which delineates the corneal stroma from the endothelium. If Descemet's membrane is damaged, its regeneration is dependent on the corneal endothelium. Corneal endothelium is a single layer of cells that maintains normal detergescense of the corneal stroma.[11]

Corneal sensation is provided by ciliary nerves, which are branches of the ophthalmic division of the fifth (trigeminal) cranial nerve. These sensory fibers run parallel to the epithelium, along with adrenergic nerve endings.[7,11] Any abrasion or denudement of the epithelium exposes these nerve fibers and causes the patient pain and discomfort.

The sequence of events of corneal disease involves loss of corneal transparency, edema, invasion of neutrophils, vascularization at the level of direct insult, fibroblastic infiltration, pigmentation, change in corneal contour, and often, cellular deposits along the endothelium and aqueous humor.[16]

In the discussion of corneal surgical techniques, it must be stated that corneal surgery, particularly keratoplasty, is facilitated by the use of the operating microscope. Special instrumentation and suture material are also necessary for optimal results.

Superficial Keratectomy

INDICATIONS

Excision of the superficial corneal layers is indicated in certain disease processes, such as dermoids, feline eosinophilic granulomatous keratitis, canine chronic superficial keratitis (pannus), feline corneal sequestration, viral papillomatosis, cholesterolosis, squamous cell carcinoma, and histiocytoma.[2,13]

SURGICAL TECHNIQUE

The degree of corneal tissue excised varies, depending on the dimensions of the disorder. The margins of the excised tissue should extend at least 1 to 2 mm into "healthy" tissue. The method used will depend on the surgical instruments available and the veterinary surgeon's preference.

Required instruments are a No. 15 Bard-Parker blade and handle or a No. 64 Beaver blade and handle, an eyelid speculum, a Castroviejo corneal trephine, scleral fixation forceps, a Martinez corneal dissector, Colibri forceps*, and 4-0 nylon or silk suture.

The patient is positioned after the induction of general anesthesia. A protective ophthalmic ointment or protective contact lens is placed in the conjunctival sac prior to clipping the eyelid hair. The conjunctival sac should be flushed several times with an irrigating solution to remove all debris. The eyelids are washed several times with an antibacterial skin cleanser; one must be careful to minimize skin irritation. A lateral canthotomy is used if greater exposure is necessary. Global fixation is achieved by scleral fixation forceps or stay sutures.

If the corneal lesion is central, a Castroviejo corneal trephine can be used. Various depth settings are obtainable, depending on the depth of the lesion. Because the canine and feline cornea is less than 1 mm thick, superficial lesions can be successfully removed when the depth of the trephine guard is set at 0.3 to 0.4 mm. The trephine is positioned over the lesion, perpendicular to the curvature of the cornea, with evenly distributed pressure. The cornea is incised with a smooth, rotating motion. The edge of the corneal incision is grasped with Colibri forceps, and the superficial layer is separated from the deeper stromal layers by blunt dissection with the corneal dissector; gentle traction should be placed on the tissue to be removed. The cutting edge of the corneal dissector is held parallel to the corneal surface at all times to prevent perforation. The cornea is intermittently moistened throughout the procedure with sterile balanced salt solution.

If the corneal trephine is not available, the cornea is incised with the No. 15 Bard-Parker or No. 65 Beaver blade, outlining the margins of the corneal disease. Colibri forceps are used to grasp the margin of the tissue to be excised. The blade is then held parallel to the corneal surface, to establish the plane of dissection. With a smooth, sweeping motion, the cutting edge of the blade is passed over the stromal surface, and the diseased corneal tissue is removed from the deeper stromal layers.

In some pathologic processes, such as canine chronic superficial keratitis (pannus), the entire corneal surface is involved, and all superficial corneal layers must be removed. This excision is possible by removing the tissue in quadrants (Fig. 6-75). The wedge method facilitates total superficial keratectomy.

POSTOPERATIVE CARE

Each postoperative medical regime varies, although the criteria for evaluation are the same. Topical iridocycloplegic agents and broad-spectrum antibiotics are applied for approximately 7 to 10 days postoperatively. The rate of re-epithelization depends on both the surface area of the surgical wound and the concurrent corneal condition. Once re-epithelization has occurred, as detected by the fluorescein dye test, a topical antibi-

*Instruments available from Storz Instrument Co., 3365 Tree Court Industrial Blvd., St. Louis, MO 63122

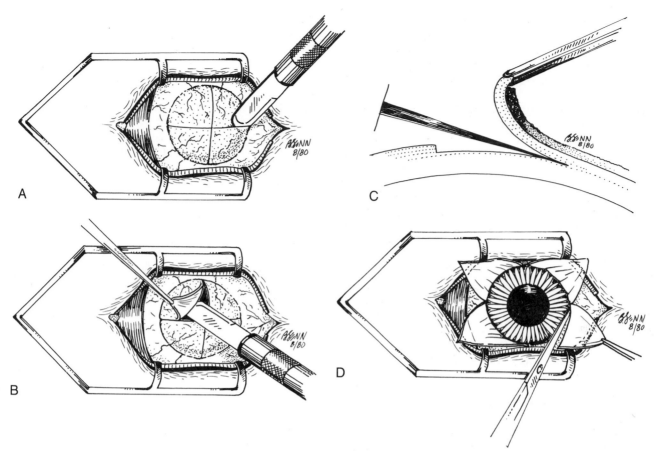

Fig. 6-75. A, *Initial corneal incisions, dividing the corneal surface into four equal parts. A No. 64 Beaver blade is utilized, penetrating through the superficial, diseased corneal stroma.* B, *Colibri corneal forceps are used to stabilize the corneal tissue, as the plane of dissection is established. Note that the blade is held parallel to the corneal surface, as the undermining process is completed.* C, *A diagrammatic representation illustrating the position of the surgical blade during the removal of the superficial corneal stroma.* D, *the diseased corneal tissue at the limbus is severed with small scissors.*

otic and corticosteroid agent may be used to reduce corneal scar formation.

Corneoscleral Transposition

A sliding pedicle graft of cornea and sclera can be used to repair large corneal defects. Adjacent corneal and scleral tissue are undermined and are transposed to cover the corneal defect. This method eliminates the need for donor tissue and the immune-mediated graft rejection process. That the curvature of the cornea is maintained facilitates corneal optics.

The integrity of the cornea is evaluated preoperatively. Control of the septic process is absolutely necessary before and after the operation for this process to succeed. It may be necessary to administer topical antibiotics, antimycotics, and iridocycloplegics.

SURGICAL TECHNIQUE

When general anesthesia has been induced, the lids and periorbital area are prepared as described previously. Required instruments include a wire lid speculum, Colibri forceps, corneal lamellar knife, fine needle holder, Halstead mosquito forceps, Beaver scalpel handle, No. 64 and No. 65 Beaver blades, Barraquer iris scissors, iris spatula, Steven's tenotomy scissors, and 9-0 and 4-0 nylon or silk suture. Balanced salt solution* is used throughout the surgical procedure to keep the cornea moist.

The corneal lesion usually involves a large, deep defect, with necrotic margins commonly accompanied by neovascularization, corneal edema, and conjunctivitis. The corneal ulcer is often accompanied by uveitis, iris prolapse, and adherent leukomas.

The ulcerated area is carefully debrided, using the No. 64 Beaver blade to remove the necrotic tissue and to prepare the corneal bed for the autogenous corneoscleral graft. With the No. 64 Beaver blade, 2 diverging linear partial thickness incisions are made, extending into healthy cornea and sclera. These incisions should extend from each side of the corneal defect (Fig. 6-76A). The corneal incisions are approximately 0.5 mm deep (Fig. 6-76B). The size of the graft should be slightly wider than the corneal defect, thereby allowing for contraction of the graft tissue[13] (Fig. 6-76A).

*Available from Alcon Surgical Products Division, Alcon Laboratories, Inc., Ft. Worth, TX 76134

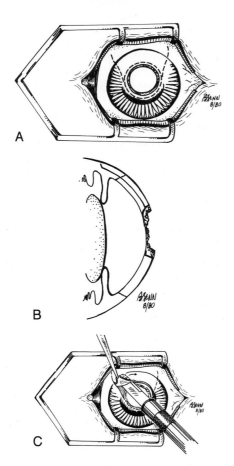

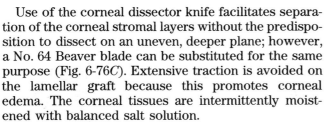

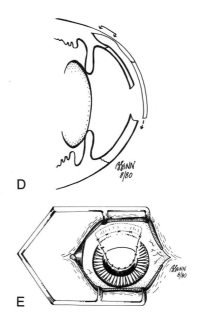

Fig. 6-76. A, *Dotted lines represent the circumference of the corneal disease.* B, *A sagittal diagrammatic representation depicting the deep corneal disease centrally.* C, *Colibri forceps are used to manipulate the corneal tissue as the superficial corneal layer is separated from the deeper layer.* D, *Transposition of the pedicle flap.* E, *After proper apposition of the lamellar graft to the new "corneal bed," stabilization is obtained.*

Use of the corneal dissector knife facilitates separation of the corneal stromal layers without the predisposition to dissect on an uneven, deeper plane; however, a No. 64 Beaver blade can be substituted for the same purpose (Fig. 6-76C). Extensive traction is avoided on the lamellar graft because this promotes corneal edema. The corneal tissues are intermittently moistened with balanced salt solution.

The linear incisions are extended into the limbus and sclera to permit the transposition of the pedicle flap into the corneal defect (Fig. 6-76D). The size of the scleral portion should be large enough to replace the cornea that surgically precedes it.[13] The lamellar graft is then trimmed to fill the corneal defect uniformly. Inaccurate and uneven apposition may predispose the patient to wound dehiscence and failure.

The lamellar graft is apposed to the new "corneal bed" with continuous or simple interrupted suture patterns, interchangeably (9-0 nylon with a General Surgical-9 (GS-9) needle). The sutures should *not* penetrate the entire thickness of either the cornea or the graft (Fig. 6-76E).

POSTOPERATIVE CARE

Postsurgical management varies, depending on the preexisting corneal disease. Topical or systemic antibiotics and even anti-inflammatory agents may be indicated. Iridocycloplegic agents are usually necessary for management of the secondary uveitis and miosis.

Postoperative results are influenced, in part, on the viability of the cornea at the time of the surgical procedure. In large corneal defects, more scleral tissue is necessary to cover the lesion, and a distorted limbus with a dense peripheral leukoma thereby results.

Keratoplasty

Corneal transplantation involves the removal of a diseased portion and replacement with healthy tissue from a suitable donor. There are two types of keratoplasty: lamellar (nonpenetrating) and penetrating (full-thickness). Success of the superficial keratectomy procedure in small animals has minimized the need for lamellar keratoplasty in clinical ophthalmology.

The veterinarian is often faced with corneal disease of the deeper layers, resulting in a permanently opaque, scarred, and pigmented area. Certain corneal dystrophies, such as in the Airedale terrier, beagle, Boston terrier, Chihuahua, dachshund, Siberian husky, and Manx cat, are usually brought to the veterinarian for bilateral ocular disease, resulting in poor vision, compromising their ability to be an active pet.

Reports on the practicality and results of penetrating corneal grafts in dogs, conflict in the literature.[1,8,10] Successful corneal grafts have been recognized for the past 30 years in man, related in part to improvements in surgical techniques, improved instrumentation (including the operating microscope), new suture materials and needles, more selective criteria of the donor grafts, and progress in the diagnosis, prevention, and management of complications.

Indications for penetrating keratoplasty in dogs consist of chronic deep pigmentation, central full-thickness leukoma, limbal tumors, certain types of keratitis, and deep corneal dystrophies.

SURGICAL TECHNIQUE

Proper handling of both the donor and recipient tissues is important for the success of full-thickness keratoplasty. A functional graft depends on a viable endothelial layer on the donor disc. **The endothelium is fragile and is adversely affected by slight mechanical trauma, changes in the pH of the surrounding medium, and normal saline solution.**

Instrumentation required for this surgical procedure are Castroviejo trephine, Colibri forceps, corneal section scissors, needle holder for fine suture, eyelid speculum, scleral fixation forceps or ring, balanced salt solution, No. 65 Beaver blade or No. 15 Bard-Parker blade and handles, 10-0 silk or nylon, 4-0 nylon, and cellulose cell sponges.

Preoperative topical medications include pilocarpine 1% for miosis, topical and systemic antibiotics, and usually corticosteroids.

Proper magnification and positioning of the eye are imperative. The patient is placed in dorsal recumbency with the surface of the iris parallel to the operating table. Proper immobilization of the globe is mandatory

and can be achieved by stay sutures of 4-0 nylon or silk, by the use of scleral fixation forceps, or by a fixation ring. A lateral canthotomy may be necessary to provide greater exposure. The donor dog can be prepared for operation simultaneously with the recipient dog; this procedure maximizes the viability of the graft.

The diameter of the trephine should be 0.5 mm larger for the donor button than for the recipient's defect. With the trephine blade exposed for a depth setting varying from 0.7 to 1.5 mm, a smooth incision is made. Even pressure is applied to the trephine as it is held perpendicular to the cornea and the instrument is swiftly rotated (Fig. 6-77A). The donor button can be removed by use of the trephine only; however, curved corneal scissors can be used to complete the incision (Fig. 6-77B). Alternately, a partial penetrating trephination can be performed by entering the anterior chamber with a No. 11 Bard-Parker blade or a No. 65 Beaver blade at the base of the trephination and by completing the incision with corneal scissors (Fig. 6-77C). A single fine suture of double-armed 10-0 nylon is placed through the anterior half of the corneal stroma, at the 12 and 6 o'clock positions of the donor button, to facilitate easy manipulation and to minimize trauma to the endothelium and the graft edge (Fig. 6-77C).

The trephine (0.5 mm smaller than the donor graft) is used to enter the anterior chamber of the host. The depth of the trephine blade can be adjusted, depending on the degree of corneal disease, for example, 1.5 mm for an edematous cornea or 0.8 mm for a nonedematous cornea. The principles mentioned previously re-

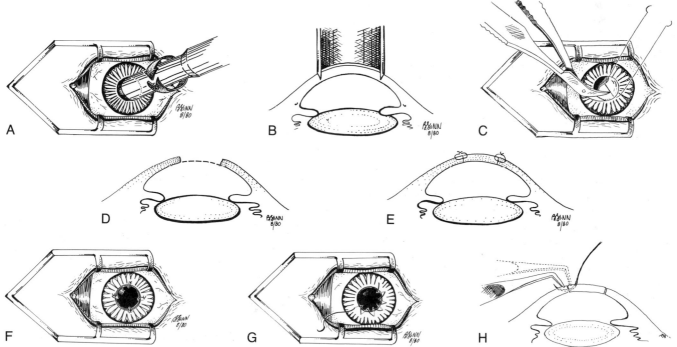

Fig. 6-77. A, *Even pressure is applied to the trephine blade.* B, *The donor button is prepared with complete corneal penetration.* C, *The anterior chamber can be entered with a No. 65 Beaver blade after partial trephination.* D, *The "host" cornea, when the central button has been removed.* E and F, *Stabilization of the "donor button,"* G, *Sutures are passed circumferentially around the donor and recipient graft edge.* H, *During the suturing process, the needle should be passed through the margin of the donor tissue first, after which the host tissue is stabilized for exit of the needle. Dotted lines indicate forceps stabilizing the donor tissue.*

garding the positioning and manipulation of the tre-phine apply to the host tissue. When the anterior chamber has been entered, the button is excised with the curved corneal scissors. One must be careful to avoid the iris. It is essential to make a clean incision and to leave no tags of tissue. As soon as the anterior chamber is opened (Fig. 6-77D), 0.1 to 0.2 ml of heparin sodium (1000 units/ml) is instilled into the anterior chamber to prevent the formation of fibrin clots in the aqueous humor.

Proper placement of the donor button in the recipient bed is the next critical step. The previously placed double-armed suture in the graft are cut, and simple nonpenetrating interrupted sutures are placed opposingly at the 12 and 6 o'clock positions. The needle is passed through the host tissue at the same depth of entry as the donor button. Additional simple interrupted sutures are placed at the 3 and 9 o'clock positions for further stabilization (Fig. 6-77E and F). Sutures of 10-0 nylon are passed circumferentially around the donor and recipient graft edge (approximately 16 to 20). These sutures should penetrate only the anterior half to two-thirds of the corneal tissues (Fig. 6-77G). Clinical research[6] has indicated the canine cornea can become more edematous and softer than the human cornea resulting in greater suture tension; hence the point of entrance of the suture should be approximately 1 mm from the edge of the donor graft and should exit 2 mm from the margin of the hosts' cornea. The needle should be passed through the donor tissue first; the margin should be stabilized with Colibri forceps, after which the forceps are moved over to the recipient (host) corneal edge to secure the tissue for the exit of the needle (Fig. 6-77H). The double-armed suture should terminate in the dorsotemporal quadrant and should be tied securely in a surgical knot.

The graft should be inspected carefully for any evidence of leaking of aqueous humor or for lack of continuity between the margins of the host's cornea and donor graft. The anterior chamber is re-established with sterile physiologic fluid, preferably a balanced salt solution.

POSTOPERATIVE CARE

Postoperative treatment and daily observations are essential for successful keratoplasty. Daily slit-lamp biomicroscopic examinations are used to ascertain the dosage of corticosteroids required. In addition, iridocycloplegic agents and antibiotics are instilled postoperatively for the first 3 weeks. With graft vascularization, therapy with topical corticosteroids is intensified. The alternate interrupted sutures may be removed on the seventh to ninth days; the remaining continuous suture can remain in place for 3 to 8 weeks postoperatively. I anticipate penetrating keratoplasty in small animals will be used increasingly in clinical veterinary ophthalmology in the near future.

References and Suggested Readings

1. Bernis, W. O.: Partial penetrating keratoplasty in dogs. Southwest Vet., 15:30, 1961.
2. Bistner, S., Aquirre, G., and Batik, G.: Atlas of Veterinary Ophthalmic Surgery. Philadelphia, W. B. Saunders, 1977.
3. D'Amico, R. A., and Castroviejo, R.: Suppression of Immune Response in Keratoplasty. Am. J. Ophthalmol., 68:829, 1969.
4. Dice, P. F.: Primary corneal disease in the dog and cat. Vet. Clin. North Am. [Small Anim. Pract.], 10, 1980.
5. Duane, T. (ed.): Clinical Ophthalmology. Corneal Surgery, Vol. 5, Chapter 6. p. 1-10. Hagerstown, MD, Harper & Row, 1981.
6. McEntrye, J. M.: Experimental penetrating keratoplasty in the dog. Arch. Ophthalmol., 80:372, 1968.
7. Gwin, R. M., Gelatt, K. N., and Chiou, C. Y.: Adrenergic and cholinergic innervation of the anterior segment of the normal and glaucomatous dog. Invest. Ophthalmol. Vis. Sci., 18:674, 1979.
8. Holt, J. R.: Corneal graft in a dog. Vet. Rec., 69:454, 1957.
9. Khodadoust, A. A., and Silverstein, A. M.: The survival and rejection of epithelium in experimental corneal transplants. Invest. Ophthalmol., 8:169, 1969.
10. Massey, J. Y., and Hanna, C.: Penetrating keratoplasty with use of through and through nylon sutures. Arch. Ophthalmol., 91:382, 1974.
11. Moses, R. A. (ed.): Adler's Physiology of the Eye. 5th Ed. St. Louis, C. V. Mosby, 1970.
12. O'Neill, P., Moeller, F. O., and Trevor-Roper, P. D.: On the preservation of cornea at −196° C for full thickness homografts in man and dog. Br. J. Ophthalmol., 51:13, 1967.
13. Parshall, C.: Lamellar corneal scleral transposition. J. Am. Anim. Hosp. Assoc., 9:220, 1973.
14. Paton, D.: Penetrating keratoplasty—advocation of microscopic management and an arbitrary selection of incision and suturing techniques. Highlights Ophthalmol., 14:176, 1972.
15. Schmidt, G. M.: Superficial keratectomy for lesions of the cornea. In Current Techniques in Small Animal Surgery. Edited by M. J. Bojrab. Philadelphia, Lea & Febiger, 1975.
16. Severin, G. A.: Veterinary Ophthalmology Notes, 1976.
17. Startup, F. G.: Diseases of the canine eye. Pt. II. Vet. Rec., 72:675, 1960.

Lens

Cataract Surgery

by ROBERT M. GWIN

Cataract removal in veterinary medicine is traditionally one of the most demanding and difficult surgical procedures. In recent years, however, refinement of surgical technique has improved success rates. In contrast to man, intraoperative and postoperative inflammation and fibrin production are copious. The iris bleeds readily when cut or torn, and mydriasis is difficult to maintain. Exposure is frequently poor, owing to rotation of the globe, a prominent muzzle, and the tendency of the globe to sink deeply into the orbit.

Thus, the sensitivity of canine cataract surgery demands a thorough knowledge and understanding of ocular anatomy, physiology, pharmacology, pathology, and the eyes' response to varying insults. This prerequisite in-depth knowledge may challenge the limits of the average student or veterinarian who is untrained in the pitfalls of intraocular surgery. This discussion is meant to be a reference and a review of technique for the student of ophthalmic surgery. The discussion assumes the availability of proper instruments for cataract surgery and, most important, the guidance of an accomplished, well-trained veterinary ophthalmologist.

Selection of Surgical Patients

Poor case selection is a significant cause of cataract surgery failure. Both eyes should be examined before and after instillation of a topical mydriatic. Pupillary responses should be observed, although the presence of normal pupillary response to light does not rule out retinal disease. Slow or incomplete pupillary light reflexes are signs that raise suspicion of retinal degeneration, particularly in toy and miniature poodles. Poor or incomplete mydriasis following administration of a short-acting mydriatic agent, such as tropicamide, is often indicative of uveitis. Anterior uveitis may be seen in association with a hypermature (more common in older dogs) or resorbing (more common in younger dogs) cataract. The lens *must be examined* under wide mydriasis before it can be adequately evaluated. Any evidence of uveitis is a contraindication to routine cataract surgery.

The cataract should be mature enough to cause functional loss of vision, and the anterior lens capsule should appear smooth and convex. The position of the lens is carefully observed.

Fundus examination is attempted in evaluation of the cataract patient. In some cases, the fundus may be observed through small, clear portions of the lens. Obviously, any sign of retinal degeneration is a definite contraindication to lens removal. Additionally, a history of poor vision in a subdued or darkened environment (night blindness) prior to cataract formation is frequently indicative of progressive retinal atrophy. Thus, an electroretinogram should be performed on any dog with suspected retinal disease and on all miniature and toy poodles when the fundus is not observed. A large percentage (60 to 70%) of toy and miniature poodles with cataracts have concurrent retinal disease (progressive retinal atrophy) and are not suitable candidates for cataract surgery.

Preoperative Medical Treatment

In the dog, two difficult areas of management are (1) obtaining a widely dilated pupil and (2) controlling inflammation. Mydriasis is mandatory to successful cataract surgery. Atropine sulfate 1% is administered topically 3 to 4 times daily for 1 to 2 days prior to the surgical procedure. Atropine sulfate 1% provides wide mydriasis, is long acting, and is nonirritating. Another frequently used sympathomimetic-parasympatholytic combination is phenylephrine hydrochloride 10% and scopolamine hydrobromide 0.3% (Muracol No. 2*).

The use of systemic corticosteroids (prednisolone, 2 mg/kg) 24 hours preoperatively significantly reduces the amount of postoperative inflammation. The oral administration of aspirin (10 to 25 mg/kg) has also been used just prior to and following intraocular surgical procedures. Although not approved for use in small animals, flunixin megumine† (1 mg/kg, sid) is a potent antiprostaglandin with fewer side effects than aspirin.

Extracapsular Extraction

Following routine induction for general inhalation anesthesia, the hair around the eye is gently clipped, and the patient placed on his back with the jaw tilted at a 45° angle to the side. The eyelids are retracted with a thin wire speculum. A lateral canthotomy may be necessary to increase exposure. A limbal-based conjunctival flap is performed from the 9 to the 3 o'clock position. The flap should not incorporate any of the underlying fibrous tissue of Tenon's capsule. The flap is continued down until the "blue zone" of the limbus is observed. A partial-thickness groove is made in the limbus for 160 to 190° with a No. 64 Beaver blade to facilitate opening of the surgical wound (Fig. 6-78).

A No. 65 Beaver blade is inserted into the anterior chamber through the limbal groove parallel to the iris. Care is taken not to damage the cornea or iris by improper blade insertion. Once the anterior chamber is entered, aqueous humor rushes out. The incision is enlarged with corneal section scissors to the desired width, usually 160 to 190° (Fig. 6-79).

The anterior lens capsule is grasped with widely opened Schweiger's extracapsular forceps. The teeth are pressed against the anterior lens capsule and are compressed slowly, tearing the capsule in the equatorial region (Fig. 6-80). This capsular material is then removed. After extraction of the lens capsule, the lens cortex and nuclear material should be removed without disturbance of the posterior lens capsule. Delivery of this cortex and nuclear material may be accomplished with the use of a small loop and a muscle hook. The muscle hook is gently pressed against the limbus at the 6 o'clock position. At the 12 o'clock position, a lens loop is placed against the posterior lip of the wound. The pressure from the muscle hook is increased to move the lens upwards over the lens loop. The loop and lens are then extracted from the globe (Fig. 6-81). Gentle irrigation of the anterior chamber with a balanced salt solution removes any remaining cortical material.

The limbal wound is closed with simple interrupted 5-0 to 7-0 ophthalmic absorbable polyglycolic acid‡ or polyglactin 910§ suture. These sutures should be buried beneath the overlying conjunctiva and placed approximately 1.5 mm apart. The conjunctival incision is closed with a continuous pattern using absorbable suture (Fig. 6-82).

*Muro Pharmacal Laboratories, Inc., Tewksbury, MA 01876
†Banamine, Schering Corp., Kenilworth, NJ 07033
‡Vicryl, Ethicon, Inc., Somerville, NJ 08876
§Dexon, Davis & Geck, Inc., Manati, PR 00701

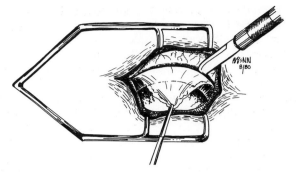

Fig. 6-78. *Preparation of limbal groove with a No. 64 Beaver blade.*

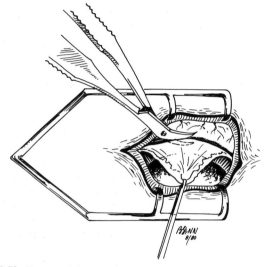

Fig. 6-79. *Enlargement of limbal wound with corneal section scissors.*

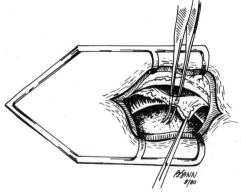

Fig. 6-80. *Tearing of anterior lens capsule with forceps through a dorsal limbal wound.*

Phacoemulsification

Phacoemulsification is a method using high-frequency vibrations to fragment and emulsify the lens into a solution or emulsion that can then be aspirated from the anterior chamber. Phacoemulsification is most easily performed in younger animals with softer lens material, but can be used in older animals in many instances.

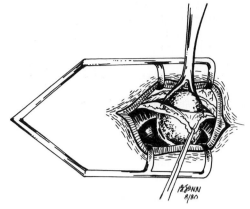

Fig. 6-81. *Delivery of lens material with lens loop.*

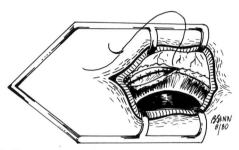

Fig. 6-82. *Closure of limbal-based conjunctival flap with a continuous suture.*

Two small stab incisions in the cornea adjacent to the limbus are necessary for the surgical approach. The first incision can be made with a 20- to 22-gauge needle connected to an irrigating solution* system. This system allows the anterior chamber to be maintained during the operation, and inflow may be varied according to the amount of fluid leaving the eye.

A second incision, approximately 2 to 3 mm wide, is made in the peripheral cornea 160 to 180° away from the infusion needle with a No. 65 Beaver blade. A cystotome introduced into the anterior chamber is extended across the pupil and engages the anterior lens capsule ventrally. The cystotome is then pulled across the lens to remove a large portion of the lens capsule and to permit exposure of the lens cortex (Fig. 6-83). The cystotome is used to manipulate the lens cortical and nuclear material into the anterior chamber. The cystotome is then removed, and the ultrasonic tip is placed into the anterior chamber. Emulsification and aspiration are then performed (Fig. 6-84). The ultrasonic tip is withdrawn following removal of all lens material. The anterior chamber is reformed with irrigating solutions and an air bubble. The surgical wound may be closed with 2 simple interrupted sutures, using a 6-0 or 7-0 absorbable suture material.

The most obvious advantage of phacoemulsification is the small incision necessary for the procedure. This advantage lessens the postoperative complications associated with a large wound and also decreases the

*Balanced Salt Solution (BSS), Alcon Laboratories, 6201 South Freeway, Fort Worth, TX 76134

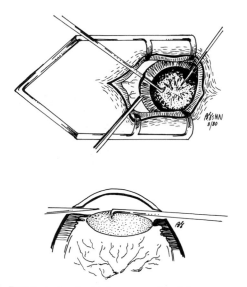

Fig. 6-83. *Rupture of anterior lens capsule with a cystotome.*

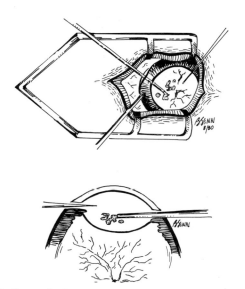

Fig. 6-84. *Removal of cortical and nuclear lens material through emulsification and aspiration.*

amount of postoperative medical therapy. This procedure is becoming more popular in veterinary medicine. When used in the proper cases, the results are superior to a standard extracapsular procedure. Although the cost of the phacoemulsification units usually limits their use to veterinary ophthalmologists, the practitioner should be aware of the availability of this new and promising procedure.

Discission and Aspiration

In young animals (under one year of age), the lens material is soft enough to allow a different type of lens removal. The technique of discission and aspiration is similar to phacoemulsification in that the eye is entered through a small incision, the anterior lens capsule is torn, and the lens cortex and nucleus are removed by suction. The softness of the lens material in the young animal allows removal of lens material without the use of an ultrasonic device.

Preoperatively, the animal should be treated in the same manner as previously described for any cataract procedure and with the same consideration for general systemic health and possible concomitant ocular disease. The pupil should be maximally dilated, and a lateral canthotomy may be performed to increase exposure when necessary. The globe is stabilized with a Flieringa fixation ring* or conjunctival-scleral stay sutures. A fornix-based or limbal-based conjunctival flap 6 to 8 mm wide is made in the dorsal or dorsotemporal region of the globe. The limbus may be entered with a discission knife needle (Barkan knife†). A wide, cruciate incision in the anterior lens capsule may be made. The knife needle may then be used to whip the lens material into a softer mass. Care must be taken to avoid rupturing the posterior lens capsule, collapsing the anterior chamber, or traumatizing the iris and cornea.

The knife needle is withdrawn from the anterior chamber, and the incision is enlarged slightly to permit introduction of the aspirating needle. A 2-way cataract aspirating needle or an 18- to 22-gauge blunted needle attached to a 3-way stopcock may be used for this purpose. Intermittent aspiration and injection of an intraocular irrigating solution into the anterior chamber allow removal of the lens material without collapse of the anterior chamber. The needle tip is transferred from one area of the lens to another as the lens protein is removed. As much lens material as possible should be aspirated, leaving the posterior capsule intact.

Following removal of the lens material, the limbal wound may be closed with 6-0 to 7-0 simple interrupted absorbable polyglycolic acid or polyglactin 910 sutures. Prior to placement of the final suture, an air bubble may be placed into the anterior chamber if it has collapsed during the suturing process. The conjunctiva is then resutured with an absorbable 5-0 or 6-0 suture.

Discission and aspiration of cataracts in young animals requires few instruments and does not involve many of the complicated techniques necessary in a conventional cataract procedure. The small incision used in this procedure, as in phacoemulsification, reduces the postoperative complications associated with a larger wound.

Postoperative Medications

Postoperatively, topical mydriatics and antibiotic and corticosteroid medications are continued 3 to 6 times daily, depending on the severity of the inflammation. Antibiotics are given systematically for 7 to 10 days. Antiprostaglandins such as aspirin or flunixin meglumine are administered for several days postoperatively. Oral prednisolone is continued at 2 mg/kg, then is slowly tapered off as inflammation subsides.

*Sparta Instruments Corp., Hayward, CA 94545
†American V. Mueller, 6600 Touhy Avenue, Chicago, IL 60648

Postoperative Complications

The most commonly observed complication is associated with the inability to control postoperative inflammation and pupil size. Other complications, including corneal edema, corneal ulceration, flat anterior chamber, secondary glaucoma, and wound incarceration of uveal tissue are associated with poor surgical technique and must be treated on an individual basis.

References and Suggested Readings

Bistner, S. I., Aguirre, G., and Batik, G.: Atlas of Veterinary Ophthalmic Surgery. Philadelphia, W. B. Saunders, 1977.

Gelatt, K. N.: Veterinary Ophthalmology. Philadelphia, Lea & Febiger, 1981.

Girard, L., and Hawkins, R.: Cataract extraction by ultrasonic aspiration; vitrectomy by ultrasonic aspiration. Trans. Am. Acad. Ophthalmol. Otolaryngol., 78:50, 1974.

Jaffe, N. S.: Safeguards in cataract surgery. South. Med. J., 61:859, 1968.

Surgical Procedures for the Glaucomas

by Kirk N. Gelatt

Glaucoma is a group of ocular diseases in which intraocular pressure (IOP) is elevated above normal levels and damages the optic nerve head and retina. The posterior fundic changes can result in visual impairment and eventually blindness. Glaucoma occurs in 1 of 204 (0.5%) dogs brought to the veterinary medical teaching hospitals of the colleges of veterinary medicine in North America.

The canine glaucomas usually require a combined medical and surgical approach. Medical treatments include the use of miotics, adrenergics, carbonic anhydrase inhibitors, and osmotic agents. The drugs are used singularly as well as in combination. Medical treatments are frequently necessary postoperatively when IOP does not return to acceptable levels.

Both medical and surgical treatments for the glaucomas in dogs and cats require classification of the type of glaucoma by thorough ophthalmic examination including gonioscopy. Observation of the aqueous outflow pathways is the predominant factor in ascertaining the preferable mode of therapy. Routine use of gonioscopy for all glaucoma patients before and after medical or surgical treatment and throughout the course of the disease optimizes preservation of vision.

Surgical procedures for the treatment of the glaucomas are divided into two types: those to improve the outflow of aqueous humor by creating new pathways of drainage within or to the outside of the eye; and those that decrease the rate of formation of aqueous humor. Procedures to increase outflow of aqueous humor include iridencleisis, corneoscleral trephination, cyclodialysis, combined iridencleisis-cyclodialysis, posterior sclerectomy, and anterior chamber implants. Procedures to reduce the rate of aqueous humor formation by partial destruction of the ciliary body are cyclocryothermy and cyclodiathermy.

Removal of the lens, although not commonly considered a glaucoma surgical procedure, may be necessary in the clinical management of the canine glaucomas. Lens removal may be indicated for glaucomas associated with lens-induced uveitis and cataract resorption, intumescent cataracts, anterior and posterior lens luxations, and subluxations. When the lens is displaced from its patella fossa, maintenance of IOP within normal limits by medical treatment may necessitate removal of the lens.

The success rate of glaucoma surgical procedures in the dog is about 30 to 50% with 1-year follow-ups. A number of factors may contribute to this less-than-desirable success rate. Selection of patients for the surgical procedures may be biased because surgical procedures are usually performed in those glaucomatous eyes in which medical treatment has been unsatisfactory or unsuccessful. These advanced glaucomatous eyes may have extensive peripheral anterior synechiae, complete iridocorneal angle closure, displaced lenses, and intraocular inflammation. The gradual sophistication of intraocular surgery using the operating microscope may facilitate improvement of existing procedures and the development of new techniques. Hemorrhage is a common problem in canine intraocular surgery; incision of the iris, especially near its base, may be accompanied by varying amounts of hemorrhage. The inflammation following entry into the anterior chamber and the extensive amounts of fibrin in the plasmoid aqueous humor of the postoperative iridocyclitides frequently obstruct the new surgical exits. Administration of corticosteroids preoperatively as well as postoperatively and the use of antiprostaglandins, such as salicylic acid acetate (aspirin), have facilitated the medical management of postoperative inflammations.

Preoperative Preparation

Considerations for surgical candidates for glaucoma procedures include: preoperative control of IOP, suppression of concurrent anterior segment inflammation, maintenance of pupil size, and dehydration of the vitreous. IOP must be reduced to the normal range prior to a glaucoma operation. Combinations of miotics, osmotics, adrenergics, and carbonic anhydrase inhibitors may be necessary to reduce IOP to 10 to 15 mm Hg. Miotic agents, such as 2% pilocarpine, are instilled every 15 to 30 minutes for several hours. Osmotic agents, such as mannitol (1 to 2 g/kg intravenously) or glycerol (1 to 2 ml/kg), may be administered 2 to 3 times in a 24-hour period. Acetazolamide (10 mg/kg intravenously) may be necessary to treat acute glaucomas (in excess of 50 to 60 mm Hg) that are nonresponsive to miotics. A Schiotz tonometer should be included with the glaucoma surgical pack; tonometry is used to estimate IOP before entry into the anterior chamber. If IOP is 20 mm Hg or higher, additional vigorous massage and hypotensive medical treatment, such as an additional dose of osmotic agents, should be initiated before the eye is entered. A glaucomatous eye without satisfactory ocular hypotension may upon entry exhibit choroidal hemorrhage, choroidal edema, vitreous protrusion through the pupil, and forward displacement of the anterior segment; the risk of intraocular hemorrhage is also increased in these globes.

Many of the canine glaucomas also exhibit a concurrent iridocyclitis; this disorder may be a primary or a secondary factor in the genesis of the glaucoma. Topical and systemic corticosteroids are indicated to suppress the inflammation and to reduce inflammatory cells and proteins in the aqueous humor.

Control of pupil's size immediately before the operation contributes to the overall success rate of intraocular procedures. For most types of glaucoma, miosis is desired at the time of operation. The pupil is usually constricted for iridencleisis, cyclodialysis, iridencleisis-cyclodialysis, and cyclocryothermy. The pupil's size, when displaced lenses are removed, is dependent on the position of the lens. For anterior-luxated lenses, the pupil is constricted to maintain the lens within the anterior chamber. A combination of 2% pilocarpine and 10% phenylephrine is recommended to provide a pupil of moderate size; a miotic pupil can aggravate the glaucomatous process by creating an acute pupil block related to the anterior-luxated lens or adherent vitreous. Before removal of the subluxated and posterior-luxated lenses, the pupil is dilated with several instillations of 10% phenylephrine and 1% atropine. At the time of mydriasis, IOP must be within normal limits.

In most types of glaucoma, the vitreous frequently undergoes partial liquefaction (syneresis). Hence, during many glaucoma surgical procedures, presentation of the vitreous may occur. To minimize vitreous disturbances, osmotic agents are essential not only to reduce IOP, but also to dehydrate the vitreous to reduce its size. Mannitol (1 to 2 g/kg intravenously) is injected at the time of induction of general anesthesia to insure maximum reduction in IOP and vitreous size. Carbonic anhydrase inhibitors reduce IOP, but do not affect the vitreous.

Iridencleisis

In the iridencleisis procedure, a radial section of the iris is permanently positioned through a limbal incision into the subconjunctival spaces beneath the bulbar conjunctiva. The reduction in IOP after iridencleisis is primarily related to the improvement in aqueous humor outflow through this area. Aqueous humor may escape between the two pillars of iris as well as through the iris stroma.

Iridencleisis has been used successfully for narrow- and closed-angle glaucoma, acute iris bombé associated with annular posterior synechiae, and glaucomas associated with peripheral anterior synechiae. When the iris is thin, atrophied, or adhered to the lens with focal posterior synechiae, the iridencleisis procedure is not recommended.

The eyelids and external eye are prepared in a standard fashion. The conjunctival fornices are cleaned with sterile Dacron swabs and 0.9% sterile isotonic saline solution. The animal is draped, leaving only the palpebral fissure exposed. The iridencleisis procedure is usually performed at the 12 o'clock position. If additional surgical procedures are necessary, other positions are used. With curved blunt-tipped standard eye scissors, a limbal-based 10-mm bulbar conjunctival flap is constructed. The flap is usually 12 to 18 mm long. Tenon's capsule is identified and is excised from the overlying bulbar conjunctiva and the sclera in the area of the limbal incision.

The anterior chamber is entered through the limbus with a No. 11 Bard-Parker or a No. 67 Beaver blade (Fig. 6-85A). The limbal incision is usually 8 to 10 mm long. A 1- to 2-mm wide section of the sclera in the caudal aspect of the limbal incision is carefully excised (posterior sclerectomy). Hemostasis and limited tissue destruction are achieved by judicious electrocautery. Wet-field cautery is superior in this region because of the frequent presence of aqueous humor. Limited application of electrocautery on the scleral aspect of the incision may facilitate maintenance of an open fistula and may reduce the possibility of closure by healing.

During the limbal incision and subsequent posterior sclerectomy, the iris may protrude into the incision. A blunt iris hook or serrated iris forceps is carefully manipulated into the anterior chamber to grasp the dorsal pupillary margin and to protract the iris into the limbal incision (Fig. 6-85B). Using two serrated forceps, the iris is protracted external to the limbal incision to its base. Using the small forceps with the wet-field cautery, the iris is cauterized radially to minimize hemorrhage. Traction is then applied with both iris forceps to slowly tear the iris radially to its base and to create two separate iridal pillars (Fig. 6-85C). Each section of the iris, with its pigmented epithelium dorsally, is manipulated into the respective end of the limbal incision. To minimize the possibility of the iris's retracting back into the anterior chamber, each tag of the iris is apposed to the sclera with a single interrupted 6-0 chromic collagen suture. The anterior chamber is carefully irrigated with balanced salt solution to remove fibrin or blood. With successful manipulation of the iris and judicious use of electrocautery, hemorrhage and fibrin in the anterior chamber at the conclusion of the surgical procedure are generally avoided. The bulbar conjunctival flap is apposed with a continuous 6-0 chromic collagen suture (Fig. 6-85D).

Postoperative treatment consists of maintaining a pupil of normal position (neither dilated nor constricted) and a normal range of IOP, as well as suppressing the postoperative iridocyclitis with topical or systemic corticosteroids. Topical and systemic antibiotics are also frequently administered to prevent postoperative infections. Phenylephrine (10%) and pilocarpine (2%) are often instilled alternately to facilitate movement of the pupil and to minimize the possibility of focal posterior synechiae. The ratio of these drugs depends on the pupil's size. For instance, if the pupil is

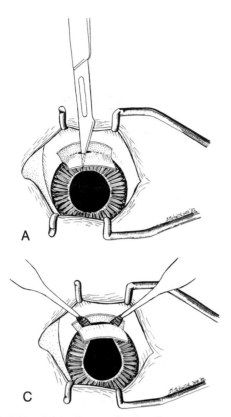

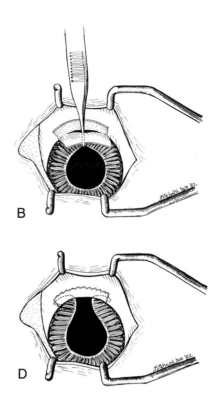

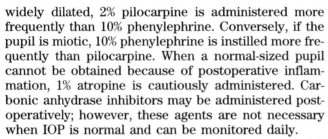

Fig. 6-85. *Iridencleisis. See text for details.*

widely dilated, 2% pilocarpine is administered more frequently than 10% phenylephrine. Conversely, if the pupil is miotic, 10% phenylephrine is instilled more frequently than pilocarpine. When a normal-sized pupil cannot be obtained because of postoperative inflammation, 1% atropine is cautiously administered. Carbonic anhydrase inhibitors may be administered postoperatively; however, these agents are not necessary when IOP is normal and can be monitored daily.

Complications of iridencleisis include excessive iridocyclitis, hyphema, posterior synechia, iris deposition of pigment on the anterior lens capsule, and cataract formation. Subconjunctival blebs usually occur following iridencleisis in the area of the limbal incision. These blebs may eventually flatten, but still appear to be functional. The bulbar conjunctiva in the area of the limbal incision usually demonstrates increased vascularity. Failure of the iridencleisis to control IOP satisfactorily is usually related to the closure of the limbal incision with either inflammatory products, associated with the postoperative iridocyclitis, or eventual fibrosis several months later. Gentle massage of the eye postoperatively and the postoperative administration of corticosteroid agents may increase the success rate of the iridencleisis procedure.

Cyclodialysis

In this procedure, an artificial fistula is created between the anterior chamber and the subconjunctival spaces. The "fistula" connects anteriorly through the suprairidociliary space and through an opening in the sclera into the subconjunctival spaces. Cyclodialysis is thought to lower IOP by facilitating the outflow of aqueous humor from the anterior chamber into the suprachoroidal space (uveoscleral outflow) and through the sclera into the subconjunctival spaces. The rate of aqueous humor formation may also be reduced in the early postoperative period, probably associated with separation of the ciliary body from the sclera and some of its vascular supply. The cyclodialysis procedure may be performed posteriorly through the scleral incision or anteriorly from the anterior chamber, usually in conjunction with removal of the lens.

The cyclodialysis procedure is used for narrow-angle glaucoma, glaucoma associated with extensive peripheral anterior synechiae, goniodysgenesis glaucoma (congenital glaucoma), and glaucoma associated with iris atrophy.

The eye is prepared by the standard surgical method. The operation is usually performed at the 12 o'clock position. With blunt-tipped, slightly curved standard eye scissors, a fornix-based bulbar conjunctival flap, measuring 10 mm deep by 10 mm wide, is fashioned. Tenon's capsule is excised in the area. A linear scleral incision is made 4 to 5 mm from and parallel to the limbus for approximately 10 mm using the No. 15 Bard-Parker scalpel blade (Fig. 6-86A). Hemorrhage is controlled by point electrocautery.

The block of sclera is carefully excised by sharp dissection; the scleral block measures 3 by 8 mm. The depth of the scleral incision should be carefully con-

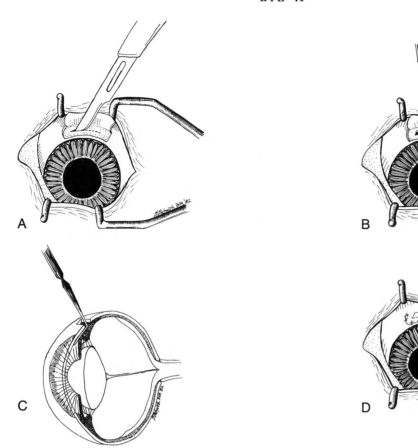

Fig. 6-86. *Cyclodialysis. See text for details.*

trolled so that the ciliary body is not penetrated. When pigmentation of the ciliary body becomes evident, the scleral block is carefully excised. The sides of the scleral defect are lightly cauterized to reduce the possibility of the defects healing closed. A cyclodialysis spatula is carefully inserted into the anterior part of the scleral incision between the sclera and ciliary body and is manipulated forward into the anterior chamber (Fig. 6-86*B*). When the anterior chamber is entered, aqueous humor usually escapes along the sides of the spatula. The spatula is moved medially and laterally to enlarge the artificial fistula approximately 8 to 10 mm. A sagittal view of the placement of the spatula is shown in Figure 6-86*C*. Choice of the cyclodialysis spatula is important in the dog. The slightly rounded cyclodialysis spatulas penetrate this area with difficulty in the dog and often contribute to excessive hemorrhage; hence a flat, smooth-edged, 10-mm spatula is preferred.

A cyclodialysis needle may be used instead of the spatula; its advantage is that at the conclusion of the sweep, the anterior chamber may be gently irrigated with balanced salt solution, removing any hemorrhage or fibrin. The scleral incision is left open, and the bulbar conjunctival flap is apposed with a simple interrupted 6-0 chromic collagen suture (Fig. 6-86*D*).

Postoperative treatment consists of control of the iridocyclitis with topical or systemic corticosteroids and antibiotics, maintenance of normal IOP by carbonic anhydrase inhibitors, and maintenance of a normal-sized pupil (neither constricted or dilated). The pupil's size is controlled by alternate instillations of a mydriatic (10% phenylephrine) and a miotic (2% pilocarpine) agent. The ratio of these drugs depends on the pupil's size. The intensity of the medications postoperatively is dependent on the IOP and the postoperative iridocyclitis; dosage is gradually reduced over several weeks.

Possible complications include hyphema, excessive iridocyclitis, iatrogenic corneal damage with the spatula, and return of the glaucoma. Hyphema is minimized by proper surgical techniques and by the use of the cyclodialysis spatula. Corneal damage is minimized in the procedure if the spatula does not exceed 10 mm in length. The scleral defect may close because of fibrosis and incorporation of inflammatory debris from the iridocyclitis. Closure of this defect may occur either in the immediate postoperative period or months later. Carefully massaging the globe 2 or 3 times daily may promote patency of the cyclodialysis fistula.

Combined Iridencleisis-Cyclodialysis

The iridencleisis-cyclodialysis procedure attempts to combine these two methods for the frequently advanced canine glaucomas. A portion of the iris is positioned through the scleral defect beneath the ciliary body into the subconjunctival space. The combination

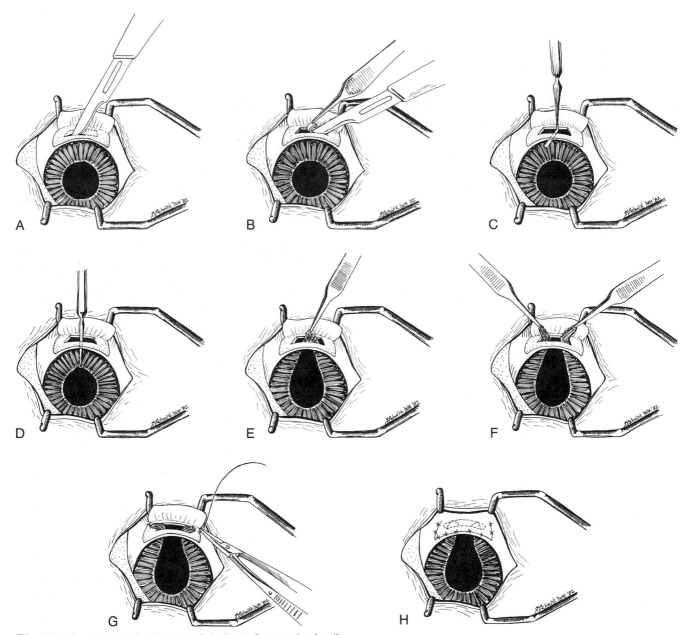

Fig. 6-87. *Combined iridencleisis-cyclodialysis. See text for details.*

of iridencleisis and cyclodialysis is used for narrow-angle glaucoma, closed-angle glaucoma, and the glaucomas with associated iridocyclitis and iris bombé.

After routine preparation for intraocular surgery, a fornix-based conjunctival flap is prepared using slightly curved standard eye scissors. The conjunctival flap is started about 8 mm from the limbus and is continued for about 12 mm. Tenon's capsule is carefully excised from the overlying bulbar conjunctiva (Fig. 6-87A). The sclera is excised as a section 2 by 6 mm with a No. 15 Bard-Parker or a No. 65 Beaver blade about 3 to 4 mm from the limbus (Fig. 6-87B). Hemorrhage is controlled by point electrocautery.

As the scleral incision approaches the underlying ciliary body, the pigment of the ciliary body is observed. The scleral block is separated from the underlying cili-

ary body by careful sharp dissection. A 10-mm cyclodialysis spatula is carefully manipulated forward between the iris-ciliary body and sclera into the anterior chamber. Upon entry into the anterior chamber, aqueous humor begins to flow into the incision. With the cyclodialysis spatula, the fistula is enlarged by lateral and medial movements (Fig. 6-87C). A broad, blunt iris hook is moved carefully through the newly created fistula into the anterior chamber and is manipulated to the pupillary margin of the dorsal iris. The iris is carefully protracted by the iris hook to the scleral wound (Fig. 6-87D). The iris is grasped with 2 pairs of serrated iris forceps at the pupillary margin (Fig. 6-87E and F).

Electrocautery is applied between the forceps at the pupillary margin of the iris and is continued to its base, by using either the electroscalpel or wet-field cautery.

Hemorrhage is usually minimal when electrocautery is used. The iris is gradually teased apart, creating 2 separate pillars that are attached at each end of the scleral defect with a single interrupted 6-0 chromic collagen suture (Fig. 6-87*G*). The anterior chamber is reformed with balanced salt solution using a cyclodialysis needle. Hemorrhage and fibrin within the anterior chamber may be carefully irrigated from the anterior chamber. The anterior chamber is again reformed with balanced salt solution, and an air bubble approximating one-fourth the volume of the anterior chamber is injected. The scleral defect is not sutured closed. The bulbar conjunctiva is apposed with a simple interrupted 6-0 chromic collagen suture (Fig. 6-87*H*).

Postoperative treatment for and possible postoperative complications of the combined iridencleisis-cyclodialysis procedure are similar to that described for both procedures. The success rate for this procedure, with 6- to 12-month follow-ups, is approximately 50%.

Cyclodialysis-Iridocyclectomy

In the combined cyclodialysis-iridocyclectomy procedure, a portion of the anterior uvea is excised immediately beneath the standard cyclodialysis procedure. The iridocyclectomy is performed to minimize the possibility of the obstruction of the cyclodialysis fistula by incorporation of uveal tissue. This procedure is used for narrow- and closed-angle glaucomas in the dog.

Following standard surgical preparation, a limbal-based conjunctival flap is prepared by blunt-tipped, slightly curved, standard eye scissors, approximately 8 mm from the limbus. The conjunctival flap and Tenon's capsule are reflected rostrally to expose a large area of the sclera. Tenon's capsule is carefully excised from the overlying bulbar conjunctiva. A rectangular block of sclera measuring 2 to 3 by 7 to 9 mm is excised approximately 6 mm posterior to the limbus. Hemostasis is maintained by point electrocautery. A 10-mm cyclodialysis spatula is manipulated forward into the anterior chamber through the suprairidociliary space. The spatula is moved from side to side for approximately 90°. A sharp iris hook is manipulated through the suprachoroidal space into the anterior chamber to grasp the peripheral iris and to protract it into the scleral incision. The peripheral iris and ciliary body are retracted into the scleral window and are excised using electrocautery. The cautery unit should be of sufficiently high power to cut the iris and ciliary body cleanly with minimal coagulation. With a cyclodialysis needle positioned in the anterior chamber, fibrin and hemorrhage are irrigated from the anterior chamber. The anterior chamber is restored with balanced salt solution and a small air bubble. The scleral window is allowed to remain open. The conjunctival flap is apposed with a continuous 6-0 chromic collagen suture (Fig. 6-88).

Postoperative treatment is similar to those operations previously discussed. This procedure, like others,

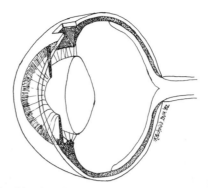

Fig. 6-88. *Combined cyclodialysis-iridocyclectomy. See text for details.*

has approximately a 50% success rate with 6- to 12-month follow-ups in the dog. Electrocautery is essential for this procedure, to excise the section of iris and ciliary body with minimal hemorrhage. The postoperative complications of this operation are similar to those previously discussed.

Removal of Subluxated and Luxated Lenses for the Glaucomas

Although the role of lens displacement and lens luxation in the canine glaucomas is not totally understood in the pathogenesis of glaucoma, the presence of the displaced subluxated lens with elevated IOP frequently complicates medical treatment of the disease; hence removal of the luxated lens in glaucoma frequently simplifies medical treatment of the disease and permits more uniform control of IOP. Removal of the subluxated lens in some dogs, particularly the wire-haired and smooth fox terriers and Sealyham terrier, may result in complete resolution of early glaucoma.

Removal of the subluxated and luxated lenses is more difficult than routine extraction of cataracts. The anterior hyaloid membrane is often ruptured by the displaced lens, and vitreous presentation is frequent during removal of the lens.

The surgical procedure is similar to that described in the cataract section of this chapter. However an intracapsular technique is planned and is usually possible. Preoperative treatment of these eyes includes control of IOP by carbonic anhydrase inhibitors, dehydration of the vitreous by osmotic agents, and control of the pupil, depending on the lens position.

Preoperative management of anterior lens luxation is usually achieved by the instillation of 2% pilocarpine; miosis assists in maintaining the anterior-luxated lens within the anterior chamber. Care must be taken not to induce an intense miosis, which may create an iris bombé resulting from incarceration and obstruction of the pupil by the lens or vitreous. Removal of the subluxated and posterior-luxated lenses (those within the vitreous) is preceded by preoperative mydriasis from the instillations immediately before the operation of 10% phenylephrine and 1% atropine. Hypodermic needles (22 or 23 gauge) can also be placed at right

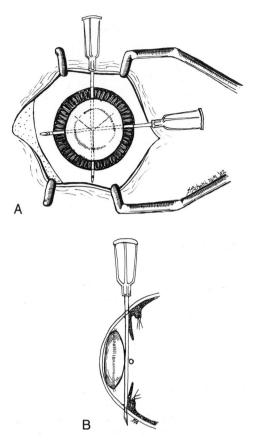

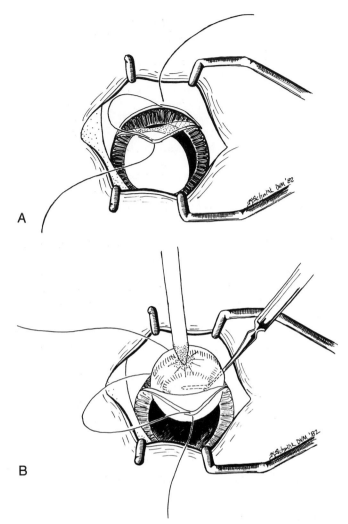

Fig. 6-89. *Removal of an anterior-luxated lens. A, Insertion of needles. B, Sagittal view. See text for details.*

angles to each other to fix the luxated lens in place. For instance, for anterior-luxated lenses, the needles may be positioned through the limbus and posterior to the anterior-luxated lens (Fig. 6-89). For subluxated or posterior-luxated lenses, the 2 needles are positioned through the sclera and the pars plana of the ciliary body about 6 to 7 mm from the limbus, to trap the subluxated lens and to prevent migration into the vitreous body prior to and during removal (Fig. 6-90).

We prefer to use cryoprobes to remove these lenses. The carbon dioxide cryoprobes achieve a temperature

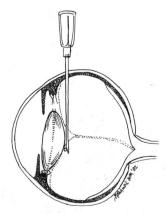

Fig. 6-90. *Removal of subluxated or posterior-luxated lens. See text for details.*

Fig. 6-91. *Removal of luxated lens with a cryoprobe. See text for details.*

of −40 to −50° C to provide excellent cryo-lens attachment. These powerful cryoprobes perform well in the presence of aqueous humor and/or vitreous. The cryoprobe is touched to the luxated lens for a few seconds, and the lens is carefully slid from the anterior chamber. A cyclodialysis spatula is positioned posterior to the lens to remove any adherent vitreous. A single preplaced limbal suture, prepositioned for extraction of the luxated lens, closes the limbal incision rapidly as the lens is removed (Fig. 6-91). Use of intra- or extracapsular forceps to grasp the free-floating luxated lenses is difficult and may further disturb the vitreous.

Management of anterior vitreous presentation is critical during removal of the displaced lens. When vitreous is presented during the limbal incision, a blunt 18-gauge hypodermic needle is inserted through the pupil into the upper aspect of the vitreous body to remove liquid vitreous (Fig. 6-92). Frequently, 0.1 to 0.5 ml of liquid vitreous can be aspirated, permitting the protruding gel fraction to fall behind the pupil. Alternately, the Kaufman Vitrector* can be used to remove vitreous

*American V. Mueller, 6600 West Touky Avenue, Chicago, IL 60648

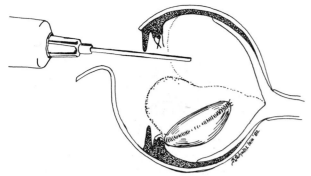

Fig. 6-92. *Management of anterior vitreous presentation during removal of luxated lens. See text for details.*

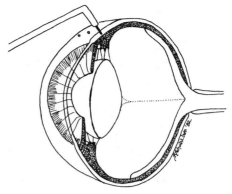

Fig. 6-93. *Cyclodiathermy. See text for details.*

from the anterior chamber. Loss of liquid vitreous appears to be well tolerated by the eye; excision or loss of gel vitreous is not desirable. Once the lens has been removed from the eye and the anterior chamber has been partially reformed, an air bubble, approximately one-fourth to one-third of the volume of the anterior chamber (0.25 to 0.3 ml), is injected to maintain the gel vitreous behind the pupil during the immediate postoperative period.

Postoperative medical treatments after lens removal in glaucomatous eyes are similar to those described in the cataract section of this chapter. In addition, IOP must be carefully monitored. If necessary, carbonic anhydrase inhibitors are added to the regimen to maintain IOP within normal limits. Other glaucoma surgical procedures, such as cyclodialysis and iridencleisis, are often used in addition to removal of the luxated lens.

Cyclodiathermy

Cyclodiathermy is the application of intense heat within the ciliary body to produce focal destruction of the structure and to reduce the rate of aqueous humor formation. Cyclodiathermy in the dog has not been highly effective. The procedure is usually reserved for buphthalmic blind glaucomatous eyes because phthisis bulbi often may occur.

Following standard preparation, a fornix-based conjunctival flap is prepared. The conjunctival flap of approximately 120° is extended caudally for approximately 8 mm with blunt-tipped, slightly curved, standard eye scissors. After adequate exposure of the sclera and hemostasis, a special diathermy needle is applied 5 to 6 mm from the dorsal limbus through the sclera directly into the ciliary body at 6 to 10 different sites. Aqueous humor may escape as the diathermy needle is withdrawn (Fig. 6-93).

Diathermy has the objectionable effect of producing necrosis of the sclera overlying the ciliary body. The postoperative inflammation of the sclera and the ciliary body is intense following cyclodiathermy and necessitates vigorous topical and systemic corticosteroid administration. The results of cyclodiathermy are unpredictable because of the variability of the regenerative powers of the ciliary body epithelium.

Cyclocryothermy

Cyclocryothermy is the application of intense cold directly through the bulbar conjunctiva and sclera to the ciliary body to reduce the rate of aqueous humor formation. The advantages of this procedure are that it may be repeated without adversely affecting the bulbar conjunctiva and sclera, and the canine patient need only be sedated. We have used cyclocryothermy primarily in advanced glaucomatous eyes to reduce IOP in the presence of persistent pain or to induce a degree of phthisis bulbi, a cosmetically acceptable alternative to the buphthalmic eye. Cyclocryothermy has also been used with considerable promise for less-advanced canine glaucomas.

The cryoprobe is applied 5 mm from the limbus directly on the dorsal bulbar conjunctiva. Three to 5 sites are frozen to approximately −60 to 90° C for 60 seconds to 2 minutes each (Fig. 6-94). Conjunctival hyperemia and chemosis follow cyclocryothermy and may be intense. Administration of topical and systemic corticosteroids is indicated to suppress the cryogenic inflammation. IOP is maintained within normal limits with carbonic anhydrase inhibitors. In approximately 6 weeks, the eventual result of cyclocryothermy can usually be ascertained. If IOP is still elevated, cyclocryothermy can be repeated.

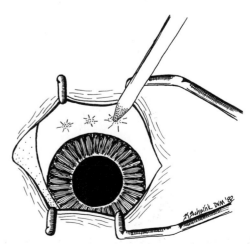

Fig. 6-94. *Cyclocryothermy. See text for details.*

References and Suggested Readings

Armaly, M. F., et al.: Symposium on Glaucoma. St. Louis, C. V. Mosby, 1967.

Fasanella, R. M. (ed.): Complications in Eye Surgery. 2nd Ed. Philadelphia, W. B. Saunders, 1965.

Gelatt, K. N.: Veterinary Ophthalmology. Philadelphia, Lea & Febiger, 1981.

Gelatt, K. N.: Veterinary Ophthalmic Pharmacology and Therapeutics. Bonner Springs, KS: Veterinary Medicine Publishing, 1970.

Gelatt, K. N., and Ladds, P. W.: Gonioscopy in dogs and cats with glaucoma and ocular tumors. J. Small Anim. Pract., 12:105, 1971.

Gelatt, K. N., Wyman, M., and Lavignette, A.: Symposium on cataract surgery in the dog. Proceedings of the American Society of Veterinary Ophthalmology, Louisville, KY, 1966.

Knight, G.: The indications and technique for lens extraction in the dog. Vet. Rec., 74:1065, 1962.

Kolker, A. E., and Hetherington, J.: Becker's-Shaffer's Diagnosis and Therapy of the Glaucomas. 3rd Ed. St. Louis, C. V. Mosby, 1970.

Lawson, D. D.: Luxation of the crystalline lens in the dog. J. Small Anim. Pract., 10:461, 1969.

Magrane, W. G.: Cryosurgical lens extraction: uses and limitation. J. Small Anim. Pract., 9:71, 1968.

Magrane, W. G.: Canine Ophthalmology. 2nd Ed. Philadelphia, Lea & Febiger, 1971.

Paton, R. T., Smith, B., Katzin, H. M., and Stilwell, D.: Atlas of Eye Surgery. 2nd Ed. New York, McGraw-Hill, 1962.

Stack, W. F.: Posterior sclerotomy—a surgical procedure for treatment of glaucoma. J. Am. Vet. Med. Assoc., 136:453, 1960.

Startup, F. G.: Low temperature cataract extraction. Vet. Rec., 77:978, 1965.

Vierheller, R. C.: Surgical treatment of glaucoma: a reappraisal of recommended operative techniques in veterinary practice. Proceedings of the American Society of Veterinary Ophthalmology, Dallas, TX, 1967.

Wyman, M.: Ophthalmic system. In Pathophysiology in Small Animal Surgery. Edited by M. J. Bojrab. Philadelphia, Lea & Febiger, 1981.

Surgery of the Iris and Ciliary Body

by ROBERT L. PEIFFER, JR.

Indications for operation on the iris and ciliary body are infrequently encountered by the veterinary ophthalmic surgeon, outside of glaucoma procedures that involve manipulation of these tissues; these techniques are elaborated upon in the section of this chapter on glaucoma and are not considered here. This discussion examines techniques of iridotomy as a means of controlling the pupillary aperture; iridectomy to remove localized tumors of the iris; iridocyclectomy for excision of more extensive anterior-segment neoplasms, pupillary membranectomy to manage the most common complication of cataract surgery; and aspiration of epithelial cysts.

Surgical Anatomy and Physiology

The iris and ciliary body consist of loosely woven connective tissue of mesodermal origin lined posteriorly by a bilayered epithelium of neuroectodermal origin. The iris epithelium is heavily pigmented with melanin in both layers; only the outermost layer of the ciliary body epithelium is pigmented. The iris epithelium is pigmented even in blue-eyed individuals, and only in true albinos is the pigmented epithelium devoid of melanin granules. It is the amount of stromal melanin that imparts to the iris its characteristic hue. Deeply pigmented irides react less readily to topical autonomic agents, both in terms of pupillary and intraocular pressure responses.

The iris and ciliary body receive their vascular supply via the anterior ciliary arteries, which are continuations of the muscular branches of the ophthalmic artery, and the long posterior ciliary arteries, which originate from the ophthalmic artery near the posterior pole and follow a transscleral and intrachoroidal route to the anterior segment. The anterior ciliary arteries, which enter the globe at the insertions of the extraocular muscles, contribute less significantly to anterior uveal perfusion in the dog than in primates. The two long posterior ciliary arteries traverse the globe in the nasal and temporal horizontal plane and give rise to the major arterial circle of the iris. This vascular circle is located in the peripheral iris approximately one-fourth the distance from the iris base to the pupil. The arterial circle is incomplete at 6 and 12 o'clock. From the major arterial circle, radial branches supply the central iris and ciliary body. These radiating vessels lack the perivascular connective tissue sheaths that minimize surgical hemorrhage in primates; significant bleeding is usually avoided, however, if the major arterial circle is not transected. Unfortunately, fibrinous exudation from the iris vasculature in response to surgical trauma is not uncommon.

The sphincter muscle runs circumferentially within the iris stroma and extends from the pupillary margin toward the base of the iris for 1.5 mm in the dog and cat to 2.0 mm in the horse. It is a cholinergic smooth muscle that, upon stimulation constricts to produce miosis; this phenomenon can be induced pharmacologically with parasympathomimetic drugs administered topically or intracamerally. Miosis also occurs in response to release of prostaglandins and other mediators of inflammation. The dilator muscle is a broad, flat, fan-shaped muscle found just anterior to the pigmented epithelium; it responds as an alpha-adrenergic smooth muscle, and pharmacologic agents such as epinephrine can be used by the veterinary surgeon to enlarge the size of the pupil.

In addition to autonomic innervation, the iris receives sensory branches of the ophthalmic branch of the fifth nerve. Anesthesia that is adequate for corneoscleral incision may need to be deepened when the iris is manipulated.

Ciliary body landmarks important to the veterinary surgeon include the ora ciliaris retinae, or junction between the pars plana of the ciliary body and the peripheral retina; this area in the dog is located 8 mm posterior to the limbus superiorly and temporally, but only 4 mm inferiorly and nasally. Iridocyclectomy posterior to the ora, which is a linear structure in subprimates, causes peripheral retinal dialysis and detachment. The ciliary body epithelium is responsible for the production of aqueous humor; although it is not known to what extent this tissue can be excised without impairing aqueous humor dynamics, it is most likely less than 90°. The veterinary surgeon must also be aware of the zonules, which arise from the pars plana and the pars plicata. Manipulations that result in extensive zonular disruption lead to dislocation of the lens. Zonular traction may also result in ciliary body hemorrhage.

Surgical Pharmacology

The control of both pupillary size and iris exudation is an important consideration for the anterior segment operation both intra- and postoperatively. Preoperative treatment with systemic corticosteroids, antiprostaglandins, and topical mydriatics minimizes fibrinous exudation and the tendency for the pupil to constrict during the operation. Intraoperative, intracameral acetylcholine (.5 to 2 ml 1:100 solution), or epinephrine (.5 ml 1:10,000 solution) can be employed to constrict or to enlarge the pupil, respectively. Judicious use of intracameral heparin may be used to inhibit fibrin clotting. Topical, subconjunctival, and systemic corticosteroids and topical mydriatics are employed postoperatively to temper the surgically induced inflammation, which, although variable, is always an important factor.

Surgical Techniques

IRIDOTOMY

The veterinary ophthalmic surgeon has traditionally avoided incision or excision of iris tissue because of the common knowledge that hemorrhage results. Significant hemorrhage can almost always be prevented if the major arterial circle is avoided; in some instances this is not possible, but even this complication can often be managed without disastrous results. Surgical iris hemorrhage can be largely prevented by the use of wet-field cautery to incise uveal tissue, but care must be taken to avoid the lens when using intraocular cautery. If hemorrhage does occur, closure of the incision and re-establishment of the anterior chamber to increase intraocular pressure will hasten clotting. In several minutes, hyphema and clots may be gently irrigated or extracted from the anterior chamber.

Indications for sphincter iridotomy include enlargement of the pupil during or following a cataract operation; if the pupil constricts prior to lens extraction or is less than 3 mm in diameter following extraction, 1- to 4-quadrant sphincterotomy is performed as necessary to enhance exposure or to achieve at least a 5-mm pupil. The technique is described and illustrated in Figure 6-95. Making an incision to a depth of 2 to 3 mm with scissors is preferable to grasping and tearing because it is less traumatic and is more readily con-

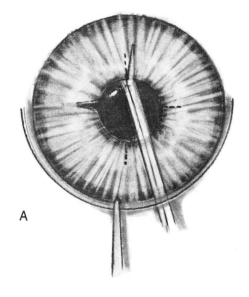

A

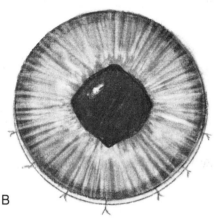

B

Fig. 6-95. *Sphincter iridotomy. A, Enlargement of the pupillary aperture may be achieved by incising the sphincter muscle of the iris. The procedure is best performed with sharp scissors and a formed anterior chamber in the superior and lateral quadrants; gentle retraction of the cornea and an "open sky" technique are necessary to incise the iris at 12 o'clock. Minimizing the incision to a depth of 2 mm prevents significant hemorrhage. B, The resultant pupil will appear diamond-shaped rather than round if 4-quadrant sphincterotomy is performed.*

trolled. The technique is performed through the corneoscleral incision with a chamber formed by an air bubble in the inferior, temporal, and nasal quadrants and by an "open sky" method, reflecting the cornea inferiorly, in the superior quandrant. As in all anterior segment surgical procedures, utmost respect must be held for the corneal endothelium; elevation and retraction of the cornea must be gentle, irrigation should be minimal and diverted away from the endothelium, and instruments within the anterior chamber must not come into contact with the endothelial surface. The use of viscous intracameral hyaluronic acid, recently popularized in human ophthalmology to protect the cornea during insertion of intraocular lenses, provides a physical protective cushion in any procedure in which anterior chamber manipulations are required.

IRIDECTOMY

Sector iridectomy is indicated for excisional biopsy of iris stromal lesions, most frequently pigmented tumors, to create a pupil subsequent to inflammatory disease with synechia or membrane formation, and to manage acute inflammatory posterior synechia with iris bombé and secondary glaucoma. A preferable technique in the latter situation is a combined posterior sclerectomy-cyclodialysis-transcleral iridencleisis. This operation provides not only a restoration of normal pathways of aqueous flow, but also a filtering procedure to alleviate the possibility of persistent glaucoma from peripheral anterior synechiae, which are likely to develop with iris bombé of any duration. If simple iridectomy is elected, the technique described

in Figure 6-96 for excisional biopsy is modified only by initially freeing the adherent pupillary margin with a blunt iris hook or a cyclodialysis spatula.

IRIDOCYCLECTOMY

Excision of the iris and ciliary body is an infrequently used technique indicated for tumors that can be localized within the anterior uvea. Ciliary body adenomas, which usually involve only the ciliary processes, may be removed with this technique. Anterior uveal malignant melanomas and ciliary body adenocarcinomas frequently are diagnosed only when they have been present for some time and likely have extended posteriorly into the choroid and retina or into the outflow pathways or deep sclera. The ideal surgical candidate has an uninvolved iridocorneal angle upon gonioscopy, a discrete, well-defined lesion confined to the anterior uveal structures, and absence of secondary uveitis or glaucoma. A thorough clinical examination,

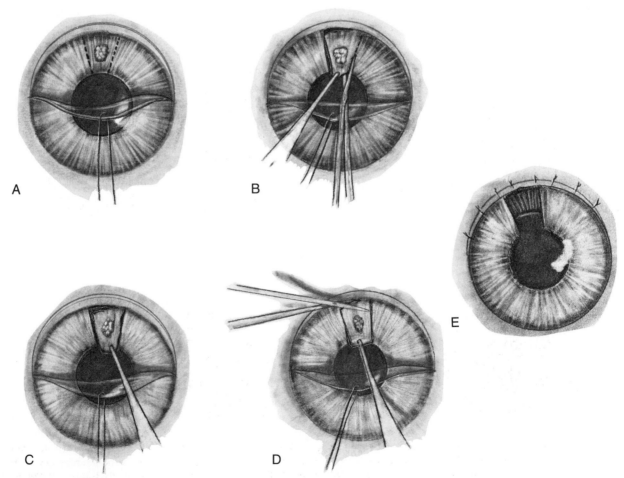

Fig. 6-96. *Sector iridectomy for excisional biopsy of a superior iris lesion. A, Following a superior 180° corneoscleral incision, the cornea is gently retracted. Lesions in the inferior quadrants are excised with a similar incision and a formed anterior chamber. Dotted lines indicate area of planned excision; note that liberal margins of grossly uninvolved tissue are allowed. B, While exerting gentle traction on the pupillary margin, the lateral iris margins are incised with scissors or cautery. If hemorrhage does occur, the corneal flap is replaced, the anterior chamber is formed, and the bleeding vessels are allowed to clot before irrigating the anterior chamber and proceeding. C and D, The base of the iris can be transected by tearing (C) or by incision (D). E, Postoperative appearance. The corneoscleral incision is closed with interrupted sutures of 7-0 polyglactin 910 (Vicryl), and the anterior chamber is reformed with lactated ringers or similar solution. Through the keyhole pupil, the lens equator, zonules, and ciliary processes are seen.*

including indirect ophthalmoscopy with scleral depression (with the patient anesthetized), critical transillumination, and ultrasonic imaging, facilitates this challenging clinical diagnosis. In most cases, 45 to 60° is the maximum tolerable extent of uveal excision. Although invasive melanomas and adenocarcinomas with angle involvement may be removed with this technique, because the angle structures and deep sclera are excised, it is difficult to define the extent of such tumors. The possibility of residual neoplasm with potential for metastasis is high. In addition, manipulation during the surgical procedure may enhance seeding or metastasis of the tumor. Thus, unless unusual circumstances exist, such as a blind fellow eye, enucleation is the procedure of choice in these cases. Iridocyclectomy is illustrated in Figure 6-97.

PUPILLARY MEMBRANECTOMY

The formation of pupillary iridocapsular membranes is a common sequela to cataract operations in the dog. If extensive, these membranes may impair vision or may precipitate secondary glaucoma. Less frequently, membranes may occur with anterior uveitis, especially lens-induced uveitis. If the animal is aphakic, sector iridectomy is indicated. In an aphakic animal, however, membranectomy is a simple, effective secondary procedure that frequently provides a satisfactory visual result, when contrasted to a cataract extraction that otherwise is relegated to failure.

The important criteria for performing pupillary membranectomy are a formed anterior chamber and near-normal intraocular pressure. The technique is illustrated in Figure 6-98. This procedure is accomplished by inserting a short infusion needle through the limbus 90 to 180° from the entrance of the membranectomy needle. The infusion needle is inserted slightly corneally to the limbus to avoid contact with the iris and is connected to a bottle of lactated Ringer's solution suspended 50 cm above the patient. The membranectomy knife is made from a disposable 25- or 27-gauge needle, bent 90° at the tip with a needle holder, and is inserted through a 2-mm limbal incision made with a pointed blade.

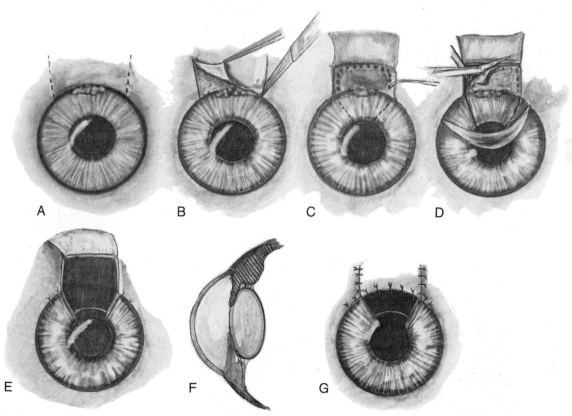

Fig. 6-97. *Iridocyclectomy for excision of an anterior uveal tumor. A, Hatched area indicates the tissues to be excised, which include deep sclera and peripheral cornea, the iridocorneal angle structures, and the iris and ciliary body. B, A broad, fornix-based conjunctival flap is prepared and retracted; conjunctiva will not be depicted in order to simplify the drawings. Lines indicate lateral margins of planned scleral flap and deeper excision. With sharp dissection, a half-thickness posterior-based scleral flap is prepared. C, Cautery is placed around the margins of the excised flap to minimize hemorrhage when the underlying ciliary body is excised. Dotted lines indicate the extent of planned iris excision. D, A corneoscleral incision is made beyond the extent of planned excision to allow mobility of the corneal flap. Scissors are used to excise the iris and the deep corneosclera and ciliary body along the area delineated by the flap. A suction-cutter is used to remove vitreous if it appears through the wound. E, Appearance after tissue has been excised. F, Cross-sectional view of eye illustrating the excised tissues. G, The flap and corneoscleral incision are closed with interrupted sutures of 7-0 polyglactin 910 (Vicryl), and the anterior chamber is reformed with lactated Ringer's or similar solution. The conjunctival flap may be sutured in place or may be allowed to reposition and heal without sutures.*

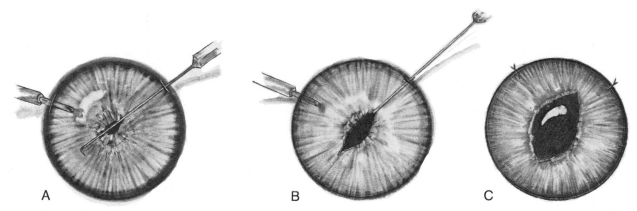

A   B   C

Fig. 6-98. *Pupillary membranectomy. A, Two 2-to-3-mm limbal incisions are made at 10 and 2 o'clock. An infusion port is placed through one and a 27-gauge needle with its tip bent 90° is placed through the other. B, The needle is rotated and its tip manipulated to engage iris; the needle is then gently depressed and is drawn across the membrane. C, The instruments are withdrawn and the incisions are closed with interrupted sutures of 7-0 polyglactin 910 (Vicryl).*

Generally, the longer after the primary operation that membranectomy is performed the better; I prefer to wait several weeks until the surgically induced inflammation has resolved. The procedure described carries approximately a 50% success rate; those that fail do so because of pupillary membrane reformation. The procedure can be repeated, but satisfactory results become less likely with successive operations, and I perform sector iridectomy if a single membranectomy is unsuccessful.

ASPIRATION OF EPITHELIAL CYSTS

Cysts of the iris and ciliary body epithelium may develop spontaneously or may occur subsequent to trauma or inflammation; they may be attached to the ciliary processes or pupillary margin, or may be observed free-floating in the anterior chamber. These cysts are identified clinically by their regular margins and their ability to transilluminate. Although they are benign, these cysts may be aspirated if they become excessively large, or to obtain a definitive diagnosis to differentiate them from malignant melanomas or cystic ciliary body adenomas when clinical distinction is not possible.

The surgical technique is identical to that used for membranectomy, with the exception that a straight 20-gauge needle is used for aspiration (Fig. 6-99). As the cyst is aspirated, the bevel of the needle is used to transect the base of the cyst if it is fixed to uveal tissue.

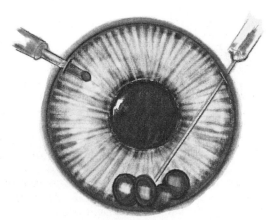

Fig. 6-99. *Aspiration of pupillary cysts. Incisions identical to those described for membranectomy are made and the infusion port is placed. A straight 25-gauge needle is used to aspirate the cystic epithelium.*

Evisceration with Implantation of Intrascleral Prosthesis

by E. DAN WOLF

The predominant goal in veterinary ophthalmology is to maintain a visual, nonpainful, and cosmetically acceptable eye. When vision is irreparably lost, persistent pain and gross buphthalmia, as in advanced glaucoma, may necessitate surgical alleviation. Enucleation may be the choice of the veterinary surgeon, but many owners find this procedure objectionable. With practice and proper instrumentation, the veterinary surgeon can offer intrascleral prosthesis implantation as an alternative to enucleation in the majority of patients with painful or buphthalmic eyes.

Prosthesis implantation involves the removal of the intraocular contents leaving only the fibrous coat (sclera and cornea) as an outer shell. The internal ocular tissues, aqueous humor, and vitreous are replaced by a silicone sphere implant. The corneoscleral shell eventually conforms to the implant. Therefore, the procedure can be used to attain a globe of nearly normal size in cases of extreme buphthalmia or to maintain the globe's size in cases of impending phthisis bulbi. When clinical conditions permit, the pleasing cosmetic appearance of patients postoperatively makes this procedure preferable to enucleation.

Indications

The sequelae of glaucoma are the most common indications for intrascleral prosthesis. Increased intraocular pressure in an irrevocably blind eye, resulting in pain and not responding to appropriate medical therapy, is a frequent indication for intrascleral prosthesis. This procedure relieves the pain by removing intraocular fluids and their source. Chronic glaucoma with marked buphthalmia can lead to chronic corneal exposure, keratitis, and degenerative pannus. Regardless of the current intraocular pressure or the presence of pain, a normal-sized, comfortable globe can be attained by inserting an intrascleral prosthesis.

Severe trauma to the globe, whether blunt or penetrating, can cause intraocular hemorrhage and severe damage to the ciliary body resulting in hypotony and eventual phthisis bulbi. If the condition is diagnosed before the fibrous tunic begins to contract, evisceration with implantation of a snugly fitting, intrascleral prosthesis can also maintain a normal-sized globe. This procedure prevents the complications and cosmetic disfigurement associated with a shrunken globe.

Contraindications

Although this procedure is often the treatment of choice in patients with severe intraocular problems, certain contraindications exist. An eye with any possibility of vision should not be considered for either enucleation or evisceration. An eye should not be eviscerated if there is orbital inflammation or involvement of the sclera such that healing might be impaired or the underlying condition not corrected. Intraocular infection (endophthalmitis) and intraocular neoplasia are additional but uncommon contraindications. Intraocular hemorrhage and panuveitis (without infection) are not treated with intrascleral prosthesis unless it can be determined that vision is definitely lost and that the condition is nonresponsive to aggressive medical therapy. Active corneal ulceration or corneal weakness is substantial justification for postponing this operation. The cornea may also be protected postoperatively by a nictitating membrane flap, a conjunctival flap, or tarsorrhaphy.

Surgical Technique

The technique described here is modified from the method described by Brightman and associates.[1] Presurgical preparations should be performed with the same fastidious attention to the details of aseptic technique dictated by other intraocular surgical procedures. In rare cases, an extensive laceration through the outer fibrous tunic may provide a direct entry site for removal of intraocular contents and insertion of the prosthetic sphere. Usually, however, an incision is made through the conjunctiva concentric with and 4 to 6 mm posterior to the limbus. The bulbar conjunctiva and fascia are freed from underlying sclera and are reflected from the incision site. A partial, penetrating

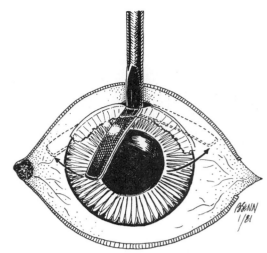

Fig. 6-100. *Separation of the uvea and sclera beginning at the midpoint of the scleral incision.*

scleral incision is performed with a No. 64 Beaver blade or a No. 15 Bard-Parker blade; this incision is extended to a length 1½ to 1¾ times the diameter of the implant. With few exceptions, a sphere that is 18 to 20 mm in diameter results in a globe that is nearly normal in size for most average dogs and cats. Black spheres are uniformly satisfactory in postoperative appearance. Other sizes and colors are also available from the manufacturer.*

Centrally, the scleral incision is gradually deepened until the ciliary body is exposed in the central 3 to 4 mm of the incision. If care is taken not to lacerate the choroid, hemorrhage is minimal and removal of the uvea in its entirety is facilitated. Following exposure of the choroid centrally, a cyclodialysis spatula is inserted between the uvea and the sclera to separate these structures bluntly. This separation is extended as far as possible in all directions. The choroid is loosely attached to the sclera, usually separating easily. The anterior attachment of ciliary body, trabecular meshwork, and base of the iris to the sclera is firmer; separations in this area result in the loss of aqueous humor (Fig. 6-100).

When the choroid has been separated from the sclera, the scleral incision is completed with small blunt dissection scissors (Steven's tenotomy scissors are applicable). The blunt tip of the scissors should be advanced in close apposition to the inner scleral surface to maintain the scleral and uveal separation.

When the scleral incision is complete, the uveal body can be further separated, often with retina, vitreous, and lens contained within the uveal tunic. A curved lens extraction loop facilitates this separation (Fig. 6-101). Applying gentle traction while alternately advancing two hemostats allows the gradual separation of uvea from sclera. Direct contact with the cornea is avoided during the dissection (Fig. 6-102).

With the uvea completely freed, the only point of attachment of intraocular contents to the sclera is at

*Jardon Plastics Research Corp., Southfield, MI 48076

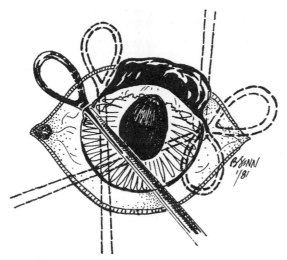

Fig. 6-101. *Insertion of a curved lens loop completes the separation between uvea and sclera.*

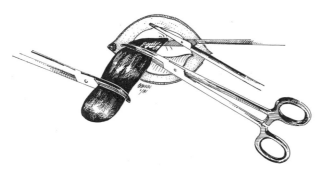

Fig. 6-102. *Hemostats alternately advanced to extract the uvea, retina, and lens in toto. The uveal and retinal attachment posteriorly at the optic nerve is severed leaving an intact but empty corneoscleral shell.*

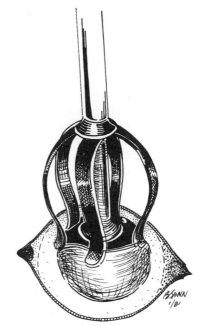

Fig. 6-103. *Silicone sphere implant is placed in the basket portion of the sphere introducer and is "plunged" into the scleral shell.*

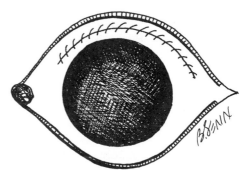

Fig. 6-104. *A simple, continuous conjunctival closure covers the scleral incision to minimize suture irritation.*

the optic nerve head; continued traction usually disrupts this attachment cleanly. To avoid leaving residual choroid in the globe, however, this attachment can be severed with curved scissors. Intraocular hemorrhage usually arises from the anterior and posterior ciliary arteries and varies considerably, depending on preexisting ocular conditions, but extensive attempts at hemostasis are generally unnecessary.

The chosen silicone sphere implant is inserted into the scleral shell. This implantation can be accomplished by grasping either side of the scleral incision with fine forceps, removing any significant amount of blood that has pooled in the globe, and gently manipulating the implant into the scleral shell. The sphere slides into position more easily if the surface is premoistened. This insertion is facilitated by using a sphere introducer,* essentially an expandable basket and plunger, to "inject" the implant into the scleral shell (Fig. 6-103).

The scleral incision is apposed with simple interrupted, through-and-through 5-0 to 6-0 synthetic absorbable sutures. Before placing the final suture, ex-

cessive blood should be irrigated from the scleral shell. An antibiotic, such as 2 to 3 mg gentamycin† diluted to 5 mg/ml, is injected to bathe the inner surface of the scleral shell. With the loss of the natural "flushing" effect of aqueous drainage, the presence of blood provides an excellent medium for bacterial growth. Therefore, meticulous surgical technique and antibiotic infusion help to minimize intraocular infection. The conjunctival incision is apposed with a simple continuous pattern (Fig. 6-104). If lateral canthotomy is necessary, this incision is also closed in a routine fashion.

Postoperative Management

The postoperative appearance, the extent of swelling, and the degree of pain are variable and depend on the preoperative condition of the globe, operative trauma, and autotrauma by the patient during the postoperative period. Mild swelling of the eyelids and

*Storz Instruments, St. Louis, MO

†Gentocin Injectable, Schering Corp., Kenilworth, NJ 07033

periorbita usually lasts 2 to 4 days and benefits from treatment with warm compresses. Discomfort manifested when the orbital area is handled excessively or when pressure is applied subsides within 1 to 2 days postoperatively. The use of analgesics may be indicated if severe pain initiates autotrauma.

The moderate to severe corneal edema that often follows sphere implantation is usually associated with a combination of surgical trauma to the endothelium and, more significantly, to a loss of the major source of nutrients to the cornea, the aqueous humor. The corneal edema may be extensive centrally, resulting in central corneal erosion and ulceration. Peripheral corneal neovascularization commonly occurs and may involve the entire cornea. Once the postoperative inflammation resolves, the cornea usually clears, with a few small blood vessels remaining at midstromal depth. These vessels are seldom noticeable to the patient's owner, unless associated with considerable fibrovascular scarring. In some patients, protection of the cornea is necessary during the first 10 to 14 days postoperatively using either a nictitating membrane flap or tarsorrhaphy. This protective procedure can be performed at the time of the operation or may be postponed a few days until the swelling and pain subside and the specific need is ascertained.

Topical antibiotics are instilled 4 to 6 times daily. Corticosteroids can be used topically to reduce swelling, but should be used judiciously if the condition of the cornea is compromised. Systemic antibiotics and corticosteroids are administered at the discretion of the veterinary surgeon. Warm compresses assist in alleviating orbital swelling and in cleansing the eyelid margins. Analgesics may be indicated if pain is severe during the first few postoperative hours. An Elizabethan collar or other restraining device is occasionally necessary to prevent autotrauma to the eye. Sutures in the lateral canthotomy are removed in 10 to 14 days. Within 2 weeks after the operation, the patient is usually comfortable, and topical medication is discontinued.

Complications

Application of meticulous surgical technique, careful attention to tissue handling and closure, and adequate postoperative treatment result in few complications with a high level of comfort for the patient and satisfaction for the owner. Complications usually result from exogenous or hematogenous localization of infection within the scleral shell around the implant and are minimized by aseptic technique and antibiotic infusion during the operation. Inflammation within and around the globe can result from residual uveal tissue left in the globe or from a reaction to foreign material such as glove powder. Additionally, the sphere may contain residual material from the sterilization process. Silicone spheres should be steam-autoclaved to avoid chemical or gas residues, then rinsed well with sterile saline solution prior to implantation.

Other complications such as disruption of the suture line can result from inadequate closure or from inadequate restraint of the patient and autotrauma. The result can be inflammation and swelling of the globe and surrounding structures, damage to the central cornea, and possibly extrusion of the implant. If marked inflammation or discomfort occurs, enucleation may be necessary.[2] Delayed (several months after the surgical procedure) extrusion of the prosthesis may result from gradual breakdown of the scleral incision. This complication is not painful, nor is it associated with inflammation; it may occur more frequently in the brachiocephalic breeds of dogs.

In summary, the intrascleral silicone sphere implant can provide a cosmetically pleasing alternative to enucleation in many patients. Although the surgical procedure is not difficult, attention to tissue handling, proper instrumentation, and adequate postoperative management are necessary to ensure a high percentage of successful prosthesis implantations, comfortable patients, and satisfied clients.

References and Suggested Readings

1. Brightman, A. H., Magrane, W. G., Huff, R. W., and Helper, L. C.: Intraocular prosthesis in the dog. J. Am. Anim. Hosp., 13:481, 1977.
2. Koch, S. A.: Intraocular prosthesis in the dog and cat. In Transactions of the Eleventh Annual Scientific Program of the American College of Veterinary Ophthalmology. Chicago, November 2 to 3, 1980.

Enucleation of the Globe

by E. Dan Wolf

Enucleation involves the surgical removal of the entire globe of the eye, including its outer fibrous coat, thereby differentiating this procedure from evisceration. Although specific indications for enucleation exist, the veterinary surgeon is often faced with choosing between enucleation and evisceration with intrascleral prosthesis implantation. Experience with the two procedures, as well as factors involving both patient and client, enter into this decision, but I now perform few enucleations when conditions permit a choice. With this bias in mind, the indications and techniques for enucleation are discussed.

Indications

Ocular disease without involvement of other orbital contents and for which no alternate medical or less-radical surgical therapy exists should be the only case for which enucleation is the treatment of choice. The specific indications for enucleation include: (1) congenital microphthalmia or acquired phthisis in which no possibility of vision exists and which is causing the patient chronic problems such as keratitis, conjunctivitis, or entropion; (2) inflammatory conditions involving the sclera or cornea that are not responsive to medical therapy and because of which vision is lost; (3) intraocular infection that is not responsive to medical therapy, or that may serve as a source of future systemic dissemination, and in which vision is lost; (4) intraocular neoplasm of sufficient size or location that it is not amenable to local excision or other treatment; (5) ocular discomfort not ameliorable by other medical or surgical therapy; (6) trauma to the globe severe enough that internal contents are lost and the outer fibrous coat cannot be reconstructed; and (7) proptosis of the globe with severance of muscle attachments and vascular supply and optic nerve damage.

Notably absent from the list of indications is glaucoma. Certain types of glaucoma, such as secondary to intraocular neoplasm or panophthalmitis, may require enucleation. Evisceration with intrascleral prosthesis implantation should also be considered in a painful or grossly buphthalmic, glaucomatous eye with irrevocable vision loss.

Several surgical approaches for enucleation include the transconjunctival,[1,3] the transpalpebral with en bloc removal,[1-3] and the lateral.[2,3] Factors such as the species of animal, the depth of the orbit, the presence of conjunctival or intraocular infection, postoperative environment, and compliance of the owner in postoperative care may influence the choice of techniques. Regardless of the technique selected, the intent of the operation is to remove the entire globe intact while leaving as much extraocular tissue as possible in the orbit to minimize the cosmetic deformity. Secreting surfaces should also be removed including the lid margins, the conjunctiva (both bulbar and palpebral) and the gland of the nictitating membrane. No matter which surgical approach is taken, the periorbital facial skin and lids are clipped and prepared as for any aseptic procedure. The surface of the skin and the conjunctival cul-de-sacs should be cleansed thoroughly with surgical solution (dilute aqueous iodine).

Transconjunctival Method

This surgical approach involves separating conjunctiva and Tenon's capsule from the globe just behind the limbus by making a 360° conjunctival incision and extending the dissection posteriorly to free fascia and conjunctiva from sclera (Fig. 6-105). Blunt scissors (curved tenotomy, strabismus, or enucleation scissors) are helpful in separating fascia from sclera. As the tendinous insertions of the extraocular muscles and the ventral oblique muscle are exposed, they can be elevated with a muscle hook or one blade of the scissors and severed as near the scleral insertion as possible (Fig. 6-106). This technique minimizes tissue loss and hemorrhage from the vessels supplying the extraocular muscles. As the rectus and oblique muscles are severed, the globe is partially released and can be displaced slightly anterior. This movement tenses the retractor bulbi muscle and facilitates the individual severing of the insertions of this muscle to the sclera. Excessive manipulation (tension or torsion) of the extraocular muscles should be avoided because this initiates the oculocardiac reflex and leads to bradycardia.

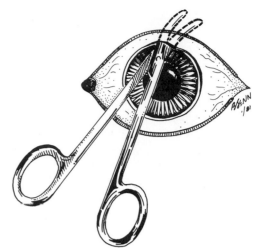

Fig. 6-105. *Initial incision in transconjunctival enucleation.*

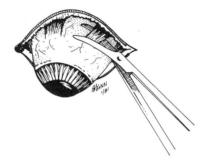

Fig. 6-106. *Dissecting posteriorly to separate sclera and overlying fascia (Tenon's capsule), one encounters the extraocular muscle insertions.*

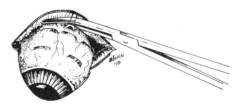

Fig. 6-107. *The optic nerve stump is grasped, ligated and severed to complete the enucleation. The conjunctiva, nictitating membrane, and lid margins are removed.*

Atropine, in the proper dose, administered preoperatively, mitigates this reflex.

Severing the extraocular muscles leaves the globe attached only by the optic nerve, nerve sheaths, and fascia. Contained within this bundle are the arteries to the globe, the posterior ciliary arteries; although the vessels are not large, ligation of this "optic nerve" stump is recommended. A curved hemostat may be slipped behind the globe and may be clamped over the optic nerve bundle (Fig. 6-107). With curved scissors, the globe may then be freed and removed by incision between the posterior globe wall and the hemostat. Care must be taken not to incise too closely to the globe because the posterior wall can be opened inadvertently and may thereby allow residual ocular tissue and vitreous into the orbit. A ligature is placed deep to the hemostat to control hemorrhage from the optic nerve stump.

The extraocular muscles and orbital fascia can be apposed to partially obliterate the tissue space in the orbit and to contain some of the expected vessel "seepage." Alternatively, a silicone sphere prosthesis* (18 to 20 mm) may be implanted into the orbit and the tissue drawn over it. Because the prosthesis is spherical with a smooth surface, several knifemarks or slices into its surface may enhance fibrous tissue infiltration and may lessen the chances of extrusion.

Following closure of the deeper layers of the orbit, the eyelid margins, nictitating membrane, and conjunctiva are removed. These secreting surfaces are removed to avoid the formation of intraorbital cysts, fistulas, and unhealing incision margins. Care should be taken in dissecting the medial canthus, which firmly attaches to the skull by the short medial canthal ligament. The eyelid margins and skin of the medial canthus must be completely excised, but the angular vein, located just medial to the ligament, should be avoided. The conjunctiva is dissected from the underlying tissue; a minimum of subconjunctival tissue should be removed.

As a concession to expediency, the nictitating membrane can be removed totally, rather than meticulously separating conjunctiva from both surfaces and then excising the gland of the nictitating membrane. The outer layer of the orbit is closed with 2-0 or 3-0 absorbable sutures; the anterior orbital rim is apposed with vertical sutures. Fascia of the orbit, ligamentous tissue of the rim of the orbit, and subcutaneous fascia are included in these sutures to provide a nearly complete anterior orbital wall. If it is not possible to construct this "wall" completely with tissue, a network of sutures can provide a matrix for fibroblastic tissue growth, to provide some protection against the "sinking in" that is a common sequela to enucleation (Fig. 6-108).

Closure of orbital and periorbital tissue following enucleation involves the apposition of intraorbital tissue, then closure of the anterior orbital fascia and periorbital tissue. Closure should therefore not be limited to a given number of sutures or prescribed layers; rather, the final goals of obliterating tissue space and providing a barrier to "sinking in" of the surface skin should dictate the extent of suturing. The skin is easily apposed and sutured in the manner preferred by the veterinary surgeon.

An alternate approach to the transconjunctival method of enucleation is the lateral approach. The lateral approach is useful in the dolichocephalic breeds of dogs and involves opening the lateral canthus prior to subconjunctival dissection and severing the extraocular muscles and optic nerve from the lateral aspect. This procedure is a modification of the transconjunctival method; the advantages and disadvantages of the transconjunctival approach also apply to the lateral approach.

*Jardon Plastics Research Corp., Southfield, MI 48076

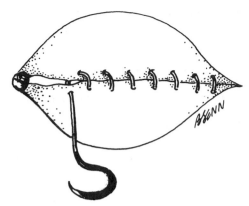

Fig. 6-108. *Multiple layered closure provides protective wall of tissue at the anterior orbit.*

Transpalpebral Method (En Bloc)

The technique I generally prefer is the en bloc or transpalpebral approach. In this method, the conjunctival cul-de-sacs are cleansed and rinsed with aqueous antiseptic solution. The lid margins are apposed with a continuous suture pattern. Closure of the lids minimizes the possibility that fluid from the conjunctival surfaces will enter the operative site. The surface skin is then thoroughly prepared for aseptic surgery. Figure 6-109 illustrates the line of incision for enucleation by this method.

Incisions are made parallel to the lid margins far enough from the margins to avoid the meibomian glands (4 to 6 mm). These incisions are extended medially and laterally until they intersect, thereby encircling the closed palpebral fissure (Fig. 6-110). Dissection is then continued deep in these incisions until the subconjunctiva is encountered. Forward traction on the

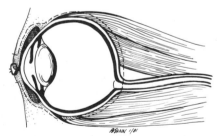

Fig. 6-109. *Schematic diagram of the incision line followed to enucleate by the transpalpebral or en bloc method. Dotted line indicates the level of dissection.*

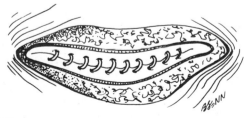

Fig. 6-110. *Initial incision of the en bloc enucleation consists of two cutaneous incisions parallel to the eyelid margins which connect just beyond the canthi.*

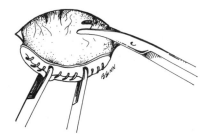

Fig. 6-111. *Dissection to, but not through, the conjunctiva and then posterior between sclera and Tenon's capsule exposes extraocular muscle insertions.*

eyelids facilitates this dissection. The conjunctiva is identified as freely movable and translucent; the corneoscleral limbus is often visible through the conjunctiva. Once bulbar conjunctiva has been identified, dissection is continued posteriorly just outside the conjunctiva until the sclera is encountered. With forward traction applied to the lid margins, the conjunctiva, now free from the sclera, is attached at the limbus. Dissection is continued posteriorly along the globe to separate the sclera from overlying tissue, as in the transconjunctival method (Fig. 6-111). The technique for severing the extraocular muscles, for hemostasis, for ligation of the optic nerve stump, and for closure of the orbital tissue is also identical to the transconjunctival procedure. Excised tissue consists of the globe, lid margins, conjunctiva, and nictitating membrane as an en bloc specimen. The nonsterile conjunctival surface is enclosed by the preoperatively performed tarsorrhaphy. To ensure sequestration of the conjunctival contents from the surgical site, perforation of the thin conjunctiva must be avoided.

Advantages and Disadvantages of the Two Surgical Procedures

Each of the previous methods for enucleation has certain advantages. The advantages of the transpalpebral method are, in general, the disadvantages of the transconjunctival method, and vice versa. Ease of dissection through better visualization is the basic advantage of the transconjunctival method. Improved exposure of the globe for the posterior dissection and a more nearly sterile environment are advantages of the transpalpebral method. The transpalpebral method is preferable when conjunctival or intraocular infection may contaminate the orbit. The transpalpebral procedure is also recommended when an intraocular neoplasm involves the aqueous drainage apparatus or has penetrated the fibrous tunic (cornea or sclera), although a more complete exenteration of the orbit is probably the treatment of choice for the majority of such cases.

Postoperative Management

Orbital hemorrhage is a common postoperative occurrence and can result in swelling of the surgical site as well as serum discharge at the site of incision. Warm compresses help to reduce swelling, ease the patient's discomfort, and cleanse the incision site. Serosanguinous discharge from the nostril can occur for 1 to 2 days postoperatively as serum drains from the orbit into the nasolacrimal system. Administration of antibiotics and corticosteroids is left to the discretion of the veterinary surgeon, but is usually unnecessary.

Complications

Complications that may occur in the first few hours following the surgical procedure include hemorrhage within the orbit. Topical pressure bandaging and tranquilization are effective control for hemorrhage. Orbital infection and autotrauma to the incision may also occur and require appropriate antibiotic therapy and physical restraint devices, respectively. Prevention of these complications includes careful hemostasis during the operation, careful attention to aseptic technique, and restriction of the patient's ability to traumatize the surgical site.

Complications can occur weeks to months after the surgical procedure. These include an unhealing portion of the incision, usually caused by the incomplete removal of the medial canthal skin. A draining fistula from the incision site may result from residual secretory tissue (conjunctival goblet cells), which proliferates to produce a seromucoid discharge. Residual secretory tissue that has not fistulated to the outside, or accidental trauma to the zygomatic salivary gland at the time of the operation, may produce fluid-filled cysts in the orbit. Focal infection and reaction to buried suture material are other possible complications.

References and Suggested Readings

1. Keller, W. F.: Enucleation of the eyeball. *In* Current Techniques in Small Animal Surgery. Edited by M. J. Bojrab. Philadelphia, Lea & Febiger, 1975.
2. Bellhorn, R.: Enucleation technic: a lateral approach. J. Am. Anim. Hosp. Assoc., *8*:59, 1972.
3. Bistner, S. I., Aguirre, A., and Batik, G.: Atlas of Veterinary Ophthalmic Surgery. Philadelphia, W. B. Saunders, 1977.

Exploratory Surgery of the Orbit

by E. DAN WOLF

Retrobulbar abscess, exploration for foreign bodies, repair of fractures of the orbital area, orbital cysts, and neoplasia may require surgery of the orbit. The "orbitotomy" procedure is therefore variable and influenced by the location and type of lesion. Approach through the posterior oral cavity to drain an orbital abscess is described elsewhere[1,2] and is not included. This section describes surgical approaches to areas inferior, superior, medial, and posterior to the globe.

Indications

The indications for orbitotomy are varied. Trauma may result in fractures to the zygomatic arch or the orbital extension of the frontal bone and sinus. Foreign bodies can lodge anywhere in the orbit and may require surgical removal. Orbitotomy may be necessary to gain access to the globe to repair a scleral laceration or a detached retina. Mass lesions, probably the most common indication for orbitotomy, include cysts of the zygomatic salivary gland or lacrimal gland, granulomas from foreign bodies, parasites, or localized infection (usually mycotic), and neoplasms.

The most common presenting clinical sign of an orbital mass is deviation of the globe position. The direction of deviation usually reflects the size and location of the mass. The origin of deviation of the globe and involvement of adjacent bony structures (zygomatic arch, bones of the medial orbit, temporal process of the mandible) can usually be determined by careful palpation of the orbit, examination of the oral cavity and ocular fundus, and proper radiographic studies (multiple views and contrast studies as required). Reduced airflow through the nasal cavity (evaluated by alternately obstructing the external nares and estimating airflow through the open nostril) is sometimes associated with an orbital mass extending into or arising from the nasal sinuses.

Involvement of the nasal cavity, frontal or maxillary sinus, and the orbit with a neoplasm is not an absolute contraindication to orbital exploration. The veterinary surgeon and the owner must be aware, however, of the possibility of an extensive surgical procedure to obliterate the abnormal tissue and the cosmetic defect thereby created. An estimation of prognosis for saving vision or for saving the globe can be more accurately determined by complete preoperative evaluation. Long-term prognosis for the patient can also be estimated preoperatively, but a more accurate prognosis depends upon the extent and invasiveness of the lesion, the pathologic process, and the thoroughness of the surgical procedure.

Contraindications

An accurate assessment of the prognosis of orbital lesions with and without an operation causes many clients to elect against surgical invasion. Few absolute contraindications to orbitotomy exist, assuming that the condition of the patient and the experience of the veterinary surgeon are adequate. As with any other treatment, orbitotomy is not indicated in conditions that do not benefit from surgical drainage or removal. Myositis of the temporal or pterygoid muscles, orbital pseudotumor, retrobulbar cellulitis, orbital lymphosarcoma, and orbital metastases are examples of conditions that usually do not benefit from orbitotomy. These conditions are often specifically diagnosed only after orbital exploration and a biopsy of affected tissue, however.

Surgical Technique

The surgical approach is determined by the suspected location of the orbital lesion. The extent of the incision is dictated by the size of the lesion and the exposure needed to effect removal. Each orbitotomy becomes an individual improvisation once the initial exposure is made.

The patient is usually placed in lateral recumbency, although an oblique head position may be useful in certain circumstances. A wide area around the orbit should be prepared for an aseptic surgical procedure. If possible the eyelids should be apposed with sutures prior to the procedure, unless a transconjunctival (anterior) approach is planned.

ANTERIOR APPROACH

The orbit may be approached anteriorly if the lesion is located anterior to the equator of the globe. In these cases, the lesion would likely be visible or palpable and only minimally deviate the globe. If exophthalmus is a prominent feature, the lesion, although it may be visible and palpable, probably extends posterior to the globe.

The orbit can be approached anteriorly through the conjunctiva or through the lid surface. The transconjunctival approach often eliminates or lessens the need for a skin incision. If necessary the incision can be extended through the lateral canthus posteriorly. This approach compromises sterile technique slightly as the conjunctival surface is open to the surgical site. Inferiorly, the incision can be made through the fornix between the globe and the nictitating membrane or between the nictitating membrane and the lower lid. The incision is extended as needed to gain adequate exposure of the lesion. Dissection is continued posteriorly at whatever plane is necessary to expose the lesion for biopsy or removal. Dissection close to the sclera frees Tenon's capsule and fascia from the globe and exposes the insertions of extraocular muscles to the sclera. More superficial dissection provides access to the anterior orbit outside the fascial layer.

Alternatively, the transcutaneous approach involves an incision parallel to the lid margin along either the superior or inferior orbital rim. Extending this incision posteriorly along the zygomatic arch provides access to the anterior and lateral orbit. Dissection to the depth desired, isolation and biopsy or removal of the lesion is the goal. The transcutaneous approach also facilitates a subperiosteal plane of dissection and permits separation of periosteum from the orbital bones until the lesion is located and excision or biopsy is performed through a small periosteal window. This technique avoids surgical trauma to vital structures because the contents of the orbit, as a whole, are displaced until the lesion is located. Closure of these anterior approaches simply requires reapposing fascial, periosteal, subcutaneous, conjunctival or skin layers. No serious consequences arise from severing the fibers of the levator

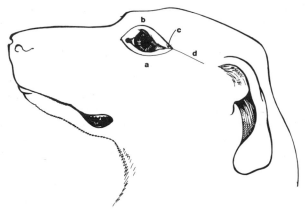

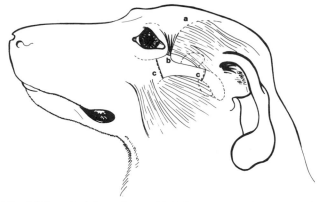

Fig. 6-112. *a, Incision along ventral orbital-rim-transcutaneous approach; b, Incision along dorsal orbital-rim-transcutaneous approach; c, Incision extended through lateral canthus—extension of dorsal or ventral transconjunctival approach; d, Incision extended along zygomatic arch for increased lateral exposure of any of the approaches.*

Fig. 6-113. *a, Incisions along orbital ligament to gain access to the orbit; b, Incision through orbital ligament combined with vertical portions of "a" to allow dorsal reflection of orbital ligament; c, Osteotomy incisions to allow reflection of zygomatic arch (do not sever orbital ligament at "b" if osteotomy is anticipated).*

muscle, and minimal hemorrhage results from an incision parallel to the lid margin. Skin incision locations for this approach are illustrated in Figure 6-112.

MEDIAL APPROACH

Lesions arising from the nasal cavity or sinuses can extend laterally to invade the orbit. The clinical appearance generally includes exophthalmus and lateral or upward deviation of the globe. Approach to the medial orbit is difficult. The medial wall of the orbit is bony, the medial canthus is firmly attached by the medial canthal ligament, and the angular vein is located just medial to the canthus. Dorsal anterior approach or an approach via the sinuses following removal of a portion of the outer bony plate usually provides better access to a mass in this area.

LATERAL APPROACH

In contrast to the medial aspect of the orbit, the lateral aspect is easily accessible. An incision is made along either the dorsal or ventral orbital rim and posteriorly along the dorsal rim of the zygomatic arch. Following reflection of the skin, entry into the orbit can be gained by several methods depending upon location and extent of the lesion. These are illustrated in Figure 6-113 and include the following:

A vertical incision along the anterior or posterior aspect of the orbital ligament extended anteriorly or posteriorly at the level of the zygomatic arch often provides access to a small lesion (Fig. 6-113, a); Severing and reflecting the orbital ligament opens the lateral orbit more extensively (Fig. 6-113, b); Maximum exposure of the orbit can be achieved by separating (by osteotomy) the zygomatic arch and by reflecting it dorsally at the attachment of the orbital ligament (Fig. 6-113, c). Periosteum of the zygomatic arch is reflected, and the bone is removed with rongeurs. Regeneration of the arch occurs inside the reapposed periosteum.

Alternatively, the arch may be removed with a bone saw, and then it may be returned to position after the operation and stabilized with wire. Removal of the zygomatic arch is also helpful in gaining access to the zygomatic salivary gland, but is generally not necessary. The extent of the incision should be determined by the size of the lesion.

Every attempt should be made to maintain the globe if not directly involved in the disease process, especially if the eye is visual. Incision or actual removal of a section of lateral orbital fascia provides access to the posterior muscle cone. Orbital fat can be retracted or removed to enhance visualization of structures. Forward traction or rotation of the globe, using preplaced sutures or fine forceps, may be helpful in exposing and in identifying retrobulbar structures.

In certain situations, a large surgical field may be necessary to expose areas of the retrobulbar orbit or optic nerve. The location of the coronoid process of the mandible should be noted. Occasionally, the presence of fractures, osteomyelitis, or neoplasia of this dorsal extension of the mandible requires a lateral orbitotomy. For increased exposure, the zygomatic arch may be transected at the anterior and posterior aspects and reflected by its orbital ligament attachment dorsally. If necessary, the temporal muscle overlying the orbit may be reflected posteriorly from its attachment to the parietal bone. This extensive orbitotomy, illustrated in Figure 6-114, has been reported in the dog.[3]

On occasion, it may be desirable to increase access to the orbit without removing the zygomatic arch. An incision along the ventral margin of the zygomatic arch and reflection of the masseter muscle ventrally increases exposure of the lateral and ventral orbit.

Closure of the orbital fascia, repair of the zygomatic arch, reapposition of the orbital ligament, apposition of muscle sheaths, and closure of the subcutaneous tissue and skin complete the procedure. It may be advisable to insert a rubber drain into the orbit during the closure. Drainage can be accomplished laterally through the incision or, less desirably, into the oral cavity.

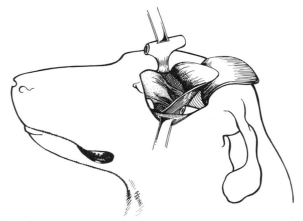

Fig. 6-114. *Reflected zygomatic arch exposing caudal orbit. Skin layer and temporal muscle are reflected dorsocaudally. (Modified from Slatter, D. H., and Abdelbaki, Y.: Lateral orbitotomy by zygomatic arch dissection in the dog. J. Am. Vet. Med. Assoc., 175:1179, 1979.)*

Postoperative Course and Complications

The degree of swelling, the duration of discomfort, and the likelihood of infection are partially related to the extent of the orbitotomy and the duration of the surgical procedure. Some difficulty with mastication, swelling of the facial area around the orbit, discharge from the incision, and discomfort are to be expected. Postoperative autotrauma may disrupt the incision, may damage the globe, and may delay healing of the zygomatic arch (if transected). Infection of the surgical site is best prevented by careful technique and postoperative administration of antibiotics. Other complications related to the surgical procedure itself include: corneal damage either from direct trauma during the operation or from exposure and drying of the corneal surface; ocular damage or reduced mobility of the globe from direct surgical trauma, indirect trauma, or swelling of periocular tissues following the operation; damage to the optic nerve directly by trauma or traction or indirect damage from a compromised blood supply; the development of retrobulbar fat necrosis; damage to the lacrimal gland or zygomatic salivary gland causing cyst formation; damage to the palpebral branch of the facial nerve resulting in lagophthalmus (usually temporary) with subsequent corneal exposure, and postoperative orbital emphysema if the thin bones of the sinuses are disrupted.

The most significant complication of orbitotomy is recurrence of the original problem, especially in cases in which neoplasia was not totally removed. Although the globe and other orbital structures should not be sacrificed unless necessary, it is more critical to remove abnormal tissue completely, especially if neoplastic. Similarly, in cases of multifocal foreign bodies, diffuse granuloma, and localized mycotic granuloma, as much offending material as possible is excised.

Postoperative treatment is not essential with orbitotomy, but the need for antibiotics, corticosteroids to reduce swelling, analgesics, tranquilizers, mechanical restraint devices, warm compresses, and topical ocular medications is based upon the extent and the duration of the surgical procedure. All tissue removed at orbitotomy should be evaluated histopathologically, especially if neoplasia is suspected.

In summary, orbitotomy is usually an individualized procedure in which the basic approach is determined by the best preoperative clinical assessment of the size, the location, and the extent of the lesion. Although the technique may vary, the basic principles of orbitotomy include: (1) maintenance of meticulous sterility; (2) adequate exposure; (3) careful handling of tissue and avoidance of unnecessary manipulation, especially of the globe and optic nerve; (4) removal of all abnormal tissue; (5) removal of the globe only if absolutely necessary; and (6) attempt at a complete assessment of the problem prior to the surgical procedure, to allow realistic prognosis and expectations on the part of the owner and the veterinary surgeon.

References and Suggested Readings

1. Magrane, W. G.: Canine Ophthalmology. 3rd Ed. Philadelphia, Lea & Febiger, 1977.
2. Bistner, S. I., Aguirre, A., and Batik, G.: Atlas of Veterinary Ophthalmic Surgery. Philadelphia, W. B. Saunders, 1977.
3. Slatter, D. H., and Abdelbaki, Y.: Lateral orbitotomy by zygomatic arch dissection in the dog. J. Am. Vet. Med. Assoc., 175:1179, 1979.

7 * Ear

Pinna

Cosmetic Ear Trimming

by KENNETH W. SMITH

Cosmetic ear trimming is done to give a dog the characteristic appearance of its breed. The length and style of the trim varies in different parts of the country and in various countries of the world. The cropped ear should conform to the prevailing height and style for the breed and should complement the size and shape of the head of the dog. Individual preference is also a consideration. The principal requirements are knowledge of the surgical technique, experience, artistic ability, and meticulous attention to detail. The veterinarian with experience can become proficient in trimming the ears of average pets; however, the owners of show dogs are often demanding.

Some veterinarians are opposed to this type of surgical procedure because they feel it is unnecessary and inhumane. If they refuse to do it, however, others who are less qualified will do it much less humanely. Cosmetic ear trimming is prohibited in the Commonwealth of Massachussetts and in some foreign countries.

Selection of Patients

The best age for trimming ears in large breeds of dogs is 8 to 10 weeks. For small breeds, it is about 12 weeks. Disadvantages in older dogs include more hemorrhage, greater difficulty in keeping braces in place, more self-trauma, greater difficulty in maintaining proper position of the ears, and adverse psychologic effects.

The first step in ear trimming is proper communication with the owner, who should understand the type of procedure he is requesting, the necessary aftercare, and the possible problems in obtaining proper carriage of the ears. When the puppy is brought to the veterinarian, it should receive a routine physical examination and a careful evaluation of the ears to determine whether they are likely to stand. Ears that are low set, abnormally large, excessively thick, or with abnormal

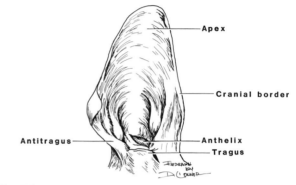

Fig. 7-1. *Anatomy of the ear.*

bending of the cartilage may fail to stand. These problems should be brought to the attention of the owner at the time of the initial examination.

Figure 7-1 illustrates the anatomy of the canine ear.

Surgical Technique

Following administration of a preanesthetic tranquilizer, the puppy is anesthetized with intravenous thiopental and placed on methoxyflurane or halothane inhalation anesthesia. The tranquilizer sedates the puppy during recovery from anesthesia and thereby eliminates head shaking, which may cause postoperative hemorrhage. The ears and top of the head are clipped and are prepared for an aseptic surgical procedure. With the dog in sternal recumbency, the ears and top of the head are draped, and the ears are marked at the proper length (Table 7-1). Several different methods exist for determining proper ear length, but the one that gives the most consistent results in the various breeds is measuring with a ruler. The end of the ruler rests gently on the head just medial to the base of the ear, and the measurement is made at the cranial border of the ear while it is held in normal standing position without traction (Fig. 7-2). The ear is marked at the proper length with indelible pencil. The skin must be slightly moist to mark with indelible pencil. Each ear is

Table 7-1. *Canine Ear Trimming*

Breed	Age	Length of Trim (inches)
Boxer	9 weeks	2½ to 2¾
Great Dane	9 weeks	3½ to 3¾
Doberman pinscher	9 weeks	2¾
Standard schnauzer	9 weeks	2¼ to 2½
Miniature schnauzer	12 weeks	2 to 2¼
Miniature pinscher	12 weeks	1¾
Boston terrier	6 months	as long as possible

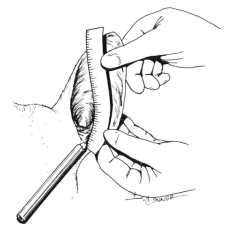

Fig. 7-4. *An assistant marks the ear while the veterinary surgeon holds the flexible ruler in the proper position.*

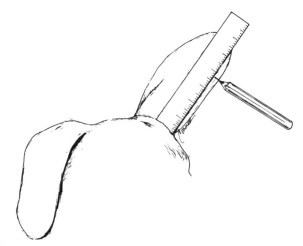

Fig. 7-2. *Measuring the ear with a 6-inch plastic ruler, and marking it at the proper length with an indelible pencil.*

measured separately, and the lengths are compared for equality by placing the tips in apposition (Fig. 7-3). If the lengths do not match, the procedure is repeated because the two ears may be congenitally unequal in size or the cartilage of one ear may be bent so that it measures short.

The length and style of the trim varies with the breed, the dog's size, and the shape of the head. The wishes of the owner are also considered, provided ex-

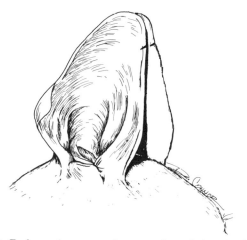

Fig. 7-3. *Each ear is measured separately and then is placed in apposition to compare the lengths.*

tremes in length are avoided. The length must be increased in older puppies to compensate for the increase in size (see Table 7-1).

When each ear has been measured and marked at the proper length, the pattern for the trim is marked on the inner skin surface with an indelible pencil (Fig. 7-4). This marking is done with the aid of a lightweight flexible plastic ruler bent concavely to conform to the inner surface of the ear. The medial edge of the ruler forms the approximate line for the incision between the mark at the tip and the notch formed by the tragus and antitragus at the base. The bent ruler is held firmly in position facing forward while an assistant marks the ear along the medial edge of the ruler. From this base line, deviations are made for different breeds and styles of trims. When the base lines have been placed in both ears, they are again compared for height and width.

With heavy, sharp scissors (some prefer serrated), each ear is cut while an assistant stabilizes the ear by holding the portion to be removed at the tip and near the base (Fig. 7-5). The veterinary surgeon holds the ear medial to the incision in order to prevent the loose skin on the back of the ear from pushing ahead of the scissors. In order to make forehanded incisions, a right-handed person incises the left ear from the base toward the tip, and the right ear from the tip toward the base. Otherwise, the left ear must be trimmed backhanded, which is not only awkward, but also causes discrepancies in the appearance of the two ears.

The shape of the ear trim varies according to breed. The ears of schnauzers are trimmed by following closely the line marked on the ear. Those of Great Danes are shaped by following the base line in the lower quarter of the ear and then by deviating medially from the line to give a concave shape to the upper two-thirds of the cut (Fig. 7-5). This procedure gives a graceful appearance to the ear and, in addition, improves its ability to stand by reducing the weight toward the tip. If the tip is too long and slender, however, it may curl medially. Boxers and Doberman pinschers are given the same general shape as the Great Dane,

skin from inside the ear above the anthelix. The incisions are made vertically, and the size of the section removed is about ¼- to ⅜-inch wide by 1- to 1 ½-inches long, tapering at both ends. The wound is closed with simple interrupted 4-0 nonabsorbable skin sutures, which should be placed close together for a strong suture line. As the incision is closed, tension on the inner skin of the ear should be sufficient to cause the ear to cone. A slim, tubular shape adds additional rigidity to the ear.

The ear is then immobilized in the normal standing position, with an inside soft roll splint held in place with adhesive tape around the ear. The ear bases are then anchored around the head and throat to further stabilize the ear. In 9 or 10 days, the support and the skin sutures are removed. The coned position is maintained by encircling tapes for another week. Additional support may be necessary until the ear muscles shorten and regain normal function. This same technique can be used higher up on the ear when only the tip is involved.

Ear Implants

Among the prosthetic aural implants, porous polyethylene* has been most widely used. The principal disadvantage to all prosthetic implants is the formation of sinus drainage tracts and scar tissue that can irreparably distort the shape of the ear. When such problems occur, removal of the implant can be difficult and time-consuming, with poor final cosmetic results. The other objection to implants is that even though the ears may stand, they are not always carried erect. The carriage is often more horizontal than vertical, especially in low-set ears. Ear implants are indicated to correct defects in the ear cartilage, as well as curled ears, in which a narrow implant is used.

The affected ear is clipped and is prepared for an aseptic surgical procedure. The anesthetized dog is placed in lateral recumbency and draped. A vertical incision is made through the inside skin of the ear directly above the anthelix and across the break in the

*Biopor canine ear implant, Porex Materials Corp., Fairburn, GA 30213

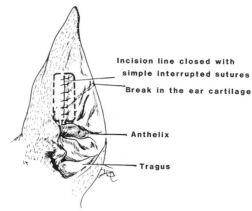

Fig. 7-13. *Surgical technique for ear implant. See text for details.*

Labels: Incision line closed with simple interrupted sutures; Break in the ear cartilage; Anthelix; Tragus

cartilage (Fig. 7-13). The skin along both margins is carefully dissected from the underlying cartilage; one must stay as close to the cartilage as possible in order to leave adequate blood supply to the skin. The objective is to make a pocket that is exactly the same size as the implant to be used. The size of the implant is usually about an inch long and half to five-eighths of an inch wide. When the implant has been inserted, the incision is closed with 4-0 nonabsorbable skin suture. An inside roll is then placed in the ear and is held there with tape around the ear to immobilize it during the healing period. This procedure has been described in my discussion of cocked ears. The skin sutures and support are removed in about 10 days, and the ear is taped in the coned position for another week.

References and Suggested Readings

Cawley, A. J., and Archibald, J.: *In* Canine Surgery. 2nd Ed. Edited by J. Archibald. Santa Barbara, CA, American Veterinary Publications, 1974.

Hancock, W. B.: Ear cropping technique. VM SAC, *63*:860, 1968.

Knecht, C. D.: Cosmetic otoplasty. *In* Current Techniques in Small Animal Surgery. Edited by M. J. Bojrab. Philadelphia, Lea & Febiger, 1975.

Vine, L. L.: Corrective ear surgery. VM SAC, *69*:1014, 1974.

Williams, E. A.: Ear trimming techniques. VM SAC, *56*:208, 1961.

External Ear

Lateral Ear Canal Resection

by Mark J. Dallman *and* M. Joseph Bojrab

Otitis externa is an inflammation of the epithelium of the external ear canal characterized by an increased production of ceruminous and sebaceous material, desquamation of epithelium, pruritis, and pain. Otitis externa is caused by one or more etiologic agents including parasites, bacteria, and fungi. In addition, allergy and trauma may play a role in otitis externa.

The conformation of the ear canal and that of the pinna are factors in the cause of otitis externa and in the development of chronic otitis externa. The incidence of the disease per breed of dog indicates that the pendulous pinna of spaniels and hounds and the pendulous pinna and hair-filled external ear canal of poodles are predisposing factors in otitis externa. A high relative humidity has been found in the external ear canal. This factor, in addition to the warmth, darkness, and enclosed nature of the ear canal of some breeds of dogs, provides an excellent environment for the growth of infective agents. Chronic otitis externa may permanently change the size and character of the external ear canal. The epithelium becomes thickened and fibrous and may become ulcerated. The ear canal may become stenotic if the epithelium becomes excessively scarred or undergoes metaplastic proliferation.

A complete otoscopic examination of each ear, including visualization of the tympanum, is imperative for proper diagnosis and assessment of the lesion. Otitis externa may be treated medically or surgically. The initial treatment of this disease consists of irrigation and cleaning of the external ear canal. Additional treatment consists of the use of ceruminolytic agents and, depending on the origin of the otitis, antibiotics (aqueous solutions) locally or parenterally, antifungal agents or parasiticides locally, and pH alteration. Binding the ears over the top of the head allows better ventilation of the ear canal. Culture and sensitivity tests, in cases of severe or repeated occurrences of otitis externa, may preclude the need for a future ear canal operation by identifying a bacterial etiologic agent and the antibiotic that should effectively eliminate that agent. Chronic otitis externa must be treated more vigorously. "Swimmers solution" (three parts isopropyl alcohol and one part white vinegar) is useful for instillation for long-term treatment that provides a cleaning-drying action and lowers the pH of the ear canal.

When otitis externa becomes unresponsive to medical therapy, a lateral ear canal operation is indicated. Other indications for lateral ear canal resection are frequent recurrence of otitis externa, chronic otitis externa due to inadequate treatment or lack of treatment, and external ear canal thickening that does not concurrently obstruct the horizontal portion of the external ear canal. The purpose of lateral ear canal resection is to provide environmental alteration by means of ventilation so that moisture, humidity, and temperature are decreased. Lateral ear canal resection also provides drainage for exudates and moisture in the ear canal.

Surgical Technique

The patient is placed in lateral recumbency, and the animal is draped so that the pinna and external ear canal region are left exposed. The veterinary surgeon is initially positioned ventral to the patient. A probe is inserted into the vertical ear canal to determine its depth. Two skin incisions are extended ventrally, parallel to each other, from the intertragic notch and tragohelicine notch. These vertical incisions are 1½ times the length of the vertical ear canal. A transverse incision joins the vertical incisions ventrally (Fig. 7-14). The skin is reflected to its dorsal attachment on the dorsal rim of the vertical ear canal. An incision is made through the subcutaneous tissue on the lateral surface of the cartilagenous vertical canal. Using scissors, the subcutaneous tissue is reflected rostrally and caudally off of the vertical ear canal (Fig. 7-15). In similar fashion, the parotid salivary gland is reflected ventrally.

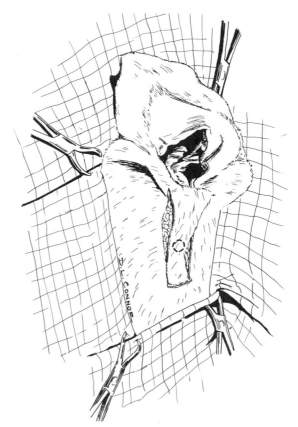

Fig. 7-14. *The three skin incisions used to expose the vertical portion of the external ear canal.*

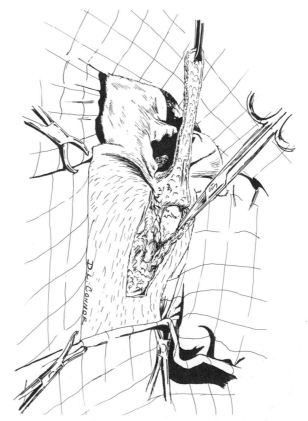

Fig. 7-15. *The reflecting of the subcutaneous tissue from the ear canal.*

The lateral aspect of the vertical ear canal should be exposed at this point.

The next portion of the surgical procedure is best performed from the dorsal aspect of the head. With scissors, two incisions are made in the cartilagenous vertical canal, one along the rostrolateral aspect of the canal and one along its caudolateral aspect. To allow the incisions to be made properly, the pinna and the skin flap are pulled dorsally, and the vertical portion of the ear canal is visualized. One blade of the scissors is placed into the vertical canal, which is then incised from the tragohelicine notch ventrally approximately half the length of the vertical ear canal. The scissor blades are angled approximately 30° rostrally, and the tip of one blade is kept pressed against the rostral wall of the vertical ear canal.

Similarly, while the pinna and skin flap are pulled dorsally, one blade of the scissors is placed into the vertical ear canal, which is then incised ventrally from the intertragic notch (Fig. 7-16). The scissor blades are inclined approximately 30° caudally, and the tip of one blade is pressed against the caudal wall of the vertical ear canal. Both the rostral and caudal incisions should be alternately extended until the floor of the horizontal ear canal limits further advancement of the scissors. The lateral wall of the vertical ear canal is now reflected ventrally. If the incisions have been made properly, the lateral wall will have a base of attachment equal to the width of the floor of the horizontal ear

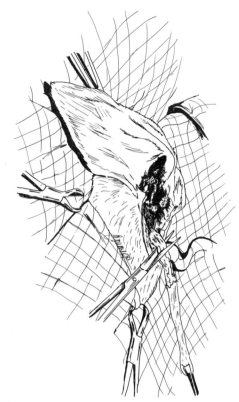

Fig. 7-17. *The "drain board" flap is created from the vertical portion of the external ear canal.*

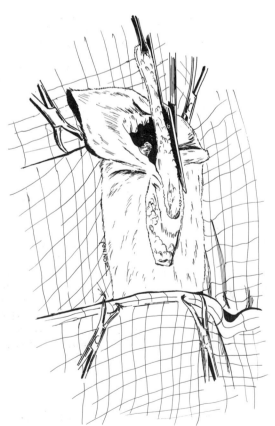

Fig. 7-16. *The caudal incision in the cartilage of the vertical portion of the ear canal.*

canal. Next, the skin flap and all but the proximal 2 cm of the lateral wall are removed (Fig. 7-17). This section will be used as the "drain board" flap.

The lateral flap is pulled ventrally. Nonabsorbable, preferably swaged-on suture material is used to suture the lateral ear canal flap and remaining vertical ear canal to the adjacent skin in a simple interrupted pattern (Fig. 7-18). A suture is placed through the rostroventral edge of the epithelium and cartilage of the "drain board." The suture is angled rostroventrally and is sutured to the skin. Similarly, a suture is placed through the caudoventral edge of the flap and is sutured caudoventrally to the skin. The skin is adjusted prior to the placement of this suture, so that no redundant skin persists between these two sutures. The next two sutures should anchor the skin to the rostral and caudal walls of the opening of the horizontal ear canal. Additional interrupted sutures are placed to join the lateral ear canal flap to the skin and the edges of the vertical ear canal to the skin in cosmetic fashion (Fig. 7-19).

The ear is placed approximately in its normal position, and the ear canal is checked for possible obstruction to drainage and ventilation by the anthelicine tubercle or proliferative ridges of tissue. If these tissues cause obstruction, they should be excised, and the resultant wound should be allowed to heal by second intention. When the incisions have been closed, the pinna needs to be anchored over the head of the dog to provide ventilation and to prevent damage from head

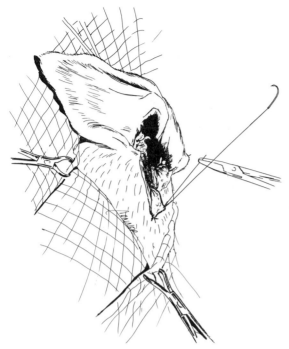

Fig. 7-18. *The first two sutures are placed to anchor the "drain board" flap.*

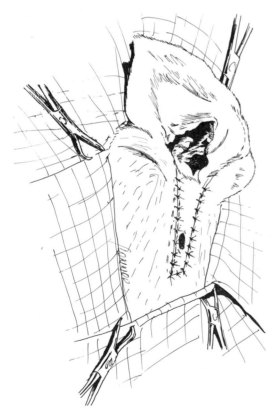

Fig. 7-19. *The finished lateral ear canal resection.*

shaking. A porous bandage may be placed over the surgical site to protect it from scratching. Paw pads may be fashioned or the patient's legs may be hobbled as additional measures to protect the ear from scratching (see Chap. 3).

Postoperative considerations include treatment with appropriate systemic antibiotics, management of self-trauma and ear movement, and coping with prolonged healing time. Healing time averages 10 to 14 days, and if the suture line breaks down, healing may take longer. If the lateral ear resection fails to control the problem of otitis externa, ear canal ablation needs to be considered.

References and Suggested Readings

Coffey, D. J.: Observations on the surgical treatment of otitis externa in the dog. J. Small Anim. Pract., *11*:265, 1970.

Fraser, G.: Factors predisposing to canine internal otitis. Vet. Rec., *73*:55, 1961.

Fraser, G.; Withers, A. R., and Spruell, J. S. A.: Otitis externa in the dog. J. Small Anim. Pract., *2*:32, 1961.

Fraser, G., et al.: Canine ear disease. J. Small Anim. Pract., *10*:725, 1970.

Grono, L. R.: Otitis externa. *In* Current Veterinary Therapy VII. Edited by R. W. Kirk. Philadelphia, W. B. Saunders, 1980.

Grono, L. R.: Studies of the microclimate of the external auditory canal in the dog. I, II, III. Res. Vet. Sci., *11*:307, 1970.

Ott, R. L.: Ears. *In* Canine Surgery. 2nd Ed. Edited by J. Archibald. Santa Barbara, CA, American Veterinary Publications, 1974.

Singleton, W. B.: Aural resection in the dog. *In* Advances in Small Animal Practice. Vol. II. Edited by B. V. Jones. Oxford, Pergamon Press.

Zepp, C. P.: Surgical correction of diseases of the ear in the dog and cat. Vet. Rec., *61*:643, 1949.

Ear Canal Ablation

by Mark J. Dallman *and* M. Joseph Bojrab

Chronic otitis externa may cause extreme connective tissue proliferation and bony metaplasia of cartilage in response to long-standing inflammation. Lateral ear resection is not indicated in many of these cases because the lumen of the horizontal portion of the external ear canal may be obliterated. Conventional excision or electrosurgical removal of the proliferative tissue can remove the obstruction, but it does not relieve the conditions leading to extensive proliferation of tissue. Cryosurgery may be effectively used to remove this proliferative material and to avoid the postoperative complications of ear canal ablation. The granulomatous tissue in the ear canal either may be reduced or may be totally removed. If cryosurgery or other methods prove ineffective, the last resort is ear canal ablation. Ear canal ablation is indicated when severe granulomatous or metaplastic changes obliterate the ear canal. This procedure is also indicated when lateral ear canal resection fails to relieve chronic otitis. Other indications for ear canal ablation are neoplasia of and severe trauma to the ear canal.

Surgical Technique

A transverse incision extending from the tragohelicine notch to the intertragic notch is made through the skin along the dorsal rim of the vertical

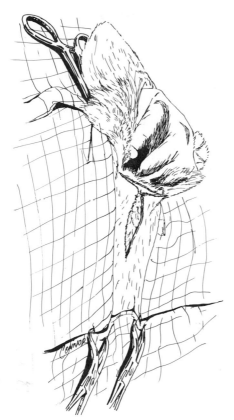

Fig. 7-20. *The skin incisions used to approach the cartilaginous ear canal.*

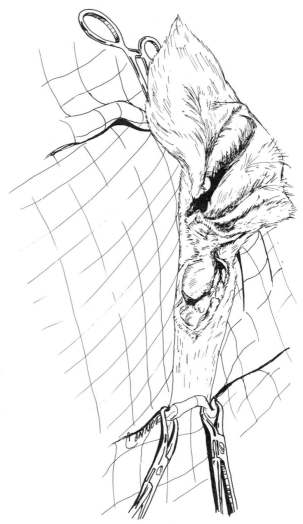

Fig. 7-21. *The connective tissue and parotid gland are reflected from the vertical portion of the ear canal.*

portion of the ear canal (Fig. 7-20). A second incision is made perpendicularly from the midpoint of the first incision to a point 1 cm ventral to the horizontal portion of the external ear canal. The connective tissue along the ear canal is incised and is reflected rostrally and caudally until the ear canal is free of subcutaneous tissue (Fig. 7-21). The parotid gland is reflected ventrally, and the horizontal ear canal is exposed. The attachment of the ear canal to the petrous temporal bones should be visible.

Blunt dissection is undertaken medial to the vertical ear canal, so that the vertical canal is freed of the surrounding tissues. A transverse incision is made through the skin and the cartilage of the medial wall of the vertical portion of the ear canal. This incision connects with the previously made transverse incision between the tragohelicine and intertragic notches. The dorsal portion of the ear canal should now be totally free (Fig. 7-22). The entire cartilaginous ear canal is excised by making an incision between the petrous temporal bone, at the external auditory meatus, and the annular cartilage that forms the horizontal ear canal (Figs. 7-23 and 7-24). If the ear canal has undergone bony metaplastic changes, this procedure may be difficult to do. In making this incision, it is necessary to stay as close to the petrous portion of the skull as possible. It is also important to be aware that the facial nerve exits from the stylomastoid foramen just caudal to the external auditory meatus and curves rostrally, ventral to the horizontal part of the ear canal.

The reflected flaps of skin are now replaced. With a simple interrupted suture pattern and nonabsorbable suture, the skin flaps are sutured laterally to each other on the midline and dorsally to the skin lining the concave surface of the ear (Fig. 7-25). Failure to remove the entire horizontal ear canal leads to postoperative complications. The ear canal epithelium continues to produce its characteristic secretions, which collect in a subcutaneous pouch that may rupture to form a fistulous tract. Other postoperative complications associated with ear canal ablation include self-trauma and impaired hearing in the operated ear.

Postoperatively, the pinna is placed over the head and is anchored with tape to prevent damage to the incision from head shaking. Measures to prevent damage from self-trauma need to be taken. These may include protective covering, hobbling, or protective pads over the paws (see Chap. 3).

The inflammatory products of otitis media must drain to the pharynx by means of the auditory tube. If the exudative process is severe, the exudate may rupture through the tympanum. In the intact ear, the exu-

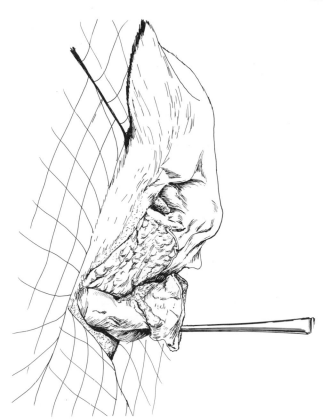

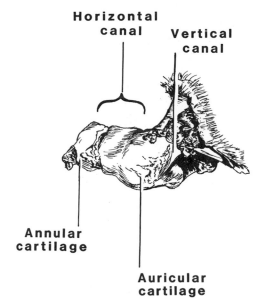

Fig. 7-24. *The excised cartilaginous ear canal.*

Fig. 7-22. *The ear canal has been excised dorsally and reflected ventrally.*

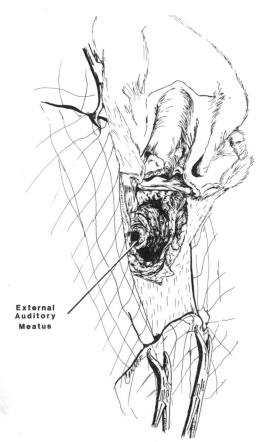

Fig. 7-23. *The complete excision of the cartilaginous ear canal.*

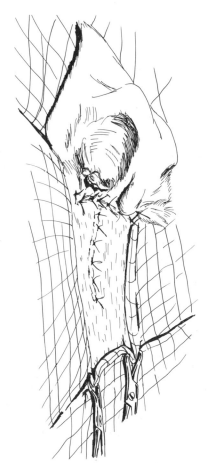

Fig. 7-25. *The appearance of the completed ear canal ablation after closure of the skin incision.*

date from otitis media may rupture through the tympanum and drain into the ear canal. After ear canal ablation, a similar rupture of the tympanum will cause a draining tract beginning in the region of the former external meatus.

References and Suggested Reading

Fraser, G., et al.: Canine ear disease. J. Small Anim. Pract., *10*:725, 1970.

Singh, G. B., and Rao, M. M.: Otitis externa in canines. Its medicinal and surgical treatment. Indian Vet. J., *36*:236, 1959.

Ablation of the External Ear Canal

by ANTHONY SCHWARTZ

Surgical ablation of the canine external ear canal was first described by Singh and Rao in 1959.[5] The procedure, which has changed little since then, involves complete excision of the vertical and horizontal portions of external ear canal and primary skin closure. Ablation is an infrequently indicated and radical procedure that generally has been reserved (1) as a salvage procedure when lateral resection or complete excision of the vertical canal has failed to correct severe chronic deep otitis externa, (2) to treat malignant tumors of the deep external ear canal, and (3) to treat severe proliferative otitis externa.

Presurgical Considerations

Most veterinarians agree that ablation of the external ear canal should not be performed in the presence of active otitis media because ablation prevents drainage from the middle ear to the outside. Owing to swelling or scarring, the eustachian tube often is functionally closed, and septic exudates thereby become trapped in the middle ear. Aggravation of otitis media can result, as can extension of the septic process either to the inner ear or by the external acoustic meatus to surrounding soft tissues, with consequent postoperative cellulitis or abscess. Therefore, it is essential that the clinician perform a thorough presurgical otoscopic examination. The existence of otitis media is indicated by finding the tympanic membrane ruptured or intact but bulging. Radiography is also a helpful tool for determining the presence of otitis media, especially when presurgical otoscopy is impossible because of obstruction of the ear canal. Radiographs may reveal the fluid density within the tympanic cavity or sclerotic changes of the osseous tympanic bulla. In certain instances, it is necessary to perform ablation of the ear canal even in the presence of otitis media. I describe a technique for ingress-egress drainage of the middle ear that has been successful in such situations.

Another presurgical concern is that ablation, especially if performed bilaterally, diminishes a patient's hearing. If a severe hearing deficit already exists prior to the surgical procedure, this objection would not obtain.

Surgical Anatomy

Several important structures must be identified and avoided during the surgical procedure. The parotid salivary gland is "V" shaped, with the apex of the "V" pointing ventrally. The two dorsal limbs of the gland are situated closely to the rostral and caudal aspects of the vertical part of the auricular cartilage (see Fig. 7-26 *B*). Major cranial nerves and blood vessels are found in the area. The deep part of the parotid salivary gland is related to the facial nerve and its branches. The facial nerve emerges from the facial canal of the petrous temporal bone, caudal to the external acoustic meatus, by means of the stylomastoid foramen (see Fig. 7-27, inset). The nerve then runs rostroventrally and, along with some of its branches, becomes associated with the ear canal. The main facial nerve trunk itself is intimately associated with the ventral aspect of the horizontal ear canal (see Fig. 7-26 *C* and *D*). The auriculopalpebral and dorsal buccal branches of the facial nerve are found near the auriculotemporal branch of the mandibular portion of the trigeminal nerve (sensory) on the rostral aspect of the auditory tube. Thus, several major nerves may be damaged by poor dissection technique. Owing to the ample collateral blood supply, severing a large arterial branch generally does not lead to avascularity.[1]

Surgical Technique

Prior to the operation, chronic infection should be brought under control by local cleansing in conjunction with local and systemic antibiotic therapy for several days. Following induction of anesthesia, the ear canal is flushed and is cleansed thoroughly, and the surgical area is prepared for an aseptic operation. The patient should be placed in a lateral recumbent position with its head supported on an elevating platform.

A scalpel is used to make a "T"-shaped incision over the external ear canal (Fig. 7-26 *A*). The vertical portion of the "T" is parallel to the vertical portion of the ear canal. The ventral end of the vertical canal can be located by using a probe (Fig. 7-26 *B*). The horizontal portion of the "T" is parallel to and just below the upper edge of the tragus cartilage. The horizontal incisions are extended medially around the rostral and caudal aspects of the external ear opening (Fig. 7-26 *B*). The incision in the concave surface of the pinna is made carefully just through the full thickness of the auricular cartilage. The two arms of the "T" thereby meet and circumscribe the entrance to the vertical portion of the ear canal.

Rostral and caudal skin and fascial flaps are developed and are reflected from the surface of the ear canal by sharp and blunt dissection (Fig. 7-26 *B*). During the dissection of the vertical and horizontal portions of the ear canals, it is especially important to avoid the parotid salivary gland and cranial nerves and blood vessels (Fig. 7-26 *C* and *D*). The entire ear canal is then excised by amputating the annular cartilage, from the petrous temporal bone, at the bony acoustic meatus (Fig. 7-26 *D*). All cartilage should be removed because residual contaminated cartilage may serve as a nidus for deep infection. The epithelial lining of the external acoustic meatus is removed by curettage.

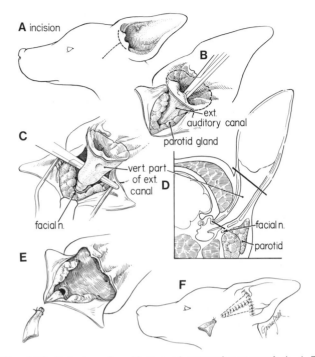

Fig. 7-26. *Technique for ablation of external ear canal. A, A T-shaped skin incision over the external ear canal. B, Ventral end of the vertical portion of the external ear canal is probed. The parotid salivary gland has been dissected for the purpose of anatomical orientation. The dotted line indicates the continuation of the horizontal arm of the skin incision, in order to circumscribe the opening of the external ear canal. C, By dissecting close to the auricular and then the annular cartilage the entire external ear canal is exposed to the level of the external acoustic meatus. The facial nerve, for the sake of description, is shown more exposed than is necessary. D, Schematic of cross-section of the surgical site. The thick diagonal lines indicate the sites of severence of the ear canal between the external acoustic meatus and the annular cartilage (lower left) and the approximate extent of excision of the auricular cartilage of the vertical ear canal (upper right). E, Completed ablation with demonstration of the position of the Penrose drain. F, Sutured skin incision. Dotted lines indicate optional wedge-shaped skin excisions performed so that skin closure increases support of erect ears. See text for further details.*

Some of the deep tissue should be saved for culture and antibiotic sensitivity testing as well as for histologic examination. The area is thoroughly flushed with physiologic saline solution, and the tympanic membrane is closely examined for evidence of otitis media prior to closing the incision.

Following complete control of hemorrhage, a Penrose drain is placed in the incision, with one end near the external acoustic meatus and the other tunneled to an opening made ventral to the ventral end of the vertical skin incision (Fig. 7-26 *E*). The drain is held in place by a single skin suture. In dogs with erect ears, it may be helpful to remove wedge-shaped pieces of skin (apex of each wedge on the ventral end) on both the rostral and caudal edges of the vertical incision (dotted lines, Fig. 7-26 *F*). By doing so, closure of the skin results in greater tension across the incision that enhances support to ear carriage. Deep closure of the

wound is accomplished with simple interrupted absorbable sutures, and the skin is closed routinely with nonabsorbable simple interrupted sutures (Fig. 7-26 *F*). A sterile gauze pack and a head and neck bandage, similar to one described by Knecht and associates,[3] is placed over the incision.

Postoperative Care

The wound is examined and redressed daily. The Penrose tube drain is removed after 3 or 4 days or when drainage has stopped. A broad-spectrum systemic antibiotic is given for at least 7 days following the operation. The therapy is changed if indicated by the results of intrasurgical bacterial culture and antibiotic sensitivity testing. Skin sutures are removed after 10 to 14 days.

Ingress-Egress Drainage for Otitis Media Following Ear Canal Ablation

In certain instances, such as in severe, chronic external ear infection, it may be necessary to perform ear canal ablation in the presence of nonresponding otitis media. In addition, I have had to treat subcutaneous sepsis, resulting from extension of inadequately managed otitis media, after ear ablation. The strategy described here has been devised because drainage of the middle ear by previously published methods (bulla osteotomy) provides for neither adequate removal of septic discharge nor a sufficiently high local level of antibacterial agent. The technique involves insertion of two catheters into the middle ear prior to wound closure. A dorsal catheter is employed to flush solutions into the middle ear through the acoustic meatus, and a ventral catheter allows for dependent drainage of septic exudates and lavage solutions (Fig. 7-27).

Following ear canal ablation, if otitis media exists, myringotomy is performed, and the middle ear is curetted and is thoroughly debrided and flushed. The middle ear is exposed for curettage by the careful use of rongeur forceps to remove the ventral and ventrocaudal portions of the bony external acoustic meatus. This bony excision also includes a slot 3 to 5 mm wide and 4 to 8 mm long, extending caudoventrally into the osseus bulla; an estimation of the extent to which bone is removed, at the level of this slot, is indicated by hatched lines in Figure 7-27. This slot allows better access to the tympanic cavity for curettage and debridement. It also helps one to avoid the sensitive inner ear structures because the surgeon can approach curettage from a more ventral position. The tubing may be placed in the slot, to avoid the auditory ossicles.

Material flushed from the middle ear should be saved for histologic examination and for culture and antibiotic sensitivity testing. At this point, one end of each of 2 sterile silicone rubber* tubes is fenestrated for a distance of .5 to 1 cm, and the fenestrated ends of both are inserted into the tympanic cavity. Each tube is then

*Silastic, Dow Corning Corp., Midland, MI 48640

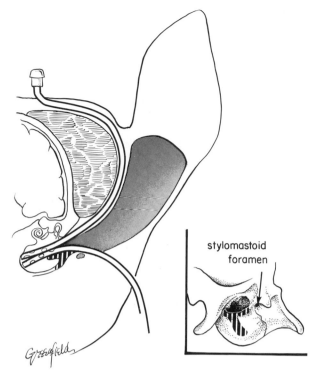

stylomastoid foramen

Fig. 7-27. *Ingress-egress drainage of the middle ear for otitis media or interna. The main portion of the figure schematically shows the placement of fenestrated catheters. The inset shows a lateral view of the left tympanic bulla. Hatched areas of both indicate the extent of removal of the bony rim on the ventral aspect of the external acoustic meatus, and the full thickness slot into the middle ear made with rongeur forceps. See text for further details.*

tunneled subcutaneously and is exteriorized away from the incision. One tube, which is tunneled rostral to the ear, exits near the dorsal midline of the skull and is used for flushing the middle ear. The second catheter, which exits just below the ventral end of the vertical skin incision, serves for drainage (Fig. 7-27). By placing an injection cap on the dorsal tube, a pressure lock is created, so that at the completion of a flushing procedure, fluid remains in the middle ear. If the tubes are sized properly, that is, if they are of large enough diameter, it may not be necessary to hold them in place with deep sutures. It may, however, be required to tie each catheter lightly to the region of the acoustic meatus. One should use absorbable sutures, which surround but do not enter the catheters; similar nonabsorbable sutures are used at the points of exit through the skin. In order to protect the catheters and the incision, a sterile pediatric urine collection bag is placed over the ventral drainage tube exit and the head and neck are bandaged.

Following the surgical procedure, the bandage is removed twice daily, and the middle ear is irrigated with liberal quantities of warm physiologic saline solution. A 1% povidone-iodine solution* or an indicated antibiotic can be employed locally in conjunction with

*Betadine solution, Purdue Frederick Co., 50 Washington Street, Norwalk, CT 06856

systemic antibiotic therapy. After irrigating, the selected antibiotic may be injected into the middle ear and may be allowed to remain. The local lavage can usually be accomplished without apparent discomfort to the animal and without sedation. Flushing and local instillation of antibiotics should be continued at least 24 to 48 hours after termination of abnormal discharge from the middle ear. Systemic antibiotic therapy should be continued for a minimum of 3 weeks following the operation.

A modification of this procedure uses a ventral bulla osteotomy approach, to allow examination and debridement of the tympanic bulla. (See the final section of this chapter, "Surgical Treatment for Middle and Inner Ear Infections," by Bojrab and Robertson.) The ventrally placed drainage tube originates from the middle ear through the new opening in the bulla. Flushing, in this case, is still accomplished by a tube inserted through the external acoustic meatus, as previously described.

Several methods for surgical drainage of the tympanic bulla have been presented previously in the literature. These procedures include myringotomy, or lateral, ventral, medial, or caudal approaches to the tympanic bulla. Parker and associates[4] described a technique for treatment of otitis media and interna in dogs. These workers performed lateral aural resection for drainage, followed by myringotomy and curettage of the bulla. I feel that the addition to this technique of external drainage and repeated flushing and local antibiotic therapy may be critical to complete recovery in many of the more established infections. The placement of indwelling tubes through the external auditory meatus probably should be reserved for those cases of otitis media in which hearing is already destroyed by chronic infection, because disruption of the auditory ossicles results from the procedure. Lavage might also be considered, without external ear ablation, for those cases of otitis interna or media associated with osteomyelitis extending to adjacent positions of the skull. In such instances, control of infection is more critical than the maintenance of hearing.

Acknowledgments

I wish to thank Ms. Harriet Greenfield of the Educational Media Center, Tufts New England Medical Center, who prepared the illustrations, and Ms. Sylvia D. Lewis, who typed the manuscript.

References and Suggested Readings

1. Evans, H. E., and Christensen, G. C. (eds.): Miller's Anatomy of the Dog. 2nd Ed. Philadelphia, W. B. Saunders, 1979.
2. Fraser, G., et al.: Canine Ear Disease. J. Small Anim. Pract., *10*:725, 1970.
3. Knecht, C. D., et al.: Fundamental Techniques in Veterinary Surgery. 2nd Ed. Philadelphia, W. B. Saunders, 1981.
4. Parker, A. J., Schiller, A. G., and Cusick, P. K.: Bulla curettage for chronic otitis media and interna in dogs. J. Am. Vet. Med. Assoc., *168*:931, 1976.
5. Singh, G. B., and Rao, M. M.: Otitis externa in canines—its medicinal and surgical treatment. Indian Vet. J., *36*:236, 1959.

Modified Ablation Technique

by M. JOSEPH BOJRAB

An alternate surgical technique for chronic otitis externa has been used when the entire vertical canal is grossly distorted or is filled with hyperplastic mucosa. This technique combines the advantages of ablation (removal of the chronically infected vertical canal) with those of lateral ear canal resection (maintenance of drainage and hearing).

The preparation of the patient (Fig. 7-28), skin incision, and vertical canal isolation are the same as described previously for lateral ear canal resection (see the corresponding earlier section of this chapter by Dallman and Bojrab). The vertical canal isolation is continued medially until the entire canal is isolated (Fig. 7-29). The auricular cartilage and skin are then cut just dorsal to the opening of the vertical canal at the base of the pinna (Fig. 7-30). This method allows complete mobilization of the vertical canal, which remains attached only at the ventral end. The vertical canal is cut approximately 2 cm dorsal to the horizontal canal

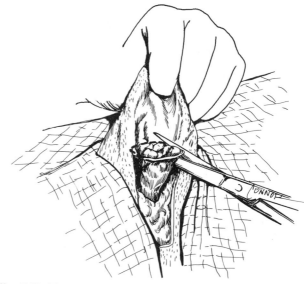

Fig. 7-30. *The auricular cartilage and skin are cut dorsal to the opening of the vertical canal.*

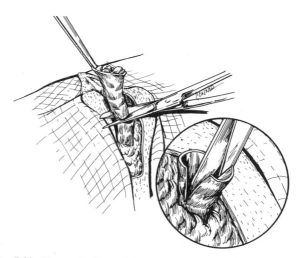

Fig. 7-31. *The vertical canal is cut dorsal to the horizontal canal. Inset, incision of the remaining vertical canal, rostrally and caudally, down to the horizontal canal.*

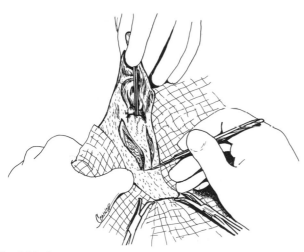

Fig. 7-28. *Skin incisions for this modified ablation technique.*

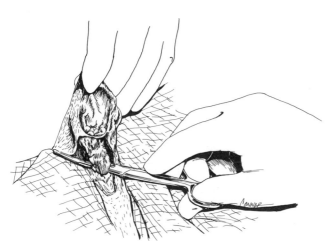

Fig. 7-29. *Isolation of the vertical ear canal.*

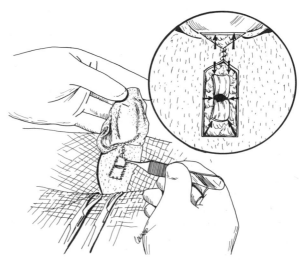

Fig. 7-32. *Suturing of the dorsal and ventral rectangular flaps.*

(Fig. 7-31) and is discarded. The remaining vertical canal is incised both rostrally and caudally down to the horizontal canal (Fig. 7-31, inset), thus creating two rectangular flaps, a dorsal and a ventral flap (Fig. 7-32). The ventral flap is sutured as described earlier for lateral ear resection. The dorsal flap is sutured as depicted in Figure 7-32.

Aftercare consists of bandaging the ear over the head for one week and administering systemic antibiotics as determined by culture and sensitivity tests.

Middle and Inner Ear

Surgical Treatment for Middle and Inner Ear Infections

by M. Joseph Bojrab *and* John J. Robertson

Clinical Signs and Diagnosis

The clinical signs of otitis externa often mask otitis media, and unless the tympanic membrane is visualized, a diagnosis of otitis media may be overlooked. In dogs, most otitis media infections are extensions of external ear infections; signs are ear drainage, pawing and rubbing of the affected ear, shaking of the head, and evident pain. More severe signs such as head tilt toward the affected side, circling, and ataxia will develop as the inner ear and vestibular apparatus are involved. Radiology may be a helpful aid to diagnosis by visualizing the bulla. Lateral, dorsoventral, and open-mouth views may show an increase in density of the petrous temporal bone with new bone formation in the wall or floor of the bulla. Lysis of the bone or a combination of osteogenesis and osteolysis may also be evident. Moreover, new bone formation around and adjacent to the temporal mandibular joint is sometimes characterized by pain upon opening the mouth. Radiology alone should not be relied upon to diagnose this condition, however, because these radiographic signs may not be evident.

Therefore, in all cases of otitis and especially in intractable ones, the tympanum must be visualized. If general anesthesia is required, the membrane may be visualized, and the ear canal may be lavaged to remove debris. The debris in chronic otitis externa includes hair, exfoliated tissue, exudate, and possibly foreign material. This debris lies next to the tympanum and may cause necrosis or eventual rupture of the membrane. The middle ear then becomes involved, and as the condition becomes chronic, the tissue lining the bulla becomes metaplastic, hyperplastic, and hypersecretory. This chronic reactive tissue then becomes resistant to medical treatment by its physical makeup; drugs have difficulty in penetrating this keratinized epithelium while bacteria are harbored in its crypts.

Pharyngitis is another source of middle ear infection, and young dogs are prone to otitis media by retrograde infection through the eustachian tube. The signs of this disease are the same as previously described, except the ear canal is not always involved, a moderate fever is usually noted, and pain is present at the base of the ear. In general, the organisms seen in middle and inner ear infections are similar to those in otitis externa: staphylococcus, pityrosporon, pseudomonas, and proteus, in that order of frequency.

Myringotomy

The purpose of a surgical approach to otitis is to establish drainage, whether by lateral ear resection, myringotomy, or bulla osteotomy. In all cases, surgical drainage is the radical approach and should be used only when intensive medical management fails to cure the condition. The first attempt to gain access to the middle ear, if the tympanum is not ruptured, is myringotomy. The normal tympanic membrane is transparent or of a pearl gray translucence, with an onionskin texture. This membrane is composed of a dorsal portion or pars flaccida, which is a loose, opaque membrane. Ventrally, the membrane is termed the pars tensa and is clear and striated. The manubrium of the malleus is sickle shaped, and this ossicle extends into the pars tensa (Fig. 7-33). Small blood vessels course this membrane and, during infection, become dilated. Bulging of the membrane often occurs because of exudate in the middle ear. This exudate may or may not be visualized, depending upon the opacity of the membrane. Sometimes, a thickened and necrotic white tympanum appears corrugated with dark, wrinkled markings.

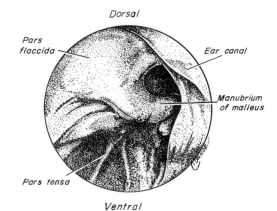

Fig. 7-33. *The tympanic membrane as viewed through the otoscope.*

Piercing the tympanum is easy and safe when done properly. Myringotomy is used routinely in human medicine for middle ear infection, and any reduction in hearing is usually due to the effects of the infection rather than the myringotomy. This membrane usually regrows into a smooth, scar-like structure within 3 to 4 weeks, and good hearing is reported. Sounds are detected by dogs without tympanic membranes; therefore, sound-wave conduction through the bones of the skull probably plays a significant role in the hearing of the dog.

While the patient is under general anesthesia and in lateral recumbency, an otoscope is passed down the ear canal until the pars tensa is visualized. A small Steinmann pin or alligator forceps is used to penetrate the membrane in the lower quadrant ventral to the manubrium of the malleus. Care should be taken to remain ventral to this structure because fracture of this ossicle impairs hearing. At this point, a culture is taken, and a sensitivity test is subsequently done. Povidone-iodine* flushes are then initiated in an attempt to clean the bulla. A blunt needle on a syringe or a Water-Pik† is used to flush out dirt and debris. The lavage is repeated until clean fluid is aspirated. Whereas this technique is successful in man, the vertical ear canal in the dog does not allow adequate drainage. Therefore, some veterinary surgeons report good results with myringotomy and lateral ear resection coupled with flushing.

Bulla Osteotomy

The middle ear is a pear-shaped cavity within the petrous temporal bone. The tympanic membrane, auditory ossicles, eustachian tube, and inner ear lie within the neck of this pear-shaped bone while the tympanic bulla is at its base. Several methods have been used to gain entry into and drainage from this area. One of the first described involves passing a Steinmann pin with an eyelet in the tip down the external auditory canal, performing a myringotomy, and then forcing the tip through the wall of the bulla into the pharynx. Steel suture is then placed through the eye in the tip, and the pin is withdrawn from the ear. A perforated rubber tube is secured to the wire and is pulled through the ear canal from the oral cavity. The end of the tubing is then sutured to the roof of the pharynx.

Another technique used to drain the middle ear is lateral ear resection followed by curettage of the bulla to debride and remove all debris. A lateral surgical approach has also been described, in which the bulla is entered between the parotid salivary gland ventrally and the horizontal ear canal dorsally. A drain is secured and flushed daily. All these surgical procedures have varying degrees of difficulty and interference with normal structures; therefore, it is our preference to enter the bulla through a ventral approach by which few important anatomic structures are encountered, and if done properly, the vital structures of the middle and inner ear are not invaded.

*Betadine, Purdue Frederick Co., 50 Washington Street, Norwalk, CT 06856

†Teledyne Aquatec Corp., Fort Collins, CO 80521

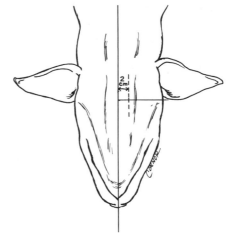

Fig. 7-34. *With the patient in dorsal recumbency, a 7-cm incision is centered 2 cm from midline at the level of the angle of the mandible.*

The anesthetized dog is placed in dorsal recumbency, and the area between the cranial third of the mandible and the caudal third of the trachea is prepared for the surgical procedure. Before draping the patient, the incision site should be located using the following anatomic landmarks. First, one should palpate the angle of the mandible as it becomes the vertical ramus. From here, one should draw a line perpendicular to the midline of the dog. The next step is to fall off this line toward the affected side 2 cm from the midline. At this point, the incision should be made directly over the bulla. A 7-cm incision should be centered over this point and made parallel with the midline (Fig. 7-34). After incising the skin, the lingual facial vein is retracted, and deeper dissection is continued between the digastricus muscle laterally and the hyo- and styloglossus muscles medially (Fig. 7-35). Spread-

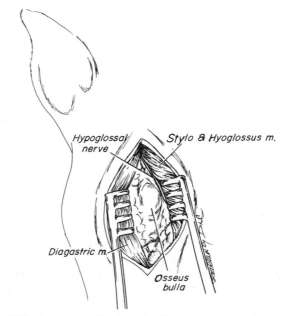

Fig. 7-35. *On incising the skin, the digastricus muscle is retracted laterally, and the stylo- and hyoglossus muscles medially. The hypoglossal nerve is visualized medially.*

ing these muscles with blunt dissection, the hypoglossal nerve can be seen running across the lateral aspect of the hyo- and styloglossus muscles. An effort should be made to preserve this nerve because it supplies innervation to the intrinsic muscle fibers of the tongue.

At this point, self-retaining retractors are used to open the surgical site by spreading between the digastricus and glossus muscles. The veterinary surgeon's finger is used to locate the cornu of the hyoid, and the bulla is palpated just cranial and medial to the tip of this cornu, and caudal and medial to the angle of the mandible. Closed Metzenbaum scissors are used as a blunt probe to dissect the soft tissue from the bony bulla. A small osteotome is then used to chip a four-sided window in the bulla. The bone of the ventral bulla is thin and may even be dissolved if infection is long-standing. One should carefully remove this bony flap and expose the middle ear.

A swab for culture and sensitivity tests is taken, and ventral drainage is established with sterile silicone rubber* tubing. This tube is inserted directly into the bulla and should be long enough to extend to the outside of the incision. The tube is then stapled into place with 2-0 synthetic absorbable† suture. This "staple" method uses a large horizontal mattress stitch: it enters the hyo- and styloglossus muscles, crosses the incision line, enters the digastricus muscle, passes around the tubing, and exits again through both muscles. The suture is then tied and holds the tube in place by friction. This suture is repeated in the subcutaneous tissues and again in the skin. Stainless steel 2-0 suture is used in the skin to crimp the tube, and a simple interrupted pattern is used to close the remaining skin incision.

* Silastic, Dow Corning Co., Midland, MI 48640
† Vicryl, Ethicon, Inc., Somerville, NJ 08876

If not done previously, a myringotomy should be performed at this time. Betadine is flushed into the external ear and is allowed to drain through the Silastic tubing. The ear is flushed in this manner twice daily for 5 days. The patient should receive 50,000 IU per pound of procaine penicillin G intramuscularly per day until the sensitivity test reveals the antibiotic of choice.

Most dogs tolerate this drain well; however, an Elizabethan collar can be placed on the dog if necessary. The drain is pulled on the fifth postoperative day provided the clinical signs indicate no inner ear involvement. In the case of inner ear involvement, the flush should be continued for at least 10 days, and the prognosis for complete recovery is not as favorable.

References and Suggested Readings

Barrett, R., and Rathfon, B.: Lateral approach to bulla osteotomy. J. Am. Anim. Hosp. Assoc., 2:203, 1975.

Bojrab, M. J.: The ear, in surgical techniques in small animal practice. Vet. Clin. North Am., 5:507, 1975.

Denny, H. R.: The results of surgical treatment of otitis media and interna in the dog. J. Small Anim. Pract., 14:585, 1973.

Knecht, C. D.: Diseases of the middle and inner ear in the dog and cat. Small Anim. Vet. Med. Update Series, 1, 1972.

Krogh, H. V.: Otitis externa in the dog—A clinical and microbiological study. Nord. Vet. Med. 27:285, 1975.

Lane, J. G.: Canine middle ear disease. Vet. Annu., 16:160, 1976.

Parker, A. J., Schiller, A. G., and Cusick, P. K.: Bulla curettage for chronic otitis media and interna in dog. J. Am. Vet. Med. Assoc., 168:931, 1976.

Spreull, J. S. A.: Tympanotomy, bulla, osteotomy and vestibular osteotomy. In Current Techniques in Small Animal Surgery. Edited by M. Joseph Bojrab. Philadelphia, Lea & Febiger, 1975.

Spreull, J. S. A.: Otitis media. Anim. Hosp., 2:89, 1966.

Spreull, J. S. A.: Treatment of Otitis Media in the Dog. J. Small Anim. Pract., 5:107, 1964.

Section C: Digestive System

8 * Palate

Repair and Reconstruction of Cleft Palate and Other Oronasal Fistulas

by DONALD R. HOWARD

A distinction has been made between a primary cleft or harelip and a secondary cleft or cleft palate.[7] Any cleft rostral to the incisive foramen and involving the lip is considered a primary cleft, whereas clefts caudal to the incisive foramen are considered secondary. The chronologic embryologic development of the premaxillas and maxillas are responsible for this terminology in man. It is known that the shelves rostral to the incisive foramen close between the fourth and seventh week of gestation and the more caudal area closes between the seventh and twelfth week of gestation.[4]

The true values for the incidence and epidemiologic presence of this disease may never be known. Natural selection and kennel (management) selection almost eliminate the possibility of determining true genetic accountability. It is, however, recognized that strong evidence supports a genetic origin in the dog and cat.[14–17] The alert kennel manager and the veterinarian recognize palate deformities by routine physical examination.

Purebred dogs are more prone to the disease, and species frequency is more common in the brachycephalic breeds and in schnauzers.[9,10] The incidence epidemiology and etiology of cleft palate disease in dogs and cats may be found elsewhere.[3,4,11]

Secondary Cleft Palate and Oronasal Fistula Repair

When secondary cleft palate and oronasal fistulas are detected at an early age, supplemental feeding by pharyngostomy or stomach tube is required. Preparation for the surgical procedure can be well controlled because this is an elective operation. Presurgical oral and nasal cultures may be obtained for aerobic and anaerobic culture and sensitivity testing. Clinical pathologic evaluation of the patient may be made, and the operation can be planned when surgical risk is mini-

mized. It is advisable to place a pharyngostomy tube and to initiate oral hyperalimentation 2 days prior to the surgical procedure. Pharyngostomy alimentation is used to minimize foreign-body lodgment in the nares, to decrease inflammatory activity of nasal tissues, and to help decrease adverse postoperative pharyngeal reflexes upon anesthetic recovery. Surgical intervention for palate repair is best done when the patient is 7 weeks of age or more.

For long-range results, it is desirable to provide a viable tissue barrier (pedicle flap), as opposed to the various dental appliances that have been recommended.[19] A recent adaptation of a vomer flap procedure in man has enabled the veterinarian greater rates of surgical success in cleft palate repair.[6] The secondary cleft palate involves a midline fissure of the soft and hard palate areas. Traumatic oronasal fistulas may result from blunt trauma, foreign body penetration, or surgical excision of neoplasms.

Prior to anesthetic induction, carefully controlled intravenous fluid therapy is initiated and is continued throughout the procedure. A buffered lactated Ringer's solution is recommended because hemorrhage during the procedure is inevitable. The patient is positioned in dorsal recumbency with an endotracheal tube in place (largest size possible). Halothane-oxygen inhalation anesthesia is recommended. The endotracheal tube is secured in place by tying gauze around the endotracheal tube and mandible. Care is taken to prevent kinking or dislodgment of the endotracheal tube. Gauze sponges may be packed deep into the pharyngeal region to help prevent aspiration of fluids and blood. Water-soluble povidone-iodine is used liberally to flush the oral and nasal cavities free of purulent exudate and debris. Following oronasal lavage, aspirating the nares with suction and changing the pharyngeal gauze sponges are recommended.

MUCOPERIOSTEAL FLAP TECHNIQUE

The purpose of the mucoperiosteal flap is to create a hinged tissue pedicle with an intact blood supply. The hinge is located at the cleft's edge. The mucoperiosteal flap technique calls for two incisions of the mucoperiosteal tissue. It is recommended to create the bed for

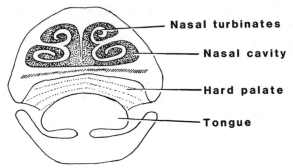

Fig. 8-1. *A schematic cross-sectional view of the normal canine nasal and oral cavities.*

the mucoperiosteal flap first. A right-angle keratome or a small surgical knife is used to separate the periosteum and the alveolar bone on one side of the cleft. At the beginning of the soft palate tissue, the bed should be created at least 2 mm greater than the distance of the cleft itself toward the dental arcade. Hemorrhage at this point is usually minimal, and the elevated mucoperiosteum is allowed to rest on the alveolar bone.

Creating the mucoperiosteal flap requires extremely careful manipulation of the periosteum. The width of the flap should be at least 2 mm wider than the measured width of the cleft. See Figure 8-1 for normal anatomy. If an error is made, it should be toward a wider flap. A perpendicular incision is made down to the alveolar bone and is parallel in most cases to the dental arcade (Fig. 8-2A). As the incision makes the transition from the hard to the soft palate, it is carried only halfway through the thickness of the soft palate. Care should be taken not to penetrate the nasopharynx. The mucoperiosteum is separated by elevating the periosteum from the palatine bone (Fig. 8-2B).

Hemorrhage is copious during the flap rotation procedure, and liberal flushing with saline solution and suction improve visualization of the manipulated tis-

sue. In the young animal, the palatine artery may usually be identified as an entity, and hemostasis may be achieved by ligation or electrocauterization. The mucoperiosteum should be elevated right up to the edge of the alveolar cleft. Once the flap has been harvested, the tissue may be secured within the bed site by 4-0 polyglycolic suture. Simple or vertical mattress sutures may be used to stabilize the wound closure. Liberal flushing after suturing helps to remove all clots. Prior to recovery from anesthesia, inspection of the pharyngostomy tube is warranted to ensure its proper position. Gauze previously inserted in the pharyngeal area should be removed when the head has been lowered, to accommodate residual fluid drainage. Recovery from anesthesia should be uneventful, but careful observation for aspiration is necessary. Feeding by pharyngostomy tube may begin within 3 hours of complete anesthetic recovery.

The surgical wound is inspected daily. If a fistula develops, the wound should be left alone because small oronasal fistulas have been reported to heal by granulation.[1] Suture removal is not necessary; the polyglycolic acid suture is absorbable. The pharyngostomy tube may be removed after 7 days, and normal feeding and drinking may be initiated. In young puppies, the open palatine bed heals quickly, and alveolar surfaces are covered with fibroblastic activity within 2 days. Epithelialization is complete in 3 weeks. Genetic counseling and animal neutering are recommended.

ORONASAL FISTULAS

Most oronasal fistulas are caused by blunt traumatic injury, necrosis due to electrical shock, or foreign body penetration. The principles of surgical closure of oronasal fistulas are similar to those for secondary cleft palate repair. Presurgical placement of a pharyngostomy tube helps to arrest any inflammatory processes due to food debris and affords the veterinarian the opportunity to prepare the animal nutritionally for the elective surgical procedure. Maintaining the objective of positioning a viable tissue to separate the oral and nasal cavity necessitates gentle tissue handling. Regardless of the location of the fistulas, the pedicle flap must be larger than the defect and must have a noncompromised vascular supply at its base. If the defect is circular, the diameter of the harvested pedicle or rotating flap must be at least 2 mm larger than the measured defect. Similar to the technique of creating the mucoperiosteal flap, a bed is created with a small surgical knife by elevating the periosteum from the alveolar bone. Tension on the flap that might compromise venous drainage at the pedicle base must be considered in advance. In cases in which a pedicle-based flap is advanced forward to close defects, it is always advantageous to consider positioning the base of the flap at the caudal area of the soft palate.[12] It is possible in some patients to maintain the integrity of the palatine artery. In most cases of transpositioning or rotating oral pedicle flaps, however, the integrity of the palatine artery is compromised by severing or stretching.

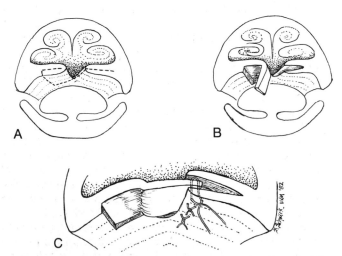

Fig. 8-2. A, *Cross-sectional view of a canine cleft palate. Incision lines are shown creating the mucoperiosteal flap and receiving bed site within the soft tissue of the hard and soft palates. B, Separation of the mucoperiosteum. C, The mucoperiosteal flap should be elevated right up to the edge of the alveolar cleft edge.*

As with the secondary cleft palate technique, the primary source of vascular integrity should be directed to maintaining viable periosteal tissue.

Large or gross shifts in tissue from the caudal aspect of the oronasal cavity have been reported and are successful in most instances.[13] Preplanning the rotation or advancement flap is most important to surgical success.[8,18] Interrupted suturing must be done meticulously and must afford a watertight seal in order for any oronasal repair operation to succeed. Polyglycolic acid suture retains suitable sustained tensile strength and tension on the wound for complete surgical healing. Stainless steel or nylon sutures may be preferable, however, when infection exists or when orthopedic stabilization is the combined objective in closure. Positioning of the patient, anesthetic conditions, and postsurgical care are as for secondary cleft palate repair.

Primary Cleft Palate (Harelip) Repair

Anatomically, repair of primary cleft palate in puppies is less exacting than in man because the reconstruction of the columella is easy. The columella, for all practical purposes, is nonexistent in the dog, and because little mucocutaneous tissue (vermilion) is externally visible in the puppy, and an excess of skin exists lateral and medial to the cleft, this reconstruction is simplified when compared to that in man. The ideal age to operate on these puppies is 6 weeks to 2 months.

Halothane-oxygen anesthesia is induced and maintained. Tracheal intubation offers no surgical approach obstructions as with secondary cleft palate repair. Once anesthesia is instituted, intravenous fluids are started (buffered lactated Ringer's solution). The puppy is placed in ventral recumbency, with its head elevated by placing sterile towels under the mandible. No hair clipping is necessary. The nasal floor, mucocutaneous tissues, and rostral premaxillas are cleansed six times with diluted povidone-iodine solutions. The tissue preparation is similar to that described for secondary cleft palate repair.

All tissue handling should be gentle. To facilitate tissue retraction, fine tissue hooks or stay sutures should be used. The first step is to close the floor of the nasal orifice so that it is confluent with the mucosal side of the lip closure. A nasal pedicle flap is mobilized from the medial side of the floor of the nares and is reflected laterally to the lateral lip mucosal side of the cleft (Fig. 8-2B). This maneuver may be compared to the mucoperiosteal flap maneuver in a previously described repair technique for secondary cleft palate.[9] The nares flap is rotated and sutured with 5-0 polyglactin* into a prepared bed site (incision) of the lateral side (Fig. 8-2C). Care should be taken to maintain a large pedicle base for proper vascular viability of the rotated flap. This maneuver is perhaps the most difficult of the entire repair procedure. Once four or five interrupted polyglactin sutures have secured the rotated pedicle flap, the cutaneous closure may be easily performed.

The simplicity of a rotation flap[5,20] repair, with its even distribution of wound tension, is most useful in veterinary surgery. A limited mucocutaneous margin cleft edge resection is made with sharp scissors. Care to remove only the superficial portion of this tissue should be emphasized, because excessive discarding of tissue is dangerous. It is not necessary to undermine or to separate the three lip layers as described for other repairs.[4] An incision through the skin and subdermis on the medial side is made perpendicular to the philtrum of the nose at a level within the hairy cutaneous lip (Fig. 8-3A). This incision should be expanded by blunt dissection so that it opens and will be the future bed site for an advancement pedicle flap from the lateral lip edge (Fig. 8-3B). When the bed site has been prepared, the lateral lip advancement flap is prepared (Fig. 8-3C and D). A triangular flap is created using the broad-based pedicle flap toward the lateral nasal floor (Fig. 8-3E). The apex of the flap should be almost at the tip of the lower cleft edge. Again, as with the bed site, this skin incision is to be carried through the dermis and only partially into the subdermis.

The lip muscle fascia should be included with the incision, even though it is most difficult to distinguish it as an entity. The triangular flap is then rotated medially and is sutured with two subdermal polyglactin 5-0 sutures into the prepared bed site (Fig. 8-3E). Tissue handling must be gentle at this point. The triangular flap is then cutaneously sutured in place with nonabsorbable sutures, preferably 4-0 nylon. Once the flap is securely sutured, the ventral-subcutaneous margins of the cleft edge may be closed with interrupted polyglactin 5-0 sutures (Fig. 8-3F). Usually enough redundant tissue is present so that apposition is not a problem. A cosmetic skin coaptation may be made with interrupted 4-0 nylon sutures. The area is cleansed by flushing with saline solution, and the puppy is allowed to recover from anesthesia. No advantage exists in the previously recommended epinephrine injections to control hemostasis.[2,7] Hemostasis is rapid once tissue apposition is complete. Suction effectively maintains the visual field.

Puppies are fed soft diets and water the day after the operation. Neither pharyngostomy tubes nor intravenous feeding is required. The most frequently observed adverse behavior is licking of the wound margin. If the cutaneous closure is complete and secure, vigorous licking should not affect healing. Sutures should be left at least 2 weeks, and only skin sutures should be removed at that time. General anesthesia is recommended for removal of sutures because puppies are active, and tissue dehiscence is possible from physical struggling. Under anesthesia, if evidence suggests closure failure at any site in the repair, it may be resutured without fear of total dehiscence of the wound.

Primary cleft closure must be performed with several principles in mind if it is to be successful and cosmetic. No "water" leaks or tissue gaps can be tolerated from the ventral nasal area. A shelf or nasal floor closure is the single most important maneuver for successful repair.

When primary and secondary clefts are present in

---

*Vicryl, Ethicon, Inc., Somerville, NJ 08876

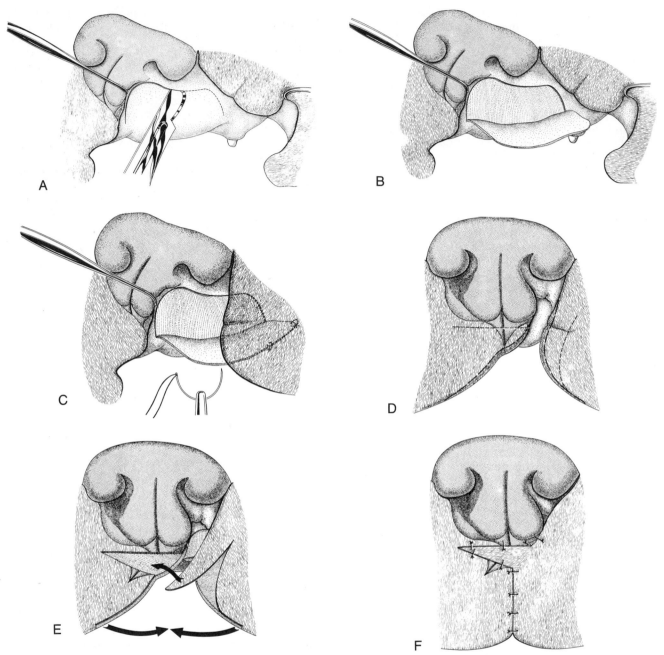

Fig. 8-3. A, *Incision of medial nasal wall for creation of a broad-based nasal floor pedicle flap.* B, *Nasal wall pedicle flap rotated toward lateral lip.* C, *Nasal wall pedicle flap sutured to the mucosal side of the left lip; when in place, this flap forms the nasal floor or shelf.* D, *Dotted lines indicating cutaneous incision line; note the perpendicular incision across the columella and the triangular shape of the pedicle flap.* E, *The mobilized position of the triangular pedicle flap rotated into the opposite cleft area.* F, *Cutaneous closure following placement of sutures.* (*From Howard, D. R., et al.: Primary cleft palate (harelip) and closure repair in puppies. J. Am. Anim. Hosp. Assoc., 12:636, 1976.*)

the same animal, the secondary cleft should take precedence in surgical intervention, and a later date should be scheduled for the primary cleft palate reconstruction. Genetic counseling should be undertaken, so that genetic carriers of the disease can be eliminated from breeding programs.

References and Suggested Readings

1. Berkman, M. C.: Early non-surgical closure of post-operative palate fistulae. Plast. Reconstr. Surg., *62*:537, 1978.

2. Cawley, A. J., and Archibald, J.: Plastic surgery. *In* Canine Surgery. 2nd Ed. Edited by J. Archibald. Santa Barbara, CA, American Veterinary Publishers, 1974.

3. Dreyer, C. J., and Preston, C. B.: Abnormal behavioral patterns in dogs with cleft palates. S. A. J. Med. Sci., *38*:13, 1973.

4. Evans, H. E., and Salk, W. O.: Prenatal development of domestic and laboratory mammals: growth curves, external features and selected references. Anat., Histol., Embryol., *2*:11, 1973.

5. Grabb, W. C., Rosenstein, S. W., and Bzoch, K. R. (eds.): Cleft Lip and Palate. Boston, Little, Brown, 1971.

6. Grabb, W. C., and Smith, J. W.: Plastic Surgery. 3rd Ed. Boston, Little, Brown, 1979.

7. Hammer, D. L., and Sacks, M.: Clefts of the primary and secondary palate. *In* Current Techniques in Small Animal Surgery. Edited by M. J. Bojrab. Philadelphia, Lea & Febiger, 1975.

8. Howard, D. R.: Principles of pedicle flaps and grafting techniques. J. Am. Anim. Hosp. Assoc., *12*:573, 1976.

9. Howard, D. R., et al.: Primary cleft palate (harelip) and closure repair in puppies. J. Am. Anim. Hosp. Assoc., *12*:636, 1976.

10. Howard, D. R., et al.: Mucoperiosteal flap technique for cleft palate repair in dogs. J. Am. Vet. Med. Assoc., *165*:352, 1974.

11. Jurkiewicz, M. J.: A genetic study of cleft lip and palate in dogs. Plast. Reconstr. Surg., *16*:472, 1965.

12. Lammerding, J. J., et al.: Repair of an acquired oral-nasal fistula. J. Am. Anim. Hosp. Assoc., *12*:64, 1976.

13. Leonard, M. S.: Repair of oronasal fistula with mucoperiosteal flap: report of case. J. Oral Surg., *37*:511, 1979.

14. Loevy, H. C., and Fenyes, V.: Spontaneous cleft palate in a family of Siamese cats. Cleft Palate J., *5*:57, 1968.

15. Loevy, H. T.: Cytogenetic analysis of Siamese cats with cleft palate. J. Dental Res., *53*:453, 1974.

16. Mulvihill, J. J., et al.: Epidemiologic features of cleft lip and/or cleft palate (CL ± P) in domestic animals. Teratology, *13*:31A, 1976.

17. Patterson, D. F., and Medway, W.: Hereditary diseases of the dog. J. Am. Vet. Med. Assoc., *149*:1741, 1966.

18. Swaim, S. F.: Surgery of Traumatized Skin: Management and Reconstruction in the Dog and Cat. Philadelphia, W. B. Saunders, 1980.

19. Thoday, K. L., et al.: The successful use of a prosthesis in the correction of a palatal defect in a dog. J. Small Anim. Pract., *6*:487, 1975.

20. Yules, R. B.: Atlas for Surgical Repair of Cleft Lip, Cleft Palate, and Noncleft Velopharyngeal Incompetence. Springfield, IL, Charles C Thomas, 1971.

9 * Teeth and Oral Cavity

Oronasal Fistula Repair

by DONALD L. ROSS

Extraction of a maxillary canine tooth may cause an oronasal fistula when previously existing periodontal disease resulted in the resorption of the lingual alveolar bone. The fistula is usually established prior to loss of the canine tooth, and its extraction makes the fistula visible. The signs include chronic nasal inflammation, nasal discharge, and food impaction.

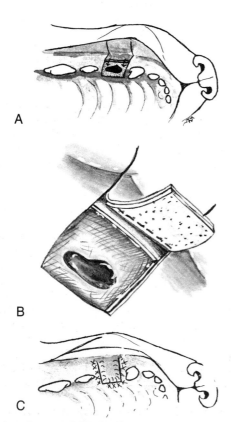

Fig. 9-1. A, *A mucosal flap is of sufficient length to cover the fistula without tension. Arrows indicate the direction of flap advancement.* B, *The area immediately adjacent to the fistula is prepared to receive the flap; incisions are placed lateral, medial, and distal to the fistula, and tissue is excised to the periosteum.* C, *The flap is sutured with nonabsorbable material in a vertical mattress pattern.*

Construction of a periosteal flap is the treatment of choice (Fig. 9-1). The procedure is begun by making incisions on the medial and distal surface of the fistula. A periosteal flap of sufficient length to cover the fistula without tension is elevated dorsally. The edges of the fistula are prepared by excision of tissue to the periosteum. The periosteum of the flap is incised at its apex. The flap is positioned over the fistula and is sutured in place. Small nonabsorbable sutures are placed in a vertical mattress pattern to prevent air passage during healing.

Healing is more likely when the periosteum of the flap contacts healthy bone all around the fistula and when no tension is placed on the flap. If small parts of the suture line open and the fistula is reestablished, attempted reclosure should be delayed for 3 to 6 months.

Dental Prophylaxis and Dental Surgery

by BEN H. COLMERY, III

Periodontitis

The most common dental disease of companion animals is periodontal disease. Periodontitis is caused by the toxins excreted by bacteria in dental plaque and results in alveolitis and bone resorption around teeth. Histopathologic examination of inflamed gingiva reveals few, if any, invasive bacteria, and antibiotics are unable to control any causative organism in dental plaque. This illustrates why antibiotics alone do not cure or control periodontitis. A complete dental prophylactic program is required to control periodontitis, with its sequela of alveolar bone resorption, and to promote general oral and gingival health.

PROPHYLACTIC SURGICAL TECHNIQUE

Thorough prophylactic scaling in companion animals requires general anesthesia and endotracheal intubation. The selection of an anesthetic agent is based on the animal's general health and the preference of the practitioner. Halothane and nitrous oxide combinations allow minimum recovery time and duration of hospitalization.

Once the animal is anesthetized, dental prophylaxis begins with ultrasonic removal of dental calculus on the crowns and exposed root surfaces (see Table 9-1 for a list of dental equipment). Although the ultrasonic scaler is a useful tool, potential dangers of this instrumentation include microetching of the tooth's surface and the production of damaging heat. The proper use of the ultrasonic scaler requires setting the power control to the lowest effective setting and applying the tip with the least amount of pressure. It is important to keep the cooling water spray dispersing as close to the working tip as possible. When using the ultrasonic scaler subgingivally, the cooling effect of the water spray may be lost, and the energy of the working tip may damage the periodontium and may microetch the

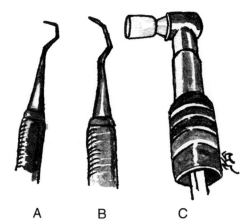

Fig. 9-2. *Dental instruments. A, Universal scaler; B, Columbia No. 13-14 curette; and C, prophy angle with cup.*

subgingival root surface. This damage allows greater ease of attachment of future subgingival calculus formation, unless the root is then properly planed by manual instrumentation.* When properly used, the ultrasonic scaler decreases procedure time (important in the geriatric animal) and facilitates calculus removal.

Once the major pieces of dental calculus have been removed, the crevices and exposed roots are cleaned with a Universal scaler. This instrument has three working surfaces on each tip and allows fine scaling in areas too small to allow access of the ultrasonic tip (Fig. 9-2A). This instrument is held in the hand like a pencil. The fourth or fifth fingers are fulcrumed on the animal's head, or other stable surface, to allow precision in scaling. Hand scaling is done on all exposed tooth surfaces.

Next, the gingival sulcus and periodontal pockets are cleaned (see Fig. 9-3). This procedure is best accomplished with a curette. I prefer the Starlite Columbia No. 13-14 curette (Fig. 9-2B). This instrument has 2 cutting surfaces on each working tip and allows root planing and subgingival curettage. The instrument is held in a manner similar to that for the scaler. The working tip enters the sulcus against the gingiva and is pushed to the bottom of the pocket. Next, the cutting surface is turned against the root, and, with gentle but firm pressure, the tip is pulled out of the pocket (Fig. 9-3). Care is taken to prevent pushing calculus deeper into the pocket. Although the goal is not to cause gingival bleeding, hemorrhage usually occurs as the opposite cutting surface debrides the subgingival tissue. In advanced cases of periodontitis, gingival hemorrhage may be impressive, but direct pressure on the gums usually stops the bleeding. The mouth is irrigated periodically with fluid to maintain a visible operative field. All subgingival surfaces are curetted, and the root is planed.

The final step in dental prophylaxis is crown polishing. The amount of polishing required to smooth the enamel and exposed root surfaces varies from animal

Table 9-1. *Equipment for Veterinary Dentistry*

Periodontal Equipment
    Emesco bench-model engine, No. 90NPB Piccolo arm—black (*Note:* Can be used for endodontic, orthodontic, and other dental procedures.)
    Handpieces—Schein-Doriot type 30,000 R.P.M. ball bearing model 30,000—heavy duty
    Periodontal instruments
        Universal scaler
        Columbia double-end Starlite curette—Columbia No. 13-14
    Prophy angle—screw type is best
    Prophy cups—screw type
    Prophy pumice—coarse
    Nupro prophy paste—medium grit
    Sharpening stone or wheel
    Ultrasonic scaler (*Note:* This should be your last purchase. This instrument should never be used subgingivally for it severely damages the periodontium. It is recommended for use on animals with heavy calculus formation.)
    Kodak dental film—periapical ultraspeed film, DF-58 (*Note:* Technique is usually on box. Use 16-inch FFD, 65-75 KVP, 10 MAS.)
    Dental film developing hanger No. 7

Orthodontic Equipment
    Jeltrate fast-set alginate
    Vel Stone mix stone
    Assorted impression trays
    Durelon cement

Endodontic Equipment
    Inverted cone burs—steel, assorted sizes
    Round burs—carbide, assorted sizes
    Standard human root-canal files for premolars, molars, and small incisors
    50-mm root canal files, for large canine teeth
    Tubli-seal (Kerr)
    Dycal caulk
    Wiggle-bug amalgamator
    Single- and double-spill spheralloy amalgam (Kerr)
    Amalgam carrier
    Packer and plugger
    Dust-off compressed "air"

Source for equipment and materials
    Any human dental supply house
    Henry Schein, Inc., 5 Harbor Park Drive, Port Washington, N.Y. 11050

*Root planing is a process in which a curette is used to debride subgingival calculi from the root of the tooth within the periodontal pocket.

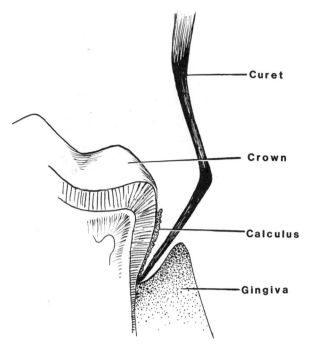

Fig. 9-3. *Gingival sulcus and periodontal pockets being cleaned with a curette.*

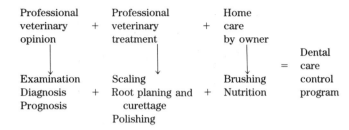

Table 9-2. *Dental Care Control Program*

The veterinarian, as well as the client, must understand that controlling the oral environment is not a one-step procedure, but requires the cooperation of the veterinarian, the animal and the owner.

Professional veterinary opinion	+	Professional veterinary treatment	+	Home care by owner		Dental care control program
↓		↓		↓	=	
Examination Diagnosis Prognosis	+	Scaling Root planing and curettage Polishing	+	Brushing Nutrition		

Preventing the cause of oral disease is more important than treating the disease. An oral examination should be included every time a cat or dog is seen by a veterinarian.

(From Dietrich, V.: Dental care: prophylaxis and therapy. Canine Pract., *3*:44, 1976.)

to animal. The goal is to leave the crown surfaces as smooth as possible. Crown polishing requires the use of pumice in a polishing cup. The most versatile, and least expensive device, is a dental engine with a prophy angle attachment (Fig. 9-2C). I prefer to use medium-grit prophy paste similar to that used in human dentistry for polishing. The prophy cup should be filled with paste and applied with direct pressure to the crown. The engine is started, and the abrasive action of the paste in the cup smoothes out the enamel. When the cup empties, it is refilled with more paste. If the prophy cup is allowed to remain empty, the friction of the latex rubber against the enamel generates damaging heat and fails to polish properly. While all exposed tooth surfaces are polished, particular attention is paid to exposed tooth roots. The cementum and dentinal layers are more porous than enamel and require more aggressive polishing. Bifurcated teeth are polished between the roots with polishing brushes. Periodic rinsing with clear solution helps to clear the operative field.

Postdental recommendations to the client include feeding dry dog food and furnishing chew toys that provide oral exercises and stimulation of the periodontium.

Depending on the rate of plaque accumulation in the animal's mouth, some amount of teeth brushing is required. The areas needing more frequent attention are those adjacent to the openings of the parotid salivary duct. The frequency of teeth brushing may be as high as twice weekly during active episodes of periodontal disease. Toothpaste is not necessary, but a salt and soda dentifrice may be useful. With proper home care, the older animal may require dental prophylaxis on a yearly basis. If the owners fail to brush the pet's teeth

at home, more frequent professional prophylaxis may be required. Table 9-2 outlines a dental care control program for companion animals.

DENTAL EXTRACTIONS

The criterion for determining whether a periodontally involved tooth is salvageable is that at least a third of the periodontium of each root must be healthy. Intraoral radiographs of the affected tooth reveal the status of bone surrounding each tooth root. If one root has abscessed, the whole tooth is lost unless the practitioner is willing to perform endodontic treatment on the salvageable roots after amputating the abscessed root.

The technique for extraction of multirooted teeth involves, first, the isolation of each root. Diamond cutting wheels in the dental engine cut through the enamel crown with ease (Fig. 9-4). Small roots, such as the lingual root of the maxillary fourth premolar, are isolated from the crown with a No. 1 round carbide bur (Fig. 9-5). Next, the gingiva is reflected away from each root, and, if necessary, a small portion of bone is burred away from the cemental enamel junction of the root. Each root is elevated free of its alveolus. Any apical portions left behind are burred out with a No. 4 or 5

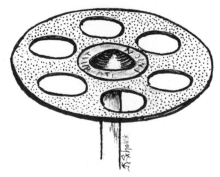

Fig. 9-4. *Diamond cutting wheel.*

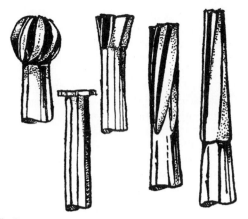

Fig. 9-5. *Basic bur shapes. Left to right, round, wheel, inverted cone, straight plain fissure, and tapered plain fissure.*

round bur or are extracted with root elevators. Recommended closure of the alveolus is with absorbable suture material.

Maxillary or mandibular canine teeth are special situations and are extracted using the following technique: A single incision is made through the gingiva on the buccal surface in the center of the root parallel to the long axis of the root. The incision starts at the gingival sulcus and stops approximately half to two-thirds up the length of the root towards the apical end (Fig. 9-6). The gingiva is reflected laterally. Hemorrhage is usually minimal. Next, a No. 1 round bur in the dental engine is used to remove approximately one-third of the alveolar bone, starting from the cement enamel junction on the buccal surface. Bone is also removed on the mesial and distal surfaces of the root in a similar fashion. Once completed, the periodontium loses a substantial amount of its lateral support. A dental elevator is then used to work around the tooth in its alveolus (Fig. 9-7). With patience, the tooth is "rocked" free and is removed intact (Fig. 9-8). Premature torquing with dental forceps may result in breaking the apical end. Once extracted, the alveolus is closed using a simple interrupted pattern with absorbable suture material

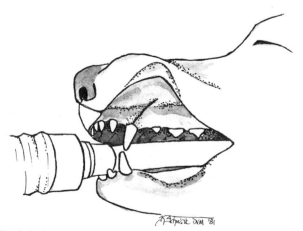

Fig. 9-6. *Canine tooth extraction. The line indicates the incision site along the long axis of the tooth root.*

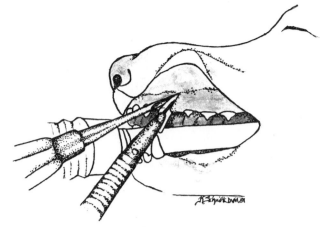

Fig. 9-7. *Canine tooth extraction. A dental elevator and bur are used to work around tooth in its alveolus.*

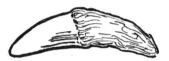

Fig. 9-8. *Extracted canine tooth.*

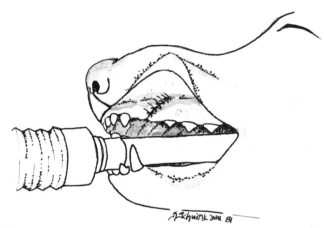

Fig. 9-9. *Canine tooth extraction. The alveolus is sutured closed.*

(Fig. 9-9). Postsurgical antibiotics may be used following dental prophylaxis or extraction when the gingiva is particularly inflamed or infected.

ENDODONTIC TECHNIQUE FOR

CANINE TEETH IN THE DOG

Endodontic therapy following pulpal death is necessary to salvage fractured teeth and prevent apical abscess formation. A major consideration is the cost-effectiveness to the animal's owner.

Inhalation general anesthesia is maintained, and intraoral radiographs of the involved tooth must be taken. If the apical end is intact, an apicoectomy is not performed. An access hole is burred into the mesial surface of the crown, approximately 2 to 4 mm above the gingiva (Figs. 9-10 and 9-11). A small round carbide bur is employed in the low-speed dental engine to

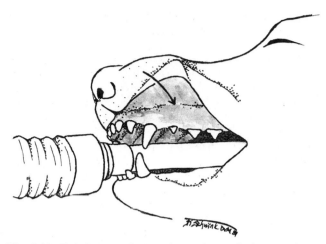

Fig. 9-10. *Endodontic technique for canine teeth. Arrow points to apical abscess draining site.*

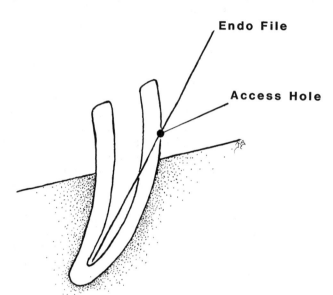

Endo File

Access Hole

Fig. 9-11. *Endodontic technique for canine teeth. Schematic drawing depicts location of access hole and angle of placement of endodontic files for reaming of the pulp chamber.*

create the access hole. Once the access hole is open, reaming of the pulp chamber begins with 50-mm endodontic files. One starts with a No. 10 or No. 15 file and finishes with up to a No. 140 file. Periodically, the tooth is alternately flushed with sodium hypochlorite, then hydrogen peroxide, then saline solution. Reaming continues until all pulp tissues are removed. Next, the tooth is dried with paper points; long type-A points work best. Once the chamber is dried, Tubli-Seal* is mixed on a pad and then is placed in a 3-ml syringe (Luer-Lok) with a 1-inch 22-gauge needle. Approximately .5 to 1 ml of mixture is required to fill the average tooth. The animal's head is placed so the apical end of the tooth is on the "downhill side." The needle is inserted into the access hole as far as it will go, and the Tubli-Seal mixture is expressed into the tooth until full. The needle is slowly backed out of the hole; the Tubli-

*Kerr Manufacturing Co., 28200 Wick Road, Romulus, MI 48174

Seal must fill the pulp chamber. The mixture is then allowed to air dry for approximately 5 minutes. An inverted cone bur is used to carve a seat for amalgam fillings in both the access hole and the fracture site in the crown.

A variation of this technique is employed in the young dog whose tooth has a large pulp chamber, thin dentinal walls, and a closed apical end. Tubli-Seal is used only to fill the apical end. The remaining space is filled with Dycal† to provide additional strength to the crown. The working time with Dycal is short, and a 20-gauge needle is needed to allow delivery, so the practitioner must move quickly. Amalgam is used to finish the procedure as described.

Other Dental Conditions

FRACTURE REPAIR USING
SUBGINGIVAL FIGURE-8 WIRES

Fractures of the maxilla may be repaired with 18-gauge stainless steel wire when premolars or canine teeth are present. Under general anesthesia, the maxillary displacements are manually reduced. A length of heavy stainless steel wire (approximately 2½ times the distance from one fourth premolar around the dental arcade to the other) is measured and cut. Using a 22- or 20-gauge hypodermic needle, a hole is made through the gingiva, up against the bone in the interdental space between the fourth premolar and first molar. Next, a similar hole is placed on the medial side of the canine tooth on the same side of the patient's mouth. A straight line is visualized between these 2 points, and similar holes are placed in the intervening interdental spaces. The wire is passed through the interdental holes in a figure-8 pattern, and this process is continued from one canine tooth to the other by looping wire between every other incisor tooth (Fig. 9-12). A similar technique may be used between the canine tooth and

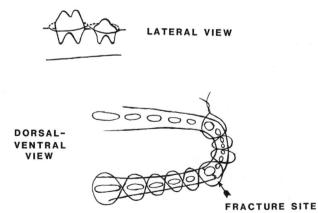

LATERAL VIEW

DORSAL-VENTRAL VIEW

FRACTURE SITE

Fig. 9-12. *Repair of fractured maxilla or mandible using subgingival figure-8 wire.*

†Available from Henry Schein, Inc., 5 Harbor Park Drive, Port Washington, NY 11050

the fourth premolar-first molar interdental space to support more lateral fractures.

After final reduction of maxillary fracture fragments, the wires are tightened until the maxilla is stabilized. The ends of the wires are then twisted together, are trimmed, and are bent flush against the gingiva. If necessary, additional wires are placed diagonally across the hard palate to provide further stability. As the maxilla heals, function returns, and the animal may break some of the wires. Healing generally occurs within 4 to 6 weeks, and the wires are then removed. Normal occlusion is generally maintained with minimal difficulty.

Many fractures of the cranial mandible may be repaired with a similar technique, using the first molars as the anchor points. Care is taken in placing wire so that the maxillary canine teeth do not break the mandibular wire when the animal closes its mouth.

ORONASAL FISTULA

Oronasal fistula formation can occur between the mouth and nose as a result of advanced periodontal disease and tooth loss. The maxillary canine tooth is commonly involved. If the practitioner discovers a deep periodontal pocket on the lingual surface of the root, a "bloody nose test" is performed. Aggressive root planing is started. If the alveolear septal bone is intact, root planing will not cause nasal hemorrhage. If the bone is eroded, however, root planing results in a "bloody nose." Without the septal bone, no chance for periodontal healing exists, and tooth loss is certain. It is then better to extract the tooth and to suture the alveolus closed than to allow the destructive process to continue. If the tooth passes the bloody nose test, and the owner is willing, a program of frequent root planing and home care may maintain the tooth for a considerable time.

Those animals with a large and established fistula may require several operations to close the fistula. The basic technique involves creating a periosteal-mucosal flap and is described in the previous section of this chapter.

References and Suggested Readings

1. Colmery, B.: Pathophysiology in Small Animal Surgery. Edited by M. Joseph Bojrab. Philadelphia, Lea & Febiger, 1981.
2. Dietrich, V.: Dental care: prophylaxis and therapy. Canine Pract., *3*:44, 1976.

Surgical Management of Selected Neoplasms of the Canine Oral Cavity

by KENNETH M. GREENWOOD

An organized approach, coupled with good communication between client and veterinarian, is necessary for the satisfactory management of oral neoplasia. Often, the animal is not presented to the veterinarian until tissue involvement is extensive and the possibility of metastasis is great. The client may still strongly desire to attempt some form of treatment, even if it is only palliative.

Each case of oral neoplasia must be managed individually. Considerations include the type of neoplasia present, the site and extent of tissue involvement, and the willingness of the patient's owner to agree to treatment regimens that can, in some cases, be lengthy and expensive. Most animals do not die of the direct effect of neoplasia in the oral cavity or of metastatic spread, but rather as a result of euthanasia performed either because they are uncomfortable and are eating poorly or because the neoplastic mass has become foul smelling and unsightly. If surgical excision is possible, the results are generally acceptable to the client and frequently relieve the animal's discomfort. The object of excisional surgery is to remove as much neoplastic tissue as possible while maintaining functional oral anatomy. Total excision may sometimes be accomplished, but even if the operation is only palliative, euthanasia can often be delayed for as much as 6 months to a year. The following surgical techniques outline possible ways for the veterinary surgeon to attempt excision of oral neoplastic masses.

In many instances, tissue involvement is so extensive that surgical excision cannot be employed. For example, neoplasia of the periodontal tissues of the upper dental arcade that invades underlying maxillary bone often cannot be surgically excised, nor can infiltrating pharyngeal masses. Radiation therapy, chemotherapy, immunotherapy, and cryosurgery should be considered when planning a management regimen. Their use as primary treatment or in conjunction with surgical excision has been described elsewhere. General application to specific tumor types is indicated in this discussion, and the reader is encouraged to consult specific references for details.[1,4,5,7-9,12]

Common Oral Neoplasms

The two oral tumors that are generally classified as benign are viral papilloma and epulis. Viral papillomas are seen primarily in dogs less than a year old. Treatment is generally unnecessary because regression is spontaneous. If large growths interfere with mastication, they can be removed using a scalpel, electroscalpel, or cryosurgical techniques.[2] Epulides arise from periodontal tissue. These tumors are generally easily excised with a scalpel or an electroscalpel. A form known as acanthomatous epulis has been shown to have the potential to infiltrate locally into bone.[3] Surgical excision must include the removal of all involved bone and soft tissue. If total excision is not possible, radiation therapy can be employed with satisfactory results.

Odontogenic neoplasms such as adamantinoma and ameloblastic odontoma are occasionally seen. Tissue involvement can be extensive locally, but metastasis is not a problem.[10] If total en bloc excision is possible, a surgical cure can be accomplished. These tumors are also radiosensitive.[8]

Squamous cell carcinoma, malignant melanoma, and fibrosarcoma are the most commonly seen malignant oral neoplasms. Unfortunately, it is rare to eradicate any of these three tumors completely with any treatment regimen. The client must be made aware of the high probability of local recurrence and metastasis. Primary surgical excision should be attempted if possible. Squamous cell carcinomas are sensitive to radiation therapy, and postsurgical irradiation can be helpful. When surgical excision is not possible, radiation alone can be employed.

Malignant melanomas respond poorly to either radiation or chemotherapy. Cryosurgery has been used, but recurrence is common.[5] Melanomas metastasize early, and even if total excision is possible, the animal will likely have complications from metastasis. Successful excision, however, can allow the dog to live comfortably until complications arise from metastatic lesions. Fibrosarcomas do not tend to metastasize. These tumors are extremely invasive locally, and total excision is difficult. Cryosurgery, chemotherapy, and radiation therapy also are rarely effective. Unless the growth is detected early and total excision is possible, treatment can only be aimed at palliative management of the local lesion.

Initial Management

The initial physical examination of the animal presented because of an oral mass should include close inspection of the entire oropharyngeal cavity and palpation of all regional lymph nodes. Thoracic radiographs should be taken to evaluate the lung tissue for metastatic lesions. It is imperative to know whether distant metastasis is present when talking to the client about any treatment regimen.

A complete blood count should be obtained. It is most important to know the hematocrit and plasma total solids if an operation or even just a biopsy is planned. Hemorrhage can be expected during surgical manipulation, and the patient's initial blood values may be lower than normal owing to previous bleeding episodes from an ulcerated neoplastic mass. If the initial hematocrit is lower than 30%, whole blood should be available for transfusion.

Biopsy and Radiography

Prognosis and possible treatment regimens can be formulated only when an accurate diagnosis has been made. Histopathologic examination of the oral neoplasia is necessary for proper identification of the tumor type. Because it is also necessary to know whether adjacent bone is involved, a radiographic study of the region should be made.

General anesthesia is necessary when attempting to obtain a diagnostic biopsy and radiographic study. Anesthetic maintenance with an inhalation agent by means of endotracheal intubation is suggested. Care

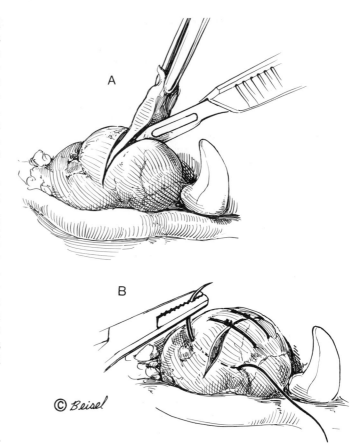

Fig. 9-13. A, *A deep incisional biopsy specimen is removed from the mass.* B, *Large simple interrupted sutures are placed to control hemorrhage and to close the defect.*

should be taken to ensure that the endotracheal tube is not superimposed on the neoplastic lesion when the radiographs are taken. It may be necessary to remove the endotracheal tube for short periods when radiographs are exposed.

A deep incisional biopsy is necessary for accurate histopathologic diagnosis. A biopsy that consists only of superficial tissue may include nothing more than granulation tissue and inflamed mucosa. A narrow wedge biopsy should be taken using a scalpel blade. The incisions should extend a minimum of 1 cm into the neoplastic tissue (Fig. 9-13A). The electroscalpel should not be used because the heat from this instrument destroys cellular architecture. When the tissue has been removed, hemorrhage is controlled using direct pressure and electrocautery. Large simple interrupted sutures of 2-0 polyglactin 910* are used to close the defect (Fig. 9-13B). Sutures are placed directly into neoplastic tissue. This tissue is usually friable, and a large amount of tissue should be included in each suture. The tension placed on the tissue by the sutures also controls any residual bleeding from the biopsy site.

*Vicryl, Ethicon, Inc., Somerville, NJ 08876

Planning Surgical Management

The type of tumor, the extent of infiltration, and the location of the tumor within the oral cavity all must be considered when formulating a treatment regimen. Small masses involving the periodontal tissue, hard palate, soft palate, or gingiva can often be totally excised at the time of biopsy. Soft- and hard-palate masses of larger proportions can be excised as described in the next few paragraphs. Neoplasia that invades the bony structure of the maxilla or is deep into the pharyngeal region generally cannot be managed surgically. Mandibular neoplasia that arises from periodontal tissue can often be managed surgically. The two mandibular techniques described in the following paragraphs maintain functional jaw anatomy. Although not discussed here, satisfactory results have been obtained with total and hemimandibulectomies.[13]

Anesthesia and Presurgical Preparation

General anesthesia is maintained with an inhalation agent by means of a cuffed endotracheal tube. When the endotracheal tube interferes with surgical manipulation, the tube can be made to exit through a pharyngotomy incision (Fig. 9-14).[6] This incision is made as described in Chapter 11, in the section on pharyngostomy. At the completion of the surgical procedure, the tube is removed and the incision is allowed to heal by second intention.

Lactated Ringer's solution should be administered intravenously during the procedure. A hematocrit may be obtained at least once during the operation and again during recovery. If hemorrhage is extensive, intravenous administration of whole blood may be necessary. When the endotracheal tube has been placed, the oral cavity is flushed with copious amounts of 1 part

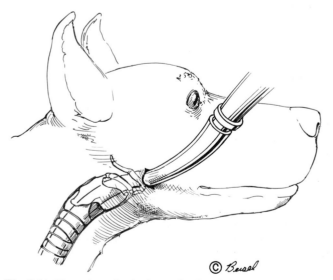

Fig. 9-14. *The endotracheal tube can be placed through a pharyngotomy incision.*

1% organic iodine complex solution* to 20 parts sterile saline solution. The patient's chin and muzzle should be clipped and scrubbed in routine surgical fashion.

Excision of Soft- and Hard-Palate Tumors

Masses located within the soft palate can best be removed by palatectomy. Any amount of the palate can be removed. A margin of normal tissue at least .5-cm wide should be removed with the tumor mass.

Temporary stay sutures of 3-0 chromic gut are placed in the soft palate to aid in retracting the tissue into the oral cavity to allow surgical manipulation (Fig. 9-15A). The entire soft-palate incision should not be made at one time. A 1- or 2-cm full-thickness incision is made and is then closed with a continuous suture pattern of 4-0 polyglactin 910.† This process is continued until the entire length of the soft palate incision has been made (Fig. 9-15B and C). Exact apposition of the mucosal edges is not necessary. Hemorrhage is controlled as sutures are placed. When excision and suturing are complete, any remaining bleeding may be controlled by direct pressure. Removal of large portions of the entire soft palate allows reflux of food and water into the nasopharynx. The dog may have a chronic nasal discharge as a result of the absence of the soft palate; however, this complication is rarely life-threatening.

When a hard-palate mass appears to be localized and does not invade the underlying bone, an elliptical incision should be made .5 to 1 cm away from the edge of the tumor. This incision should extend down to the underlying bone. An electroscalpel should be used if available. A periosteal elevator is then used to lift the involved section of palate tissue from the bone (Fig. 9-16). Hemorrhage is controlled by electrocautery and direct pressure. The large palatine vessels arising from the palatine foramina must be ligated if they are severed during the dissection. The wound cannot be closed and is allowed to heal by granulation.

The animal should be fed a gruel during the healing period. When the animal has eaten, the mouth should be flushed with fresh water to remove all food debris from the surgical site. When the defect is massive, alimentation by means of a pharyngostomy tube can be beneficial during the first 2 weeks following the operation.

Excision of the Rostral Mandible

Neoplastic masses that arise from the region of the lower incisor teeth and invade mandibular bone can be excised by removing the entire rostral portion of the mandible. The mandibular symphysis extends caudally to the level of the first root of the second premolar teeth. The rostral mandible can be amputated just caudal to the first premolar teeth. The remainder of the

*Prepodyne solution, West Chemical Products, Inc., New York, NY
†Vicryl, Ethicon, Inc., Somerville, NJ 08876

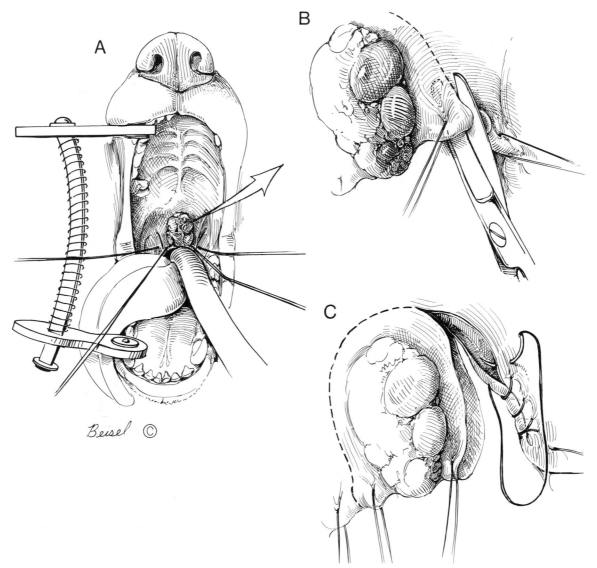

Fig. 9-15. A, *Stay sutures in the caudal edge of the soft palate retract the soft palate into the oral cavity.* B, *A portion of the excision is made using scissors.* C, *A continuous suture pattern is placed in the cut edge of the soft palate followed by a stepwise completion of the remaining excision.*

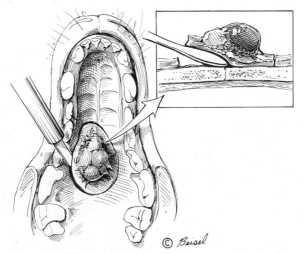

Fig. 9-16. *A circumferential incision is made around the hard palate mass, and the tissue is elevated from the underlying bone.*

jaw is left in a functional state, and the results are cosmetically acceptable.

An incision is made in the buccal mucosa around the rostral lip. At the level of the first premolar tooth on each side, the incision is extended over to the alveolar ridge of the mandible. The chin skin is then reflected from the rostral mandible using sharp dissection along a shallow subcutaneous plane (Fig. 9-17A). As much subcutaneous tissue as possible should be left with the rostral mandible to increase the chance of excising the neoplasia totally. Hemorrhage is best controlled by electrocautery. Large mental vessels will be encountered and may require ligation.

An incision is then made in the mucosa of the floor of the mouth on a line between the first premolar teeth. This incision crosses rostral to the lingual frenulum. The base of the lingual frenulum must be avoided because it contains the orifices of the mandibular and sublingual salivary ducts (Fig. 9-17B). The mucosa is

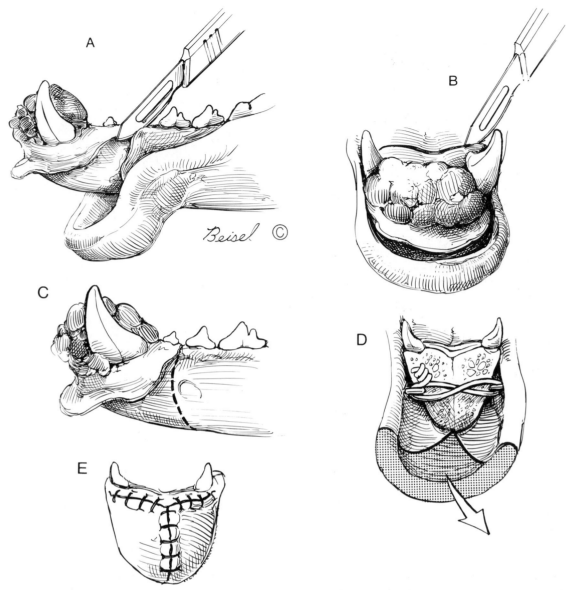

Fig. 9-17. A, *When an incision has been made in the rostral buccal mucosa, the chin skin is reflected ventrally.* B, *An incision is made across the floor of the oral cavity rostral to the lingual frenulum.* C, *The rostral mandible is excised caudal to the first premolar teeth.* D, *The mandibular bodies are fixed to each other. A pie-piece wedge of chin skin is removed to allow cosmetic closure.* E, *Chin skin is apposed using simple interrupted nonabsorbable sutures. The buccal mucosal edge is sutured to the mucosal edge of the floor of the oral cavity.*

reflected from the mandible for a short distance caudal to the incision.

A bone saw, Gigli wire, or air-driven bur is then used to amputate the rostral mandible en bloc immediately caudal to the first premolar teeth (Fig. 9-17C). Any remaining portion of the canine teeth root tips should be removed using a tooth root elevator. Hemorrhage from mental and alveolar vessels is controlled by electrocautery and ligation. The rostral ventral edge of the mandibular bodies is rounded using a rongeur or air-driven bur, to give a more cosmetic look to the reconstructed chin.

The mandibular bodies must be fixed to one another because a majority of the symphysis has been removed. This fixation is accomplished by placing a Kirschner wire horizontally across the 2 mandibular bodies. The

Kirschner wire is allowed to protrude approximately 2 mm on each side. Twenty- or 22-gauge wire is then placed in a figure-8 fashion to give compression across the stabilized symphysis (Fig. 9-17D).

The chin skin is then prepared for coverage of the shortened mandible. A "pie-piece" wedge is removed from the rostral center of the skin flap (Fig. 9-17D). Enough skin is left to allow the rostral most points to meet when the skin is brought back up around the mandible. The skin edges are sutured with 3-0 nonabsorbable suture material in a simple interrupted pattern. Mucosal surfaces are apposed using simple interrupted sutures of 4-0 polyglactin 910 (Fig. 9-17E). Complete intraoral closure of all mucosal surfaces should be achieved, and ventral drainage is rarely necessary.

The animal is allowed oral intake of water and soft gruel the day after operation. The surgical site should be kept free of debris by flushing the mouth with fresh water a minimum of 3 times a day. The client should be warned that the dog's tongue will hang out more than normal, and a minor amount of drooling may occur. The animal adjusts to the shortened jaw without problems, and the results should be acceptable to the owner. Skin sutures are removed 14 days after the surgical procedure. The mucosal sutures are allowed to be absorbed and are sloughed with time.

Excision of Periodontal Mandibular Body Neoplasia

Periodontal neoplasia in the region of the mandibular premolar and molar teeth can be excised en bloc with surrounding alveolar bone and associated teeth. If at least the ventral third of the mandibular body appears normal on radiographs, then excision can be attempted and a functional jaw will be maintained.

An incision is made in both the lingual and labial mandibular mucosa .5 cm outside the margins of the neoplastic mass. These incisions should join rostrally and caudally over the alveolar ridge at interdental spaces free of neoplastic tissue. The mucosa is reflected from the mandibular body using a periosteal elevator. An air-driven bur is then used to cut completely across the mandibular body in an arc below the neoplastic tissue (Fig. 9-18A). The amount of tissue removed is determined by visual inspection and the extent of bone infiltration as seen radiographically. The segment of bone, teeth, and soft tissue is removed en bloc (Fig. 9-18B). Excessive hemorrhage can be expected from alveolar vasculature. Once the resected segment is removed, hemorrhage is controlled by electrocautery and ligation. Any remaining tooth root tips are extracted using a tooth root elevator.

The labial mucosal edge is mobilized and is pulled medially so as to cover the exposed defect in the mandibular body. The labial and lingual mucosal edges are then apposed using simple interrupted sutures of 4-0 polyglactin 910* (Fig. 9-18C). Postsurgical care is the same as after amputation of the rostral mandible. The client should be warned that the animal's jaw is weaker than normal and that bone chewing and rough playing should not be allowed.

Postsurgical Monitoring

The animal should be examined at 2-week intervals during the first 2 months after the operation and then at intervals of no longer than 2 months. Any return of the neoplasia will be detected early, and an additional surgical procedure is sometimes possible. Local and regional submandibular and retropharyngeal lymph nodes should be palpated for the presence of tumor metastasis.

*Vicryl, Ethicon, Inc., Somerville, NJ 08876

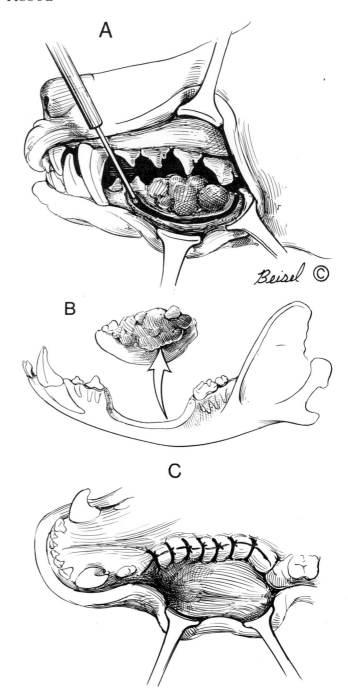

Fig. 9-18. A, *When the lingual and labial mucosal incisions are made and the mucosa is reflected from the bone, an air-driven bur is used to cut the mandibular body.* B, *The entire segment of involved mandible is removed en bloc.* C, *The labial mucosal edge is sutured to the lingual mucosal edge.*

Surgical cure of benign oral neoplasms is possible. Total local excision of malignant oral neoplasia is also possible; however, metastasis present at the time of operation often eventually causes the death of the animal. An excisional surgical procedure alone or in combination with other cancer therapy techniques offers the advantage of eliminating unsightly neoplastic masses that might otherwise be the reason for early euthanasia of the afflicted pet.

References and Suggested Readings

1. Banks, W. C., and Morris, E.: Results of radiation treatment of naturally occurring animal tumors. J. Am. Vet. Med. Assoc., *166*:1063, 1975.
2. Clifford, D. H., and Clark, J. J.: The mouth. *In* Canine Surgery. 2nd Ed. Edited by J. Archibald. Santa Barbara, CA, American Veterinary Publications, 1974.
3. Dubielzeg, R. R., Goldschmidt, M. H., and Brodey, R. S.: The nomenclature of periodontal epulides in dogs. Vet. Pathol., *16*:209, 1979.
4. Gillette E. L.: Radiation Therapy. Current Veterinary Therapy VI: Small Animal Practice. Edited by Robert W. Kirk. Philadelphia, W. B. Saunders, 1977.
5. Goldstein, R. S., and Hess, P. W.: Cryosurgery of canine and feline tumors. J. Am. Anim. Hosp. Assoc., *12*:340, 1976.
6. Hartsfield, S. M., et al.: Endotracheal intubation by pharyngotomy. J. Am. Anim. Hosp. Assoc., *13*:71, 1977.
7. Hess, P. W.: Principles of cancer chemotherapy. Vet. Clin. North Am., *7*:21, 1977.
8. Langham, F. R., Mostosky, U. V., and Schirmer, R. G.: X-ray therapy of selected odontogenic neoplasms in the dog. J. Am. Vet. Med. Assoc., *170*:820, 1977.
9. MacEwen, E. G.: General concepts of immunotherapy of tumors. J. Am. Anim. Hosp. Assoc., *12*:363, 1976.
10. Moulton, J. E.: Tumors in Domestic Animals. Los Angeles, University of California Press, 1978.
11. Theilen, G. H., and Madewell, B. R.: Veterinary Cancer Medicine. Philadelphia, Lea & Febiger, 1979.
12. Thrall, D. E., and Biery, D. N.: Principles and application of radiation therapy. Vet. Clin. North Am., *7*:35, 1977.
13. Withrow, S. J.: Mandibulectomy in treatment of oral cancer. J. Am. Anim. Hosp. Assoc. In press.

$10 *$ Salivary Glands

Salivary Gland

by JOHN J. LAMMERDING

Diseases of the salivary gland in small animals can be classified generally as inflammatory, neoplastic, or traumatic.

Sialadenitis is seen occasionally in dogs and cats. If the gland is abscessed, ventral drainage becomes necessary. Infrequently, inflammation or abscess formation can be associated with foreign body migration. In this case, removal of the foreign body with establishment of drainage is indicated.

Salivary gland tumors are not common in small animals. Salivary gland adenocarcinoma has been reported infrequently, and I have seen it in only two dogs, in association with salivary mucoceles. In these two cases, the tumor involved the mandibular salivary gland and responded to gland removal and drainage of the mucocele. The mandibular and parotid salivary glands are reportedly the most commonly involved with neoplasia in dogs and cats. Mandibular gland adenocarcinomas carry a favorable prognosis with complete surgical removal if metastasis has not occurred. Preoperative chest radiographs and intraoperative biopsy of the mandibular lymph nodes are indicated in these animals. Parotid salivary gland tumors are more difficult to remove completely surgically and, therefore, have a more guarded prognosis.

Trauma to the parotid duct from bite wounds is seen occasionally in cats and dogs. Subsequent to wounding, a small fistula develops and produces a serous salivary secretion. A primary anastomosis may be attempted, but simple ligation of the duct proximal to the fistula with 4-0 monofilament nylon or polypropylene is an effective treatment. The wound should also be properly drained.

Mucoceles and Ranulas

It is believed that rupture of the sublingual salivary ducts results in the formation of a salivary mucocele. The injury may be due to trauma or to unknown causes. These mucoceles, or accumulations of saliva, can occur in various ways. A ranula is a sublingual mucocele. A cervical mucocele is first seen as an external swelling, which may vary in size, in the ventral neck area. A pharyngeal mucocele, which develops as a swelling in the pharyngeal wall that may cause airway obstruction, may require emergency evacuation and marsupialization. Mucoceles are usually seen as painless, fluctuant swellings. Initially, some pain may exist from tissue irritation by saliva, but this phase is rarely part of the clinical presentation.

DIAGNOSIS

The diagnosis of salivary mucocele is not always easy, especially if the swelling has been previously aspirated or injected. In these cases, it may be difficult to differentiate between a mucocele and a cervical abscess. Diagnosis should depend on the patient's medical history, a complete physical examination, and the character of the fluid obtained after aseptic aspiration of the swelling. This fluid may be straw-colored to blood-tinged and is viscid.

A consistently effective treatment for cervical salivary mucocele is removal of the affected mandibular and sublingual glandular chain and duct. Therefore, it is necessary to determine on which side the lesion appears. This determination may be obvious, or it may require careful observation and palpation of the mucocele with the animal under anesthesia in dorsal recumbency. Application of pressure to the ventral swelling may also cause the sublingual area to swell and may help to locate the lesion.

If the lesion cannot be located physically, sialography by cannulation of the sublingual ducts may be helpful. Leakage from the duct is sometimes demonstrated by radiographic contrast studies. Alternately, the mucocele may be incised and evacuated, and the side may be determined by observation of communication between the mucocele and the salivary tissue. One may also elect to remove the mandibular, sublingual chains bilaterally without locating the side on which the lesion appears. Sufficient saliva from the zygomatic and parotid salivary glands is present to allow proper chewing and swallowing.

SURGICAL TECHNIQUE

It is wise to review the important and complex anatomy of this area before performing the operation. The surgical procedure for removal of the mandibular and sublingual salivary glands and their duct requires general anesthesia, wide clipping of the mandibular and cervical areas, and preparation for an aseptic operation. The dog is positioned in oblique lateral recumbency with a sandbag directly under the proposed incision line. A linear incision is made between the linguofacial vein and the maxillary vein near the point at which they join to form the jugular vein at the angle of the jaw (Fig. 10-1). The platysma muscle is divided, and the common capsule of the mandibular and sublingual glands is identified deep to the veins. A branch of the second cervical nerve crosses the capsule and should be preserved. The capsule is opened, and the mandibular gland is grasped with an instrument. Caudolateral traction is carefully applied (Fig. 10-2) while

sharp and blunt dissection around the sublingual glandular chain and salivary duct is also conducted in a craniomedial direction.

The major blood supply to the mandibular gland is from the glandular branch of the facial artery, which enters the gland where the mandibular duct leaves it. The dorsal part of the deep surface of the gland also accepts branches from the great auricular artery. The major vein also leaves the deep surface of the gland. All these major vessels require ligation.

The dissection is carried to the digastricus muscle. At this point, if the communication of the glandular tissue with the mucocele is not obvious, the sublingual glandular chain may be passed from lateral to medial beneath the digastricus muscle and the dissection continued rostrally (Fig. 10-3). Care must be taken to avoid

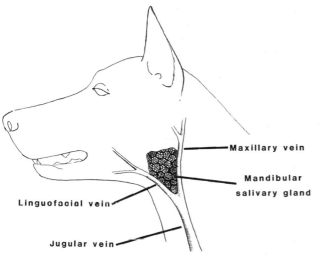

Fig. 10-1. *Schematic drawing of anatomic relationships in mandibular and cervical area. A linear incision is made between the linguofacial vein and the maxillary vein near the point where they join to form the jugular vein.*

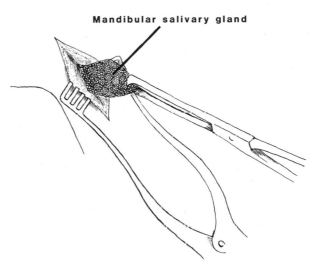

Fig. 10-2. *The platysma muscle is divided, and the common capsule of the mandibular and sublingual glands is opened to allow caudolateral retraction of the mandibular salivary gland.*

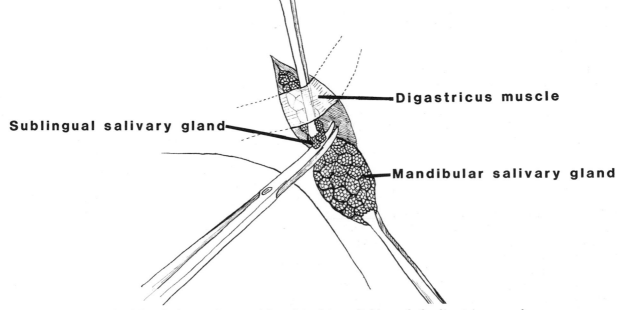

Fig. 10-3. *The sublingual glandular chain may be passed from lateral to medial beneath the digastricus muscle.*

injury to the hypoglossal and lingual nerves as well as to the external carotid and lingual arteries. The common salivary duct is ligated after passing a ligature as far rostral to the termination of the sublingual chain as possible.

It is not necessary to remove the mucocele, which is technically a foreign body granuloma, because it does not have a secretory epithelial lining. A quarter-inch Penrose drain may be placed to drain both the primary incision and the mucocele. Closure consists of absorbable interrupted sutures in the platysma muscle or subcutaneous tissue, and skin closure. The drain may be removed in 3 to 5 days. Complications can include seroma formation, recurrence of the mucocele, and local infection.

MARSUPIALIZATION FOR INTRAORAL MUCOCELES

Marsupialization has also been reported to be an effective treatment for ranulas and pharyngeal muco-celes. Mandibular and sublingual gland and duct removal are performed in case of failure of the marsupialization. The technique is performed by simply removing a section of the mucocele wall in an effort to create a permanent fistula from the ranulas or mucocele to the oral cavity. This procedure seems to be more effective in treating pharyngeal mucoceles than ranulas.

References and Suggested Readings

Evans, H. E., and Christensen, G. C.: Miller's Anatomy of the Dog. 2nd Ed. Philadelphia, W. B. Saunders, 1979.

Harvey, C. E., and Obrien, J. A.: Disorders of the oropharynx and salivary glands. *In* Textbook of Veterinary Internal Medicine: Diseases of the Dog and Cat. Edited by S. J. Ettinger. Philadelphia, W. B. Saunders, 1975.

Harvey, H. J.: Pharyngeal mucocoeles in dogs, J. Am. Vet. Med. Assoc., *178*:1282, 1981.

Hoffer, R. E.: Surgical treatment of salivary mucocoele. Vet. Clin. North Am., *5*:333, 1975.

11 * Esophagus

Conservative Management of Esophageal Foreign Bodies

by MAX G. EASOM

Esophageal foreign bodies are commonly seen in veterinary practice. Many of these cases present a unique challenge to the veterinarian, who must understand appropriate current surgical techniques and aspects of conservative treatment. Most recent literature indicates that veterinary and human surgeons prefer conservative management to surgical removal of esophageal foreign bodies in their patients.[2,4-7,11-16]

Signs and Diagnosis

Signs of esophageal obstruction can vary, depending on the location and the length of time the foreign body has been in place. Initially, patients usually exhibit drooling, gagging, and recurrent retching. In acute cases, regurgitation can occur 5 to 15 minutes after eating. As the obstruction becomes more chronic, the attitude of the animal may become anxious or depressed. Anorexia, dehydration, and weight loss are often seen. In chronic cases of partial obstruction, electrolyte disturbances or infections can be life-threatening. Secondary effects of esophageal foreign bodies may be mucosal lacerations, esophagitis, esophageal necrosis, pleuritis, mediastinitis, pyothorax and pneumothorax.[15] Such complications generally present a life-threatening therapeutic dilemma.

A routine data base of a complete blood cell count, blood chemistry and electrolyte evaluations, and radiography is mandatory for all seriously ill patients. Radiography is useful in assessing both the location and type of foreign body. Contrast studies of the esophagus are needed to depict mucosal tears and radiolucent foreign bodies. If a mucosal tear is suspected, an aqueous iodinated contrast medium is used for the examination.

Esophageal foreign bodies commonly lodge in 4 sites: the pharyngeal esophagus, the thoracic inlet, the base of the heart, and the esophageal hiatal region. The cervical region of the esophagus appears to be most prone to obstruction in the dog. The "closed" approach to dislodgment and retrieval of an esophageal foreign body should always be attempted before surgical intervention.[5-7,11,13-15] One study of 66 cases revealed that only 6 actually required surgical removal.[15] One report from the human literature showed a 38% mortality rate in a group treated surgically, as opposed to a 9% mortality rate in a conservatively treated group.[13]

The most important aspect of conservative management of this disorder is a complete evaluation of the patient. Some animals may not be able to tolerate therapeutic procedures that necessitate general anesthesia. In these animals, intravenous fluids and antibiotics are initial, lifesaving therapy.

Surgical Procedures

The treatment of choice for esophageal foreign bodies is esophagoscopy and forceps delivery. With the aid of an endoscope, the veterinarian can assess the character of the foreign body and, more important, the extent of damage to the esophagus. This direct examination should be correlated with the patient's medical history, physical findings, and radiographic examinations.

Numerous techniques of esophagoscopy have been reported.[3,8,15,16] Regardless of technique employed, careful instrumentation of the esophagus is necessary to prevent iatrogenic injury. Many surgical supply companies offer flexible fiberoptic scopes that are excellent for use in animals. With flexible scopes, the veterinarian can evaluate the clinical condition of his patient both quickly and safely. In some areas, local veterinary associations have purchased endoscopes for use by members; this practice reduces the expense to individual veterinarians and makes a valuable diagnostic tool accessible. Rigid-scope endoscopy is also useful for visualizing obstruction. Alligator forceps passed through rigid tubular endoscopes are useful in dislodgment and retrieval.

Another technique is retraction of the esophageal wall by a Foley urethral catheter.[7,11,12] In general, this procedure should be reserved for blunt esophageal foreign bodies. The procedure consists of passing a Foley catheter with a stylet in place past the foreign body and inflating the catheter bulb with radiographic contrast media. Radiographs ascertain the correct position of the inflated cuff. In some cases, gentle retraction of the catheter dislodges blunt foreign bodies and pulls them forward into the oral cavity. Another method of conservative care is to use a rigid endoscope or a large-bore plastic tube to push obstructions into the stomach. This technique must be elected with extreme care in the case of sharp objects, for obvious reasons.

The key to successful conservative therapy for esophageal obstruction is prompt recognition of complications. If a mucosal laceration is diagnosed within 24 hours of occurrence, a surgical procedure is indicated in most instances. During this period, the patient is at less of an anesthetic risk, and secondary complications from contamination may be minimized with aggressive therapy. In 36 to 48 hours, a more conservative approach is indicated. One study indicated a mortality rate greater than 50% in patients operated after 24 hours of esophageal perforation.[6] Complications from foreign bodies located in the thoracic esophagus are more serious than those in the cervical esophagus because diffuse mediastinitis, pleuritis, pyothorax, and pneumothorax are commonly seen with thoracic esophageal perforations.

The essence of treatment is supportive care; all oral intake should be stopped. Dehydration and electrolyte disturbances should be adjusted with appropriate fluid therapy. Antibiotics are routinely given to these patients. Clindamycin and cephalosporins are effective against the aerobes and anaerobes commonly encountered in the oral cavity and gastrointestinal tract. Corticosteroids may be necessary in the critically ill patient. If the pleural space is contaminated, chest drainage by tube thoracostomy must be instituted and may be lifesaving in many cases. Pharyngostomy tubes have been found to be useful in maintaining a positive nitrogen balance in animals and in providing esophageal bypass, so that infection can be controlled and wound healing encouraged.[1,4,6,10] Once a patient's condition is stabilized and the foreign body is removed, more definitive surgical procedures may be considered, although such procedures are not usually necessary.

References and Suggested Readings

1. Balkany, T. J., and Bloustein, P. A.: Cervical esophagostomy in dogs; endoscopic, radiographic, and histopathologic evaluation of esophagitis induced by feeding tubes. Ann. Otol. Rhinol. Laryngol., 86:588, 1977.
2. Behar, J.: Reflux esophagitis; pathogenesis, diagnosis, and management. Arch. Intern. Med., 136:560, 1976.
3. Berry, H. L.: Gastrointestinal Panendoscopy. Springfield, IL, Charles C Thomas, 1974.
4. Böhning, R. H., et al.: Pharyngostomy for maintenance of the anorectic animal. J. Am. Vet. Med. Assoc., 156:611, 1970.
5. Brown, R. H., and Cohen, P. S.: Nonsurgical management of spontaneous esophageal perforation. JAMA, 240:140, 1978.
6. Cameron, J. L., and Kieffer, R. F.: Selective nonoperative management of contained intrathoracic esophageal disruptions. Ann. Thorac. Surg., 27:404, 1979.
7. Campbell, J. E., and Davis, W. S.: Catheter technique for extraction of blunt esophageal foreign bodies. Radiology, 108:438, 1973.
8. Demling, L., and Otterjann, R.: Endoscopy and Biopsy of the Esophagus and Stomach: A Color Atlas. Philadelphia, W. B. Saunders, 1972.
9. Dodman, N. H., and Baker, G. J.: Tracheoesophageal fistula as a complication of an oesophageal foreign body in the dog—a case report. J. Small Anim. Pract., 19:291, 1978.
10. Freeman, D. E., and Naylor, J. M.: Cervical esophagostomy to permit extraoral feeding of the horse. J. Am. Vet. Med. Assoc., 172:314, 1977.
11. Henry, L. N., and Chamberlain, J. W.: Removal of foreign bodies from esophagus and nose with the use of a Foley catheter. Surgery, 71:918, 1972.
12. Kretschmer, K. P.: Another useful application of the balloon tipped Fogarty catheter. Am. J. Surg., 122:417, 1971.
13. Lyons, W. S., et al.: Ruptures and perforations of the esophagus: the case for conservative supportive management. Ann. Thorac. Surg., 25:346, 1978.
14. Mengoli, L. R., and Klassen, K. P.: Conservative management of esophageal perforation. Arch. Surg., 91:238, 1965.
15. Ryan, W. W., and Greene, R. W.: The conservative management of esophageal foreign bodies and their complications. J. Am. Anim. Hosp. Assoc., 11:243, 1975.
16. Wirtschafter, M. Z.: Successful recovery of a foreign body from the forestomach of a dolphin by preoral endoscopy. Gastrointest. Endosc., 23:156, 1977.

Cricopharyngeal Dysphagia

by Eberhard Rosin

Cricopharyngeal dysphagia, although an uncommon condition, is considered in the differential diagnosis of persistent dysphagia of young dogs. This condition is characterized by inadequate or asynchronous relaxation of the cricopharyngeal sphincter that prevents the normal movement of food from caudal portions of the pharynx into the cranial esophagus. The etiologic basis of this failure of reflex relaxation has not been established. Dogs with cricopharyngeal dysphagia usually have a history of dysphagia persisting since weaning. Attempts to swallow solid food result in anxiety, gagging, and expulsion of food from the mouth by forward movements of the tongue. After repeated ingestion of the masticated food, the entire meal passes into the stomach.

Diagnosis

Except for slight nasal exudate and occasional coughing, physical examination reveals no abnormality. Examination of the pharynx reveals no inflammatory or obstructive lesions. Under anesthesia, an esophagoscope can be passed into the stomach without difficulty. The resting pressure provided by the closed sphincter, as encountered by passage of the endoscope and as measured by manometry, is normal.

Radiographs of a barium swallow study reveal contrast material remaining in the pharynx. In some dogs, barium is aspirated into the lungs. Fluoroscopic examination of a barium swallow demonstrates normal movement of the barium bolus into the oropharynx by elevation of the tongue and contraction of the pharyngeal musculature. Despite the presence of sufficient force to distend the caudal pharyngeal wall, inadequate or asynchronous relaxation of the cricopharyngeal sphincter prevents normal movement of the barium bolus into the proximal esophagus. The thin stream of barium that passes through the sphincter moves into the stomach with no evidence of failure of reflex relaxation of the gastroesophageal sphincter. This cycle is repeated in rapid succession until all the barium is swallowed. As the epiglottis, which closes the glottis in normal fashion during swallowing attempts, opens during inspiration, the residual barium filling the caudal pharyngeal region may be aspirated into the trachea and discharged by coughing.

Immediate relief of the dysphagia is achieved by cricopharyngeal myectomy. Complete division of muscle fibers of the cricopharyngeal muscle is essential for permanent elimination of the condition.

Technique for Cricopharyngeal Myectomy

The dog is anesthetized, intubated, and placed in dorsal recumbency. A midline incision is made from the cranial aspect of the larynx to the thoracic inlet. Exposure of the trachea and esophagus is by midline dissection of the ventral neck musculature. Partial incision of the insertion of fibers of the sternohyoid muscle on the basihyoid bone may be necessary. The bisected sternohyoid muscle is retracted with Allis tissue forceps to expose the trachea. Dissection is continued to the left of the trachea by transection of the insertion of the left sternothyroid muscle to the lateral surface of the thyroid lamina. The left thyroid gland is exposed between the trachea and the sternothyroid muscle. Several small branches of the cranial thyroid artery that supply the upper aspect of the left thyroid gland are ligated and transected (Fig. 11-1). The left recurrent laryngeal nerve should be preserved.

The cricopharyngeal muscle and dorsal proximal esophagus can be exposed by grasping the larynx and rotating it. The cricopharyngeal muscle can be identified as a bundle of transverse muscle fibers converging on the dorsal midline and blending into the longitudinal muscle fibers of the cranial esophagus. Two parallel incisions, approximately 2 mm apart, are made on the dorsal midline through the cricopharyngeal muscle and onto the cranial esophageal musculature (Fig. 11-2).

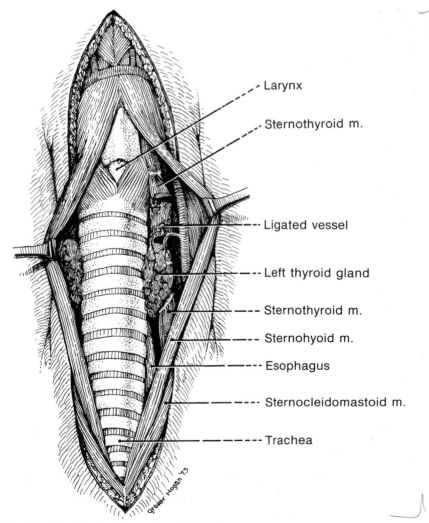

Larynx

Sternothyroid m.

Ligated vessel

Left thyroid gland

Sternothyroid m.

Sternohyoid m.

Esophagus

Sternocleidomastoid m.

Trachea

Fig. 11-1. *Mobilization of the left side of the trachea and cranial esophagus.*

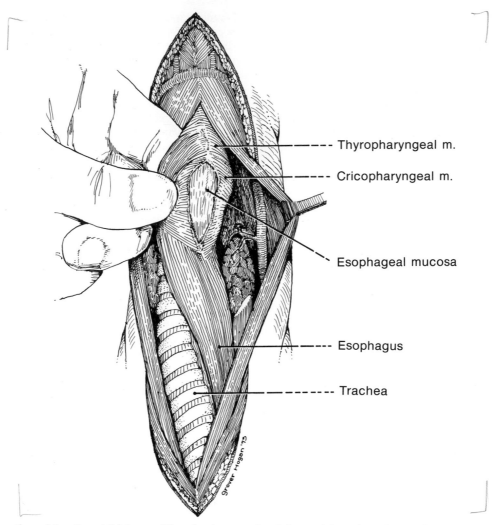

Thyropharyngeal m.

Cricopharyngeal m.

Esophageal mucosa

Esophagus

Trachea

Fig. 11-2. *Myectomy through length and thickness of the cricopharyngeal and the cranial esophageal musculature. The esophageal mucosa is not incised.*

The esophageal mucosa is not incised. The incised muscle fibers are separated from the mucosa and excised. Bleeding is controlled by use of gauze and pressure; the myectomy is not sutured.

Closure of the incision is initiated by apposition of the sternohyoid muscle with simple interrupted 3-0 absorbable sutures. It is unnecessary to suture the transected insertion of the sternothyroid muscle. The subcutaneous tissue and skin are sutured routinely. Although other tissue planes that were separated for exposure are not sutured, seroma formation is uncommon.

Postoperative Care

No special postoperative care is required. Patients tolerate solid food the day following the operation. Recurrence of dysphagia because of fibrosis and constriction at the myectomy site is prevented by adequate removal of sphincter muscle fibers during the original surgical procedure.

References and Suggested Readings

Hurwitz, A. L., and Duranceau, A.: Upper esophageal sphincter dysfunction: pathogenesis and treatment. Am. J. Digest. Dis., *23*:275, 1978.

Lund, W. S.: The functions of the cricopharyngeal sphincter during swallowing. Acta Otolaryngol. (Stockh.), *59*:497, 1965.

Pearson, H.: The differential diagnosis of persistent vomiting in the young dog. J. Small Anim. Pract., *11*:403, 1970.

Rosin, E., and Hanlon, G. F.: Canine cricopharyngeal achalasia. J. Am. Vet. Med. Assoc., *160*:1496, 1972.

Seaman, W. B.: Functional disorders of the pharyngoesophageal junction. Radiol. Clin. North Am., *11*:113, 1969.

Sokolovsky, V.: Cricopharyngeal achalasia in a dog. J. Am. Vet. Med. Assoc., *150*:281, 1967.

Suter, P. F., and Watrous, B. J.: Oropharyngeal dysphagias in the dog: a cinefluorographic analysis of experimentally induced and spontaneously occurring swallowing disorders. I. Oral stage and pharyngeal stage dysphagias. Vet. Radiol., *21*:24, 1980.

Cervical and Thoracic Esophageal Resection and Anastomosis

by DON R. WALDRON

The esophagus serves to carry food, water, and saliva from the pharynx to the stomach. Interruption of this function by partial or total obstruction results in dysphagia and regurgitation. Obstruction may be caused by foreign bodies, masses, strictures, or compression by adjacent structures. Esophageal perforation is a potential sequela to foreign bodies and neoplasia. Perforation can be caused iatrogenically by esophagoscopy, instrumentation, or stomach tube passage.

Diagnosis of esophageal disorders is based on the patient's medical history and clinical signs and is confirmed by radiology, possibly including contrast studies. Careful examination of the esophagus with an endoscope may be of value prior to surgical intervention.

Surgical Anatomy and Physiology

The esophagus begins at the level of the first cervical vertebra (C1) where it lies dorsal to the trachea. From its origin, the cervical esophagus courses to the left of the trachea until the thoracic inlet is reached, where it again passes dorsal to the trachea. In the thorax, the esophagus continues dorsally and to the left of the trachea and to the right of the aortic arch. From the tracheal bifurcation to its termination at the stomach, the esophagus lies slightly to the right of midline.

The wall of the esophagus is made up of four coats: tunica mucosa, tela submucosa, tunica muscularis, and tunica adventitia.[3] Esophageal mucosa consists of stratified squamous epithelium that forms numerous folds in the undistended esophagus. The importance of this tissue layer to the veterinary surgeon lies in that it is the strongest layer for placement of sutures. The tela submucosa contains the nerves and blood supply to the esophagus. The muscular coat consists of two layers of striated muscle in the dog, whereas part of this muscle is smooth in the cat. The tunica adventitia of the esophagus consists of contributions from cervical fascia, pleura, and tissue of surrounding organs.

Several reported factors pose significant problems to normal tissue healing in the esophagus following a surgical procedure.[4] First, no serosal covering exists to help form a fibrin seal and to prevent leakage at the surgical site. The esophagus is subject to constant movement by swallowing and normal respiratory excursion; this movement may contribute to leakage at the suture line. Surgical invasion of the esophagus, especially resection and anastomosis, carries the risk of postoperative stricture, which necessitates further treatment.

Adherence to general principles of intestinal and soft tissue surgery enhances the success rate of esophageal anastomosis: (1) handling esophageal tissue with instruments is discouraged; instead, stay sutures and preplaced sutures are used (see Fig. 11-6); for manipulation (2) one should use the smallest number of sutures needed to appose tissue precisely; (3) sutures are tightened only to appose tissue, not to strangulate it; and (4) the esophagus is "rested" following the surgical procedure.

Clinical Signs and Diagnosis

The predominant clinical sign of esophageal disorder is dysphagia. Regurgitation, hypersalivation, and repeated attempts to swallow are frequent presenting signs. The patient's appetite may be normal, ravenous, or depressed. When esophageal obstruction is complete, the patient constantly regurgitates undigested food in the form of a tubular cast. If the obstruction is incomplete or is caused by an enlarging mass of surrounding structures (mediastinal mass), regurgitation may be intermittent, and progressive emaciation may be noted by the patient's owner. Coughing caused by aspiration pneumonia is a frequent complication of esophageal disorders.

On physical examination, one may note a fetid oral odor caused by food accumulation in the obstructed esophagus. If the obstruction is located in the cervical esophagus, a ballooning of the esophagus proximal to the obstruction may be seen. The presence of fever and depression, along with the described clinical signs, suggests esophageal perforation.

Diagnosis is suggested by the patient's medical history and is confirmed by radiologic, endoscopic, or surgical procedures. Plain radiographs of the esophagus extending from the caudal portion of the oral cavity to the stomach should be made. Radiopaque foreign bodies and the presence or absence of aspiration pneumonia may be seen on plain radiographs. The presence of mediastinitis, pneumomediastinum, or pleural effusion suggests esophageal perforation.

Contrast examination of the esophagus is indicated if plain radiographs are nondiagnostic. In most cases, a barium paste such as Esophotrast* provides an adequate study. If perforation is suspected, an aqueous organic iodine such as Gastrografin† should be used in order to avoid spilling barium into the mediastinum or pleural space.[5]

Esophagoscopy has been found to be useful in the diagnosis of esophageal disorders. A rigid esophagoscope or a small gastroscope allows examination of the esophagus and manipulation of foreign bodies with alligator forceps. Flexible endoscopes are needed for evaluating the extent of esophageal stricture and biopsy of possible neoplastic lesions. Suction is useful to remove excessive mucus and debris from the esophagus, to allow better visualization of the lumen and mucosal surface. Extreme care is taken when any esophagoscopy is performed because the risk of iatrogenic perforation is increased when diseased tissue is present. Instruments should be gently passed and rotated if resistance is encountered; force is never used.

*Esophotrast, Barnes-Hind Diagnostics, Sunnyvale, CA 94086
†Gastrografin, E. R. Squibb & Sons, Princeton, NJ 08540

Other than foreign bodies, the most common cause of esophageal disorder, in my experience, is idiopathic megaesophagus. It is essential that this condition be ruled out diagnostically because the role of surgery in this condition is controversial. The reader is referred to Chapter 12 for further details.

Surgical Indications

These indications include foreign bodies, esophageal strictures, and neoplasia or granulomas. Most esophageal foreign bodies can be treated with conservative management. (See the section of this chapter by Easom.) Surgical treatment is indicated when conservative techniques fail or when the esophagus is perforated. Early diagnosis of esophageal perforation is critical because an operation performed more than 24 hours following perforation is associated with high mortality rates.[7] Esophagotomy by longitudinal incision is the preferred technique for removal of foreign bodies. If the esophagus is grossly necrotic, or if a large perforation has occurred, esophageal resection and anastomosis should be performed.

Theoretically, any injury to the esophagus may result in esophageal stricture. The most common causes of esophageal stricture include foreign body with or without perforation and iatrogenic injury caused by esophagoscopy, stomach tube passage, or surgical procedures. An additional cause of stricture is associated with previous general anesthetic administration. It is theorized that postanesthetic stricture is due to the reflux of acidic gastric contents. Most strictures caused by gastric reflux occur at or near the thoracic inlet.

The majority of strictures, especially those involving a considerable length of esophagus, should be treated by dilatation of the affected segment. This dilatation is accomplished by the passage of progressively larger diameter bougies until the stricture is stretched enough to dilate the esophageal lumen. Surgical resection of a stricture and anastomosis should be contemplated if the stricture is unresponsive to bougienage or if a danger of perforation exists owing to esophageal fragility.

Neoplastic or granulomatous disease of the esophagus is usually secondary to Spirocerca lupi infection. Carcinomas and leiomyomas have been reported as primary esophageal tumors.[6] Spirocerca lupi infection may produce granulomas or osteosarcomas that can obstruct the esophagus. These masses are usually located in the esophagus at the heart base or caudal thorax. Spirocerca infection should be considered in the presence of any tissue mass in the esophagus causing signs of obstruction. Diagnosis is based on finding the Spirocerca ova in the feces.

If technically possible, esophagoscopy and biopsy are useful aids in formulating a surgical plan and prognosis regarding soft-tissue masses.

Preoperative Considerations

Patients with esophageal obstruction are first seen in varying degrees of fitness. Prolonged dysphagia and regurgitation may result in cachexia and dehydration. Aspiration pneumonia is a common complication of esophageal disease. If perforation has occurred, mediastinitis, pneumomediastinum, pneumothorax, and pleural effusion are present.

Prior to operation, dehydrated patients should be treated with intravenous lactated Ringer's solution. The surgical procedure should be performed as soon as the patient's fluid deficit has been replaced. Because the esophagus contains the normal bacterial flora of the oral cavity, I give all patients parenteral antibiotic therapy prior to the operation. Bacteriocidal antibiotics such as ampicillin or the cephalosporins are preferred.

Inhalation anesthesia is preferred for all esophageal operations. The endotracheal tube should have a functional cuff to prevent aspiration of fluids during the procedure. An esophageal stethoscope or a stomach tube is useful for surgical manipulations. If thoracotomy is to be performed, chest tubes should be available for postoperative drainage.

Surgical Approaches

CERVICAL ESOPHAGUS

The cervical esophagus is approached through the ventral midline. A skin incision is made from the larynx to the manubrium (Fig. 11-3). The subcutaneous tissues are sharply incised, and the thin median raphe of the

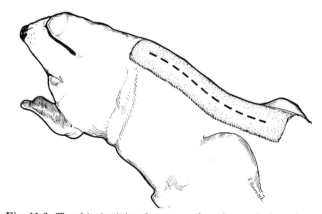

Fig. 11-3. *The skin incision for approach to the cervical esophagus extends from the larynx to the manubrium.*

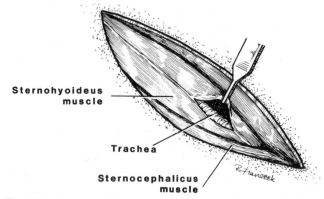

Sternohyoideus muscle

Trachea

Sternocephalicus muscle

Fig. 11-4. *Exposure of the trachea by division of the sternohyoideus muscles on their midline.*

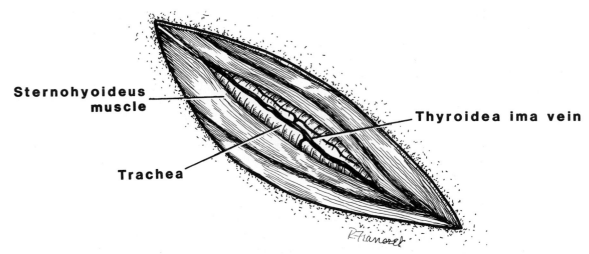

Sternohyoideus muscle

Thyroidea ima vein

Trachea

Fig. 11-5. The thyroidea ima lies on the ventral surface of the trachea.

sternohyoideus muscle is identified and incised (Fig. 11-4). As the sternohyoideus muscle bellies are separated, the thyroidea ima, a large vein on the ventral surface of the trachea, is seen (Fig. 11-5). This vein should be preserved, although collateral branches have to be severed. The trachea is then retracted to the right, and the left carotid artery sheath is identified. Moistened laparotomy pads are used to protect the trachea and the left carotid artery sheath. Exposure is maintained by the use of Balfour or Weitlander self-retaining retractors. The left recurrent laryngeal nerve should be identified on the ventromedial aspect of the esophagus and should be preserved. Passage of a stomach tube helps to immobilize the esophagus and to allow aspiration of esophageal and stomach contents. Once the stomach tube is passed, the appropriate length of esophagus is exposed by blunt dissection. Mobilization should not exceed 4 to 5 cm proximal or distal to the diseased portion, in order to preserve blood supply to the cut ends.

Exposure of the caudal cervical esophagus from C6 to the second thoracic vertebra (T2) is more difficult. To expose the esophagus adequately as it approaches the thoracic inlet requires elevation of the sternocephalicus muscle from its origin on the manubrium. Additional exposure may be obtained by splitting the first two sternebra. Prior to closure, the operative field is flushed with normal saline solution. Penrose drains are placed in the operative field and exit the skin lateral to the incision. The sternohyoideus muscle bellies and subcutaneous tissues are closed with absorbable suture and the skin with nonabsorbable suture of the verterinary surgeon's choice.

THORACIC ESOPHAGUS

Thoracotomy is required for exposure of the esophagus between T2 and its termination at the stomach. Intermittent positive pressure ventilation is required, as well as chest-tube drainage following the surgical procedure.

The cranial thoracic esophagus extending from the thoracic inlet to the heart base is exposed by thoracotomy through the left fourth intercostal space (see Chap. 20). Once the thorax is entered, the ribs are spread and are held in place with self-retaining retractors (Fig. 11-6). Moistened laparotomy pads are used to pack lung lobes caudally. The vagus nerve is identified as it passes over the origin of the aorta and should be protected throughout the procedure. Identification of the esophagus, which is located in the mediastinum just dorsal to the brachiocephalic trunk, is aided by passage of a stomach tube. In the cranial thorax, the large costocervical vein, a branch of the internal thoracic vein, crosses the esophagus and should be avoided or protected throughout the operation (Fig. 11-7). The appropriate length of esophagus is exposed by blunt and sharp dissection of mediastinum and surrounding tissue.

If the esophageal disorder is located at the heart base, the approach of choice is through the right fifth intercostal space. The lung lobes are packed off caudally with moistened laparotomy pads. The esophagus is located just dorsal to the trachea in the mediastinum. The large azygos vein must be bluntly isolated and retracted to allow adequate exposure of the esophagus (Fig. 11-8).

The caudal thoracic esophagus between the heart and gastroesophageal junction is exposed by thoracotomy through the left eighth or ninth interspace. To expose the esophagus, the caudal lung lobes are packed off cranially with moistened laparotomy pads. Adequate mobilization of the caudal lobes necessitates cutting the pulmonary ligament that attaches the lung lobe to the mediastinal pleura. The esophagus is identified just ventral to the aorta. A trunk of the vagus nerve is seen coursing over the lateral aspect of the esophagus. This trunk, as well as dorsal and ventral vagal branches, should be protected throughout the procedure (Fig. 11-9).

All patients undergoing thoracic esophageal operations should have chest tubes placed before the thoracotomy incision is closed. If mediastinitis or pyothorax is present as a result of esophageal perforation, more than one tube may be necessary to drain both the mediastinum and thorax adequately.

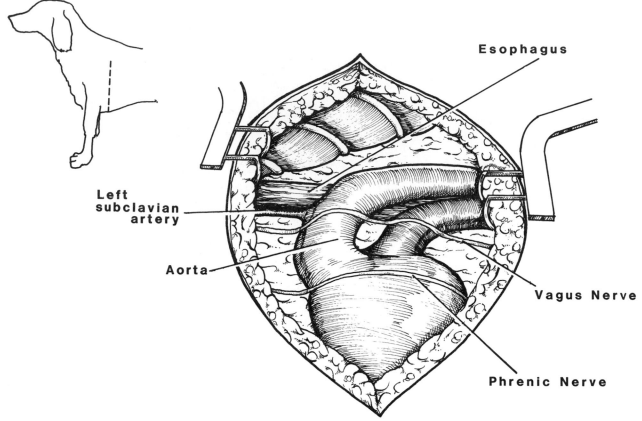

Fig. 11-6. *Exposure of the cranial thoracic esophagus through the left fourth intercostal space. The lung lobes have been packed off caudally.*

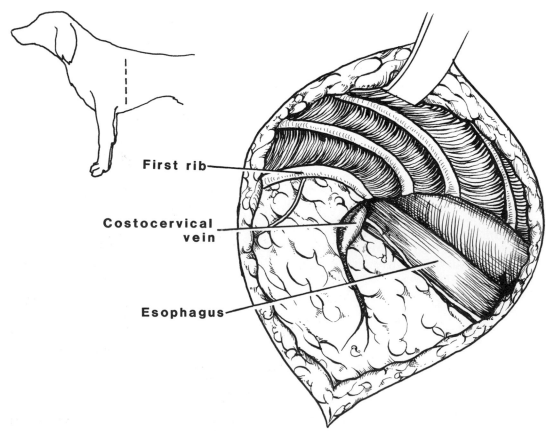

Fig. 11-7. *The large costocervical vein crosses the esophagus just caudal to the thoracic inlet.*

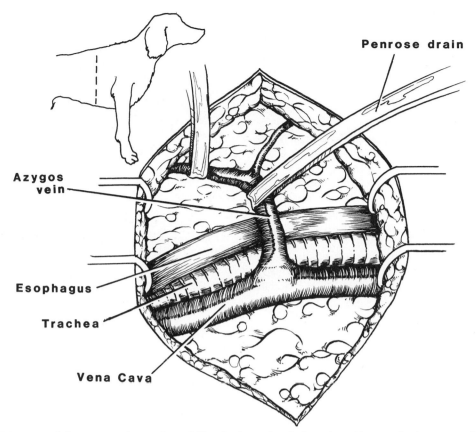

Fig. 11-8. *Right fifth intercostal thoracotomy for esophageal disorder located at the heart base. Penrose drains are used to retract the azygos vein overlying the esophagus.*

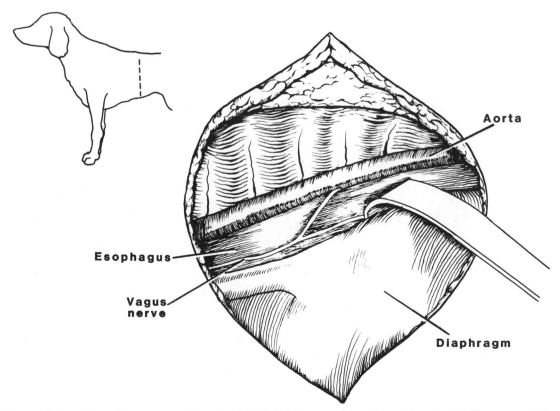

Fig. 11-9. *The caudal thoracic esophagus as seen through a left ninth interspace thoracotomy. The retractor lies on one of the crura of the diaphragm. The vagus nerve and its branches lie on the esophagus and should be preserved.*

Surgical Technique

The technique for esophagotomy or esophageal resection and anastomosis is the same in both the cervical and thoracic portions of the esophagus.

ESOPHAGOTOMY

Esophagotomy is indicated for the removal of foreign bodies if conservative techniques fail. When the appropriate approach to the esophagus has been selected and the esophagus has been identified, the operative field is packed off with moistened laparotomy pads. If esophageal tissue appears normal, a longitudinal incision is made directly over the foreign body. If the esophagus is damaged, but tissue is viable, the incision should be made in healthy tissue caudal to the foreign body. Necrotic tissue or extensive perforations with necrosis are indications for resection and anasto-

mosis. Perforations that involve less than one-fourth the circumference of the esophagus and are surrounded by healthy tissue may be debrided and closed primarily. Gentle traction and rotation are used to extract the foreign body and to avoid further tissue damage. The mucosa is now closed with 4-0 polypropylene suture* on a tapered needle. Knots of the mucosal sutures should be within the lumen (Fig. 11-10). The muscular layer is closed with horizontal mattress sutures of 3-0 polyglactin 910† on a tapered needle (Fig. 11-11).

ANASTOMOSIS

Once adequate exposure has been obtained, the operative field should be packed off with moistened laparotomy pads to prevent contamination with esophageal

*Prolene, Ethicon, Inc., Somerville, NJ 08876
†Vicryl, Ethicon, Inc., Somerville, NJ 08876

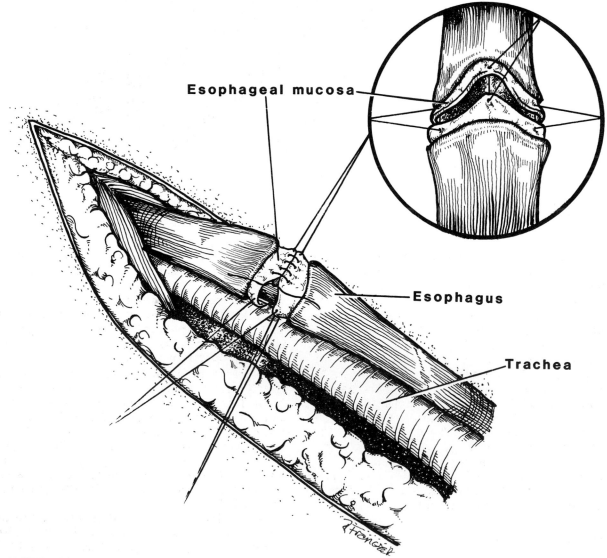

Esophageal mucosa

Esophagus

Trachea

Fig. 11-10. *When the esophagus is cut, the tunica muscularis and mucosa retract from the mucosa. Stay sutures are placed in the mucosa to facilitate gentle handling. The mucosa is closed and the knots of the sutures lie within the lumen.*

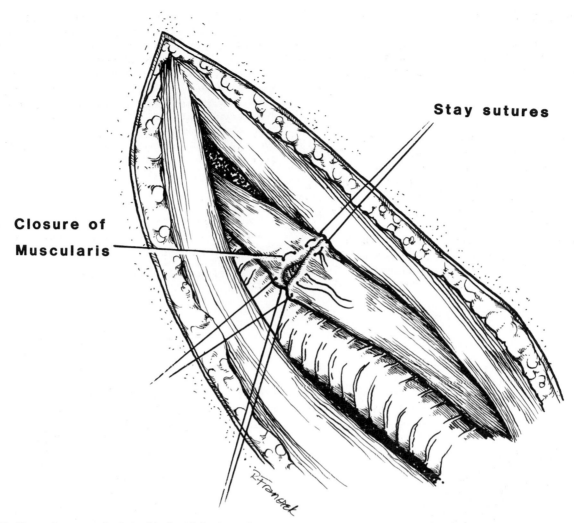

Fig. 11-11. *The tunica muscularis is closed with horizontal mattress sutures.*

contents. The esophagus is then stabilized by an assistant who uses the index and middle fingers of each hand to "clamp" the esophagus and thereby to minimize contamination. The diseased portion of esophagus is resected using a new scalpel blade. All necrotic tissue should be excised, and shreds of tissue and muscle should be carefully debrided to expose healthy tissue. Three stay sutures are placed at equal distances around the esophagus in healthy tissue. These sutures facilitate gentle handling of the esophagus and help to maintain apposition of the cut ends. The mucosa is now closed with simple interrupted sutures of 4-0 polypropylene on a tapered needle. The sutures should be about 2 mm apart and include a 2-mm bite of mucosa. All knots of the mucosal sutures should lie in the lumen. Because the muscular layer is thin and tears easily, it is closed with simple interrupted horizontal mattress sutures of 3-0 polyglactin 910.

Postoperative Care

At the conclusion of the operation, a pharyngostomy tube is placed. (See the next section of the chapter.)

The patient is fed a liquid diet through the pharyngostomy tube for 5 days. Several feedings daily are needed to meet the water and caloric needs of the patient. Caloric needs are calculated on the basis of 70 kcal/kg/day, whereas water maintenance requirements are calculated at 80 ml/kg/day.[2] On removal of the pharyngostomy tube, a semiliquid diet is fed for 48 hours, and then solid food may be given.

Drains placed at the time of a cervical esophageal operation may usually be removed within 72 hours. If a thoracotomy has been performed, the chest tubes should be aspirated frequently during the first 24 hours postoperatively. The amounts of air or fluid removed from the thorax should be recorded. Chest tubes may be removed within 24 hours if drainage is minimal. Patients who have been operated on for esophageal perforation and subsequent mediastinitis may need drains for 5 to 7 days.

Patients showing signs of dysphagia and regurgitation following an esophageal operation should be suspected of having esophageal stricture, and follow-up esophagoscopy and radiographic contrast studies are indicated.

References and Suggested Readings

1. Akiyama, H.: Esophageal anastomosis. Arch. Surg., *107*:512, 1973.
2. Crane, S. W.: Placement and maintenance of a temporary feeding tube gastrostomy in the dog and cat. Compend. Contin. Ed. Practicing Vet., *2*:770, 1980.
3. Evans, H. E., and Christensen, G. C.: Miller's Anatomy of the Dog. 2nd Ed. Philadelphia, W. B. Saunders, 1979.
4. Hoffer, R. E., and Hunt, C. E.: A practical suture technic for esophageal closure in the dog. Small Anim. Clinician, 75, 1963.
5. Kleine, L. J.: Radiologic examination of the esophagus in dogs and cats. Vet. Clin. North Am., 663, 1974.
6. Lawson, D. D., and Pirie, H. M.: Conditions of the canine oesophagus, II: vascular rings, achalasia, tumors, and periesophageal lesions. J. Small Anim. Pract. *7*:117, 1966.
7. Schwartz, A.: Esophageal Foreign Bodies. In Ear, Nose and Throat Section. American College of Veterinary Surgeons Surgical Forum, 1978, pp. 72–79.
8. Sumner-Smith, G.: Oesophagotomy and oesophageal resection. J. Small Anim. Pract., *14*:429, 1973.

Pharyngostomy for Oral Maintenance

by RICHARD H. BÖHNING, JR.

It is often necessary to assist the anorectic preoperative and postoperative patient in maintaining proper nutrition. Hypodermoclysis or forced oral administration are the methods most frequently employed. Restraint during oral feeding can be a problem and is often difficult without adding to the discomfort of the animal. Pharyngostomy is a useful surgical procedure to minimize the difficulties encountered when forced oral alimentation is indicated.

Indications

Pharyngostomy may be indicated in animals that are unable or unwilling to eat, such as those with pneumonitis, uremia, or acute mandibular or maxillary fractures or both. Other indications for pharyngostomy are when healing would be otherwise difficult after oral or esophageal operations. In animals with gastric dilatation or dilatation-volvulus syndrome, the pharyngostomy tube can be used as a means of removing gas accumulation and liquid material from the stomach during and after surgical intervention.

Surgical Technique

The animal is anesthetized with a short-acting general anesthetic agent, or a local anesthetic may be used if the animal is severely depressed. The animal is placed in lateral recumbency, and an area caudal to the angle of the mandible is prepared for the surgical procedure. The mouth is held open using a conventional mouth speculum, and the index finger is inserted into the pharynx near the base of the tongue. The epiglottis, thyroid, arytenoid cartilages, and hyoid apparatus may then be palpated.

Flexing the finger toward the lateral aspect of the neck, one can find a natural retropharyngeal pouch, the piriform fossa of the pharynx, which is located caudal to the base of the tongue and lateral to the hyoid apparatus (Figs. 11-12 and 11-13). Pressure is gently applied to the lateral wall of the pouch with large curved forceps so that a bulge is externally visible. A small incision is made through the skin at the center of the bulge.

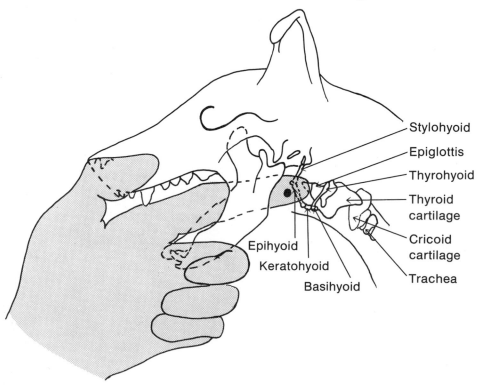

Fig. 11-12. *Schematic drawing showing proper placement of index finger lateral to hyoid apparatus. (From Böhning, R. H.: Pharyngostomy for oral maintenance of the anorectic animals. J. Am. Vet. Med. Assoc., 156:612, 1970.)*

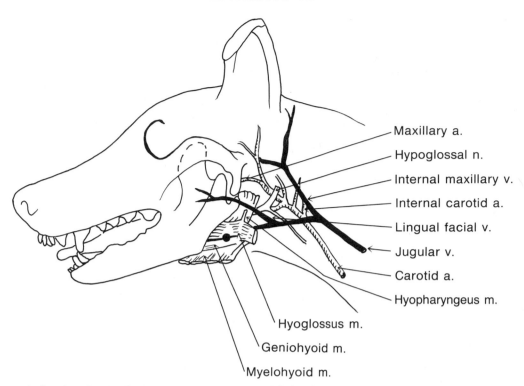

Maxillary a.

Hypoglossal n.

Internal maxillary v.

Internal carotid a.

Lingual facial v.

Jugular v.

Carotid a.

Hyopharyngeus m.

Hyoglossus m.

Geniohyoid m.

Myelohyoid m.

Fig. 11-13. *Schematic drawing showing basic anatomic structures and their relation to surgical site for pharyngostomy. (From Böhning, R. H., et al.: Pharyngostomy for oral maintenance of the anorectic animal. J. Am. Vet. Med. Assoc., 156:612, 1970.)*

The forceps is then pushed firmly through the incision to the external surface (Fig. 11-14). A flexible plastic or rubber stomach tube is grasped with the forceps and is drawn into the pharynx through the pharyngostomy incision. The length of the tube is determined by the distance between the ramus of the mandible and the thirteenth rib. The tube is then directed over the arytenoid cartilages, down the esophagus, and into the stomach (Fig. 11-15).

A strip of adhesive tape is used to form a cuff around the proximal end of the tube (Fig. 11-16). Stainless steel suture is placed through both the skin and the cuff to prevent the animal from swallowing the tube or from dislodging it by scratching. If a longer external section of the tube is selected, a wide tape collar is used to secure the tube; this is the method of choice (Fig. 11-17). The tube may be either open or closed at the distal end. Blockage of the tube is less likely to

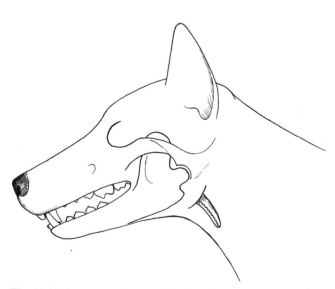

Fig. 11-14. *Schematic drawing showing forceps in proper position through incision site.*

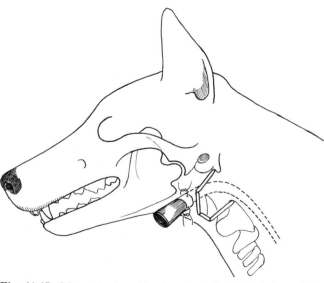

Fig. 11-15. *Schematic drawing showing tube in position within the pharynx and esophagus.*

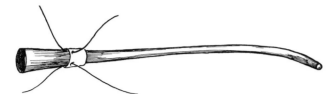

Fig. 11-16. *Drawing of pharyngostomy tube with tape cuff and suture placement.*

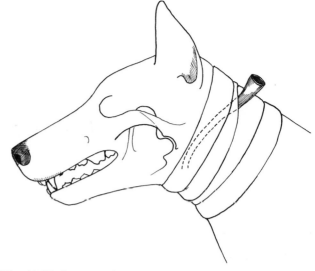

occur with the open-ended type. The tube can be capped when not in use to prevent loss of gastric contents or to prevent intake of air. When the tube is no longer required, it can be removed. Sutures are not needed to close the wound.

Reference and Selected Reading

Böhning, R. H., Jr., DeHoff, W. D., McElhinney, A., and Hofstra, P. C.: Pharyngostomy for maintenance of the anorectic animal. J. Am. Vet. Med. Assoc., *156*:611, 1970.

Fig. 11-17. *Drawing showing wide tape collar used with longer tube.*

12 * Stomach

Feeding and Drainage Tube Gastrostomy

by JOHN PARKS

Gastrostomy, the establishment of an artificial opening into the stomach, was once primarily an investigative procedure. Now, however, gastrostomy is considered to be useful in the surgical management of the gastric dilatation-volvulus syndrome and has therapeutic applications in bowel obstruction and peritonitis, as well as in oral, pharyngeal, and esophageal diseases.

Indications

Gastrostomies may be indicated for the purposes of gastric decompression, gastric fixation (gastropexy), and feeding of certain patients.

GASTRIC DECOMPRESSION

Gastric decompression by gastrostomy is a comfortable, safe method by which to drain gastric fluid and gas for both therapeutic and investigative purposes. Decompression by gastrostomy may also be indicated in both the emergency and postoperative management of the patient with gastric dilatation-volvulus syndrome. In addition, gastric decompression may be indicated in certain patients with peritonitis and intestinal obstruction to reduce bowel distension and to aid the early return of function.

FEEDING GASTROSTOMIES

Feeding gastrostomies are indicated in patients that cannot eat normally because of traumatic, inflammatory, neurologic, or neoplastic disease of the oral or pharyngeal cavities or the esophagus.[2]

ADJUNCT TECHNIQUES

Gastropexy, the surgical fusion of the stomach to the abdominal wall, is indicated in the surgical management of the gastric dilatation-volvulus syndrome, to prevent recurrence. A permanent method of gastropexy has been described, but an alternate and simpler tube gastrostomy procedure has also been found effective in preventing gastric migration.

Two basic types of gastrostomies may be seen, temporary and permanent. Temporary gastrostomy procedures generally involve gastric catheterization in which the catheter leaves the abdominal wall through a stab wound. This type of gastrostomy requires adjacent serosal surfaces and interposed omentum to seal the catheter from leakage into the abdomen. Catheters are generally left in place for several days, and the gastrocutaneous fistula closes shortly after catheter removal. A gastric wall marsupialization procedure, located in the flank, is also useful as a temporary emergency decompression procedure for patients with gastric dilatation-volvulus syndrome. This procedure necessitates a second operation to repair the gastrostomy.

Permanent gastrostomy procedures are more extensive. These gastrostomies are usually formed by a mucosa-lined tube of stomach wall brought out through the abdominal wall. Catheters are only inserted during feeding or sampling of gastric contents. A second surgical procedure is necessary to obliterate the mucosal tube.

Surgical Techniques

FLANK GASTRIC MARSUPIALIZATION

This procedure is usually performed for emergency decompression in the gastric dilatation-volvulus syndrome. The bloated patient is gently restrained in left lateral recumbency, or it may be permitted to remain standing. The right flank and pericostal regions are surgically prepared, and an inverted "L" block is performed with 2% lidocaine. If additional sedation is required, meperidine or oxymorphone is administered systemically. A 6-cm vertical skin incision is made 4 to 6 cm caudal to the costal arch and 10 cm lateral to the epigastric vessels (Fig. 12-1). The subcutaneous tissues are divided in line with the skin incision to expose the abdominal muscles. By blunt separation of muscles in the direction of their fibers, the incision is continued through the external, internal, and transverse abdominal muscles in a "grid" manner (Fig. 12-2A). A

143

is also constructed to prevent external reflux of gastric juice. Thus, an important feature of this tubulovalvular gastrostomy is the development of an antireflux valve within and parallel to the lesser curvature of the stomach.

After midline laparotomy, the valve is created by infolding 4 cm of the stomach wall over a 14-French catheter and suturing the apposed serosal surfaces with interrupted 3-0 nylon sutures (Fig. 12-3A). The catheter is then removed, and a flap of stomach wall for construction of the tube is outlined from the 4-cm base of the valve toward the greater curvature. The flap should be of sufficient length to form a tube long enough to pass through the abdominal wall and to reach the skin without excessive tension.

When the flap incision has been made, bleeding is controlled by ligature or point electrocoagulation of gastric vessels. The flap is retracted upward, exposing the mucosal aspect of the folded stomach wall that will form the valve at the base of the tube (Fig. 12-3B). Each side of the infolded mucosa is approximated, and the sides are united with interrupted 3-0 nylon seromuscular sutures. The defect in the stomach wall is repaired with a mucosal layer of 3-0 chromic catgut or absorbable synthetic suture material placed in a continuous pattern and reinforced with a continuous seromuscular oversew closure with 3-0 nylon (Fig. 12-3C and D).

The remainder of the flap is now converted into a tube by approximating the opposite edges of the flap (started at the base) with mucosal and seromuscular sutures (Fig. 12-3E). The last suture placed near the mouth of the tube is left long so that it may act as a guide in bringing the tube through the abdominal wall. A wide body-wall wound is created by blunt, grid dissection through the abdominal wall. The location of the stoma is chosen where passage to the origin of the tube is straightest.

The gastric tube is drawn through the abdominal wound, and the stomach at the base of the tube's end is anchored to the peritoneum with 3-0 nylon (Fig. 12-3F). Finally, a circular piece of skin the size of the tube is excised, and the mucosa of the gastrostomy stoma is united to the skin with 4-0 nylon interrupted sutures. Careful approximation is required to achieve primary healing of the new mucocutaneous junction and to preclude postoperative stricture formation. When the operation is completed, the tube should accommodate a 14-French catheter.

Postoperatively, the catheter or suitable obturator is passed into the stomach for a few minutes every 6 to 12 hours for several days, to insure patency of the valve and the tube. Thereafter, the catheter is only inserted for feeding or decompression, after which it is removed.

References and Suggested Readings

1. Betts, C. W., Wingfield, W. E., and Rosin, E.: Permanent gastropexy—as a prophylactic measure against gastric volvulus. J. Am. Anim. Hosp. Assoc., 12:177, 1976.

2. Crane, S. W.: Placement and maintenance of a temporary feeding tube gastrostomy in the dog and cat. Compend. Contin. Ed. Practicing Vet., 2:770, 1980.

3. Parks, J. L., and Greene, R. W.: Tube gastrostomy for the treatment of gastric volvulus. J. Am. Anim. Hosp. Assoc., 12:168, 1976.

4. Pass, M. A., and Johnson, D. R.: Treatment of gastric dilatation-torsion in the dog: gastric decompression by gastrostomy under local analgesia. J. Small Anim. Pract., 14:131, 1973.

5. Rosi, P. A.: Gastrostomy, pyloroplasty and operative treatment of perforated peptic ulcer. In The Craft Of Surgery. Vol. II. Edited by Philip Cooper. Boston, Little, Brown, 1964.

Gastroesophageal Cardiomyotomy

by ROBERT L. LEIGHTON

The surgical procedure of incising the musculature at the gastroesophageal junction is performed for relief of congenital or acquired megaesophagus. This disorder has also been labeled achalasia, esophageal dilatation, cardiospasm, hypomotility, aperistalsis, and esophageal paralysis.

To clarify definitions, achalasia is a disease of man and is not comparable to megaesophagus in the dog.[17] It has been shown that no spasm of the cardia is present and that it functions normally.[14,19] The cardia fails to open because of the lack of a stimulating contractile wave from the esophagus.[11] Certain diseases such as Spirocerca infestation in the cardia,[3] heart disease,[18] functional strictures,[1] and neuromuscular disease[9] may be similar in appearance and signs, but the true cause of congenital and acquired megaesophagus is unknown. Hence the term idiopathic is consequently used to describe this disorder.

Considerable speculation and interesting observations exist as to the cause and effect of destruction of the nucleus ambiguus.[9,19]

Diagnosis

The clinician must rule out other causes of regurgitation such as vascular ring anomalies and cricopharyngeal dysphagia. Congenital megaesophagus is probably a hereditary disease[2] and usually becomes evident when the young animal begins to ingest solid foods. The puppy may not be presented to the veterinarian for treatment until maturity.[10] The bolus of food is regurgitated after a varying period of time. It is often covered with foamy saliva and is not sour smelling because it has never reached the stomach. The material is usually reingested. The actual solid food intake is limited, and as a result, the animal is unthrifty and small. Although ravenously hungry, the animal may hesitate to eat out of certain knowledge that it will regurgitate the food.

Acquired megaesophagus occurs in young mature to late-middle-aged dogs usually after stress,[5] the cause of which stress may be as simple as being boarded in a kennel or undergoing an operation. Acquired megaesophagus may also be a manifestation of systemic neuromuscular disorders. The previously normal animal now begins to regurgitate its food and to show the same signs as in the congenital form. The diagnosis of both types of the disease has been well described.[7,15]

The radiographic appearance of the esophagus, especially using contrast media, is a great diagnostic aid. The typical appearance of the dilated esophagus caudal to the heart, filled with contrast material coming to a point at the diaphragm with little in the stomach, is not pathognomonic, but it is suggestive.[13]

Medical treatment is directed toward varying the consistency of the food and feeding the animal in an upright position. Medication has also been suggested.[4] Improvement and total recovery have been reported either spontaneously or from medical management.[4] Reports on the effectiveness of surgical procedures vary.[1,2,8,17] Treatment by bougienage has been recommended.[2] Varying results from gastroesophageal cardiomyotomy may reflect differences in surgical procedure, technique, case selection, duration of observation, and postoperative care. In my experience, animals with congenital megaesophagus may require up to 3 months after the surgical procedure to become free of signs, whereas animals with the acquired disorder improve much sooner.

Surgical Procedure

The esophagus should be empty of food. Inhalation anesthesia with manual or mechanically assisted ventilation is required. With the animal in right lateral recumbency, the area of the left chest wall is prepared for the operation. Toweling and surgical draping are centered over the left eighth intercostal space.

An incision is made with a scalpel through the skin and subcutaneous tissue in the space between the eighth and ninth ribs. Hemorrhage is controlled. The incision is continued through the cutaneous trunci and the latissimus dorsi muscle dorsally to the iliocostalis muscle and ventrally through the obliquus externus abdominis muscle to the rectus abdominis using sharp and blunt dissection with scissors. The external and internal intercostal muscles and the pleura are incised. The anesthetist now begins the positive pressure ventilation. The edges of the incision are protected with moist sponges, and a Finochietto or other suitable rib retractor is inserted. As wide an exposure as possible is obtained.

The left caudal lung lobe is packed off cranially with a moistened laparotomy pad (Fig. 12-4). The distal esophagus is grasped and is retracted cranially. Avoiding the ventral branch of the vagus nerve, one should insert a piece of umbilical tape, to be used in retraction, through a hole made in the mediastinum close to the esophagus.

An incision is made with Metzenbaum scissors through the left side of the phrenicoesophageal ligament at the point of entry of the esophagus through the diaphragm (Fig. 12-5). When the diaphragm is entered, the stomach is recognized. A considerable number of engorged blood vessels are typically present on the gastric surface. The cranial wall of the stomach is grasped by an assistant who maintains traction on the

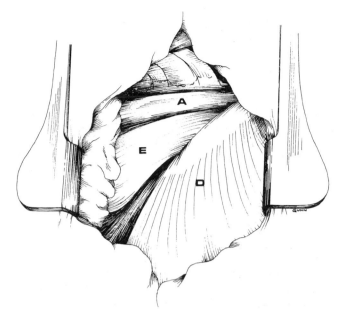

Fig. 12-4. *Exposure from the left eighth to ninth intercostal space showing the aorta (A), the esophagus (E), and the diaphragm (D).*

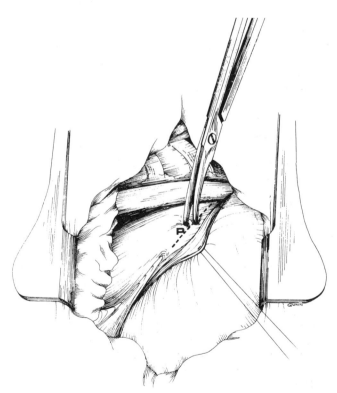

Fig. 12-5. *Phrenic pleural reflection and incision in the phrenicoesophageal ligament (P) to show the gastroesophageal junction.*

esophagus with the umbilical tape and holds firmly onto the exposed portion of the stomach. The cardia is well exposed.

A longitudinal incision is made through the tunica serosa and tunica muscularis with a scalpel 3 cm caudal to the cardia onto the stomach and an equal distance cranially into the esophagus (Fig. 12-6). Continued gentle dissection is made in order to cut all the

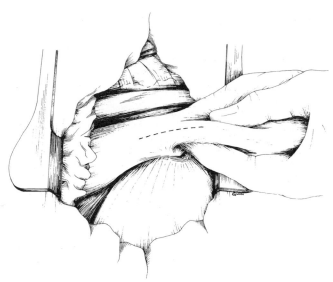

Fig. 12-6. *Proposed myotomy site with the stomach prolapsed through the diaphragmatic incision.*

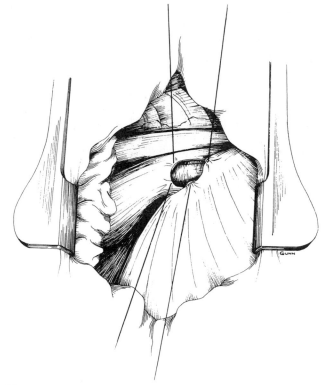

Fig. 12-8. *Placement of sutures from the muscular incision in the esophagus to the diaphragm.*

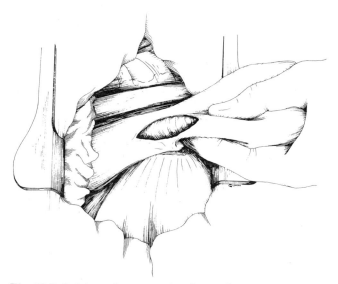

Fig. 12-7. *Bulging submucosa after the esophagomyotomy.*

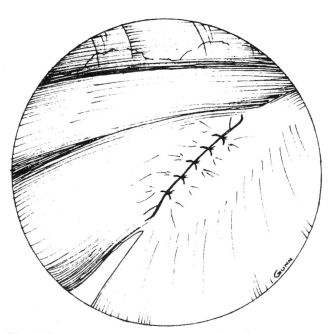

Fig. 12-9. *A close-up view of the closed incision.*

muscle fibers and to allow the mucosa to bulge out (Fig. 12-7). The gastric mucosa separates easily and is much stronger than that of the esophagus. A number of small blood vessels need to be incised and ligated with 4-0 chromic catgut.

The incision through the diaphragm is closed using simple interrupted sutures of 2-0 chromic catgut. A suture is placed in the tunica muscularis of the esophagus at the most cranial position of the incision and is secured to the middle of the incision in the diaphragm (Fig. 12-8). Additional sutures are placed to secure the tunica muscularis of the esophagus to the diaphragmatic incision (Fig. 12-9). In effect, the cranial (esophageal) portion of the incision in the tunica muscularis has been changed from longitudinal to horizontal. The exposed mucosa is now in the abdominal cavity. This step reduces gastric acid reflux and increases the angle

of entry of the esophagus into the stomach, thus facilitating a valvular effect.[6] The abdominal incision through the diaphragm is next closed.

The umbilical tape and the laparotomy pad are removed. The caudal lung lobe is checked for atelectasis. All blood clots and fluid are removed. The rib retractor is removed along with the protecting sponges. The site of entry into the chest is closed by placing sutures around the opposing ribs and approximating them to their normal position. The incisions in the muscles over the ribs are closed with 2-0 chromic catgut suture. When the closure of the muscles has been made, air is expelled from the thoracic cavity either by use of a previously placed drain or through a small hole held open at the incision site by mosquito forceps. This small hole is then closed with a mattress suture while the lungs are held inflated. The anesthetist now may allow the animal to breathe on its own. The subcutaneous tissues and the skin are routinely closed.

Postoperative Care

Because many of these patients have a chronic foreign body inhalation pneumonia, antibiotics are usually administered. Hydration and nutrition are maintained with intravenous fluids. Feedings with slurried dog food can be started in 24 hours with the animal eating in an upright position. Recovery from the operation is usually speedy and uneventful. Nursing and home care is centered on determining an acceptable diet that provokes the least amount of regurgitation. Patience and the prevention of scavenging are necessary. No radiographic changes in the size of the dilated portion of the esophagus is to be expected.

The benefit of the operation is that the cardia, which normally remains closed until stimulated to open by a chain of stimuli down the esophagus, remains open, and the food bolus is thereby able to enter the stomach more readily. The benefit is especially marked if gravity is used by feeding the animal in an upright position.

A review of 38 cases of radiographically confirmed megaesophagus at the Veterinary Medical Teaching Hospital at Davis, operated on in the manner described since 1968, showed 21 to have had good or satisfactory results.

Three were classified as fair with eventual recovery. Five results were poor. Nine patients died or were subject to euthanasia, but 3 of these deaths were caused by errors in feeding just after the operation, 1 patient died of distemper, 4 died of overwhelming inhalation pneumonia, and 1 died of rupture of the esophagus.

Almost all except the youngest puppies with congenital megaesophagus suffered from varying degrees of inhalation pneumonia. In those with the acquired form of the disorder, inhalation pneumonia was a problem when the condition was especially severe or when it had been present for longer than 2 or 3 months. A history of stress prior to the onset of signs was not obtained in earlier acquired cases, but has been obtained in most of those cases seen recently.

What constitutes a good result is empirical, because it depends mostly upon the owner's evaluation. A beneficial result is assumed when the dog is apparently well and its behavior no longer seems to demand veterinary attention. In a few cases long-term follow-up was possible for as long as 8 years, and the dogs remained well. In spite of varied reports of the efficacy of the operation, the procedure appears to have merit.

References and Suggested Readings

1. Boothe, H. W., Jr.: Acquired achalasia (megaesophagus) in a dog: clinical features and response to therapy. J. Am. Vet. Med. Assoc., 173:756, 1978.
2. Clifford, D. H.: Management of esophageal achalasia in miniature schnauzers. J. Am. Vet. Med. Assoc., 161:1012, 1976.
3. Dessinis, A.: A case of megaesophagus in a dog resulting from achalasia of the cardiac orifice of the stomach caused by Spirocerca lupi. Hellenic Vet. Med., 14:105, 1971.
4. Diamant, N., Szczepanski, M., and Mici, H.: Idiopathic megaesophagus in the dog, reasons for spontaneous improvement and a possible method of medical therapy. Can. Vet. J., 15:66, 1974.
5. Erbeck, D. H., and Hagee, J. H.: Achalasia or acquired megaesophagus in a 10 year old dog. VM SAC, 68:887, 1973.
6. Gourley, I. M., and Leighton, R. L.: Esophagotomy and pyloromyotomy in the dog. Practicing Vet., 43:19, 1971.
7. Guffy, M. M.: Esophageal disorders. In Textbook of Veterinary Internal Medicine. Edited by S. J. Ettinger. Philadelphia, W. B. Saunders, 1975.
8. Harvey, C. E., et al.: Megaesophagus in the dog. A clinical survey of 79 cases. J. Am. Vet. Med. Assoc., 165:443, 1974.
9. Higgs, B., Kerr, F. W. L., and Ellis, F. H.: The experimental production of esophageal achalasia by electrolytic lesions in the medulla. J. Thorac. Cardiovasc. Surg., 50:613, 1965.
10. Hinko, P. J., et al.: Congenital achalasia in a 2 year old dog. VM SAC, 67:660, 1976.
11. Janssens, J., et al.: Studies on the necessity of a bolus for the progression of secondary peristalsis in the canine esophagus. Gastroenterology, 67:245, 1974.
12. Kipnis, R. M.: Megaesophagus: remission in two dogs. J. Am. Anim. Hosp. Assoc., 14:247, 1978.
13. O'Brien, T. R.: Radiographic Diagnosis of Abdominal Disorders in the Dog and Cat. Philadelphia, W. B. Saunders, 1978.
14. Rogers, W. A., Fenner, W. R., and Sherding, R. G.: Electromyographic and esophagomanometric findings in clinically normal and in dogs with idiopathic megaesophagus. J. Am. Vet. Med. Assoc., 174:181, 1979.
15. Schepper, J. De: Recent concepts on the nature and treatment of esophageal achalasia in the dog and cat. Tijdschr. Diergeneesk., 43:293, 1975.
16. Schwartz, A., et al.: Congenital neuromuscular esophageal disease in a litter of Newfoundland puppies. J. Am. Vet. Radiol. Soc., 17:101, 1976.
17. Sokolovsky, V.: Achalasia and paralysis of the canine esophagus. J. Am. Vet. Med. Assoc., 160:943, 1976.
18. Sternberg, J. C.: Megaesophagus caused by congenital heart disease. VM SAC, 72:196, 1977.
19. Strombeck, D. R., and Troya, L.: Evaluation of lower motor neuron function in two dogs with megaesophagus. J. Am. Vet. Med. Assoc., 169:411, 1976.

Acute Gastric Dilatation-Volvulus Syndrome

by WAYNE E. WINGFIELD

Acute gastric distension in the immature animal often results from overeating and is relieved by vomiting. In the mature, large breed dogs, acute gastric dilatation may eventually result in a life-threatening syndrome characterized by cranial abdominal distension with tympany, splenomegaly, and retching with nonproductive vomiting. Accumulated gas and fluid are unable to pass into the esophagus or duodenum and initiate a series of pathophysiologic events that may culminate in the death of the animal if they are not promptly recognized and vigorously treated.

Pathologic Anatomy

With gastric dilatation in the mature, large breed of dog, the stomach develops a flaccid character and a laxity of the gastrohepatic ligament. With further episodes, the stomach may rotate on its mesenteric attachments and may produce a volvulus. These animals require surgical intervention, and their anatomic features are described.

In gastric volvulus, the dilated fundus is displaced from left to right and ventrally in the abdomen. The pylorus moves caudodorsally, and the greater curvature lies along the ventral abdomen. The pylorus gradually moves dorsally, cranially, and toward the left. The spleen follows the greater curvature toward the right. Radiographically, a large gas or fluid-filled stomach is generally seen, with a soft-tissue density separating the pylorus from the fundus.[5,6] These displacements cause the fundus to be covered by two layers of omentum (Fig. 12-10). The spleen passively moves with the rotation of the fundus because of splenic and vascular attachments to the stomach. These attachments include the gastrosplenic ligament (part of the greater omentum) and short gastric arteries. In gastric volvulus, the spleen may be seen in various locations. These include the spleen located outside the omental bursa, the dorsal part of the spleen within the omental bursa, and the spleen pulled within the omental bursa and covered by the greater omentum.[5] Occasionally, the stomach is in

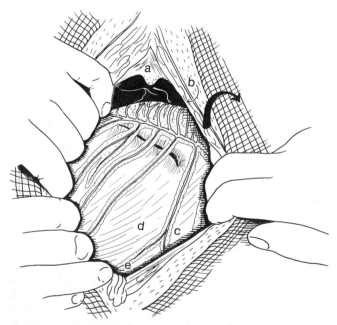

Fig. 12-10. *Abdominal anatomy of a dog in dorsal recumbency with gastric volvulus: a, xiphoid cartilage; b, liver; c, greater omentum; d, greater curvature of stomach; e, pylorus—located cranially, dorsally, and toward the dorsal midline.*

a normal position and the spleen is displaced at the time of celiotomy. This phenomenon may be important in the etiopathogenesis of *splenic torsion.* (See "Surgical Techniques of the Spleen," in Chapter 36.)

Vascular changes, ranging from fundic hyperemia through necrosis with a central perforation, are usually observed. Vascular lesions are always found on the area of the greater curvature, where the short gastric arteries anastomose with the left gastroepiploic artery.

Indications for Surgical Treatment

Gastric dilatation-volvulus syndrome necessitates surgical intervention. This syndrome is diagnosed through clinical signs, physical findings, and confirmation of the volvulus through abdominal radiography.

CLINICAL SIGNS. Large breed, deep-chested dogs are most frequently affected with gastric dilatation-volvulus syndrome, although 28 breeds have been reported.[9] Dachshunds, Pekingese, and other breeds that do not conform to the generalization of a large breed, deep-chested dog are also affected. Domestic cats have also been reported with gastric dilatation-volvulus syndrome. Van Kruiningen and associates[10] who reviewed other species with acute gastric dilatation, include the monkeys, foxes, mink, captive wild carnivores, rabbits, guinea pigs, and other rodents. Most dogs with this syndrome are mature, middle-aged, or older.[9] Males predominate over females by a 2 : 1 ratio.[1]

Retching with an inability to vomit is an important clinical finding in gastric dilatation-volvulus syndrome. With increased retching and aerophagia, dogs with acute gastric dilatation have cranial abdominal distension with tympany. The abdomen is tensed upon palpation. Increased respiratory efforts, hyperpnea, and open-mouthed panting are frequently seen. The abdomen appears asymmetrical if viewed dorsally to ventrally while the dog is standing. Most of this abdominal asymmetry is on the dog's right side. As the gastric dilatation syndrome progresses, shock develops. Scleral vessels become injected, and the dog may be unable to rise or walk. Salivation and respiratory grunting progressively increase and suggest pain.

PHYSICAL FINDINGS. Abdominal palpation may reveal splenomegaly, with the spleen oriented along a cranial-to-caudal plane. A weak femoral pulse, tachycardia, and prolonged capillary refill time are commonly noted. Passage of an orogastric tube decompresses the stomach. This technique is *not* a diagnostic test for gastric dilatation-volvulus syndrome, as was once believed. Even though a gastric tube may be passed, this result does *not* rule out gastric volvulus.

RADIOGRAPHY. A definitive diagnosis of gastric volvulus is made with abdominal radiography. Radiographs are taken following initial shock therapy and gastric decompression. A lateral projection and one in dorsal recumbency are necessary for assessment of gastric positioning. Barium is occasionally administered to better visualize the stomach.

Following gastric decompression, patients vary in their radiographic course of events. Sometimes, the stomach returns to a normal position immediately or within several hours. In other cases, the stomach remains malpositioned for days or weeks without functional disturbance.[5] Gastric volvulus is diagnosed when the pylorus is located dorsal, cranial, and to the left of the midline.

Physiologic Effects[13]

Following gaseous distension, the stomach does not evacuate, owing to abnormal gastroesophageal angulation that interferes with belching or vomiting. Compression of the duodenum by the dilated stomach may prevent passage of gas into the small bowel. Disturbed extrinsic innervation of the stomach may also be a factor in gastric atony. As the stomach dilates, the spleen is passively moved. Eventually, the splenic vessels become partially obstructed; this obstruction leads to venous congestion and a secondary splenomegaly. As the stomach dilates, it also exerts pressure upon the caudal vena cava and causes the venous return to be shunted through the ventral vertebral sinuses and the azygos vein to the cranial vena cava. Rotation of the stomach also actively occludes the portal vein and leads to serious venous congestion of abdominal splanchnic viscera and decreased cardiac output. Portal venous occlusion may initiate septic shock in dogs with gastric dilatation-volvulus syndrome. When the portal vein is experimentally occluded, a high mortality rate is noted in the dog. This mortality rate results from hypovolemia, a neurogenic enhancement of the shock state, or a failure of the reticuloendothelial system's capability to neutralize endotoxins. Gram-negative bacteria within the gut release their endotoxins with portal venous occlusion. This endotoxin enters the circulatory system either through the peritoneal surface or through the lymphatic channels.

Neurogenic stimulation of the splanchnic sympathetic nerves by the distended stomach results in hypotension. The consequences of hypotension and decreased circulating blood volume are a low velocity of flow. At low velocity, blood increases in viscosity, and the ability to perfuse tissues efficiently decreases. This sludging also promotes disseminated intravascular coagulation.

As intragastric pressures increase, the peristaltic activity decreases because of ischemic hypoxia. Severe damage to the ganglion cells of Auerbach's plexus may result and may contribute to the patient's large, atonic stomach. If the hypoxia is corrected within 3.5 to 4.0 hours, however, the neurologic insult is reversible. Whereas arterial pressures to the stomach are maintained during gastric dilatation, venous compromise results in subepithelial hemorrhage, edema, erosions, and ulcers. With continued gastric distension, the systemic arterial pressures fall while the caudal vena caval pressure rises. With the sequestration, oxyhemoglobin desaturation occurs in the blood within the caudal vena cava and right atrium. The encroachment of the dilated stomach on the thoracic space initially decreases tidal volume and increases respiratory rate in order to maintain minute volume. Lung compliance decreases with gastric dilatation and may result in a compromised ventilation-perfusion ratio.

In summary, gastric dilatation-volvulus syndrome alters many organ systems. Recognition of the complexity of the pathophysiologic features of this disorder should be adequate incentive for the veterinary surgeon to provide aggressive, prompt therapy.

Preoperative Care

Shock is the most important preoperative consideration. The treatment of shock involves medical therapy and gastric decompression. Medical therapy of shock is initiated with fluid therapy. The type of isotonic fluid is not as important as the volume and route of administration. Lactated Ringer's solution is readily available and is usually selected.

Survival of the patient often depends on the rapid intravenous infusion of large volumes of fluid. An initial loading volume of 90 ml/kg body weight is given.[3] The resultant hemodilution increases the patient's total oxygen transport capacity because of the increased cardiac output and improved flow characteristics.[7]

Corticosteroids are useful in the early treatment of shock, but are *always preceded* by conventional shock therapy, that is, the administration of fluids. In pharmacologic doses, corticosteroids enhance endothelial integrity, particularly in capillaries. Lysosomal membranes are stabilized and thus interfere with the degranulation of polymorphonuclear leukocytes and possibly decrease the formation of ancillary shock enhancing factors such as the myocardial depressant factor. Corticosteroids have an alpha-like blocking action that results in vasodilation and improved perfusion. High doses of corticosteroids protect against activation of unbalanced coagulation-fibrinolytic pathways and thereby protect against disseminated intravascular coagulation. Of potential importance in the gastric dilatation-volvulus syndrome, corticosteroids inhibit complement activation by endotoxin, a process that mediates many of the adverse effects and high mortality rates associated with systemic endotoxin circulation.

Bowen[2] lists the principal glucocorticoids and doses in shock therapy as follows: (1) hydrocortisone sodium succinate (Solu-Cortef), 50 mg/kg; (2) prednisolone sodium succinate (Solu-Delta Cortef), 40 mg/kg; (3) methylprednisolone sodium succinate (Solu-Medrol) 30 mg/kg; and (4) dexamethasone (Azium) 5 mg/kg. Because economic factors are important, it is noted that methylprednisolone, the most expensive, costs over 16 times more per kg of body weight than dexamethasone, the least expensive.

Antibiotics are used in the treatment of septic shock. Selection of bacteriocidal versus bacteriostatic agents is still controversial. At this time, the bacteriocidal drugs are favored. The mortality rate of septic shock patients is considerably higher when antibiotics are unaccompanied by corticosteroids.

Gastric decompression is achieved most quickly by passing a stomach tube or by gastrocentesis (trocarization). A well-lubricated, colt-sized,* stiff stomach tube can frequently be passed, and the gastric contents may be removed with warm-water lavage. Trocarization is occasionally required with a 12- to 16-gauge needle passed into the right paracostal area. With this partial release of gastric gas, passage of the orogastric tube may be successful.

Gastrostomy can be used as a decompressive procedure.[11] Tissue viability of the stomach may be checked through the gastrostomy, and complete decompression will result. In order to realign the stomach anatomically, the gastrostomy must be dismantled. Gastric decompression improves cardiovascular function and thus enhances the rapid fluid replacement. Surprisingly, clinical patients with gastric dilatation-volvulus syndrome have *not* proved to be in the severe metabolic acidosis seen in animals with the experimentally induced syndrome.[14] At present, bicarbonate therapy is *not* recommended in the initial management of this disorder.

Baseline laboratory parameters should be collected prior to fluid administration. Packed cell volume (PCV) and total solids (TS) determinations are useful in assessing fluid replacement. Complete blood count (CBC) and blood glucose tests are useful in assessing septic shock. In sepsis, a leukopenia with significant immature granulocytes and hypoglycemia (<60 mg/dl) suggest septicemia. Prior to administering fluids, a urine specific gravity determination is useful in assessing renal function.

Surgical Techniques

Chronic recurring gastric dilatation or gastric volvulus is an indication for surgical exploration. The dog is placed in dorsal recumbency, and a midventral abdominal incision is made from the xiphoid cartilage caudally to the umbilicus. Upon entry into the peritoneal cavity, the stomach with volvulus is covered ventrally by the greater omentum (see Fig. 12-10).

The stomach and spleen must first be anatomically realigned. This procedure requires an understanding of the anatomic features described previously. With realignment, the stomach wall is assessed for areas of necrosis. With necrosis or questioned viability the affected area is excised. The gastrectomy is closed as a routine gastrostomy (see the first section of this chapter).

Thrombi of the splenic vessels are occasionally noted. These thrombi prevent the spleen from returning to normal size and require splenectomy (see Chap. 36). It is important to note that splenectomy does *not* prevent the recurrence of gastric dilatation-volvulus syndrome.[12]

Pyloromyotomy or pyloroplasty is used to relieve gastric retention or gastric obstruction (see the final section of this chapter). This operation alters terminal antral contractions and disrupts antral retropulsion of solid particles, thus accelerating gastric emptying of solids.

Numerous operative techniques have been attempted to prevent recurrence of this syndrome. These include gastropexy, gastrocolopexy, "permanent gastropexy," tube gastrostomy, and circumcostal gastropexy.[4] Open gastrostomy is described in the following section of this chapter. Currently, the tube gastrostomy is favored. It provides a continuous method for postoperative decompression and medicating the stomach. A firm adhesion develops between the stomach and abdominal wall, and this adhesion appears to be adequate to prevent rotation of the stomach with additional bouts of gastric dilatation.

TUBE GASTROSTOMY

The tube gastrostomy may be placed as an emergency decompression technique or at the time of open gastric repositioning. The approach for the former is as

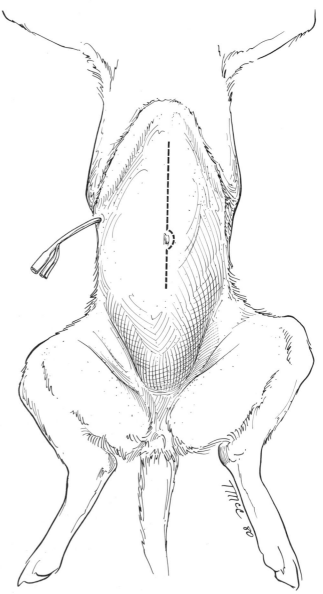

Fig. 12-11. *The animal is placed in dorsal recumbency and is prepared for operation to accommodate a ventral incision and the exit of the Foley catheter in the right paracostal area.*

*PVC plastic colt stomach tube, Jensen-Salsbury Laboratories, 520 West 21st Street, Kansas City, MO 64141

in the "grid" incision described previously. For the latter, the animal is placed in dorsal recumbency and is prepared for an aseptic operation. Hair clipping, surgical preparation, and draping include the right paracostal area for exit of the Foley catheter. A midventral abdominal incision is made from the xiphoid cartilage extending caudal to the umbilicus (Fig. 12-11).

A 26-French Foley catheter is used in the tube gastrostomy. Carmalt forceps are passed through the abdominal wall in the right paracostal area (Fig. 12-12) near the tip of the thirteenth rib. It is important to move dorsally from the ventral midline in tube placement to provide a proper adhesion site between the stomach and body wall when the dog returns to full alimentation and activity. The exit hole through the skin should be smaller than the tube diameter in order to ensure a tight fit.

When the Foley catheter has been carefully retrieved through the paracostal hole (Fig. 12-13), nonabsorbable suture material is used to place a full-thickness pursestring suture in the pyloric antrum. The position of this suture is usually two-thirds of the distance toward the pylorus and away from the fundus. A small incision is made within the circumference of the pursestring suture, and the Foley catheter is passed through the greater omentum into the stomach lumen through the incision within the antral pursestring suture (Fig. 12-

14). The balloon portion of the catheter is inflated, using the appropriate quantity of saline solution. The pursestring suture is tightened against the Foley catheter. This suture must be tight enough to prevent leakage, but not so tight as to prevent removal of the tube. By pulling on the inflated catheter, the stomach can now be moved to a position adjacent to the peritoneal wall.

A local gastropexy using nonabsorbable sutures is placed in the abdominal wall and stomach (Fig. 12-15). Each gastropexy suture extends to the submucosa to achieve holding strength. With the greater omentum entrapped between the stomach and peritoneum and the gastropexy sutures, any leakage that may result is localized. A pursestring suture is placed in the skin around the Foley catheter. Adhesive tape may be placed as a butterfly around the tube and may be sutured to the skin to restrict the tube's motion.

An alternative gastrostomy technique is preferred by some veterinary surgeons. A Witzel technique is employed in this procedure. With this technique, a tunnel provided for the Foley catheter is believed to lessen the occurrence of leakage complications around the catheter. Leakage has not been a major complication with the previously described gastrostomy, but for the sake of completeness, the Witzel technique is described here.

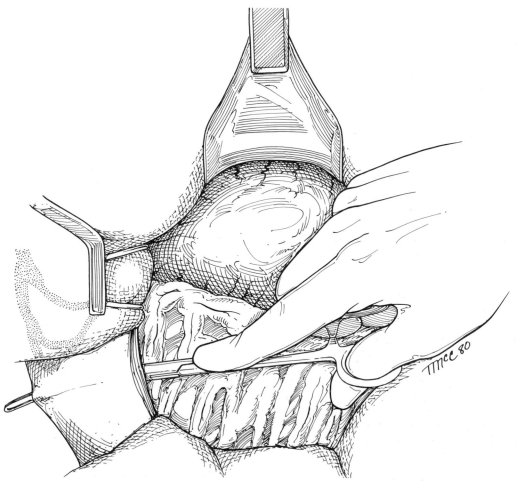

Fig. 12-12. *Forceps are passed through the abdominal wall just ventral to the tip of the thirteenth rib.*

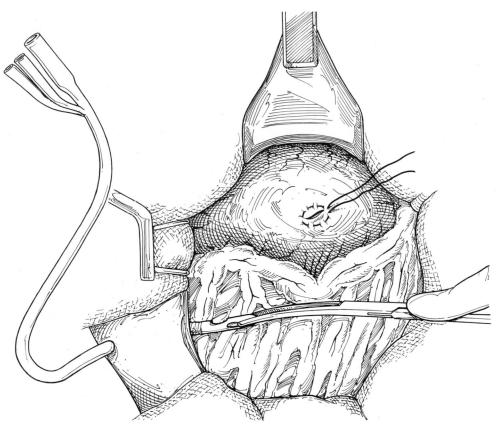

Fig. 12-13. *The Foley catheter is pulled through the abdominal wall, and a full-thickness pursestring suture is placed in the pyloric antrum.*

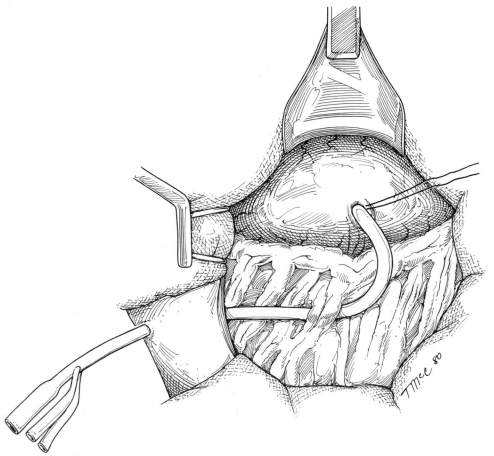

Fig. 12-14. *The Foley catheter is passed through the greater omentum and is introduced into the stomach.*

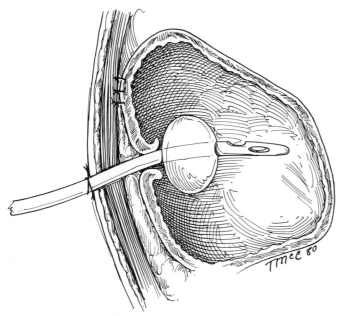

Fig. 12-15. *Cross-sectional view of the stomach and abdominal wall. The Foley catheter has its balloon inflated. Gastropexy sutures are used to hold the stomach adjacent to the peritoneum while an adhesion forms. A pursestring suture is placed in the skin around the Foley catheter.*

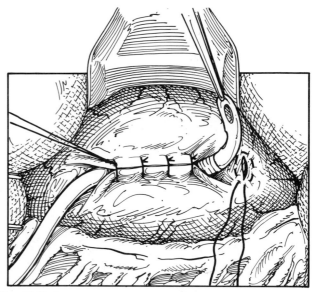

Fig. 12-17. *Lembert sutures are placed along the catheter. A full thickness pursestring suture is inserted into the pyloric antrum.*

The initial abdominal incision and tube entry are essentially the same as previously described. With the Witzel technique, an incision is made in the right paracostal area. The tube is laid over the pyloric antrum, and full-thickness sutures are used to place a Lembert pattern over the Foley catheter (Fig. 12-16). A full-thickness pursestring suture using nonabsorbable material is placed in the antrum (Fig. 12-17). The Foley catheter is inserted into the gastric lumen, and the balloon is inflated with saline solution. One last Lembert suture is placed to cover the tube, and the catheter is

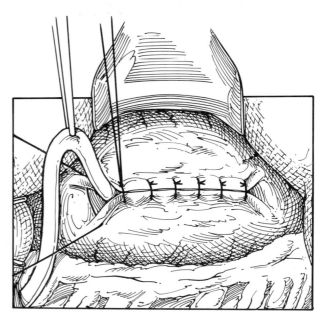

Fig. 12-18. *The Foley catheter is inserted into the stomach lumen and the area is covered with one last Lembert suture. Retraction of the catheter assures a tight fit.*

retracted to ensure a tight fit (Fig. 12-18). The stomach is sutured through the various abdominal wall structures. Sutures grasp the stomach to peritoneum, muscle, and subcutaneous tissues (Fig. 12-19). A pursestring suture is placed in the skin and is tightened around the Foley catheter. A tape butterfly is used to keep the tube from slipping. The abdominal incision is closed in the routine manner.

Postoperative Care

The tube gastrostomy must be protected from the animal. Bandaging of the abdomen, to include the Foley catheter, is usually adequate. Occasionally, other restraint devices are required (see Chap. 3).

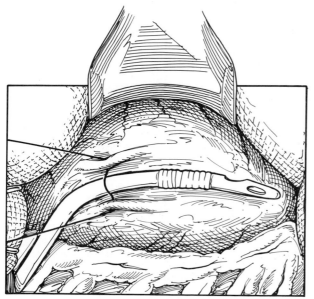

Fig. 12-16. *A Witzel gastrostomy, with the Foley catheter laid over the pyloric antrum. A Lembert suture is placed over the catheter in order to form a tunnel from which the tube will exit.*

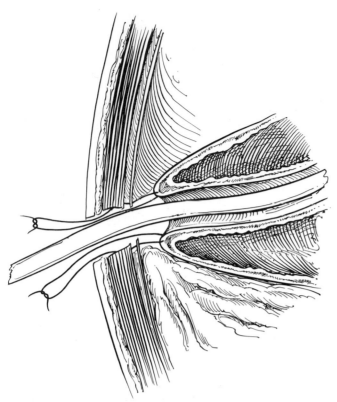

Fig. 12-19. *The Foley catheter is retracted laterally, and the stomach is sutured to the peritoneum, abdominal muscles, and subcutaneous tissue.*

Table 12-1. *Guidelines for Potassium Replacement*

Serum (Extracellular) Potassium (K) (meq/L)	Potassium Chloride (KCl) Replacement (meq) per 250 ml Fluids*
2.0	20
2.0–2.5	15
2.5–3.0	10
3.0–3.5	7.5
3.5**	5

*Do not exceed 0.5 mEq/kg/hr
**If serum potassium levels are unavailable, replace at least 5 meq KCl/250 ml fluids

10 days. When removing the tube, one merely removes the pursestring skin suture, deflates the balloon (the balloon is often broken from reaction with gastric acid), and pulls out the tube. The gastrostomy heals by second intention (granulation) within 2 to 3 days. This area should be kept clean and bandaged. Premature tube removal may cause peritonitis, which requires immediate laparotomy and medical management. Leakage around the tube occasionally results in cellulitis, which requires surgical drainage and replacement of the tube gastrostomy.

Prevention

In that the cause of gastric dilatation-volvulus syndrome is unknown, it is difficult to advocate exact preventive measures. Foodstuffs are not the cause, and the syndrome has been noted in dogs fed free-choice or multiple feedings. Soybean-based and soybean-free diets and postprandial exercise may or may not be associated with this disorder. No specific foodstuff or feeding practice is presumed to be incriminated in the etiology of gastric dilatation-volvulus syndrome. Prophylactically, it is important to note that frequent, small quantities of food decrease gastric distension. Moistening foods and eliminating postprandial exercise or excitement may help to control aerophagia. Antifoaming antacids are *not* important because the dog does not experience a frothy bloat.

In summary, gastric dilatation-volvulus syndrome is a potentially life-threatening disease requiring prompt recognition, aggressive medical and surgical therapy, and close postoperative monitoring. The rate of recurrence of this syndrome is decreased with newer operative procedures. When the exact cause of this disorder is identified, more specific recommendations may be offered for its prevention.

Postoperative complications are associated with shock, hypokalemia, cardiac dysrhythmias, and gastrostomy complications. Fluid therapy and monitoring of the patient are important. Owing to the gastritis caused by gastric dilatation-volvulus syndrome, nothing is offered by mouth for 24 to 48 hours. It is important to maintain the patient's fluid and electrolyte balance during this period. Cardiac dysrhythmias are important in this syndrome.[8] Supraventricular dysrhythmias include atrial premature contractions, junctional rhythms, and atrial fibrillation. Ventricular premature contractions, paroxysmal ventricular tachycardia, ventricular tachycardia, and multifocal ventricular tachycardia also occur. These dysrhythmias may or may not respond to antiarrhythmic drug therapy. Lidocaine and procainamide or quinidine are most useful in managing serious ventricular dysrhythmias. An intracellular hypokalemia is apparently present in dogs with gastric dilatation-volvulus syndrome, probably owing to the pathophysiology of shock and significant fluid therapy. Muscle weakness and cardiac dysrhythmias are frequently seen postoperatively, but if potassium chloride is supplemented in the fluids and is carefully administered, both problems are less frequent. Table 12-1 lists guidelines for potassium replacement in intravenous fluids, based on extracellular potassium levels.

Gastrostomy complications usually result from the premature removal of the Foley catheter. This tube must be left in place at *least* 5 days and preferably 7 to

References and Selected Readings

1. Betts, C. W., Wingfield, W. E., and Green, R. W.: A retrospective study of gastric dilatation-torsion in the dog. J. Small Anim. Pract., *15*:727, 1974.
2. Bowen, J. M.: Are corticosteroids useful in shock therapy? J. Am. Vet. Med. Assoc., *177*:453, 1980.
3. Brasmer, T. H.: Fluid therapy in shock. J. Am. Vet. Med. Assoc., *174*:475, 1979.

4. Fallah, A. M., et al.: Circumcostal gastropexy in the dog. A preliminary study. Vet. Surg., *11*:9, 1982.

5. Funkquist, B.: Gastric torsion in the dog—I. Radiological picture during nonsurgical treatment related to the pathological anatomy and to the further clinical course. J. Small Anim. Pract., *20*:73, 1979.

6. Kneller, S. K.: Radiographic interpretation of the gastric dilatation-volvulus complex in the dog. J. Am. Anim. Hosp. Assoc., *12*:154, 1976.

7. Messmer, K.: Hemodilution. Surg. Clin. North Am., *55*:659, 1975.

8. Muir, W. W., and Lipowitz, A. J.: Cardiac dysrhythmias associated with gastric dilatation-volvulus in the dog. J. Am. Vet. Med. Assoc., *172*:683, 1978.

9. Todoroff, R. J.: Gastric dilatation-volvulus. Compend. Contin. Ed., *1*:142, 1979.

10. Van Kruiningen, H. J., Gregoire, K., and Meuten, D. J.: Acute gastric dilatation: a review of comparative aspects, by species, and a study in dogs and monkeys. J. Am. Anim. Hosp. Assoc., *10*:294, 1974.

11. Walshaw, R., and Johnston, D. E.: Treatment of gastric dilatation-volvulus by gastric decompression and patient stabilization before major surgery. J. Am. Anim. Hosp. Assoc., *12*:162, 1976.

12. Wingfield, W. E., Betts, C. W., and Greene, R. S.: Operative techniques and recurrence rates associated with gastric volvulus in the dog. J. Small Anim. Pract., *16*:427, 1975.

13. Wingfield, W. E., Betts, C. W., and Rawling, C. A.: Pathophysiology associated with gastric dilatation-volvulus in the dog. J. Am. Anim. Hosp. Assoc., *12*:136, 1976.

14. Wingfield, W. E., et al.: Acid-base and electrolyte values in dogs with acute gastric dilatation-volvulus. J. Am. Vet. Med. Assoc., *180*:1070, 1982.

Gastrotomy

by MARY L. DULISCH

A gastrotomy is usually made in a hypovascular area on the ventral aspect of the stomach between the lesser and greater curvatures. The most common indications for gastrotomy are to remove foreign bodies, to inspect the gastric mucosa for ulcers, neoplasms, or hypertrophy, and to obtain a biopsy.

Preoperative Considerations

Prior to the surgical procedure, the entire gastrointestinal tract should be examined thoroughly by physical examination and radiographs to determine whether additional lesions are present. The patient should be evaluated for fluid and electrolyte imbalances; these should be corrected prior to the operation.

Surgical Technique

The patient is placed in dorsal recumbency, and a ventral midline incision is made extending from the xiphoid to the umbilicus. Moistened laparotomy pads are placed on either side of the incision line and are folded over the cut edges. A Balfour retractor is used to retract the body wall. The stomach is grossly inspected and then is elevated from the abdomen with the use of Babcock forceps (Fig. 12-20). The forceps are placed in

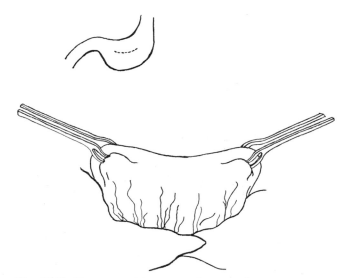

Fig. 12-20. *Placement of forceps on the stomach.*

the least vascular area of the body of the stomach and approximately 10 cm apart. Following exploration, the surrounding abdominal structures are packed off with moistened laparotomy pads. Using a No. 10 Bard-Parker scalpel blade with the cutting edge up, a stab incision is made into the lumen of the stomach (Fig. 12-21). This incision is extended with Metzenbaum scissors toward the forceps (Figs. 12-22 and 12-23). After inspection of the lumen, the stomach is closed in a two-layer inverting seromuscular pattern. The first layer consists of a Cushing pattern using 2-0 chromic

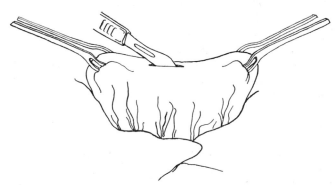

Fig. 12-21. *Stab incision into the stomach.*

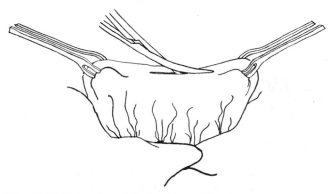

Fig. 12-22. *Extension of the incision with scissors.*

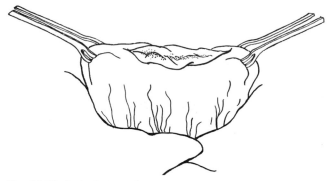

Fig. 12-23. *Incised stomach.*

catgut. The sutures begin at the serosal surface and penetrate to, but not through, the mucosa (Figs. 12-24, 12-25, and 12-26). The second layer consists of a Lembert pattern also using 2-0 chromic catgut (Figs. 12-27 and 12-28). Omentum may be placed over the incision if desired. Two simple interrupted sutures of 3-0 or 2-0 chromic catgut are sufficient for local omental attachment. Synthetic absorbable sutures can be used in place of the chromic catgut.

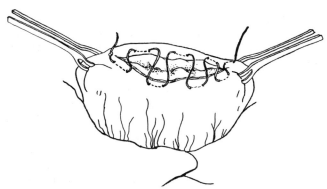

Fig. 12-24. *Cushing suture line in the stomach.*

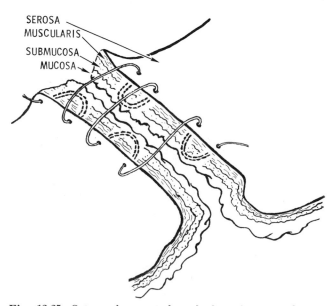

SEROSA
MUSCULARIS
SUBMUCOSA
MUCOSA

Fig. 12-25. *Suture placement through the submucosa, but not through the mucosa.*

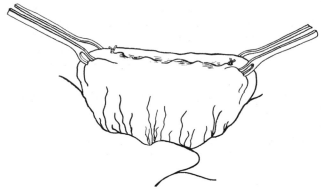

Fig. 12-26. *Closed incision line.*

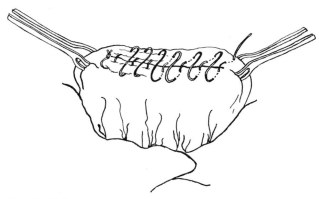

Fig. 12-27. *Lembert suture line in the stomach.*

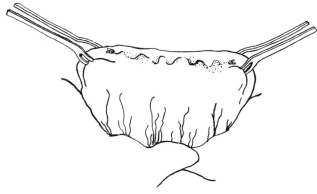

Fig. 12-28. *Closed incision line.*

Pyloromyotomy and Pyloroplasty
by MARY L. DULISCH

Pyloromyotomy (Fredet-Ramstedt) and pyloroplasty (Heineke-Mikulicz) are two surgical techniques used to increase the diameter of the pyloric lumen.[1] This change results in a decreased gastric emptying time. The pyloroplasty is a permanent technique, whereas a pyloromyotomy may scar over and may allow the clinical problem to recur. These techniques are indicated in patients with a diagnosis of pylorospasm, pyloric stenosis, gastric dilatation, or gastric dilatation-volvulus syndrome. Pylorospasm is usually seen in toy and miniature breeds of dogs. The disease is characterized by intermittent projectile vomiting after eating. Probably neurogenic in origin, there is a failure of the pyloric sphincter to relax in coordination with propulsive peristaltic contractions of the pyloric antrum.[2] Pyloric stenosis may be either acquired or congenital and is characterized by persistent projectile vomiting after eating. The stenosis is usually due to hypertrophy of the pyloric sphincter muscle or hypertrophied mucosal folds following chronic gastritis. This hypertrophied pyloric tissue may increase gastric emptying time and may predispose a patient to gastric dilatation.[2,3]

Surgical Techniques

The surgical approach for pyloric operations is the same as for a gastrotomy. When the stomach and pylorus have been located, it may be useful to transect the gastrohepatic ligament to increase pyloric mobilization (Fig. 12-29). The gastrohepatic ligament is a thin band of tissue extending from the pyloric region to the hilus of the liver. Care is taken not to cut the common bile duct, which is cranial and dorsal to the ligament. The abdominal structures are packed off with moistened laparotomy pads so that the stomach, pylorus, and descending duodenum are the only structures visible.

PYLOROMYOTOMY

When performing a pyloromyotomy, the pylorus can be elevated into view with the use of Babcock forceps (Fig. 12-30). An incision approximately 4 cm long is

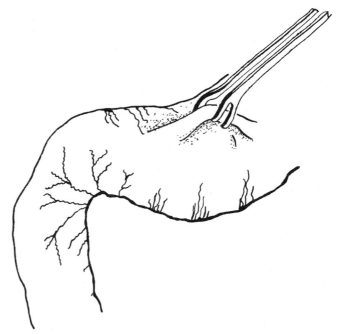

Fig. 12-30. *Placement of Babcock forceps on the stomach.*

made into the least vascular area of the pyloric canal, pylorus, and proximal duodenum. The pylorus is the midpoint of the incision. The incision extends through the tunica serosa and the muscle layer (Fig. 12-31). The muscle layer is cut and separated by sharp and blunt dissection using Metzenbaum scissors. All muscular bands should be identified and severed. Care is taken not to cut through the tunica mucosa (Fig. 12-32). If a small hole is made in the tunica mucosa, it can be closed with a single, simple interrupted suture using 2-0 or 3-0 chromic catgut. If a larger hole has been made, the incision should be converted into a pyloroplasty. When the muscle bands have been completely severed, the tunica mucosa will bulge out of the incision site (Fig. 12-33).

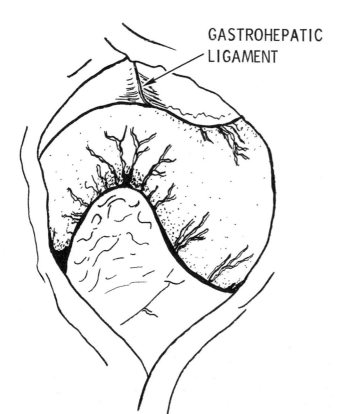

Fig. 12-29. *Relation of the gastrohepatic ligament to the pylorus.*

GASTROHEPATIC LIGAMENT

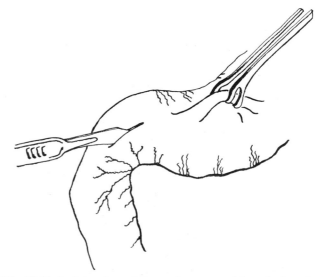

Fig. 12-31. *Incision through the tunica serosa of the pyloric region.*

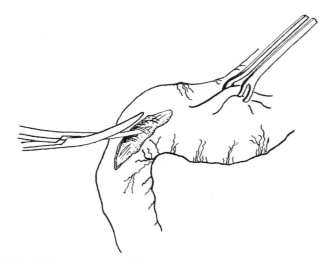

Fig. 12-32. *Dissection of muscle from the pyloric region.*

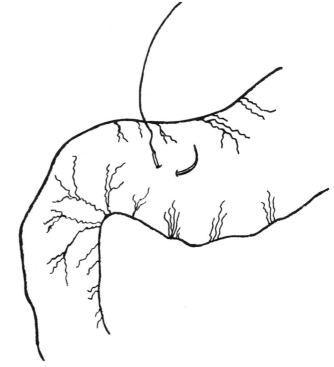

Fig. 12-34. *Stay suture in the least vascular area of stomach.*

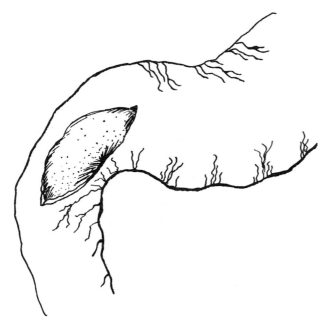

Fig. 12-33. *Bulging of the tunica mucosa through the incision line.*

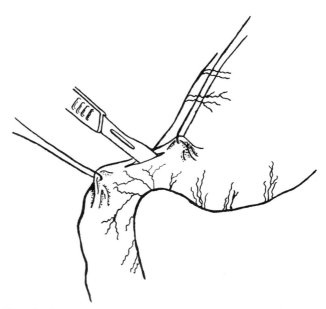

Fig. 12-35. *Incision into the pyloric region.*

PYLOROPLASTY

When performing a pyloroplasty, temporary stay sutures of 2-0 chromic catgut are placed in the least vascular portions of the ventral stomach and the proximal duodenum (Fig. 12-34). These sutures are approximately 10 cm apart, with the pylorus as the midpoint. Using a No. 10 Bard-Parker scalpel blade with the cutting edge up, a stab incision is made into the lumen and is extended with scissors to span a distance of 1 to 2 cm on either side of the pylorus (Figs. 12-35, 12-36, and 12-37). When the stay sutures have been removed, the longitudinal incision is closed transversely (Fig. 12-38) using 2-0 chromic catgut suture in a simple interrupted crushing pattern (Fig. 12-39) or in a Gambee suture pattern. If the animal is hypoalbuminemic or if slow healing is anticipated, 2-0 nylon or polypropylene

should be used. Omentum is placed over the incision area to act as a seal and may be tacked down with 1 or 2 simple interrupted sutures of 3-0 chromic catgut. Abdominal closure is performed in a routine manner.

Postoperative Care

Postoperative care is the same for both procedures. No food, water, or oral medication should be given for 24 hours. Maintenance fluid requirements are sustained

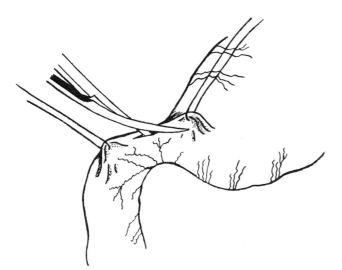

Fig. 12-36. *Extension of the incision with Metzenbaum scissors.*

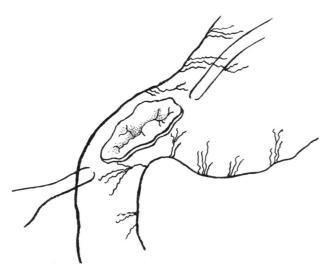

Fig. 12-37. *Pyloric incision.*

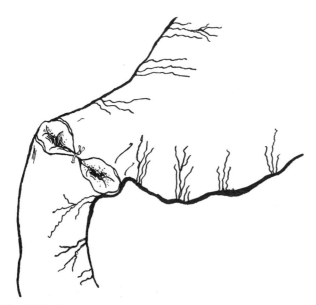

Fig. 12-38. *Stay sutures are removed, and the pyloric incision is sutured transversely.*

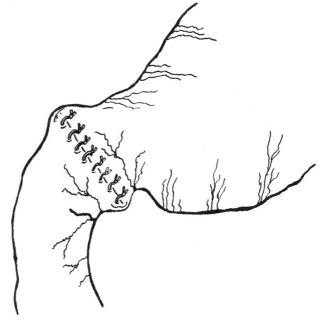

Fig. 12-39. *Complete view of closure.*

with intravenous fluids. Antibiotics, given prophylactically, are administered intravenously prior to the surgical procedure and for the first 24 hours postoperatively. Antibiotics are administered orally for 7 to 10 days. A soft diet consisting of small amounts of baby food or a soft dog-food gruel can be fed 24 hours after the operation. This diet should be fed in small amounts several times a day. The consistency of the food can be thickened with each succeeding day. Once the patient has started to drink on its own, the intravenous fluids are gradually discontinued.

References and Suggested Readings

1. Ewing, G. O.: Pyloric stenosis. *In* Current Veterinary Therapy IV. Edited by R. W. Kirk. Philadelphia, W. B. Saunders, 1971.
2. Arnoczky, S. P., and Ryan, W. W.: Gastrotomy and pyloroplasty. Vet. Clin. North Am., *5*:343, 1975.
3. DeHoff, W. D., and Greene, R. W.: Gastric dilatation and gastric torsion complex. Vet. Clin. North Am., *2*:150, 1972.

13 * Intestines

Surgery of the Small Intestine

by D. J. KRAHWINKEL, JR. *and*
DANIEL C. RICHARDSON

Although intestinal surgery has been performed since the days of Hippocrates (460 B.C.), significant advances were not made until the 1800s. The introduction of intestinal healing by Lembert in 1826 and of ether by Long in 1842 opened the doors to the field of intestinal surgery. Many different techniques were advocated, but Halsted promoted the principle of a one-layer closure and the importance of sutures in the submucosal layer. Parker and Kerr introduced the closed anastomosis, and great strides were made in intestinal closure in the early 1900s. Aseptic technique reduced infection rates, the use of antibiotics facilitated a return to an open technique of anastomosis, and simple intestinal clamps were devised to aid the surgeon.

Controversies have continued, however, with regard to preferred techniques of intestinal closure: the one-layer versus the two-layer closure, everting versus inverting versus appositional techniques, open versus closed, and absorbable versus nonabsorbable suture. Many variations of anatomic alignment, such as end-to-end, end-to-side, and side-to-side, have also been advocated. The recent development of intestinal stapling has added another alternative. It is now accepted that simple appositional end-to-end anastomosis produces excellent results.

All these current techniques have been evaluated biomechanically and clinically. Because every technique has its advantages and disadvantages, veterinary surgeons must decide which is best for their particular needs. Despite controversy, it is probably safe to say that in the hands of a competent veterinary surgeon using sound surgical principles, any one of the many different techniques is usually successful. The techniques of small intestinal surgery described are simple, rapid to perform, require no special instrumentation, and provide excellent results when properly executed. Although technique has changed in recent decades, the principles proposed over a hundred years ago by Halsted, Travers, and Lembert still apply. These principles are to: (1) incorporate the submucosal layer in the anastomosis; (2) anastomose to provide serosa-to-serosa contact: (3) minimize trauma and contamination; (4) maintain an adequate blood supply; and (5) avoid tension across the anastomosis.

Intestinal Resection and Anastomosis

INDICATIONS

Sections of small bowel are removed when damage to the intestinal wall is irreversible. This damage can occur with an intraluminal foreign body, traumatic injury to the bowel or mesentery, obstruction from an intraluminal or intramural neoplasm, strangulation of a loop of gut from herniation or volvulus, or irreducible intussusception.

The decision to excise or to repair a segment of bowel should be made after thorough examination and complete exploration of the abdominal cavity. Only then should attention focus on the affected bowel segment. For years, the decision to excise has been based on color, presence of peristalsis, and pulsation of the mesenteric vessels to the segment. The decision to resect should not be hasty because relieving a strangulation and bathing the gut with warm, sterile saline solution for several minutes may dramatically improve the appearance of the affected bowel. Contractility may be checked by gently compressing the gut to see whether a local spasm develops. A small stab wound on the antimesenteric border of the intestine can help to verify a functional blood supply.

More recently, intravenous fluorescein and Doppler scanning have been used to determine the viability of intestine. Intraoperatively, fluorescein is administered intravenously (10 mg/kg), and the bowel is scanned with a Wood's light to determine whether the segment is being perfused. A loop of normal bowel should be used for comparison. Doppler ultrasound can be used to determine the adequacy of the blood supply to the bowel. A sterilized Doppler Flowmeter* is used to scan the antimesenteric border of the affected intestinal segment, to determine the presence of audible arterial signals. Again, the affected bowel should be compared with a normal segment. These two techniques should be used to supplement, but not to replace, clinical judg-

*Model 810, Parks Electronics, Beaverton, OR

ment. If in doubt, it is better to resect viable bowel than to leave a questionable segment.

INTESTINAL FOREIGN BODY. Common foreign bodies include stones, children's toys, bones, plastic food packaging, and household fabrics. Many of these objects pass through the gastrointestinal tract without incident; others require surgical intervention. Medical treatment of an obstruction due to foreign body is seldom curative. Most foreign bodies can be removed by enterotomy; however, on occasion, the extent of damage requires resection. Removal by enterotomy may be performed, and the intestine may be bathed and observed to see whether viability returns. If not, then resection should be performed.

INTUSSUSCEPTION. The telescoping of one portion of the gut into another usually causes bowel obstruction. Occasionally, an intussusception occurs at multiple sites. Puppies and kittens are most commonly affected, and any portion of the bowel may be involved. The ileocecal area predominates in frequency, however. The exact cause of this disorder is unknown, but it is probably due to abnormalities of peristalsis. Many intussusceptions may be manually reduced by gentle traction on the internal segment while softly "milking" the external segment (Fig. 13-1). If the lesion cannot be reduced, resection is required. If the intussuscepted segment is substantially devitalized following reduction, resection and anastomosis are necessary. Following reduction, the affected bowel is bathed with warm saline solution and is observed. Treatable predisposing factors, such as parasitic infection, should be determined and eliminated.

STRANGULATION. A loop of small intestine that herniates through an abdominal wall defect or undergoes internal herniation occluding the vascular supply is said to be strangulated. This phenomenon is most com-

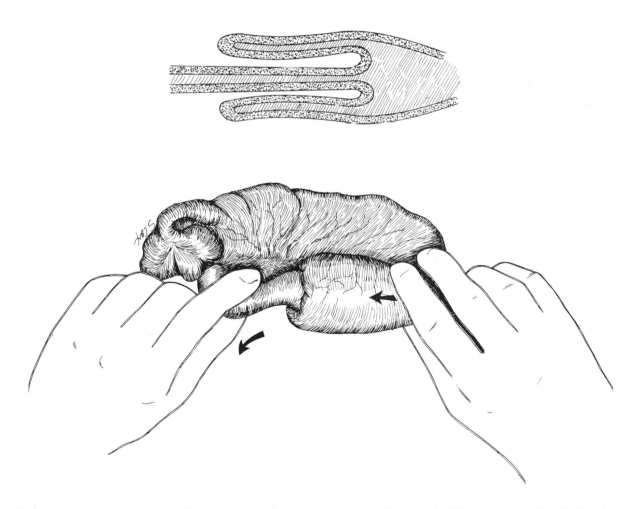

Fig. 13-1. *An intussusception is reduced by applying gentle pressure on the invaginated end while simultaneously "milking" the opposite end.*

monly seen with inguinal and traumatic ventral hernias. Umbilical hernias rarely cause bowel strangulation. Occasionally, a diaphragmatic hernia manifests with signs of intestinal obstruction secondary to the strangulation of a loop of small intestine through a tear in the diaphragm. With strangulation, the venous supply is obstructed, followed by intestinal congestion, ischemia, arterial stasis, changes in capillary permeability, and loss of fluid and electrolytes into the bowel. If corrected early in the disease process, the segment may be salvaged by relieving the strangulation, bathing the segment in warm saline solution, and determining the viability of the injured segment by the previously mentioned criteria.

TRAUMATIC INJURIES. Penetrating abdominal wounds and blunt abdominal trauma commonly injure the intestine or the mesentery and associated vasculature. Penetrating wounds, such as gunshot wounds, of the abdomen should be explored immediately, and the entire bowel should be examined. Intestinal resection is rarely required unless the intestinal vasculature is compromised. Blunt abdominal trauma, as from motor vehicle accidents, may directly injure the bowel with resulting contusion, bruising, and hematoma. Occasionally, the mesentery is torn from the intestine, and the result is an avascular loop of bowel. Blunt injury is difficult to diagnose unless the bowel is ruptured or significant hemorrhage occurs. In these instances, diagnostic peritoneal lavage confirms the injury. Evisceration and self-induced trauma following abdominal surgical procedures are all too common an indication for intestinal resection. Proper surgical technique and aftercare minimize this complication.

INTESTINAL NEOPLASMS. The intestine is occasionally the site of neoplasia in small animals. Adenocarcinoma, leiomyoma, and lymphosarcoma are the most common neoplasms. Clinical signs are commonly those of partial obstruction. Metastasis often occurs to regional lymph nodes, liver, spleen, and peritoneum. Early diagnosis, followed by wide resection of the affected bowel and histopathologic confirmation, should be the surgical goal. Prognosis in cases of intestinal neoplasia is poor to guarded because of the frequency of nonresectable lesions and metastasis.

VOLVULUS AND TORSION. Axial rotation of a loop of intestine (volvulus) or a twist in the mesentery (torsion) are uncommon in the small animal because of the short mesenteric attachments. When these disorders do occur, the jejunum and ileum are the usual sites. The length of time present and the extent of involvement dictate whether the lesion can be manually reduced or whether a resection is required. Adhesions may be present and must be broken down before manual reduction may be performed. As with neoplasms, the clinical signs are commonly associated with a partial obstruction.

CLINICAL SIGNS OF INTESTINAL LESIONS

Clinical signs depend upon the location of the intestinal lesion and whether the lesion has totally or partially occluded the intestinal lumen. Nausea, anorexia, restlessness, depression, abdominal pain, and abdominal distension are all signs of partial or total intestinal obstruction. The accumulation of gastrointestinal fluids and ingesta distends the gut and causes intestinal reflux and vomiting. Obstructions of the proximal small bowel cause vomiting much earlier in the disease process than distal obstructions. With some distal small intestinal obstructions, vomiting may not occur.

The onset of obvious signs with distal obstruction may be delayed for several days, and the severity of these signs may be much less than when the lesion is in the proximal small bowel. Abdominal distension is less noticeable because the majority of the fluids have been absorbed proximal to the obstruction. The vomitus is more likely to be fetid with distal obstructions because of increased food breakdown and bacterial action. The distal obstruction may take the form of a chronic disease, whereas the proximal obstruction is usually more acute and life-threatening. One may observe generalized weakness due to the loss of body fluids and electrolytes. Panting occurs as the animal attempts respiratory compensation for metabolic acidosis; however, severe vomiting usually results in a metabolic alkalosis because of the loss of gastric fluids.

The signs of incomplete obstruction mimic those of distal obstruction in that they are variable and chronic. Feces are usually present and may appear normal, or they may contain blood and excessive mucus. A fetid diarrhea may result from the increased fluid accumulation proximal to the lesion and the bacterial action favoring gas and fluid production. In prolonged cases of obstruction, the clinical signs are those of hypovolemic shock due to the loss of body fluids by vomiting and transudation into the bowel lumen.

DIAGNOSIS OF INTESTINAL LESIONS

Diagnosis of an intestinal lesion begins with a thorough physical examination. Abdominal pain and distension may prevent accurate palpation. Foreign bodies and tumor masses are often palpable in the cooperative patient, however. An intussusception has the feel of an elongated "sausage" in the abdomen. Strangulated intestine may be palpable as distended, painful gas- and fluid-filled loops of bowel leading to a hernia ring. Even without a palpable mass, gas- and fluid-distended gut can be construed as a clue to obstruction.

Dehydration, as evidenced clinically by increased skin turgor and dry mucous membranes or by elevated packed cell volume and total plasma protein, is commonly observed. Leucocytosis and elevation of the blood urea nitrogen are also common laboratory findings.

Radiography is a useful adjunct to diagnosis. Radiodense foreign objects, abnormal soft-tissue masses, and ileus evidenced by grossly distended gas- and fluid-filled loops of bowel of nonuniform caliber suggest intestinal obstruction. Contrast studies are required to demonstrate the radiolucent object or the partial obstruction due to soft-tissue masses. If barium is used as a contrast medium, the veterinary surgeon must remember that peritoneal contamination can lead to a fatal peritonitis. If the bowel has been perforated and peritonitis is present, or when bowel injury is accompanied by hemorrhage, a diagnostic peritoneal lavage is a useful diagnostic aid.

Exploratory celiotomy is one of the most useful diagnostic techniques. When clinical evaluation and radiographic procedures suggest intestinal disease that requires surgical treatment, exploration should not be unduly postponed because mortality rates increase rapidly with time.

PREOPERATIVE PREPARATION

Preparation of the patient with complete proximal intestinal obstruction is an emergency procedure. In partial or distal obstruction, more time may be spent in ensuring that the patient is in optimum condition for anesthesia and the surgical procedure. In all cases, the patient should be "physiologically balanced" as much as possible to decrease surgical risk.

Food and water should be withheld preoperatively to reduce ingesta in the gut. Because many patients are dehydrated due to vomiting, diarrhea, and the transudation of body fluids into the bowel, intravenous fluids are administered. Acute and persistent vomiting commonly causes hypochloremic alkalosis. More chronic disease leads to acidosis from starvation and ketosis. If blood gas and pH determinations are not possible, sodium bicarbonate should be administered to the patient with a chronic disorder, but not to the vomiting patient with an acute disorder. Electrolyte determinations are also helpful for proper preoperative replacement therapy. If not readily available, then a balanced electrolyte solution such as lactated Ringer's solution should be used.

Because prerenal uremia is common, sufficient intravenous fluids are administered to promote a mild diuresis. Animals in shock from complete obstruction must receive large fluid loads to combat hypovolemic shock. In those cases of endotoxic shock, intravenous corticosteroids are beneficial. Broad-spectrum parenteral antibiotics are administered to combat septicemia arising from a devitalized bowel. If vomiting is not persistent, oral antibiotics such as neomycin or kanamycin have value in reducing the bacterial flora, especially when a distal intestinal operation is anticipated.

OPERATIVE PROCEDURE

The operation is performed as soon as the patient is in optimum physiologic condition. Anesthesia is critical because the patient may have a compromised cardiovascular system with impending shock. Preanesthetic and anesthetic agents must be administered cautiously and with constant monitoring. Phenothiazine tranquilizers are given in reduced doses, if at all, because of their propensity to produce hypotension. Barbiturates are given slowly and to effect, because they are much more active in the acidotic patient. Inhalation anesthetics such as methoxyflurane and halothane are favored for general anesthesia; they are more easily controlled than injectable agents and do not depend on metabolism for recovery of the patient. Nitrous oxide should not be used in patients with obstruction in that it diffuses into gas-filled spaces and aggravates bowel distension. Hypothermia develops rapidly when the abdomen is opened, especially in the small patient; therefore, a warming device should be used. Excessive wetting of the anesthetized patient while preparing for the surgical procedure also promotes hypothermia.

The abdomen is prepared for a midline abdominal incision of adequate length to explore the entire gastrointestinal tract. The incision edges are draped with saline-moistened laparotomy sponges, and a self-retaining Balfour* retractor is used to visualize the abdominal viscera. The entire abdominal cavity must be explored before the veterinary surgeon's attention is turned to any obvious lesion. A systematic exploration beginning at the stomach and working down the intestinal tract ensures finding the subtle lesion. A short segment of bowel is exteriorized, examined, and replaced, and the next distal segment is treated thus until the entire tract has been examined. The abdominal viscera must always be handled gently to prevent shock and postoperative ileus. The patient may be able to overcome either contamination or trauma, but the combination may be fatal. The veterinary surgeon must attempt to minimize both complications.

The affected bowel segment is isolated from the remainder of the viscera and is packed off with saline-moistened laparotomy sponges to prevent accidental contamination. The area to be resected and a short segment of normal intestine on either side are left exposed. The remainder of the gut is replaced in the abdomen to prevent desiccation and hypothermia. The segment of bowel in question should be carefully examined before resection is begun. If any doubt about the viability of the intestine exists, it is bathed in warm saline solution for 5 minutes and is critically examined by the criteria mentioned previously.

When resection and anastomosis are decided upon, the mesenteric vessels to the affected area are isolated and are ligated. A short segment of normal intestine on either side of the diseased area is included in the resection. Next, the arcadial vessels within the mesenteric fat along the intestine are isolated and are ligated (Fig. 13-2). Within minutes, the section of bowel bounded by the ligatures becomes cyanotic. It is imperative that the entire discolored segment be excised. Crushing clamps are placed at approximately a 60° angle to the long axis of the bowel just inside the arcadial ligatures. This clamping ensures that when the bowel is transected, the remaining ends will have an adequate blood supply from the vasa recta vessels. The ingesta are gently milked away from the crushing clamps for a distance of 3 to 5 cm, and a noncrushing clamp, such as Doyen or rubber-shod Allis forceps,* is placed to prevent

*American V. Mueller, 6600 West Touhy Avenue, Chicago, IL 60648

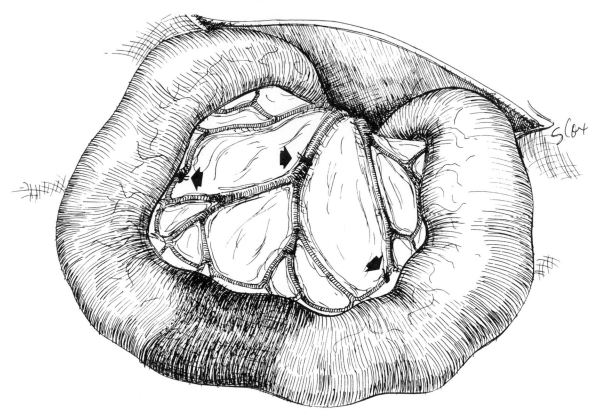

Fig. 13-2. *The segment of bowel to be resected along with a short section of normal bowel on either side is isolated from the remaining viscera. The mesenteric and arcadial vessels are ligated (arrows).*

gross contamination of the surgical site (Fig. 13-3). The noncrushing clamp should not obstruct blood flow in the arcadial vessel supplying the ends of the intestine.

A less traumatic method is to have an assistant gently hold the intestine between the thumb and fore-finger (Fig. 13-4). A sharp scalpel is used to excise the

bowel along the outside edge of the crushing clamp, and the mesentery is transected with fine tissue scissors (Fig. 13-5). Care is taken not to excise the ligatures on the arcadial vessels along the intestinal margin. If the surgical field becomes soiled from the bowel lumen, the soilage is wiped away with moistened gauze

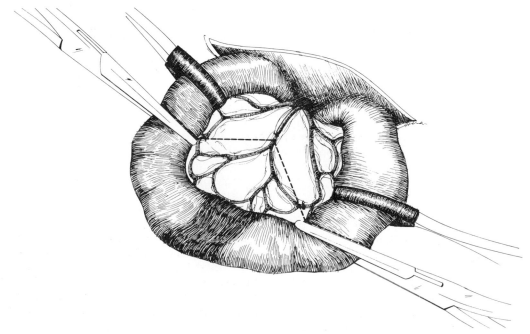

Fig. 13-3. *Crushing clamps are placed across the point of excision (broken line). Noncrushing clamps are used to prevent spillage of ingesta.*

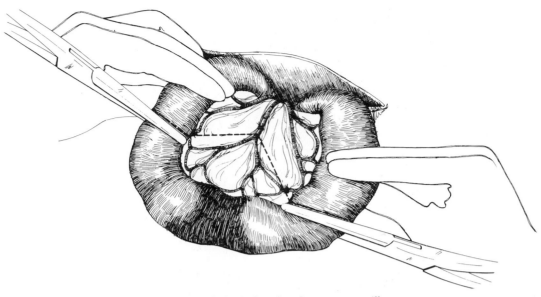

Fig. 13-4. *An assistant's fingers can also be used to occlude the bowel and to prevent spillage.*

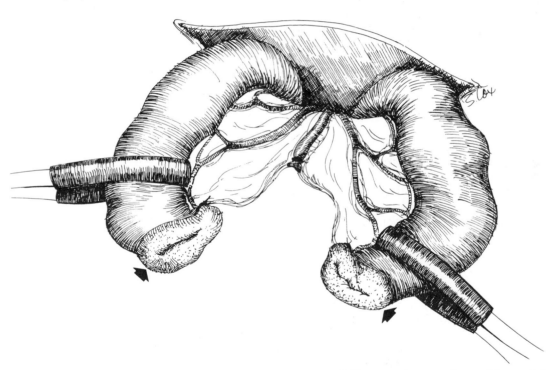

Fig. 13-5. *The diseased segment of bowel and its mesenteric attachment are resected. The everted mucosa (arrows) is resected with scissors before the ends are anastomosed.*

sponges. The excised portion of the intestine is discarded, and the ends to be anastomosed are examined to assure viability. The outwardly rolled mucosal collar around the transected ends is resected with sharp scissors to ensure that the individual layers of the bowel wall are accurately apposed. If the intestinal ends differ in lumen size, then the small end can be cut at a more acute angle to increase its lumen size (Fig. 13-6). Should this maneuver still not provide approximately equal lumen sizes, the antimesenteric edge of the small end can be incised longitudinally to increase its lumen size.

The anastomosis is carried out using atraumatic thumb forceps and either 3-0 or 4-0 polyglycolic acid* or polyglactin 910† suture. Because of the difficulty of penetrating the submucosal layer, a trocar point or taper-cut swaged-on needle is preferred. The bowel is approximated with 10 to 16 simple interrupted through-and-through sutures. The sutures can be pulled down until they "crush" through all layers of the bowel except the dense submucosa (Fig. 13-7). We have found that simply tightening the sutures until the

*Dexon, Davis & Geck, Inc., Manati, PR 00701
†Vicryl, Ethicon, Inc., Somerville, NJ 08876

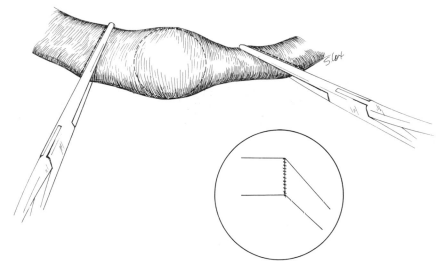

Fig. 13-6. *To accommodate unequal lumen sizes, the small end is cut at an acute angle and the large end at nearly 90° (broken lines). The resulting anastomosis is at an angle (inset).*

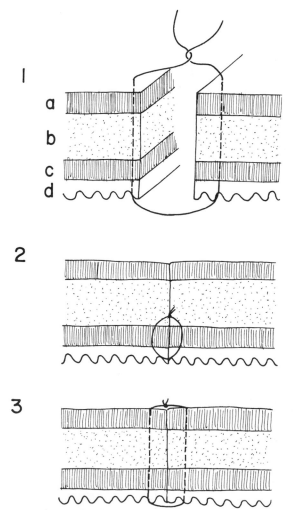

Fig. 13-7. *The anastomosis made with simple interrupted sutures (1) encompasses all layers of the intestinal wall: serosa (a), muscularis (b), submucosa (c), and mucosa (d). The "crushing" technique (2) requires that the suture be tightened to cut through all layers except the submucosa. The simple appositional technique (3) opposes the layers into anatomic alignment.*

tissues are gently apposed but not crushed is adequate for apposition of tissue.

The first suture is placed at the mesenteric border because this area is the most likely to leak. Care must be taken to ensure that this suture incorporates the full thickness of the bowel; fat in this area obscures the veterinary surgeon's view. The second suture is placed 180° away, at the antimesenteric margin (Fig. 13-8). This technique divides the suture line equally into halves and allows one to determine whether the ends are approximately equidiameter. The ends of these first 2 sutures can be left long, to aid in the manipulation of the anastomotic site and to prevent trauma by digital manipulation. Sutures are placed approximately 3 mm apart along one side of the anastomosis. Each suture should include 2 to 3 mm of the cut end of the bowel, to ensure that all layers of the intestinal wall (serosa, muscularis, submucosa, mucosa) are included in the suture line. Three throws on synthetic absorbable suture materials are adequate.

When the suture line on one side is complete, the bowel is rotated 180°, and the second side is sutured to finish the anastomosis. Mucosa is not allowed to protrude through the suture line because it would impede proper healing and promote adhesion formation. The anastomotic site is inspected, and additional sutures are placed if needed. Manipulation of the suture line must be kept to a minimum, to avoid trauma and to avoid disrupting the fibrin clot that helps to seal the anastomosis.

Sponges moistened with saline solution are used to remove spillage and blood from the surgical field, and the occluding clamps are removed. Instruments used on the open bowel should be kept separate from sterile instruments and should be discarded when the anastomosis is complete. The veterinary surgeon either may wear two sets of gloves at the beginning of the procedure and discard one set after the anastomosis or may change gloves at the appropriate time to minimize contamination. Spillage from the distal bowel is more seri-

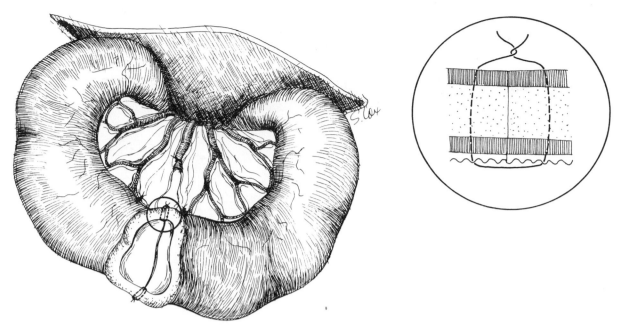

Fig. 13-8. *The first suture is placed at the mesenteric edge and the second at the antimesenteric edge. Inset, our preferred technique for simple apposition, including 2 to 3 mm of the cut end of the bowel.*

ous than from the proximal bowel because of the increased bacterial flora. Laparotomy sponges are removed, and the defect in the mesentery is closed using a 3-0 or 4-0 absorbable suture. One must be careful not to accidentally ligate or puncture a mesenteric vessel supplying additional intestine (Fig. 13-9).

Occasionally, it is not possible or feasible to remove a sufficient amount of intestine to provide healthy ends for an anastomosis. In these instances, a pedicle of

omentum may be placed around the anastomosis and may be sutured to the intestine (Fig. 13-10), to help prevent leakage and subsequent peritonitis (see the section of this chapter on serosal patching.) This technique must never be used as a substitute for a properly performed anastomosis.

If gross abdominal contamination occurs, then abdominal lavage with saline solution is useful. Two or 3 cycles of irrigation and suction with 250 to 1000 ml

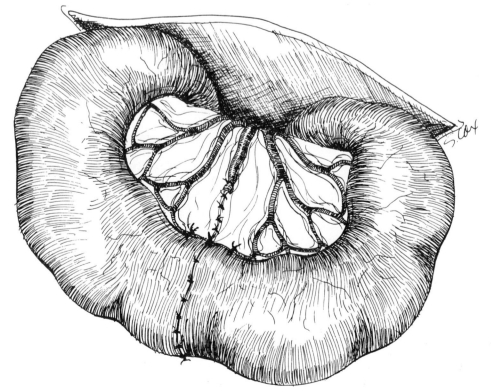

Fig. 13-9. *Additional sutures are placed to complete the anastomosis, and the mesenteric defect is closed.*

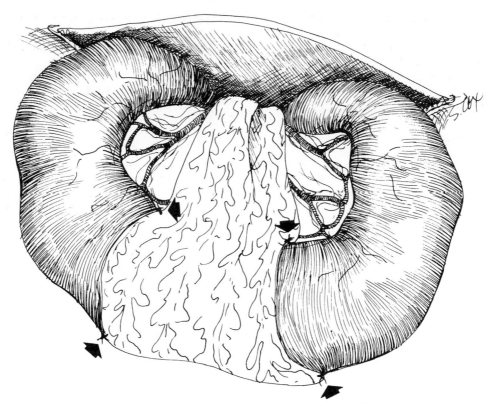

Fig. 13-10. *A pedicle of omentum can be used to reinforce the anastomosis. Sutures are used to hold the omentum in place (arrows).*

warm saline solution or lactated Ringer's solution usually suffice. If peritonitis is present preoperatively, antibiotics such as kanamycin or neomycin or 10% povidone-iodine may be included in the final irrigation and may be suctioned in a few minutes. The abdomen is closed in either 3 or 4 layers; one must take precautions for accurate peritoneal and muscle fascia closure. Absorbable suture material is adequate for most cases. In the face of severe infection, however, monofilament nonabsorbable suture is preferred. The diagnosis and treatment of local and generalized peritonitis are covered in Chapter 16.

POSTOPERATIVE CARE

Intravenous fluids are continued in the postoperative period to ensure rehydration and renal function. Usually, 20 ml/kg/hr during the operation and the early postoperative period are adequate. The animal should be placed on a warm surface and should be covered with a blanket until totally recovered from anesthesia. Feeding should resume within 24 hours to prevent ileus. Water should be freely offered the day following the operation, unless the patient is vomiting. Multiple meals of an easily digestible food are preferred for the first 3 to 5 days. Normal feeding patterns are gradually resumed. Parenteral antibiotics are administered prophylactically for 5 to 7 days following the surgical procedure. Longer antibiotic therapy is advocated in patients with peritonitis.

Enterotomy

INDICATIONS

The primary indication for performing an enterotomy is the ingestion of a foreign body. Ingested foreign bodies seldom penetrate the bowel wall. Straight pins, sharp metal objects, glass, open safety pins, fish hooks, and splintered bones commonly pass without causing clinical signs. In the event of penetration, rapid sealing of the wound prevents leakage in most cases; however, localized or remote abscesses may form with foreign body penetration and migration.

Not all intestinal foreign bodies require surgical intervention. Many pass without much difficulty. The progress of radiopaque objects can be followed with serial radiographs. If the object ceases to move along the intestinal tract, surgical intervention and removal of the object are indicated. The area most likely for a foreign body to lodge is in the intestinal flexures along the tortuous route of the jejunum or at the ileocecocolic junction. Symptoms depend upon the duration, degree, and location of the obstruction. Long-standing obstruction may lead to perforation of the bowel segment due to ischemia and pressure necrosis around the foreign body.

Linear foreign bodies such as bologna casings, sewing thread, or fishing line present further problems. Rarely does a linear foreign body of substantial length pass through the intestinal tract unimpeded. The trailing end is often caught around the tongue base or in the stomach and acts as an anchor. Normal peristaltic movement increases in an effort to move the string along the tract. The result is bowel plication or intussuception. With continued hyperperistalsis, the string may cut through the gut wall on the mesenteric border and may cause peritonitis.

OPERATIVE PROCEDURE

The surgical approach and the isolation of the involved bowel segment are similar to those described for resection and anastomosis. After isolating and packing off the segment of bowel containing the for-

eign body, the intestinal contents are gently "milked" out of the surgical field both proximal and distal to the obstruction. An assistant's fingers or intestinal clamps are applied on either side of the foreign body to aid in manipulation of the bowel and to keep the intestinal contents out of the surgical field. An incision is made on the antimesenteric border in healthy tissue on the dilated portion of the bowel proximal to the obstruction. A longitudinal or transverse incision may be used. The foreign body is then "milked" out the enterotomy site (Fig. 13-11).

Linear foreign bodies often require multiple enterotomies for complete removal (Fig. 13-12). Initially, the anchoring point should be identified and released. This

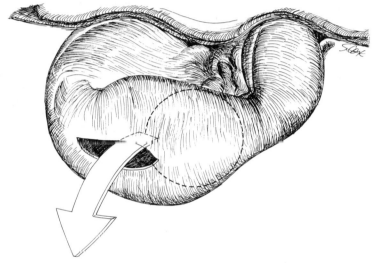

Fig. 13-11. *A longitudinal enterotomy is performed in the dilated intestine proximal to the obstruction. Arrow indicates how the foreign body is "milked" through the incision.*

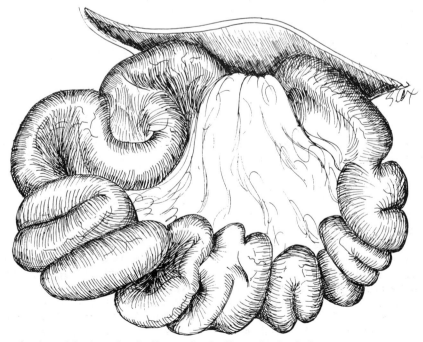

Fig. 13-12. *The accordian pleating of the intestine is diagnostic of a linear foreign body.*

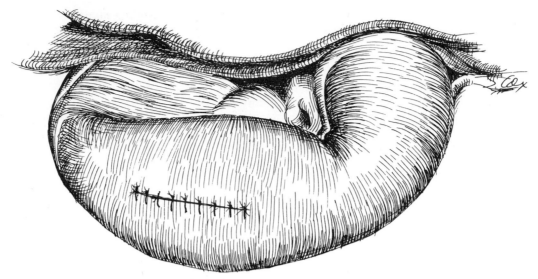

Fig. 13-13. *A longitudinal enterotomy can be closed using a simple interrupted suture pattern.*

point is usually under the base of the tongue or at the pylorus. An enterotomy is then performed several centimeters distal to what is thought to be the proximal end of the linear foreign body. At this point, the string proximal to the enterotomy is pulled through the incision. This procedure is repeated until the distal extent of the linear foreign body is extracted. Gentle traction on the string through the enterotomy site aids in determining at what point the string is entrapped and where the next enterotomy will be necessary.

The enterotomy incisions in the antimesenteric border may be closed with a simple appositional or crushing pattern, an inverting pattern, or a transverse closure. Simple interrupted appositional sutures, placed 3 to 4 mm apart and 2 to 3 mm from the cut edge, incorporate all layers of the intestinal wall (Fig. 13-13). If inversion is desired, it is obtained through a Connell, Cushing, or Lembert pattern. Submucosa must be incorporated into each "bite" of the suture pattern. The degree of inversion is determined by the distance from the suture penetration to the cut edge, usually 2 to 3 mm (Fig. 13-14). Transverse closure of a longitudinal incision is performed to avoid luminal constriction. A simple interrupted suture is placed to incorporate all layers of the bowel wall and to pull the two ends of the incision together. The edges are then closed with interrupted appositional sutures placed 2 to 3 mm from the cut edge and 3 to 4 mm apart (Fig. 13-15). Transverse enterotomy incisions are best used for intestine with a small lumen (Fig. 13-16).

Absorbable suture material, such as polyglycolic acid or polyglactin 910, in a 3-0 to 4-0 size with a swaged-on needle is best for enterotomy closure. A trocar-type needle aids in penetrating the submucosal layer. Atraumatic, smooth thumb forceps or a totally "nontouch" technique are indicated for handling the bowel to avoid iatrogenic trauma to the tissues. Abdominal lavage with or without antibiotics or antiseptics is not indicated unless intestinal contents have spilled. Systemic antibiotics are generally sufficient.

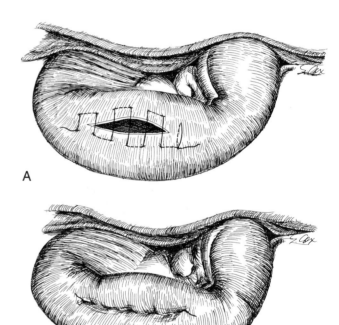

Fig. 13-14. A, *The enterotomy may also be closed with a continuous inverting suture pattern.* B, *Serosa-to-serosa contact is achieved with this pattern.*

Treatment of Perforation

Intestinal perforations from ingested foreign bodies generally create clinical signs compatible with localized peritonitis and may even remain undetected. Obstruction by a large foreign body with associated necrosis and perforation, however, may result in generalized peritonitis from intestinal leakage. If perforation is suspected or is thought to be imminent, an exploratory celiotomy and an enterotomy are indicated.

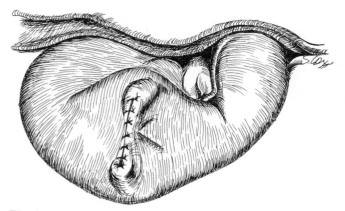

Fig. 13-15. *A transverse closure of a longitudinal enterotomy prevents luminal constriction.*

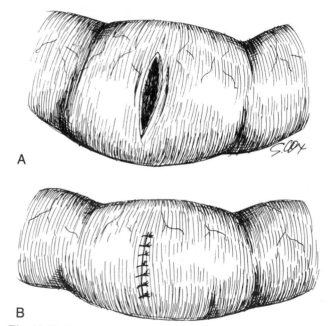

Fig. 13-16. *Transverse enterotomy (A) and closure (B) are beneficial in intestine with a small lumen.*

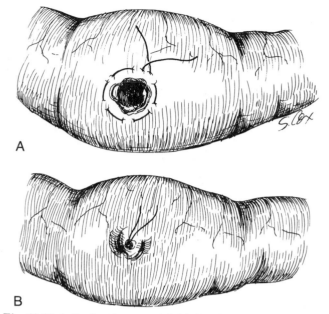

Fig. 13-17. A, *Perforations are debrided and a pursestring suture placed in the bowel wall.* B, *The suture is firmly tightened to ensure that no leakage occurs.*

Perforations are debrided to healthy, bleeding tissue. Defects up to 5 mm in diameter can be closed with a pursestring suture (Fig. 13-17). If intestinal wall viability is questionable or if the defect is larger than 5 mm, a simple interrupted appositional or an inverting suture pattern is used for closure after appropriate debridement.

Biopsy

Removal of a portion of the bowel wall is frequently indicated as a diagnostic procedure. Excisional biopsies are curative as well as diagnostic if the lesion is focal and is entirely removed. Diffuse disorders of the small intestine requiring surgical biopsy are usually associated with maldigestion or malabsorption. Surgical intervention with removal of a specimen for histopathologic study and culture is used to rule out or to diagnose a physical disorder.

Because diagnostic biopsy is usually performed in diseased areas of the bowel, each biopsy site is isolated and is packed off as for enterotomy. Once the bowel is entered, a full-thickness, 2- to 3-mm wedge section is excised. Incisions are on the antimesenteric border and may be either longitudinal or transverse. Closure is the same as for enterotomy incisions. If gross pathologic features are not seen, or if a diffuse disorder is suspected, multiple biopsies are required throughout the duodenum, jejunum, ileum, cecum, and colon.

Acknowledgments

We wish to thank Mrs. Robbyn Wilhite and Ms. Amy Shaver for typing the manuscript and Ms. Sue Cox for providing the medical illustrations.

The intestinal tract occupies the major portion of the abdomen; thus, it is often the recipient of several perforations from penetrating objects such as sharp sticks, wires, knives, gunshot, and arrows. Small wounds, such as from shotgun BBs, may seal themselves and require little or no surgical repair. Damage from larger high-velocity missiles varies, depending on size and velocity. Penetration into the abdomen by any high-velocity missile should be explored as soon as possible, however. Careful systematic evaluation is necessary during exploration in order to avoid missing multiple sites of penetration and subsequent leakage. Clinical signs vary with the amount of leakage and blood loss, showing varying degrees of peritonitis and shock.

References and Suggested Readings

Anderson, N. V.: Disorders of the small intestine. *In* Textbook of Veterinary Internal Medicine: Diseases of the Dog and Cat. 2nd Ed. Edited by S. J. Ettinger. Philadelphia, W. B. Saunders, 1975.

Butler, H. C.: Surgery of the small intestine and colon. Vet. Clin. North Am., 2:155, 1972.

DeHoff, W. D.: Small intestinal anastomosis. Vet. Clin. North Am., 5:551, 1975.

DeHoff, W. D., Nelson, W. and Lumb, W. V.: Simple interrupted approximating technique for intestinal anastomosis. J. Am. Anim. Hosp. Assoc., 9:483, 1973.

Grier, R. L.: Techniques for intestinal anastomosis. *In* Current Techniques in Small Animal Surgery. Edited by M. J. Bojrab. Philadelphia, Lea and Febiger, 1975.

Hunn, D. H., and Buchwald, H.: Gastrointestinal anastomoses: facts and fiction. *In* Gastrointestinal Surgery. Edited by J. S. Najarian and J. P. Delaney. Chicago, Yearbook Medical Publishers, 1979.

Larsen, L. H., and Bellenger, C. R.: Stomach and small intestines. *In* Canine Surgery. 2nd Ed. Edited by J. Archibald. Santa Barbara, CA, American Veterinary Publications, 1974.

McLachlin, A. D., and Denton, D. W.: Omental protection of intestinal anastomosis. Am. J. Surg., 125:134, 1973.

Combined Thoracoabdominal Approach Through the Ventral Midline

by DENNIS T. CROWE

A ventral midline abdominal approach from the xyphoid process to the os pubis affords adequate exposure to most organs and regions of the abdominal cavity including the hilus of the liver, the diaphragmatic-hepatic junction, and the esophagogastric region. By continuing cranially with the ventral midline approach through the chondrosternal articulation (or through the midline of the sternebra) and by dorsally incising the diaphragm, however, exposure to the cranial abdominal region is enhanced. Such exposure is particularly beneficial in the surgical management of severe liver injuries, damage to deep abdominal vascular structures, and thoracoabdominal injuries in which quick exposure to both abdomen and chest is necessary. In combined thoracoabdominal trauma or in other situations that may require increased abdominal exposure, generous midline and lateral preparation of the thorax and abdomen is performed.

Surgical Technique

A routine entry exposes the midline ventral aspect of the abdominal cavity. The midline skin incision is then extended cranially to at least the midsternal area. If further exposure is necessary, the incision is continued to the manubrium. A deeper incision is then made to reflect the origins of the superficial pectoral muscle bilaterally. Hemorrhage is controlled by electrocoagulation or ligature. Following identification of the sternebrae, the incision is directed either on the midline or to the parasternal area. An oscillating bone saw or a combination of osteotome and mallet is used for sternal osteotomy.

The chondrosternal articulations are cut through for the parasternal approach (Fig. 13-18). The chondrosternal articulations are best divided with a sharp scalpel (No. 10 Bard-Parker scalpel blade). In patients in which the incision continues just lateral to the sternum, it is important to stay as close to the sternebra as possible to avoid the internal thoracic artery and vein. If the artery or vein is cut, pressure with a finger, followed by placement of a tight suture ligature, controls hemorrhage. Midline sternotomy affords the advantages of a secure closure and of less likelihood of injuring the internal thoracic vessels. The disadvantages of sternal splitting procedure are that more time and special equipment are often necessary. Generally, the narrowness of the sternebra necessitates that the median sternotomy be performed only in animals over 20 kg, whereas the chondrosternal disarticulation is recommended in animals under 20 kg.

Following initiation of controlled ventilation upon entry into the thorax, the diaphragm is incised to allow retraction of the wound edges and further opening of the thoracic cavity. When approaching deep liver trauma, the incision is commonly extended dorsally to the hiatus of the caudal vena cava (Fig. 13-19). If the gastroesophageal area is involved, then the incision through the diaphragm extends to the esophageal hiatus. Small phrenic arteries are ligated as needed. This ligation is best accomplished with a transfixation suture that incorporates the cut edge of the diaphragm itself. The thin, ventral mediastinal tissue is removed or is retracted as necessary for visualization. Self-retaining retractors help to maintain exposure into the chest and abdomen. After covering the exposed cut edges of the incision with saline-moistened laparotomy sponges or towels, a Finochietto or other retractor is placed in the incision through the sternum, and the blades are spread apart (Fig. 13-19). In smaller patients, a variety

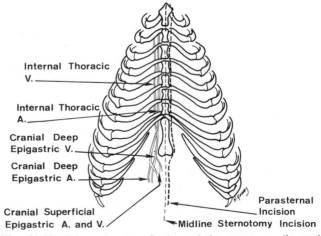

Internal Thoracic V.

Internal Thoracic A.

Cranial Deep Epigastric V.

Cranial Deep Epigastric A.

Cranial Superficial Epigastric A. and V.

Parasternal Incision

Midline Sternotomy Incision

Fig. 13-18. *Schematic ventral view of the sternum, ribs and chondrosternal articulations demonstrating the incisional pathway taken for the midline sternotomy and the parasternal approach as a cranial extension from the abdominal wound.*

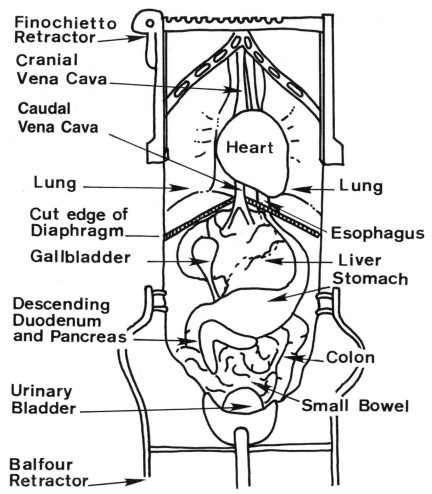

Finochietto Retractor

Cranial Vena Cava

Caudal Vena Cava

Heart

Lung

Lung

Cut edge of Diaphragm

Esophagus

Gallbladder

Liver

Stomach

Descending Duodenum and Pancreas

Colon

Urinary Bladder

Small Bowel

Balfour Retractor

Fig. 13-19. *Schematic ventral view of the completed thoracoabdominal incision and positioning of the Finochietto and Balfour retractors.*

of self-retaining retractors work well if caution is taken to avoid injury from instrument blades or points. If self-retaining retractors are not available, wedging a needle holder or a sterile plastic syringe between manually retracted edges of the sternal incision can be effective in maintaining exposure.

Closure is initiated after the insertion of a chest tube, which may exit from either side of the thorax. Because of the disruption of the ventral mediastinum, one tube is sufficient to drain both sides. The diaphragm is closed, beginning with the dorsal (deepest) portion point of the incision. I prefer to use 2-0 or 3-0 polypropylene on a taper-point swaged-on needle, but other nonabsorable materials may be used. A simple continuous single-layer closure is the pattern generally selected for repair of the diaphragmatic defect. At least 2 mm of tissue in small dogs or cats and 3 mm in larger patients should be included in each suture.

Large stainless steel monofilament orthopedic wire is used to appose the bisected sternebra or the chondrosternal disarticulation. Simple interrupted sutures placed through predrilled holes or encircling the entire sternebra are used to repair the sternal osteotomy. A cruciate pattern around the end of the rib and sternebra is used to repair the parasternal approach

(Fig. 13-20). With the parasternal approach, wire sutures should penetrate or come near the cranial aspect of the costal cartilage and should then be directed to encircle the sternebra. A second pass with the suture is made caudal to the rib and then encircles the same sternebra (Fig. 13-21). Care is taken to avoid the internal thoracic vein and artery. Intercostal vascular injury is also possible. I prefer to use tapered needles for this reason. Hemorrhage from these vessels can be difficult to locate and is best controlled with a cruciate suture ligature of chromic catgut (Fig. 13-22).

It is important that adequate apposition and stable fixation be attained with either method of closure. Eighteen- to 20-gauge wire is used in large dogs, and 20- to 24-gauge wire is recommended for smaller animals. All wire loops used for fracture stabilization must be smoothly passed, not kinked, and twisted tightly, and the ends must be bent over. Often, more sutures are necessary than are shown in the figures. The sternal and parasternal incised surfaces must be sufficiently closed to ensure an airtight and stable closure.

Following the preplacement of all of the sutures, control of hemorrhage from the internal thoracic and intercostal vessels is ensured. The preplaced sutures are apposed by an assistant and are twisted beginning

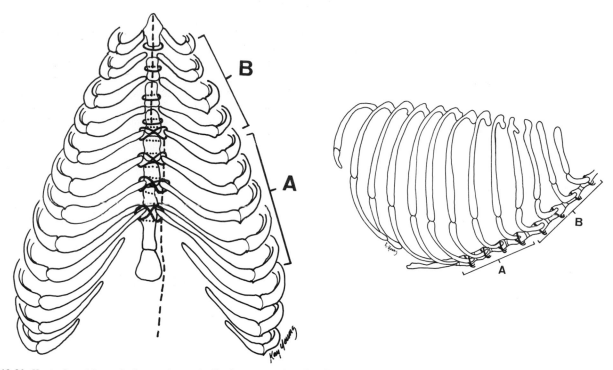

Fig. 13-20. *Ventral and lateral views schematically demonstrating the placement of the suture used in a cruciate pattern (A) to close the parasternal incision. With this type of pattern, approximation and fixation of the chondrosternal articulation are accurate. In both views, B indicates the placement of the suture used to close the midline sternotomy incision.*

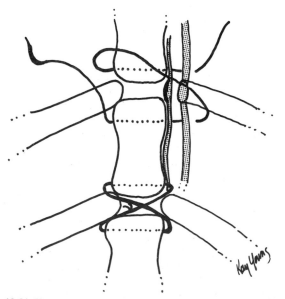

Fig. 13-21. *Ventral view schematically demonstrating proper placement of the cruciate suture used to reapproximate the chondrosternal articulations in closure of the parasternal incision.*

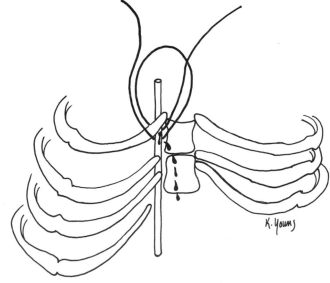

Fig. 13-22. *Ventral view schematically demonstrating cruciate suture ligature placement for controlling hemorrhage from the internal thoracic artery or vein. The suture is passed through the adjacent soft tissues and the bleeding area twice, and then it is tightened and tied.*

in the center of the incision (Fig. 13-23). These steps are repeated until all wires are twisted. This method eliminates the need for holding the sternabrae together with a towel clamp or a similar traumatic method that may damage the internal thoracic artery. Nonabsorbable sutures other than stainless steel are also suitable for parasternal closures. Polypropylene, nylon, and Dacron are most commonly used. Regardless of material used, it is important to keep the knots as lateral as possible and covered with subcutaneous tissue to avoid irritation from pressure placed on the sternebra, particularly in the deep-chested or thin dogs.

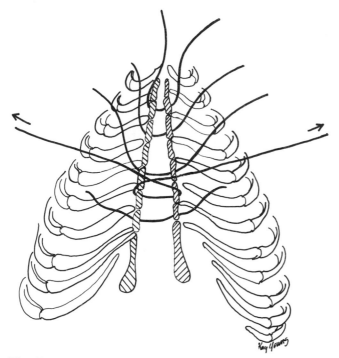

Fig. 13-23. *Following preplacement of all the sutures, the cut surfaces of the sternebra are approximated by having an assistant cross one of the sutures and apply tension. The nearest preplaced suture is then tightened and tied or twisted while the assistant maintains the apposition.*

Pectoral fascia and subcutaneous tissue are closed using the material and pattern of the veterinary surgeon's choice. I prefer chromic catgut or synthetic absorbable material in an inverted vertical mattress pattern. Because the dog or cat may put pressure on the wound during recovery, it is important to obliterate dead space and to provide a tension-free skin closure. This goal is accomplished with an effective subcutaneous-subdermal closure. Steel is not recommended as a skin closure material for the sternal area. The abdominal cavity is then closed in a routine fashion. (See the section of this chapter entitled "Simple Continuous Suture Closure of Abdominal Incisions.")

Postoperative Considerations

Because of the possible presence of a chest tube and the exposed location of the wound, a sterile gauze dressing is recommended, followed by a gently compressive torso bandage. The dressing is removed or is changed approximately 24 hours postoperatively or at the time of chest-tube inspection or removal. Analgesics are often required postoperatively, but are generally not required past the second postoperative day if rigid fixation of the sternebra has been achieved.

The combined thoracoabdominal approach does increase the surgical time and the morbidity rate. These acknowledged liabilities must be balanced against the dangers and technical frustrations inherent in an inadequate surgical approach. For example, pulling on the patient's duodenum and stomach while trying to ex-

pose the hilus of the liver adequately enough to visualize and repair a deep hepatic laceration can result in tearing the common bile duct or tearing the original laceration further. By using the combined approach and by splitting the diaphragm in a dorsal direction to the postcaval hilus, excellent exposure and accessibility can be attained without causing serious iatrogenic harm.

References and Suggested Readings

Archibald, J., and Harvey, C. E.: Thorax—sternum splitting incision (median sternotomy). *In* Canine Surgery. 2nd Ed. Edited by J. Archibald. Santa Barbara, CA, American Veterinary Publications, 1974.

Crouch, J. E.: Text-Atlas of Cat Anatomy. Philadelphia, Lea & Febiger, 1969.

Evans, H. E., and Christensen, G. C.: Miller's Anatomy of the Dog. 2nd Ed. Philadelphia, W. B. Saunders, 1979.

Hurov, L., Knauer, K., Playter, R., and Sexon, R.: Handbook of Veterinary Surgical Instruments and Glossary of Surgical Terms. Philadelphia, W. B. Saunders, 1978.

Lipowitz, A. J., and Schenk, M. P.: Surgical approaches to the abdominal and thoracic viscera of the dog and cat. Vet. Clin. North Am., 9:169, 1979.

Serosal Patching and Jejunal Onlay Grafting

by Dennis T. Crowe

Serosal "patching" uses the antimesenteric border of the small bowel or other hollow viscus for serosal reinforcement in situations in which conventional suture closure must be done in marginally viable tissue or in closures that are otherwise unreliable. Although the use of omentum as a serosal sealing agent has been effective in many clinical situations, its use may be limited because elevated intraluminal pressure may cause an omental seal to leak. If a healthy serosal surface can remain in contact with the questionable serosal surface, however, significant fibrin sealing is seen. The advantages of mechanical reinforcement by the submucosal and muscular tunics of the small bowel "patch" are also realized. This technique has been used successfully to close many intestinal perforations caused by gunshot and dog bites, for example. The procedure has been used in the management of pyloroplasty dehiscence and in the buttressing of other organ closures involving the small bowel, stomach, urinary bladder, colon, pancreatic stump, uterus, and diaphragm.

Surgical Technique for Serosal Patching

One row of interrupted nonabsorbable 3-0 or 4-0 sutures are placed at 3- to 5-mm intervals to sew normal viscera over the area of perforation or "questionable" area. The technique is demonstrated in cases of perforating injury to the duodenum (Fig. 13-24), urinary

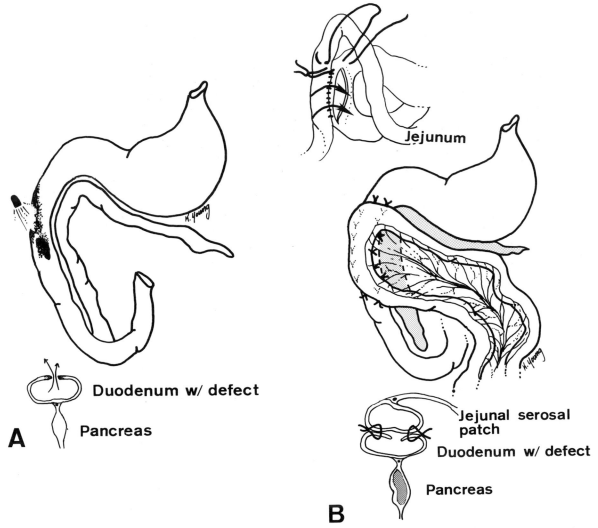

Fig. 13-24. *Diagrammatic representations of* (A) *a gunshot wound to the descending duodenum and* (B) *the resultant repair using a serosal patch from a loop of jejunum.*

bladder (Fig. 13-25), and colon (Fig. 13-26). I prefer to use polypropylene on a fine, swaged-on, taper-point needle. The sutures should include the submucosa of both the viscera used as the patch and the viscera being repaired. The area selected for suture placement in the perforated or questionable area should be far enough away from the edges of the defect to permit their placement into healthy viable tissue with an adequate blood supply. In other words, *the patch is not sewn to the edges of the defect.* When using the technique for buttressing a closure in which viability of the tissues is uncertain and leakage may occur, the placement of the sutures remains the same. Linear wounds are the easiest to patch, but irregular areas are also reinforceable.

It is, of course, important not to disrupt the major blood supply to organs as they are repositioned for reinforcement purposes. This disruption may happen if the bowel is stretched, twisted, or kinked, or if the mesentery is incorporated into sutures. The bowel chosen for the patch should be gently looped to preclude par-

tial luminal obstruction. Gentle back-and-forth looping has been used along the entire length of the bowel to close multiple perforations caused by gunshot wounds. In this situation, the lateral aspect of the bowel between the mesenteric and antimesenteric surfaces is used, as well as the antimesenteric border for the patching surface.

Surgical Technique for Jejunal Onlay Grafting

Jejunal onlay grafting is a variant of serosal patching and is useful for closure of large defects. For example, in neoplasia or extensive wounds of the duodenal walls, a complete or partial pancreaticoduodoenectomy may be required. If the mesenteric border of the duodenum, including the common bile duct, the pancreatic ducts, and the pancreas can be preserved, the duodenum can be preserved by using an interposed sec-

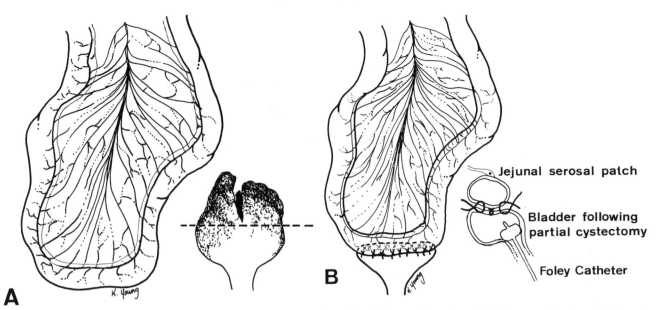

Fig. 13-25. A, *Diagrammatic representation of a severe blow-out and crushing injury to the urinary bladder necessitating partial cystectomy.* B, *A loop of jejunum was used to buttress the suture line where the viability of the sutured edges of the bladder remained under suspicion.*

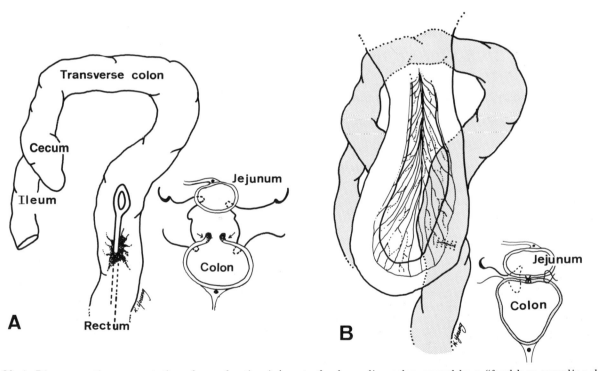

Fig. 13-26. A, *Diagrammatic representation of a perforating injury to the descending colon caused by a "fecal loop sampling device."* B, *Following debridement and suture closure of the wound, a serosal patch with a loop of jejunum was used as a buttress.*

tion of jejunum. The antimesenteric border of jejunum is opened, and by appositional single-layer closure, the edges of the jejunum are apposed against the duodenum (Fig. 13-27). The advantage of the technique over a total or partial pancreaticoduodenectomy is obvious. The advantage of the "jejunal onlay graft" over simple serosal patching is that devitalized mucosa is replaced with healthy mucosa, and mucosal continuity does not have to be reestablished by "creeping" substitution, as

occurs with serosal patching. Full reconstruction of the bowel circumference is also possible and thereby precludes partial obstructions.

References and Suggested Readings

Ballinger, W. F., McLaughlin, E. D., and Baranski, E. J.: Jejunal overlay closure of duodenum in the newborn: lateral duodenal tear caused by gastrostomy tube. Surgery, *59*:150, 1966.

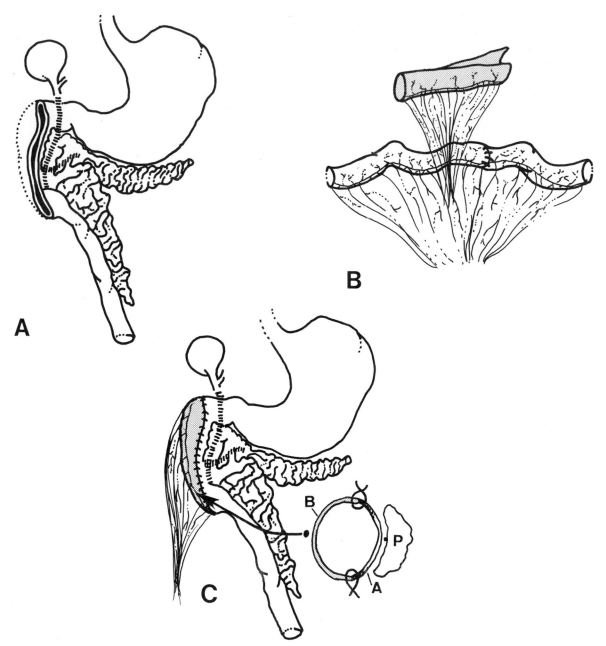

Fig. 13-27. *Diagrammatic representations of a large antimesenteric duodenal defect being managed with a jejunal onlay graft. A, The defect before reconstruction, which originated following resection of an adenocarcinoma involving the duodenum. B, Removal of a segment of the jejunum, retaining its blood supply and cutting its antimesenteric border. C, Placement of the jejunal onlay pedicle graft (B, portion of jejunal wall acting as onlay graft; A, mesenteric portion of duodenum remaining after resection; P, pancreas.)*

Barnett, W. O.: Investigation regarding the management of the duodenal stump. Surg. Gynecol. Obstet., *113*:197, 1961.

Bender, H. W., Sebor, J., and Zuidema, G. D.: Serosal patch grafting for closure of posterior duodenal defects. Am. J. Surg., *115*:103, 1968.

Jones, S. A., Gazzaniga, A. B., and Keller, T. B.: The serosal patch. Am. J. Surg., *126*:186, 1973.

Jones, S. A., and Joergenson, E. J.: Closure of duodenal wall defects. Surgery, *53*:438, 1963.

Jones, S. A., and Steedman, R. A.: Management of chronic infected intestinal perforations by the serosal patch technique. Am. J. Surg., *117*:731, 1969.

Kobold, E. E., and Thal, A. P.: A simple method for the management of experimental wounds of the dog. Surg. Gynecol. Obstet., *116*:340, 1963.

Simple Continuous Suture Closure of Abdominal Incisions

by DENNIS T. CROWE

In all surgical closures of the abdominal cavity, the primary objective is to gain a good purchase on fascia external to the rectus muscle or the fascia and aponeurosis of the external and internal abdominal oblique muscles. Simple continuous, single-layer abdominal wall closure using a monofilament, inert polypropylene*

*Prolene, Ethicon, Inc., Somerville, NJ 08876

suture material has proved satisfactory in its clinical application in over 700 dogs and cats. The incidence of dehiscence is negligible (less than 0.1%), and the savings in operating time is substantial in long incisions. The technique is best and most commonly used for midline (median) ventral incisions of the abdominal cavity. It may also be used successfully in paramedian, pararectus, or paralumbar incisions however. In these situations, the veterinary surgeon may elect a two-layer continuous closure if the patient's musculature is well developed.

Surgical Technique

Following the completion of the intra-abdominal procedure(s), the abdominal wall of each patient is closed using a synthetic suture material. Recommended materials that have proved effective include polypropylene,* nylon,† polyglactin 910,‡ and polyglycolic acid.§ Dacron and stainless steel are not recommended. The material of choice is polypropylene or monofilament nylon, especially in patients with contaminated wounds or systemic disease. In my opinion, chromic catgut and silk should not be recommended for use in dogs and cats owing to the unreliability and reactivity of these suture materials.

Ideally, suture material should be swaged onto a taper-point, general-closure needle. The size of the suture material is based on the patient's body weight. Size 3-0 is selected for patients up to 5 kg, 2-0 for animals under 10 kg, and 1-0 for those up to 50 kg. For giant breeds of dogs, size 1 suture material is selected.

The simple continuous suture pattern is begun at either end of the abdominal wall incision and is continued to the opposite end if the incisions are short. In incisions over 20 cm long, the suture is begun at both ends of the incision, and closure is commenced toward the center until the ends meet and are then interlocked with a knot (Fig. 13-28). Care is taken to incorporate clearly a substantial portion of rectus fascia. At the end of the closure, two passes through the fascia on each side of the incision are recommended before the knot is tied (Figs. 13-28 and 13-29).

From 3 to 5 mm of both external and internal rectus fascia should be obtained with each needle "bite" when closing the canine abdomen. Inclusion of only the external rectus fascia is necessary in the feline abdominal closure, however. Muscle is easily avoided (Figs. 13-30 and 13-31). Parietal peritoneum is not closed specifically, but sutures in the internal rectus sheath in dogs usually do approximate the peritoneal edges.

When nearing the end of the fascial closure, the last few throws should be placed loosely in a "preplacing fashion." This technique allows continued visualization of the deeper structures and incision edges and elimi-

*Prolene, Ethicon, Inc., Somerville, NJ 08876
†Ethilon, Ethicon, Inc., Somerville, NJ 08876
‡Vicryl, Ethicon, Inc., Somerville, NJ 08876
§Dexon, Davis & Geck, Manati, PR 00701

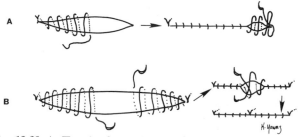

Fig. 13-28. A, *The simple continuous closure of a short incision.* B, *In incisions over 20 cm in length or in those in which its "corners" are difficult to visualize, the suturing is begun at both ends of the incision.*

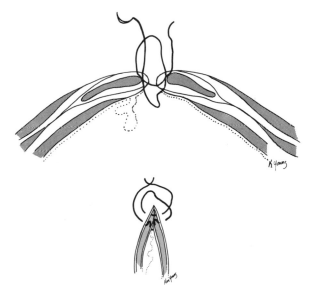

Fig. 13-29. *Two passes through the fascia on each side are recommended before the knot is tied.*

nates the "blind" placement of the suture into the fascia. Following penetration of the last "preplaced" suture, the suture is tightened and the knot is tied.

Because of the "slippery" nature of most synthetic sutures, a surgeon's knot is used in the beginning of each tie with 5 or 6 flat, square throws placed on top. When the last throw has been made, both ends of the suture are pulled tightly to cause elongation and internal locking of the knot structure. The ends are then cut to 1 or 2 mm to avoid skin irritation over the top of the knot. The suture ends should not be cut directly on the knot, however, because this technique predisposes the knot to untying.

Subcutaneous tissue is closed over the closure of the external rectus sheath. It is important to ensure a good subcutaneous closure over the knots in the abdominal fascia. Failure to accomplish this goal may lead to irritation of the skin and may predispose the patient to a chronic inflammatory reaction over the knots and potential sinus formation. The skin is closed using a simple interrupted or continuous pattern with a nonabsorbable suture of the veterinary surgeon's choice.

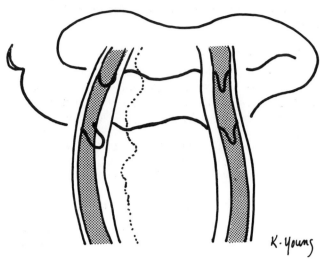

Fig. 13-30. *Care is taken to incorporate large bites of external rectus fascia in the closure.*

References and Suggested Readings

Archibald, J. (ed.): Canine Surgery. 2nd Ed. Santa Barbara, CA, American Veterinary Publications, 1974.

Coles, J. C., Carroll, S. E., and Gergely, N.: An improved method of abdominal closure. Can. J. Surg., 5:233, 1962.

Crowe, D. T.: Closure of abdominal incisions using a continuous polypropylene suture: clinical experience in 550 dogs and cats. Vet. Surg., 7:74, 1978.

Douglas, P. M.: The healing of aponeurotic incisions. Br. J. Surg., 40:79, 1952.

Evans, H. E., and Christensen, G. C.: Miller's Anatomy of the Dog. 2nd Ed. Philadelphia, W. B. Saunders, 1979.

Everett, W. G.: The Choice of Suture Materials for Abdominal Closure: International Symposium—Sutures in Wound Repair. London, Ethicon, 1972.

Herrmann, J. B.: Changes in tensile strength and knot security of surgical sutures in vivo. Arch. Surg., 106:707, 1973.

Holmland, E. E. W.: Physical properties of surgical suture materials stress-strain relationship, stress relaxation and irreversible elongation. Ann. Surg., 184:189, 1976.

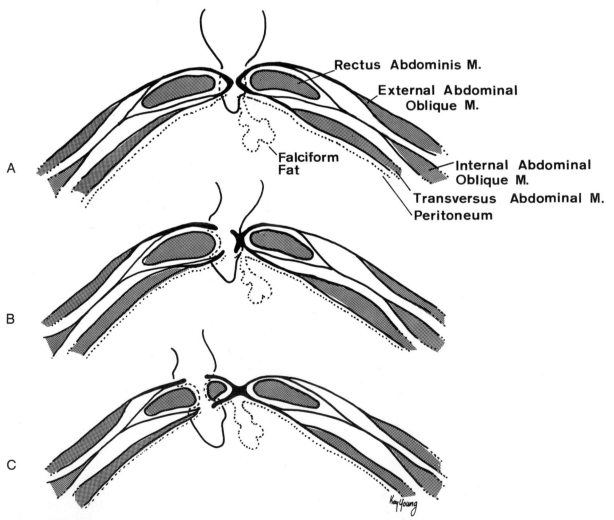

Fig. 13-31. *Muscle itself is easily avoided by angling the point of the needle to exit at the fascial-muscular junction with penetration of the internal and external rectus fascia. Note the amount of fascia included in each bite (approximately 3 mm to 5 mm, depending on the patient's size) and that the falciform ligament is avoided by careful suture placement. Closure of (A) median, (B) paramedian, and (C) perrectus incisions. Another acceptable method of abdominal wall closure is to place sutures only through the external rectus fascia. This method is particularly advantageous in animals under 35 kg, which do not require the extra holding strength afforded by including the internal rectus fascia.*

Bowel Plication for Preventing Recurrent Intussusception

by MARK H. ENGEN

Intussusception of the small intestine is a common clinical entity. Recurrence may follow resection of the intussusception and bowel anastomosis. Although the biomechanics of the condition is poorly understood, it is most commonly seen in young animals with hyperperistalsis due to heavy parasite infestation, linear foreign bodies, or severe enteritis such as occurs in canine distemper.

The primary treatment for intussusception is usually intestinal resection and anastomosis because of serious devitalization of bowel segments. Recurrent intussusception can be prevented by bowel plication. Adhesions form between the plicated loops of bowel and prevent telescoping of the bowel due to hyperperistalsis.

Surgical Technique

The procedure is performed by laying the bowel side by side to form a series of gentle loops that are sutured together at the antemesentric borders with absorbable suture material (Fig. 13-32). It is recommended that three loops of plicated bowel be used proximal and distal to the anastomosis. Closure of the abdomen is routine, and normal postoperative care after intestinal anastomosis should be provided.

Reference and Suggested Reading

Chambers, J. N.: Diseases of the intestine. *In* Pathophysiology in Small Animal Surgery. Edited by M. J. Bojrab. Philadelphia, Lea & Febiger, 1981.

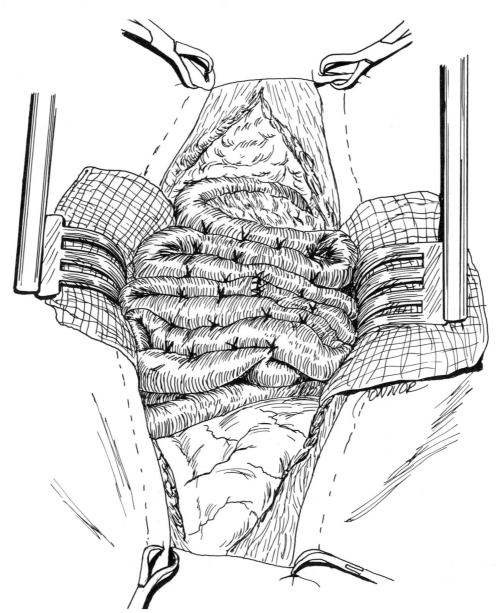

Fig. 13-32. *Bowel plication after resection and anastomosis.*

Management of Rectal Prolapse

by Mark H. Engen

Rectal prolapse can occur with any condition that causes prolonged tenesmus. It is most commonly seen in heavily parasitized animals that have severe diarrhea and tenesmus. Other causes of straining resulting in rectal prolapse are dystocia, urolithiasis, intestinal neoplasia and foreign bodies, prostatic disease, perineal hernia, constipation, and congenital defects.

Diagnosis

The diagnosis is made by visual observation of a tube-like mass, of varying length, protruding from the anus. If diagnosed early, the prolapse may be of short length and the prolapsed mucosa will appear bright red and nonulcerated. Rectal prolapse of long duration will be of greater length; the mucosa will appear red or black and will be either ulcerated or necrotic.

It is important to differentiate a true rectal prolapse from a prolapsed intussusception of the intestine or colon. The diagnosis can be determined by passing a probe between the anus and the prolapsed mass. If an intussusception is present, the probe can be passed; the probe cannot be passed if a rectal prolapse has occurred.

The cause of straining must be corrected to achieve a permanent cure, such as removal of intestinal parasites by worming.

Treatment

Treatment to correct the prolapse depends on the viability of the exposed tissue and the size of the prolapse. A small prolapse with viable-appearing mucosa may be replaced by using a finger or bougie to reposition the bowel. Topical application of hypertonic sugar solution for 20 to 30 minutes may be helpful in relieving edema, so that the prolapse may be reduced more easily. When the prolapse has been reduced, an anal pursestring suture is used to prevent recurrence. General anesthesia or epidural analgesia is used in some patients to facilitate the reduction of the prolapse and the placement of the anal pursestring suture (Fig. 13-33).

Following reduction of the prolapse, epidural analgesia prevents straining for several hours. Periodic rectal application of a local anesthetic ointment (1% dibucaine)* may be done initially and after removal of the anal pursestring suture to prevent further straining. The anal pursestring suture is left in place for a minimum of 24 to 48 hours, and the animal is given only fluids orally during this time.

When the rectal prolapse cannot be reduced by manipulation, and the lack of tissue viability contraindicates reduction, rectal resection and anastomosis are performed (Fig. 13-34). This procedure is performed

*Nupercainal ointment, Ciba Pharmaceutical, Ciba-Geigy, 556 Morris Avenue, Summit, NJ 07901

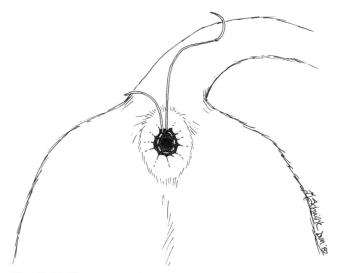

Fig. 13-33. *Placement of the anal pursestring suture.*

under general anesthesia or epidural analgesia. A tube is placed into the lumen of the bowel to prevent fecal contamination. Three stay sutures are placed through the full thickness of both layers of the prolapse to form a triangle (Fig. 13-34C and D). The prolapse is then resected 1 to 2 cm from the anus. The anastomosis is performed with a single-layer closure using a simple interrupted suture pattern (Fig. 13-34E). Synthetic absorbable or chromic gut suture of 3-0 or 4-0 size is preferred. The sutures are placed through the full thickness of the incised ends of the bowel. It is essential that the suture passes through the submucosa to ensure proper holding strength. The stay sutures are then removed, and the anastomosis is reduced manually inside the anus.

When the rectal prolapse cannot be reduced by external manipulation, and the rectal tissue is still viable, a celiotomy is performed and the prolapse is manually reduced by gentle traction on the colon.

A colopexy is performed, after reduction of the prolapse, to prevent recurrence (Fig. 13-35). A colopexy may also be performed in cases of recurrent rectal prolapse that can be reduced by external manipulation. Such a colopexy is rarely needed, however, if the cause of straining has been diagnosed and eliminated.

Topical anesthetic (1% dibucaine) ointment is instilled rectally after correction of any rectal prolapse to prevent further tenesmus. The patient may be fed on the day after the operation. A diet of soft food and a fecal softener (dioctyl sodium sulfosuccinate) may also be administered for one week postoperatively. Diarrhea should be treated with neomycin, intestinal coating agents, and anticholinergic drugs. Feces should be examined, and antihelmenthic agents should be administered, based on results of fecal examinations for parasitic ova.

In conclusion, once the rectal prolapse has been corrected, recurrence of the rectal prolapse is rare if the cause of the tenesmus has been diagnosed and resolved.

A

B

C

D

E

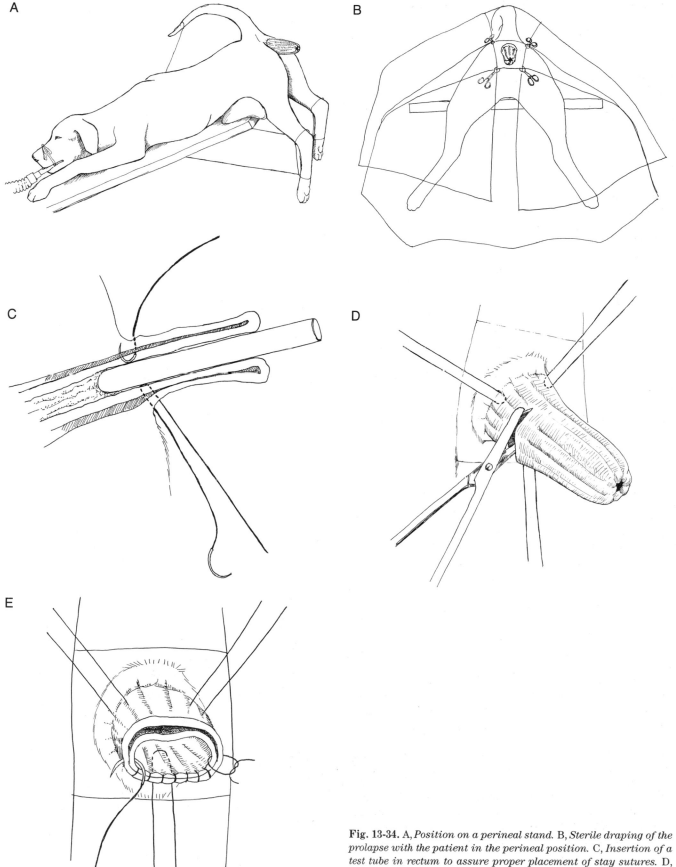

Fig. 13-34. A, *Position on a perineal stand.* B, *Sterile draping of the prolapse with the patient in the perineal position.* C, *Insertion of a test tube in rectum to assure proper placement of stay sutures.* D, *Excision of the prolapsed mass.* E, *Full-thickness anastomosis of the rectal lumens.*

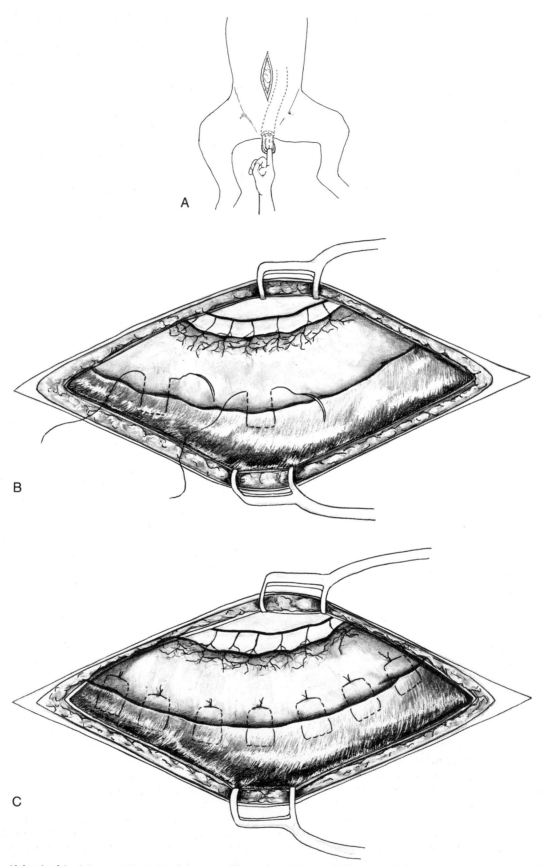

Fig. 13-35. A, *Abdominal incision and digital replacement of the prolapsed tissue.* **B,** *Placement of colopexy mattress sutures.* **C,** *Six to eight mattress sutures are placed to complete the colopexy.*

References and Suggested Readings

Annis, J. R., and Allen, A. R.: An Atlas of Canine Surgery. Philadelphia, Lea & Febiger, 1967.

Archibald, J.: Canine Surgery. 2nd Ed. Santa Barbara, CA, American Veterinary Publications, 1974.

Evans, H. E., and deLahunta, A.: Miller's Guide to the Dissection of the Dog. Philadelphia, W. B. Saunders, 1971.

Greiner, T., and Christie, T.: The cecum, colon, rectum, & anus. *In* Current Techniques in Small Animal Surgery. Edited by M. J. Bojrab. Philadelphia, Lea & Febiger, 1975.

LeRoux, P. H.: Dilation of the cecum in dogs. J. S. Afr. Vet. Med. Assoc., *33*:73, 1962.

Markowitz, J., Archibald, J., and Downie, H. G.: Experimental Surgery. 5th Ed. Baltimore, Williams & Wilkins, 1964.

Sabiston, D. C.: Davis-Christopher Textbook of Surgery. 12th Ed. Philadelphia, W. B. Saunders, 1982.

Schiller, A. G., Helper, L. C., and Knecht, C. D.: Repair of rectocutaneous fistulas in the dog. J. Am. Vet. Med. Assoc., *50*:758, 1967.

Stockman, V., and Stockman, M. R. J.: Cecal impaction in the dog. Vet. Rec., *73*:337, 1961.

Swenson, O. and Bill, A. H.: Resection of rectum and rectosigmoid with preservation of the sphincter for benign spastic lesions producing megacolon. *In* Surgery 24. St. Louis, C. V. Mosby, 1948.

Walshaw, R., and Harvey, C. E.: The rectum and anus. *In* Pathophysiology in Small Animal Surgery. Edited by M. J. Bojrab. Philadelphia, Lea & Febiger, 1981.

Surgery of the Colon

by Daniel C. Richardson *and*

D. J. Krahwinkel, Jr.

Colonic disorders requiring surgical intervention in the dog and cat are not common, and such intervention is frequently avoided because of a historical fear of operative and postoperative complications.

The major function of the colon is absorption of sodium and water and the addition of potassium and bicarbonate to the colonic contents. Bacteria comprise more than 10% of feces on a dry-weight basis. Although these bacteria can be detrimental to surgical techniques involving the colon, they synthesize riboflavin, nicotinic acid, biotin, folic acid, and vitamin K, which the colon absorbs. Most absorption occurs in the proximal colon, whereas the distal colon functions mainly for fecal storage and evacuation.

Blood supply to the colon is through the cranial and caudal mesenteric arteries. The cranial mesenteric artery supplies all parts of the colon, and the caudal portion of the descending colon and rectum are supplied by the caudal mesenteric artery. Venous drainage of the ascending colon is through the right colic and ileocecocolic veins. The middle colic vein drains the cranial portion of the descending colon and transverse colon, and the left colic vein drains the descending colon. Lymph nodes are located within the mesocolon, and their efferent vessels drain into the intestinal lymphatic trunks.

Clinical Signs of Colonic Disorder

Colonic disease classically presents with tenesmus and frequent small amounts of stools containing fresh (red) blood and mucus. Tenesmus becomes less common as the disorder occurs further proximally in the colon. Most absorption and digestion of nutrients takes place in the small bowel; therefore, with the exception of histiocytic colitis, colonic disorders rarely result in weight loss. Flatulence is usually associated with small bowel disorders, but may occur with constipating disorders of the colon. Vomiting has also been reported on rare occasions with colonic disease. The associated cause may be chronic blockage from intussusception or a possible reversal of the gastrocolic reflex. Clinical and ancillary findings are compatible with low intestinal obstruction, ranging from partial to complete blockage.

Indications for Surgical Treatment

Surgical treatment of disorders of the colon usually requires anastomotic or biopsy techniques. Resection and anastomosis is usually required in cases of intussusception, neoplasia, or trauma. Biopsy is an important aid in clinical diagnosis in cases refractory to other diagnostic techniques.

Intussusception of the colon occurs most commonly at the ileocecocolic junction. Rarely does the colon invaginate on itself. Simple, uncomplicated intussusceptions may be handled as described for the small bowel. (See the first section of this chapter, "Surgery of the Small Intestine.") Complications of ischemia and necrosis following intussusception may dictate resection and anastomosis.

Neoplasia of the colon is rare when compared to the integumentary system, mammary glands, or testis. Benign tumors of the colon include adenomatous polyps, leiomyomas, and papillary adenomas. Adenomatous polyps are thought in man to precede the development of carcinoma of the colon. This may also be the case in the dog. Malignant tumors are usually carcinomas or adenocarcinomas of a mucous or cirrhous type. Metastasis occurs most commonly to the regional lymph nodes, the peritoneal cavity, and the liver. Neoplasia involving the feline large bowel is uncommon; adenocarcinoma and lymphosarcoma have been reported.

Injury to the large bowel may result from external or intraluminal trauma. Blunt external trauma occasionally results in contusion, avulsion of the mesocolon, or thrombosis of mesenteric vessels leading to an ischemic segment of colon. Intraoperative Doppler ultrasound is an adjunct to clinical evaluation and aids the decision whether to excise the segment. Penetrating external trauma may also perforate the colon. More commonly, the colon becomes traumatized from within the lumen during passage of sharp foreign bodies or iatrogenically through transrectal instrumentation.

Preoperative Preparation

The basic principles discussed in the first section of this chapter, "Surgery of the Small Intestine," are appropriate for the colon. The increased complications of colonic surgery have long been recognized, however. Healing is delayed because of surgical stimulation of a high collagenase activity of the submucosa. This activity weakens the suture line for 5 to 7 days postoperatively. The bacterial population is much higher in the colon and consists of many pathogenic aerobes and anaerobes.

Elective colonic surgical procedures allow for a planned approach. Emergency procedures of the colon, as for penetrating wounds, necessitate operating in a contaminated field without the benefit of adequate preparation. Time permitting, bowel preparation should begin 24 to 48 hours prior to the surgical procedure. Food is withheld during this period. It may be necessary, owing to the animal's condition, to maintain low-residue liquid intake of high caloric content. A mild laxative (milk of magnesia) along with warm, soapy water enemas are administered each day. An enema with warm water and 10% povidone-iodine is advocated 2 to 3 hours prior to the operation.[*]

Emptying of the bowel helps to protect against large fecal masses disrupting a colonic surgical site. Although mechanical cleansing is probably the most important aspect in preparation for colon operations, reduction of bacterial flora is also crucial. Natural flora in the colon consist of a mixture of anaerobic and aerobic bacteria.

The history of colonic surgery emphasizes the need for achieving a clean surgical field for surgical success. Preoperative intestinal antisepsis has been attempted with antibiotics and antiseptics used alone or in combination. Fear of producing resistant bacterial and fungal flora has moderated the use of these compounds. An additional hazard is that too much emphasis may be placed on prophylactic therapy rather than on surgical skill and attention to detail. Short-term antibiotic therapy is beneficial in that it lowers bacteria's ability to colonize and to establish themselves and thus suppresses or avoids infections. Oral neomycin (20 mg/kg tid) is the drug of choice for reduction of aerobic bacteria within the colon. Although this drug is usually not absorbed, intestinal disease or an overdose can result in nephrotoxicity. Kanamycin sulfate,[†] an aminoglycoside (11 mg/kg bid), has a high degree of activity in the colon against aerobic organisms and may be used alone or in combination with other agents. Metronidazole[‡] (60 mg/kg sid) may be used to control the anaerobic bacterial population, especially the predominant Bacteroides species. These drugs should be used 24 to 48 hours prior to the surgical procedure. Unless peritonitis or septicemia is present, systemic antibiotics are not indicated.

Emergency situations requiring immediate surgical intervention to repair the colon preclude the adequate preoperative preparation. Oral neomycin and metronidazole will have little time to be of benefit, and systemic antibiotics such as ampicillin or a cephalosporin are indicated in these situations. A cleansing enema may be contraindicated because of its liquifying effect on the colonic contents that predisposes a patient to leakage. If an enema is to be given, a 10% povidone-iodine solution is the agent of choice.

Surgical Techniques

Surgical techniques for the colon parallel those for the small intestine. Under general anesthesia, the animal is placed in dorsal recumbency, is widely clipped, and is aseptically prepared from midthorax to the caudal end of the pubis. A ventral midline incision is made from 2 to 3 cm cranial to the umbilicus caudally to the pubis. The actual length of the incision depends upon exposure necessary in each individual case. Laparotomy sponges moistened with saline solution are placed along the abdominal incision, and a Balfour or Gossett retractor§ is positioned. All the abdominal viscera are examined to identify coexisting disease processes. The involved segment of colon is gently manipulated and is exteriorized. Laparotomy sponges moistened with saline solution are placed to prevent gross spillage into the abdominal cavity. If present, colonic contents are gently "milked" away from the proposed surgical site. Doyen intestinal clamps, umbilical tapes, or an assistant's fingers are used to keep the contents from the surgical field.

Segmental instillation of a 10% Betadine solution‖ can be used to enhance other methods of bowel preparation. This is done by isolating the proposed surgical site between 2 occluding umbilical tapes and injecting a 10% povidone-iodine solution intraluminally with a 20-gauge needle and syringe. A 20-minute contact time is advocated.

BIOPSY

Biopsy techniques of the colon are similar to those of the small intestine. Upon entering the lumen, a full-thickness wedge section 2 to 3 mm in width is excised from the antimesenteric border. Closure is carried out with 3-0 or 4-0 chromic catgut or synthetic absorbable material in a simple interrupted appositional or inversion pattern.

Because the colon is distensible, inverting patterns to achieve serosa-to-serosa contact allow a rapid, secure seal with minimal stenosis. Cushing, Connell, or Lembert patterns are adequate and do not require a second layer. The inverting pattern should be consid-

---

[*] Editor's note: Some veterinary surgeons prefer to avoid administering preoperative enemas, in order to minimize the chance for liquid fecal matter to escape during the surgical procedure and thereby to contaminate the patient's abdomen and the sterile operating field.
[†] Kantrim, Bristol Laboratories, Bristol-Myers Co., Thompson Road, Syracuse, NY 13201
[‡] Flagyl, Searle & Co., San Juan, PR 00936

§American V. Mueller, 6600 West Touhy Avenue, Chicago, IL 60648
‖ Purdue Fredrick, 50 Washington Street, Norwalk, CT 06856

ered the preferred method when disease processes impede healing or when the integrity of the bowel wall is questionable.

Biopsy of the colonic mucosa is often carried out intraluminally with a rigid proctoscope or with flexible fiberoptics equipment. Full-thickness samples require abdominal exposure to ensure accurate samples and a secure closure. Biopsy is a straightforward diagnostic procedure, but should be approached and carried out with the same meticulous preparation and technique as a resection and anastomosis.

Prior to closure, the laparatomy sponges within the abdomen should be removed, and the abdomen should be irrigated twice with warm saline and 10% povidone-iodine solutions. A change of gloves and instruments is advocated before the abdominal cavity is closed.

RESECTION AND ANASTOMOSIS

Preoperative preparation, surgical approach, and isolation of the bowel segment are similar to that described for biopsy. Small vasa recti (straight vessels) are segmentally given off perpendicularly from the hemorrhoidal vessels. When a portion of the colon is to be excised, the vasa recti must be isolated individually and ligated, preserving the major arterial supply coursing parallel to the colon (Fig. 13-36). The involved segment is excised as in the small bowel to ensure an adequate blood supply to the entire circumference.

During the surgical procedure, local irrigation of the abdominal cavity with 10% povidone-iodine solution aids in reducing bacterial contamination. This solution should be warm to avoid further hypothermia of the patient. Another technique is to irrigate the cut ends of resected colon with 5 to 10 ml of 10% povidone-iodine solution prior to anastomosis. This technique does not interfere with healing and aids in further reducing the bacterial population at the surgical site.

Healing of colonic anastomoses depends on both local and systemic factors. Absolute requirements include good nutritional status of the patient, correct suture placement through the submucosa, adequate blood supply to the cut ends, and an absence of tension at the anastomotic site.

End-to-end closure of a colonic anastomosis may be carried out with interrupted sutures in a crushing or simple apposition technique, as described for the small intestine. Swaged-on synthetic absorbable suture such as polyglycolic[*] or polyglactic acid[†] with a trocar-point needle makes penetration of the tough submucosa less traumatic. Sutures are first placed at the mesenteric and antimesenteric borders; additional sutures are placed every 2 to 3 mm. Excessive flaring of mucosa from the cut ends may be excised back to the serosal edge.

An inverting end-to-end closure of a colonic anastomosis is best accomplished with interrupted sutures in a Connell pattern. Sutures are placed 2 to 3 mm apart and incorporate approximately 2 to 3 mm of the cut edge (Fig. 13-37). These sutures are tightened to give serosa-to-serosa contact for a quick seal, but one must avoid causing ischemic necrosis from strangulating the tissue (Fig. 13-38). A second layer is not used.

Each pattern has its own advantages and disadvantages. Either technique results in a healed, functional bowel resistant to disruption in most cases. The end-to-end crushing or apposing pattern allows for the best anatomic alignment; however, it is more prone to leakage and disruption if the normal healing process is interrupted for any reason. Inversion of the cut ends allows for a rapid serosal seal with a minimum of leakage, but the lumen of the bowel may be compromised, depending on the amount of tissue inverted. Clinically, this does not pose a problem because of the high degree of distensibility of the large bowel. Theoretically, stricture formation could be a long-term postoperative complication with either method. Tests of bursting strength 30 days after the anastomosis have

[*]Dexon, Davis & Geck, Inc., Manati, PR 00701
[†]Vicryl, Ethicon, Inc., Somerville, NJ 08876

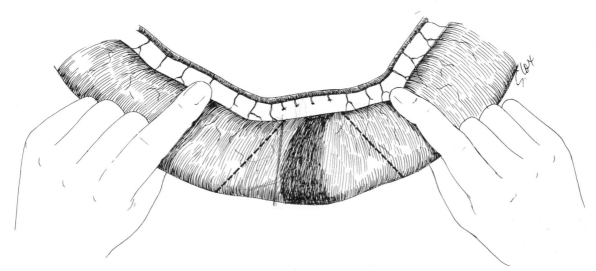

Fig. 13-36. *Short straight vessels to the bowel segment are ligated, preserving the vessel parallel to the colon. Dotted lines indicate the proposed line of incision.*

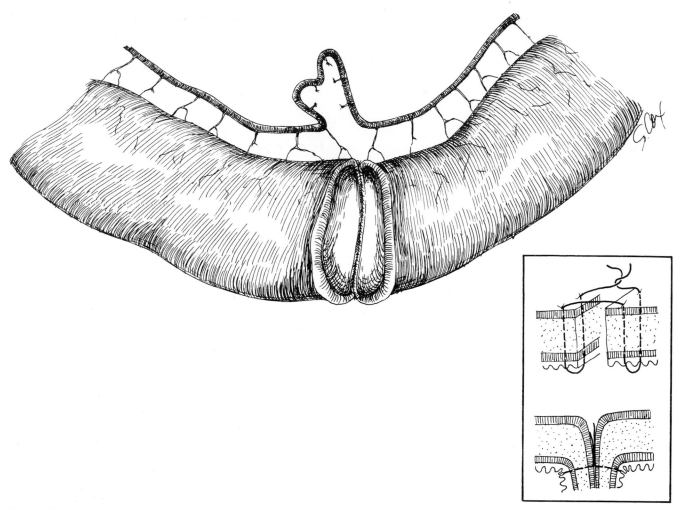

Fig. 13-37. *Sutures are first placed at the mesenteric and antimesenteric borders, and inversion is begun. A simple interrupted inverting suture pattern is used (inset).*

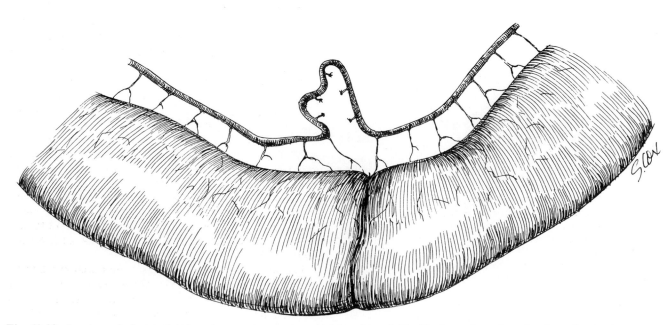

Fig. 13-38. *Anastomosis is completed, and serosa-to-serosa contact is achieved. The blood supply to the colon is maintained.*

shown end-to-end closures to be slightly weaker than inverted closures.

Inversion is advocated if the patient is debilitated or if the bowel wall's integrity is in question. Owing to the relative infrequency of performing anastomotic techniques on the colon, we feel that inversion is probably the quickest and safest technique.

Postoperative Care and Complications

Drainage of the abdominal cavity postsurgically has been advocated to monitor for early leakage. Placement of a drain in contact with the surgical site increases the risk of anastomotic breakdown, however, because it prevents the omentum and other body defenses from combating contamination. Drains are indicated for continued flushing and drainage if gross fecal spillage was encountered during the operation.

The patient should return to a liquid diet within 24 hours. Normal intake of food should begin in 48 hours. A stool softener is continued for 5 days, along with any oral or systemic medication begun prior to or at the time of the surgical procedure. Further antibiotic therapy is contingent on the animal's overall condition and must be decided on daily, on an individual basis. Any disruption of the surgical site usually occurs within the first 5 days. Monitoring of white blood cell counts, rectal temperature, and abdominal tenderness aids in evaluating for possible leakage. These aids are inconsistent, however, and should not be relied upon totally. Absence of stool, vomiting, depression, and anorexia during the first 5 postoperative days may indicate the need for a "second-look" operation before the animal becomes terminally ill.

Acknowledgments

We wish to thank Ms. Robbyn Wilhite and Ms. Amy Shaver for typing the manuscript and Ms. Sue Cox for providing the medical illustrations.

References and Suggested Readings

Brass, C.: The effect of metronidazole on the incidence of postoperative wound infection in elective colon surgery. Am. J. Surg., *135*:91, 1978.

Chen Chijen, et al.: The use or abuse of antibiotics in surgery of the colon. Surg. Clin. North Am., *53*:603, 1973.

Dunn, D. H., and Buchwald, H.: Gastrointestinal anastomoses: facts and fiction. *In* Gastrointestinal Surgery. Edited by J. S. Najarian and J. P. Delaney. Chicago, Year Book Medical Publishers, 1979.

Dunphy, J. E.: Preoperative preparation of the colon and other factors affecting anastomotic healing. Cancer, *28*:181, 1971.

Evans, H. E., and Christensen, G. C.: Miller's Anatomy of the Dog. 2nd Ed. Philadelphia, W. B. Saunders, 1979.

Greiner, T., and Christie, T.: The cecum, colon, rectum and anus. *In* Current Techniques in Small Animal Surgery. Edited by M. J. Bojrab. Philadelphia, Lea & Febiger, 1975.

Horney, F. D., and Archibald, J.: Colon, rectum, and anus. *In* Canine Surgery. 2nd Ed. Edited by J. Archibald. Santa Barbara, CA, American Veterinary Publications, 1974.

Jiburn, H., et al.: Healing of experimental colonic anastomoses—III. collagen metabolism in the colon after left colon resection. Am. J. Surg., *139*:398, 1980.

Lorenz: Disorders of the large bowel. *In* Textbook of Veterinary Internal Medicine: Diseases of the Dog and Cat. Edited by S. J. Ettinger. Philadelphia, W. B. Saunders, 1975.

Perianal Fistula in the Dog

by Richard Walshaw

Before considering this disease and its treatment, a brief review of the anatomy of the anal and perianal regions of the dog is essential.[1,7]

Anatomic Features

The anal canal is about 1 cm in length and is surrounded by the internal and external anal sphincter muscles. The anal canal, anus, and perianal region can be divided into four zones: columnar, intermediate, inner cutaneous hairless, and outer cutaneous hairbearing.

The columnar zone begins cranially at the anorectal line. It contains the anal columns (longitudinal ridges), which run caudally and are united at the anocutaneous line. The anal sinuses are formed by the converging of the anal columns. The intermediate zone (anocutaneous line) is less than 1 mm wide and is lined by squamous epithelium. It is an irregular, sharp-edged scalloped fold. The inner cutaneous hairless zone contains the anus. The zone varies considerably in width, owing to glandular development that changes with age, especially in the male dog. The outer cutaneous hairbearing zone merges with the surrounding skin.

A number of important glandular structures are found in these zones. The circumanal (perianal, hepatoid) glands are located subcutaneously, surrounding the anus, in the inner cutaneous hairless zone. Each gland consists of two distinct portions: an upper, sebaceous portion that opens to the surface by a duct, and a major, deeper, nonsebaceous portion. The nonsebaceous portion is a solid mass of large polygonal cells without secretory ducts that is sex-hormone dependent. Apocrine and sweat glands are also present in this zone. The anal glands are tubuloalveolar glands located around the anus; their ducts open onto the surface of the intermediate zone. The glands of the anal sacs lie on the wall of the sacs and open into them. The anal sacs are paired sacs that lie on each side of the anal canal between the internal and external anal sphincter muscles. Their ducts open onto the lateral margins of the anus adjacent to the intermediate zone. The sacs themselves serve as reservoirs for the secretions of the anal sac glands.

The important musculature to be considered is that comprising the anal sphincters. The internal anal sphincter muscle is the terminal, thickened portion of the circular smooth muscle of the rectum and anal canal. The external anal sphincter muscle is a circular band of striated muscle that attaches dorsally to the coccygeal fascia and rectococcygeus muscles. Ventrally, approximately 50% of its fibers decussate to join the bulbocavernous and urethral muscles in the male and the constrictor vulvae in the female. Laterally, the muscle is united with the muscles of the pelvic diaphragm by fascia.

The major blood supply to this region comes from two branches of the internal pudendal artery, the caudal rectal and perineal arteries. The caudal rectal artery supplies the perianal structures and glands. The perineal artery supplies the cutaneous and subcutaneous structures of the ischiorectal fossa. The venous drainage parallels the arterial supply.

The sensory and voluntary motor innervation is derived from the pudendal nerve. Its function is motor to the external anal sphincter muscle and sensory to the skin of the anus and perineal region. The smooth muscle of the anal canal is innervated by components of the pelvic plexus.

It is important to be familiar with the arrangement of the anatomic structures in these regions in the dog so that the disease processes discussed in this and following sections of this chapter, their treatment, and possible complications may be clearly understood.

Perianal Fistula

The common term used for this disease as seen in the dog is inaccurate because true fistulous tracts from the rectoanal canal to the perianal skin are extremely rare. Although perianal sinuses would be a better term, the term "perianal fistula" is commonly used to describe this disease syndrome.

The disease is seen most commonly in the German shepherd breed; dogs of either sex and of a wide age range are affected. It is seen less frequently in Irish setters and retrievers. Few other breeds appear to be affected.[2,7]

This specific disease of dogs is characterized by ulcerating skin and draining tracts, with a malodorous purulent discharge around the anal orifice. The tracts are lined by chronic inflammatory tissue and are invariably infected. Only in the most severe, long-standing cases do the tracts extend to the lumen of the rectoanal canal and thereby become true fistulas. The diseased skin surrounding the draining tracts is frequently discolored.[7]

Patients are presented with a spectrum of severity of the disease, ranging from only a few superficial draining tracts (Fig. 13-39), to severe, widespread multiple lesions all around the anal opening and extending deeply into the perianal and perirectal tissues (Fig. 13-40).

ETIOLOGY

Gross and histopathologic examinations of dogs with perianal fistula reveal that the disease may result from superficial contamination of the perianal region. This contamination leads to infection and abscessation

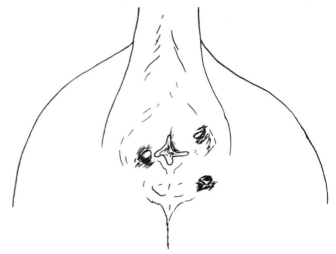

Fig. 13-39. *A few superficial draining tracts are seen in a mild case of perianal fistula.*

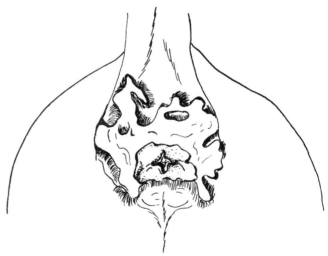

Fig. 13-40. *Extensive, widespread lesions, deep in the perirectal tissues, are seen in a severe case of perianal fistula.*

of circumanal glands, hair follicles, and other glands in the perianal skin and results in necrosis, ulceration, and both acute and chronic inflammation of the perianal skin and subcutaneous structures. The anal sacs are only secondarily involved in the disease process. The infected tracts can extend deeply into the perianal and perirectal tissues, often causing significant damage to the external anal sphincter muscle. Rarely do the tracts extend to the bowel lumen.[2,7]

It is important to realize that this disease in the dog does not have the same origin as a similar problem seen in man. The disease in man characterized by perirectal abscesses and anal fistula has a definite cryptoglandular origin, is not multiple in presentation, and is associated with true fistulization from the bowel lumen to the perianal skin. No anatomic, histopathologic, or gross evidence suggests that the two diseases are the same, as has often been suggested in the veterinary literature.[3,7]

Conformation of the German shepherd dog, with its broad-based tail held close to the anal region, is probably a significant factor in maintaining a film of fecal material and anal sac secretion over the perianal region. This conformation, along with the poor ventilation that is afforded by such tail carriage and the tendency for German shepherds to have soft stools or diarrhea, provides a suitable environment for the establishment of infection in the perianal region. These factors probably account for the high incidence of perianal fistula in this particular breed.[3,6,7] Many of these dogs have generalized skin problems and are hypothyroid, and some have poor T-cell function. It is suggested, therefore, that perianal fistula may be one expression of a generalized skin and systemic problem in these dogs.[8,9]

CLINICAL PRESENTATION AND DIAGNOSIS

The primary clinical signs associated with this disease are tenesmus, constipation, dyschezia, licking, and biting at the anal area. Weight loss, decreasing appetite, lethargy, and diarrhea are also reported. A mucopurulent, odoriferous discharge is seen, and hemorrhage may also be present.[2,3,7]

The severity of the clinical signs is usually correlated with the severity of the disease, which depends upon the extensiveness of the problem, the amount of scar tissue formation, and the length of time the patient has had the disorder. Occasionally, a dog with mild perianal fistula appears to be in extreme pain; and therefore, some individuality in presentation is found.

Diagnosis is made by direct visual examination of the perianal region and by finding multiple draining tracts. It is important to differentiate this disease from primary anal sac disease that has led to abscessation, followed by rupture and fistula formation. Anal sac disease in German shepherds and other large breeds of dogs is extremely rare. The lesions associated with anal sac fistulas are confined to the ventrolateral perianal regions, whereas perianal fistula lesions can be found 360° around the anus. Therefore, differentiation is usually not difficult.

Rectal examination is essential, but may have to be performed under anesthesia because of the patient's severe discomfort. An assessment should be made of the depth of the lesions, the extent of circumferential involvement, and any degree of anal stricture that may be present due to the chronicity of the disease. These factors obviously affect the extensiveness of surgical intervention and possibly the prognosis for the case.

TREATMENT

Many different surgical methods of therapy have been described for perianal fistula in the dog.[2,3,4,5,6,7] Owing to the nature of the disease, no treatment is entirely effective at the present time. Some of the previously described methods are associated with minor problems, such as recurrence of the disease, which requires further therapy. Others have potentially serious

sequelae, for example, fecal incontinence and severe anal stricture, which can lead to the death of the patient.

Medical therapy is ineffective in the control of the disease and may in fact increase the severity of the problem by preventing early institution of more effective therapeutic measures.

The treatment regimen that I currently use is described and discussed. At the present time, this technique gives the most consistent results with the least number of complications, when compared with previously described techniques.[7]

PREOPERATIVE PREPARATION

Routine physical and laboratory evaluations are performed on all patients prior to anesthesia and the surgical procedure. T_3 and T_4 values should also be obtained. Food is withheld before the operation for approximately 12 hours. If an enema is indicated, it should be a warm water, cleansing enema and should be given the day before the surgical procedure. An enema given on the morning of the operation allows liquid fecal material to escape during the surgical procedure. I do not routinely give these patients enemas, unless they are severely constipated. The majority of these patients are in great pain, and giving an enema can be stressful.

Following anesthetic induction, the whole perianal region is carefully clipped from beneath the tail to the level of the scrotum or vulva, and as far laterally on each side of the anus as necessary to allow complete exploration of the draining tracts. A tampon,* or a number of gauze sponges, is placed into the rectum to prevent leakage of fecal material during the procedure. Routine preparation of the surgical area is performed using a povidone-iodine† surgical scrubbing solution. The patient is moved into the operating room and is positioned on a well-padded surgical table in ventral recumbency. The table is tilted at the required angle, in a head-down position, and the patient's rear legs are hung over the end of the table and secured. The tail is taped over the back of the dog. The operative area is finally prepared with a povidone-iodine solution† in a sterile manner and, following the veterinary surgeon's preparation, is draped.

SURGICAL TECHNIQUE

The goal of this method of therapy is to preserve healthy tissue and vital structures, for example, the external anal sphincter, as much as possible. The diseased areas are explored, are debrided, and are allowed to heal by wound contraction and epithelialization.[7]

The first step is identification of the anal sac duct openings. A probe is inserted into each anal sac to ascertain its position, or to determine whether it has been

*Tampax super tampons, Tampax Co., Palmer, MA 01069
†Betadine, Purdue Fredrick Co., 50 Washington Street, Norwalk, CT 06856

destroyed secondarily by the inflammatory tissue and scarring. If the anal sacs are still present, a bilateral anal sacculectomy is performed. (See the next section of this chapter.) It is essential to dissect and remove the entire anal sac carefully. Any remnants that remain will cause the development of new draining tracts or the persistence of tracts already present. If the primary disease is extensive in the area of the anal sacs, sac dissection may be difficult because of the presence of chronic granulation tissue. Care must be taken to prevent further damage to the external anal sphincter muscle and its nerve supply.

Each of the draining-tract openings is identified and is probed to determine its depth and direction (Fig. 13-41). Using an electroscalpel, the overlying diseased tissue and periphery of the lesions are excised to open up the tracts (Fig. 13-42). The draining tracts are all explored to their fullest extent, and chronic granulation tissue and excessive scar tissue are removed in order to create an open, saucer-shaped wound (Fig. 13-43). All the tracts should be thoroughly explored and opened, so that no pockets of residual infection remain. This step may require, in severe cases, incising through portions of the external anal sphincter muscle and into the deeper perirectal tissues. No attempt is made to dissect and completely remove the base of the lesions. In this way, portions of the anal sphincter muscle are not removed, its nerve supply is not damaged, and therefore, postoperative fecal incontinence is not a problem.

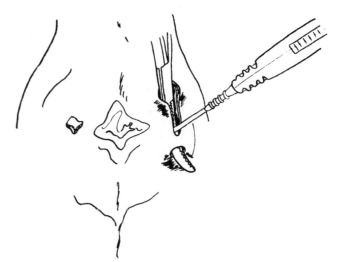

Fig. 13-42. *The electroscalpel is used to open all the draining tracts to allow complete exploration.*

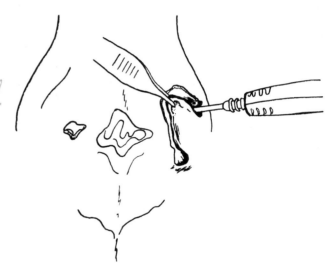

Fig. 13-43. *Saucer-shaped, open wounds are created by excising the superficial diseased tissue, using the electroscalpel.*

The electroscalpel is used to perform the dissection because excellent hemostasis can be achieved during the procedure in what would otherwise be a hemorrhagic area of diseased tissue. The overall desired effect is to leave the diseased areas open. The base of each lesion is then fulgurated using electrocautery (Fig. 13-44). A controlled killing of the diseased tissue is achieved without damage to deeper, often vital, structures. Moreover, adequate postoperative hemostasis is obtained. Occasionally, one finds deep tracts that are difficult to fulgurate because of their location. In these cases, an 80% liquified phenol solution is applied carefully with cotton-tipped applicators. Hemorrhage, however, occurs with phenol cauterization, and therefore, the patient should be carefully monitored in the immediate postoperative period.

At the end of the surgical procedure, the rectal packs are removed, and the perianal region is washed with a povidone-iodine solution.

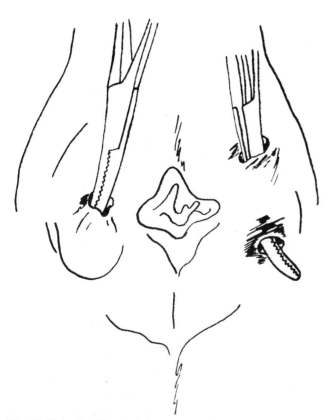

Fig. 13-41. *Each of the draining tracts is probed, using a mosquito hemostat, to determine its extent.*

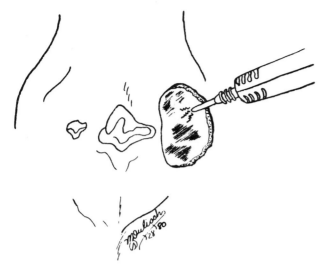

Fig. 13-44. *The base of each lesion is thoroughly fulgurated to kill the diseased tissue without damaging deeper, often vital, structures.*

POSTOPERATIVE CARE

The dog is usually hospitalized for 3 to 4 postoperative days. The patient is started on broad-spectrum antibiotic therapy, using oxacillin. The perianal region is washed carefully and thoroughly 3 times daily and after the dog defecates with povidone-iodine solution, diluted 4-to-1 with water. The patient should be walked 3 times daily and carefully observed for problems with defecation. A soft-food, low-bulk diet is fed. If severe dyschezia or tenesmus is present, a stool softener such as Metamucil* is added to the food. Once normal defecation has returned and healing is progressing, the patient is discharged. Continued nursing care at home is required. The owners should continue to wash the perianal region 3 times daily and to report problems with defecation. Oxacallin antibiotic therapy is continued for 6 to 8 weeks until healing is complete.

Re-examination at 2- to 4-week intervals is essential. It is important to examine the patient to determine that healing by wound contraction and epithelialization is progressing without complication. If the dog is having any functional problems, suitable symptomatic therapy, such as dietary adjustment or stool softeners, is instituted if required. Nursing care at home and repeat examinations should be continued until the perianal lesions are completely healed.

If the dog is hypothyroid, this disorder should be treated appropriately.

COMPLICATIONS

Two main postoperative problems are encountered: persistence of the infection and severe scarring that causes anal stricture.

PERSISTENCE OF DRAINING TRACTS. This problem should be detected as early as possible during the regularly scheduled postoperative reexaminations. During the

*Searle Consumer Products, Box 5110, Chicago, IL 60680

process of wound healing, a smooth, healthy granulation tissue bed is formed in the open wound. Areas of persistent infection appear as chronically inflamed tissue, often where deep pockets of infection were previously located. A purulent discharge is frequently associated with these lesions.

Early detection followed by repeated exploration, debridement, and fulguration are essential to prevent further progression. Perianal washing is continued until healing is complete. Problem cases may require

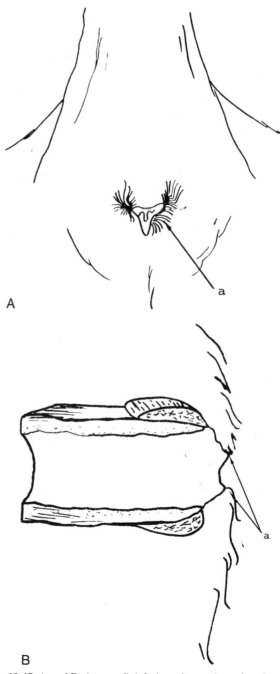

A

B

Fig. 13-45. A and B, *A superficial ring of scar tissue has formed at the junction of the skin and anal mucosa (a) as a result of the considerable contraction that has occurred during the closure of an extensive wound.*

two or three repeat procedures until all pockets of infected tissue have been successfully treated.

SEVERE SCARRING AND ANAL STRICTURE. Patients with long-standing, extensive lesions are likely to have considerable amounts of scar tissue already associated with the chronic inflammatory process. Some degree of anal stricture may already be present at the time of presentation. Little can be done about this problem

A

B

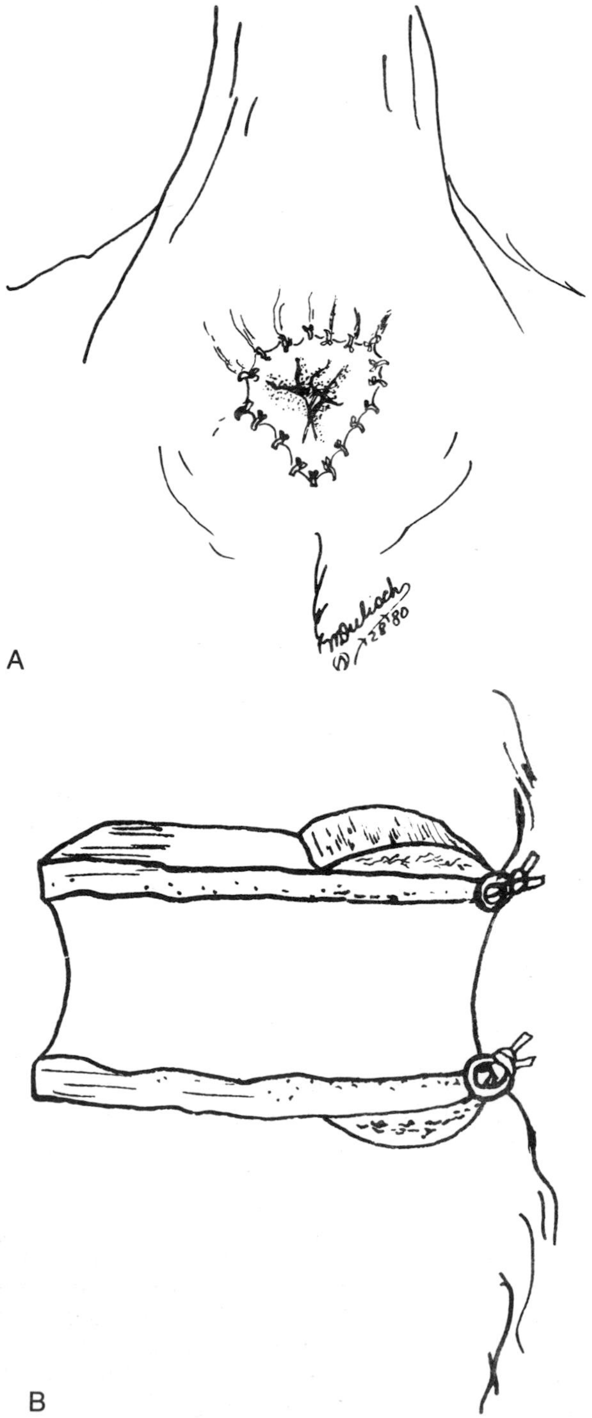

Fig. 13-46. A and B, *Following scar resection, the wall of the anal canal has been brought caudally and is sutured to the surrounding skin. Primary wound healing is the result.*

until the chronic inflammation and infection have been successfully treated. Diet changes and the use of stool softeners provide symptomatic relief.

Wound healing by contraction and epithelialization also results in some scar tissue formation. In patients with wide, extensive lesions, considerable contraction must occur to close the wound. A resulting superficial ring of scar tissue at the skin-anal mucosal junction may cause stricture of the anal opening (Fig. 13-45). If possible, surgical correction of the stricture is delayed until the infected tracts have healed. Resection of the skin-anal mucosal junction, with careful dissection and resection of the scar tissue, may be performed. Care is taken to avoid dissecting deeply into the external anal sphincter muscle. The resection is performed circumferentially over the affected area until an anal opening of functional size is created. The wall of the anal canal is brought caudally and is sutured to the skin (Fig. 13-46).

Postoperative care in these patients consists of administering antibiotics and stool softeners, to prevent tenesmus and dyschezia, and restraining the dog from licking or biting its perianal area. If nonabsorbable sutures were used, these are removed in 10 to 14 days. Once healing has occurred, the patient may be weaned, slowly, from the stool softener, until normal bowel movements are obtained.

References and Selected Readings

1. Evans, M. E., and Christensen, G. C.: Miller's Anatomy of the Dog. 2nd Ed. Philadelphia, W. B. Saunders, 1979.
2. Griener, T. P., and Betts, C. W.: Diseases of the rectum and anus. *In* Textbook of Veterinary Internal Medicine: Diseases of the Dog and Cat. Edited by S. Ettinger. Philadelphia, W. B. Saunders, 1975.
3. Harvey, C. E.: Perianal fistula in the dog. Vet. Rec., *91*:25, 1972.
4. Lane, J. G., and Burch, D. G. S.: The cryosurgical treatment of canine anal furunculosis. J. Small Anim. Pract., *16*:387, 1975.
5. Liska, W. D., et al.: Cryosurgery in the treatment of perianal fistula. Vet. Clin. North Am., *5*:449, 1975.
6. Robins, G. M., and Lane, J. G.: The management of anal furunculosis. J. Small Anim. Pract., *14*:333, 1973.
7. Walshaw, R., and Harvey, C. E.: The rectum and anus. *In* Pathophysiology in Small Animal Surgery. Edited by M. J. Bojrab. Philadelphia, Lea & Febiger, 1981.
8. Rosser, E. J.: Personal communication.
9. Walshaw, R.: Case records at Michigan State University.

Anal Sac Disease

by RICHARD WALSHAW

Anal sac disease is the most common disorder of the anal region of the dog seen in veterinary practice. Small, purebred dogs, when compared to the general canine population, have a high incidence of the disease. The problem is rarely seen in large or giant breeds.[3,6,8]

The function of the anal sacs is unknown, although their association with behavioral and social patterns has been suggested. The normal secretion is a slightly granular, brownish, serous or viscid fluid with a distinctive odor. Normal expression occurs by the action of the external anal sphincter muscle during defecation.[1,6,8]

Etiology

Anal sac disease can be divided into two presenting types, (1) impaction and (2) infection and abscessation. Possible predisposing causes of impaction are a change in the character of the glandular secretion, abnormal bowel elimination failing to empty the sacs, hypersecretion associated with generalized seborrhea, and poor muscle tone in obese dogs. Retention of anal sac secretion may result in fermentation, inflammation, or secondary infection with the possibility of abscess formation.[6,8]

Clinical Presentation and Diagnosis

Clinical signs associated with anal sac disease are related to the discomfort associated with the disease. These include tenesmus, dyschezia, discomfort in sitting, licking or biting the anal area, and tail chasing.[1,2,5,8]

On examination of the perianal region, firm masses in the area of the anal sacs are palpated in cases of impaction. If infection and abscessation are present, the patient experiences severe pain when the veterinarian attempts to examine the perianal region. Hyperemia and discoloration of the overlying perianal skin may be present. Abscessation, with rupture to the skin, results in the formation of fistulous tracts in the area of the anal sacs, with a purulent discharge. These lesions must be differentiated from perianal fistulas.

In dogs with chronic anal sac problems, other clinical signs have been noted, for example, skin irritation of the abdomen, groin, and axilla, otitis externa, periorbital dermatitis, interdigital dermatitis, and areas of alopecia due to self-trauma. Thus, chronic anal sac disease may be one expression of a more generalized problem.[2,5,8]

Diagnosis of anal sac disease is made by considering the patient's medical history, the presenting signs, the breed of dog, and the results of the physical examination of the perianal region. Rectal examination is essential to determine the degree of involvement and duct patency. During the rectal examination, the sacs can be expressed, atraumatically, and their contents may be evaluated.

Indications for Surgical Treatment

Anal sac impaction is treated by digital expression. Correct early treatment may prevent more serious forms of anal sac disease from developing. Education of the client regarding the clinical signs of anal sac disease is important. The differences between simple impaction, infection, and abscessation should be explained.[1,4]

If infection is present, the sacs should be expressed and flushed with an antiseptic solution. Systemic antibiotic therapy may be indicated.[1,4]

The indications for surgical intervention in anal sac disease are: recurrent episodes of impaction or infection in which medical therapy is becoming ineffective, abscessation, with or without fistulous tracts, and anal sac gland adenocarcinoma.

Anal sac gland adenocarcinoma is a malignant neoplasm of the glands that surround the anal sacs. It is locally invasive, and metastases to sublumbar lymph nodes and distant sites occur. Therefore, careful staging is essential prior to consideration of local resection. Adjunctive therapy may be required.

Preoperative Preparation

Routine physical and laboratory evaluations are performed on all patients prior to anesthesia and the surgical procedure. Food is withheld for approximately 12 hours preoperatively. Preparation for the operation is identical to that for perianal fistula. The rectum is packed with a tampon or gauze sponges. The patient is placed in the perineal position on the operating table. (See the previous section of this chapter.) The anal sacs are expressed prior to the surgical procedure.

Surgical Technique

ANAL SACCULECTOMY*

Many different procedures have been described for anal sacculectomy.[1,4] Some authors describe packing the sacs with various materials to aid in identification during surgical dissection. Both open and closed resection techniques have been described. I prefer a closed technique, with duct ligation, and I do not pack the sacs with any materials prior to removal.

The duct opening of one of the anal sacs is identified (Fig. 13-47), and a mosquito hemostat is inserted through the duct into the sac. The hemostat is used to push up the overlying structures and skin to identify the position of the sac. A curved skin incision is then made in the hairless perianal skin immediately overlying the sac (Fig. 13-48).

Dissection is continued through the subcutaneous tissues until the tip of the sac, containing the hemostat, is identified (Fig. 13-49). A second mosquito hemostat is then used to grasp the sac. The hemostat that was inserted into the sac is removed and is replaced on the instrument tray, so that it does not contaminate the other surgical instruments. It may then be used for the same procedure on the other side. Using fine Metzenbaum scissors, the fibers of the external anal sphincter muscle are carefully, bluntly and sharply, dissected from the anal sac. The veterinary surgeon must keep the dissection on the surface of the anal sac, to prevent excessive damage to the external anal sphincter muscle (Fig. 13-50). Additional hemostats are employed to aid in retraction of the sac during dissection. The dissection is continued until the duct is identified and is isolated (Fig. 13-51). The duct is ligated and is tran-

*See editor's note at end of section.

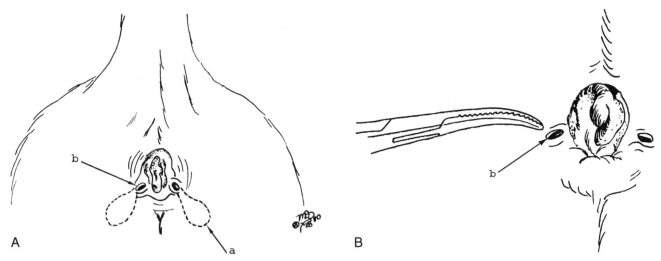

Fig. 13-47. A and B, *The position of the anal sacs (a) and their duct opening (b).*

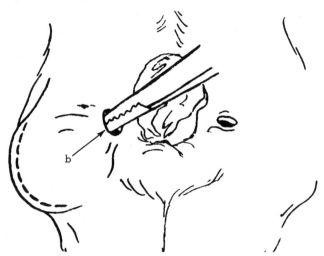

Fig. 13-48. *A mosquito hemostat is inserted into the anal sac to identify its position. The curved skin incision over the sac is indicated by the dotted line; b indicates the duct opening.*

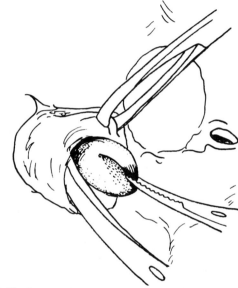

Fig. 13-50. *A mosquito hemostat is used to retract the anal sac while it is being dissected from the external anal sphincter muscle.*

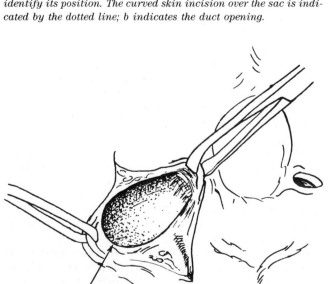

Fig. 13-49. *Following dissection through the subcutaneous tissues, the tip of the anal sac (a) is identified.*

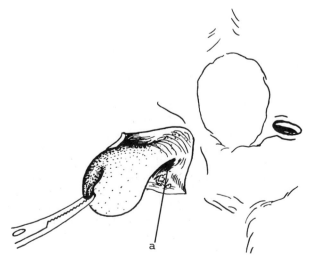

Fig. 13-51. *Dissection is continued until the sac is free and the duct (a) has been identified and isolated.*

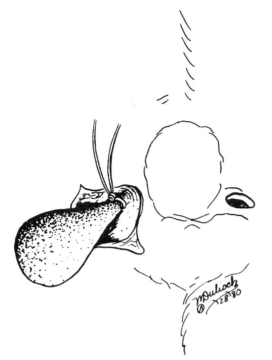

Fig. 13-52. *The duct is ligated prior to transection and removal of the anal sac.*

sected (Fig. 13-52). The sac should be examined to ensure that removal is complete.

The muscle fibers are then carefully apposed with simple interrupted sutures of fine chromic catgut. The subcutaneous tissues and skin are closed in a routine manner, and the procedure is repeated on the opposite side. If the anal sac has been inadvertently punctured during the dissection, the wound should be carefully flushed with saline solution, to which povidone-iodine solution has been added, prior to closure, in order to remove any contamination.

FISTULOUS TRACTS FOLLOWING RUPTURE OF

AN ABSCESSED ANAL SAC

The basic principles of surgical treatment of this problem are identical to those for the treatment of perianal fistula. This problem usually occurs unilaterally, but occasionally may be bilateral.

A bilateral anal sacculectomy is the first procedure to be performed. If all the remnants of the ruptured anal sac are not removed, a chronic fistula develops. Careful dissection is required to identify the remaining pieces of this structure and to remove them without excessively damaging the external anal sphincter muscle. The fistulous tracts are explored to their fullest extent. The electroscalpel is useful for this procedure and allows adequate hemostasis during the dissection. Once debridement has been completed and an open wound has been created, the base of the lesion is fulgurated by electrocautery. The wound is washed with a povidone-iodine solution.

Postoperative Care

A patient with a routine anal sacculectomy requires little specific postoperative care. An Elizabethan collar may need to be used to prevent self-trauma to the operative sites. If anal sac infection was present, or if the operative site was contaminated during the procedure, systemic antibiotic therapy should be instituted. Sutures should be removed 10 to 14 days postoperatively.

In the case of a dog with anal sac rupture and a fistulous tract that now has an open wound in the perianal region, postoperative care is similar to that for a perianal fistula. Broad-spectrum antibiotics are administered for 5 days postoperatively. The perianal region is washed 3 times daily with povidone-iodine solution, diluted 4-to-1 with water. A soft-food diet to which a stool softener has been added may be required if dyschezia is noted postoperatively. The patient should be seen regularly by the veterinarian until complete healing of the wound by contraction and epithelialization has occurred. It is essential that nursing care, that is, washing the perianal region, is continued at home until wound healing is complete.

Complications

Three main problems are associated with anal sac disease and its surgical treatment. These are: fecal incontinence, formation of chronic fistulas, and tenesmus from scar formation.

FECAL INCONTINENCE. This complication results from damage to the caudal rectal branch of the pudendal nerve. This nerve is the sole motor supply to the external anal sphincter muscle. If damaged bilaterally, complete incontinence occurs. Electromyography reveals complete denervation of the external anal sphincter muscle. Treatment of this complication is difficult, but consists of (1) diet control to ensure a firm, formed stool and (2) a surgical procedure that uses a fascial sling to occlude the anal opening, except at the time of voluntary defecation.[7]

CHRONIC FISTULA FORMATION. This complication results from incomplete removal of the anal sacs. It can especially be a problem when the sac has ruptured because of abscessation. Reoperation is required to find and to remove the sac remnants, followed by wound healing by contraction and epithelialization.

TENESMUS DUE TO SCAR FORMATION. Scar formation from excessive surgical trauma may occur in and around the external anal sphincter muscle. If extensive enough, significant anal stricture occurs and causes some degree of tenesmus. This disorder is usually minimal, however, so that symptomatic medical therapy often eliminates the problem.

A possible complication of anal sac abscessation and rupture is perirectal stricture formation. The patients are presented with moderate to severe tenesmus and a history of previous anal sac disease. Evidence of persistent abscessation or fistula formation may still be present, or the disease process may have completely resolved itself. Scar formation extends 360° around the rectal and anal canals, with varying degrees of involvement of the external anal sphincter muscle. Surgical intervention is required, but such an operation may be associated with the complications of incontinence or further scar formation.

References and Selected Readings

1. Griener, T. P., and Betts, C. W.: Diseases of the rectum and anus. *In* Textbook of Veterinary Internal Medicine: Diseases of the Dog and Cat. Edited by S. Ettinger, Philadelphia, W. B. Saunders, 1975.
2. Halnan, C. R. E.: The diagnosis of anal sacculitis in the dog. J. Small Anim. Pract., *17*:527, 1976.
3. Halnan, C. R. E.: The frequency of occurrence of anal sacculitis in the dog. J. Small Anim. Pract., *17*:537, 1976.
4. Halnan, C. R. E.: Therapy of anal sacculitis in the dog. J. Small Anim. Pract., *17*:685, 1976.
5. Halnan, C. R. E.: Anal sacs of the dog. Royal College of Veterinary Surgeons Thesis, 1973.
6. Harvey, C. E.: Incidence and distribution of anal sac disease in the dog. J. Am. Anim. Hosp. Assoc., *10*:573, 1974.
7. Lumb, W. V.: Surgical treatment of fecal incontinence. J. Am. Anim. Hosp. Assoc., *12*:666, 1976.
8. Walshaw, R., and Harvey, C. E.: The rectum and anus. *In* Pathophysiology in Small Animal Surgery. Edited by M. J. Bojrab, Philadelphia, Lea & Febiger, 1981.

Editor's Note

An alternate procedure for anal sacculectomy has been used successfully by the editor for a number of years. This procedure consists of incising the lateral wall of the anal sac and dissecting the sac free from the underlying external anal sphincter.

The incision is made by placing one scissor blade into the duct and cutting (Ed. note Fig. 1). It is helpful to pull the duct up onto the scissor blade with forceps, to ensure a complete cut of all structures. This procedure then opens the sac for visualization and identification of the grayish sac lining (Ed. note Fig. 2). Laterally,

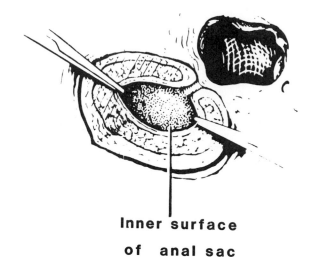

Inner surface of anal sac

Ed. note Fig. 2. *Once the incision is completed, the sac lies open.*

the sac is covered by the external anal sphincter muscle. The caudal third of this muscle is divided when the initial incision is made. Two mosquito hemostats are placed on the sac lining to hold the sac open and curved.

Metzenbaum scissors is used to dissect and to lift the sac from the external anal sphincter (Ed. note Figs. 3 and 4). The caudal rectal artery lies medial to the anal sac duct and should be preserved in the dissection process. When the dissection is completed and the sac is removed, one or two deep sutures of 3-0 synthetic

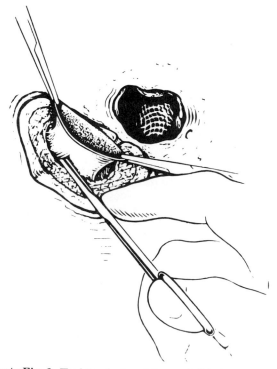

Ed. note Fig. 3. *The lateral edge of the sac is lifted with mosquito hemostats, and the sac is carefully dissected by the use of scissors.*

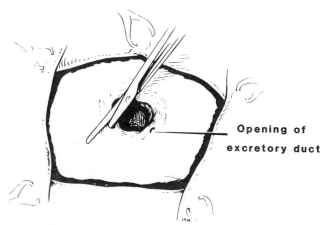

Opening of excretory duct

Ed. note Fig. 1. *The incision is made by placing one blade of the Metzenbaum scissors into the duct and opening the duct and sac in one stroke.*

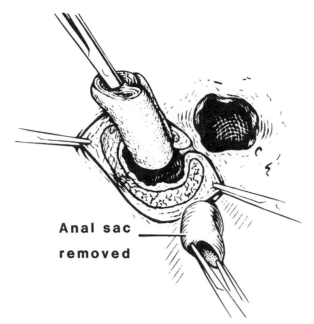

Ed. note Fig. 4. *After complete dissection from the sphincter muscles, the anal sac is removed.*

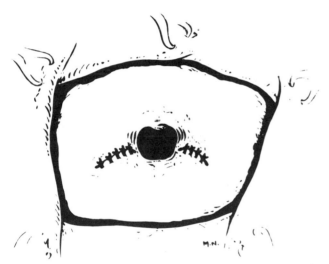

Ed. note Fig. 5. *The cavity is closed by drawing the sides together with two or three interrupted sutures. The skin is closed with interrupted sutures. (Ed. note Figs. 1 to 5 from Leonard, E. P.: Fundamentals of Small Animal Surgery. Philadelphia, W. B. Saunders, 1968.)*

absorbable suture are placed in the subcutaneous tissue. The skin is closed with 2-0 nonabsorbable sutures (Ed. note Fig. 5).

Rectoanal Strictures in the Dog

by RICHARD WALSHAW

Strictures associated with the rectal and anal canal of the dog[1,2] are of two types, benign and malignant. Benign strictures are usually secondary to anal sac disease, perianal fistula, trauma, or inflammatory proc-

esses. Iatrogenic complications of rectoanal operations are also observed as a cause of anal stricture.

Adenocarcinoma of the rectum and anus is frequently initially seen as a scirrhous, infiltrating, "napkin ring" lesion resulting in a severe stricture of the bowel lumen. Other neoplastic lesions also found in the pelvic region narrow the bowel lumen.

Surgical Treatment

Treatment of superficial strictures of the anal opening is accomplished by local resection and anastomosis of the anal mucosa to the skin. (See the section of this chapter on perianal fistula.) Because the lesion is superficial, interference with deeper vital structures is avoided, and postoperative problems with incontinence therefore should not be encountered.

Deeper strictures often require extensive perirectal dissection, and bilateral incisions may be required to enter the perirectal space. The scar is released by incision or excision of the affected tissue. Postoperative incontinence may be caused by damage to the external anal sphincter muscle and its nerve supply. Further scar formation can result from the surgical procedure and may lead to recurrence of the problem.

If the stricture is extensive, it may be necessary to resect a portion of the rectal or anal canals, using a rectal pull-through procedure. (See the next section of this chapter.) This procedure is associated with a number of potentially serious complications, including restricture at the anastomosis.

Malignant lesions are frequently inoperable by the time they are brought to the veterinarian's attention. Associated with these lesions are the possibilities of metastases to local lymph nodes and the liver. Careful staging of these lesions is essential prior to any attempts at therapy. Malignant lesions confined to the mucosa and submucosa may sometimes be excised by prolapsing the rectum and performing a submucosal resection. If the lesion is more extensive, but still operable, then a rectal pull-through operation is required. Adjunctive antineoplastic therapy is necessary in most cases.

In benign strictures of the rectal and anal canal, adjunctive medical therapy plays an important role in the treatment plan. Diet changes and the use of a stool softener may be required, often for extended periods of time. Treatment of rectoanal strictures ideally should result in a patient that is continent, yet able to defecate without any problems.

References and Selected Readings

1. Griener, T. P., and Betts, C. W.: Diseases of the rectum and anus. *In* Textbook of Veterinary Internal Medicine: Diseases of the Dog and Cat. Edited by S. Ettinger. Philadelphia, W. B. Saunders, 1975.
2. Walshaw, R., and Harvey, C. E.: The rectum and anus. *In* Pathophysiology in Small Animal Surgery. Edited by M. J. Bojrab. Philadelphia, Lea & Febiger, 1981.

Editor's Note

An alternate method of anal stricture (Ed. note Fig. 1) repair involves cutting the stricture in four places (dorsal, ventral, and left and right lateral), so that half of each incision extends outward through the skin with the other half extending inward through the mucosa (Ed. note Fig. 2). Each incision is sutured in the opposite direction (Ed. note Fig. 3) with three 3-0 synthetic absorbable sutures.

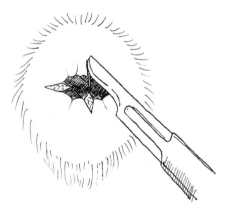

Ed. note Fig. 1. *Stricture of anus.*

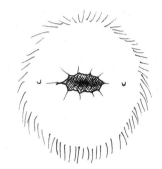

Ed. note Fig. 2. *Scalpel cutting stricture on right lateral side of anus. The dorsal and left lateral incisions are already made. Note the diamond configuration of the incised sites.*

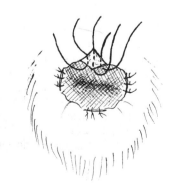

Ed. note Fig. 3. *Suturing of stricture incisions. Note the three sutures placed in each incision.*

Rectal Pull-Through, Resection, and Anastomosis

by C. W. Betts

Indications

The rectal pull-through procedure is indicated for excision of lesions that would be difficult to remove through an anal or an abdominal approach. Although infrequent in occurrence, multiple polyps, sessile growths, or an infiltrating mural lesion may be removed by this technique. Isolated perianal or perineal fistulas communicating with the rectum and lacerations secondary to foreign bodies or pelvic fracture are good indications for the pull-through technique. The terminal bowel may be advanced through the anal ring to the level of the caudal mesenteric lymph node and caudal rectal artery. Tissue cranial to this would be approached through a celiotomy incision. The technically more difficult combined abdominal-anal pull-through is indicated for lesions difficult to remove by either approach alone. The distinct advantage of the combined approach is access to the abdominal cavity to inspect for metastasis.

Preoperative Evaluation and Preparation

Many of these animals are middle-aged or older, and a thorough medical history, a physical examination, and a laboratory profile are mandatory. Careful systematic palpation of abdominal structures, regional lymph nodes, and the pelvic canal precedes proctoscopy and radiographic evaluation of the abdomen and thorax. This technique is not satisfactory if there is palpable or radiographic evidence of adhesions or extension of neoplasia into adjacent structures. Metastatic lesions in the abdomen should be evaluated by celiotomy prior to the pull-through procedure.

A urinalysis is always indicated. Urine specific gravity and urine protein are important in determining anesthetic and fluid management. Total protein may be low from inappetence, chronic blood loss, and mucoid stools. If contrast radiography is used to evaluate the colon, electrolyte loss or imbalances may be present from lack of food and administration of cleansing enemas.

If possible, a low-bulk diet should be started a few days prior to the surgical procedure, and a warm water enema should be administered the evening before. Studies in man substantiate the value of preoperative antibiotics in colorectal surgery in conjunction with mechanical cleansing of the bowel. Oral antibiotics should be started 12 to 16 hours before the operation. Systemic antibiotics, when used, are given 1 to 6 hours prior to the operation; this schedule reflects the time necessary for effective blood levels. Erythromycin, administered orally at 10 mg/kg t.i.d., or neomycin, at 20 mg/kg q.i.d., is recommended for dogs. Erythromycin and neomycin in combination provide broad-spectrum coverage and protection against aerobes and anaerobes. Antibiotics exert no beneficial effect when the wound has been sealed with fibrin and should not be continued longer than 24 to 48 hours after the surgical procedure.

Anesthetic Considerations and Intraoperative Management

Inhalation anesthesia is recommended, although sedation, supplemental oxygen, and an epidural anesthetic are satisfactory for high-risk cases. The operation may be performed with the animal in a perineal position, but dorsal or lateral recumbency facilitates respiratory support. Intravenous fluids should be administered prior to induction of anesthesia at a level sufficient to promote diuresis. These fluids are maintained throughout the procedure.

Surgical Technique

After a standard clipping and scrubbing, the anus and a small area of the circumanal region are draped with 3-corner draping or a fenestrated drape. Stay sutures are placed an equidistance apart in the anorectal junction. The rectum is then circumferentially incised through all layers 6 to 8 mm cranial to the sutures, which can now be used to evert and widen the anal ring (Fig. 13-53). Traction on the incised proximal end of the rectum is applied by grasping the tissue with Allis or Babcock tissue forceps. By means of blunt dissection between the rectum and the medial aspect of the external anal sphincter, the freed rectum is carefully exteriorized through the anal ring (Fig. 13-54). The nerve supply to the cranial rectum is the hypogastric nerve. The

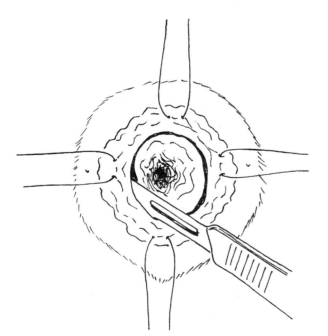

Fig. 13-53. *Rectum is circumferentially incised through all layers cranial to preplaced stay sutures.*

pelvic nerves, from the pelvic plexus supply the medial and caudal rectum. This portion of the innervated rectum is to be excised, and identification or preservation of the nerve supply is not attempted. Strict attention to careful dissection and gentle tissue handling is essential to minimize damage to adjacent structures and deprivation of innervation. A considerable amount of tension is required to maintain adequate traction to facilitate dissection. The reflection of the peritoneum at the pararectal fossa occurs at the lateral aspects of the terminal rectum, and entry into the peritoneal cavity usually occurs. Sufficient distal bowel is brought out to assure adequate healthy tissue cranial to the lesion for anastomosis. Lesions with well-defined margins can be palpated through the rectal tube. Multiple lesions necessitate incising the rectum linearly (Fig. 13-55) to determine when normal tissue has been exteriorized. The tunica serosa and tunica muscularis of the prolapsed segment and the anorectal cuff are then sutured with closely placed, simple interrupted sutures of 3-0 or 4-0 polyglycolic acid* or polyglactin 910† (Fig. 13-55). The colorectal segment containing the lesion is then incised just caudal to the first row of sutures. A simple interrupted or continuous pattern of 3-0 or 4-0 polyglycolic acid or polyglactin 910 is placed in the mucosal and submucosal layers. Simultaneous incision and anastomosis using a through-and-through, simple interrupted technique are also effective. Relaxation of caudal tension and release of the stay sutures re-establishes the continuity of the terminal bowel and draws the anastomotic line into the pelvic canal.

Postoperative Considerations

The entire tissue specimen should be submitted for histopathologic examination. Postoperative straining is kept to a minimum with a low-bulk diet, stool softeners, supervised exercise, sitz baths, and glycerin suppositories if necessary. Topical anesthesia with lidocaine suppositories may be used if the animal evidences extreme discomfort initially. Supervised feeding should resume as soon as the animal wishes to eat. Postoperative antibiotics are discontinued in 3 to 4 days maximum.

Follow-up Evaluation

The main advantage of the rectal pull-through procedure is reduction of anesthetic and surgical time. The major disadvantage is the lack of access to the abdominal cavity to inspect for primary or metastatic lesions. It is imperative that these animals be followed carefully on a scheduled basis to evaluate bowel function, possible recurrence, metastasis, or stricture and to maintain contact with the client. Gentle rectal palpation and direct inspection of the anastomosis through an anoscope or similar instrument may be done safely 8 to 10 days after the operation.

*Dexon, Davis & Geck, Inc., Manati, PR 00701
†Vicryl, Ethicon, Inc., Somerville, NJ 08876

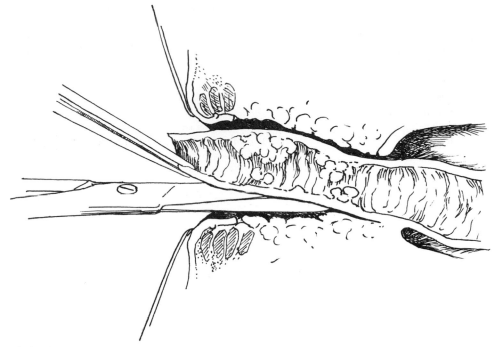

Fig. 13-54. *Rectum is freed by blunt dissection and is exteriorized.*

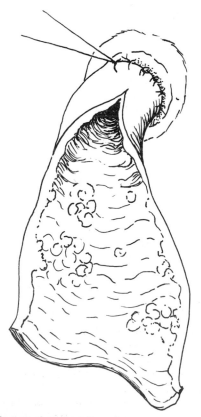

Fig. 13-55. *Rectum is incised linearly to determine extent of normal tissue and is sutured with simple interrupted sutures—the serosa and muscularis of the prolapsed segment to the anorectal cuff.*

Postoperative complications include wound dehiscence and cicatricial stenosis. Incontinence should not be a problem because this technique preserves both sphincteric and reservoir continence. Sphincteric continence is disrupted when the internal anal sphincter is excised and the external anal sphincter is resected bilaterally. Reservoir continence, defined as a storage function of the colon until the need for mass evacuation, may still be anticipated, and coordinated with feeding and exercise schedules.

References and Selected Readings

Greene, J. A., and Knecht, C. D.: Pull-through resection of the rectum. Canine Pract., *2*:43, 1977.

Greiner, T. P., and Betts, C. W.: Diseases of the rectum and anus. *In* Textbook of Veterinary Internal Medicine: Diseases of the Dog and Cat. Edited by S. J. Ettinger. Philadelphia, W. B. Saunders, 1975.

Jonsell, G., and Edelmann, G.: Single-layer anastomosis of the colon. A review of 165 cases. Am. J. Surg., *135*:630, 1978.

Hurley, D. L., et al.: Perioperative prophylactic antibiotics in abdominal surgery. A review of recent progress. Surg. Clin. North Am., *59*:191, 1979.

14 * Liver, Biliary System, and Pancreas

Surgery of Hepatic Vascular Tissues

by EUGENE M. BREZNOCK

Anatomy of the Hepatic Blood Supply

In classic developmental anatomy, blood flow to the fetal liver is via the right and left omphalomesenteric veins. At approximately the sixth week of fetal development, the right omphalomesenteric vein is obliterated and the left persists, developing ultimately as the main portal vein. Blood flow of the umbilical vein becomes encompassed by the developing liver and shifts from the sinus venosus to a simple intrahepatic pathway, which is the ductus venosus. The ductus venosus exists in the dog up to the birth of the fetus, providing the channel to carry oxygenated blood directly to the heart. Physiologic changes induced by postpartum respiration and a lowering of the umbilical vein pressure close the ductus venosus. Although the time of closure of the ductus venosus varies among animal species, in the dog it closes off entirely between the second and third day of extrauterine life.[5] The umbilical vein persists as the round ligament.

The hepatic artery originates from the celiac artery. The common hepatic artery in the dog may divide from one to five or more times, to supply each liver lobe with one or more proper hepatic arteries. In the cat, the hepatic artery usually divides into three branches supplying the right, left, and middle hepatic divisions. The portal vein is a confluence of smaller splanchnic veins (gastroduodenal, splenic, left gastric, caudal mesenteric, cranial mesenteric, iliocecocolic, and jejunal veins). The portal vein is the only major venous channel that allows blood to traverse another organ before returning to the heart. In the dog and cat, the portal vein and its branches are predictable in location (Fig. 14-1). The portal vein of the dog is divided into right and left major divisions. The right main division supplies afferent splanchnic blood to the caudate and right lateral liver lobes (right hepatic division). The left main portal division divides into five branches to the papil-

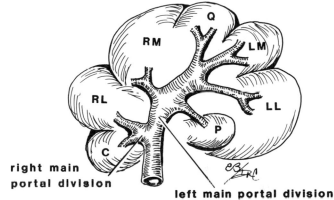

Fig. 14-1. *Schematic diagram of the usual portal vein distribution of the dog. Lobes of the liver: C, caudate; RL, right lateral; RM, right medial; Q, quadrate; LM, left medial; LL, left lateral; P, papillary process of caudate.*

lary process of caudate lobe and the left lateral, left medial, quadrate, and right medial liver lobes (central and left hepatic divisions). In the cat, there are usually three branches of the portal vein, dividing into the right, central, and left divisions of the liver. The number of major hepatic veins draining the liver varies between six and eight. Two large hepatic veins, one draining the left and one draining the central hepatic division, are consistent in location. The remaining hepatic veins are less consistent in location, size, and portion of the liver they drain.

Nearly 25% of the total cardiac output is carried through the liver. Three quarters of the hepatic blood flow are transported in the portal vein under low pressure (6 to 12 mm Hg); the remainder is transported in the hepatic artery under systemic arterial pressure (>90 mm Hg). The portal vein of the dog is septic and has a low oxygen tension when compared to that of the cat and other species. In the dog and cat, sudden ligation of the portal vein is fatal within a few hours. Death results not from liver failure, but from trapping of blood in the congested splanchnic bed behind the obstruction. Interruption of the mesenteric arterial blood supply eliminates portal flow, and death results from intestinal infarction rather than from liver failure. The portal vein of the dog and cat may be completely obstructed if the procedure is performed slowly over several weeks before complete obstruction is realized. In addition, certain diseases such as hepatic cirrhosis, splenomegaly, and malignant tumors may cause intrahepatic or extrahepatic occlusion of the portal vessels that results in portal vein hypertension. With portal hypertension, part of the impeded portal blood is forced into collateral portosystemic communications in which blood bypasses the liver and is directed into the systemic circulation. In the dog and cat, the portosystemic communications are normally small, insignificant vessels present at certain intra-abdominal locations. These vessels may undergo considerable dilation in cases of portal obstruction and may become vitally important collateral pathways.

The liver fails to develop or atrophies after congenital or acquired diversion or reduction of portal blood flow and has a diminished capacity to regenerate. The patient becomes sensitive to protein ingestion, a disorder referred to as meat or ammonia intoxication. Nonetheless, hepatic parenchymal function is usually adequate to sustain life, although under restricted conditions.

Two anomalies of the hepatic vascular system are amenable to surgery, hepatic lobe arteriovenous fistulas and portosystemic shunt. The portosystemic shunt may be classified as either single or multiple and extrahepatic or intrahepatic. The radiographic and clinicopathologic diagnostic methods for these anomalies are considered elsewhere.[7]

Surgical Pharmacology

In the dog and cat, common hepatic artery ligation ordinarily is not fatal; sufficient collateral blood flow is derived from the gastroduodenal and pancreaticoduodenal circulations. If high doses of antibiotics (penicillin) are administered concomitantly, the dog survives proper hepatic artery ligation. Normally, the elevated hepatic arterial O_2 tension prevents anaerobic organism overgrowth; following hepatic artery ligation, the administered antibiotic prevents bacterial overgrowth. Antibiotics probably need not be administered to the cat following proper hepatic arterial ligation(s) because this species has a higher portal venous oxygen tension than the dog. I have occasionally ligated hepatic arterial and portal venous branches to selected lobes in dogs and cats without fatal outcome. In both species, antibiotics were concomitantly administered, and portal venous pressure was measured during the ligation process.

Hepatic Arteriovenous Fistulas

An arteriovenous fistula of the liver may be congenital or acquired. An acquired fistula may be secondary to penetrating or blunt trauma, surgical procedures, or degeneration and rupture of arteries into accompanying veins. Systemic signs include tachycardia, decreased diastolic pressure, and a wide pulse pressure. Hemodynamic data usually reveal an increased blood volume and an increased cardiac output. Cardiomegaly may occur if the fistula is large or chronic, and high-output heart failure may result.

Intrahepatic fistulas between the hepatic artery and the portal vein have been reported in both the dog and cat. The origin of these lesions in man and probably in the dog includes trauma, rupture of hepatic artery aneurysms, congenital defects (vascular hamartomas), hepatic vein obstruction, and cirrhosis with extreme portal hypertension. Fistulas from the hepatic artery to the portal vein usually result in lethargy, anorexia, poor growth, emaciation, and ascites. At operation, large, tortuous vessels may extend from the affected liver surfaces. Fremitus can be palpated in these vessels. Temporary occlusion of the proper hepatic arteries to the specifically affected lobes may decrease or eliminate the fremitus. Most cases of hepatic-arterial-to-portal-vein fistula also cause enough portal hypertension to result in the formation of multiple portosystemic shunts.

When the arteriovenous shunt(s) involve a single liver lobe, resection of the liver lobe should be performed. (See the next section of this chapter.) If the arteriovenous fistulas extensively involve multiple liver lobes, or if the hepatic lobe cannot be resected, selective dearterialization of the affected lobe(s) should be performed. (See the next section of this chapter.) The multiple portosystemic shunts (portal vein to caudal vena cava) should also be ligated. During ligation, portal venous pressure should be monitored and should not be allowed to exceed 20 to 25 cm H_2O. If dearterialization is performed, systemic collateral vessels may allow the recurrence of the disease. Selected dearterialization by embolization, employing angiocatheterization techniques, of acrylic, Gelfoam, muscle, polyurethane foam, or similar substances may be effective for hepatic arteriovenous fistulas. This technique has been used with limited success in other organs, such as the kidney.

Portosystemic Shunts

Many clinical and clinical pathologic alterations are seen in dogs with anomalous portosystemic shunts.[1,3,8] Although rarely reported in cats, portosystemic shunts do occur. Portosystemic communications are observed in the normal cat, and gradual increases in feline portal vein pressure result in the dilation of these anastomoses.[4]

SINGLE SHUNTS

Single extrahepatic and intrahepatic shunts are probably congenital; multiple extrahepatic shunts arise from portal hypertension (neoplasms, arteriovenous shunts, hepatic fibrosis, or cirrhosis) and are probably acquired. Medical therapy and dietary management of hepatic encephalopathy caused by portosystemic shunts are valuable, but are currently palliative rather than curative.

EXTRAHEPATIC. The recommended treatment for single extrahepatic portosystemic shunts is surgical attenuation or obstruction of the anomalous vessel. *A procedure to obstruct the shunting vessel completely should only be performed if portal vein pressure is measured by a water manometer or a strain gauge transducer.* If portal pressure does not rise above 20 to 25 cm H_2O with the anomalous vessel completely occluded, the vessel is permanently ligated.

Most single extrahepatic portosystemic shunts appear to originate in the gastrosplenic or splenic vein prior to their entry into the portal vein. The single portosystemic shunt usually terminates in the caudal vena cava between the left phrenicoabdominal and renal vein. Identification of a single extrahepatic portosystemic shunt is not difficult because few large veins normally drain to the abdominal caudal vena cava. Small venous tributaries from a single extrahepatic portosystemic shunt should be ligated.

Prior to attenuation or ligation of the large extrahepatic portosystemic shunt, a 4-0 prelubricated cardiovascular silk suture is placed in a pursestring pattern in a prepared area of the portal vein (Fig. 14-2A), or a small mesenteric vein is isolated, is sacrificed, and is prepared for catheterization (Fig. 14-2B). A needle incision is made, and the catheter is connected to a water manometer or a strain gauge transducer for monitoring portal pressure during manipulation of the portosystemic shunt (Fig. 14-2C). The portosystemic shunt often bypasses the abdominal caudal vena cava, traverses the diaphragm, and enters the azygos vein, right atrium, or thoracic caudal vena cava. Preoperative portal venograms aid but are not essential for diagnosis. The portocaval shunt is identified and is skeletonized

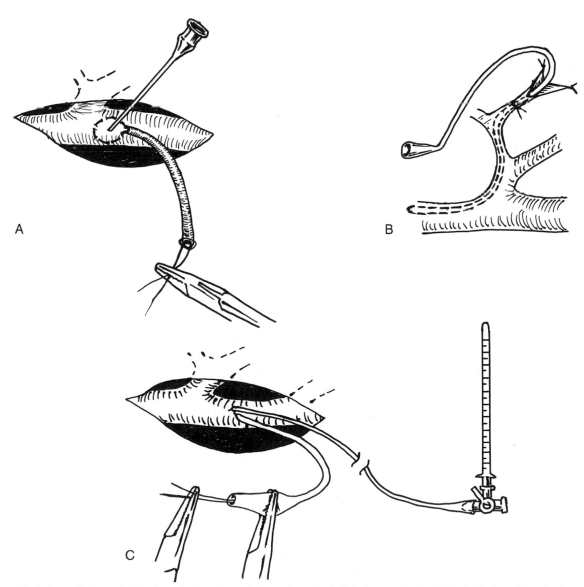

Fig. 14-2. A, *A needle is used to incise, within a pursestring suture, the isolated segment of portal vein.* B, *A catheter is placed in a segment of mesenteric vein and advanced into the portal vein.* C, *The pursestring suture is tightened around a catheter placed into the portal vein and is connected to a water manometer.*

as close to the diaphragm as possible. A silk ligature is passed around it, and the shunt is gradually obstructed while portal venous pressure is monitored. If central venous pressure is monitored during the surgical procedure, this water manometer may be temporarily used to measure portal venous pressure. Normal portal pressure is equal to approximately 13 cm water. If intrahepatic portal venous circulation is unable to handle the increased splanchnic blood flow following complete occlusion of the anomalous shunt, portal venous pressure will rise above 40 cm water. Portal venous pressure above 25 cm water may result in compromised splanchnic perfusion, severe portal hypertension, ascites, and death. As mentioned previously, the dog cannot survive complete, sudden obstruction of the portal vein, and some dogs cannot survive even acute, moderate portal hypertension. Following attenuation or obstruction of the anomalous shunt, several patients have died, even though the measured portal venous pressure did not exceed 25 cm water.

When the anomalous vessel has been attenuated or obstructed, the portal vein catheter may be removed, the pursestring suture may be tied, and the abdomen may be closed in a routine manner. If the catheter is placed in the mesenteric vein, the veterinary surgeon may elect to exit the catheter outside the abdomen for postoperative portal venous pressure monitoring or angiography; the catheter can simply be pulled without ligation when the procedures are complete.

During manipulation of the portosystemic shunts, whether extrahepatic or intrahepatic, other parameters of the patient should be monitored in addition to portal venous pressure; these include heart rate, central venous pressure, systemic arterial pressure, and color of the splanchnic viscera. One should not rely solely upon observation of the splanchnic viscera for signs of congestion or hypoxia when deciding whether to obstruct completely or attenuate the anomalous shunt. Several patients have died 12 to 24 hours following the surgical procedure from severe splanchnic congestion, even though the splanchnic viscera had an apparently normal circulation as judged by the color of the serosal surface of the abdominal viscera.

INTRAHEPATIC. Surgical manipulation of intrahepatic single portal systemic shunts (including patent ductus venosus) is technically more difficult than the extrahepatic single shunt. Two surgical techniques have been employed for surgical attenuation or obstruction of intrahepatic portosystemic shunts in dogs. Through a median incision, the entire extrahepatic portal vein is

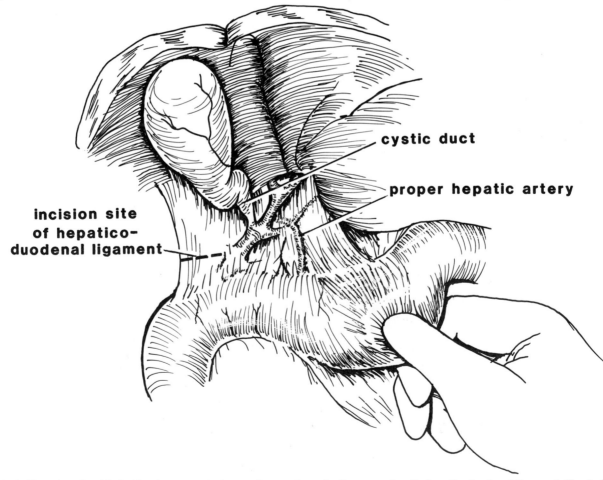

Fig. 14-3. *The stomach with duodenal segment is retracted away from the liver exposing the hepaticoduodenal ligament. The dashed line indicates the incision line.*

identified and is skeletonized by careful sharp and blunt dissection. The small liver normally seen with portal systemic shunts makes possible identification of the portal branches as they enter their respective hepatic lobes (Figs. 14-3 and 14-4). A catheter is placed in the portal vein to monitor portal pressure (see Fig. 14-2). The ductus venosus or intrahepatic shunt may arise from the left (more common) or right main branch of the portal vein and has been seen to communicate with a hepatic vein draining the left, central, and right divisions. The location of the intrahepatic shunt varies. Therefore, if difficulty is encountered in determining the location, segmental isolation and obstruction of portal vein branches, while monitoring portal pressure, usually indicate the area of the shunt. If the shunt is of moderate size, hepatic portal resistance will be negligible, and portal venous pressure will be nearly or equal to central venous pressure (-3 to $+3$ cm H_2O).

Obstruction of a portal vein branch not intimately connected with the shunt does not change portal venous pressure. When the portal vein intimately connected to the shunt is obstructed, portal venous pressure increases. Once the area of the shunt is located, the portal vein supplying this particular area should be isolated (Fig. 14-5). The veterinary surgeon should make every attempt to isolate by ligature only that portion of the portal vein that supplies the portosystemic shunt. One must take care to avoid portal vein branches not associated with the shunt. The hepatic

arterial and biliary ducts to all lobes of the liver, including the lobe or lobes in the shunt, should also be protected.

The elevated portal venous pressure seen following attenuation or ligation of portosystemic shunts (extrahepatic or intrahepatic) usually decreases to normal within several weeks.

Following recovery from operation and anesthesia, dramatic and immediate clinical improvement is usually observed. Antibiotics are administered for 2 weeks postoperatively. A second surgical procedure has not been performed on any patient in which attenuation only of the portosystemic shunt was performed because all survivors were clinically normal. Although most clinical abnormalities return to normal within weeks, the results of certain tests (ammonia tolerance) may continue to be abnormal for more than a year.[1]

Another method developed for closure or attenuation of intrahepatic portosystemic shunts does not compromise portal blood flow to liver lobe(s).[2] A median linea alba incision extends into a median sternotomy with the incision of three to four sternebrae. The diaphragm is incised down to and partially around the caudal vena cava at the vena cava hiatus. Umbilical tapes are passed around the thoracic caudal vena cava near the border of the pericardial sac, the abdominal caudal vena cava just caudal to the liver and cranial to the renal veins, and the portal vein just proximal to the first hepatic branch (Figs. 14-5 and 14-6). The umbilical

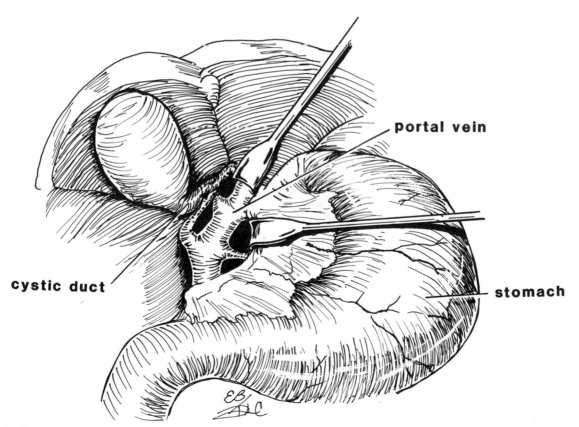

Fig. 14-4. *The hepaticoduodenal ligament is incised, and by careful sharp and blunt dissection, the ligament and enclosed structures, such as the cystic duct, common bile duct, and hepatic artery, are retracted off the portal vein.*

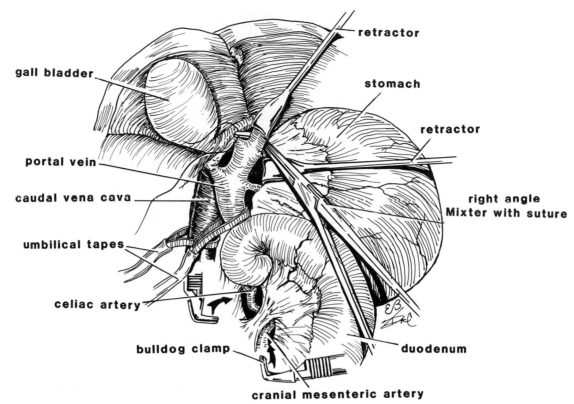

gall bladder

portal vein

caudal vena cava

umbilical tapes

celiac artery

bulldog clamp

cranial mesenteric artery

retractor

stomach

retractor

right angle
Mixter with suture

duodenum

Fig. 14-5. *Right-angle Mixter angular clamp forceps are used to carry a ligature around the segment of portal vein. Umbilical tapes within rubber tubing and bulldog clamps can be used to control hepatic blood flow.*

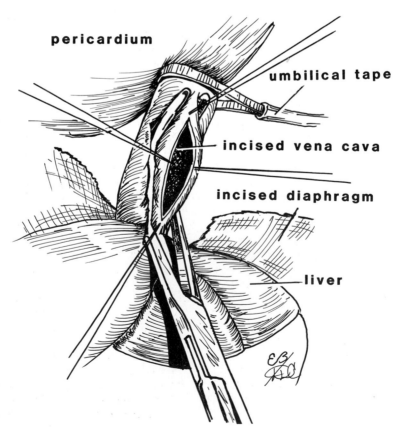

pericardium

umbilical tape

incised vena cava

incised diaphragm

liver

Fig. 14-6. *An umbilical tape is placed around the caudal vena cava at the level of the heart. A partial occluding clamp on, and traction sutures in, the vena cava permit incision of the vessel.*

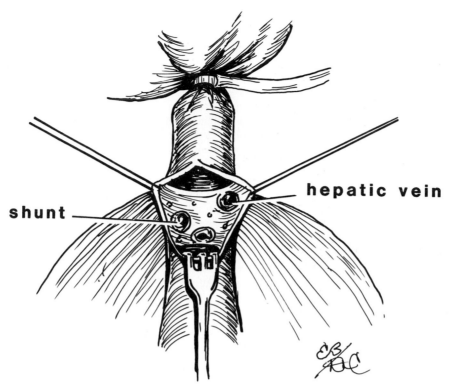

Fig. 14-7. *With the occlusion of afferent and efferent blood vessels, the partial occluding clamp on the vena cava is removed and the incision edges are retracted open to expose the hepatic veins and intrahepatic portosystemic shunt.*

tapes are passed through rubber tubing to obstruct blood flow when needed. The phrenicoabdominal veins, whether they drain into the portal vein or the caudal vena cava, should be identified, skeletonized, and ligated. The celiac artery and the cranial mesenteric artery should be isolated and prepared for obstruction with umbilical tape and rubber tubing or a bulldog clamp (see Fig. 14-5). I prefer a bulldog clamp for obstruction of the arterial supply to the splanchnic viscera.

Regional hypothermia of the splanchnic viscera with an ice slush of dextrose or saline solution may protect the abdominal organs during venous occlusion. Intravenous antibiotics should be instituted prior to interruption of the vascular blood supply to the liver. Traction sutures are placed in the vena cava at the most cranial and caudal portions of the anticipated longitudinal incision line. With slight elevation of the traction sutures, the vena cava is elevated, and a vascular partial-occluding clamp* is placed as close to the liver as possible. Between the confines of the partial-occluding clamp and the traction sutures, a longitudinal incision is made with a scalpel and Potts scissors.* Two additional traction sutures are placed at the edge of the incised vessel in the middle of the longitudinal incision (Fig. 14-6). Placement of the bulldog clamps to obstruct the celiac and cranial mesenteric arteries results in a

portal venous pressure near zero. The umbilical tapes are tightened, and the rubber tubing completely obstructs their encompassed vessel. The partial-occluding clamp is removed, and the remaining hepatic blood is aspirated.

The intravascular defect, although variable in location, is visible. Little confusion exists in distinguishing this intravascular defect from the normal hepatic veins (Fig. 14-7). The defect may be sutured closed with simple interrupted or cruciate stitches, or a Dacron patch may be sutured over the defect. Slight traction is placed on the sutures in the vena cava, and the partial-occluding clamp is placed to confine the limits of the vessel incision. The clamp should be placed loosely over the caudal vena cava to allow the escape of air from within the vascular channels of the liver and vena cava when the portal vein, the abdominal caudal vena cava umbilical tapes, and the celiac and cranial mesenteric bulldog clamps are released. The thoracic caudal vena cava tape is released last.

Although evidence suggests that hepatic vascular obstruction can be performed for periods of up to 20 minutes, during this procedure, splanchnic blood flow is interrupted for no longer than 5 to 10 minutes.[6] If additional time is needed for the complete correction, the partial-occluding clamp may be replaced on the caudal vena cava, and the vascular obstructing tapes and instruments may be released for 10 to 15 minutes. Once the animal's condition has stabilized, the splanchnic circulation may again be obstructed, and

*American V. Mueller, 6600 West Touhy Ave., Chicago, IL 60648

intracaval manipulations upon the shunt may be performed a second and third time if needed. With obstruction of the splanchnic circulation, systemic arterial pressure decreases to a mean of 30 mm Hg, whereas abdominal caudal cava pressure increases to a mean of 25 mm Hg.

Autoregulatory vascular dilation of the hypoxic splanchnic and distal peripheral circulations may require the administration of large volumes of fluid or an alpha-stimulating drug such as phenylephrine in order to elevate systemic arterial pressure following removal of the obstructing tapes and instruments. When the defect has been repaired, the caudal vena caval incision is closed with a simple continuous suture pattern, using one of the preplaced traction sutures placed in the vena cava. The diaphragm, median sternotomy, and median epigastric abdominal incisions are repaired in a routine manner. The portal vein catheter is treated as previously described. The animal is given postoperative antibiotics and is treated symptomatically if digestive dysfunction associated with splanchnic hypoxia (pancreatitis, bloody diarrhea) occurs.

MULTIPLE SHUNTS

Most multiple extrahepatic portocaval shunts do not respond to surgical treatment. All the patients with multiple extrahepatic portocaval shunts, in my experience, have had moderate elevations in portal venous pressure (15 to 18 cm water). Ligation of the multiple shunts until portal pressure approaches 20 to 22 cm water has not cured any patient.

Several experimental procedures have been attempted on dogs with multiple shunts. These procedures involved an end-to-end anastomosis from the splenic artery to the portal vein or periotonealization of a raw liver surface using a flat neurovascular pedicle graft of jejunum without mucosa. Both these techniques have failed to improve hepatic function or to alleviate signs of ammonia intoxication or hepatoencephalopathy.

References and Suggested Readings

1. Breznock, E. M.: Surgical manipulation of portosystemic shunts in dogs. J. Am. Vet. Med. Assoc., *174*:419, 1979.
2. Breznock, E. M., et al.: Surgery of intrahepatic portosystemic shunts (including patent ductus venosus in dogs). J. Am. Vet. Med. Assoc. In press.
3. Ewing, G. O., Sutur, P. F., and Bailey, C. S.: Hepatic insufficience associated with congenital anomalies of the portal vein in dogs. J. Am. Anim. Hosp. Assoc., *10*:463, 1974.
4. Khon, I. R., and Vitarus, A.: Portosystemic communications in the cat. Res. Vet. Sci., *12*:215, 1971.
5. Lohse, C. L., and Suter, P. F.: Functional closure of the ductus venosus during early postnatal life in the dog. Am. J. Vet. Res., *38*:839, 1977.
6. Raffucci, F. L.: The effects of temporary occlusion of the afferent hepatic circulation in dogs. Surgery, *33*:342, 1953.
7. Rubin, G. J., and Jones, B. D.: The liver. *In* Pathophysiology in Small Animal Surgery. Edited by M. J. Bojrab. Philadelphia, Lea & Febiger, 1981.

Surgery of Hepatic Parenchymal and Biliary Tissues

by EUGENE M. BREZNOCK

Detailed descriptions of the comparative gross and microscopic anatomy, embryology, and physiology of the liver can be found in standard textbooks of anatomy, embryology, and physiology. Only selected anatomic, embryologic, and physiologic information particularly pertinent to the problems encountered by the veterinary surgeon is included here.

Surgery of the liver, the largest glandular organ in the body, involves manipulations of parenchymal, biliary, and vascular tissue. Hepatic parenchymal damage is inevitable during surgical resection, incision, and biopsy. Major biliary and vascular structures to unaffected hepatic tissues must be preserved in order to avoid hepatic insufficiency.

Surgical Anatomy

Five liver lobes are described in the cat and six in the dog. The six lobes of the canine liver are arranged in three major divisions: the right division, caudate and right lateral lobes; the central division, right medial and quadrate lobes; and the left lateral division, left medial and left lateral lobes and papillary process of the caudate lobe. The liver has two afferent blood supplies through the portal vein and hepatic artery, and one efferent blood supply through the hepatic vein. In the dog, the portal vein and the hepatic veins are consistent in number, size, and location.[7] The proper canine hepatic arteries and their branches vary in number, size, distribution, and point of origin.[6,7] The portal vein and the hepatic arteries of the cat are also consistent and have three branches (right, middle, and left) distributed to the respective hepatic divisions.[1] Major differences in hepatic anatomic, physiologic, and pathophysiologic features among animal species and between animals and humans make it difficult for the veterinarian to extrapolate research data from one species when considering a surgical procedure on another. For example, differences among species in microbial and quiescent oxygen tensions in the portal vein and the capacity to form vascular or bile duct collateral vessels are important considerations.

Hepatic Pharmacophysiology: An Overview

Anesthetics should be administered cautiously to patients undergoing liver operations. Any drugs that may be hepatotoxic or that require hepatic conjugation prior to elimination should be avoided if possible. Many drugs have a profound effect on the physiologic and pathophysiologic features of the liver, and it is necessary to consider the benefits of certain pharmacologic interventions. For example, phenothiazine derivatives may be hepatotoxic in patients with compromised liver function. Morphine and morphine-like narcotics increase portal venous pressure in the dog and cat by constricting hepatic sphincters. In addition, morphine and tranquilizers have the added disadvantage of interfering with the elimination of bile.

Glucagon can hemodynamically enhance splanchnic blood flow by increasing portal venous circulation by 100%. When portal venous flow is reduced by hemorrhage, injection of glucagon restores splanchnic blood flow to nearly prehemorrhage values.[8] Glucagon causes glycogenolysis and increases hepatocyte oxygen needs, however. Thus, the hemodynamic benefit of intravenous glucagon may be desirable, but the glycogenolytic response is undesirable. Because the consumption of oxygen by hepatocytes is constant over a wide range of blood flow and oxygen delivery, glucagon does not improve hepatocyte function in the hypoxic liver. As long as this increased demand by hepatocytes for oxygen does not exceed the availability of oxygen in the afferent blood, hepatic function is not likely to be endangered by pharmacologic doses of glucagon. Should the amount of oxygen available to the liver be suddenly reduced, as it is by hypotension and hypovolemia in shock, glucagon may cause hepatic failure.

Sympathomimetic drugs have a direct and often profound effect on the hepatic sphincter of the dog and cat. The alpha-mimetic phenylephrine increases the hepatic sphincter tone and thereby increases portal venous pressure. Conversely, beta-stimulation with isoproterenol relaxes the hepatic sphincters and reduces portal venous pressure to 50% of normal. It is apparent that the veterinarian contemplating hepatic parenchymal, vascular, or biliary surgical procedures should select pharmacologic agents with discretion, to avoid misinterpretation of intraoperative physiologic data that may result in a fatal outcome.

Hepatic Parenchymal Surgical Procedures

Hepatic segmental anatomy of the dog and cat has been well defined; however, resection of a major liver lobe that is not pedunculated and is of normal or increased size (from neoplasia or abscessation) is difficult. Surgical exploration and manipulation of the liver is usually accomplished through a median epigastric incision extended cranially, by a median sternotomy, or caudally as far as necessary. The left or right divisions of the liver may be better exposed by turning and extending the epigastric incision paracostally to the appropriate side.

LIVER TRAUMA REPAIR

Hepatic parenchymal operations are often undertaken for repair of hepatic trauma with concomitant hemorrhage or resections of liver masses. Being protected by the ribs and the vertebrae, the liver is safe from direct trauma. Concussion from contact with its bony envelope following blunt impact, however, may result in contusion, avulsion, or laceration of liver lobe(s). Hemorrhage is the most immediate threat to life associated with trauma to the liver. Arterial hemorrhage, although less common, is more serious and is more difficult to control than venous hemorrhage. Avulsion of a hepatic lobe from the vena cava is usually fatal. Penetrating wounds from displaced fractured ribs or low-velocity firearm projectiles usually cause localized damage with varying hemorrhage. Following hemorrhage and hepatic trauma, bacterial toxemia (Clostridia) may become a life-threatening complication. The portal vein of the dog is septic, unlike in man and primates, and harbors both aerobic and anaerobic bacteria. Following trauma, anaerobic bacteria usually proliferate in portions of liver that become hypoxic.

Treatment of liver injuries depends upon the nature and the degree of the injury. Little or no surgical intervention is indicated for hepatic parenchymal trauma with no apparent active hemorrhage. Arterial hemorrhage should be controlled before venous hemorrhage. Small arterial hemorrhage in a lacerated or contused liver lobe may be controlled by ligation of vessels if the end of the vessel can be visualized. If disrupted small arterial branches deep within the hepatic tissue cannot be visualized, skeletonized, and ligated, selective dearterialization of an injured lobe usually controls the hemorrhage. The specific hepatic arteries supplying the affected lobe are identified and are doubly ligated with silk suture or a Hemoclip*. In the dog, as in man, translobar collateral vessels eventually rearterialize the lobe. Antibiotic therapy should be instituted intraoperatively and postoperatively to prevent hepatic necrosis and bacterial toxemia. I do not recommend overlapping deep sutures within the liver parenchyma for control of hemorrhage or for approximation of wound edges (Fig. 14-8). In most instances, placement of such hepatic parenchymal sutures requires a degree of tension sufficient to disrupt liver parenchyma. In addition, hepatic parenchymal sutures have been shown to lead to necrosis, sepsis, and abscess formation. Infrequently, bleeding into the bile radicals and into the digestive tract (hemobilia) also occurs.[4]

Following hepatic trauma, I do not use gauze packs, absorbable hemostats, peritoneal drains, choledochal tubes, or sutures (except vascular ligatures). Arterial and venous hemorrhage should be controlled, but deep wounds in hepatic parenchyma should remain open and unsutured to permit adequate drainage of sloughing hepatic parenchymal tissues.

LIVER LOBECTOMY

Neoplasia, focal abscessation, cysts, uncontrolled hepatic hemorrhage, arteriovenous fistulas, and other hepatic disorders may require partial or total amputation of a liver lobe. Partial hepatectomy in the larger patient (>10 kg) is usually performed by bluntly fracturing the hepatic parenchyma with the fingers, followed by ligation of interparenchymal vessels and

*Edward Week & Co., Inc., 49-33 31st Place, Long Island City, N.Y. 11101

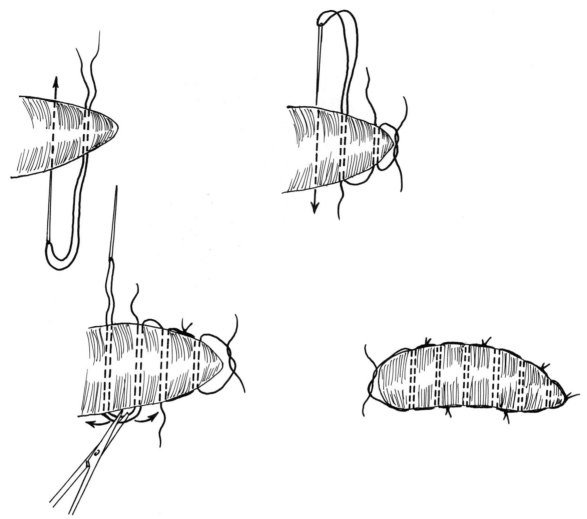

Fig. 14-8. *Technique for hepatic hemostasis during partial hepatectomy.*

ducts (Fig. 14-9). For the smaller patient, serrated tissue forceps may be used instead of the veterinary surgeon's fingers for interparenchymal dissection. The narrow forcep blades are closed and are placed carefully within the tissue; relaxation of the forceps allows its spring to open the liver parenchyma without trauma to blood vessels or biliary ducts (Fig. 14-10). Hepatic tissue is carefully removed from the ducts and vessels, which are then ligated and severed. I prefer Hemoclips for ligation of both vascular and biliary vessels. No attempt is made to cover the raw surface of the liver. If hemorrhage during partial hepatectomy is severe, it may be temporarily controlled (<5 to 8 minutes) by umbilical tape obstruction of the celiac and cranial mesenteric arteries and the portal vein.

Amputation of liver lobe(s) in the dog or cat may be performed quickly and with control of hemorrhage by careful and specific, isolation, skeletonization, and ligation of all afferent and efferent vessels and ducts (portal vein, hepatic artery, and bile ducts, respectively). First, umbilical tapes should be passed around afferent and efferent blood vessels of the liver: the caudal vena cava in front of and behind the liver, the portal vein

prior to its entry into the liver, and the celiac and cranial mesenteric arteries. The umbilical tapes are passed through rubber tubing and are used to occlude the hepatic blood supply should hemorrhage become uncontrollable. Pedunculated liver lobes of the dog and the cat are easy to remove in this manner; however, lobes intimately surrounding the vena cava require careful sharp and blunt dissection to identify, skeletonize, and ligate the hepatic vein(s) of the lobe to be removed. Mass ligation of the hepatic pedicle should be avoided.

LIVER BIOPSY

Biopsy of hepatic tissue may be safely performed through a laparotomy incision, by simple catgut ligation of a tapering edge of a liver lobe. The strangulating ligature is pulled tightly to fracture the small piece of hepatic parenchyma and to occlude vessels and bile ducts. The ligated portion of the lobe is amputated with scalpel or scissors 1 to 2 mm away from the ligature.

Because of the disadvantages of burying significant quantities of suture material deep within hepatic paren-

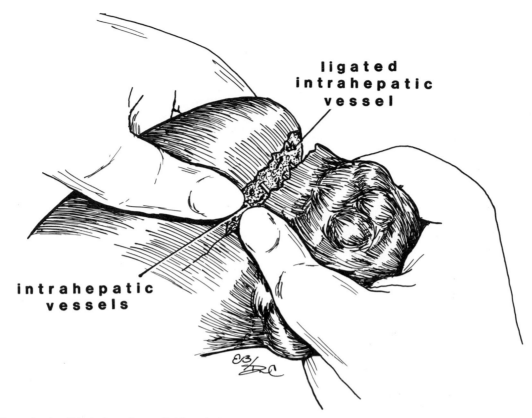

ligated
intrahepatic
vessel

intrahepatic
vessels

Fig. 14-9. *"Finger-fracture" technique for partial hepatectomy.*

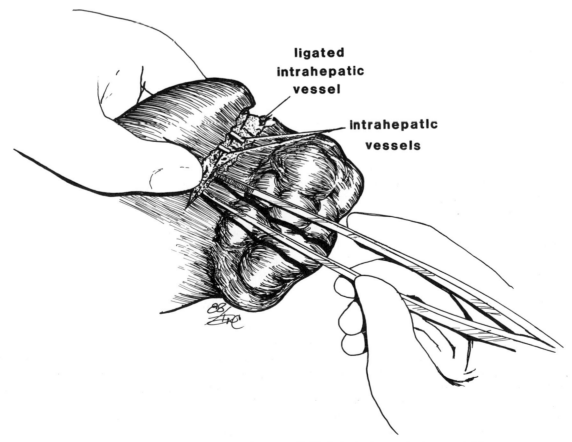

ligated
intrahepatic
vessel

intrahepatic
vessels

Fig. 14-10. *Fracture technique employing a serrated tissue forcep to divide hepatic tissues during partial hepatectomy.*

chyma, I do not perform hepatic wedge resections between two strangulating interlocking suture lines. A wedge resection is performed using a technique similar to that described for partial hepatectomy. No attempt is made to approximate the cut edges of the liver. No sutures need to be passed deep within parenchymal tissue.

Surgical Procedures of the Biliary System

The gallbladder of the dog and cat is consistent in its location, its attachment to the liver, and its conformation. It is connected to the extrahepatic bile duct (the common bile duct) by a single cystic duct. The common bile duct of the dog has three, or more commonly four, major proximal tributaries (Fig. 14-11). Usually, one major collection duct for the right hepatic division, one major collection duct for the left hepatic division, and two major collection ducts for the central hepatic division exist.[7] Within the framework of three or four divisional collection ducts, the basic pattern of bile drainage from the lobes of the liver varies little. In the dog, an auxiliary retroportal network of bile ducts is present. Tiny collateral channels connect the intrahepatic bile ducts of adjacent lobes and are capable of providing adequate drainage of bile when the primary pathways are obstructed.[7]

The major diseases of the biliary tract amenable to surgical treatment are usually divided into neoplastic, traumatic, and inflammatory conditions. Although primary diseases of the gallbladder do exist in the dog and cat, biliary dysfunction in animals is usually associated with other diseases.

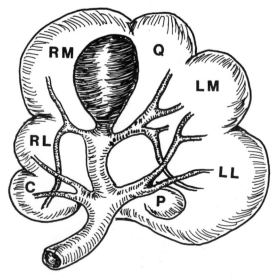

Fig. 14-11. *Schematic diagram of the usual bile duct distribution of the dog. Lobes of the liver are indicated as follows: C, caudate; RL, right lateral; RM, right medial; Q, quadrate; LM, left medial; LL, left lateral; P, papillary process of caudate.*

CHOLECYSTOTOMY

The principal indications for cholecystotomy are internal decompression of the biliary tract, gangrenous cholecystitis, drainage of inspissated bile from within the gallbladder, tube exploration of the extrahepatic biliary tree, biliary flukes (in cats), and cholelithiasis. Most of my patients that undergo cholecystotomy are operated on for tube exploration of the extrahepatic biliary tree. Cholelithiasis does occur in the dog and cat. The stone most commonly encountered is the pigmented stone composed of calcium bilirubinate. Inspissated bile, frequently observed in the geriatric or anoretic dog or cat, may require surgical exploration and drainage.

Stay sutures or noncrushing intestinal clamps are placed over the fundus of the gallbladder, and the cholecystotomy is performed. Inspissated or normal bile is removed, and tube exploration of the extrahepatic biliary tract is undertaken, employing appropriately sized soft latex or polyvinyl tubing (3½-French infant feeding tube for cats and small dogs). The collecting ducts or cystic duct may arise at an acute angle to the common bile duct, and catheter placement may be difficult in one or another duct. In this case, several milliliters of 11% patent blue violet dye may be injected through the catheter to determine patency and the anatomic location of the hepatic, cystic, and common bile ducts. If attenuation of the common bile duct is suspected as it courses within the duodenal wall or at its entry into the intestinal lumen, a 50% dextrose solution may be injected through the catheter to estimate resistance along the extrahepatic biliary tract. Elevated resistance to flow without visually apparent extrahepatic biliary tract disease is an indication for enterotomy and exploration of the common bile duct hillock within the duodenum (see the discussion following on choledochotomy and choledochostomy). The gallbladder is closed with interrupted 3-0 chromatic catgut sutures and a second layer of inverting Lembert or Connell sutures of 3-0 chromic catgut.

CHOLECYSTECTOMY

Tumors, trauma, cholecystitis, and gallstones are potential indications for excision of the gallbladder. A median epigastric incision extending to the xiphoid process is preferred in deep-chested dogs. An incision curved paracostally to the right side may aid in exposure. To palpate the structures in the hepaticoduodenal ligament, the veterinarian's left index and middle fingers are passed through the epiploic foramen into the left lesser omental cavity; with the aid of the left thumb, one may palpate the common bile duct, the portal vein, and the hepatic artery (portal triad) (Fig. 14-12). Closed intestinal artery forceps or traction sutures are applied to the fundus of the gallbladder, and traction is exerted upward. After attaining adequate exposure, the gallbladder may or may not be decompressed prior to the dissection. The advantages of the immediate decompression are: (1) the gallbladder is smaller

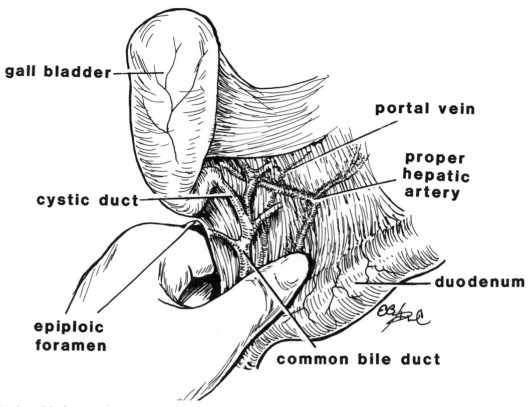

Fig. 14-12. *Palpation of the hepaticoduodenal ligament and intimate portal vein, common bile duct, and proper hepatic arteries. (Redrawn from Nora, P. F. (ed.): Operative Surgery. Philadelphia, Lea & Febiger, 1972.)*

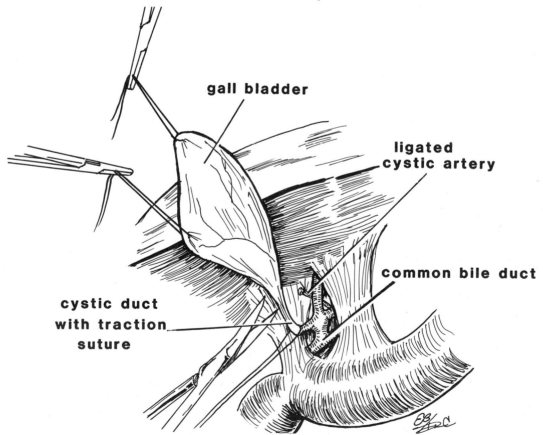

Figure 14-13. *Sharp and blunt dissection isolates the cystic duct with traction sutures; the cystic artery is doubly ligated and transected between ligatures. (Redrawn from Nora, P. F. (ed.): Operative Surgery. Philadelphia, Lea & Febiger, 1972.)*

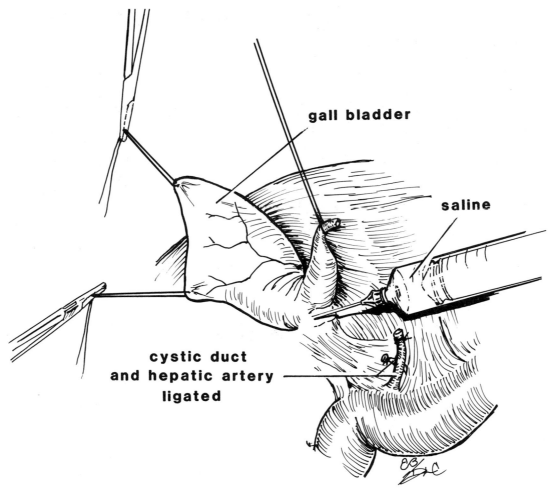

Fig. 14-14. *Saline solution injected subserosally where the gallbladder adheres to the liver aids dissection during cholecystectomy. (Redrawn from Nora, P. F. (ed.): Operative Surgery. Philadelphia, Lea & Febiger, 1972.)*

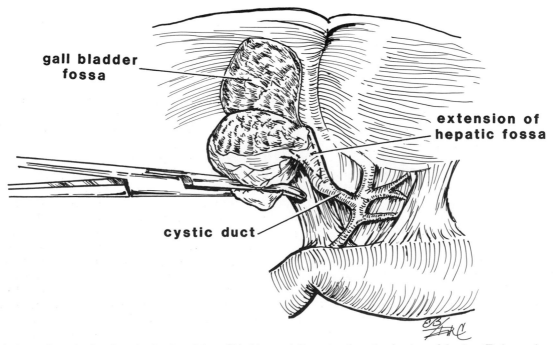

Fig. 14-15. *A tissue clamp is placed on the fundus of the gallbladder, and dissection from fundus to neck begins. (Redrawn from Nora, P. F. (ed.): Operative Surgery. Philadelphia, Lea & Febiger, 1972.)*

and occupies less of the surgical field, and (2) less danger exists of spillage of bile (resulting in biliary peritonitis) during operative dissection. The primary disadvantage to immediate removal of the bile is that the cleavage plane is less discernible between the liver and gallbladder fossa.

The gallbladder may be removed by identifying the cystic duct and cystic artery with the initial dissection and working toward the fundus (Figs. 14-13 and 14-14) or by starting the dissection at the fundus and moving toward the cystic duct (Fig. 14-15). I prefer the former method whenever visualization of important structures is obvious. The cystic artery is identified, is skeletonized, and is ligated near the gallbladder (see Fig. 14-13). The junction of the cystic and common bile duct is identified. At this time, the veterinary surgeon may wish to slip a catheter into the cystic duct near the junction of the common bile duct for tube exploration and patency confirmation of the entire extrahepatic biliary system. Following tube exploration of the extrahepatic biliary tree, the cystic duct is clamped with forceps, is ligated, and is transected between transfixed ligatures (see Fig. 14-14). By sharp and blunt dissection the peritoneal attachments of the gallbladder to the liver are divided. In carrying out this phase of the operation, the veterinary surgeon must proceed cautiously while observing anatomic relationships for arterial and ductal anomalies. If any accessory vessels or ducts are encountered between the gallbladder and the liver, they should be individually ligated. To allow better development of the surgical plane, saline solution may be injected subserosally where the gallbladder and liver adhere (see Fig. 14-14); such a maneuver may leave serosa attached to the liver and may thus prevent a raw liver surface. The serosal edges of the gallbladder bed are left open.

In the dog, extrahepatic biliary ducts dilate after cholecystectomy.[3] The intramural portion of the common bile duct is surrounded by a double layer of smooth muscle, and the discharge of bile depends to a large extent on the activity of the duodenum. After cholecystectomy, the intraductal tension increases until it overcomes the powerful sphincter mechanism at the intramural portion of the common bile duct.

CHOLEDOCHOTOMY AND CHOLEDOCHOSTOMY

Tube exploration of the entire extrahepatic biliary system is considered in the foregoing discussion. Open exploration of the common bile duct in companion animals is infrequently performed because of the small size of the common bile duct and the high risk of developing strictures. If the common bile duct is dilated, however, exploration can be readily performed. I prefer tube exploration through a cholecystotomy. If tube exploration of the extrahepatic biliary tree indicates an abnormal resistance, the cause of which cannot be visualized, a duodenotomy is performed (Fig. 14-16), and the common bile duct hillock is explored. Noncrushing intestinal clamps may be applied to the proximal and distal duodenum to minimize intestinal spillage.

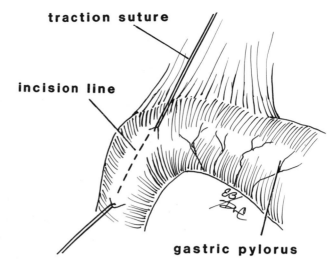

Fig. 14-16. *Duodenotomy site is just distal to the pylorus of the stomach. (Redrawn from Nora, P. F. (ed.): Operative Surgery. Philadelphia, Lea & Febiger, 1972.)*

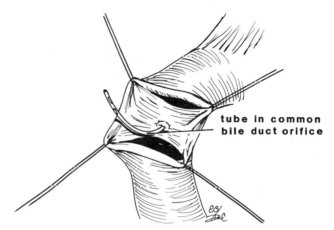

Fig. 14-17. *The duodenal incision is opened with four traction sutures. A choledochal tube passed into the duodenum identifies the common duct orifice.*

Passage of the choledochal tube into the duodenum aids in the identification of the common bile duct hillock (Figs. 14-17 and 14-18). Choledochotomy is usually only performed on patients with a dilated bile duct (>5 mm in diameter). If adhesions prevent the identification of the common bile duct, a sterile syringe and a 25-gauge needle may be used to aspirate the structure in question (Fig. 14-19), but if bile is inspissated, aspiration through a 25-gauge needle may be difficult. Following identification and isolation of the common duct, two traction sutures are placed in the common duct prior to its incision (Figs. 14-20 and 14-21). Proximal and distal tube explorations of the common duct, collecting ducts, and cystic duct are performed.

Following choledochotomy, a choledochal tube (T-tube) may be placed within the incision of the common duct to act as a stent to support the sutured incision. (See the discussion following on reconstruction of the biliary tract.) If decompression is required or is determined to be advantageous at the time of the operation, a temporary cholecystostomy tube is placed and is

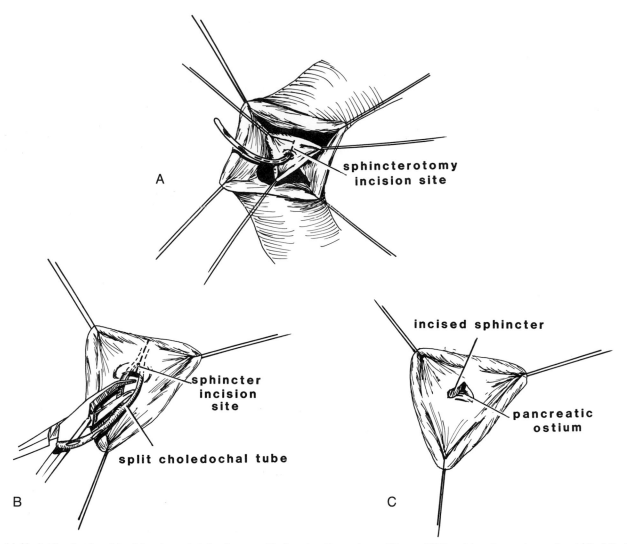

Fig. 14-18. A, *The duodenal incision is maintained open with four traction sutures. Three additional traction sutures elevate the bile duct hillock containing a choledochal tube in the bile duct orifice. Dashed lines on hillock and tube indicate incision lines. B, The choledochal tube is split and retracted into the common bile duct. A mosquito forcep spreads the split tube in and out of the common duct. Sphincterotomy can be easily performed along the split tube (dashed line). C, Sphincterotomy is complete. The ventral pancreatic duct may be present within the common bile duct hillock.*

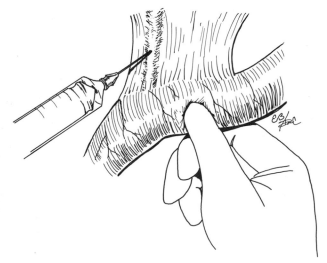

Fig. 14-19. *Syringe aspiration will identify the common bile duct if fibrosis of the hepaticoduodenal ligament prevents easy identification. (Redrawn from Nora, P. F. (ed).: Operative Surgery. Philadelphia, Lea & Febiger, 1972.)*

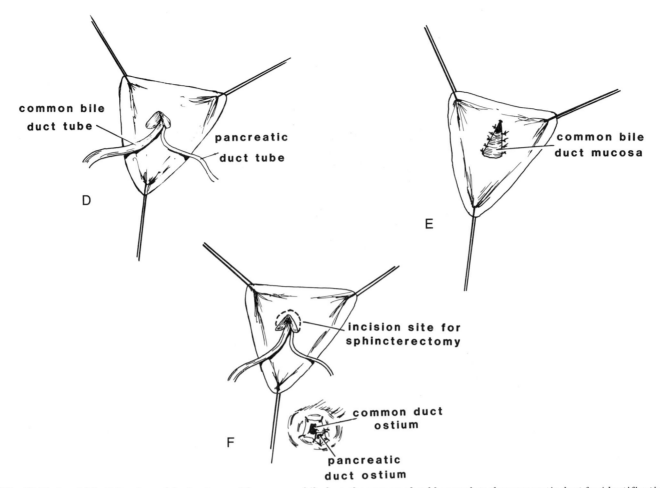

common bile duct tube

pancreatic duct tube

D

common bile duct mucosa

E

incision site for sphincterectomy

common duct ostium

pancreatic duct ostium

F

Fig. 14-18. *(cont.)* D, *Following sphincterotomy of the common bile duct, the surgeon should cannulate the pancreatic duct for identification during other manipulative techniques. E, Sphincteroplasty completed with simple interrupted fine catgut sutures. (Redrawn from Nora, P. F. (ed.): Operative Surgery. Philadelphia, Lea & Febiger, 1972.) F, Sphincterectomy (dashed line) following sphincterotomy can be performed after identification of the pancreatic ostium in the common bile duct hillock. Two ostia (common and pancreatic ducts) may need to be constructed after excision of the bile duct sphincter.*

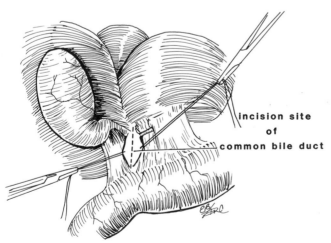

incision site of common bile duct

Fig. 14-20. *The common bile duct is isolated below the cystic duct. Two traction sutures stabilize the common duct prior to incision (dashed line). (Redrawn from Nora, P. F. (ed.): Operative Surgery. Philadelphia, Lea & Febiger, 1972.)*

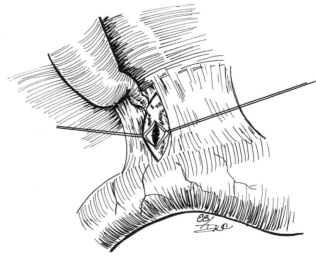

Fig. 14-21. *The common bile duct is incised for intraluminal exploration. (Redrawn from Nora, P. F. (ed.): Operative Surgery. Philadelphia, Lea & Febiger, 1972.)*

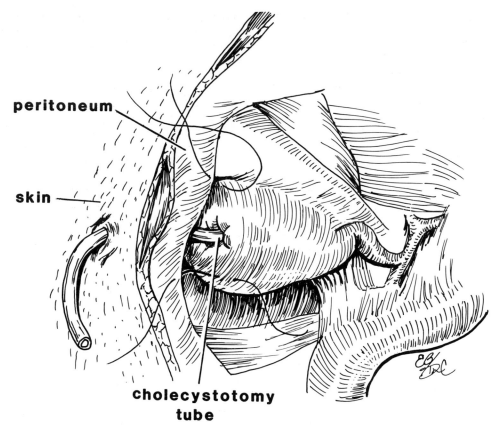

peritoneum

skin

cholecystotomy tube

Fig. 14-22. *A cholecystostomy tube is maintained in the gallbladder with a pursestring suture. Two (of five or six) chromic catgut sutures are placed through the serosa of the gallbladder and peritoneum at the place of exit through the skin.*

brought to the exterior through a small abdominal incision (Fig. 14-22). If choledochotomy or tube exploration of the extrahepatic common bile duct determines that an obstruction exists at the common duct sphincter or as the common duct courses intramurally within the duodenum, an enterotomy incision is made through the antimesenteric wall of the duodenum. Traction sutures are used to retract the severed edges of the duodenal wall and mucosa (see Figs. 14-17 and 14-18). Probe or tube exploration of the common bile duct ostium is performed if visual inspection of the opening reveals obvious intrinsic disease causing stricture. Depending on the nature of the disease, sphincterotomy, sphincterectomy, or sphincteroplasty may be required to alleviate the obstruction. The longitudinal duodenotomy is closed in a transverse fashion.

BILIARY-INTESTINAL ANASTOMOSIS

If fibrosis is the determined cause of the obstruction, an easier technique, especially in small patients, and one that I prefer is a bypass procedure such as a cholecystogastrointestinal anastomosis or a choledochointestinal anastomosis. Treatment of tumors in this area depends on the extent, location, infiltration, and kind of tumor. A biopsy is usually in order to determine whether a simple excision, a bypass procedure, or a radical pancreaticoduodenectomy is to be performed.

Sphincterotomy can be safely performed if a tube or groove director is passed through the gallbladder into the intraluminal common duct and the incision is made through the sphincter onto the preplaced guide (see Figs. 14-18A, B, and C). Sphincteroplasty requires the excision of a wall of duodenum and intramural common bile duct; the edges of the incised tissue are sutured in a simple interrupted suture pattern with 4-0 or 5-0 chromic catgut (see Figs. 14-18A, D, and E). The common bile duct of large dogs runs intramurally a distance of 1.5 to 3 cm prior to entering the duodenum; excision of intestinal and bile duct wall can therefore be performed with minimal risk of dehiscence and bile leakage. In small patients, size precludes sphincterotomy or sphincteroplasty and requires a bypass procedure.

During a sphincterotomy, a sphincterectomy, or a sphincteroplasty, great care must be taken to avoid the left pancreatic duct. This pancreatic duct empties into the duodenal hillock with the common bile duct in approximately 50% of dogs and cats. To perform a sphincterotomy, a sphincteroplasty, or a sphincterectomy, tube exploration and identification of the pancreatic duct should be done (see Figs. 14-18C, D, and F). Although the left and right pancreatic ducts do intercommunicate in the majority of dogs, the veterinary surgeon cannot assume that iatrogenic surgical obstruction of the left pancreatic duct will result in normal pancreatic function.

BYPASS PROCEDURES FOR BILIARY TRACT DISEASE

Malignant or benign obstructions of the biliary tract, trauma, the patient's size, and other conditions may necessitate biliary bypass procedures. Bile stasis, fibrosis of the common bile duct sphincter, erosion of the common bile duct with peritonitis and fibrosis of surrounding tissues, tumors involving the common bile duct, or traumatic injuries may require some type of biliary bypass. Biliary-to-intestinal diversion procedures include cholecystogastrostomy, cholecystoduodenostomy, cholecystojejunostomy, choledochoduodenostomy, and choledochojejunostomy. Although anastomoses involving the gallbladder are less complicated procedures than those involving the common duct, if the common duct is notably dilated, the difference is minimal. Using the gallbladder rather than the common bile duct for an anastomosis may result in associated inflammation or in kinking of the cystic duct and inadequate flow of bile.

The technique is similar for all three types of gallbladder-gastrointestinal anastomoses. The fundus of the gallbladder is grasped with noncrushing intestinal clamps or is retained by traction sutures. If mobility of the gallbladder is minimal, the fundus can be dissected and partially freed as described for cholecystectomy. The serosa of the intestinal tract (jejunum or duodenum) is approximated to the serosa of the gallbladder by a row of interrupted 3-0 or 4-0 polypropylene or silk sutures (Fig. 14-23). Noncrushing intestinal clamps should be applied to the proximal and distal jejunum (not needed for duodenum or stomach) to minimize

intestinal spillage. An incision is made in both the gallbladder and the intestine close to the previously placed serosal suture line. The gallbladder-to-intestine anastomosis is approximated by continuous Connell sutures of 4-0 chromic catgut. The remaining serosal layers are further approximated with interrupted sutures of 4-0 silk or polypropylene. To prevent intestinal reflux into the biliary tree, a jejunojejunostomy may be placed distally after the biliary-jejunal anastomosis. Occlusion of the afferent limb of jejunum may be accomplished with inverting mattress sutures (Fig. 14-23).

Choledochoenterostomy can be performed if the common bile duct is large enough to permit such an anastomosis (commonly observed after chronic bile duct obstruction) (Fig. 14-24). An oblique or longitudinal incision is made in the common duct for purposes of exploration and anastomosis (Fig. 14-25). Assuming that the bypass procedure is for a benign condition with a dilated common bile duct, the adjacent intestinal serosa and common bile duct serosa are approximated by interrupted 4-0 sutures. A parallel incision is made in the intestine adjacent to the common duct incision (Fig. 14-25). The mucosa of the common bile duct and intestine are approximated with 4-0 continuous chromic catgut suture started on the back half of the midline and continued toward the veterinary surgeon. The near aspect of the mucosal anastomosis is reinforced with 4-0 interrupted sutures by a Cushing stitch through the serosa (Fig. 14-26).

RECONSTRUCTION OF THE BILIARY TRACT

The biliary tree may be injured by trauma or by iatrogenic surgical errors. Small peripheral hepatic ducts may be ligated without consequence because of interlobular communications of the biliary tree. The identification of lacerations or transections of major bile

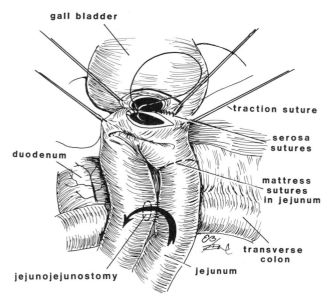

Fig. 14-23. *A serosal suture line joins the gallbladder to the jejunum. The mucosa of the gallbladder and the jejunum are united with a simple continuous suture line. Traction sutures maintain apposition of the organs during colecystoduodenostomy. Mattress sutures across the ascending limb of the jejunum together with a jejunojejunostomy prevent reflex of intestinal content into the biliary system. (Redrawn from Nora, P. F. (ed.): Operative Surgery. Philadelphia, Lea & Febiger, 1972.)*

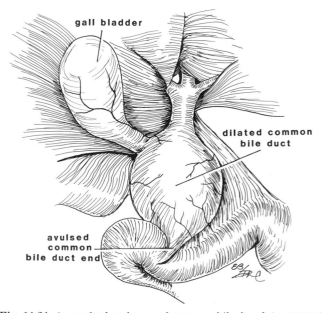

Fig. 14-24. *An avulsed and scarred common bile duct has occurred in a common bile duct and collecting ducts.*

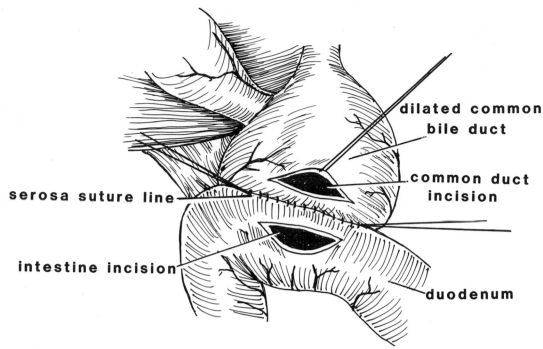

Fig. 14-25. *The dilated common bile duct is united by a simple interrupted serosal suture line to the intestine, and a gallbladder incision and enterotomy are made close to the serosal suture line. (Redrawn from Nora, P. F. (ed.): Operative Surgery. Philadelphia, Lea & Febiger, 1972.)*

duct(s) may be difficult, especially in cases of bile peritonitis. An attempt should be made to salvage large ducts of the distal biliary tree, however. Cholecystotomy tube exploration and dye infusions aid in identifying ductal trauma and leakage in all divisions of the bile excretory system. If the cystic duct is not open, or if extensive obliteration of the common bile duct has

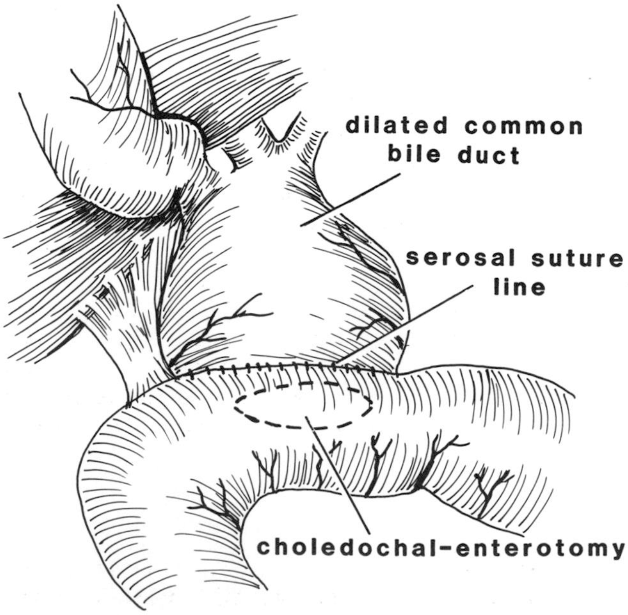

Fig. 14-26. *The choledochoenterostomy is completed when the initial serosal suture line is extended completely around the enterotomy suture line. (Redrawn from Nora, P. F. (ed.): Operative Surgery. Philadelphia, Lea & Febiger, 1972.)*

taken place, conversion must be made to a transduodenal entry into the common bile duct to see whether it is salvageable.

After identification of trauma, leakage, stricture, or fibrosis, serial sectioning of the junction of normal and pathologic tissue is used to isolate viable and patent duct tissue. This step is essential for the anastomosis to succeed. The length of bile duct is usually not important because the distal common duct or duodoneum may be moved to the hiatus of the liver to accept the anastomosis and may be anchored to the stomach. The effects on the reconstructive outcome of suture type, of the manner in which the suture is placed, and of the number of layers used is equivocal at this time. The surgical goal, however, should always be a technically accurate mucosal repair using fine, well-spaced sutures with absolutely no tension on the suture line.

The effect of choledochal tubes (T-tubes) as supportive stents within the anastomosis is controversial. Although clinical data indicate less scar contraction with long-term as opposed to short-term placement of supportive stents, laboratory studies indicate that such stents act as a stimulus for fibrosis and delay healing.[2,5] Appropriately sized stents decompress the anastomosis, and their use remains a matter of judgment. If bile is drained externally during convalescence, bile salt replacement tablets will be necessary.

Maturation of any scar follows an exponential curve and is most pronounced during the first phase of healing.[5] A duct that is anastomosed with a larger diameter shows less chance for recurrent stricture. Thus, certain plastic procedures may be employed to increase the diameter of the proximal duct before anastomosis (Fig.

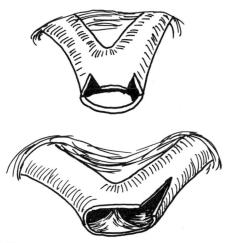

Fig. 14-27. *Plastic procedures for increasing the diameter of vessels or ducts prior to anastomosis. (Redrawn from Braasch, J. W. In Operative Surgery. Edited by P. F. Nora. Philadelphia, Lea & Febiger, 1972.)*

14-27). Following long-term (weeks) bile duct obstruction, the proximal duct usually has a large diameter, and the anastomosis is less likely to close by scar contraction.

Although the lumen size of the postoperative biliary duct affects bile transit, it is recognized that bile flow may be retarded in a visually patent bile duct. Fibroblastic proliferation surrounding the anastomosis may render a segment of the bile duct rigid and may thus impair the transit of bile to the intestine.

Lacerations located in the common duct proximal to the cystic duct may be anastomosed to the gallbladder more easily than to a smaller portion of the duct itself. If the common duct is available for anastomosis only above the cystic duct, the situation becomes difficult. The best option is probably a choledochojejunostomy into a 12-inch Roux loop of jejunum. Because reflux is not harmful, a simple loop of jejunum, with or without an enteroenterostomy at its base, is satisfactory for the biliary drainage in the course of biliary tract reconstruction (see Fig. 14-23).

Finally, the use of autologous tissues such as vein or small bowel allografts for reconstruction of the biliary tract has no real clinical application. The use of autologous tissues requires one suture line to be replaced by two suture lines. Such a maneuver increases the risk of failure from fibroblastic contraction or dehiscence and bile leakage.

Although alternatives are available to the veterinary surgeon for reconstruction of a diseased biliary tract in companion animals, the size of the patient often precludes the use of certain techniques.

References and Suggested Readings

1. Crouch, J. E.: Text-Atlas of Cat Anatomy. Philadelphia, Lea & Febiger, 1969.
2. Madden, J. L., and McCann, W. J.: Reconstruction of the common bile duct by end-to-end anastomosis without the use of an internal splint or stent support. Surg. Gynecol. Obstet., *112*:305, 1961.
3. Mahour, G. H., Wakin, K. G., Soule, E. H., and Ferris, D. O.: Effect of cholecystectomy on the biliary ducts in the dog. Arch. Surg., *97*:570, 1968.
4. Mays, E. T.: The hazards of suturing certain wounds of the liver. Surg. Gynecol. Obstet., *143*:201, 1976.
5. Peacock, E. E., and Van Winkle, W. V.: Wound Repair. 2nd Ed. Philadelphia, W. B. Saunders, 1976.
6. Schmidt, S., Lohse, C. L., and Suter, P. F.: Branching patterns of the hepatic artery in the dog: arteriographic and anatomic study. Am. J. Vet. Res., *31*:1090, 1980.
7. Sleight, D. R., and Thonford, N. R.: Gross anatomy of the blood supply and biliary drainage of the canine liver. Anat. Rec., *166*:153, 1970.
8. Witte, C., Witte, M. H., and Kintner, K.: Effects of glucagon on hepatic lymph (tissue) PO$_2$ after ligation of the hepatic artery: an experimental study. J. Trauma, *18*:27, 1978.

Closed Biopsy Techniques of the Liver

by Edward C. Feldman *and*

David F. Edwards

A complete medical history and physical examination, in conjunction with appropriate laboratory data and radiographs, often provide the veterinarian with enough information to conclude that a patient has a disease involving the liver. It is the morphologic examination of hepatic tissue, however, that may confirm a clinical diagnosis or may change a clinical impression.[16] In dogs or cats, the diagnosis of a specific type of liver dysfunction can seldom be made without histologic examination of tissue. Without such evaluation, the treatment of liver disease becomes supportive and nonspecific, whereas when a precise diagnosis is made, specific therapeutic measures or a prognosis (or both) may be given.

In our experience, the blind percutaneous biopsy is a safe, reliable, inexpensive, simple, and valuable tool. The specific advantages to the veterinarian are that the procedure takes little time (minutes), requires inexpensive instruments, and is simple to learn. The advantages to the patient with potential liver disease are that it is nonstressful and does not require anesthesia, which may further compromise a diseased liver. In our opinion, if a patient is anesthetized for this procedure, a major advantage has been by-passed, and an exploratory celiotomy may as well be performed. The advantage to the client is that the procedure is less expensive than surgery and thereby enables more clients to afford better care for their pets.

Indications

The indications for blind percutaneous liver biopsy can be broadly stated as any situation in which histologic evaluation of the liver may establish a diagnosis, determine the type of therapy, or indicate a prognosis, provided the risks are acceptable in light of the alternatives.[9] More specific indications [5,7,11,12] include the following: (1) differential diagnosis of hepatomegaly; (2)

differential diagnosis of decreased size of the liver; (3) clarification of abnormal liver function test (BSP) results; (4) clarification of abnormal liver enzyme test results; (5) differential diagnosis of jaundice; (6) differential diagnosis of fever of unknown origin; (7) differential diagnosis of suspected neoplasia or granulomatous disease; (8) assessment of the degree of continued hepatic disease, such as fibrosis or hepatitis; (9) evaluation of the success or failure of treatment measures; and (10) clinical research.

Contraindications

Complications are inevitable with any procedure, but these can be minimized during blind percutaneous liver biopsy if proper technique is combined with appropriate case selection for biopsy. Conditions that represent a contraindication to blind percutaneous liver biopsy[3,5,7,12] include the following: (1) the uncooperative patient; (2) anemia; (3) peritonitis; (4) high-grade extrahepatic jaundice; (5) bleeding disorders; (6) suspected vascular tumor, cyst, or abscess; (7) pleural effusion (transthoracic approach); (8) right-sided pneumonia (transthoracic approach); (9) ascites (transthoracic approach); and (10) microhepatia (transabdominal approach).

Many contraindications are relative in that they can be avoided. The uncooperative patient can be sedated. In our experience, most cats require sedation, whereas, most dogs do well with only local anesthesia. The anemic patient can be transfused prior to the biopsy procedure. The presence of pleural effusion, right-sided pneumonia, or ascites precludes the use of a transthoracic biopsy approach because perforation of the diaphragm allows transfer of fluid or infection from one body cavity to another. By the same token, one must be careful not to perforate the diaphragm while using the transabdominal approach when these disorders are present. The existence of peritonitis is an absolute contraindication to percutaneous liver biopsy by any route because thoracic or intrahepatic dissemination of infection is a likely sequela. The small liver is generally well recessed within the thoracic cavity and is therefore better suited to biopsy by the transthoracic approach.

The procedures described here are modifications of the method first outlined by Menghini[8] and can be performed by two approaches, transthoracic or transabdominal. The use of one approach over the other may be dictated by the presence of complicating factors, but generally, the veterinarian should use that approach with which he is most familiar and proficient. Both techniques are described and, in our experience, are equally effective; however, the transthoracic approach to liver biopsy is technically easier to master.

The Menghini needles* used to obtain the biopsy specimens are 16-, 17-, and 18-gauge thin-walled needles, 2⅔ and 4¾ inches long (Fig. 14-28).

*Model Nos. 1483, 1484, and 1485, Becton Dickinson and Co., Rutherford, NJ

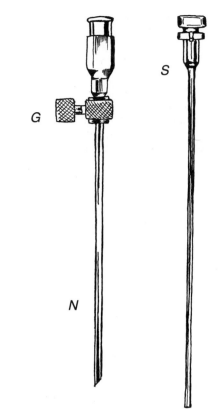

Fig. 14-28. *The Menghini biopsy needle (N), with guard (G) in place, and blunt-ended stylet (S).*

A brief review of the functional anatomy of the thorax and liver is given to clarify the concepts presented in the description of the transthoracic and transabdominal approaches to liver biopsy.

Functional Anatomy of the Thorax and Liver

Knowledge of the location of the diaphragm, with respect to the lateral wall of the thorax, is important when planning transthoracic percutaneous biopsy of the liver. By dissection through the rib cage, the major portion of the diaphragm extends dorsally from the thirteenth rib forward to the sixth intercostal space. Laterally, the diaphragm is attached to the lower (horizontal) part of the ninth cartilage, to the tenth and eleventh cartilages a little below the junction with the rib, to the twelfth rib at its ventral end, and to the last rib, below its middle.[6] From this origin, the diaphragm extends almost directly cranially, forming a slit-like space or recess within the thorax. This recess is formed by the diaphragm centrally and the ribs and intercostal structures peripherally. Because the recess is never totally filled by the lungs, even on forced inspiration, this region is safer for the transthoracic approach (Figs. 14-30 and 14-31). The distance an object must travel from the sixth or seventh intercostal space at the costochondral junction to the diaphragm, when the thorax has been entered, is usually less than two rib spaces.

The lungs are in contact with the lateral wall of the thorax. A blunt object gently thrust into the pleural space displaces the lung, rather than penetrates it. This displacement must be assumed, inasmuch as the transthoracic liver biopsy technique, in our experience, rarely results in the recovery of pulmonary tissue, although the needle always passes through the thorax.

The heart extends from approximately the third rib to the eighth rib.[6] The cardiac border only presents a hazard during the biopsy procedure when severe cardiomegaly or cardiac displacement is present. Lateral recumbency also causes the heart to fall away from the site of biopsy.

The liver is the largest gland in the body and lies almost entirely within the thoracic portion of the abdomen. The diaphragmatic surface of the liver is extremely convex. Most of this parietal surface of the liver faces laterally and dorsally; much less liver tissue faces cranially or ventrally.

In the dog and cat, the left lateral liver lobe is the largest lobe, but more actual liver tissue lies to the right of the midline. The greatest diaphragmatic contact is associated with the surface of the right lobes; the right side is thus better suited to transthoracic percutaneous biopsy.[7] The fundus of the stomach forms a large depression in the left lateral lobe of the liver. The proximity of the stomach and diaphragm on the left side (the liver is relatively thin) is the major drawback to the use of the left side for transthoracic percutaneous biopsy.

The gallbladder lies in a deep depression on the visceral surface of the liver, at the level of the eighth and tenth intercostal spaces, and is usually in contact with the pylorus of the stomach. The body of the gallbladder is on the level of the costal arch and lies to the right of the midline. Because bile is irritating to the peritoneum, the gallbladder must be avoided during any biopsy procedure.

Preoperative Preparation

The patient should be fasted for 12 hours prior to the procedure. A mixture of vegetable oil* and syrup† (or a commercial product‡) is administered orally 30 to 60 minutes prior to the procedure to stimulate contraction of the gallbladder.[9] A 50:50 mixture is used at a dose of 2.2 ml/kg of body weight in small dogs and cats, and less total volume is administered to larger dogs.

Whole blood clotting time is determined by drawing approximately 1.5 to 2 ml of blood into a clean, siliconized tube and by tilting the tube back and forth until a solid clot forms. The time from venipuncture to clot formation is the whole blood clotting time;[4] clotting

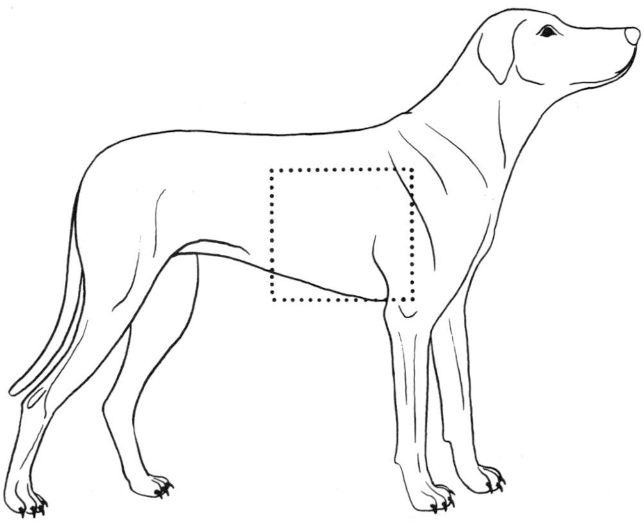

Fig. 14-29. *The dotted line indicates the area typically shaved prior to performing the transthoracic percutaneous liver biopsy.*

should occur within 12 minutes. A more accurate assessment of clotting time may be obtained by use of an activated clotting tube. The reader is referred to another source for details on this procedure.[1] Because the liver produces most clotting factors, clotting dysfunction must be ruled out before a liver biopsy is performed. A platelet count is also obtained from each patient. Any abnormality in whole blood clotting time, activated clotting time, or platelet count should preclude the biopsy procedure until the nature of the clotting disorder is corrected.

For transthoracic liver biopsy, the patient's right thoracic wall is clipped and prepared for an aseptic surgical approach. The clip extends caudally from the scapula to slightly beyond the tip of the xyphoid process. It extends from the upper third of the ribs dorsally on the right to the ventral midline (Fig. 14-29). For transabdominal liver biopsy, the cranial aspect of the patient's left ventrolateral abdominal wall is prepared in a similar manner. The area should encompass the "V" outlined laterally and cranially by the left costal arch and medially by the xyphoid process.

If sedation is necessary in the dog, a mild tranquilizer (a preanesthetic dose of acetylpromazine§) may be given 30 to 60 minutes prior to the biopsy. The small liver of the cat is more suited to biopsy by the transthoracic approach, and owing to the nature of the animal, sedation is generally required. Cats should be premedicated with atropine‖ (0.05 mg/kg) subcutaneously 30 minutes before the biopsy procedure. Immediately prior to the biopsy procedure, the cat should be given a light dose of ketamine hydrochloride# (2 mg/kg) intravenously.

---

*Mazola Oil, Best Foods, Englewood Cliffs, NJ
†Karo Syrup, Best Foods, Englewood Cliffs, NJ
‡Dyne, Biolab Corp., Norborne, MO

§ Acetylpromazine, Ayerst Laboratories, 685 Third Avenue, New York, NY 10017
‖ Atropine sulfate, Butler Co., Columbus, OH
#Vetalar, Parke-Davis, 201 Tabor Road, Morris Plains, NJ 07950

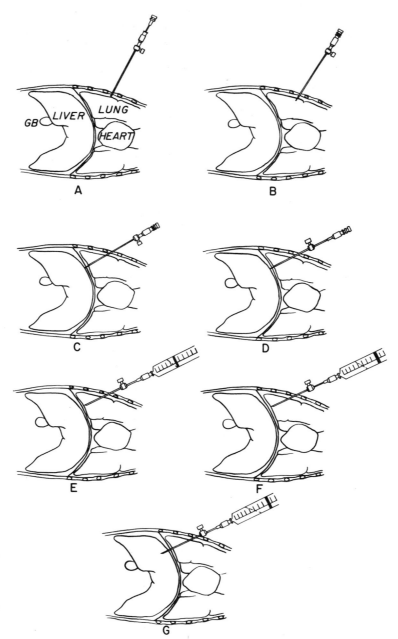

Fig. 14-30. *Sequential representation of biopsy technique. A, As the Menghini needle is passed into the pleural space, the stylet is not completely within the needle hub. The guard is near the hub at this time. GB, gallbladder. B, Immediately after penetration, the stylet is advanced into the hub of the needle, allowing the blunt edge of the stylet to protrude beyond the cutting edge of the needle. C, With the stylet in the lead, the needle is passed caudally until it rests against the diaphragm. D, The guard is adjusted so that it lies approximately half an inch (13 mm) from the skin. E, The stylet is removed and the syringe is securely fastened to the needle hub. F, Holding the end of the syringe in one hand, negative pressure is produced by partially withdrawing the plunger. G, In one even motion, the needle is passed caudally into the liver, using the guard to determine the appropriate depth. This thrust is followed by quick withdrawal of the biopsy apparatus from the body. The biopsy specimen is thereby sucked through the needle and into the fluid-filled syringe.*

Surgical Techniques

TRANSTHORACIC BIOPSY APPROACH

The site for biopsy is determined by evaluating two radiographic views of the thorax and abdomen. Usually, the needle is passed through the fifth, sixth, or seventh intercostal space, slightly dorsal to the costochondral junction. Individual variation in liver size and shape, or configuration of the thorax and its contents, may alter the site of the biopsy.

The dog or cat is positioned in *left* lateral recumbency. The limbs are held in extension, with the forelimbs stretched slightly cranially. For the safety of the handler, dogs should be muzzled. The skin incision site is infiltrated with 1 to 2 ml of 2% lidocaine hydrochloride‡ from the skin to the parietal pleura. When the local

‡ Lid-o-cain, Butler Co., Columbus, OH

anesthetic has been administered, the area is covered with a 1- to 2-inch fenestrated surgical drape.

The biopsy procedure may be divided into two phases: the extrahepatic phase, when the veterinarian may want to ascertain the needle's location, the patient's welfare, and the diaphragm excursion; and the second phase, involving the intrahepatic thrust and withdrawal of the biopsy apparatus. The intrahepatic phase of the biopsy procedure should be a *split-second maneuver*. The risk to the patient is directly related to the length of time the biopsy apparatus remains within the liver.[8]

To prevent dulling of the biopsy needle, a skin incision is made at the desired location, using a No. 11 Beaver blade. The skin incision should be just large enough to accommodate the Menghini needle. The Menghini needle should be clean and sterile. The guard should be on the needle and as close to the hub as possible. A 12-ml syringe containing 5 or 6 ml of sterile physiologic saline solution should be available. The solution is used as a temporary means of protection for the biopsy specimen.

The needle, with the stylet almost to its tip, is then placed in the incision site (Fig. 14-30A). With moderate, even pressure, the needle is advanced. As soon as the needle penetrates the parietal pleura (associated with a popping sensation), the stylet is fully advanced so that its tip extends beyond the tip of the needle (Fig. 14-30B). Trauma to the lung is thus prevented, and the risk of pneumothorax is minimized.

The entire instrument is then directed caudally, almost parallel to the wall of the thorax. The veterinarian knows that he has contacted the diaphragm when the instrument advances back and forth in accompaniment to the diaphragmatic movements associated with respiration (Fig. 14-30C). On making contact, one should adjust the needle guard to a point approximately half an inch (13 mm) from the skin (Fig. 14-30D). The needle guard prevents the veterinarian from advancing the needle too far when the biopsy thrust is made.

The veterinarian then removes the stylet and attaches the syringe (Fig. 14-30E). This step must be done quickly if pneumothorax is to be avoided. During this procedure, the tip of the biopsy needle should be resting gently against the diaphragm, to reduce further the chance of pneumothorax. The entire apparatus is now held with one hand. Negative pressure corresponding to approximately 3 ml of fluid volume is produced by drawing on the syringe plunger (Fig. 14-30F).

When the patient has completed full exhalation, the needle is thrust caudally, quickly, and smoothly up to the guard (Fig. 14-30G). The biopsy apparatus is then removed from the patient, and negative pressure is maintained throughout the procedure. *This last entire step should take place in a split second.* The thrust and extraction should be rectilinear only, without rotation or "arcing" to reduce the chance of trauma to the liver and thoracic structures. Timing penetration of the diaphragm with height of expiration adds to the ease and safety of securing the biopsy.

The biopsy specimen rests in the fluid within the syringe. The plunger is gently removed from the syringe barrel, and the contents of the barrel are poured into a small vial containing formalin. Formalin solution is then pulled through the needle to recover any fragments of hepatic tissue that may have remained within the needle.[7]

TRANSABDOMINAL BIOPSY APPROACH

Liver biopsy by the transabdominal approach is technically similar to that described for the transthoracic approach; therefore, only the differences between the approaches are considered.

The dog or cat is placed in *right* lateral recumbency. The skin incision site is located equidistant from the left costal arch and xyphoid process (Fig. 14-31A). Slight cranial or caudal displacement can be made to suit the veterinarian and to adjust for the patient's liver size or position. The needle, with the stylet allowed to float freely, is placed in the incision site (Fig. 14-31B). The needle is slowly advanced until moderate resistance is felt by the abdominal wall; then a *short*, but deliberate, thrust is used to perforate the abdominal musculature and peritoneum. Too vigorous a thrusting motion may force the needle into the liver prematurely. Once the tip of the needle is inside the abdominal cavity, the stylet is fully advanced beyond the tip of the needle (Fig. 14-31C). Prior evaluation of a lateral abdominal radiograph dictates the direction in which to advance the biopsy needle. A normally positioned liver or a small liver is best approached by directing the needle cranially and dorsolaterally. Biopsy of a large or caudally displaced liver may be performed by directing the needle caudally and dorsolaterally. Once the needle is positioned correctly, it should be advanced *gently* until a mild resistance is encountered (Fig. 14-31D). By moving the needle outward and inward, the same resistance should be met at approximately the same needle depth. Aggressive advancement of the needle causes premature penetration of the liver and should be avoided.

Once the liver is palpated with the needle, the stylet is removed and the syringe is attached. If preferred, the intraluminal nail (Fig. 14-31E) can be inserted into the biopsy needle before attaching the syringe. The intraluminal nail, by holding the liver core in the needle, usually prevents the fragmentation of the biopsy specimen that frequently occurs when the tissue is aspirated directly into the syringe.

Once the syringe is attached to the needle, one should adjust the needle guard to a point approximately half an inch (13 mm) from the skin (Fig. 14-31F). Because of the pliability of the abdominal musculature, the needle guard does *not* prevent the veterinarian from advancing the needle too far when the biopsy thrust is made. The guard is, however, a useful visual guide in estimating the depth of thrust to be made with the needle.

The entire apparatus is now held with one hand. Negative pressure corresponding to approximately 3 ml of fluid volume is produced by drawing on the syringe

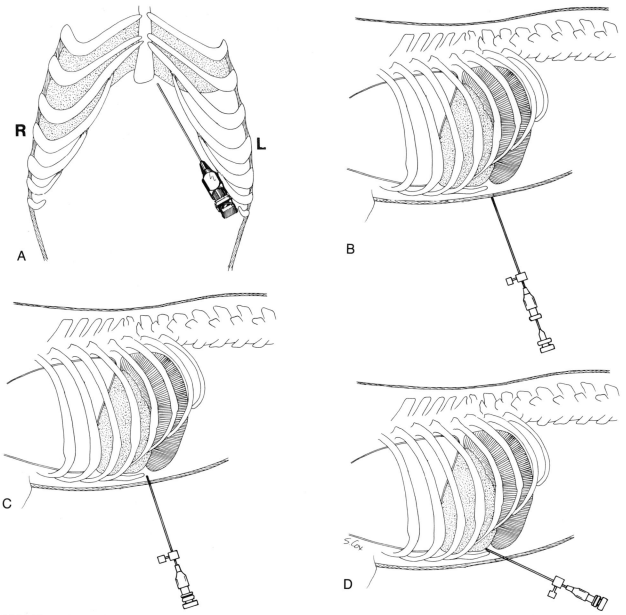

Fig. 14-31. *Ventrodorsal (A) and lateral (B) views depicting correct positioning of needle tip in the area bounded by the left costal arch and the xyphoid process. C, Immediately after penetration of the peritoneum, the stylet is advanced into the hub of the needle, and the blunt edge of the stylet is allowed to protrude beyond the cutting edge of the needle. D, With the stylet in the lead, the needle is slowly advanced in a dorsolateral plane until it rests against the liver.*

plunger (Fig. 14-31*G*). The biopsy maneuver is identical to that described for the transthoracic approach (Fig. 14-31*H*).

If the intraluminal nail is used, the biopsy specimen will occlude the needle, and negative pressure will be maintained even after the needle is withdrawn from the abdomen. To recover the liver core, one should force 2 to 3 ml of fluid through the needle, and the biopsy specimen will be ejected.

Postoperative Care and Complications

Immediately following the procedure, the dog or cat should be positioned on its right side (transthoracic

approach) or in sternal recumbency (transabdominal approach) for approximately 5 minutes; the patient's body weight should be allowed to compress the site of the wound. Following this step, the animal should be confined to a cage for approximately 8 hours and should be evaluated periodically for vomiting, dyspnea, abdominal pain or swelling, and capillary refill time.

Careful attention to technique and frequent postoperative evaluation are essential to minimizing risk. In our combined experience, liver biopsy has been performed by the Menghini technique in over 300 animals, and only 1 death has been attributable to the procedure. Complications reported in both human[12,15,17] and veterinary literature[5,7,9] include: (1) hemoperitoneum;

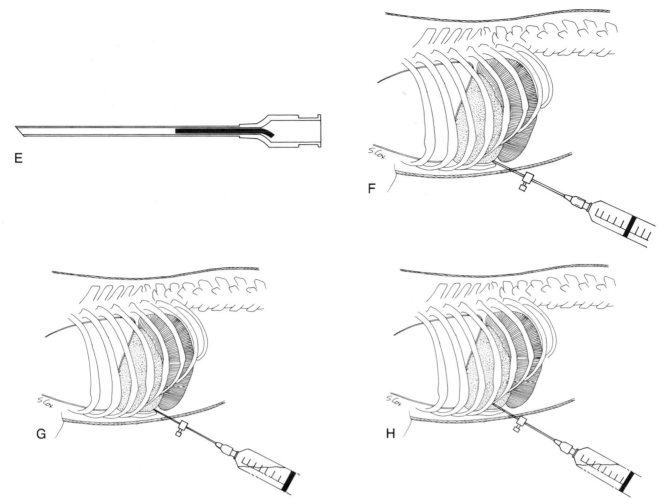

Fig. 14-31. (cont.) E, *An intraluminal nail in the needle hub prevents fragmentation of the liver biopsy.* F, *The syringe is securely fastened to the needle hub and the guard is adjusted so that it lies approximately half an inch (13 mm) from the skin.* G, *Holding the end of the syringe in one hand, negative pressure is produced by partially withdrawing the plunger.* H, *In one even motion, the needle is passed into the liver; the guard determines the appropriate depth. This thrust is followed by quick withdrawal of the biopsy apparatus from the body.*

(2) biopsy of adjacent organs; (3) bile peritonitis; (4) pneumothorax; (5) shock; (6) transfer of ascitic fluid into the thorax; (7) failure to retrieve liver tissue; (8) hemothorax and pleural effusion*; (9) bile pleuritis*; (10) hemobilia*; (11) intrahepatic arteriovenous fistula*; (12) subcapsular, intrahepatic, intradiaphragmatic, and retroperitoneal hematoma formation; (13) bacteremia and bacterial peritonitis*; and (14) tumor seeding*.

Tissue Handling

Once a liver biopsy has been obtained, the core of tissue should be placed in an appropriate fixative or culture medium. Routine histologic assessment of hepatic tissue can be performed on samples fixed in a 10% buffered neutral formalin solution. If hepatic glycogen deposition is suspected, the buffered formalin solution should be refrigerated prior to and during tissue immersion. For those samples in which electron-microscopic examination may be indicated, the dual fixative, Carson's fixative, enables both routine processing for histologic evaluation and processing for electron-microscopic study.[2]

Cultures of liver biopsies are obtained by placing the specimens in aerobic and anaerobic culture tubes† and sending the samples to a laboratory. Granulomatous hepatitis of undetermined origin should be cultured for fungal elements.

Liver biopsies have been assayed for a variety of substances. Analyses of liver samples from Bedlington terriers for copper content[14] and from hyperammonemic dogs for urea cycle enzyme activity[13] exemplify the clinical usefulness of percutaneous liver biopsy coupled with analytic technology. Unfortunately, investigations such as these are limited by the availability of appropriate equipment and technology.

*Complications documented only in human literature.

†Marion Laboratories, Inc., P.O. Box 9627, Kansas City, MO 64137

References and Suggested Readings

1. Byars, T. D., Ling, G. V., Ferris, N. A., and Keeton, K. S.: Activated coagulation time (ACT) of whole blood in normal dogs. Am. J. Vet. Res., *37*:1359, 1976.
2. Carson, F. L., Martin, J. H., and Lynn, J. A.: Formalin fixation for electron microscopy: a re-evaluation. Am. J. Clin. Pathol., *59*:365, 1973.
3. Conn, H. O.: Liver biopsy in extrahepatic biliary obstruction and in other "contraindicated" disorders. Gastroenterology, *68*:817, 1975.
4. Dodds, W. J.: Bleeding disorders. *In* A Textbook of Veterinary Internal Medicine: Diseases of the Dog and Cat. Edited by S. J. Ettinger. Philadelphia, W. B. Saunders, 1975.
5. Edwards, D. F.: Blind percutaneous liver biopsy: a safe diagnostic procedure. Cal. Vet, *31*:9, 1977.
6. Evans, H. E., and DeLahunta, A.: Miller's Guide to the Dissection of the Dog. 2nd Ed. Philadelphia, W. B. Saunders, 1974.
7. Feldman, E. C., and Ettinger, S. J.: Percutaneous transthoracic liver biopsy in the dog. J. Am. Vet. Med. Assoc., *169*:805, 1976.
8. Menghini, G.: One-second biopsy of the liver. Gastroenterology, *35*:190, 1958.
9. Osborne, C. A., Stevens, J. B., and Perman, V.: Needle biopsy of the liver. J. Am. Vet. Med. Assoc., *155*:1605, 1969.
10. Raines, D. R., Vanheertum, R. L., and Johnson, L. F.: Intrahepatic hematoma: a complication of percutaneous liver biopsy. A report on the incidence of postbiopsy scan defects. Gastroenterology, *67*:284, 1974.
11. Schaffner, F.: The clinical utilization of liver biopsy. Med. Clin. North Am., *44*:709, 1960.
12. Schiff, L.: Diseases of the Liver. 4th Ed. Philadelphia, J. B. Lippincott, 1975.
13. Strombeck, D. R., Meyer, D. J., and Freedland, R. A.: Hyperammonemia due to a urea cycle enzyme deficiency in two dogs. J. Am. Vet. Med. Assoc., *166*:1109, 1975.
14. Twedt, D. C., Sternlieb, I., and Gilbertson, S. R.: Clinical, morphologic and chemical studies on copper toxicosis of Bedlington terriers. J. Am. Vet. Med. Assoc., *175*:269, 1979.
15. Terry, R.: Risks of needle biopsy of the liver. Br. Med. J., *1*:1102, 1952.
16. Wilbur, R. D., and Foulk, W. T.: Percutaneous liver biopsy. J. Am. Vet. Med. Assoc., *202*:147, 1967.
17. Zarncheck, N., and Klausenstock, O.: Liver biopsy. II. The risks of needle biopsy. N. Engl. J. Med., *249*:1062, 1953.

Surgery of the Pancreas

by DENNIS D. CAYWOOD

Pancreatic surgery in small animals is generally limited to obtaining biopsy tissue and managing pancreatic neoplasia or trauma. Other surgical indications such as pancreatic abscesses or cysts are rarely encountered in the dog and cat. Most instances of pancreatic trauma or neoplasia can be managed by partial pancreatectomy. Because of associated postoperative insulin dependency and exocrine deficiency, total pancreatectomy should be performed only when the main excretory ducts of the pancreas have been destroyed.

Anatomy

In the embryo, the pancreas begins as an endodermal pouch on the dorsal wall of the duodenum. An additional pouch appears later, on the caudal portion of an angle formed by the duodenum and the developing hepatic buds. The latter pouch constitutes the ventral pancreas. The dorsal pancreas grows more rapidly than the ventral pancreas, and rotation of the duodenum and common bile duct carries the ventral pancreas to the right. Fusion occurs subsequently, and the ventral pancreas becomes the uncinate process.

The developed pancreas is a coarsely lobulated, elongated gland with a nodular surface. It is located caudal to the liver in the dorsal part of epigastric and mesogastric abdominal segments. The pancreas consists of three parts: right lobe, left lobe, and body (Fig. 14-32). The right lobe lies in the mesoduodenum near the dorsal portion of the right flank. It extends from the ninth intercostal space to the fourth lumbar vertebra. The left lobe lies in the greater omentum near the caudate process of the liver, portal vein, caudal vena cava, and aorta. Much of the left lobe is hidden behind the stomach. Consequently, injuries or neoplasia involving this lobe may easily escape casual exploration. The right and left lobes unite at a 45° angle to form the body of the pancreas.

The cranial and caudal pancreaticoduodenal arteries are the main vessels to the right lobe of the pancreas (Fig. 14-32). They anastamose within the gland and supply the duodenum as well as the pancreas. Loss of the vessels impairs duodenal blood supply and often leads to ischemic necrosis. The left lobe of the pancreas is primarily supplied by a branch of the splenic artery. It also receives branches from the common hepatic and celiac arteries (Fig. 14-32). The caudal pancreaticoduodenal vein drains the right lobe, whereas branches of the splenic vein primarily drain the left lobe of the pancreas.

Most sympathetic nerve fibers come from the celiac plexus, although the cranial mesenteric plexus may contribute to the caudal part of the right lobe. The vagus nerve supplies parasympathetic fibers. Fortunately, nerve supply is often of little surgical consequence.

Several groups of lymph nodes, including the duodenal, hepatic, splenic, and mesenteric, drain the pancreas. Excision of these nodes can only be accomplished by a "node picking" procedure rather than en bloc resections with wide surgical margins.

The pancreas has two excretory ducts resulting from the dual origin of the gland. The ducts usually communicate and lie within the parenchyma of the pancreas (Fig. 14-33). The ventral pancreatic duct enters the duodenum at the dorsal duodenal papilla in association with the bile duct. The dorsal duct usually enters the duodenum at the ventral duodenal papilla distal to the dorsal duodenal papilla.

Numerous variations exist in the anatomic relationship between the excretory ducts as they enter the

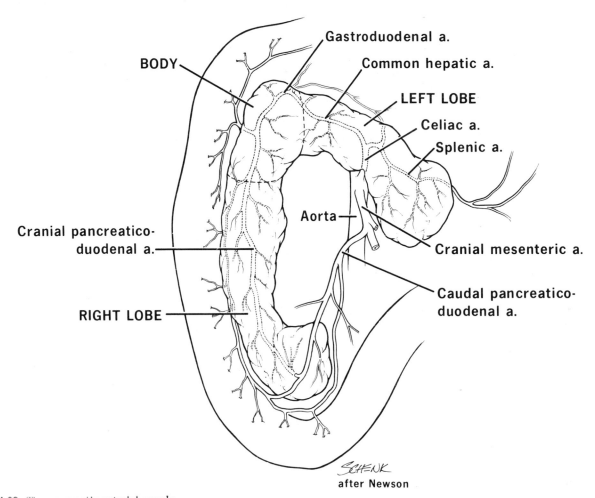

Fig. 14-32. *The pancreatic arterial supply.*

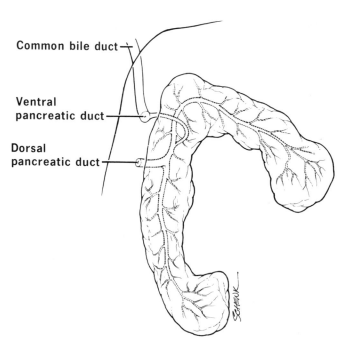

Fig. 14-33. *The pancreatic excretory ducts.*

duodenum (Fig. 14-34). At one extreme, each duct terminates in the duodenum through entirely separate papillae. At the other end of the spectrum, the two ducts join and enter the duodenum at a single papilla. Discretion is mandatory when operating on the pancreatic angle because inadvertent ligation or obstruction of a single common duct damages the remaining pancreas.

Indications

TRAUMA

The majority of traumatic pancreatic injuries come from penetrating wounds of the abdomen and are often associated with multiple-organ injuries. The aorta, caudal vena cava, cranial mesenteric artery and vein, and the splenic vessels are closely related to the pancreas. Therefore, traumatic wounds involving the pancreas are often associated with vascular injury. Failure to visualize the injured pancreas during exploratory celiotomy may lead to fatal complications.

Seldom is total pancreatectomy indicated with trauma. An edematous, lacerated, hemorrhagic portion

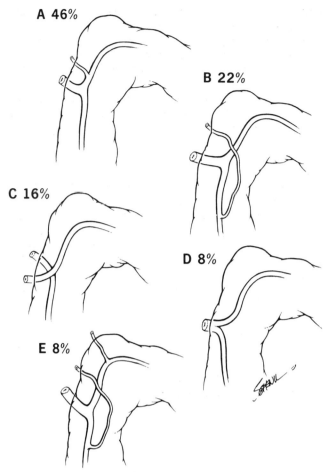

A 46%

B 22%

C 16%

D 8%

E 8%

Fig. 14-34. *Percentage of pancreatic duct variation in the dog.*

The functional pancreatic islet cell adenocarcinoma is a less commonly observed but more easily recognized pancreatic neoplasm. The neoplasm, arising from beta cells in the islets of Langerhans, begins as a small, nodular mass in the pancreatic parenchyma. Initial clinical signs are entirely related to hypoglycemia secondary to hyperinsulinism. Clinical signs include muscle tremors, muscle weakness, ataxia, collapse, and convulsions. Diagnosis is generally based on demonstrating fasting hypoglycemia and hyperinsulinism through the comparison of the ratios of fasting insulin to glucose levels. Exploratory celiotomy should include a careful inspection of the liver, mesentery, and associated lymph nodes because these structures are common sites of metastasis. These neoplasms are generally small, nodular masses in either the left or the right lobe of the pancreas and are treated by means of wide partial pancreatectomy.

Both exocrine and endocrine pancreatic neoplasms are nearly always malignant. Although considered palliative, surgical procedures may extend the normal life of the animal, particularly in patients with islet cell carcinoma. Obviously, the condition should be considered operatively noncorrectable if liver or widespread abdominal metastasis is present. The acinar carcinoma has a poorer short-term prognosis than the islet cell carcinoma because of its extensive invasion of peripancreatic tissues.

Adjunctive chemotherapy for islet cell carcinoma is sometimes useful. The reader is directed to medical texts for details.

Surgical Techniques

PARTIAL PANCREATECTOMY

A ventral midline abdominal approach is used. The incision should extend from the xiphoid process to just caudal to the umbilicus. The pancreas is exposed by isolating and exteriorizing the descending duodenum and by cranially reflecting the stomach. The remainder of the abdominal contents are reflected sinistrocaudally and are packed off with moistened laparotomy sponges. It is now possible to visualize and to palpate the entire pancreas.

The portion of the pancreas to be excised is isolated and is packed off by moistened laparotomy sponges, and the mesentery is incised along the caudal border of the gland. The serosal layer is grasped with tissue forceps and is torn away from the portion of the pancreas to be excised (Fig. 14-35A). The exposed pancreatic parenchyma is then gently separated, using Halsted mosquito forceps (Fig. 14-35B). Isolated ducts and small vessels away from the duodenum should be double-ligated with nonabsorbable suture material (Fig. 14-35C).

Pancreatic tissue adhering to the duodenum should be carefully rubbed free from the intestine and pancreaticoduodenal vessels using a moistened gauze sponge (Fig. 14-36A and B). Care should be exercised when manipulating the pancreaticoduodenal vessels to

of the pancreas may often be managed by partial pancreatectomy. Total pancreatectomy is indicated when disruption of both the major pancreatic ducts at the body of the pancreas is extensive. Partial duodenectomy with subsequent cholecystoduodenostomy and gastroduodenostomy may be necessary when the duodenum and common bile duct are also involved.

NEOPLASIA

The most common neoplasm of the pancreas is a carcinoma arising from the exocrine glands. Clinical signs are generally nonspecific, and antemortem diagnosis of acinar carcinoma is often made during exploratory celiotomy. Sometimes, impairment of hepatic function and icterus occur secondary to common bile duct obstruction, because the neoplasm frequently arises from the body of the organ. The tumor commonly invades the peripancreatic fat, duodenum, and stomach and often metastasizes to the liver and regional lymph nodes. These structures must be carefully inspected during surgical examination. When an acinar carcinoma is operable, either total pancreatectomy or a pancreaticoduodenectomy is indicated. Insulin dependency and exocrine deficiency are important consequences of these surgical procedures.

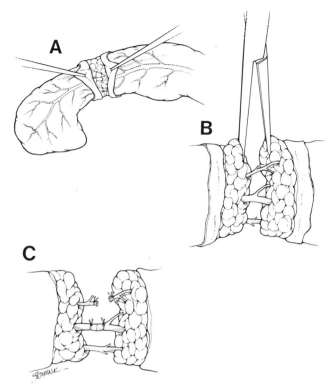

Fig. 14-35. *Pancreatectomy technique: duct and vessel ligation.*

maintain normal blood supply to the duodenum. Pancreatic branches of the pancreaticoduodenal vessel near the caudal portion of the right pancreatic lobe may be double-ligated and severed (Fig. 14-36*C*). Hemorrhage resulting from manipulation of the proximal right lobe and body may be controlled by direct pressure. When operating on the pancreatic body, exocrine duct location and variation must be considered to avoid inadvertent ligation.

TOTAL PANCREATECTOMY

The surgical approach and isolation of the pancreas are similar to those for partial pancreatectomy. An incision is made in the mesentery just caudal to the pancreas along the entire length of the gland. The pancreatic branches of the splenic vessels are isolated and are double-ligated. The mesenteric incision is extended dextrocranially around the left lobe toward the body of the pancreas. The pancreatic ducts are identified, are ligated, and are separated. As in partial pancreatectomy, the remaining portion of the body and right lobe of the pancreas is carefully separated (rubbed) from the surface of the duodenum using a gauze sponge. The pancreaticoduodenal vessels should not be ligated or clamped to avoid ischemic necrosis to the duodenum. Hemorrhage is controlled by pressure.

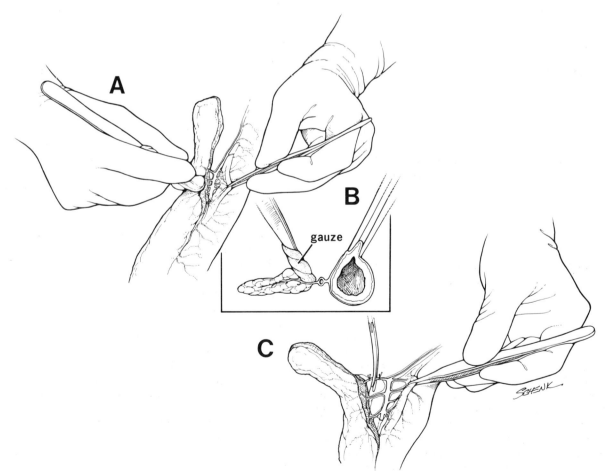

Fig. 14-36. *Pancreatectomy technique: separation of the pancreas from the duodenum.*

PANCREATICODUODENECTOMY

In man, a number of surgical techniques have been developed to manage traumatic or neoplastic diseases of the pancreas and duodenum with associated destruction of the pancreatic and common bile ducts. Acinar cell carcinoma and traumatic lesions may present a similar situation in small animal practice.

Owing to the extremely small pancreatic duct size in the dog and cat, human surgical techniques involving pancreatic duct anastamosis are probably not practical. Total pancreatectomy with partial duodenectomy can be performed, however. Complete reconstruction following pancreaticoduodenectomy should include a cholecystoduodenostomy and gastroduodenostomy.

Intraoperative and Postoperative Management

Considerable controversy exists over intraoperative management of patients with functional beta-cell neoplasms. Many clinicians have urged aggressive glucose administration during the surgical procedure to prevent hypoglycemic crises due to insulin release following tumor manipulation. The patient's intraoperative plasma glucose concentration rises to greater than normal values without glucose administration, however. Apparently, stress gluconeogenesis induced by anesthesia and the surgical procedure more than counteracts possible insulin release from tumor manipulation. Thus, glucose administration may still be advisable, but it is not mandatory. Routine intraoperative fluid management is advisable. The plasma glucose concentration and serum amylase activity should be monitored closely for the first 12 to 24 hours postoperatively, and thereafter daily for 4 to 5 days.

In anticipation of postoperative pancreatitis, some clinicians have recommended withholding all oral intake and administering atropine, glucocorticoids, and antibiotics for 3 to 5 days following pancreatic operations. Unlike in man, pancreatitis is uncommon following partial pancreatectomy in the dog and cat, and prophylactic therapy is generally considered unnecessary.

Total pancreatectomy results in insulin dependency and exocrine insufficiency necessitating dietary control and pancreatic enzyme supplementation. These patients are also "brittle" diabetics and require careful insulin therapy. It is questionable whether these patients actually qualify as pets following the surgical procedure.

References and Suggested Readings

Anderson, N. V.: The pancreas. A review. J. Am. Anim. Hosp. Assoc., 9:89, 1973.

Caywood, D. D., and Wilson, J. W.: Functional pancreatic islet cell adenocarcinoma in the dog. *In* Current Veterinary Therapy VII. Edited by R. W. Kirk. Philadelphia, W. B. Saunders, 1980.

Caywood, D. D., Wilson, J. W., Hardy, R. M., and Shull, R. M.: Pancreatic islet cell adenocarcinoma: clinical and diagnostic features of six cases. J. Am. Vet. Med. Assoc., *174*:714, 1979.

Dingwall, J. S.: The pancreas. *In* Current Techniques in Small Animal Surgery. Edited by M. J. Bojrab. Philadelphia, Lea & Febiger, 1975.

Dingwall, J. S., and McDonell, W.: Partial pancreatectomy in the dog. J. Am. Anim. Hosp. Assoc., 8:86, 1972.

Nielsen, S. W., and Bishop, E. J.: The duct system of the canine pancreas. Am. J. Vet. Res., *15*:266, 1954.

15 * Diaphragm

Repair of Diaphragmatic Rents Using Omentum

by RONALD M. BRIGHT

Omentum may be used in several surgical reconstructive applications in both dogs and cats. Indications for the use of omentum in the repair of the diaphragm include congenital hemidiaphragmatic defects or repair of large pericardial-peritoneal diaphragmatic hernias. Traumatic rents in which a large amount of the diaphragmatic musculature is devitalized or is removed are other possible indications for the use of an omental flap.[2]

To mobilize the omentum for use in diaphragmatic repair, a lengthening procedure needs to be done. An omental pedicle flap is formed to allow mobility of that portion of the omentum transferred to the diaphragm.

Surgical Technique

A ventral abdominal midline incision is made from the xiphoid cartilage to behind the umbilicus. A Balfour retractor is used to maximize exposure after packing off the wound. The spleen, greater gastric curvature, and greater omentum are exteriorized, and the blood supply to the omentum is closely examined.

The right gastroepiploic artery is located by carefully dissecting near the pancreas (Fig. 15-1A). This artery is ligated at the point at which it leaves the pancreas, at the medial surface of the duodenum (Fig. 15-1B, a). Small gastric branches of both the right and left gastroepiploic arteries, which course along the greater curvature of the stomach, are isolated and ligated using 3-0 gut suture (Fig. 15-1B, small arrows). These arteries are ligated close to the serosal surface of the stomach, in order to preserve the gastroepiploic arcade lying within the cranial border of the omentum (Fig. 15-1B, large arrow). When reaching the origin of the left gastroepiploic artery, care is taken to prevent sacrificing this artery because it now serves as the main source of blood to the left omental pedicle flap that is formed (Fig. 15-1B, open arrow). To free the omentum sufficiently for transfer, the remaining few splenic and pancreatic attachments are carefully dissected from the omentum. The omental pedicle flap that is formed is now ready to be mobilized to the site of the diaphragmatic defect (Fig. 15-1C).

Should a right omental pedicle flap be desired, the opposite gastroepiploic artery (left) is sacrificed, and the rest of the technique remains the same. The major blood supply to a right pedicle comes from the right gastroepiploic artery, which must be preserved. (Fig. 15-1D).

A double-layered free edge of omentum is now carefully handled and is placed over the diaphragmatic defect. This omentum is loosely sutured around the periphery using 1-0 or 2-0 nylon in a simple interrupted or continuous pattern (Fig. 15-1E, a). Twisting or kinking of the pedicle is avoided to prevent compromise of the blood supply to the omentum. A fold of omentum is then created and, in accordion style, is brought forward and is draped over the defect (Fig. 15-1E, b). This layer of omentum is attached to the diaphragm outside the first row of sutures, using a simple interrupted pattern. Finally, the last step is to place 6 to 8 sutures from one side of the defect to the other, coursing through the omentum in a loose, weaving pattern (Fig. 15-1E, c). Care is taken not to tighten these sutures excessively, to avoid strangulating the vessels within the omentum. The purpose of these weave-patterned sutures is to provide a scaffolding for the omentum, in order to limit excessive paradoxic movement of the omental patch in response to changing intrathoracic pressures.

The chest should be completely closed before proceeding to the midline abdominal wound closure. Following closure of the defect, a chest tube is placed from the exterior and is affixed to the skin. This tube should be removed when a negative intrathoracic pressure is obtained and when the amount of pleural fluid is minimal.

The omentum in dogs is a thin, lacey structure and should be handled carefully when performing the lengthening procedure and when transferring the flap to the site of repair. In addition, it is important to clamp and ligate omental vessels immediately, especially the small gastric branches as they leave the gastroepiploic arcade along the greater curvature of the stomach. A hemostat torn from one of these vessels usually causes

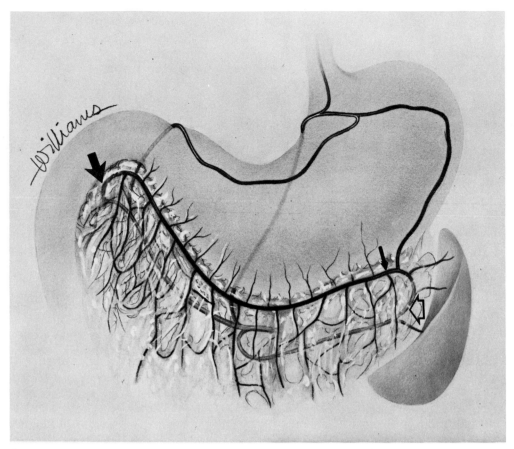

A

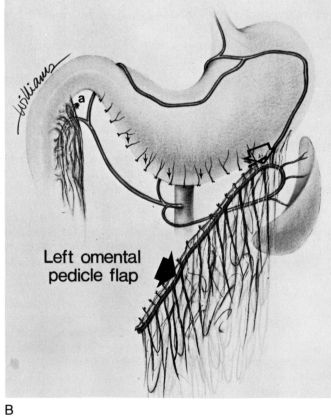

Left omental
pedicle flap

B

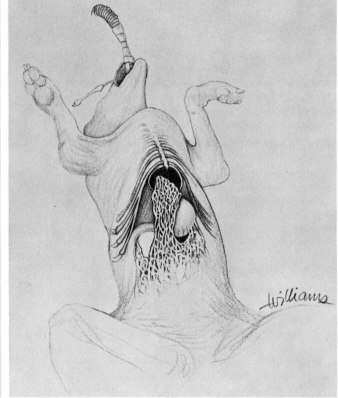

C

Fig. 15-1. *Legend on opposite page.*

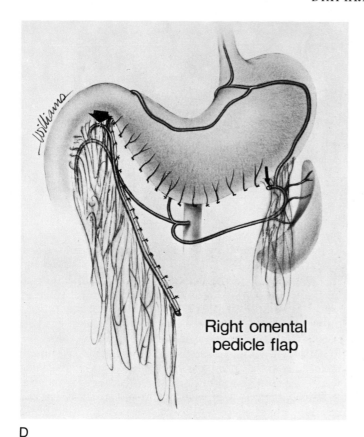

**Right omental
pedicle flap**

D

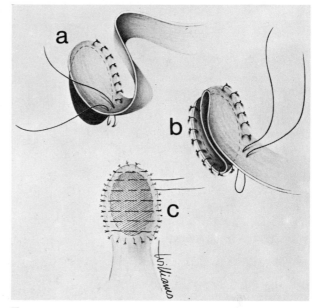

E

Fig. 15-1. A, *The large arrow points to the right gastroepiploic artery after it leaves the gastroduodenal artery. The small arrow points to the origin of the left gastroepiploic artery, the last artery to branch from the splenic artery (large open arrow). Small gastric branches of the right and left gastroepiploic arteries are seen penetrating the serosa along the greater curvature of the stomach. B, Transection and ligation of the right gastroepiploic artery are performed at the artery's origin (a). Small gastric branches are sacrificed along the greater curvature of the stomach (small arrows). The preserved gastroepiploic arcade is shown within the cranial portion of the omentum (large arrow). The remaining intact left gastroepiploic artery now serves as the main blood supply to the omentum (open arrow). Thus, a left omental pedicle flap is formed. C, This sketch demonstrates the formation of a left omental pedicle flap and its transfer to the site of the diaphragmatic defect. D, The formation of a right omental pedicle flap is possible by preserving the right gastroepiploic artery (large arrow) and by sacrificing the left (small arrow). E, The first layer of omentum is affixed to the periphery of the diaphragmatic defect using simple interrupted sutures (a). A double fold of omentum is then brought forward and tacked to the diaphragm just outside the original row of sutures (b). Six to eight sutures are now placed from side to side (c). (A to E, from Bright, R. M., and Thacker, H. L.: The formation of an omental pedicle flap and its experimental use in the repair of a diaphragmatic rent in the dog. J. Am. Anim. Hosp. Assoc., 18:283, 1982.)*

a large hematoma, which could compromise the amount of useful omentum remaining for mobilization to the site of repair.

References and Selected Readings

1. Baffi, R. R., Didolkov, M. S., and Bakamjran, V.: Reconstruction of sternal and abdominal wall defects in a case of desmoid tumor. J. Thorac. Cardiovasc. Surg., 74:105, 1977.
2. Bright, R. M., and Thacker, H. L.: The formation of an omental pedicle flap and its experimental use in the repair of a diaphragmatic rent in the dog. J. Am. Anim. Hosp. Assoc., 18:283, 1982.
3. Casten, D. F., and Alday, E. S.: Omental transfer for revascularization of the extremities: Surg. Gynecol. Obstet., 132:301, 1971.
4. Drummond, D., and Morison, R. A.: A case of ascites due to cirrhosis of the liver cured by operation. Br. Med. J., 2:728, 1896.
5. Goldsmith, H. S., and Beattie, E. J.: Carotid artery protection by pedicled omental wrapping. Surg. Gynecol. Obstet., 130:57, 1970.
6. Goldsmith, H. S., Delos Santos, R., and Beattie, E. J.: Relief of chronic lymphedema by omental transposition. Ann. Surg., 166:573, 1967.

16 * Peritoneum

Peritonitis and Intraperitoneal Drainage

by ALAN J. LIPOWITZ

Peritonitis may be either primary or secondary. Feline infectious peritonitis, in which the peritoneum is the target organ of disease, is the only known or recognized condition of primary peritonitis in small animals.[9] Secondary peritonitis results from disease or injury of intra-abdominal organs or puncture wounds of the abdominal wall. This discussion is concerned with secondary peritonitis only.

Secondary peritonitis may be of two types, local or diffuse.[5] A local peritonitis may be considered as a walled-off intra-abdominal abscess in which the affected area within the abdomen is isolated from the remaining peritoneal surfaces by the abscess walls. Diffuse or generalized peritonitis involves nearly all peritoneal surfaces. A combination of types may occur in which diffuse peritonitis is present, as well as small spaces or pockets of walled-of purulent material within the greater omentum or mesentery.

Causes of Peritonitis

Secondary peritonitis is often a sequela to gastrointestinal problems. Bowel or stomach perforation by foreign objects allows leakage of luminal contents and peritoneal contamination. Perforation may also occur as a result of neoplasia, ulcers, corticosteroid administration, or trauma.

Nonperforating gastric or bowel lesions are other causes of peritonitis. Devitalization of the gut wall, as may occur subsequent to gastric and intestinal volvulus, long-standing intestinal obstruction, or tearing of the mesenteric vessels, allows transmural migration of luminal bacteria and other deleterious substances and thus involves the peritoneum.

Genitourinary disease or injury may also cause peritonitis. Urine leakage from an injured bladder, ureter, or kidney induces a chemical peritonitis. Such a chemical peritonitis may become infected. Transmural migration of bacteria in pyometritis, rupture of a gravid or infected uterus, pyelonephritis, and bacterial prostatitis (with or without cyst or abscess formation) may all lead to peritonitis.

The liver and biliary systems are sometimes injured in the traumatized dog and cat. Bile leakage from hepatic lacerations and fractures and tears or lacerations of the common bile duct or gallbladder may cause a diffuse bile peritonitis. Bile peritonitis is due to a combination of chemical and bacterial agents. Although rarely reported, primary hepatic abscesses may also cause peritonitis. Intra-abdominal leakage of pancreatic enzymes, as seen with acute pancreatitis, trauma to the pancreas, or following pancreatic operations, may cause peritoneal irritation and inflammation.

Additional causes of peritonitis include direct peritoneal contamination at celiotomy or by perforating abdominal wounds, resulting in peritoneal infection. Iatrogenic causes of peritonitis include intraoperative spillage of visceral contents and leaving surgical instruments or sponges in the abdomen following surgical procedures. In humans, a granulomatous peritonitis caused by the powder from surgeons' gloves has been reported,[8] but this source of contamination apparently is not a major problem in small animals. The diagnosis of peritonitis may be established or aided by physical examination, abdominal radiography, abdominal paracentesis, diagnostic lavage of the peritoneum, or exploratory celiotomy.

Treatment of Peritonitis

In the treatment of peritonitis, attention must first be given to the primary causes, such as closure or resection of a leaking, hollow viscus.[5,10] Once the primary problem has been addressed, the peritoneal disease may be treated. In some cases of diffuse peritonitis, loculated areas of abscessed material exist within the greater omentum, mesentery, or in fibrinous debris. These areas must be opened, and their contents must be evacuated. A thorough debridement of the peritoneal surfaces must be performed by removing as much fibrin and debris as possible.

Following mechanical debridement, the abdominal cavity should be lavaged to aid in the further removal of deleterious materials.[5,7,10] Regardless of the type of lavage fluid used, it should be administered at body temperature and should be available in large supply. The lavage fluid is poured into the abdominal cavity and is evenly distributed throughout. All peritoneal surfaces must come into contact with the fluid. Suction is used to evacuate the fluid, and the process is repeated several times. If no indications exist for the placement of local drains, the abdomen is then closed. Lavage fluid should not be left in the abdominal cavity. Monofilament nonabsorbable suture material should be used for abdominal wall closure.

Sterile lactated Ringer's solution and physiologic saline solution are common lavage fluids and may be used unaltered or with the addition of antibiotics. The use of dilute povidone-iodine solution is advocated by some and is finding increased favor because of its bacteriocidal effects.[3,6] One part of povidone-iodine solution (not soap) in nine parts of lavage fluid is the recommended dilution. Although no adverse effects have been seen in some studies,[2,3,6] others have shown that, at least in the rat, allowing the povidone-iodine solution to remain in the abdomen has deleterious effects on intraperitoneal macrophage function.[1] This information suggests that povidone-iodine lavage should be followed by lavage with unaltered saline solution or lactated Ringer's solution.

Systemic antibiotics should be administered to all patients with peritonitis.[5,10] Until the results of bacterial cultures and sensitivity tests from the affected areas are obtained, broad-spectrum antibiotics particularly effective against gram-negative species should be used. Increased awareness of intra-abdominal anaerobic infections suggests that culture specimens should be examined for anaerobic bacteria.

Closed abdominal lavage has also been advocated as a treatment for diffuse peritonitis.[5] Lavage fluid is placed within the abdomen by needle and syringe or by a dialysis catheter. The animal is then gently rolled from side to side to distribute the fluid within the abdomen. The fluid is then withdrawn, and the procedure is repeated as necessary. Another technique of closed lavage employs ingress and egress drains.[7] Single or multiple drains are strategically placed throughout the abdomen at the time of celiotomy. After abdominal closure, lavage fluid is placed into the abdominal cavity through the more dorsally positioned drainage tubes and is expected to exit the ventral drains. The quantity of fluid recovered from the abdominal cavity varies with the type of drain used. A Penrose drain alone has the poorest recovery rate, whereas a sump drain,* combined with a Penrose drain, has the greatest rate.[10]

INTRAPERITONEAL DRAINAGE

Drainage of the abdominal cavity for the treatment of diffuse peritonitis is a topic that rarely fails to spark comment and criticism, discussion, and opinion. Surgeons have long debated the advantages and disadvantages of abdominal drainage, but all agree that the removal of contaminated intraperitoneal fluid, debris, and free secretions is mandatory.

Although opinions still exist to the contrary, most now agree that diffuse peritonitis cannot be treated adequately with multiple indwelling drains. This principle was recognized as early as 1889[4] and was restated by Yates in 1905.[11] Yates showed that abdominal drains in the dog were encapsulated by fibrous tissue within 6 hours and therefore no longer served as egress conduits for the entire abdominal cavity. Instead, they acted as local drains allowing exit of fluid only from the area immediately adjacent to the drain. It has been stated that abdominal cavity drains can serve only two purposes[4]: first, to provide egress for pus or fluid that is already walled off; and second, to remove secretions such as bile or pancreatic fluid before they can lead to further complications.

One may choose from a plethora of drains and drainage systems for evacuation of isolated areas within the abdomen. The Penrose drain is a soft, flexible, flat rubber tube available in varying lengths and diameters. It may be used individually or in clusters in one or more locations within the abdomen. This drain comes close in fulfilling three important criteria of an "ideal" drain: (1) it is soft and malleable and therefore does not exert undue pressure on adjacent blood vessels or other structures; (2) it is nonirritating to the tissues; and (3) it is of a stable composition and therefore does not decompose when subjected to prolonged heat or moisture.

Other types of drains, such as double- and triple-lumen drains, sump drains, and suction drains, have been advocated for intraperitoneal drainage. When properly applied and cared for, they may have advantages over the Penrose drain, particularly in the removal of large quantities of fluid, but for ease of application and care and for generally acceptable results, the Penrose drain is preferred.

DRAIN PLACEMENT. Although the placement of intra-abdominal drains is not a demanding procedure, several points should be emphasized to ensure maximum efficacy of the drain and to avoid complications. Drains should be placed just prior to abdominal closure, and the drain should exit the abdomen in such a manner that when the animal assumes a standing position, the drain exit is in a dependent position.[5] This positioning is critical because Penrose drains function by the gravity flow of fluid. The drain should exit through a stab incision in the abdominal wall and should not be placed through the primary abdominal incision. A drain tract through a suture line is a potential source of weakness and may lead to incisional hernia. It is recommended that the stab incision be placed lateral to the rectus abdominis muscle to avoid laceration of the cranial and caudal epigastric vessels.[4]

When the site for the drain's exit has been chosen, a small incision is made with a scalpel through all layers, from skin to peritoneum.[4] Some recommend incising only the skin and subcutaneous tissues and then forcing medium-sized forceps through the muscular layers

---

*A double-lumen drain consisting of an outer tube with a more slender tube within it, which may be attached to a suction pump. Available from American V. Mueller, 6600 Touhy Avenue, Chicago, IL 60648

and peritoneum.[5] Opening the forceps jaws enlarges the drain tract and ensures an adequate pathway for fluid flow (Fig. 16-1). The drain is then passed from within the peritoneal cavity outward through to the skin with the aid of the forceps (Fig. 16-2). The end of the drain should be placed at the appropriate site within the abdomen, and the drain should be positioned along the shortest and most direct path from the area to be drained through the stab incision. Before the drain is placed in its final position, all intra-abdominal structures are returned to the position they are to occupy during the recovery period. This positioning avoids kinking or displacement of the drain that may hinder its efficacy. If the exact position of the drain is critical, it may be anchored in place with a 4-0 or 5-0 plain gut suture. This suture is rapidly absorbed and allows the drain to be removed in 5 to 6 days.

The drain must be anchored to the skin with a nonabsorbable suture of appropriate size.[5,10] In addition, a large, sterile safety pin may be placed through the distal end of the protruding drain, to aid in preventing the drain from slipping back into the wound.[4,10] If the drain does slip into the wound, the pin will act as a radiographic marker (Fig. 16-3).

When possible, the drain's end should be covered with a soft, nonrestrictive bandage placed around the entire abdomen. The bandage serves several purposes: (1) it helps to prevent the animal from removing the drain; (2) it may act as a barrier for ascending contamination; and (3) it acts as a measuring device for the quantity of material passing through the drain. If left unbandaged, drainage material goes uncollected, and the degree of drainage is difficult to assess. By changing the bandage daily, or more frequently if necessary, the relative amount of drainage may be determined by the quantity of material absorbed by the bandage. Changes in the character of the drainage fluid may also be thus noted. At the time of the daily bandage change, the drain should be examined. Tube drains and multilumen drains should be checked for patency. Frequently, a fibrin seal forms between the drain and the skin and thus inhibits drainage. This seal may be dislodged by gently wiggling the exposed portion of the drain. This procedure is particularly important when Penrose drains are used because drainage occurs primarily around rather than through a Penrose drain.

DRAIN REMOVAL. Simply stated, drains are removed when drainage has stopped. With adequate systemic treatment of the problem, and barring complications, most abdominal drains may be removed within 5 to 6 days. Small amounts of serosanguinous fluid may be present even after drainage of the original material has ceased. This fluid is due to the presence of the drain itself and is a reliable indicator that the drain may be removed. Whereas some advocate removal of drains in stages, others feel the entire drain may be safely removed at one time. The drain is removed by releasing the sutures between the drain and the skin and by gently pulling on the drain.

Seepage of small quantities of serosanguinous material from the stab incision usually occurs for 2 to 3 days following drain removal. Therefore, the stab incision should not be sutured closed immediately following drain removal, thus maintaining some patency if drainage has not fully subsided. The stab incision is allowed to heal by granulation.

Complications associated with the use of abdominal drains are few, particularly when Penrose drains are employed.[4] Some complications, such as drain retraction into the wound and ascending contamination, have already been mentioned. Other complications include hematoma due to inadvertent laceration of a vessel when making the stab incision and herniation of abdominal viscera through the drain tract. Careful attention to the size and placement of the stab incision enables one to avoid these problems.

Tubes less flexible than Penrose drains are often used as sump or multilumen drains. If drains of this type are employed, the drain tip must be placed so that it is not adjacent to hollow viscera; it must also be well anchored. Drainage of an anastomosis site is not rec-

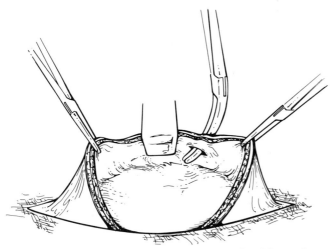

Fig. 16-1. *A stab incision through all layers of the abdomen is enlarged with forceps.*

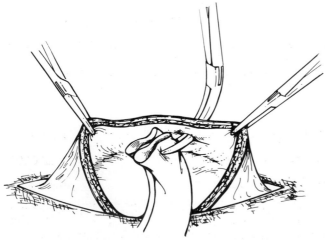

Fig. 16-2. *After placement of the proximal end of the drains within the abdomen, the distal ends are passed through the stab incision in the abdominal wall.*

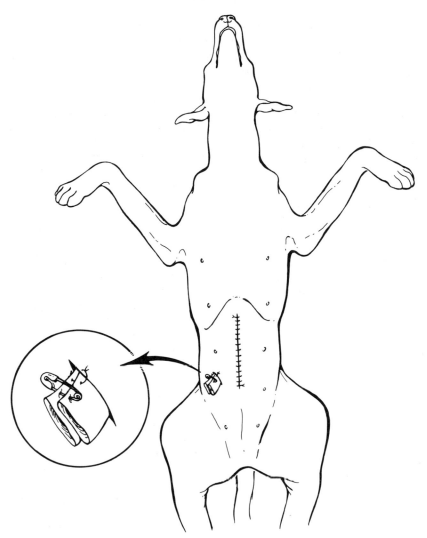

Fig. 16-3. *Drains are placed to allow gravity flow of fluid and are secured to the skin with sutures. A safety pin may be placed through the distal end of the protruding drain.*

ommended because of the increased incidence of suture line disruption associated with the placement of the drain against the anastomotic site.[4]

References and Suggested Readings

1. Ahrenholz, D. H., and Simmons, R. L.: Povidone-iodine in peritonitis I. Adverse effects of local instillation in experimental E. coli peritonitis. J. Surg. Res., 26:458, 1979.
2. Bolton, J. S., Bornvide, G. H., and Cohn, J., Jr.: Intraperitoneal povidone-iodine in experimental canine and murine peritonitis. Am. J. Surg., 137:780, 1979.
3. Gilmore, O. J. A., Reid, L., Houang, E. T., and Shaw, E. J.: Prophylactic intraperitoneal povidone-iodine in alimentary tract surgery. Am. J. Surg., 135:156, 1978.
4. Hermann, G.: Intraperitoneal drainage. Surg. Clin. North Am., 49:1279, 1969.
5. Hoffer, R. E.: Peritonitis, Vet. Clin. North Am., 2:189, 1972.
6. Lavigne, J. E., et al.: The treatment of experimental peritonitis with intraperitoneal betadine solution. J. Surg. Res., 16:307, 1974.
7. Parks, J., Gahring, D., and Greene, R. W.: Peritoneal lavage for peritonitis and pancreatitis in twenty-two dogs. J. Am. Anim. Hosp. Assoc., 9:442, 1973.
8. Perper, J. A., Pidlaon, A., and Fisher, R. S.: Granulomatous peritonitis induced by rice-starch glove powder—a clinical and experimental study. Am. J. Surg., 122:812, 1971.
9. Weiss, R. D., and Scott, F. W.: Feline infectious peritonitis. *In* Current Veterinary Therapy VII. Edited by R. W. Kirk. Philadelphia, W. B. Saunders, 1980.
10. Withrow, S. J., and Black, A. P.: Generalized peritonitis in small animals. Vet. Clin. North Am., 9:363, 1979.
11. Yates, J. L.: An experimental study of the local effects of peritoneal drainage. Surg. Gynecol. Obstet., 1:473, 1905.

Adjunct to Intraperitoneal Drainage with the Purdue Column Disk Catheter

by Jerry A. Thornhill

The column disk catheter developed by investigators at Purdue University has been shown to be an effective catheter for long-term peritoneal dialysis in man and in the dog.[1,3,4] It is successful because the disk portion of the catheter rests against the peritoneum and does not float freely in the abdominal cavity, and thus circumvents entanglement by omentum or intestinal loops.

The catheter was developed because of the failure of conventional catheters to drain the abdomen (outflow obstruction) of the dog adequately, following the fluid-filling and fluid-dwelling periods of a peritoneal dialysis cycle. An anephric dog, with a column disk catheter, was supported for 78 days by continuous ambulatory peritoneal dialysis (CAPD), using bagged dialysate and 4 to 6 exchanges per day.[5] At no time during this period did outflow obstruction from catheter malfunction occur, and no catheter replacement procedure was required.

One may appreciate the use of the disk catheter in the treatment of peritonitis and for removal of contaminated intraperitoneal fluid, debris, and free secretions, owing to the excellent flow characteristics of this catheter. Moreover, with use of the catheter, a saline-iodine flush of the abdomen, which has been successful in patients undergoing peritoneal dialysis for clearance of bacterial infection, can be employed. In this technique, 1 L saline solution is delivered to the abdominal cavity and is drained immediately, followed by the introduction of 1 L saline solution, to which has been added 0.2 ml 2% U.S.P. iodine solution, which is allowed to dwell for 4 to 5 minutes before drainage.[2] The technique may be repeated daily or twice a day, depending on the degree of infection and the therapeutic response.

Characteristics of the Catheter

The catheter* is composed of a terminal disk, approximately 2¾ inches in diameter and ⁵⁄₁₆ inch thick, which consists of silicone sheets separated by numer-

*Physio-Control Corp., Redmond, WA

ous pillars, each ¼ inch tall (Fig. 16-4). Silastic tubing (outer diameter of ¼ inch, inner diameter of ⅛ inch) enters the ventral portion of the disk and communicates with the space between the Silastic sheets. Two Dacron velour cuffs, one next to the base of the catheter and one near the free end, are positioned so that they may be placed preperitoneally and subcutaneously. The cuffs stimulate fibroblastic ingrowth, to wall off the catheter and to prevent bacterial migration along the wall of the tubing.

Catheter Placement and Removal

The catheter must be placed surgically into the lower abdominal quadrant (Fig. 16-5). Through a paramedial incision in the skin and grid separation of the external and internal abdominal oblique and rectus abdominis muscle layers, the peritoneum is exposed and is severed. The foldable disk is squeezed and is placed through the surgical opening into the peritoneal cavity. The disk is pulled firmly against the parietal peritoneum, which is then closed over the base of the catheter. Muscle layers are sewn tightly around the first Dacron velour cuff, but sutures need not enter the cuff for an adequate seal. The free end of the catheter is tunneled subcutaneously, to exit through a skin stab incision at a point beyond the second Dacron velour cuff, which is buried.

The catheter must be surgically removed when peritoneal drainage has ceased or when prophylactic or therapeutic peritoneal lavage has ended. Through a skin incision, the muscle wrapped around the first Dacron velour cuff is dissected free, and the peritoneum is severed at the entrance of the catheter into the abdomen. The disk is squeeze-clamped and is removed from the peritoneal cavity; the catheter tubing is transected above the first cuff adjacent to the disk. The exit site

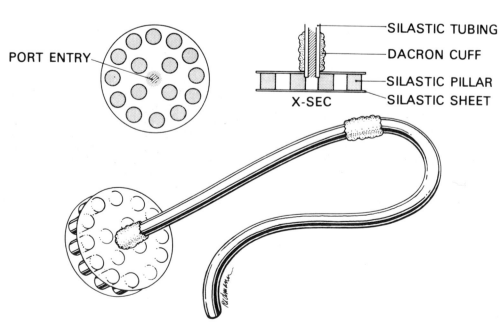

Fig. 16-4. *Purdue column disk catheter with double-layered disk separated by pillars and Dacron velour cuffs around Silastic tubing.*

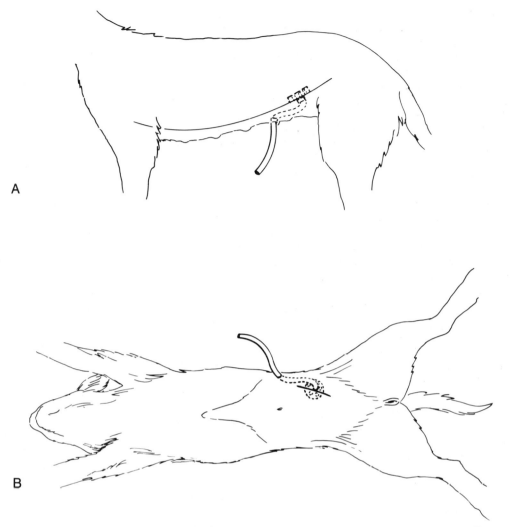

Fig. 16-5. *Schematic illustrations of disk catheter properly positioned in the abdominal cavity.* A, *Lateral view;* B, *ventral view.*

beyond the second Dacron velour cuff is surgically prepared, followed by blunt dissection in the subcutaneous tissue to free the cuff portion and to release the catheter for extraction. The peritoneum and muscle layers are closed routinely, but the catheter exit site in the skin is left open to heal by granulation. Some seepage of serosanguinous material may be expected from the catheter tract for 2 to 3 days following surgical removal. The skin incision, used for exposure of the catheter for removal, is closed routinely. To date, no complication of fibrinous deposits or fibrous encasement of the disk portion of the catheter has occurred, even in the face of active peritonitis.

References and Suggested Readings

1. Ash, S. R., et al.: The immobilized disc peritoneal catheter. A peritoneal access device with improved drainage. J. Am. Soc. Artif. Intern. Organs, *3*:109, 1980.
2. Stephen, R. L., et al.: Peritoneal dialysis. Peritonitis: saline-iodine flush. Dial. Transplant., *8*:584, 1979.
3. Thornhill, J. A.: Peritoneal dialysis in the dog and cat: an update. Compend. Contin. Ed. Practicing Vet., *3*:20, 1981.
4. Thornhill, J. A., et al.: Peritoneal dialysis with the Purdue column disc catheter. Minn. Vet., *20*:27, 1980.
5. Thornhill, J. A., et al.: Successful support of an anephric dog for 78 days with continuous ambulatory peritoneal dialysis and a new peritoneal access catheter design. Unpublished manuscript.

17 * Nasal Cavity

Surgical Management of Upper Airway Distress

by KENNETH KAGAN

Brachycephalic Airway Syndrome

Because of selective breeding, the upper airways of the brachycephalic dog only slightly resemble the functional airways of other breeds. The short and distorted soft tissues and skull create a relative restriction to the free passage of air into the nose, the trachea, and the lungs. The degree of restriction varies among individuals. Some become dyspneic with only small amounts of physical activity or increases in ambient temperature.

The brachycephalic conformation predisposes these dogs to a number of specific anatomic abnormalities, such as stenotic nares, elongated soft palate, everted laryngeal saccules, collapsed larynx, and redundant pharyngeal mucosa, which contribute to the airway obstruction.

When a dyspneic brachycephalic dog is presented to the veterinarian, all possible abnormalities must be investigated. Except for evaluation of stenotic nares, general anesthesia is necessary to perform pharyngoscopy and laryngoscopy. Because recovery from anesthesia may be difficult for these patients, owners should be advised of the nature of the syndrome and should authorize any anesthesia and indicated surgical treatment at the time of evaluation. Tracheostomy may be indicated in severe cases, in order to allow examination of the pharynx and larynx without endotracheal intubation.

STENOTIC NARES

The external nares are formed by a cartilaginous skeleton, covered with skin externally and mucosa in the lumen. The cartilage plates are so shortened and so thick in some brachycephalic dogs that the nostril is almost obliterated (Fig. 17-1A). The obstruction is accentuated by collapse on inspiration. Surgically reducing the bulk of the lateral nasal cartilage creates a nostril of larger diameter. The greatest bulk of the cartilage is at the rostral tip; the more caudal portions of the nares are less restrictive. This type of obstruction can be corrected by resecting a tissue wedge from the tip of the lateral cartilages.

SURGICAL TECHNIQUE. Under general anesthesia, a wedge of approximately one-third to half of the lateral cartilage is excised from the rostral surface (Fig. 17-1B). The depth and width of tissue excised in the wedge vary according to individual requirement. Hemostasis is accomplished with direct pressure. When first incised, the nasal cartilage bleeds freely, but with gentle pressure and a few minute's time, hemorrhage is almost completely arrested. Topical or local use of vasoconstrictors is not necessary.

Suturing the defect opens the air passage and further arrests hemorrhage. Interrupted sutures of 4-0 polypropylene are placed about 2 to 3 mm apart (Fig. 17-1C). If the nostril has not been opened sufficiently, the sutures are removed, and additional tissue is excised. Most animals do not bother the incision after recovery, but suitable restraints such as leg bandages, hobbles, and collars should be applied if indicated. Sutures may be removed in approximately 10 days. The incision site

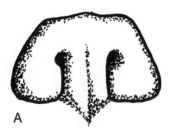 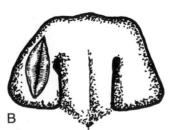 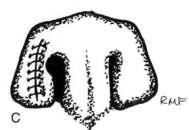

Fig. 17-1. A, *Stenotic nares.* B, *Wedge of tissue removed from lateral cartilage.* C, *Interrupted sutures to close the defect and to enlarge the naris.*

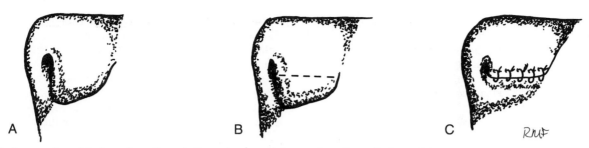

Fig. 17-2. *Amputation of the lateral cartilage. A, Lateral aspect of the nasal cartilages. B, Line of amputation across the distal extremity of the cartilage. C, Sutures placed across the incision to control hemorrhage.*

is usually depigmented at the time of suture removal. Pigment returns in 2 to 4 months in most cases.

If the nostril is obstructed to a greater depth, wedge resection may not be adequate. Amputation of the distal portion of the lateral wing gives relief, but is not always cosmetically pleasing (Fig. 17-2). Following amputation, direct pressure controls hemorrhage. If hemorrhage persists, simple interrupted or mattress sutures are effective.

ELONGATED SOFT PALATE

The soft palate partitions the oral pharynx from the nasal pharynx. It normally extends slightly caudal to the palatine tonsils, with the tip of the palate extending over the apex of the epiglottis. Brachycephalic dogs often have soft palates that extend into the laryngeal

glottis and interfere with the free passage of air from the mouth or nose into the larynx. Owing to the obstruction, increased inspiratory effort is required. This effort is accompanied by a stridulous noise as the palate vibrates and as the glottis opens and closes around the palate with the rapidly fluctuating pressure changes in the airway during inspiration. The palate responds to the turbulence and trauma by becoming thickened, edematous, inflamed, and thus even more obstructive.

DIAGNOSIS. An elongated soft palate is suspected in all brachycephalic dogs, but can only be diagnosed by inspection. After induction of general anesthesia, but prior to intubation, the mouth is held open and the pharynx is examined with a laryngoscope. A tongue depressor can be used to retract tissues to facilitate visualization of the area. The length and the presence

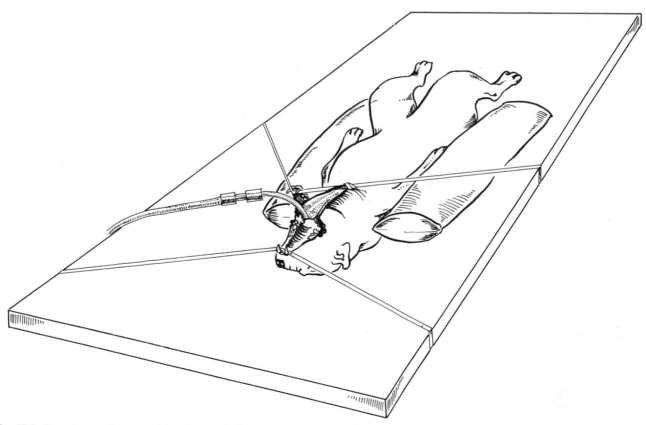

Fig. 17-3. *Dorsal recumbency position for surgical procedures of the palate.*

or absence of thickening and inflammation are evaluated. Familiarity with the normal situation can be gained while intubating patients that do not have airway obstructions. If the palate is grossly thickened and extends to the base of the epiglottis or further, it can be considered elongated. It is unusual to make a diagnosis of elongated soft palate if the palate is neither thickened nor inflamed.

SURGICAL TECHNIQUE. Soft palate resection should be performed with an oral endotracheal tube in place. The smallest size that allows adequate ventilation and protects the airway should be used to improve surgical access. The patient is positioned in dorsal recumbency (Fig. 17-3). Tape is passed over the upper canine teeth, to hold the maxilla parallel to the table. The mandible is held open maximally with another long piece of tape passed over the lower canine teeth and is secured to the sides of the table at about the level of the stifles. The endotracheal tube is brought out of the side of the mouth at the commissure of the lips and is secured against accidental displacement or kinking. If the tongue is dry, it may be drawn slightly rostrally and laterally and may be fixed to the adhesive tape holding the mandible. This position affords reasonable exposure of the oropharynx to a veterinary surgeon seated at the head of the table.

The tip of the soft palate is grasped with forceps and is drawn rostrally to fold the palate forward upon itself. Stay sutures are placed to each side of the tip, and the palate is now handled by the sutures (Fig. 17-4). The point at which to divide the palate is determined; one should remember that a palate that is left too long is far easier to correct than one that is too short. Usually, a point caudal to the palatine tonsil is selected, to place the new free edge at the tip of the epiglottis, with the larynx in its normal position.

For a right-handed veterinary surgeon, the division of the palate is started on the right lateral edge of the palate with curved tissue scissors. Approximately one-quarter to one-third the width of the palate is cut. Maintaining traction on the retention sutures allows visualization of the new edge. Bleeding is active from the incised tensor veli palatini muscle, but suturing of the incised edge establishes adequate hemostasis. Starting at the edge, a simple continuous suture is placed with 3-0 or 4-0 medium chromic gut on a tapered needle; this suture brings the nasal mucosa and oral mucosa into apposition over the edge of the muscle (Fig. 17-5). By maintaining slight tension on the suture, the adjacent edge may be visualized. As the divided segment is sutured, another interval of the palate is divided and is sutured until the elongated tip has been removed (Figs. 17-6 and 17-7). If no other laryngeal obstruction is present, the patient will be noticeably improved upon re-

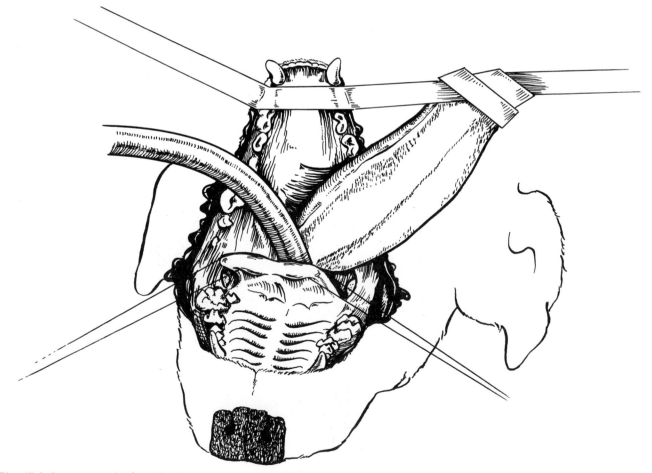

Fig. 17-4. *Stay sutures in the soft palate roll the tip rostrally.*

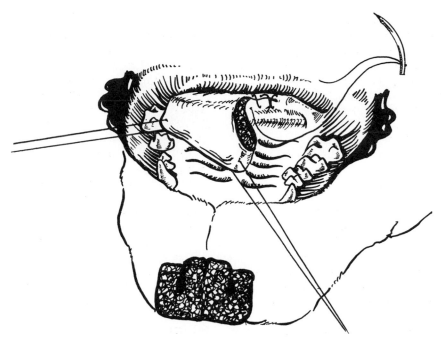

Fig. 17-5. *Palate resection is started with a partial incision, and a simple continuous suture opposes the mucosal layers and controls hemorrhage.*

covery. A single dose of intravenous corticosteroids may be given during the operation (dexamethasone 1 mg/kg), to help control postoperative edema.

The remaining components of the brachycephalic airway syndrome may occur with time; the following conditions are often secondary to the effects of chronic partial airway obstruction due to the conformation of the skull and stenotic nares or elongated palate.

EVERTING LARYNGEAL SACCULES

The laryngeal ventricle is a small pocket in the wall of the larynx lateral to the vocal fold. The entrance to the ventricle is bounded by the vocal and vestibular folds. Eversion of the mucosa of the ventricle is presumed to be a response to excessive negative pressure in the airway at the ventricular orifice that results from the increased inspiratory effort necessitated by

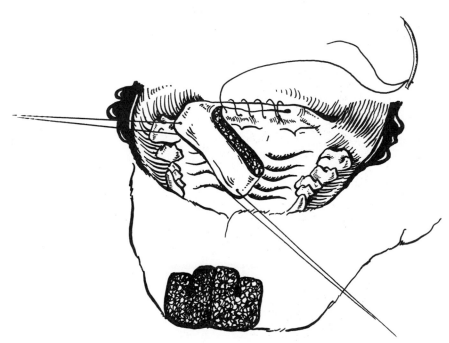

Fig. 17-6. *Incision and suturing are continued in sections across the palate.*

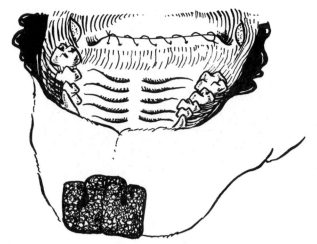

Fig. 17-7. *Resection and suturing of the palate is complete.*

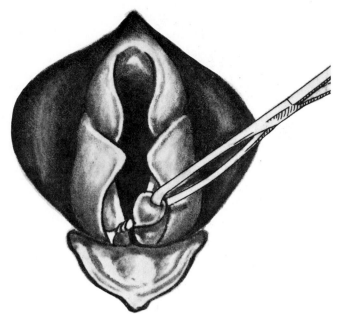

Fig. 17-9. *The everted saccule is grasped with a forcep and is twisted until it is avulsed.*

chronic partial airway obstruction. The mucosa, which becomes stretched and prolapses, contributes to further airway obstruction.

It is necessary to visualize the glottis in order to diagnose everted lateral saccules. Eversions appear as small, red, fleshy, pea-shaped masses in the ventral half of the glottis that obscure visualization of the vocal cords (Fig. 17-8).

SURGICAL TECHNIQUE. Removal is usually performed by the previously described oral approach, and the procedure is brief. Following ultrashort anesthetic induction, the everted saccule is grasped with forceps. Slight traction is exerted on the saccule, and the forceps are twisted until the saccule is avulsed (Fig. 17-9). Hemorrhage is minimal or absent in most cases. If the saccule cannot be adequately secured with forceps for traction and twisting, it is amputated at its base with forceps and narrow scissors. An endotracheal tube is placed

during recovery. The saccule may also be removed by a ventral laryngotomy incision with a tracheostomy tube in place if other laryngeal procedures are to be performed by that approach. Antibiotics and corticosteroids are usually not given.

LARYNGEAL COLLAPSE

The shape of the cartilages that form the boundary of the laryngeal orifice (rima glottidis) can change in response to chronically increased inspiratory effort. The cuneiform process of the arytenoid cartilage is the most commonly affected. Distortion and collapse of cartilage into the glottis causes luminal obstruction, stridor, and inspiratory effort. Turbulence and vibration irritate the mucosa, which becomes inflamed and edematous. The aryepiglottic fold is also weakened and is drawn into the glottis (Fig. 17-10). Collapse is seldom seen without eversion of the lateral ventricles. In chronic cases, distortion is so extreme that the corniculate processes also collapse. The net effect is an almost obliterated laryngeal orifice and a resulting severe respiratory dyspnea.

DIAGNOSIS. Laryngoscopic examination is necessary to identify the medially deviated cuneiform process(es) in the glottis. Because collapse is usually a secondary condition, the soft palate and nares should be critically evaluated.

SURGICAL TECHNIQUE. Partial laryngectomy of the collapsed cartilage and mucosa is performed by the oral approach. The procedure is similar to the oral ventriculocordectomy with an alligator-type cutting biopsy instrument. The instrument is passed and is placed with the fixed blade in the glottis and the moveable blade around the tissue to be excised. The instrument is used to remove the collapsed cuneiform process and

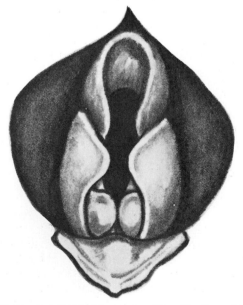

Fig. 17-8. *Everted laryngeal saccules. Visualization of the vocal cords is obscured.*

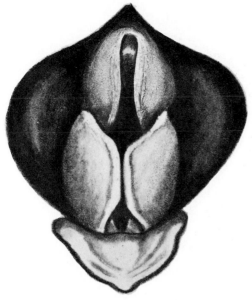

Fig. 17-10. *Obstruction of the glottis. The cuneiform processes of the arytenoid and aryepiglottic folds have collapsed medially.*

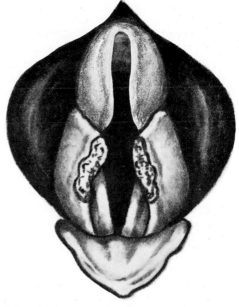

Fig. 17-12. *Partial laryngotomy allows an adequate airway.*

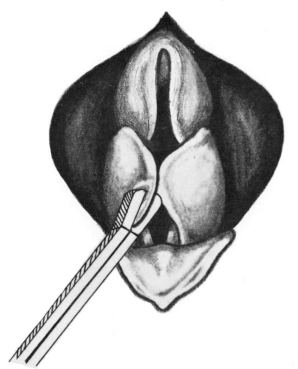

Fig. 17-11. *Biopsy forceps are used to excise pieces of the cuneiform process and the aryepiglottic fold.*

adjacent aryepiglottic fold (Fig. 17-11). Once an adequate airway is achieved, the resection is stopped (Fig. 17-12). Ventriculocordectomy can be done at the same time to enlarge the airway. Most patients usually maintain patency of the airway during recovery and postoperatively. These patients must be carefully supervised, and one should always be prepared to reanesthetize and intubate, or to perform a tracheostomy.

Smaller-breed brachycephalic dogs present special problems and are much more difficult to handle because the pharyngeal lumen is so small and crowded, even after elongated soft palate excision or removal of everted saccules. These patients should have a tracheostomy tube placed prior to the surgical procedure and maintained throughout the recovery and immediate postoperative period. Partial laryngotomy is performed as described previously, but restricted visibility and the friability of the pharyngeal and laryngeal tissues are limiting factors. Blood oozes profusely with the least trauma, and once a piece of laryngeal tissue is removed, ensuing hemorrhage obscures orientation and visualization. It is usually not possible to remove enough tissue to open the glottis adequately at one time. When a few pieces of tissue have been removed, structures are no longer identifiable; the procedure is terminated, and the animal recovers from the operation. The tracheostomy tube is maintained postoperatively as necessary. In 4 or 5 days, the procedure may be repeated. It may require 4 or 5 surgical episodes until as much tissue as practical is removed from the glottis. Antibiotics and corticosteroids are administered to these patients to alleviate laryngeal edema. (Dexamethasone, 1 to 2 mg/kg, is given intravenously at the beginning of the operation, and 0.5 to 1 mg/kg is repeated in 6 hours).

REDUNDANT PHARYNGEAL MUCOSA

Usually, the pharyngeal mucosa of brachycephalic dogs is thrown into shallow folds. Although the genesis of these folds is not currently known, it has been speculated that they are a secondary reflection either of the condensed airways or of the inspiratory stress and turbulence seen in these dogs. This phenomenon is accentuated in many dogs with marked dyspnea and with increased age and obesity. For whatever reason they occur, redundant mucosal folds occupy space in crowded air passages and may contribute to airway obstructions.

Redundant pharyngeal folds are diagnosed by inspection. Because of limited access to the pharynx, resection of these folds is not attempted. Treatment is directed toward ameliorating the inspiratory distress by correcting other components of the airway syndrome. Weight reduction may be of benefit.

Laryngeal Paralysis

Laryngeal paralysis may occur in any breed of dog and should be considered in the differential diagnosis in cases of inspiratory dyspnea, especially if a stridor is present. The Bouvier des Flandres inherits this defect as an autosomal dominant trait.

The recurrent laryngeal nerves lie along the dorsolateral edges of the trachea. Damage can occur to the nerves at any point along their path, from where they originate in the vagus in the thorax to where they enter the larynx. Practically all cases of canine laryngeal paralysis are of undetermined origin. The recurrent nerves innervate all the intrinsic laryngeal muscles except the cricothyroid muscle. Usually, owners report a change in the dog's bark preceding the onset of inspiratory dyspnea. The dorsal cricoarytenoid muscle is the only one that dilates the glottis; it is the paralysis of this muscle that causes the inspiratory dyspnea.

Direct visualization of the larynx is required. Anesthetic management during the examination is important. Anesthesia depresses spontaneous laryngeal motility, so the animal is given only enough short-acting barbiturate to allow visualization. The veterinarian watches the arytenoid cartilages and correlates the motion seen with the phase of respiration. In a normal,

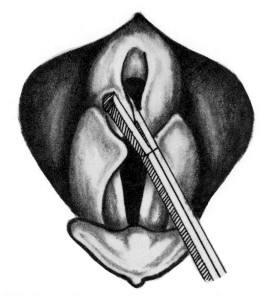

Fig. 17-14. *Biopsy forceps positioned on corniculate process.*

lightly anesthetized dog, the arytenoid cartilages spontaneously abduct during inspiration and widen the glottis. With laryngeal paralysis, the arytenoids and vocal folds are close to the midline between breaths. They adduct rather than abduct during inspiration, being drawn inward by the air stream; they abduct during expiration, being blown apart by the exhaled air stream. This pattern of motion of the arytenoid cartilages with laryngeal paralysis is passive and paradoxical. The paradoxical motion can be misinterpreted as spontaneous unless the examiner is careful about evaluating the phase of respiration. It is necessary to place one hand on the patient's chest and abdomen while watching the larynx or while an assistant calls out the inspirations.

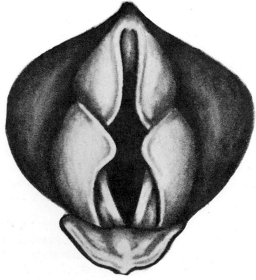

Fig. 17-13. *Narrow glottic fissure due to paralysis of dorsal cricoarytenoid muscle.*

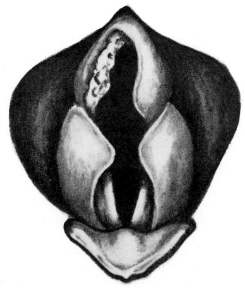

Fig. 17-15. *Glottic lumen enlarged by removal of corniculate process.*

SURGICAL TECHNIQUE. The surgical objective is to create a permanently larger glottis that will not be restrictive upon inspiration. At the same time, the veterinary surgeon is limited in the amount of tissue to be resected, so as to prevent aspiration from occurring during swallowing. Partial laryngotomy is performed through the oral cavity with biopsy forceps, as described for laryngeal collapse. The corniculate process of one arytenoid cartilage is removed (Figs. 17-13 to 17-15). Following this removal, the adequacy of the glottis is evaluated. If not satisfactory, the arytenoid cartilage is trimmed further. Both vocal cords are also removed (see Chap. 18). The glottis should now be adequate for normal activity. The opposite arytenoid cartilage is usually not disturbed for fear of causing aspiration. If the clinical results are not acceptable, the remaining arytenoid cartilage may be excised later.

References and Suggested Readings

Blackely, C. L.: Repair of nasal cartilage in dogs. North Am. Vet., *32*:628, 1951.

Bojrab, M. J. (ed.): Pathophysiology in Small Animal Surgery. Philadelphia, Lea & Febiger, 1981.

Christensen, G. C., and Toussaint, S.: Vasculature of external nares and related areas in the dog. J. Am. Vet. Med. Assoc., *13*:504, 1957.

Cook, W. R.: Observations on the upper respiratory tract of the dog and cat. J. Small Anim. Pract., *5*:309, 1964.

Leonard, H. C.: Collapse of the larynx and adjacent structures in the dog. J. Am. Vet. Med. Assoc., *137*:360, 1960.

Leonard, H. C.: Surgical relief for stenotic nares in a dog. J. Am. Vet. Med. Assoc., *128*: 530, 1956.

Trader, R. L.: Nose operation. J. Am. Vet. Med. Assoc., *114*:210, 1949.

Surgery of the Nasal Cavity and Sinuses

by COLIN E. HARVEY

Diagnosis of Nasal Disease

Confirmed diagnosis of the cause of chronic nasal disease is often difficult because the nasal mucosa and turbinate bones are confined within a rigid, bony case.

Aids to diagnosis include radiologic, microbiologic and serologic, cytologic, and histopathologic studies.

RADIOLOGIC STUDIES. Satisfactory nasal radiographs are obtained only under anesthesia because positioning and immobilization are critical to the production of diagnostic radiographs. Lateral, occlusal or open-mouth, and frontal-sinus-projection radiographs are made. Interpretation requires considerable care because of the fine bony detail of these structures and the differences among normal skulls of various shapes. Erosion of normal midline structures (nasal septum and vomer bone) or the external osseous shell of the nose is highly suggestive of nasal neoplasia. Areas of increased radiolucency in the nasal cavity suggest nasal fungal disease. Two recent reports of the inter-

pretation of nasal radiographs in the dog are listed in the references.

MICROBIOLOGIC TESTS. In my opinion, nasal bacterial cultures and sensitivity testing are rarely useful because the bacterial flora of the nose of a normal dog is so rich. Fungal culture is of more value, although up to 25% of samples taken from the nose of normal dogs in a veterinary hospital showed some growth on fungal media. False-negative results from fungal culture are common in dogs with nasal fungal disease. Staining of a smear of nasal discharge is a rapid technique that may show hyphal elements of fungi and is useful when examining cats suspected of having coccidioidomycosis. The agar gel diffusion test for serologic diagnosis of Aspergillus or Penicillium spp. infection is useful, whereas skin testing is unreliable.

CYTOLOGIC AND HISTOPATHOLOGIC EXAMINATION. Biopsy and cytologic or histopathologic examination of tissue are reliable if tissue representative of the disease is obtained. This criterion is not always easily met, however, owing to the remote location of lesions.

Several methods are available for obtaining a tissue specimen. If an external or oral mass is palpable, a limited incision and biopsy are usually satisfactory. A lesion may occasionally be visible by direct or indirect rhinoscopy, and resection of a specimen by biopsy forceps may then be possible. Vigorous flushing of the nasal passage with saline solution may provide sufficient tissue debris for biopsy. The patient is anesthetized and is provided with a well-inflated endotracheal cuff. The head should be kept below the level of the neck.

Blind biopsy, either by long-handled biopsy forceps inserted through the external naris or through a trephined opening in the frontal or maxillary bones, may also yield diagnostic tissue. The only certain way to obtain a diagnostic biopsy from the nasal cavity, however, is by nasal exploration and turbinectomy, exposing the lesion to direct vision.

OTHER DIAGNOSTIC AND PROGNOSTIC AIDS. Dogs that are presented to the veterinarian because of epistaxis occasionally are suffering from a coagulopathy or vascular disease rather than rhinitis or a nasal neoplasm. Thus, as a preliminary diagnostic step, a blood sample should be drawn for complete blood count and clotting profile.

The relationship between nasal fungal disease and the immune system is poorly understood. In dogs with suspected or confirmed nasal fungal disease, a blood sample may be sent for a lymphocyte transformation test prior to administering any drugs that affect the immune system. Dogs that show immunosuppression on the basis of this test respond poorly to treatment of the nasal fungal disease.

When prognosis of neoplastic disease is considered, thoracic radiographs are indicated. Intranasal tumors, however, regardless of cell type, rarely metastasize. The size and extent of local infiltration and histopathologic diagnosis are of more importance in assessing prognosis and therapy options.

Indications for Nasal Exploration

A nasal exploration procedure is indicated for: (1) diagnosis of intranasal disease not diagnosed by other means; and (2) resection of lesions, whether from trauma, turbinate necrosis, or foreign bodies, nasal fungal disease, idiopathic chronic rhinitis, or intranasal neoplasia (as a prelude to radiation therapy).

Surgical Technique for Nasal Exploration

The nose is richly supplied with blood vessels; hemorrhage may be massive if hemostatic measures are ignored. If the surgical procedure is to be performed unilaterally, ipsilateral ligation of the carotid artery is considered to reduce blood loss. No neurological complications result from this maneuver.

Preoperatively, a moist sponge is wrapped around the endotracheal tube in the pharynx, to prevent reflux of blood into the nasopharynx and the endotracheal cuff is appropriately inflated. The dog is placed in sternal recumbency, a sand bag is placed under the neck, and the head is secured in position with tape.

For either unilateral or bilateral surgical procedures, the skin incision is made on the midline from the caudal end of the cartilage of the external naris to the midpoint of the frontal bone (Fig. 17-16). Hemorrhage is controlled by clamping and ligation; then the incision is deepened through the periosteum of the midline by keeping the scalpel firmly pressed against the bone. Vessels cut during this maneuver are difficult to clamp, and hemorrhage is controlled by pressure. If the operation is bilateral, the periosteum is elevated intact from both dorsolateral bony surfaces of the nose. If the operation is unilateral, the periosteum is lifted for only 2 to 3 mm on the nonoperated side, so as to provide an edge for suturing.

To enter the nasal cavity, a rectangle of bone formed by parts of the nasal, maxillary, and frontal bones must be removed (Fig. 17-16). The preferred method is to use an oscillating bone saw to cut a clean bone flap on three sides (lateral, medial, and caudal), leaving it attached rostrally. This flap may be used in closing the rhinotomy if the bone is healthy. An alternate method is to enter the nasal cavity with a trephine or a Steinmann's pin mounted in a Jacob's chuck. The opening is then enlarged with a bone rongeur. The rhinotomy should be made as large as possible, compatible with the size of the skull.

Preferably, a finger should be able to palpate the interior of the nose during the operation. For unilateral nasal exploration, the medial bone incision is made lateral to the midline and is beveled laterally to avoid damaging the nasal septum. Although a unilateral bone flap is easy to elevate, a bilateral flap requires elevation of the bony midline septum of the frontal bone. The

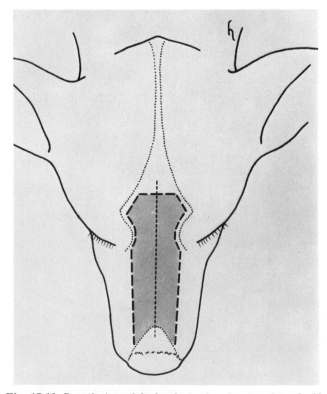

Fig. 17-16. *Dorsal view of the head of a dog showing the palpable bony landmarks (dotted line), maximum practical extent of surgical access to the nasal cavity and frontal sinuses (shaded area within long dashed line), and skin incision for nasal exploration (short dashed line).*

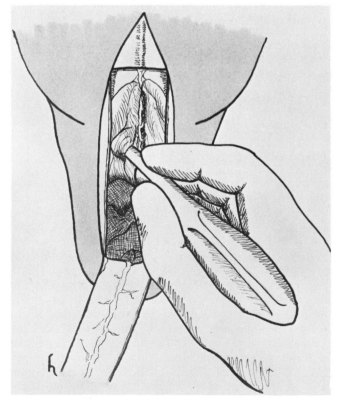

Fig. 17-17. *Nasal turbinectomy. A bilateral dorsal bone flap has been reflected rostrally, and the caudal turbinate bones are being curetted. A sponge is packed into the rostral end of the nasal cavity to achieve hemostasis.*

cartilages at the rostral end of the nose tether this area and provide resistance to elevation.

As the flap(s) is(are) raised, control of hemorrhage is of primary importance. Pressure from surgical sponges is usually sufficient for hemostasis. If the nasal cavity is mentally divided into two zones, rostral and caudal, one zone may be examined while the other zone is firmly packed with sponges (Fig. 17-17). Unless the lesion is immediately visible and is confined to the dorsal aspect of the nasal cavity (that would be unusual), the entire turbinate system should be removed. If the operation is bilateral, the cartilaginous nasal septum would be included. The turbinate bones are extirpated by avulsion and curettage. At the attachment to the rostral cartilages of the nose, the turbinate bones are severed with strong surgical scissors. The surgical procedure proceeds gradually deeper, by alternating curetting and packing, until the palatine bone is reached (Figs. 17-18 and 17-19).

The nasofrontal opening is effectively enlarged by removing the ectoturbinate scrolls that project into the frontal sinuses (Fig. 17-20). Simultaneous exploration of the frontal sinus and nasal cavity is also possible. The maxillary sinus recess is also curretted. At this point, the sphenopalatine artery may be visible on the lateral floor of the nasal cavity (see Fig. 17-18). It is sometimes possible to clamp and to ligate this vessel. The nasopharynegeal meatus, or nasopharynx, if the operation is bilateral, may be palpated by sliding caudally along the palatine bone. Any tags of tissue or bony projections should be removed to avoid obstruction (see Fig. 17-19). The ethmoturbinate bones are curetted by reaching caudally into the nasopharyngeal meatus and then curetting with an upward stroke. Curetting forcefully in a caudal direction is avoided, however, so that the cribiform plate is not penetrated (see Fig. 17-18). When resection of mucosa and turbinate bones are completed, the extent of any continuing hemorrhage is assessed. Pooling of blood that covers the palate surface within one minute indicates active bleeding and requires further packing.

In most dogs, it is unnecessary to leave a gauze pack in the nasal cavity postoperatively. If active bleeding does not cease with short-term intraoperative packing, however, a large surgical sponge is unfolded to form a long, thin pack. This sponge is then pulled through the external naris, to make sure that it can be removed by that route. It is then packed into the nasal cavity and is arranged in the cavity recesses in an accordian-pleated pattern to facilitate removal. The placement of a tube through the skin and outer table of the frontal bone into the nasal cavity is useful for delivering medication directly into the nasal cavity of dogs with nasal fungal infections and reduces postoperative subcutaneous emphysema (Fig. 17-21). Intravenous tubing is of appropriate size and stiffness. A butterfly of adhesive

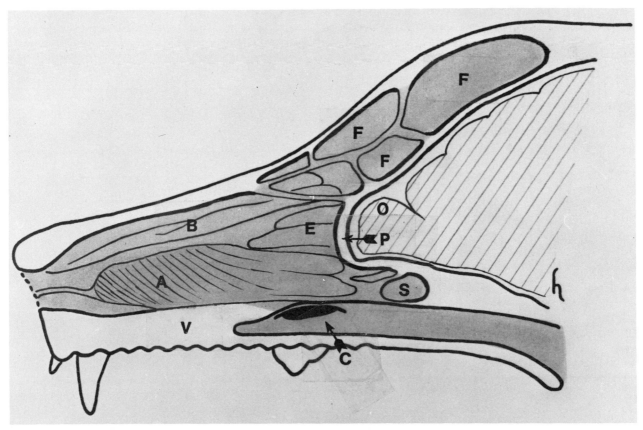

Fig. 17-18. *Section of the head of a dog just lateral to the midline. The nasal cavity, paranasal sinuses, and nasopharynx are shaded. A and B, Ventral and dorsal nasal concha; C, choana; E, ethmoidal concha; F, frontal sinus space; O, olfactory lobe of brain; P, cribriform plate; S, sphenoidal sinus; V, vomer bone.*

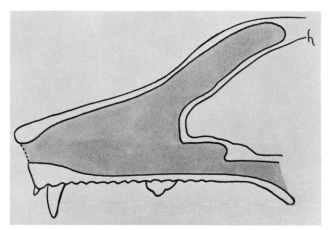

Fig. 17-19. *Section of the head of a dog showing the extent of the cleared out nasal and paranasal sinus spaces (shaded area) following complete bilateral nasal turbinectomy. Note that the entire vomer bone has been resected.*

tape on the tube is sutured to the skin (Fig. 17-21).

The wound is closed by replacing the bone flap and by attaching it to the skull with 2 or 3 sutures of 28-gauge surgical wire through holes made with Kirschner wires. The periosteum does not usually have enough elasticity to be easily sutured, but the periosteal edges may be apposed by placing surgical gut sutures through the connective tissue immediately adjacent to the periosteum. There is usually room for subcutaneous-subdermal sutures to buttress the periosteal closure. Skin sutures are placed in a routine manner.

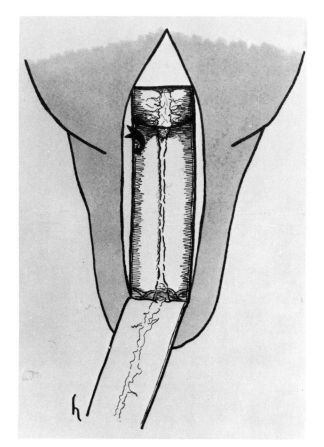

Fig. 17-20. *View of the nasal cavity of a dog at the completion of bilateral turbinectomy. The cribriform plate covered by remnants of the ethmoturbinate bones and the base of the midline septum and vomer bone insertion are visible. The arrow indicates the location of the right sphenopalatine artery on the floor of the nasal chamber.*

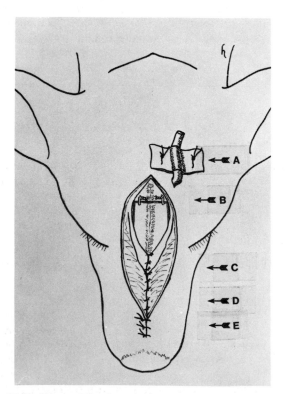

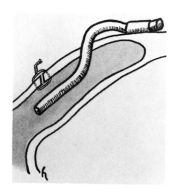

Fig. 17-21. *Closure following nasal exploration. A, Tube inserted into the frontal sinus and held in place by skin sutures placed through a butterfly of adhesive tape; B, wire sutures hold bone flap in place; C, sutures in periosteum; D, sutures in connective tissue buttressing the periosteal closure; E, skin sutures. Inset, Location of tube placed into frontal sinus.*

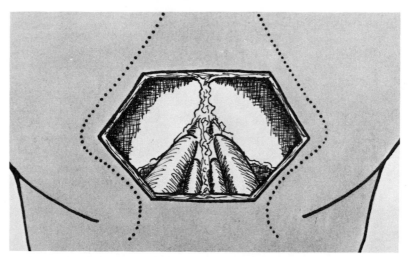

Fig. 17-22. *Dorsal view of the contents of the frontal sinuses following resection of a bilateral bone flap. The ectoturbinates of the ethmoidal conchae partially occlude the nasofrontal openings.*

Postoperative Care

Dogs tolerate turbinectomy well, but the long-term prognosis usually depends on the diagnosis and the extent of disease rather than on surgical factors.

Postoperative care includes the following: (1) observation for continued hemorrhage, including blood that may be swallowed; mucous membrane color and pulse rate and strength should be monitored; (2) removal of intranasal packing within 24 hours of the operation; and (3) removal of the frontal sinus tube 48 hours postoperatively, or at 10 to 14 days if it is being used to instill antifungal medication.

Subcutaneous emphysema may occur postoperatively and results from positive expiration against obstructed external nares. This complication is more likely to occur if a gauze pack has been left in the nose or if the turbinate bones have not been adequately removed from the rostral nasal cartilages. The emphysema is of no functional importance, although the owner may be distressed by the appearance of the dog. No treatment is necessary.

Serosanguinous discharge from the external nares may occur for 2 to 3 weeks. Excoriation of the rhinarium (nasal plane) can be reduced or prevented by gently washing the rhinarium with water and by using petroleum jelly on the area twice a day.

Frontal Sinus Exploration and Nasal Flushing

Occasionally disease is radiographically restricted to a dog's frontal sinuses. The frontal sinuses can be explored through a skin incision directly over the sinus, extended through the subcutaneous tissues and periosteum. A periosteal elevator is used to strip the periosteum, and the outer table of the frontal bone is removed with a bone saw, trephine, or Steinmann's pin and rongeurs. The internal bony pillars and baffles of the frontal sinus are resected, and abnormal mucosa is removed with a curette. The nasofrontal opening is enlarged by resecting the ectoturbinates that extend into the frontal sinus to promote drainage (Figs. 17-20 and 17-22). The nasal cavity is then flushed vigorously with saline solution to ensure patency of the nasal passages. A medication tube may be placed as previously described. The periosteum is apposed by suturing the adjacent connective tissue, and subcutaneous and skin sutures are placed.

This procedure has been described for the treatment of chronic rhinitis and sinusitis of cats, but it is of little long-term value. More satisfactory results are obtained by nasal exploration and turbinectomy, although postoperative nasal discharge may continue for a month or more.

References and Suggested Readings

Gibbs, C., et. al.: Radiological features of intranasal lesions in the dog. J. Small Anim. Pract., *20*:515, 1979.

Harvey, C. E., et. al.: Chronic nasal disease in the dog— radiographic diagnosis. Vet. Radiol., *20*:91, 1979.

O'Brien, J. A., and Harvey, C. E.: The upper airway. *In* Textbook of Veterinary Internal Medicine: Diseases of the Dog and Cat. Edited by S. J. Ettinger. Philadelphia, W. B. Saunders, 1975.

Surgical Treatment of Chronic Sinusitis in the Cat Using Autogenous Fat Implants

by Ronald M. Bright

Primary frontal sinusitis in the cat is rare; however, its occurrence secondary to rhinitis is common. Although the cause of rhinitis in cats can be either viral, bacterial, or mycotic, the most common cause of rhinitis is viral. The two primary pathogens are feline calicivirus (FCV) and feline rhinotracheitis virus (FVR).[1,2] The damage these viruses do to the mucosal and osseous portions of the nasal turbinate bones allows bacteria to "homestead." Secondary bacterial infection with some of the more common micro-organisms, such as streptococci, staphylococci, pasteurella, and Escherichia coli, may result.[2]

The sinus involvement that follows rhinitis results from a direct extension into the frontal sinus or from the obstruction of the nasofrontal duct draining the mucous secretions of the frontal sinus. This collection of secretions can produce a mucocele and, in some instances, may result in a bony deformity of the overlying frontal bones. Bacterial proliferation is enhanced by the medium provided by these trapped secretions and causes a chronic bacterial sinusitis.

Most rhinitis and sinusitis conditions are seen by the veterinarian in the acute stages and are successfully treated by conservative management. The acute disorder sometimes becomes chronic sinusitis, however.

When antimicrobial therapy is unsuccessful and the response to other therapy is unsatisfactory, surgical drainage is indicated. This allows not only drainage, but also irrigation of the frontal sinuses. Any accompanying rhinitis should always be treated concomitantly. In chronic forms of rhinitis, partial or complete turbinectomy may be necessary to achieve a final cure.

When rhinitis appears to have subsided, a periodic mucopurulent nasal exudate may still be seen, as well as occasional sneezing episodes. These signs may herald a chronic frontal sinusitis that has persisted in spite of surgical drainage of the sinuses. I have finally achieved a cure in some patients by the successful use of autogenous fat implanted into the sinus cavity(ies).

Various types of autogenous grafts and prosthetic materials have been implanted into the feline frontal sinus in an attempt to obliterate it. Osseous implants, Gelfoam, and plastic materials have been used, but none have been as successful as adipose tissue in consistently obliterating the sinuses.[3,4] The sinus cavity is obliterated satisfactorily as long as meticulous care is taken to remove the mucous membrane and periosteum lining the frontal sinus(es).[3,4,5] The purpose of mucoperiosteal obliteration is to prevent regrowth or hyperplasia of mucous membrane or the extension of the mucous membrane into the sinus from the nasofrontal area. Prevention of osteoneogenesis is also an aim of adipose tissue obliteration because osteoneogenesis into this area may compartmentalize the frontal sinus and may preclude full obliteration.

Surgical Anatomy

The sinuses of the cat can be described as diverticula of the nasal cavity. A cat has both frontal and sphenoid sinuses, the latter being of little clinical importance. In the Persian and similar brachycephalic cat breeds, the frontal sinus is small and even absent in some instances. In the dog, the ethmoturbinate scrolls usually extend into the frontal sinus; however, this extension is not seen in the cat (Fig. 17-23). Each sinus is well separated from its corresponding nasal fossa and is connected only by means of a single narrow ostium that empties into the ethmoid region of the nasal cavity.

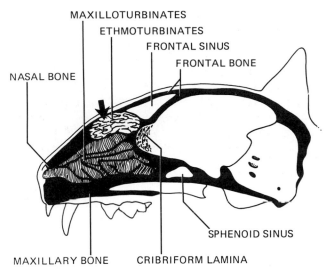

Fig. 17-23. *The ethmoturbinate bones (arrow) are not intimately associated with the frontal sinuses in the cat. No further compartmentalization is seen in the frontal sinuses of cats.*

Although a median septum separates the right and left frontal sinuses, no further division of each frontal sinus into cranial and caudal compartments occurs, as seen in the dog (Fig. 17-23). The lining of the sinus is thinner than that of the nasal cavity; the epithelium is ciliated, with streams driving toward the ostium. Removal of this mucosal lining plays an important part in ensuring the success of this procedure.[4,5]

Surgical Technique

The cat is anesthetized and is placed initially in dorsal recumbency. A short caudoventral midline incision is made, and the skin is reflected to allow the gentle harvesting of fat from the subcutaneous tissue. Sharp dissection with a scapel blade minimizes trauma. The fat is wrapped in gauze and is placed in warm saline

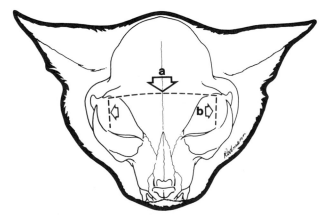

Fig. 17-24. *Halfway between the lateral canthus of each eye and the medial attachment of the pinna marks the point (a, large arrow) where a transverse incision should initially be made. The incision should extend laterally as far as the lateral canthus of each eye. From the lateral edge of this initial incision (b, small arrows), two small incisions are now made rostrally extending approximately 1.0 to 1.5 cm.*

solution. Routine closure of the abdominal wound is performed. The cat is then placed in sternal recumbency, with the head propped up on a sand bag. The head is secured in position with adhesive tape.

To locate the incision site, an imaginary line is drawn between the medial attachment of the pinna of the ear and the lateral canthus of the eye. This line is bisected with a transverse incision through the skin, extending laterally as far as the lateral canthus of each eye (Fig. 17-24). From the edge of this transverse incision, two additional incisions are made, each about 1 cm in length and extending rostrally (Fig. 17-24). The skin flap created is now reflected rostrally to expose the rim of the bony orbit, which occupies much of the feline skull (Fig. 17-25). Retraction of the skin can be maintained using a Weitlander retractor.

The periosteum is now incised transversely, directly in line with the original skin incision, but extending laterally only as far as a line drawn through the approximate center of each eye (Fig. 17-25). Two additional periosteal incisions are made, each parallel to the midline and extending forward approximately 1.00 to 1.25 cm. The periosteum is undermined and is retracted with a periosteal elevator. An osteotome or an oscillating saw can be used to make beveled cuts through the bone over the periosteal incision (Fig. 17-25). Another

transverse incision through the periosteum is now made parallel to the caudal transverse bony incision, to join the two rostrocaudal incisions. The bone along this incision, however, is only scored so that it can remain attached following the elevation of the bone flap (Fig. 17-26). This bony flap can be reflected rostrally once the medial septum of the sinus is cut with an osteotome or a small rongeur. Should the bone flap become detached, this presents no problem because it will fit snugly into the defect and may be held in place by the periosteum, subcutaneous tissue, and skin once the wound has been closed.

Following the rostral reflection of the bony flap, the mucosal lining is stripped free using forceps. To enhance the complete removal of the mucous membrane, a binocular dissecting microscope or ophthalmic head loupe should be used. This part of the procedure is tedious and should be done meticulously. A high-speed air drill with a bur tip should now be carefully used to remove the periosteum from the same surfaces that the mucous membrane was covering (Fig. 17-26). It is important that the underneath surface of the retracted bone flap is similarly freed of its mucosal lining and periosteum.

A rich blood supply is exposed following the removal of the periosteum. This exposure is important if the fat transplant is to maintain its viability. Prior to placing the fat into the sinuses, a small piece of temporalis muscle fascia is harvested and is placed into each nasofrontal ostium leading to the corresponding nasal fossa. This procedure should be done with care because it is most important to the success of this operation that there be no remaining communication with

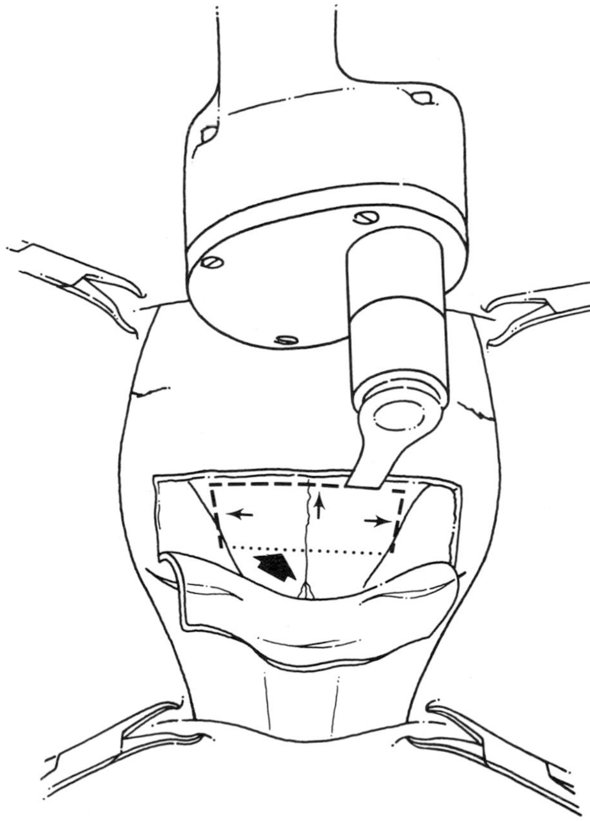

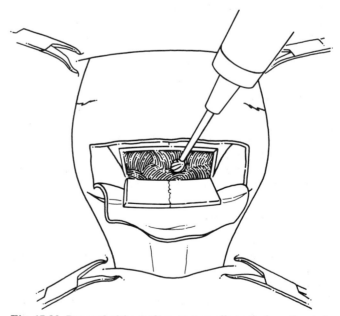

Fig. 17-25. *The skin and subcutaneous tissue are reflected rostrally exposing the frontal bone and bony rim of the orbit. Periosteal incisions are made as depicted, and the periosteum is elevated and reflected (see text). An oscillating saw or osteotome is used to cut a full-thickness bone flap (dashed line). The front edge is only scored so that the bone flap will remain attached (dotted line).*

Fig. 17-26. *Removal of the median septum allows the bone flap to be reflected rostrally. Following the meticulous removal of the mucous membrane lining the surfaces of the sinus cavities and the bone flap, a high-speed bur is used to remove the periosteal covering. A small piece of temporalis muscle fascia is harvested and is placed in the nasofrontal opening.*

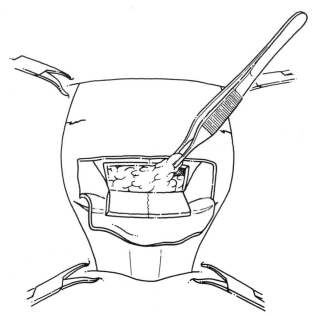

Fig. 17-27. *Fat is now gently placed in the frontal sinuses. A sufficient amount of fat is used to obliterate the sinuses; too much fat prevents the proper replacement of the bone flap.*

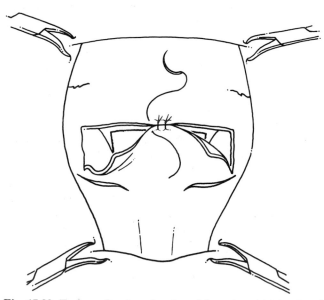

Fig. 17-28. *The bone flap is replaced, and the outer periosteum and subcutaneous tissue is sutured over it. The skin is closed from the midline laterally.*

the nasal cavity. This helps prevent the regeneration and possible migration of the mucous membrane from the ethmoid region of the nasal cavity into the frontal sinuses. The fat is now gently placed into each sinus, and one must take care to push portions of this fat into the crevices of the cavity (Fig. 17-27). Once the fat is in place, the bone flap is replaced. This replacement should be easily accomplished, with only a small amount of resistance offered by the fat. The outer periosteum, along with the fascia and subcutaneous tissue, is closed using 4-0 gut in a simple continuous suture pattern. The skin is closed using 4-0 nylon or polypropylene in a simple interrupted pattern, starting at the middle and working toward the edges (Fig. 17-28).

The postoperative period is generally uneventful except for occasional periods of sneezing.

Comment

1. This procedure should only be used in those patients that have failed to respond to the more traditional forms of medical and surgical therapy.

2. The most important part of the procedure is the complete removal of the mucosal lining and the complete obliteration of the sinuses with at least 95% viable adipose tissue.

3. Handling of the fat should be gentle during the harvesting period and when it is placed into the sinuses, to ensure maximum viability.

4. Even if a certain percentage of fat does not survive, as long as it is adequately replaced by fibrous tissue it will generally maintain a complete obliteration, and the animal most likely will be clinically free of frontal sinus disease.

References and Suggested Readings

1. Bright, R. M.: Nasal foreign bodies, tumors, and rhinitis/sinusitis. *In* Pathophysiology in Small Animal Surgery. Edited by M. J. Bojrab. Philadelphia, Lea & Febiger, 1981.

2. Lane, J. G.: Rhinitis and sinusitis in the cat. *In* Textbook of Veterinary Internal Medicine: Diseases of the Dog and Cat. Edited by S. J. Ettinger. Philadelphia, W. B. Saunders, 1976.

3. Montgomery, W. W.: The fate of adipose implants in a bony cavity. Laryngoscope, *74*:816, 1964.

4. Schenck, W. L.: Frontal sinus disease, III. Experimental and clinical features in failure of the frontal osteoplastic operation. Laryngoscope, *85*:76, 1975.

5. Tomlinson, M. J., et al.: Autogenous fat implantation as a treatment for chronic sinusitis in a cat. J. Am. Vet. Med. Assoc., *167*:927, 1975.

18 * Larynx

Devocalization Procedures

by KENNETH KAGAN

Pet owners may request devocalization for a particularly noisy and annoying animal. Barking sounds are produced by vibrations of the laryngeal folds in an expired air column. The vocal fold is a mucosal reflection along the inner surface of the lateral laryngeal wall. The fold contains the vocal ligament and the vocalis muscle. It also forms the medial boundary of the laryngeal ventricle. Devocalization procedures involve total or subtotal resection of the vocal fold performed by an oral or a ventral cervical approach.

Oral Ventriculocordectomy

Anesthesia is induced and is maintained with short-acting barbiturates administered intravenously. No endotracheal tube is used. The animal is positioned in ventral recumbency. The mouth is held open with a dental speculum, the head is extended, and the tongue is drawn forward to allow visualization of the larynx. The soft palate is elevated with an instrument, and the epiglottis is depressed with a laryngoscope to allow best visualization of the glottis. Alligator-action biopsy forceps* are used to remove part of the vocal fold. The instrument is placed over the vocal fold with the movable blade in the ventricle and the larger stationary blade in the laryngeal lumen. The forcep jaws are positioned over the vocal cord at a point one-quarter the length of the cord dorsal to the ventral midline (Fig. 18-1A and B). The forcep jaws are closed, and the piece of tissue is removed. The remainder of the vocal cord dorsal to the initial "bite" is removed as completely as possible (Fig. 18-1C). It is important to excise a sufficient amount of the vocal fold, including some of the vocalis muscle as well as the vocal ligament. If the excision is too shallow, the defect may fill quickly with scar tissue. Hemorrhage, which usually consists of free oozing from the cut surfaces or small vessels, can be controlled with direct pressure. A small sponge grasped in the jaws of the forceps is applied against the area.

*Such as Yeomans rectal biopsy forceps or Kevorkian-Younge uterine biopsy forceps, American V. Mueller, 6600 West Touhy Avenue, Chicago, IL 60648

Care must be taken to prevent aspiration of blood. Positioning the patient in a head-down posture so that blood flows away from the airway is effective. After satisfactory removal of the first vocal fold, the opposite fold is removed in a similar manner.

The ventral quarter of each vocal cord is not removed (Fig. 18-1D). It is important not to carry the resection to the ventral midline, where the folds meet, because it is impossible to excise the folds completely without leaving tags of tissue and small clots that would be a framework for scar formation across the glottis. Such scarring predisposes a patient to formation of a fibrous web that could create a functional stricture of the laryngeal opening.

When performing an oral ventriculocordectomy, the veterinarian is not completely in command of the situation. For example, the tissues are not close at hand for easy manipulation, and visibility is poor. Adequate illumination of the surgical field is difficult, and as soon as an attempt is made to use more than one instrument, the combination of instruments and hands reduces the visibility further. To control hemorrhage, more objects are brought into the surgical field, and the cycle escalates. The only way to protect the airway—to lower the patient's head—complicates visualization. A tracheotomy would protect the airway, but would negate the advantages of the oral approach, that is, speed and limited surgical incision and dissection.

Ventral Ventriculocordectomy

The procedure using the ventral approach is performed following anesthetic induction and intubation. The endotracheal tube selected is smaller than usual, but is still adequate to protect the airway and yet allow surgical manipulation in the larynx. Using the slightly smaller endotracheal tube allows removal of the vocal cord without removing the tube.

The patient is positioned in dorsal recumbency, and a small wedge is placed under the neck to extend it. The skin and subcutaneous tissues are divided in the midline directly over the hyoid bone, larynx, and cranial trachea. The sternohyoid muscles are exposed, and the two muscle bellies are separated to reveal the larynx. When dividing the two muscles, care must be

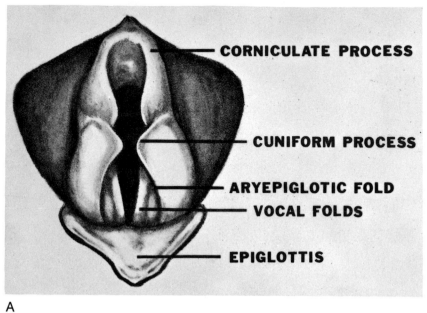

CORNICULATE PROCESS

CUNIFORM PROCESS

ARYEPIGLOTIC FOLD
VOCAL FOLDS

EPIGLOTTIS

A

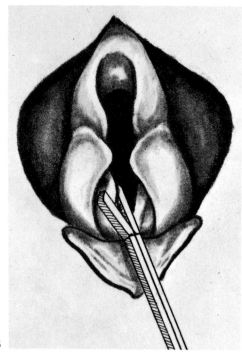

B

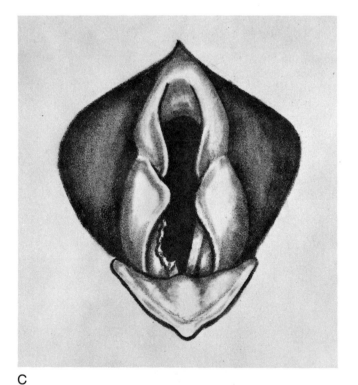

C

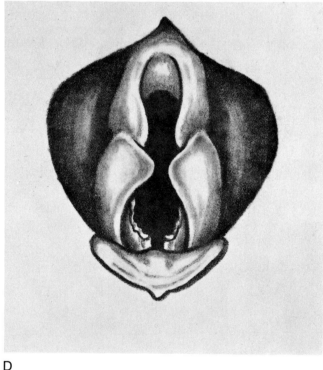

D

Fig. 18-1. A, *Oral view of glottis.* B, *Biopsy forceps on right vocal cord, fixed blade in laryngeal lumen.* C, *Cord removed except ventral quarter.* D, *Bilateral ventriculocordectomy, showing remaining ventral quarter of each cord.*

taken not to damage the hyoid venous arch. The laryngeal cartilages and the cricothyroid ligament are identified (Fig. 18-2).

The larynx is entered with a stab incision through the cricothyroid ligament. The blade should pass through the membrane and the laryngeal mucosa into lumen. The incision is carried cranially through about half the thyroid cartilage. Staying on the midline minimizes hemorrhage. The edges of the laryngotomy are separated with small retractors (spay hooks work well), and the incision is carried further cranially if necessary to expose the vocal folds (Fig. 18-3A). The base of the vocal fold is grasped with forceps, and the tip of one scissor blade is passed into the ventricle. By main-

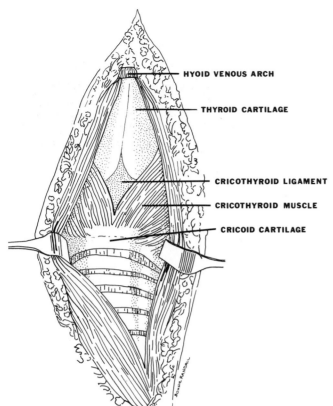

Fig. 18-2. *Ventral approach to larynx.*

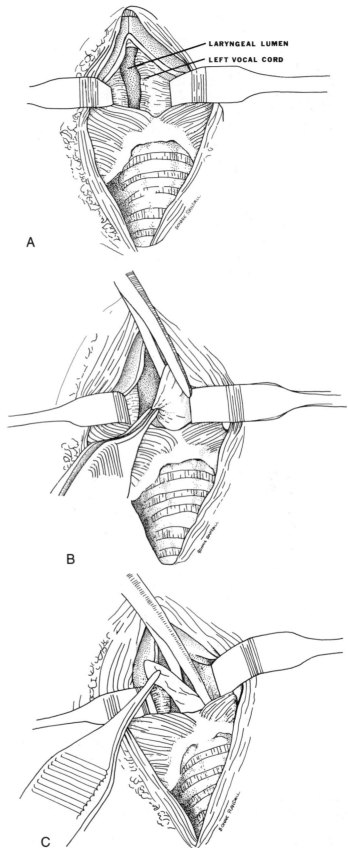

Fig. 18-3. A, *Ventral laryngotomy exposing the ventral attachment of the vocal cords. B and C, left cord grasped with forceps to facilitate trimming with scissors.*

taining traction on the fold with the forceps, the scissors may then be used to excise the vocal fold (Fig. 18-3B and C).

The vocal cord is removed completely, leaving no tags that might form adhesions or a web. Hemostasis may be achieved with direct pressure, forceps, ligatures, electrocoagulation, or Hemoclips. When hemostasis has been achieved, the laryngotomy incision is closed with interrupted sutures. Two or three interrupted sutures of 4-0 or 3-0 monofilament stainless steel are preplaced in the thyroid cartilage. The cricothyroid ligament is closed with interrupted sutures of stainless steel or polypropylene placed in the ligament, but not passing through the laryngeal mucosa. The remainder of the closure is routine.

Postoperative Care

Postoperatively, the patient is monitored closely until fully recovered. An intravenous catheter should be maintained, so that if the animal experiences any airway obstruction or hemorrhage, it can be reanesthetized to allow aspiration or reintubation. The animal is kept in a head-down posture until it starts to move around. Corticosteroids and antibiotics are not normally administered to healthy animals.

Some "voice" return can be expected after ventriculocordectomy, but the chances are greater when the oral approach is used. The ventral approach has given me more consistent and satisfactory results. Long-term complications include stricture or webbing of the glottis and are difficult to correct because strictures often recur after successive operations. If strictures are encountered, repetitive bougienage has been the most effective treatment.

Owners who request "debarking" should be advised of the possible complications. The veterinarian must be certain that clients understand the risks and limitations of the procedure before undertaking the operation.

References and Suggested Readings

Marlow, J. B.: Techniques for devocalizing small animals (a review). VM SAC, 66:129, 1971.

Palumbo, N. E., et al.: A technique for feline ventriculocordectomy. VM SAC, 60:921, 1965.

19 * Trachea

Collapsed Trachea

by Tommy L. Walker *and* H. Phil Hobson

The canine trachea is a flexible, tubular organ containing 35 to 45 semicircular hyaline cartilages and lined with a ciliated respiratory mucosa. The interannular ligaments connecting each cartilage provide an open lumen whose width is regulated by the action of the transverse trachealis muscle.[1,5] When flattening of the tracheal cartilages occurs because of a weakened, flaccid trachealis muscle, the trachea assumes a lunate configuration that severely compromises the lumen dorsoventrally (Fig. 19-1). The deformity results in the collapsed trachea syndrome most commonly reported in the toy breeds of dogs such as Chihuahuas, Pomeranians, toy poodles, and Yorkshire terriers, but occasionally seen in other breeds.[6,18]

A congenital collapsed trachea has been reported with a shallow malformation of the tracheal rings occurring at the thoracic inlet.[10] Most cases are initially seen in middle-aged to older dogs, however, as an acquired lesion in which the tracheal rings have not lost potential lumen diameter, but rather have lost their ability to remain firm. Subsequently, such affected tracheal segments collapse dorsoventrally.[8]

The origin of the collapsed trachea syndrome is unknown. One investigator considered the essential lesion to be the removal of organic matrix from the cartilage. It was thought that this disorder was congenital in origin, but required the presence of concurrent lung disease as a triggering factor before clinical signs developed.[6,7] Another study indicated a neurologic deficiency to the trachealis muscle as a primary cause of the syndrome.[9]

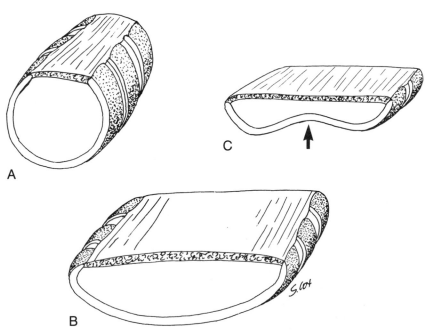

Fig. 19-1. *Schematic diagram of the trachea in a normal configuration (A), in dorsoventral collapse (B), and in a state in which the cartilaginous ring has inverted into the lumen (C). Inverted rings require partial chondrotomy at their central point (arrow) to conform to the prosthetic ring.*

Pathophysiologic Features

Many patients with collapsed trachea are asymptomatic and are able to move enough air through the narrow tracheal lumen to prevent dyspnea. When the tracheal collapse becomes clinically significant, it has been described as a "respiratory distress syndrome."[17] The affected dog is presented to the veterinarian with a long history of a harsh, dry cough producing a "goose honk" sound. This cough is easily initiated by any pressure, such as from a leash or from palpation, on the already small tracheal lumen and may become life-threatening as the dynamics of airflow through the upper conducting airways are compromised.[8]

Normally, air moves through the trachea with ease because of its open, unobstructed lumen. During inspiration, negative intrapleural pressure expands the intrathoracic airway lumen and balloons the thoracic trachea while the cervical trachea collapses. When a flaccid, collapsed cervical trachea is present, *inspiratory* dyspnea results. Upon expiration, the positive intrapleural pressure narrows the *intrathoracic* trachea while air passively moves through the cervical portion. When a collapsed intrathoracic trachea is present, air is unable to exit the lung on expiration; this situation results in a forced expiration and a "honking" cough. When both the cervical and thoracic portions of the trachea are involved, expiratory dyspnea becomes clinically predominant. Therefore, any increased physical exertion or accompanying cardiac or pulmonary disease that increases inspiratory or expiratory effort may decompensate the animal with a subclinically collapsed trachea and may lead to the clinical syndrome.[11,18]

Diagnosis

Palpation of the cervical trachea reveals weak, flaccid tracheal rings with a lumen that may be easily occluded. Slight pressure on the dorsal trachealis muscle often produces paroxysmal coughing and may completely obliterate the tracheal lumen. The caudal cervical trachea is most often noted to be wide and flattened, allowing the examiner to palpate the ends of the tracheal rings in many cases.

Radiography is the most frequently used diagnostic technique. Lateral radiographs of a collapsed trachea generally show a narrow or distorted tracheal shadow. Exposures taken during both inspiration and expiration are required to determine whether cervical, thoracic, or both areas of the trachea are involved. Dorsal flexion of the neck accentuates collapse at the thoracic inlet. Because tracheal collapse is dynamic in its location on inspiration and expiration, it is common for radiographs to depict an abnormal section of trachea as normal; that is, the cervical trachea is collapsed on inspiration, but ballooned on expiration. For this reason, fluoroscopic motion studies are most useful in locating all the affected areas. The extent and location of collapse are especially important when prognosis and treatment are evaluated.[3,8]

A definitive diagnosis may be obtained when a tracheoscopic examination is performed under general anesthesia while constant oxygenation is provided through the instrument. A bronchoscope is passed to the tracheal bifurcation and is slowly withdrawn as the veterinarian watches for flaccid dorsal musculature. The extent of cervical or thoracic collapse may thus be evaluated. This technique also allows for culturing of the tracheal mucosa, particularly when long-term tracheal infections are suspected.[3]

The list of differential diagnoses for tracheal collapse mimics the list of potential concurrent diagnoses. Such conditions as tonsillitis, laryngeal paresis or paralysis, stenotic nares, eversion of the lateral ventricles, elongation of the soft palate, tracheitis, bronchitis, and pneumonia may aggravate tracheal collapse or may cause dyspnea themselves. Decompensated mitral valvular disease and other cardiovascular diseases require consideration to determine their role in the suspected tracheal collapse. Marked hepatomegaly is an example of a concurrent metabolic problem reported in patients with collapsed trachea.[8] Congenital tracheal hypoplasia should also be considered in the differential diagnosis, when applicable.[3]

In most mild cases, treatment of the concurrent conditions results in a compensated, subclinical state of tracheal collapse. Dietary management of the obese patient should be established. Animals periodically requiring antitussives or tranquilizers during peak periods of anxiety or excitement generally do not require surgical correction. In cases of deep intrathoracic or thoracic bifurcation collapse, postsurgical improvement may be limited. Mitigating pathologic factors throughout the bronchial tree may persist even after attempted surgical correction of the collapsed intrathoracic trachea. Medical management, with bronchodilators, antitussives, and the symptomatic control of respiratory disease, is most often used in treatment.

Surgical Technique

When cases of cervical and thoracic inlet collapse do not respond to conservative therapy, surgical correction should be considered. Although a number of surgical corrections for tracheal collapse have been reported,[2-4,12-16,18,19] we have found the use of a ring prosthesis with occasional chondrotomy of the tracheal cartilage to be the most successful technique.[9] On occasion, plication of some areas of trachealis muscle is indicated.

The prosthetic tracheal rings may be made from 3-ml polypropylene syringe holders[9] (Fig. 19-2), or they may be purchased as a porous polypropylene implant.* The porous implant allows tissue to grow over its entire surface and allows suture passage at any point along the prosthesis. Implants made from syringe cases rely on holes drilled through the ring for suture placement and adequate tissue ingrowth to secure the prosthesis to the trachea. The rings may be sterilized with ethylene oxide or by autoclaving.

*Richards Manufacturing Co., Memphis, TN

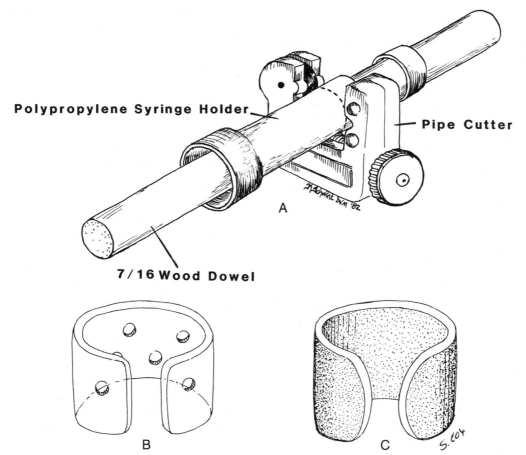

Polypropylene Syringe Holder

Pipe Cutter

7/16 Wood Dowel

A

B

C

Fig. 19-2. A, *Diagram of the prosthetic ring made from a 3-ml polypropylene syringe holder. The 7/16-inch wooden dowel is placed inside the syringe holder to give support for the cutting with a pipe cutter. This method of making the prosthetic ring ensures smooth edges and a uniform, neat cut.* B, *A ring when it has been shaped and when holes have been drilled.* C, *A porous polypropylene ring.*

Preoperative culture of the larynx or trachea and appropriate antibiotic therapy should precede any corrective technique. The placement of a cuffless endotracheal tube also requires preoperative consideration. The patient is positioned in dorsal recumbency with its front legs tied caudally and a small towel positioned between the neck and the table. A ventral midline incision is made from the larynx to the thoracic inlet. The trachea is exposed by separating the sternohyoideus and sternomastoideus muscles. The flattened, intubated trachea is then examined to locate the paired recurrent laryngeal nerves found in the loose areolar tissue on the dorsolateral surface of the trachea near the ends of the cartilaginous rings. The nerves run caudocranially, parallel to the trachea, and provide motor innervation to the larynx. They must be protected throughout the surgical procedure and must not be entrapped either in sutures or in the space between the trachea and the prosthetic ring.

A small section of trachea in the collapsed area is completely isolated by blunt dissection with a curved hemostat. This section should be only large enough to accept the plastic ring, in order to preserve the neurovascular integrity of the trachea. The curved hemostat is reintroduced dorsal to the trachea. One end of the prosthetic ring is grasped in the jaws of the hemostat,

and the ring is directed around the trachea (Fig. 19-3). The flexible rings are slightly straightened when passed, but return to their original shape. The recurrent laryngeal nerves are carefully retracted as the ring is placed. The open ends of the ring are sutured to the ventral surface of the trachea with 4-0 polyglycolic acid* sutures. The sutures are placed around the tracheal cartilage and through the plastic ring. The needle should enter the tracheal lumen only when necessary. A small hemostat is clamped to the prosthesis, and the trachea is gently rotated, first one way and then the other, in order to facilitate the placement of the more dorsal sutures. Approximately five sutures are placed on each ring, to pull the tracheal cartilages and the trachealis muscle out to the plastic ring in all directions (Fig. 19-4).

Additional rings are placed as needed, leaving approximately 1 cm between each ring. Where necessary, rings may be placed well within the thoracic inlet; one must be careful not to invade the pleural cavity. The trachea may be retracted cranially for placement of the intrathoracic rings by gentle traction on one of the plastic rings that is already sutured to the trachea (Fig. 19-5). Generally, no more than four to five rings are required to correct cervical and thoracic inlet collapse.

*Dexon, Davis & Geck, Inc., Manati, PR 00701

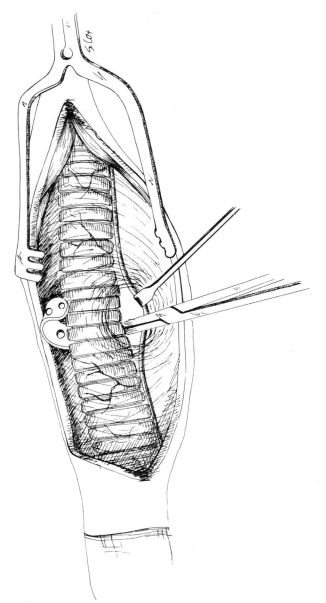

Fig. 19-3. *A small section of trachea is isolated by blunt dissection with a curved hemostat. The hemostat is then used to direct the prosthesis around the trachea; the recurrent laryngeal nerves are carefully retracted.*

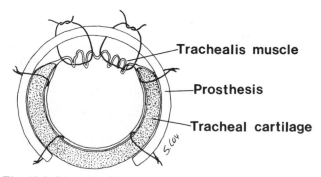

Tracheal is muscle

Prosthesis

Tracheal cartilage

Fig. 19-4. *Schematic diagram of rings and suture placement.*

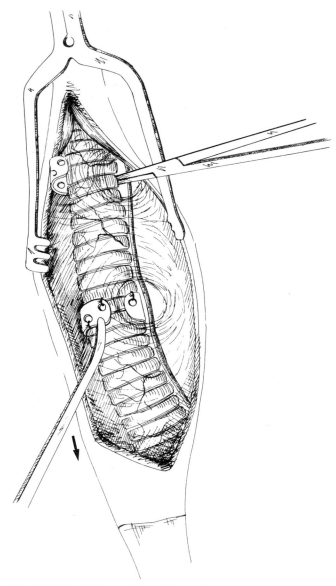

Fig. 19-5. *Cranial retraction of the trachea facilitates placement of the prosthesis on the intrathoracic trachea.*

Positioning of the rings at the thoracic inlet is critical. Care must be taken to ensure that the ring is placed flat on the trachea and in a physiologic position. If the ring does not seat on the trachea uniformly, the resulting "kink" will cause the plastic to erode through the trachea with movement. The tracheal diameter in this area is smaller than the upper cervical area; therefore, placement of too large a ring will tear the dorsal trachealis muscle as the trachea is drawn out toward the oversized ring. To correct this problem, the open ends of the plastic rings are sutured with 4-0 monofilament stainless steel to form the desired diameter. The cut ends of the wire suture should be directed into the prosthesis to prevent the sharp, free end from lacerating a major vessel in the area. When severely inverted tracheal rings are encountered (see Fig. 19-1) it may be necessary to perform a ventral chondrotomy on the tracheal cartilage in order to allow coaptation of the trachea to the prosthetic ring.

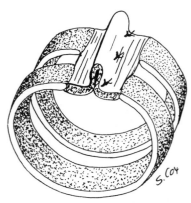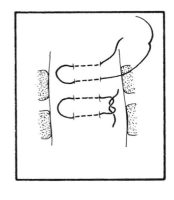

Fig. 19-6. *Schematic representation of the plicated dorsal trachealis muscle with a mattress suture (see also inset). (Redrawn from Rubin, G. J., et al.: Surgical reconstruction for collapsed tracheal rings. J. Small Anim. Pract., 14:607, 1973).*

Prior to routine closure of the sternohyoideus and sternomastoideus muscles, the endotracheal tube is withdrawn to observe for areas of redundant dorsal trachealis muscle. Additional sutures may be required to imbricate the muscle to an adjacent prosthetic ring and to ensure a patent tracheal lumen. Size 3-0 or 4-0 polyglycolic acid suture material, with a swaged-on, small, half-circle tapered needle, is used in this plication. The sutures must be placed carefully to prevent stretching of the delicate tissue to the point of tearing. Plication (Fig. 19-6) of the dorsal trachealis muscle between prosthetic rings and in the cranial cervical area is occasionally indicated to complete the tracheoplasty. Care must be taken neither to decrease the narrow tracheal lumen excessively nor to tear the trachealis muscle with plication sutures placed under extreme tension. Small air leaks at the sites of needle penetration are not a significant clinical problem.

Postoperative Care

Although complications have been minimal, strict cage rest is required immediately after the operation. Oxygen therapy is occasionally required. Gentle tracheal aspiration may be indicated for the slight bleeding into the lumen resulting from suture placement. Antitussives and corticosteroids are administered if coughing persists because of pre-existing tracheal disease or surgical irritation of the trachea. Postoperative antibiotic therapy should continue, according to the results of presurgical culture and sensitivity tests. A slight increase in coughing 2 to 3 weeks postoperatively may result from the degradation of the polyglycolic acid sutures, which pass through the tracheal mucosa.

In the absence of underlying pulmonary or cardiac disease, the persistence of a honking cough postoperatively usually indicates more extensive intrathoracic collapse that may or may not respond well to continued medical management. For this reason, careful case selection and a complete preoperative diagnostic evaluation are of the utmost importance.

References and Suggested Readings

1. Amis, T. C.: Tracheal collapse in the dog. Aust. Vet. J., 50:285, 1974.
2. Anderson, G. R.: Surgical correction of tracheal collapse using Teflon rings. Oklahoma Vet., 23:6, 1971.
3. Bojrab, M. J.: Collapsed tracheal rings. In Current Techniques in Small Animal Surgery. Edited by M. J. Bojrab. Philadelphia, Lea & Febiger, 1975.
4. Bojrab, M. J., and Nafe, L. L.: Tracheal reconstructive surgery. J. Am. Anim. Hosp. Assoc., 12:622, 1976.
5. Dellmann, H. D., and Brown, E. M.: Textbook of Veterinary Histology. 2nd Ed. Philadelphia, Lea & Febiger, 1981.
6. Done, S. H.: Canine tracheal collapse—aetiology, pathology, diagnosis and treatment. Vet. Annu., 18:255, 1978.
7. Done, S. H., and Drew, R. A.: Observations on the pathology of tracheal collapse in dogs. J. Small Anim. Pract., 17:783, 1976.
8. Ettinger, S., and Ticer, J.: Diseases of the Trachea. In Textbook of Veterinary Internal Medicine: Diseases of the Dog and Cat. Edited by S. J. Ettinger. Philadelphia, W. B. Saunders, 1975.
9. Hobson, H. P.: Total ring prosthesis for surgical correction of collapsed trachea. J. Am. Anim. Hosp. Assoc., 12:822, 1976.
10. Jubb, K., and Kennedy, P.: Pathology of Domestic Animals. New York, Academic Press, 1963.
11. Killough, J.: Protective mechanisms of the lungs; pulmonary disease; pleural disease. In Pathologic Physiology, Mechanisms of Disease. Edited by W. A. Sodeman and T. M. Sodeman. Philadelphia, W. B. Saunders, 1979.
12. Knowles, R., and Snyder, C. C.: Proceedings of the 34th Annual Meeting of the American Animal Hospital Association, 1967, p. 246.
13. Leighton, R.: Tracheal surgery. In Canine Surgery. 2nd Ed. Edited by J. Archibald. Santa Barbara, CA, American Veterinary Publications, 1974.
14. Leonard, H. C.: Surgical correction of collapsed trachea in dogs. J. Am. Vet. Med. Assoc., 158:598, 1971.
15. Leonard, H. C., and Wright, J. J.: An intraluminal prosthetic dilator for tracheal collapse in the dog. J. Am. Anim. Hosp. Assoc., 14:464, 1978.
16. Longbottom, G. M.: A case of tracheal collapse in the dog. Vet. Rec., 101:54, 1977.
17. O'Brien, J., Buchanan, J., and Kelly, D.: Tracheal collapse in the dog. J. Am. Vet. Radiol. Soc., 7:12, 1966.
18. Rubin, G. J., Neal, T. M., and Bojrab, M. J.: Surgical reconstruction for collapsed tracheal rings. J. Small Anim. Pract., 14:607, 1973.
19. Schiller, A., Helper, L., and Small, E.: Treatment of tracheal collapse in the dog. J. Am. Vet. Med. Assoc., 145:669, 1964.

20 * Bronchi and Lungs

Surgery of the Bronchi and Lungs

by A. W. NELSON

Bronchial and pulmonary operations are not routine procedures in general veterinary surgical practice. Knowledge of respiratory physiology, anatomy, and anesthesia as related to thoracic surgery are prerequisites for surgical treatment. The basic techniques of vascular surgery should also be familiar to the veterinarian.

Bronchi

Surgically treatable disease involving the main bronchi is uncommon. Intraluminal foreign bodies and mucous plugs can occur and are usually handled with bronchoscopy equipment, with flexible forceps and suction attachments. Intraluminal bronchial tumors are rarely diagnosed. Bronchial wall lacerations seldom require suturing if chest drainage equipment is available.

REMOVAL OF FOREIGN BODIES

Inhaled foreign bodies more frequently lodge proximal in the bronchial system, trachea, or larynx and are accessible to bronchoscopic examination and retrieval with flexible forceps. Grass awns may lodge deep in the bronchial tree and may create granulomatous reactions and abscesses, or they may migrate to other locations in or outside the lung. Deep bronchial foreign bodies and their initiated reaction frequently require partial or complete lobectomy rather than bronchial incision.

The nonretrievable bronchial foreign body requires at least a thoracotomy and bronchiotomy. General inhalation anesthesia is used, and the surgical site is aseptically prepared. The approach is made through a standard fifth-intercostal-space lateral thoracotomy. A chest retractor is needed for adequate exposure. The uninvolved lung lobes are packed out of the way with laparotomy pads, and the region of the involved bronchus and lung are thereby exposed. Adjacent tissues are dissected away to expose the bronchial wall. Care must be taken not to injure the many bronchial vessels,

nerves, and other structures in the area. The bronchial incision site should be additionally packed off to decrease pleural space contamination from bronchial contents. The incision is over or cranial to the foreign body, and the foreign body is removed (Fig. 20-1). Close examination is made of devitalized tissue, and debridement is completed. The incision is closed with simple interrupted sutures of a fine (4-0) nonabsorbable monofilament material (Fig. 20-1, *C* and *D*). A cutting-edge needle is used, and the stitches are placed either through or around the bronchial rings. This technique is also used if a segmental bronchial resection is necessary.

The chest is filled with warm saline solution, and the bronchial closure is checked for bubbles emanating during lung inflation (20 to 30 cm H_2O pressure). The appearance of bubbles indicates a leaking anastomosis; major leaks should be sutured. The suture line should be reinforced with a parietal pleural patch of adjacent soft tissue (Fig. 20-1*E*). The chest is lavaged, evacuated, and all lung lobes are returned to their normal positions. A standard chest drain is placed, and thoracotomy is closed in a routine manner. The drain is removed in 24 hours, or when fluid or air accumulation has stopped, or when fluid accumulation has stabilized at a few milliliters for a period of 8 hours or more. The drain itself causes some fluid accumulation (1 to 2 ml/hour), owing to pleural irritation.

EXCISION OF TUMORS

Tumors of the bronchi are rare and, if diagnosed, are seldom amenable to local bronchial excision, owing to the surrounding lung tissue. Lobectomy is generally required.

REPAIR OF LACERATIONS

Injury to a bronchus that lacerates the bronchial wall may lead to a significant tension pneumothorax and mediastinal and subcutaneous emphysema. Continuous or intermittent (every 1 to 3 hours) chest suction or underwater-seal chest drainage should be done before surgical exploration is initiated. If the pneumothorax can be reduced to a point compatible with life by suc-

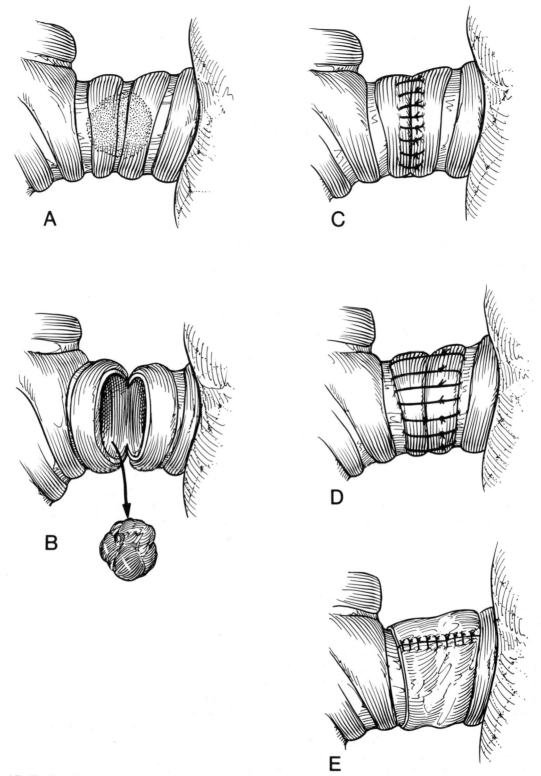

Fig. 20-1. A *and* B, *The bronchus is exposed, is incised at the site of the lesion, and the foreign body is removed.* C *and* D, *The incision is closed with simple interrupted sutures, either penetrating or encircling the bronchial cartilages.* E, *A parietal pleural patch may be placed over the incision site.*

tion or water-seal drainage, then surgical exploration may be avoided. Emergency exploration of the chest is indicated when acute pneumothorax cannot be controlled by chest suction or when the laceration has not

sealed after 3 to 4 days of chest drainage. Bronchoscopy and contrast bronchograms may be used to confirm the diagnosis of the laceration and its location prior to any surgical exploration of the chest.

The lacerated bronchus is approached through a fifth- or sixth-intercostal-space lateral thoracotomy on the involved side. The injury is exposed by dissection of the pleural tissues overlying the affected bronchus. Packing of the lungs should be as described in the discussion of bronchial foreign bodies. The wound is explored for devitalized tissue, and only healthy tissues are left to be apposed with simple interrupted sutures of fine (4-0) monofilament nonabsorbable suture. Sutures may be placed through the cartilaginous rings to increase the strength and tissue alignment of the closure (Fig. 20-1). The sutured laceration may be reinforced by suturing pleura and adjacent tissue over the site.

The suture closure of the bronchus is examined for air leaks by flooding the area with warm normal saline solution during positive-pressure respiration (20 to 30 cm H_2O pressure). Any leaks are repaired with additional sutures, and the chest is irrigated with warm normal saline solution and is suctioned clear of fluid and blood clots. A new chest drain is placed, and a standard thoroacotomy closure is completed.

Lungs

REPAIR OF LACERATIONS

Small lung lacerations may be closed by a simple suture technique (Fig. 20-2). A series of interrupted or continuous horizontal mattress sutures is placed through the lung parenchyma. The visceral pleura may be closed with a simple continuous suture pattern. Fine (5-0 or 6-0) suture material, either absorbable or nonabsorbable, should be swaged onto a fine, tapered needle for the least traumatic closure. A chest drain should be placed routinely in these patients.

THERAPEUTIC AND DIAGNOSTIC
PARTIAL LOBECTOMY

Lung biopsy and partial lobectomy may be used to diagnose pathologic conditions of the lung. Needle aspirates and biopsies of abnormal portions of the lung seldom contain adequate tissue specimens for accurate diagnoses. Moreover, the needle aspiration technique may disseminate neoplastic and infected tissue to other parts of the lung and the pleural cavity as the needle is withdrawn. Occasionally, air leakage and hemorrhage occur after needle biopsies of the lung. These conditions are rarely fatal; however, they may cause significant complications of hemorrhage into the lung and hemopneumothorax. Biopsy patients should be monitored closely during the postoperative period for the accumulation of fluid or air in the chest.

Partial lobectomy at thoracotomy is a useful procedure for therapeutic purposes in extirpating small lung lesions and in diagnosing diffuse lesions of the lung. The technique allows for direct visualization of the tissue removed and thus provides the veterinary surgeon and pathologist with representative samples of normal

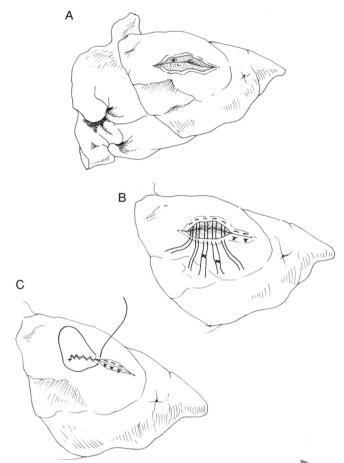

Fig. 20-2. A to C, *Lacerations of the lungs may be sutured with interrupted mattress sutures oversewn with a simple continuous layer of sutures.*

and abnormal tissue for comparison. It is the method of choice in treating patients with nonresponsive or chronic lung abscesses, deep bronchial foreign bodies, isolated tumors, and lacerations that cannot be adequately sutured.

The surgical technique for removing a portion of a lung lobe is not difficult. A standard intercostal thoracotomy is used to approach the affected lung lobe. If the area of interest is near the apex of a lung lobe, a simple wedge or distal lobe amputation may be performed. The area of the lung lobe to be removed is cross-clamped with a pair of noncrushing forceps. If a wedge is to be excised, two pair of forceps may be used to form the outline of the wedge (Fig. 20-3). The lung lobe is incised on the distal side of the forceps, the portion of the lung is removed, and the tissue is cultured or is placed in a fixative for histopathologic preparation. The incised edge of the lobe is sutured on the proximal side of the forceps in a continuous horizontal mattress pattern, which is both hemostatic and pneumostatic (Fig. 20-3B). The end of the suture is tied, and the two ends are left long, so that they may be used as tags to manipulate the lung when the clamps have been removed. The clamp(s) is (are) removed, and the edge of the lung incision is oversewn with a simple continuous suture pattern. The tag ends are cut, and

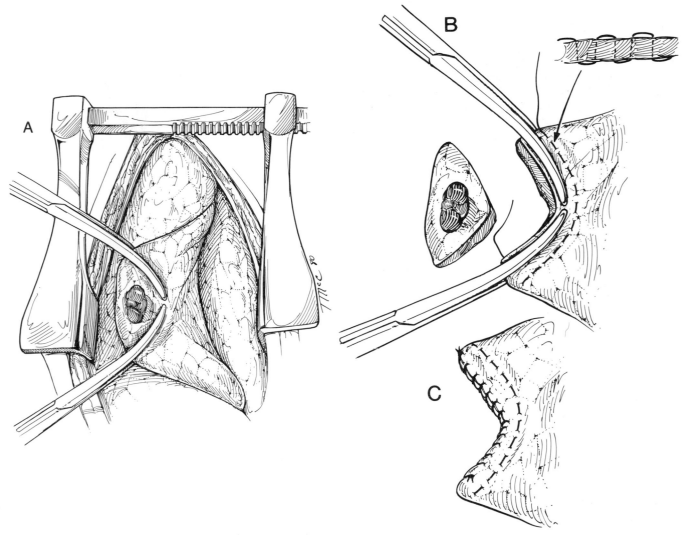

Fig. 20-3. A, *Wedge-shaped portion of lung parenchyma is excised distal to the two forceps. A combination of mattress* (B) *and simple continuous* (C) *sutures are used to close the defect.*

the lobe is allowed to drop back into the chest cavity. The chest is filled with saline solution; the lungs expanded so that the submerged suture line can be checked for leaks. If significant leaks are identified, additional sutures may be placed. The chest is evacuated of fluid and any other debris, the chest drain is placed, and the intercostal incision is closed as previously described.

A modification of this technique is the use of mechanical stapling equipment* instead of sutures. This method adds considerable expense to the procedure and is only justified when a short intraoperative time is desired because of the patient's condition or when a busy surgical schedule dictates rapid case flow. If little or no fluid or air accumulates in the chest cavity within the first 24 postoperative hours, the chest drain is removed.

*Autosuture, United States Surgical Corp., 150 Glover Avenue, Norwalk, CT 06850

LOBECTOMY

The complete removal of a lobe of the lung is necessary in such conditions as lobe torsion, severe laceration, rupture of a large emphysematous bulla, abscess, isolated neoplasm near the base of the lobe, and severe laceration or tumor involving the lobe bronchus. The contents of the entire pleural cavity are palpated and are inspected to determine the character and extent of the disease prior to initial hilar dissection.

The surgical approach is through a standard lateral thoracotomy over the hilus serving the affected lung area. It is better to be one interspace caudal, if any question exists as to the specific location of the diseased lobe. Other lung lobes are reflected and are packed out of the way with moist laparotomy sponges; the lobe to be resected is carefully elevated. The pleural surface of the hilar area is approached from a craniodorsal position, and the bronchus is located by a combination of palpation and dissection.

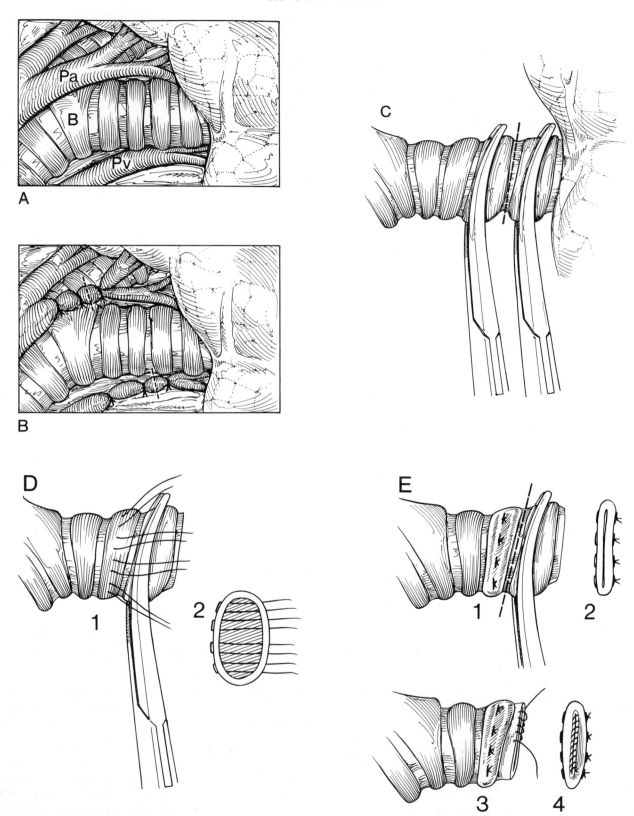

Fig. 20-4. A, *The anatomic relationship at the bronchus (B) and pulmonary artery (Pa) and vein (Pv). The artery is usually slightly dorsolateral and the vein ventromedial to the bronchus. B, The artery and vein are doubly ligated, and the vessels are transected between the distal two ligatures (dotted line). C, The bronchus is transected between crushing forceps (dotted line), and the lung lobe with the bronchial stump is discarded. D, Mattress sutures are placed proximal to the bronchial clamp (1) and are tied to collapse the cartilage ring (2). E, The crushed distal portion of the bronchus (1) is amputated (dotted line) to leave only healthy tissue at the bronchial closure, which had been collapsed by tying the mattress suture (2). The membranous portion of the bronchus is oversewn with a simple continuous suture pattern (3 and 4).*

The pulmonary artery to the affected lobe is located slightly dorsolateral to the bronchus (Fig. 20-4A). Dissection of pulmonary artery is done with curved scissors and curved or right-angle forceps to aid in vessel isolation. A piece of ⅛-inch moistened umbilical tape is passed around the artery to move the vessel while ligatures are placed and to act as an emergency ligature if the vessel is torn. A simple ligature of 2-0 or 3-0 nonabsorbable suture material is placed on the proximal end of the artery near its branch point (Fig. 20-4B). A similar suture is placed distal to the point at which the vessel is to be transected. A third transfixing suture is placed just distal to the proximal suture. This technique prevents the proximal suture (main hemostatic suture) from slipping off the vessel during the postoperative period.

When the ligatures are in place, the vessel may be transected between the distal two sutures. The lung lobe is retracted craniodorsally, and the pulmonary vein is approached on the ventrocaudal side of the bronchus. Care must be taken as the dissection is extended around the pulmonary vein to prevent laceration of this delicate vessel, which lies ventral and medial to the bronchus. Sharp dissection using scissors, combined with gentle blunt dissection with forceps, is needed to isolate the vein without rupturing it. The dissection is facilitated by a pair of right-angle forceps that help to determine when the dissection is complete around the back side of the vein. When the vein has been isolated, it is ligated as was the artery. The ligature is not near enough to the left atrium to interfere with the venous drainage from adjacent lung lobes.

The next structure to be isolated and ligated is the main stem bronchus of the lobe. By this point in dissection, the bronchus is almost isolated. Any remaining tissues are dissected free from the bronchus so that sutures may be placed. The bronchus is double-cross-clamped with crushing-type forceps at a convenient but distal point for transection. The bronchus is transected between the two forceps, and the lobe is removed (Fig. 20-4C). This method provides better exposure and more working room in the hilar region for the remaining part of the operation.

The bronchus proximal to the remaining clamp and near its branch point is sutured with interrupted horizontal mattress sutures preplaced across the trunk (Fig. 20-4D). The sutures are tied, and the bronchus is transected next to the bronchial ring held by the crushing clamp (Fig. 20-4E). Approximately 2 mm of noncrushed bronchus is left distal to the mattress sutures. When all the mattress sutures have been tied, a simple continuous suture pattern is used to complete the closure of the end of the bronchus. The bronchus is checked for air leaks by flooding the chest cavity with warm saline solution and by applying positive-pressure respiration (25 to 30 cm H_2O pressure). If any leaks occur, additional sutures may be placed. The end of the bronchus and ligated vessels are then covered with the adjacent tissue by placing simple sutures through the pleura and loose connective tissue. This maneuver aids in decreasing adhesions between the lungs and the raw

tissues exposed during the operation and helps to heal the tissue over the exposed vessels and bronchus.

An alternate technique is mechanically suturing the isolated vessels and bronchus with automatic stapling equipment. This method provides a rapid closure and seal of these tubular structures. The TA-30 tissue stapler is ideal for this purpose.

The chest is suctioned clear of all fluid and blood clots, a chest drain is placed, and the lateral thoracotomy is closed as previously described. The chest drain is removed when the production of air and fluid has essentially stopped.

PNEUMONECTOMY

Pneumonectomy is defined as the surgical removal of either the right or the left lung. This procedure is rarely done in veterinary surgical practice and is feasible only when a pathologic condition of one entire lung has not involved the remaining lung. The remaining lung will have to maintain all respiratory function.

The surgical procedure for pneumonectomy is essentially the same as for lobectomy. Bronchus and pulmonary vein closure and transection are identical to that described for lobectomy. The pulmonary artery may be double-ligated (including one fixation ligature) in some small dogs; however, it is safer to oversew the proximal end with a simple continuous suture of fine (4-0 or 5-0) nonabsorbable material.

The remaining procedures for checking for air leaks, chest drainage, and closure are as described for lobectomy.

Thoracotomy

by A. W. NELSON

Lateral Thoracotomy

Lateral thoracotomy (Fig. 20-5) is the standard approach to the chest cavity in most clinical cases. The right or left hemithorax may be approached through an intercostal incision for most intrathoracic procedures. The second and third intercostal spaces are used to approach the cranial mediastinal area, the fourth or fifth intercostal space for the heart and lung hilar area, and the eighth intercostal space for the caudal esophagus and diaphragm. Guidance for interspace selection is available from radiographs. If doubt exists as to which of two possible spaces to use, it is advisable to choose the more caudal space because the ribs cranial to an intercostal incision are much more retractable than the caudal ones.

When the interspace has been selected, the ribs are counted by palpation through the skin (counting caudal to cranial), and the location of the skin incision is determined. The incision is deepened to the latissimus dorsi muscle, and the ribs are again palpated through

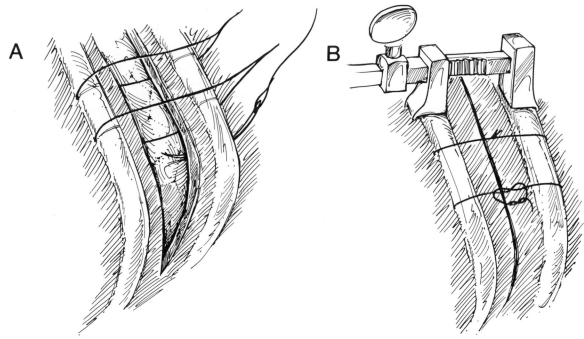

Fig. 20-5. A, *Rib sutures (catgut of 0-0 to 2-0) are preplaced around the ribs adjacent to the thoracotomy incision before the ribs are approximated. B, A rib approximator (or towel clamps in small dogs and cats) is used to hold the ribs in close approximation while the rib sutures are tied.*

the exposed tissues and counted to verify the correct intercostal space. Scissors are used to carry the dissection through the different muscle layers. The latissimus dorsi muscle, the first major muscle encountered, should be divided parallel to the intercostal space as far caudally as the exposure will permit. This technique allows the suture line in the latissimus dorsi muscle to be caudal to the sutures in the skin and deeper muscle tissue when the chest is closed. It also causes the least damage to the function of the latissimus muscle when healed.

The muscles deep to the latissimus dorsi on the ventral aspect of the lateral chest wall (scalenus and pectoral muscles) are transected perpendicular to their fibers. The serratus ventralis muscle is separated parallel to its muscle fibers at the desired interspace. Metzenbaum scissors are convenient to incise the external intercostal muscle. The scissors are pushed along the intercostal space in a half-opened position, instead of being repeatedly opened and closed. This incision should be closer to the caudal rib to avoid the intercostal artery and vein. The internal intercostal muscle is incised in a similar manner, without incising the pleura. A 2- to 3-mm incision made in the pleura during expiration allows air to flow into the chest and permits the lungs to collapse away from the chest wall. The pleural incision can then be extended without fear of incising the lung.

It is best to extend the intercostal incision ventrally past the costochondral junction, close to the sternum, and dorsally beyond the arch of the rib. This method allows the chest wall to be maximally retracted. As the intercostal incision approaches the sternum, the inter-nal thoracic artery and vein can be seen and avoided.

Moist laparotomy sponges are applied to the exposed edges of the chest incision, and a Finochietto* retractor used to spread the ribs. In small dogs and cats, Weitlaner,* Beckman,* or Gelpi* self-retaining retractors may be used instead of the larger Finochietto retractors.

Closure of the thoracotomy incision requires that the ribs be approximated with a heavy monofilament absorbable or nonabsorbable suture material (Fig. 20-5). In adult patients, the suture size may range from 0 to No. 2, depending on the animal's size. Smaller sutures (2-0 or 3-0) may be used in neonates or young patients. A series of 4 to 6 interrupted sutures is preplaced. The ribs are brought in close proximity with a rib approximator or a pair of towel clamps. All sutures are tied before the rib approximator is removed. It is desirable, but not necessary, to avoid encompassing the neurovascular bundle that lies just caudal to each rib. These sutures are tied tightly enough to bring the ribs on each side of the incision in close approximation without overlapping. The intercostal muscles are sutured with a simple continuous pattern using absorbable material. The remaining muscles are approximated with absorbable suture material using simple continuous or interrupted patterns. The retracted latissimus dorsi muscle is approximated with simple interrupted sutures placed primarily in the fascia. Each muscle layer should be sutured separately, so that the postoperative motion of the chest wall is not mechanically restricted. Skin closure is standard.

*American V. Mueller, 6600 West Touhy Avenue, Chicago, IL 60648

MODIFICATIONS

Modifications of the lateral thoracotomy procedure are useful to obtain additional exposure. Such a modification is accomplished either by approaching the chest through a periosteal rib bed with rib resection or by transecting ribs next to the intercostal incision.

RIB RESECTION. The approach is directly over the rib to be resected. Musculature is dissected as previously described, and an incision is made in the periosteum longitudinally on the lateral aspect of the exposed rib (Fig. 20-6). The periosteum is dissected with a periosteal elevator along the entire lateral, cranial, and caudal borders of the rib. A periosteal elevator or the handle of a scalpel blade is worked between the periosteum and the rib on the medial side of the rib. The instrument is pushed dorsally and ventrally to separate the

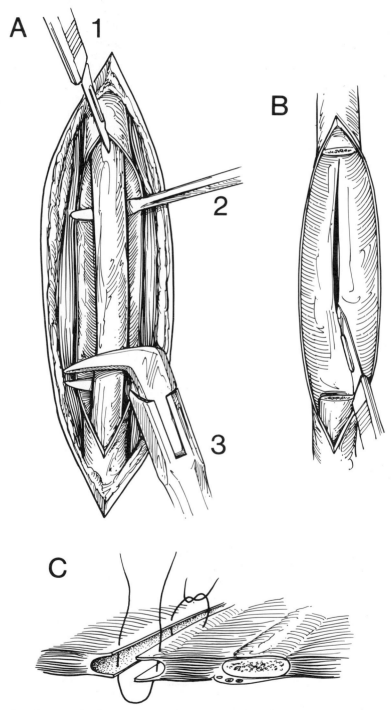

Fig. 20-6. *A, Rib resection is done by incising the periosteum (1), elevating the periosteum off the rib with a periosteal elevator (2), and transecting the rib at both ends with a rib or bone cutter (3). B, The thoracic cavity is entered by incision through the medial side of the periosteal bed and pleura. C, The thoracic cavity is closed by suturing the periosteal incisions in one or two layers.*

periosteum from the rib. It is not necessary to invade the thoracic cavity. The rib is transected at each end with bone cutters and is discarded. The perichondrium on the cartilaginous part of the rib is difficult to elevate; thus, any portion of the cartilage that is in the way is excised with bone cutters and is discarded.

When the rib has been transected and removed, the periosteal bed is exposed. The incision into the pleural cavity is made through the periosteum and pleura that were covering the medial side of the rib. This incision allows more exposure in the chest cavity than could be obtained with a single intercostal incision. Closure of the wound is simple because the periosteum may be primarily sutured with a simple interrupted or continuous suture (Fig. 20-6C). The lateral and medial aspects of the periosteal bed may be sutured either separately or together, to allow some degree of rib regeneration. The musculature superficial to the periosteal incision is closed as described previously.

RIB TRANSECTION. If the chest has been opened in a standard lateral intercostal approach, but adequate exposure is not available, a rib next to the incision can be transected. This transection provides as much exposure as a simple rib resection. The rib is transected as far dorsally as possible, and a 4- to 5-mm section of the rib is removed and is discarded along with attached soft tissue. The rib thereby heals after realignment without bone edges rubbing together during breathing, and so postoperative pain is decreased. The cartilaginous portion of the rib is transected as far ventrally as possible. Rib transection may be extended to one rib cranially or caudally without postoperative complications. The ribs need not be wired together at the cut ends during the closure of this incision. Healing takes place without loss of chest function.

The ribs on each side of the incision are approximated, and muscular tissues are sutured as described for the standard intercostal thoracotomy.

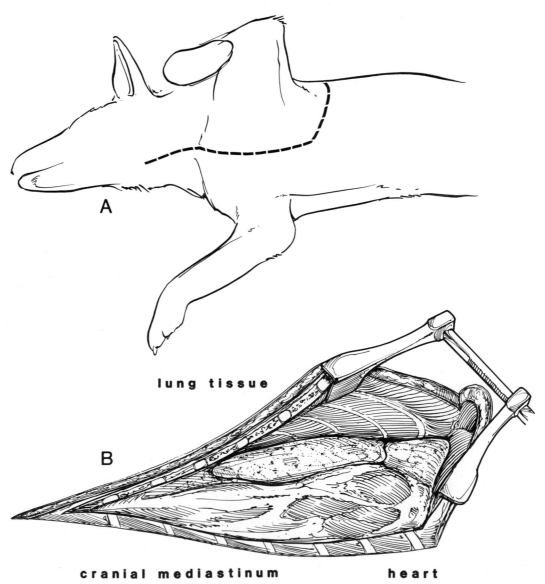

Fig. 20-7. *Cranial thoracic wall flap thoracotomy is a combined partial sternotomy and lateral intercostal incision. A, The proposed incision line. B, The incision is complete, and the rib retractor is in the proper position to retract the left cranial portion of the thoracic wall; this retraction exposes the caudal cervical and cranial mediastinal regions.*

Radical Thoracotomy

Wide exposure is possible for the cranial thoracic cavity by a combined cranial sternotomy and lateral thoracotomy (cranial thoracic wall flap). A complete sternotomy exposes the ventral aspect of all thoracic viscera.

CRANIAL THORACIC WALL FLAP

The surgical approach to the cranial thorax is obscured in the dog by the upper forelimb. This problem is circumvented with the thoracic wall flap. The dog is placed in a dorsolateral position with the sternum 8 to 15 cm above the operating table's surface (Fig. 20-7A). The axilla is exposed by elevating and abducting the forelimb with adhesive tape that extends from the table's edge, around the flexed elbow, and back to the table's edge.

A ventral midline incision begins approximately 5 cm cranial to the manubrium and extends caudally to the fourth or fifth sternebra. The skin incision is then continued dorsally in the intercostal space. When the sternum has been exposed, the intercostal and pleural incisions are completed as previously described for a standard intercostal thoracotomy. The internal thoracic artery and vein are double-ligated (standard ligature with a transfixation ligature on each cut end) as

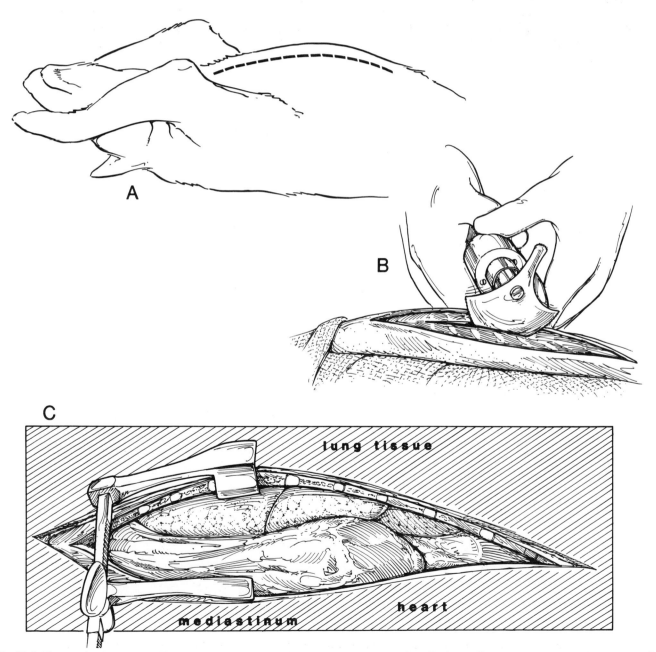

Fig. 20-8. *The standard ventral midline sternotomy incision:* A, *The proposed incision line.* B, *An oscillating saw can be used to transect the sternabrae along their midline.* C, *Both sides of the thoracic cavity can be viewed with this approach.*

they are exposed in the ventral aspect of the intercostal space.

The sternebrae are then transected longitudinally on the midline with a sternal chisel, osteotome, bone saw, bone cutters, or, in the neonate, a heavy pair of scissors (see Fig. 20-8B). With the intercostal incision completed, the internal sides of the sternebrae may be palpated as they are transected. This method ensures protection of the thoracic viscera, which is especially important when an osteotome is used. The cranial midline incision is extended between the ventral cervical muscles directly on the midline, to reduce trauma to the muscles during retraction.

Dampened gauze laparotomy pads or small towels are placed into the incision edges, and the craniolateral portion of the thoracic wall, including the forelimb, is retracted laterally (Fig. 20-7B). This retraction provides exposure of the entire cranial hemithorax and the distal cervical region. This approach exposes the entire trachea, the cranial two-thirds of the esophagus, all mediastinal tissues, and the cranial great vessels originating from the aorta.

The incision is closed by approximating the sternebrae with interrupted sutures of heavy (Nos. 0 to 2) monofilament material. The suture may either circle the sternebrae or may penetrate the sternebrae or their cartilaginous portions for better structural alignment. The intercostal incision is closed as described for standard lateral thoracotomy. All subcutaneous tissues should be closed completely to ensure an adequate thoracic seal and to prevent incision breakdown as the animal begins to lie on the incision. A standard skin closure is used for the ventral midline and intercostal approach.

STERNOTOMY

The entire chest cavity may be exposed by performing a complete sternotomy (Fig. 20-8) with the dog in dorsal recumbency (Fig. 20-8A). The technique is similar to that described for the partial (cranial) sternotomy, but the incision is continued caudally to the linea alba. The diaphragm may be incised in a ventrodorsal or costal-arch direction to allow maximal sternal retraction. This method provides adequate exposure to both sides of the thorax and thoracic viscera, except the dorsal aspects of the viscera are not easily accessible (Fig. 20-8C). The sternotomy is closed as described for the thoracic flap procedure. Standard closure techniques are used for muscle, subcutaneous tissue, and skin.

Thoracotomies in general, and this approach in particular, cause considerable postoperative discomfort for the patient, and analgesics should therefore be used as indicated.

References and Suggested Readings

Archibald, J., and Harvey, C. G.: Thorax, In Canine Surgery. 2nd Ed. Edited by J. Archibald. Santa Barbara, CA, American Veterinary Publications, 1974.

Dabell, A. R. C.: Thoracic incisions. In Gibbon's Surgery of the Chest. 3rd Ed. Edited by D. C. Sabiston, Jr., and F. C. Spencer. Philadelphia, W. B. Saunders, 1977.

Lawson, D. D.: Indication and techniques for thoracotomy. J. Small Anim. Pract., 9:389, 1968.

Pettit, G. D.: Principles of thoracic surgery. J. Am. Vet. Med. Assoc., 147:1424, 1965.

Takaro, T.: Lung infections and interstitial pneumonopathies. In Gibbon's Surgery of the Chest. 3rd Ed. Edited by D. C. Sabiston, Jr., and F. C. Spencer. Philadelphia, W. B. Saunders, 1977.

21 * Thoracic Wall

Reconstruction of Thoracic Wall Defects Using Marlex Mesh

by Ronald M. Bright

Full-thickness (en bloc) resection of the chest wall refers to the radical excision of tissue including pleura, ribs, muscles, fascia, and overlying skin. Indications for this resection include: neoplasia in which involvement of ribs and associated soft tissues renders selective resection impossible; extensive trauma to the ribs and musculature such that conservative repair or osseous fixation is impractical; and mycotic or bacterial infection with pleurocutaneous sinuses or multiple fistulas that are unresponsive to other forms of surgical therapy. Following this en bloc resection, some type of reconstructive procedure must be performed if two or more ribs are included in the excision. The goal must be to achieve chest-wall stability and a closed chest, so that adequate ventilation may begin in the immediate postoperative period.

Although numerous prosthetic implants have been used to repair thoracic wall defects, Marlex* mesh appears to be superior. The physical characteristics of this mesh fulfill many of the requirements for a reconstructive repair of this type. Marlex mesh is a nonreactive, knitted material that is resistant to infection and can be safely autoclaved. Its highly crystalline molecular structure provides excellent tensile strength. This property allows the mesh to be tightly stretched over a surgical defect, and in the thoracic wall, this ability is important because it contributes to the immediate stability of the chest wall. Marlex mesh is a porous material and, once implanted, allows adequate infiltration of its interstices with fibrous tissue. Because it forms a strong fibrous bond to surrounding tissue, Marlex mesh usually remains intact for a long time without undergoing fragmentation.[2,3,4,5]

Surgical Technique

Following chest wall excision, the technique of placing the mesh is tedious but straightforward.[1] After a chest tube has been placed, a piece of autoclaved mesh

*Davol Rubber Co., Providence, RI

is tailored to fit the defect. This mesh should be cut slightly larger than the defect, so that when it is folded over at the edge, it forms a double-thickness margin of approximately 1 cm around the periphery of the prosthesis. This double-thickness fold ensures additional strength at its point of attachment to adjacent tissue. The free edges of the folded mesh should face the exterior of the defect, to prevent possible irritation to the underlying lung.

Close attention to the proper placement of the mesh is mandatory. To achieve the best mechanical advantage and hence optimum chest-wall stability, the mesh is placed intrapleurally. The initial fixation starts along one of the vertical borders of the defect (Fig. 21-1). Sutures are first placed around and under the adjacent rib, and then are drawn through the double thickness of the mesh and back through the intercostal musculature and tied. As the suture is drawn tightly, the mesh slides under the rib; the resulting approximation of mesh and tissue is excellent (Fig. 21-2). Sutures of 1-0 or 2-0 nylon with a swaged-on cutting needle are preferred. The braided form of polypropylene that may accompany the mesh should not be used, owing to the trauma of tissue drag as it pulls through the mesh and tissue.

The dorsal and ventral borders of the mesh are now affixed to the intercostal musculature and the associated rib remnants. When placing the suture around each rib, it is important that the needle and suture pass through the double layer of the mesh on both sides of the rib (Fig. 21-3). The mesh should be under slight tension (Fig. 21-3, arrow) when placing each suture, to prevent wrinkling as one proceeds to the opposite side. Even tension around the periphery is desired (Fig. 21-4). When the opposite side of the defect is reached, the mesh is then affixed under slight tension to the adjacent rib and musculature. In most cases, a single layer of mesh is sufficient to create an adequate repair. If necessary, however, a double-layered piece of mesh may be used.

After the intrapleural placement of Marlex, the overlying soft tissue is closed. The surrounding musculature is now gently undermined where possible, to allow it to slide toward the center of the defect. The latissimus dorsi muscle is usually most suitable for this pur-

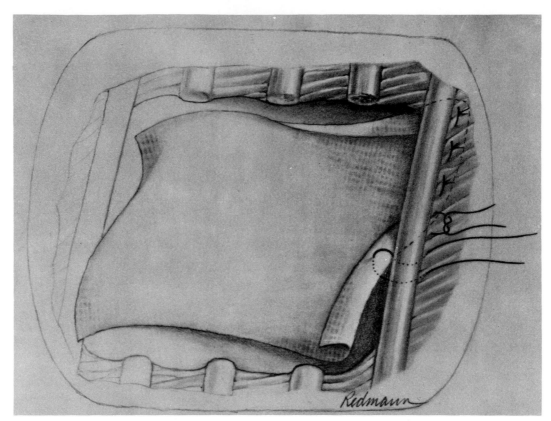

Fig. 21-1. *Nylon sutures placed under and around the rib course through the double-layered border of the mesh and return to a point adjacent to the initial entry site. This intrapleural placement allows satisfactory skeletal rigidity. (From Bright, R. M.: Reconstruction of thoracic wall defects using Marlex^R mesh. J. Am. Anim. Hosp. Assoc., 17:415, 1981.)*

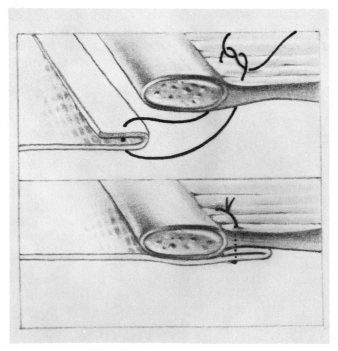

Fig. 21-2. *When the sutures around the ribs are pulled tightly, a good approximation of mesh and tissue results. (From Bright, R. M.: Reconstruction of thoracic wall defects using Marlex^R mesh. J. Am. Anim. Hosp. Assoc., 17:415, 1981.)*

pose. A four-corner interrupted suture pattern works well in closing the muscle layer of the defect (Fig. 21-5). Sutures of 1-0 or 2-0 gut or polyglycolic acid may be used. An airtight seal is usually obtained with this closure technique (Fig. 21-6). A Penrose drain is then placed subcutaneously and is allowed to exit above and below the wound. Sufficient skin exists in this region so that primary skin closure is easily accomplished, again using a four-corner type of suture pattern.

When pleural drainage is no longer necessary, the chest tube is removed. A light-pressure bandage is then applied and is changed every other day. The Penrose drain is removed on the third postoperative day, and the final bandage is removed on the fifth postoperative day.

Paradoxical movement of the chest wall (flail chest) is a potential problem. The ridigity of the Marlex mesh when placed intrapleurally and under tension, however, minimizes this effect. Any remaining paradoxical movement is usually gone in 3 days and is generally not a threat to the patient's life. The cosmetic appearance is excellent; little palpable defect is present once tissue infiltration has occurred and healing is completed.

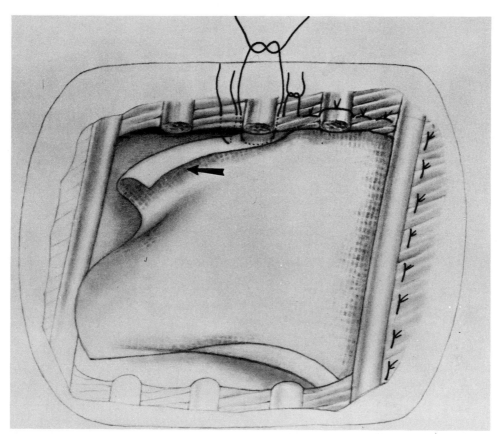

Fig. 21-3. *The dorsal and ventral borders of the mesh are also sutured in place by passing the nylon through the double-layered border of mesh and by affixing it to the underside of each rib and to the intercostal musculature, as shown. (From Bright, R. M.: Reconstruction of thoracic wall defects using Marlex^R mesh. J. Am. Anim. Hosp. Assoc., 17:415, 1981.)*

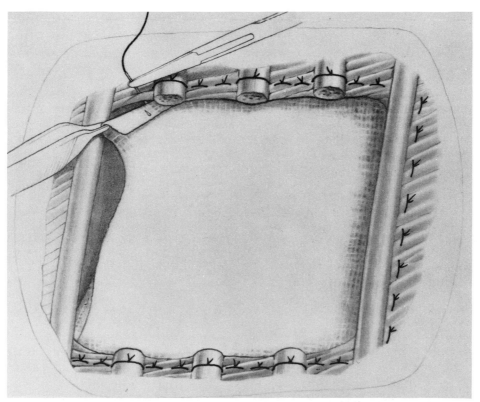

Fig. 21-4. *The dorsal and ventral borders should be repaired simultaneously to obtain even tension around the periphery of the defect. (From Bright, R. M.: Reconstruction of thoracic wall defects using Marlex^R mesh. J. Am. Anim. Hosp. Assoc., 17:415, 1981.)*

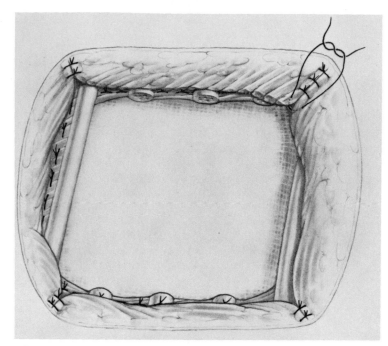

Fig. 21-5. *The opposite vertical portion of the mesh is affixed as in Figures 21-1 and 21-2. Following this procedure, the musculature surrounding the defect is freed, and a four-corner suture pattern is used to provide soft tissue cover and an airtight seal of the chest. Suture of 1-0 or 2-0 gut can be used for this layer. (From Bright, R. M.: Reconstruction of thoracic wall defects using Marlex^R mesh. J. Am. Anim. Hosp. Assoc., 17:415, 1981.)*

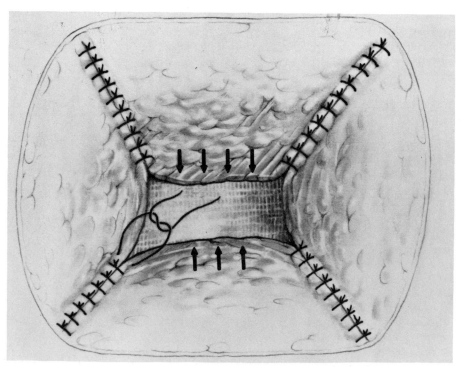

Fig. 21-6. *When the four-corner suture pattern has drawn the edges of the musculature closer together, a side-to-side simple interrupted suture pattern can be used to close the defect in the direction depicted by the arrows.*

References and Suggested Readings

1. Bright, R. M.: Reconstruction of thoracic wall defects using Marlex[R] mesh. J. Am. Anim. Hosp. Assoc., 17:415, 1981.
2. Graham, J., et al.: Marlex mesh as a prosthesis in the repair of thoracic wall defects. Am. Surg., 151:469, 1960.
3. Parrish, F. F., Murray, J. A., and Urquhart, B. A.: The use of polyethylene mesh (Marlex[R]) as an adjacent in reconstructive surgery of the extremities. Clin. Orthop., 137:276, 1978.
4. Usher, F. C., and Wallace, S. A.: Tissue reaction to plastic. A comparison of nylon, Orlon, Dacron, Teflon and Marlex. A.M.A. Arch. Surg., 76:997, 1958.
5. Usher, F. C., et al.: Marlex mesh, a new plastic mesh for replacing tissue defects. III. Clinical studies. A.M.A. Arch. Surg., 78:138, 1959.

Repair of Thoracic Wall Defects Using Marlex Mesh and an Overlying Omental Pedicle Flap

by Ronald M. Bright

When large quantities of soft tissue are removed during an en bloc resection of a portion of the lateral chest wall, it may not be possible to close this defect using only the remaining surrounding soft tissue. The resulting physiologic defect may threaten the animal's ability to resume normal ventilation. Closing this defect, therefore, may call for extensive reconstructive repair.

Omentum has been used successfully both in human and veterinary surgical procedures to reconstruct chest walls in which defects existed without sufficient soft tissue cover.[1,3,5,6] When combined with the intrapleural placement of Marlex mesh*, this repair provides excellent chest-wall stability and allows immediate and effective postoperative ventilation.[2,3] The repair is dependable, the donor defect is minimal, and the morbidity rate is low.

Skeletal support is provided by the intrapleural placement of Marlex mesh. This mesh implant not only supplies rigidity to the wall, but also acts as a "bed" for accepting the transferred omental flap. The distance one can mobilize the omentum outside the abdomen in the dog depends on the size of the dog, the amount of fat within the omentum, and how far forward on the thoracic wall the defect is. I have successfully repaired both right- and left-sided thoracic wall defects as far forward as the fourth rib. Defects up to four rib spaces in width have been successfully repaired.

For left-sided thoracic wall defects, a left omental pedicle is formed; similarly, a right-sided omental pedicle flap is formed for repair of a right lateral wall defect[4] (see Chap. 15).

Surgical Technique

Following en bloc excision of diseased tissues, a chest tube is inserted and is allowed to exit two spaces

*Davol Rubber Co., Providence, RI

cranial or caudal to the defect. Marlex mesh is tailored to the defect and is placed intrapleurally. The mesh inlay and the surrounding soft tissue are temporarily covered with towels soaked in saline solution while the veterinarian harvests the omental flap in the abdominal cavity.

A paracostal incision is used to approach the abdomen and should be of sufficient length to allow easy exposure of the stomach, greater omentum, pancreas, and spleen. Omental lengthening procedures are done, and the left omental pedicle is formed (Fig. 21-7). A subcutaneous tunnel is then made between the paracostal incision and the defect (Fig. 21-8, large arrow). The tunnel must be of sufficient width to prevent excessive pressure on the vessels within the pedicled omentum. The omentum is handled carefully, to avoid kinking or twisting as it is mobilized cranially through the subcutaneous tunnel. The omental flap is laid over the mesh so that the defect is covered and is filled with omentum. This flap is then carefully tacked to the periphery of the defect using 2-0 or 3-0 nylon or polyglactin 910 suture.† An adequate seal of the thoracic cavity is ensured before proceeding by tacking additional layers of omentum loosely over the first layer, as needed.

†Vicryl, Ethicon, Inc., Somerville, NJ 08876

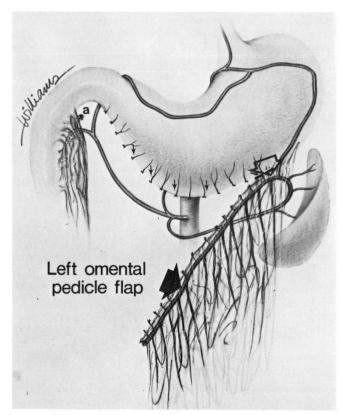

Fig. 21-7. *A left omental pedicle has been formed with the left gastroepiploic artery preserved (arrow). (From Bright, R. M., Birchard, S. J., and Long. G. G.: Repair of thoracic wall defects in the dog with an omental pedicle flap. J. Am. Anim. Hosp. Assoc., 18:277, 1982.)*

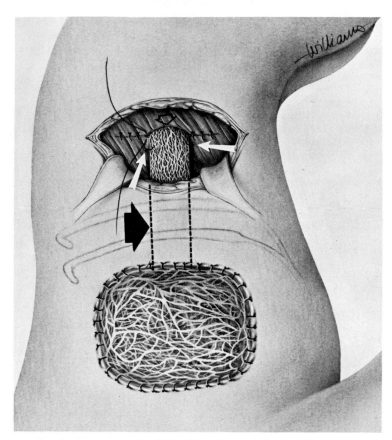

Fig. 21-8. *A defect in the paracostal musculature remains where the omental pedicle is seen to emerge from the abdominal cavity (open arrow). A subcutaneous tunnel accommodates the omentum as it courses forward to cover the thoracic defect (large arrow). The dorsal and ventral border of the omentum is affixed securely to the underlying musculature (white arrows). The omentum is laid over the Marlex mesh "bed" and is tacked to the peripheral musculature to create an airtight seal. (From Bright, R. M., Birchard, S. J., and Long. G. G.: Repair of thoracic wall defects in the dog with an omental pedicle flap. J. Am. Anim. Hosp. Assoc., 18:277, 1982.)*

The paracostal abdominal incision is then closed above and below the area where omentum exits from the abdomen (Fig. 21-8, open arrow). The purpose of this incomplete closure of the paracostal musculature and fascia is to avoid compromising the blood supply of the omentum as it passes through the incision. The defect remaining in the abdominal wall is approximately two fingers in width. With slight forward tension on the omentum, the dorsal and ventral edges of the omentum are then affixed to the underlying musculature using 3-0 nylon suture (Fig. 21-8, white arrows). This procedure stabilizes the omentum and prevents its tendency to slide back into the abdominal cavity. Penrose drains are then placed subcutaneously beneath the thoracic and paracostal incisions. Skin closure is not a problem, because of the amount of redundant skin in this region.

The chest tube is removed when the veterinarian judges it prudent to do so. Generally, 2 or 3 hours is sufficient time for chest tube placement. The Penrose drain placed under the paracostal skin incision is removed in 2 or 3 days, the thoracic drain is removed in 5 days. This delay in removal from the thoracic site is necessary to prevent a higher incidence of seroma formation. The wound sites are bandaged with a minimum of pressure. Daily bandage changes are necessary until the final Penrose drain is removed.

Results

The cosmetic appearance of the chest wall following this repair is excellent. Animals undergoing such reconstruction have an immediate return of ventilatory function. Because the omentum has a rich blood supply, it aids in combating localized infection. This ability is of particular benefit to those patients requiring resection of infected tissue in the lateral thoracic chest wall.

References and Suggested Readings

1. Baffi, R. R., Didolkov, M. S., and Bekamjian, V.: Reconstruction of sternal and abdominal wall defects in a case of desmoid tumor. J. Thorac. Cardiovasc. Surg., 74:105, 1977.
2. Bright, R. M.: Reconstruction of thoracic wall defects using Marlex[R] mesh. J. Am. Anim. Hosp. Assoc., 17:415, 1981.
3. Bright, R. M., Birchard, S. J., and Long, G. G.: Repair of thoracic wall defects in the dog with an omental pedicle flap. J. Am. Anim. Hosp. Assoc., 18:277, 1982.

4. Bright, R. M., and Thacker, H. L.: The formation of an omental pedicle flap and its experimental use in the repair of a diaphragmatic rent in the dog. J. Am. Anim. Hosp. Assoc., *18*:283, 1982.

5. Jacobs, E. W., Hoffman, S., Kirschner, P., and Danese, C.: Reconstruction of a large chest wall using greater omentum. Arch. Surg., *113*:886, 1978.

6. Jurkiewicz, M. G., and Arnold, P. G.: The omentum: an account of its use in the reconstruction of the chest wall. Ann. Surg., *185*:548, 1977.

Thoracic Drainage

by DENNIS T. CROWE

The recognition and management of the dog or cat with fluid or air accumulation in the pleural cavity is common in small animal practice. Although small accumulations may be easily tolerated and hence go undetected, larger amounts prevent normal lung expansion during the inspiratory phase of the ventilatory cycle and cause significant increases in ventilatory effort. If significant air or fluid accumulations are present, the practicing veterinarian is presented with an animal displaying signs of dyspnea, orthopnea, polypnea, and poor tolerance for exercise or stress. Immediate thoracentesis of fluid or air can be accomplished with a minimal amount of stress and may provide enough drainage to be lifesaving. Although mild conditions may require treatment only by thoracentesis, others of a more severe nature require the placement of a chest tube (tube thoracostomy) and either intermittent or continuous pleural evacuation. It is the purpose of this discussion to review these methods and their effectiveness and management.

Needle Thoracentesis

Emergency and diagnostic needle thoracentesis can be performed simply with an 18- to 20-gauge hypodermic needle, a short plastic intravenous catheter, or a bovine teat cannula. Because the less danger of iatrogenic injury exists with the catheter and the teat cannula, these instruments are preferred. A 3-way stopcock and a 25- or 60-ml syringe are attached to the needle either directly or by a 20-inch section of intravenous extension tubing. A second section of tubing, attached to the sidearm of the stopcock, is useful in directing aspirated fluids into a collection jar (Fig. 21-9). This assembled apparatus can be operated by one person.

Thoracentesis is usually performed in the seventh or eighth intercostal space, with the patient standing. Sternal or lateral recumbency are also suitable positions. The dorsoventral location of the puncture site within the intercostal space is influenced by whether air or fluid is to be aspirated. With air, the midthoracic region is preferred, with the animal in lateral recumbency. If the animal is standing or is in sternal recumbency, air is aspirated at the junction of the dorsal and middle thirds. Fluid is best removed from the middle third of the seventh intercostal space, when the animal

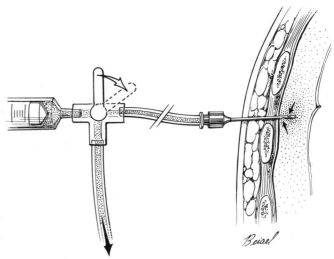

Fig. 21-9. *Apparatus for thoracentesis: an indwelling intravenous catheter or a bovine teat cannula, a three-way stopcock, a large syringe, and tubing from an intravenous administration set.*

is standing or is in sternal recumbency. Lower placement of a needle may lead to penetration of the dome of the diaphragm and or liver injury.

Inadvertent injury to the lung parenchyma with the tip of the needle may lead to pneumothorax. This complication is avoided by the use of a metal or plastic teat tube instead of a hypodermic needle. If a needle is used, a sterile hemostat should be clamped to the shaft of the needle, to prevent overpenetration as soon as the pleura has been entered.

Thoracentesis is best used as a diagnostic maneuver to remove enough fluid for diagnostic purposes and for initial treatment of acute pneumothorax and pleural effusions. This procedure may also be used for intermittent drainage of the pleural cavity in the treatment of a slow accumulation of fluid or air in the pleural space.

The surgical placement of a chest drainage tube (tube thoracostomy), however, is preferred for the removal of large volumes of fluid or continuing accumulation of air. Clinical experience has also suggested that it is impossible to drain the pleural space adequately with simple thoracenteses when accumulations of blood or pus are present.

Tube Thoracostomy

Tube thoracostomy involves the surgical placement of a rubber, polyvinyl or silicon* tube into the pleural space. The tubing should be flexible, but not collapsible. The internal diameter of the tube should be at least half to two-thirds the width of one of the larger intercostal spaces (approximate diameter of a mainstem bronchus). This is important if tension pneumothorax is being treated.

The tube's size is also especially important when draining fluid that is viscous. Other factors that influence flow rates and effectiveness are the number and

*Such as Silastic, Dow Corning Corp., Midland, MI 48640

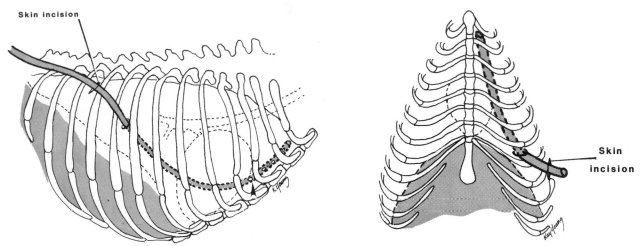

Fig. 21-10. *Line drawings from lateral (A) and ventrodorsal (B) radiographs demonstrate proper intrathoracic location of the chest drain. Arrowhead in A indicates the location of the last side hole in the catheter as seen on the radiograph (where the radiopaque line is interrupted). (Note: For best function, the tube should be placed no farther cranially than the level of the second rib; more cranial placement may obstruct the flow of air or fluid.)*

size of the holes placed in the catheter tip. Experimental flow studies on catheters indicate that when 3 side holes are present, each additional hole increases the flow rate by only 5%. Most commercially available chest tubes contain an end hole and 5 or 6 side holes. The recommended size of the hole is approximately one-fourth the circumference of the tube. Diameters exceeding one-third the circumference of the tube cause considerable weakness and predispose the tube to kinking.

Commercially available chest tubes contain a marker strip throughout their length to allow radiographic confirmation of placement. The end of a chest tube should be placed on the ventral floor of the patient's thorax and cranial to the heart or next to it. In this location, both air and fluid can be drained efficiently (Fig. 21-10).

It is, of course, imperative that all holes be within the chest cavity (Fig. 21-11). This placement can be verified radiographically with tubes that have a "sentinel eye," that is, the radiopaque marker is interrupted where the last hole is located (see Fig. 21-10A).

To place a chest tube at the time of a surgical proce-

dure, a small skin incision is made at the ninth or tenth intercostal space. With a curved hemostat, a subcutaneous tunnel is made in a cranial direction. The tip of the hemostat is bluntly forced through intercostal muscle and parietal pleura at the seventh or eighth intercostal space. The tip of the tube is positioned in its correct location within the chest cavity, and the connector end is withdrawn externally by the clamp (Fig. 21-12). At the skin's surface, long, heavy sutures are tied to the exiting tube and are secured by simple criss-cross wrapping (Fig. 21-13). Such measures have been found to be more effective than suturing through adhesive tape placed around the catheter, because moisture may loosen the tape. The exiting catheter and torso are then wrapped gently but securely with gauze and tape for further protection. The end of the catheter should be exposed somewhere near the dorsum of the animal's back, and the rest of the catheter should be covered to prevent its being damaged or dislodged.

Closed Thoracostomy

A "closed" tube thoracostomy is performed outside the operating room with the patient in lateral recumbency. Following liberal clipping of the hair and surgical preparation of the skin on the side selected, local anesthestic is infiltrated into the proposed site of tube insertion. This should include the nearby pleura and intercostal nerve. Although local anesthesia generally suffices, neuroleptanalgesia or sedation may also be used. Using aseptic technique, a small skin incision is made at the tenth-to-eleventh interspace, and a curved hemostat is used bluntly to create a tunnel cranially to the seventh-to-eighth or eighth-to-ninth interspace. This same hemostat is then used to separate the intercostal muscles and to create a small defect into the pleural space. The catheter tip is then grasped in the jaws of stout hemostatic clamps, is passed down the subcutaneous tunnel, and is forced into the chest cavity through intercostal musculature previously sepa-

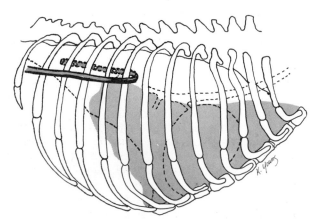

Fig. 21-11. *Line drawing of a lateral radiograph demonstrates improper placement and kinking of the chest drain.*

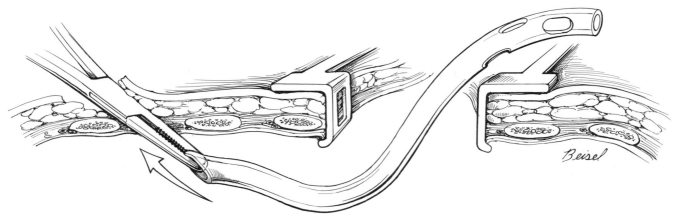

Fig. 21-12. *In pulling the chest drain out through the seventh or eighth intercostal space, cutting the end of the tube on an oblique angle facilitates its movement through the thoracic wall.*

rated by the tip of the hemostat. This maneuver is difficult and must be closely controlled to prevent overpenetration. Practice with a cadaver is recommended.

Placement can also be accomplished using a commercially available tube and trocar stylet unit, which is pushed through the chest wall. Again, *extreme care* must be taken not to penetrate viscera after placement through the pleura. The skin over the tenth-to-eleventh interspace is pulled cranially by an assistant to overlie the eighth-to-ninth interspace. The trocar-pointed stylet is then forced through the intercostal space with a controlled thrust. As soon as the tip of the tube enters the chest, the metal stylet is retracted to just within the cannula. The rigidity of the stylet aids in manipulating the tube into the correct cranioventral position. The assistant then allows the patient's skin to retract caudally to its normal position. Once released, the skin and subcutaneous tissue form a seal over the hole.

The open end of the tube must be attached to one of the following: (1) a Heimlich valve* or another one-way egress valve; (2) a three-way stopcock; (3) an underwater seal; (4) an underwater seal with controlled, continuous, low-vacuum suction drainage; or (5) an underwater seal with controlled, intermittent, low-vacuum suction drainage. The choice of device depends upon the size of the patient, the nature of the pleural fluid, and the patient's tractability. The Heimlich valve consists of a rubber one-way flutter valve that is enclosed in a clear plastic tube that is open at each end. The end of the chest tube is attached to the wide end of the flutter valve and is an excellent instrument for evacuating air, blood, and other fluids (Fig. 21-14). The valve may have to be replaced during long-term drainage of blood or other tenacious fluids because the rubber valve may become sticky and may not open freely. Although the valve has been used with success in animals weighing under 15 kg, some smaller patients may not be able to generate sufficient increases in intrapleural pressure during expiration to open the valve and to allow evacuation. One-way valves are especially useful in the initial management of tension pneumothorax.

A stopcock attached to the end of a catheter prevents air or fluid from moving either in or out without its manual operation. Its use is recommended in those animals weighing less than 15 kg and in animals that are not accumulating air or fluid rapidly in their pleural cavity. Using a large syringe for periodic aspiration, the valve is opened and closed as needed, to accomplish thoracentesis.

A disposable plastic intravenous administration set can be used to facilitate the drainage of large quantities

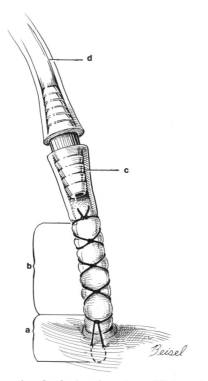

Fig. 21-13. *Securing the drain tube using a "Chinese finger trap" friction suture. First the suture is tied without tension to prevent irritation of the skin (a), then, in a criss-cross fashion, multiple surgeon's knots are tied around the tube (b); chest catheter (c); gum-rubber tubing (d).*

*Bard-Parker, Rutherford, NJ 07070

Expiration   Inspiration

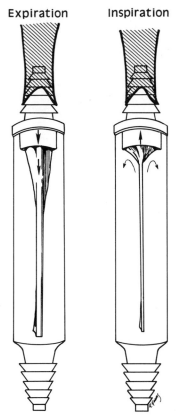

Fig. 21-14. *These diagrams demonstrate the function of the Heimlich flutter valve. During inspiration, the valve stays closed, and no air can enter the thoracic cavity. During expiration, as intrapleural pressure increases, the air or fluid is forced out of the pleural space through the chest tube and one-way valve.*

of pleural effusion. The male end of the plastic tubing is fitted to the side arm of the stopcock, and the drip chamber is cut from the other end. When the side arm tubing is filled and the stopcock is opened, drainage of the pleural space to a collecting vessel is possible by siphon action.

To make and use an underwater seal, a length of tubing connected to the chest catheter is placed 1 to 2 cm below the fluid's surface in a bowl or bottle containing 2 to 3 cm of sterile saline solution. This useful, quickly made, one-way valve is recommended only as a *temporary* measure when no other instruments or one-way valves are available and when time does not permit delayed action. When using this technique, care is taken to make sure the tube stays submerged. If the seal is broken, pneumothorax rapidly develops. Thus, constant observation of this temporary device is mandatory.

UNDERWATER SEAL AND SUCTION DRAINAGE

Suction drainage of the pleura can be easily and economically accomplished. Both 2-bottle and 3-bottle systems are adaptable to veterinary practice, and the equipment is unsophisticated and reusable. With a 2-bottle suction drainage system, the chest catheter is connected to a 500- to 2000-ml sterile glass bottle con-

taining enough sterile saline solution to fill it to a level of 2 to 3 cm from the bottom. The tube within the bottle is placed 1 to 2 cm below the surface of the saline solution. The bottle acts as both a collection reservoir and an underwater seal system to prevent air from being aspirated into the pleural space. A second bottle is partially filled with sterile saline solution and is connected to the first. A rigid plastic vent tube is open to room air, so that it permits air to be aspirated into the bottle as vacuum is applied (Fig. 21-15). Thus, by raising or lowering the tube in the second bottle, the amount of vacuum applied to the catheter extending into the patient's chest can be controlled. If the vacuum regulation tube is submerged to 10 cm, the patient will not experience more than 10 cm water transpleural suction pressure.

Experimental and clinical studies have shown that a continuous 10 to 15 cm negative pressure effectively aspirates tension pneumothorax and allows visceral and parietal pleural surfaces to be approximated. This pressure has proved to be one of the keys to the successful, spontaneous sealing of large defects in the lungs of man and animals. With the use of suction drainage, many pneumothoraces close, and the need for thoracotomy is thus obviated. This finding is in contrast to drainage without suction, experimental and clinical studies of which have shown that large leaks either do not seal or seal slowly.

With a 3-bottle suction drainage system, the first bottle is connected to the chest catheter and acts as a fluid trap. Such a system is particularly useful if hemorrhage or hydrothorax is voluminous. If traumatic hemorrhage is severe, autotransfusion may be considered from this

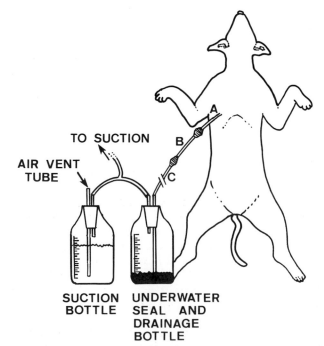

TO SUCTION

AIR VENT
TUBE

A

B

C

SUCTION
BOTTLE

UNDERWATER
SEAL AND
DRAINAGE
BOTTLE

Fig. 21-15. *Two-bottle suction drainage. A, Distal end of the chest tube exiting from the bandaged thorax; B, gum-rubber tubing (approximately half an inch in diameter), to allow "stripping" of the chest tube, about three feet long (see text); C, polyvinyl chloride "bubble" tubing.*

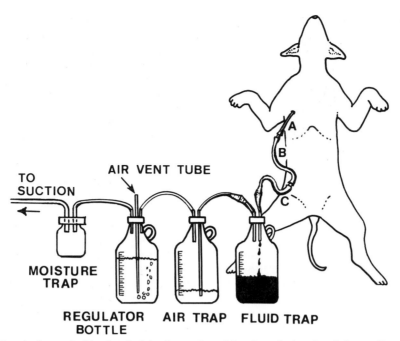

TO SUCTION

AIR VENT TUBE

MOISTURE TRAP

REGULATOR BOTTLE

AIR TRAP

FLUID TRAP

A

B

C

Fig. 21-16. *Three-bottle suction drainage. A, Distal end of the chest tube exiting from the bandaged thorax; B, gum-rubber tubing (approximately half an inch in diameter), to allow "stripping" of the tube, about three feet in length (see text); C, polyvinyl chloride "bubble" tubing.*

vessel. In this case, instead of being empty in the beginning, approximately 50 to 75 ml anticoagulant solution are added to the bottle. When 500 to 1000 ml blood have been aspirated, a second fluid-trap bottle containing anticoagulant is substituted for the first bottle and allows autotransfusion to begin. The second bottle of the 3-bottle system is connected to the first bottle and acts as the underwater seal. Its function and filling is similar to the first bottle of a 2-bottle system. The third bottle is connected to the second and again acts as suction regulator (Fig. 21-16).

Any animal whose chest catheter is connected to an underwater seal device by a tube must be watched carefully because detachment or chewing of the tubing could lead to a massive pneumothorax. This possibility is the major drawback of the use of the bottle suction systems in small animal practice. If an intensive-care unit, a 24-hour-staffed hospital, or an emergency practice is available, however, then continuous suction and drainage may be accomplished and continued for as long as necessary.

With several alternatives available, selection of a drainage system depends on: (1) the patient's size; (2) the type of material being drained and its rate of accumulation within the pleural space; (3) the facilities and staff available for monitoring; and (4) economic considerations. Without question, the underwater seal and suction drainage system is the most effective. It is also the most time consuming and complicated and is the least economical, however. Even though the glass components can be autoclaved and reused, the initial expense for a commercial 3-bottle system is approximately $30.*

Currently, the underwater seal and suction drainage system is primarily recommended for the treatment of trauma or disease conditions involving the continuous or rapid accumulation of air or fluids in the pleural space. In other situations, the use of a Heimlich valve is preferred if the patient's weight exceeds 15 kg. For patients under 15 kg, a 3-way stopcock and syringe are effective in evacuating the pleural space.

Complications

As previously mentioned, anytime the patient must be left unattended, the *entire* chest catheter and attached apparatus must be covered completely under a well-secured dressing to prevent disturbance or dislodgment.

An occasional problem is the accumulation of fibrin clots, especially when a small-lumen-diameter catheter (under 20 French) has been used or when a large amount of fibrin, blood, or other proteinaceous material is being drained. Blockage is prevented by frequent manipulations of the tubing extending from the chest catheter to the underwater seal. When using a three-way stopcock on the end of the chest catheter, a small amount of air and sterile heparinized saline solution can be infused every few hours; when using the Heimlich valve or other one-way rubber valve, it may be necessary to change the valve.

For the underwater seal and suction drainage system, at least the first three feet of the tubing leading from the chest catheter to the underwater seal should be made of gum rubber† (see Figs. 21-15 and 21-16). By grasping the tubing (B in the figures) as near to the

*Available from American Hospital Supply Corp., McGaw Park, IL 60085. A 3-bottle system is no longer available, but one may buy a 2-bottle and a 1-bottle system and combine them.

†Tomac amber latex intravenous tubing, available from American Hospital Supply Corp., McGaw Park, IL 60085

patient as possible and by pinching it closed, a stripping motion (a sliding motion, with the tube pinched off) is applied along the length of the tube for 20 to 40 cm. The stripping action creates a sudden, high negative pressure inside the tube past the area where the tube has been pinched closed. At the end of each stripping action, the pinch is released, and a surge of negative pressure is transferred to the thoracic catheter. The high negative pressure often jars loose and evacuates fibrin clots and debris inside the catheter. It is recommended that this "stripping" be done every hour when a significant amount of blood or other "sticky" fluid is encountered. The frequency of stripping may be decreased as the amount of fluid being removed decreases. Generally, by the second day, stripping is only necessary every few hours.

Another reported complication is subcutaneous emphysema as the result of a large hole in the chest wall that is not completely occluded by the presence of the drain tube. An occlusive dressing applied around the exit site helps to minimize this problem. Lung-tissue entrapment and infarction by vigorous chest suction have been reported with the use of low vacuum levels. This complication may be considered whenever a radiographic pulmonary infiltrate appears near a side or end hole of the chest tube. Unregulated, high vacuum levels, as in operating room or portable suction units (80 to 120 mm Hg), should never be used. All active suction must be regulated by a 2- or 3-bottle system.

Although infection can occur whenever any indwelling catheter is used, this problem is minimized by careful tube placement and care. In a randomized study of 120 human patients with indwelling chest drains, half were treated with prophylactic antibiotics and the other half were given a placebo. Those patients given antibiotics had the higher infection rate. Clinical results with the use of chest drains in dogs and cats also seem to indicate similar conclusions. Proper wound care at the site where the drainage catheter enters the chest and strict attention to aseptic technique and suction drainage remain the most important factors in preventing serious infection of the pleural cavity and subcutaneous tissue.

The chest drain should be removed whenever its presence is no longer needed. This time may range from the immediate postoperative period to more than a week. A rule of thumb in dogs over 20 kg is that when under 50 ml fluid is drained in a 24-hour period, the tube may be removed. In smaller patients, the amount of fluid accumulation considered significant is proportionally less. If any question exists concerning the safe removal of the chest tube, it should be clamped for 24 hours. Radiographs are then taken to determine whether any intrapleural accumulation of air or fluid is present. If there is none, the tube may be safely removed.

When the veterinarian feels that the tube is no longer needed, the sutures and bandage are discarded, and the tube is quickly removed. The hole is covered with a gauze dressing impregnated with an antibiotic ointment. The gauze is held in place with a torso bandage. Complete sealing of the wound occurs in 2 or 3 days.

Comments

Often, animals suffering from multiple injuries, including fractures, have a pneumothorax. Mild pneumothoraces do not render the animal dyspneic and are readily diagnosed by chest radiographs. If anesthesia is necessary for fracture repair, it is my opinion that a chest tube should be inserted to aid resolution of the pneumothorax, to help in lung healing, and to allow earlier and safer use of anesthesia. Positive-pressure ventilation during anesthesia may predispose the healing lung or bronchi to rupture. Without a chest tube in place, a tension pneumothorax could rapidly develop and could prove fatal.

References and Suggested Readings

Brandstetter, R. D., and Cohen, R. P.: Hypoxemia after thoracentesis. JAMA, *242*:1060, 1979.

Brasmer, T. H.: Thoracic wall reconstruction. *In* Current Techniques in Small Animal Surgery. Edited by M. J. Bojrab. Philadelphia, Lea & Febiger, 1975.

Butler, W. B.: Use of a flutter valve in treatment of pneumothorax in dogs and cats. J. Am. Vet. Med. Assoc., *155*:1997, 1969.

Creighton, S. R., and Wilkins, R. J.: Pleural effusions. *In* Current Veterinary Therapy: Small Animal Practice IV. Edited by R. W. Kirk. Philadelphia, W. B. Saunders, 1977.

Graham, J. M., Mattox, K. L., and Beall, A. C.: Penetrating trauma of the lung. J. Trauma, *19*:665, 1979.

Griffith, G. L., et al.: Acute traumatic hemothorax. Ann. Thorac. Surg., *26*:204, 1978.

Harrah, J. D., and Wangensteen, S. L.: A simple emergency closed thoracostomy set. Surgery, *68*:583, 1970.

Hopkins, J. W., and Fisk, C.: Continuous suction therapy of pneumothorax in the newborn infant: a rapid cribside technique. J. Iowa Med. Soc., *60*:631, 1970.

Krahwinkel, D. J.: Lower respiratory tract trauma. *In* Current Veterinary Therapy: Small Animal Practice IV. Edited by R. W. Kirk. Philadelphia, W. B. Saunders, 1977.

Richards, W.: Tube thoracostomy. J. Fam. Pract., *6*:629, 1978.

Sauer, B. W.: Valve drainage of the pleural cavity of the dog. J. Am. Vet. Med. Assoc., *155*:1977, 1969.

Withrow, S. J., Fenner, W. R., and Wilkins, R. J.: Closed chest drainage and lavage for treatment of pyothorax in the cat. J. Am. Anim. Hosp. Assoc., *11*:90, 1975.

Zimmerman, J. E., Dunbar, B. S., and Klingenmaier, C. H.: Management of subcutaneous emphysema, pneumomediastinum, and pneumothorax during respirator therapy. Crit. Care Med., *3*:69, 1975.

22 * Kidney

Nephrectomy

by EBERHARD ROSIN

Nephrectomy may be considered as treatment for the following unilateral conditions: (1) solitary renal cysts causing serious renal dysfunction; (2) hydronephrosis; (3) polycystic disease of the kidney complicated by pyelonephritis refractive to medical treatment; (4) infestation by Dioctophyma renale with severe degenerative changes; (5) neoplasms of the kidney if metastasis has not occurred; (6) traumatic destruction of the majority of the renal parenchyma; (7) avulsion of the renal pedicle or uncontrolled hemorrhage; and (8) abnormal kidney drained by an ectopic ureter.[1] The diagnosis of these conditions and assessment of adequate function of the contralateral kidney are described elsewhere.

Nephrectomy is seldom performed when the architecture and vascular supply of the kidney are normal. In certain chronic pathologic states, the kidney is frequently enlarged and is extensively supplied by neovascularization. The normal renal artery and vein may be present or nonexistent. Surgical technique for nephrectomy in such instances is improvised by the veterinary surgeon and may approximate the dissection required to remove any abdominal mass. The operative technique described in the following paragraphs is limited to removal of a kidney in which the gross anatomic structure is normal.

Surgical Technique

The patient is anesthetized and an endotracheal tube is placed, with the patient in the dorsal recumbent position. The abdomen is prepared for an aseptic surgical procedure.

A midline abdominal incision is made from the xiphoid process through the umbilicus. The edges of the incision are protected with moist laparotomy packs, and a Balfour* retractor is inserted.

The right kidney is exposed by lifting the descending portion of the duodenum and by positioning the other loops of intestine to the left of the mesoduodenum. The left kidney is similarly exposed, by using the mesentery of the descending colon as retractor to displace bowel loops to the right. (Fig. 22-1). The viscera are covered with moist laparotomy packs.

*American V. Mueller, 6600 West Touhy Avenue, Chicago, IL 60648

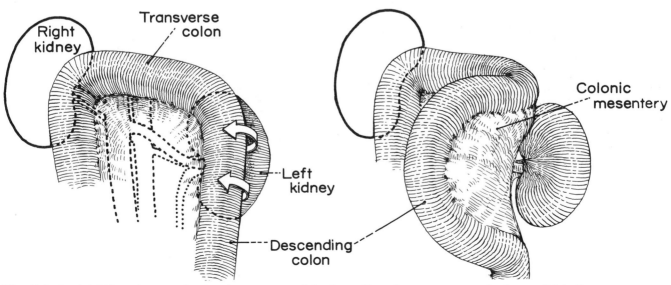

Fig. 22-1. *The left kidney is exposed using the mesentery of the descending colon as a retractor for the small intestine.*

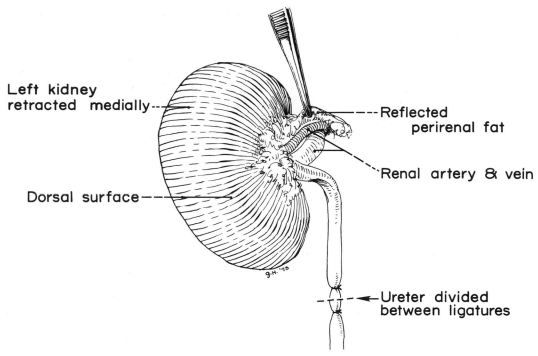

Left kidney
retracted medially

Reflected
perirenal fat

Renal artery & vein

Dorsal surface

Ureter divided
between ligatures

Fig. 22-2. *Reflection of the perirenal fat on the dorsal lateral surface of the renal hilus exposes the renal artery.*

The kidney to be removed is mobilized in the following manner: The peritoneum over the caudal pole of the kidney is grasped with tissue forceps and is incised with scissors. The veterinary surgeon inserts a finger into the opening and gently peels the peritoneum from the kidney. Occasionally, the peritoneum is firmly adhered over the kidney surface at scattered points; these attachments are severed with scissors. Bleeding generated by this reflection of the peritoneum is controlled by electrocautery. Perirenal fat is reflected from the ventromedial surface of the renal hilus to expose the renal vein and ureter. The ureter is further mobilized by dissection through the retroperitoneum, to permit ligation as close to the urinary bladder as feasible. The ureter is divided between 2-0 medium chromic catgut or synthetic absorbable ligatures.

The kidney is lifted from its bed and is retracted medially to expose the perirenal fat on the dorsolateral surface of the renal hilus (Fig. 22-2). Reflection of this fat exposes the renal artery. Care must be taken to avoid transection of *one or more branches* of the renal artery that may be present.

The exposed renal artery and vein are separated and are independently ligated with 2-0 absorbable suture material (Fig. 22-3). The artery and vein are transected distal to each ligature, and the kidney is removed. A

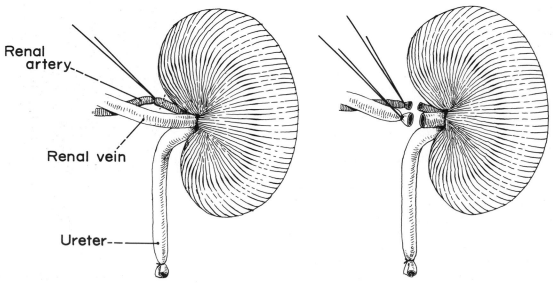

Renal
artery

Renal vein

Ureter

Fig. 22-3. *Individual ligation and transection of the renal artery and vein.*

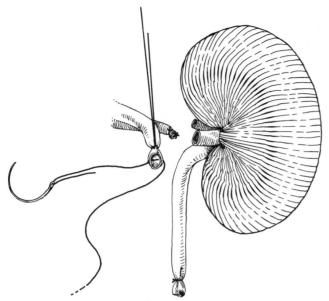

Fig. 22-4. *A ligature is passed through the lumen of the renal artery and vein, distal to the first ligature.*

separate suture ligature of 3-0 absorbable suture material is passed through the lumen of the renal artery and vein, distal to the first ligature, to transfix the distal ligature and to prevent retraction of the vessel from the ligature (Fig. 22-4).

The intestines are returned to normal position, the greater omentum is repositioned over the small intestine, and the abdomen is closed in a standard manner.

Reference and Suggested Reading

1. Osborne, C. A., Low, D. G., and Finco, D. R.: Canine and Feline Urology. Philadelphia, W. B. Saunders, 1972.

Nephrolithotomy

by ELIZABETH A. STONE

Nephrolithotomy is indicated for the removal of a calculus or calculi from a functional kidney. Nephrolithiasis is often associated with chronic or recurrent urinary tract infections. If severe pyelonephritis is present, and if the opposite kidney is normal, nephrectomy is preferred.

Although the most frequently accompanying factor is infection, metabolic defects may also contribute to stone formation. Thus, a preoperative urine sample should be collected by cystocentesis or catheterization; urinalysis, sediment examination, and a quantitative urine culture and sensitivity test should be obtained. If infection is present, appropriate antibiotic therapy should be instituted 24 hours before the surgical procedure, to establish adequate parenchymal and urinary levels of the drug. Renal calculi may cause renal hemorrhage or obstruction of the renal pelvis resulting in hydronephrosis. Plain radiographs and contrast excretory urographs help to identify the size and

shape of the kidneys and to give a crude estimate of renal function.

Serum urea nitrogen and creatinine levels should also be assessed, along with hematologic tests. If the animal is azotemic, diuresis is established before anesthesia, and urine output is monitored through a urinary catheter. A mannitol diuresis helps to prevent renal shutdown due to arterial occlusion.

Surgical Technique

A midline abdominal incision is made extending from the xiphoid process to the umbilicus. If a cystotomy is planned or becomes necessary, the incision is

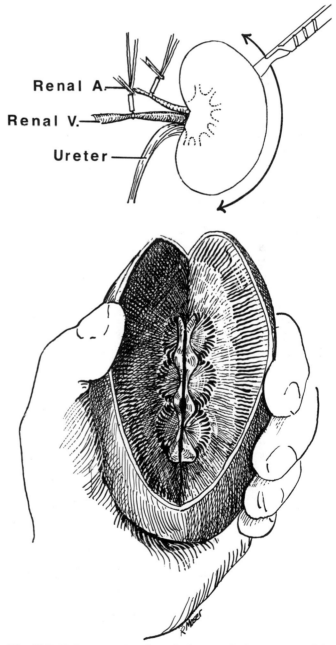

Fig. 22-5. *Midline incision through the capsule down to the pelvic diverticula.*

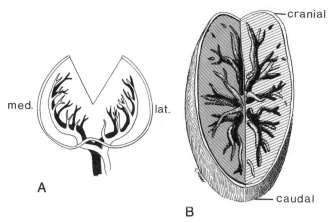

Fig. 22-6. *Distribution of the interlobar vessels, which are avoided by staying on the midline. A, Cross-section. B, Sagittal section.*

extended to the pubis. The renal vessels are located cranial to the ureter. (Their isolation is described in the previous section of this chapter.)

Silk suture (size 1-0) is passed around the renal artery and through a 2-cm length of rubber tubing. This tubing is moved down the ligature to the renal artery to occlude the artery. The procedure is repeated on the renal vein (Fig. 22-5). Thumb-finger compression of the vessels by an assistant is an alternate method. Care is taken to not damage the ureter.

When it has been gently freed from its retroperitoneal attachments, the kidney is isolated by and is packed off with laparotomy sponges, to help prevent abdominal contamination. A sharp incision with a No. 10 or No. 21 scalpel blade is made through the capsule down to the pelvic diverticula long the greater curvature of the organ. It is important to stay on the midline, to avoid damaging the interlobar vessels (Fig. 22-6). The kidney is flushed with warm lactated Ringer's solution, and calculi are carefully removed with forceps or a small curette. A culture is then taken from the renal pelvis. A 3½-French soft rubber catheter is passed down the ureter into the bladder to check for ureteral obstruction (Fig. 22-7). The nephrotomy incision is closed with 3-0 horizontal mattress polyglycolic acid* sutures through the renal cortex. The sutures should not be too tight because the returning blood will increase the size of the kidney. The capsule is then closed with 4-0 nylon† in a continuous pattern (Fig. 22-8). The tourniquets are removed, and any hemorrhage is controlled by direct pressure over the nephrotomy site. Organ ischemia should not exceed 30 minutes.

Postoperative Management

After the surgical procedure, a diuresis is maintained to remove blood clots. Hematuria may persist for a few days. Calculi are analyzed to identify their mineral content. Medical management[1] is essential to prevent recurrence of the calculi.

*Dexon, Davis and Geck, Manati, PR 00701
†Dermalon, Ethicon, Inc., Somerville, NJ 08876

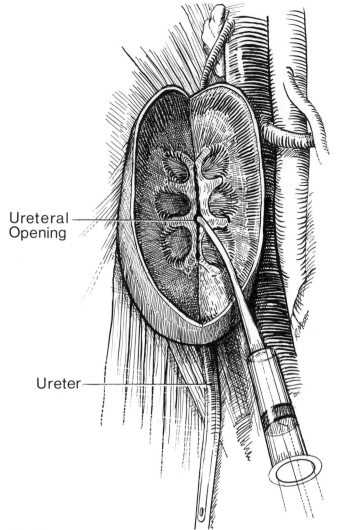

Fig. 22-7. *Catheter passed into the ureter from the renal pelvis.*

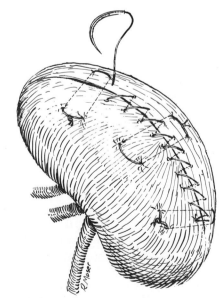

Fig. 22-8. *Closure of the incision with interrupted horizontal mattress sutures in the cortex and a simple continuous suture pattern in the capsule.*

Reference and Suggested Reading

1. Osborne, C. A., Low, D. G., and Finco, D. R.: Canine and Feline Urology. Philadelphia, W. B. Saunders, 1972.

Percutaneous Renal Biopsy

by David F. Edwards

Clinical, laboratory, and radiographic methods can establish the presence of renal dysfunction; however, the specific diagnosis often remains undetermined or is unsatisfactory in dictating management of the patient. Under these circumstances, percutaneous renal biopsy in the dog and cat has provided the veterinarian with a safe, inexpensive method of evaluating renal parenchymal disease. It must be emphasized that renal biopsy without adequate clinical evaluation of the patient represents a *dangerous abuse* of the procedure.

Indications

The indications for renal biopsy can be broadly stated as any situation in which histologic evaluation of the kidney may establish a diagnosis, may determine the type of therapy, or may indicate a prognosis, provided the risks are acceptable in light of the alternatives. More specific indications[3,4,7] include the following: (1) differential diagnosis of hematuria; (2) differential diagnosis of proteinuria; (3) differential diagnosis of renal insufficiency; (4) differential diagnosis of hypertension; (5) differential diagnosis of abnormal renal shape or size; (6) estimation of severity and potential for reversibility or progression of renal disease; (7) evaluation of the success or failure of treatment; and (8) clinical research.

Contraindications

Biopsies should not be performed when the risks of complication outweigh the potential diagnostic benefits. Conditions that represent a contraindication to percutaneous renal biopsy [1,3,4,6,7] include: (1) anemia; (2) bleeding disorders; (3) solitary functional kidney; (4) oliguria or anuria; (5) suspected perinephric abscess; (6) severe azotemia; (7) severe hypertension; (8) hydronephrosis; (9) intrarenal infection, such as pyonephrosis, abscess, or pyelonephritis; (10) suspected renal cysts, vascular tumors, or vascular anomalies; (11) scarred, contracted kidneys; and (12) obstructive uropathy.

Percutaneous renal biopsies are often performed in the presence of contraindications because the conditions are either alleviated, are not suspected, or are not considered to represent an unacceptable risk. The anemic patient can be transfused. Severe azotemia and hypertension increase the risk of postoperative bleeding, but they can be reduced by dialysis and antihypertensive therapy. In man, severe hypertension has been associated with an increased incidence of postbiopsy arteriovenous fistula formation. Conditions of decreased urine production, that is, anuric or oliguric nephropathy and obstructive uropathy, may lead to postbiopsy hematoma formation in the renal pelvis with subsequent hydronephrosis. Knowledge of renal histopathologic changes is often vital to the management of the anuric or oliguric patient, however, and the risks associated with biopsy are relative. An obstructive uropathy should be relieved prior to a biopsy procedure. Scarred, contracted kidneys have a small cortex, making inadvertent biopsy of the renal medulla or pelvis more likely, but not unavoidable.

Suspicion of hydronephrosis, renal cysts, vascular tumors or anomalies, and perirenal or intrarenal infection normally precludes the use of percutaneous renal biopsy. In questionable cases, a 22-gauge spinal needle can be passed along the proposed biopsy route. If aspiration returns an unsuspected fluid, such as blood, pus, or urine, it means other than percutaneous renal biopsy should be used to establish a diagnosis. Percutaneous renal biopsy has been performed on patients with pyelonephritis without evidence of dissemination of the infectious process.[6] The patient with only one functional kidney is better suited to a visually guided biopsy procedure. A postoperative complication resulting in transient renal dysfunction can be lethal to the patient with a solitary kidney.

Materials

Franklin-modified Vim-Silverman biopsy needles* (Fig. 22-9) and disposable Vim Tru-Cut biopsy needles† (Fig. 22-10) are used to obtain the biopsy specimens.

Surgical Anatomy

A brief review of the positional and functional anatomy[5] of the kidney in the dog and cat is given to clarify the concepts presented in the description of the biopsy techniques.

The kidneys of the dog and cat are bean-shaped retroperitoneal structures, obliquely situated on either side of the vertebral column. The right kidney is usually located between the thirteenth thoracic and second lumbar vertebra, whereas the left kidney is generally half a kidney's length caudal to the right. Both kidneys in the cat and the left kidney in the dog are freely movable. The right kidney in the dog is more firmly attached to the body wall. The renal artery and vein and the ureter join the kidney at the central depression in the medial surface (hilus). A fibrous capsule surrounds both kidneys.

The functional unit of the kidney is the nephron. Approximately 415,000 nephrons per kidney are found in the dog and 190,000 are seen in the cat. The nephron is composed of the glomerulus and tubular system. An ultrafiltrate of blood is formed in the glomerulus and

*American V. Mueller, 6600 West Touhy Avenue, Chicago, IL 60648
†Travenol Laboratories, Inc., Deerfield, IL 60015

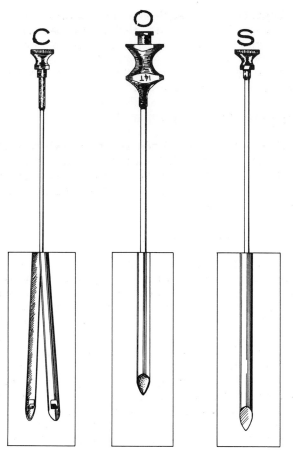

Fig. 22-9. *Franklin-modified Vim-Silverman biopsy needle. Parts include cutting prongs (C), outer cannula (O), and stylet (S).*

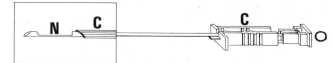

Fig. 22-10. *Vim Tru-Cut biopsy needle. Parts include inner obturator (O) with its cutting notch (N) and outer cannula (C).*

passes down the tubular system, which consists of the proximal tubule, the loop of Henle, the distal tubule, and the collecting duct, to reach the papillary ducts that empty into the funnel-shaped renal pelvis.

The kidney receives the greatest blood flow, by weight, of any organ; this blood flow amounts to 20 to 25% of cardiac output. The main renal artery arises from the dorsal aorta and branches outside the hilus. Several interlobar arteries arise from each branch of the renal artery. These branch into arcuate arteries at the corticomedullary junction. The arcuate arteries radiate toward the periphery of the cortex and give rise to interlobular arteries. Subsequent divisions in the cortex give rise to intralobular arteries and afferent arterioles. The venous return follows a pattern similar to, but not identical to, that of the arterial system.

Longitudinal bisection of the kidney reveals the cortex, medulla, and renal pelvis (Fig. 22-11). The cortical tissue forms the red-brown outer shell of the kidney and is composed predominantly of proximal and distal tubules, and glomeruli. The cortex is the target zone of a percutaneous needle biopsy. If the biopsy contains at least five-six glomeruli, it is generally considered to be

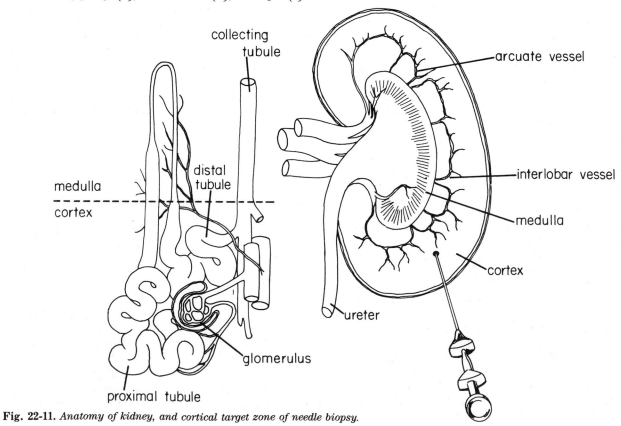

Fig. 22-11. *Anatomy of kidney, and cortical target zone of needle biopsy.*

adequate for diagnostic purposes. The medulla, which lies under the cortex, is lighter in color and is composed of loops of Henle, collecting and papillary ducts, and interstitial tissue. If the biopsy needle penetrates the medulla, the risk of hemorrhage is increased, owing to the presence of larger vessels. The renal pelvis is a funnel-shaped structure that lies central and medial to the medulla. Penetration of the pelvis with the biopsy needle is not only associated with an increased risk of hemorrhage, but also with the potential formation of subcapsular or perirenal urinomas and pyelocutaneous fistulas.

Preoperative Preparation and Anesthesia

The patient should be fasted for 12 hours prior to the procedure. Whole blood clotting time and a platelet count are obtained from each patient. (See "Closed Biopsy Techniques of the Liver," in Chapter 14.) Any abnormalities in hemostasis should preclude performing the biopsy procedure until the nature of the clotting disorder is corrected. Abnormalities in fluid and electrolyte balance and acid-base status should be corrected prior to the biopsy. When possible, an adequate rate of urine production is established by intravenous fluids or diuretics. If use of the blind biopsy technique in the dog is anticipated, the colon is cleared with a warm-water enema 2 to 3 hours prior to the biopsy, and the urinary bladder is emptied immediately preoperatively.

The type of anesthesia required to perform a kidney biopsy is largely dependent upon the level of consciousness of the patient. Biopsy may be performed on severely depressed animals after infiltrating the proposed biopsy site with 2% lidocaine (never exceeding 4.4 mg/kg). Most animals require a general anesthetic. Care must be taken to avoid drugs that are eliminated primarily through the kidney. The ultrashort-acting barbiturates such as thiopental and thiamylal may be used in the dog and cat to induce inhalation anesthesia or for the entire biopsy procedure, if it can be completed in a short enough time.

My preference for anesthesia in a dog undergoing renal biopsy is to administer atropine (0.044 mg/kg, subcutaneously or IM) and oxymorphone (0.22 mg/kg, up to a *maximum* total dose of 4 mg, IM) and to wait 15 to 20 minutes. Then one should administer halothane, place an endotracheal tube, maintain anesthesia with halothane or a halothane-nitrous oxide mixture. Biopsy may be performed on some dogs using lidocaine locally, coupled with atropine and oxymorphone. If rapid awakening is desired, the effects of oxymorphone may be reversed with naloxone (0.2 to 0.4 mg subcutaneously, IM, or IV).

Cats undergoing renal biopsy are premedicated with atropine (0.044 mg/kg, subcutaneously) and acepromazine (0.22 mg/kg, IM). If significant renal insufficiency is *not* present, the cat may then be anesthetized with a light dose of ketamine hydrochloride (2 to 4 mg/kg, IV). In the presence of significant renal insufficiency, the cat should be placed in an induction chamber and an-

esthetized with halothane. An endotracheal tube should be placed, and anesthesia should be maintained with halothane or a halothane-nitrous oxide mixture. Different anesthetic regimens have been recommended by others when obtaining percutaneous renal biopsies in the dog and cat.[6]

Surgical Techniques

Three biopsy techniques are described, two blind and one using a keyhole incision. A cat's kidney can usually be biopsied by a blind technique, whereas renal biopsy in the dog frequently necessitates the use of the keyhole technique.

BLIND BIOPSY IN THE CAT

The cat is positioned in right or left lateral recumbency, depending on which kidney is to be biopsied. The kidney is located by digital palpation of the abdomen and is gently pulled laterally; one should note the area of greatest contact with the abdominal wall (Fig. 22-12). On releasing the kidney, this area is clipped and is prepared as for any aseptic surgical approach. The kidney is again immobilized against the abdominal wall. To prevent dulling of the biopsy needle and to facilitate placement of the needle against the renal capsule, a skin incision is made at the desired location using a No. 11 Beaver blade. The skin incision should be just large enough to accommodate the biopsy needle.

The biopsy needle is then placed in the incision site and is directed in such a fashion that the long axis is pointed away from the hilus and *only* cortical tissue is penetrated (Fig. 22-13). The person who has immobilized the kidney should position the biopsy needle while an assistant performs the other maneuvers necessary to complete the biopsy.

If the Franklin-Silverman biopsy needle is used, the needle with its stylet is placed against the renal capsule

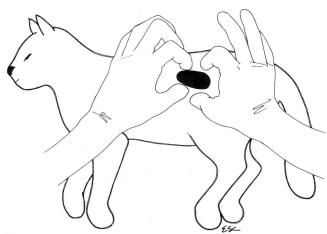

Fig. 22-12. *Schematic drawing depicting positioning of cat kidney for needle biopsy. Fingertips are on mediolateral aspect of kidney. Outward traction pulls kidney laterally.*

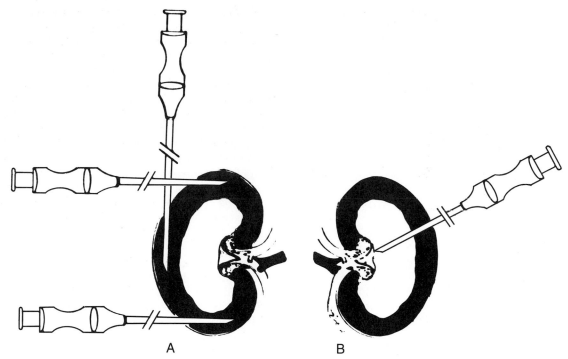

Fig. 22-13. *Pathways of biopsy needle in the kidney:* A, *Several different pathways may be used because they avoid the renal pelvis, renal artery, and renal vein.* B, *Biopsy needle incorrectly aimed and thrust into the renal pelvis. (From Osborne, C. A., Stevens, J. B., and Perman, V.: Kidney biopsy. Vet. Clin. North Am., 4:351, 1974.)*

(Fig. 22-14*A*). The stylet is removed, and the cutting prongs are *gently* inserted until they meet resistance (Fig. 22-14*B*). If no resistance is encountered, the biopsy needle is incorrectly positioned. Once resistance is encountered, the cutting prongs are advanced into the kidney with a *single, sharp, brisk* movement (Fig. 22-14*C*). The inner cutting prongs are held stationary while the outer cannula is slowly advanced in a clockwise-counterclockwise rotary motion (Fig. 22-14*D*). The proximal shaft of the cutting prongs should be permanently marked at a point identifying the depth to which the outer cannula should be advanced in order to ensure closure of the cutting prongs, yet prevent dangerous overpenetration of the renal parenchyma. When the outer cannula has been fully advanced over the cutting prongs, the two parts are removed as a unit (Fig. 22-14*E*). The biopsy specimen is retained between the distal ends of the cutting prongs (Fig. 22-14*E*). An inadequate biopsy specimen is obtained if the needle is misdirected, if the intrarenal advancement of the cutting prongs is not brisk, if the cutting prongs are inadvertently advanced with the outer cannula, or if the outer cannula is incompletely advanced.

The Tru-Cut biopsy needle is similar to the Franklin-modified Vim-Silverman needle, except the former has no stylet, and the outer cannula is fixed together with the inner obturator as a single unit (see Fig. 22-10). If the Tru-Cut needle is used, the needle is placed against the renal capsule with the outer cannula extended over the obturator and its cutting notch (Fig. 22-15*A*). The obturator is advanced into the kidney with a *single, sharp, brisk* movement (Fig. 22-15*B*). The obturator is

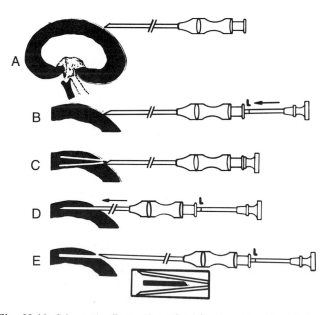

Fig. 22-14. *Schematic illustration of mechanism of action of the Franklin-Silverman biopsy needle. A, The tip of the outer cannula with stylet is in contact with the renal capsule. B, The stylet is removed and is replaced with cutting prongs. C, The cutting prongs are thrust into the kidney. The resistance imparted by the renal parenchyma forces the blades of the cutting prongs to spread apart. D, The outer cannula is advanced over the cutting prongs, forcing them into apposition. The outer cannula is advanced just beyond the landmark (L) filed in the shaft of the cutting prongs. E, The outer cannula and cutting prongs containing a biopsy sample (inset) are removed from the kidney. (From Osborne, C. A., Stevens, J. B., and Perman, V.: Kidney biopsy. Vet. Clin. North Am., 4:351, 1974.)*

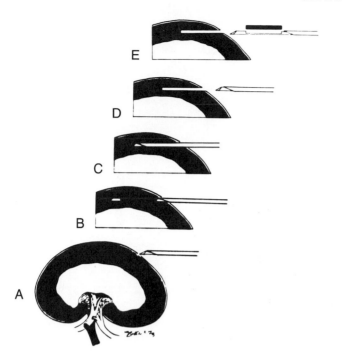

Fig. 22-15. *Schematic illustration of procedure and mechanism of action of the Vim Tru-Cut biopsy needle. A, The tips of the outer cannula and inner obturator-specimen rod are in contact with the renal capsule. B, The inner obturator-specimen rod is thrust into the renal cortex. C, The outer cannula is advanced over the specimen notch in the stationary inner obturator-specimen rod. D, The biopsy needle containing a biopsy specimen is removed from the kidney. E, The outer cannula is pulled back to expose the specimen notch containing a biopsy sample. (From Osborne, C. A., Stevens, J. B., and Perman, V.: Kidney biopsy. Vet. Clin. North Am., 4:351, 1974).*

Digital palpation is used to locate the *left* kidney and to immobilize it against the *right* abdominal wall. This maneuver requires placing the thumb and index finger of one hand against the cranial pole of the kidney and the thumb and index finger of the opposite hand against the caudal pole of the kidney (Fig. 22-16). Alternatively, the kidney may be elevated to the left lateral abdominal wall with one hand, while the thumb and index finger of the opposite hand are placed against the cranial pole of the kidney (Fig. 22-17). Depending on the maneuverability of the left kidney and the depth of anesthesia, a variable amount of force is required to immobilize the kidney. Elevation of the cranial half of the dog facilitates the palpation of the left kidney. If the left kidney is not palpable, or if it is difficult to immobilize, the keyhole technique should be used to perform the biopsy.

Once correct positioning of the kidney is ensured, the left lateral abdominal wall is clipped and is prepared as for any aseptic surgical approach. The left kidney is again fixed against the right abdominal wall. The veterinary surgeon, operator of the biopsy needle, stands on the opposite side of the table from the assistant, who has immobilized the kidney. By digital palpation with one finger, the veterinary surgeon identifies the outline and the position of the kidney. Using a No. 11 Beaver blade, a skin incision is made at the desired location, the biopsy needle is placed against the renal capsule, and the needle is directed in such a fashion that the long axis is pointed away from the hilus; *only* cortical tissue is penetrated (see Fig. 22-13). (See the discussion on biopsy technique in the cat for technical aspects of operating the biopsy needle.) I have found

held stationary while the outer cannula is slid forward over the cutting notch (Fig. 22-15C). The needle is removed, retaining the biopsy specimen in the cutting notch (Fig. 22-15D and E).

When the biopsy needle has been withdrawn from the kidney, digital pressure is applied over the biopsy site for 5 minutes as an aid to hemostasis.

BLIND BIOPSY IN THE DOG

Blind percutaneous renal biopsy in the dog is more difficult than the technique described for the cat and is applicable only to a biopsy of the *left* kidney. Approximately 50% of all dogs may undergo biopsy by the blind percutaneous technique; in the remainder, the modified, keyhole biopsy technique should be used. Dogs that are obese or ascitic, or that have large intra-abdominal masses, are not candidates for blind percutaneous renal biopsy. Prior to biopsy, the dog's colon and urinary bladder should be evacuated. The use of drugs causing splenomegaly, for example, phenothiazine tranquilizers and barbiturates, is to be avoided. Inhalation anesthesia is generally required to achieve the abdominal relaxation necessary for immobilization of the left kidney.

The dog is positioned in *right* lateral recumbency.

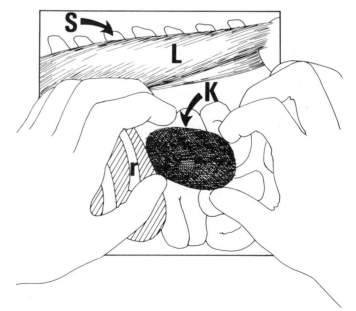

Fig. 22-16. *Schematic drawing of positioning of the dog's left kidney for needle biopsy. After localizing the kidney, the thumb and index fingers are placed on its cranial and caudal poles. Downward pressure immobilizes the kidney against the right abdominal wall. S, spinous process of vertebrae; L, lumbar musculature; K, left kidney; r, rib.*

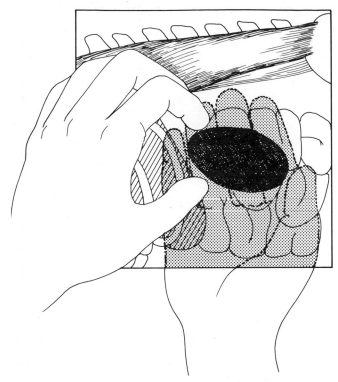

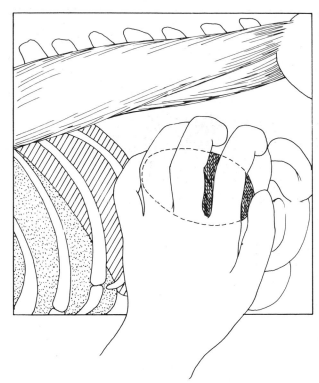

Fig. 22-17. *Schematic drawing of positioning of the dog's left kidney for needle biopsy. After localizing the kidney, the left thumb and index fingers are placed on its cranial pole while the right hand applies upward force immobilizing the kidney against left abdominal wall.*

Fig. 22-18. *Schematic drawing of positioning of the dog's left kidney for needle biopsy. After localizing the kidney, fingertips are placed on the cranial, dorsal, and caudal aspects of the kidney. Force applied in a ventrolateral direction immobilizes the kidney against the right abdominal wall.*

the Tru-Cut biopsy needle preferable to the Franklin-modified Vim-Silverman biopsy needle when performing the blind renal biopsy technique in the dog.

When the left kidney is small, it may be immobilized with one hand by placing several fingers on the dorsomedial aspect of the kidney and by pulling it ventrally while simultaneously pushing it toward the right side of the dog's abdomen (Fig. 22-18). If this one-handed procedure is possible, the veterinary surgeon's other hand is used to place and to direct the biopsy needle.

When the biopsy needle has been withdrawn from the kidney, digital pressure is applied over the biopsy site for 5 minutes, as an aid to hemostasis.

KEYHOLE BIOPSY IN THE DOG

The keyhole renal biopsy technique[6] is employed in the dog when the left kidney cannot be immobilized by abdominal palpation or when a biopsy of the right kidney is desired. Some prefer to perform a biopsy on the right kidney because its firm attachment to the body wall generally ensures its anatomic position. Others, however, including myself, prefer the left kidney because its mobility frequently permits better positioning.

The dog is positioned in lateral recumbency. The skin is clipped and is prepared as for any aseptic surgical approach. The clip extends from the dorsal midline to a point half-way down the lateral abdomen. The cranial and caudal limits of the clip extend from the level of the twelfth thoracic vertebrae to the third lumbar vertebrae, respectively.

With the dog's vertebrae facing the veterinary surgeon, an oblique paralumbar skin incision 2 to 2½ times the width of the index finger is made. The proximal third of the incision overlaps the ventral lumbar musculature, whereas the remainder of the incision lies below this plane (Fig. 22-19). The incision is caudal to the last rib in order to ensure that the intercostal artery is not transected.

An index finger is placed in the skin incision at a point immediately ventral to the lumbar muscles. The finger is gradually advanced as the subcutaneous tissue and muscle are bluntly dissected with a curved hemostat. Because the plane of dissection is immediately ventral to the lumbar muscles, a large quantity of vascular muscle tissue is avoided. A hemostat with long jaws is preferred because it makes a hole large enough to accommodate the finger's width. Constant inward pressure is applied by the index finger until a sudden loss of resistance is noted. At this point, the index finger has penetrated either the peritoneal cavity or the retroperitoneal space. Blind palpation with the index finger reveals the location of the kidney.

The kidney is immobilized by displacing it against the body wall with the index finger. If the hilar structures (renal vessels and ureter) can be hooked with the index finger, the kidney is pulled back toward the inci-

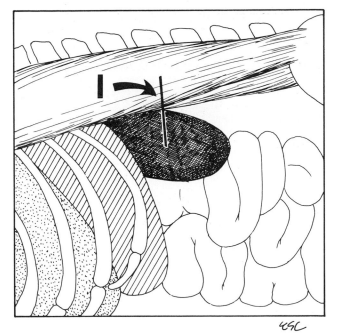

Fig. 22-19. *Schematic drawing of the landmarks for kidney biopsy via a modified, keyhole technique. The skin incision (I) is caudal to the last rib and extends above and below the ventral aspect of the lumbar musculature.*

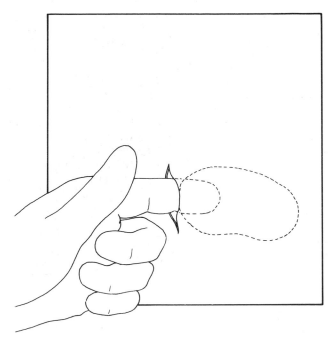

Fig. 22-21. *Schematic drawing of digital fixation of kidney. The index finger is placed against the caudal pole of kidney. Force is then applied to the immobilized kidney between the finger and the dorsolateral abdominal wall.*

sion and is fixed against the dorsolateral abdominal wall (Fig. 22-20). Digital pressure on the caudal pole of the kidney is another common method of fixation (Fig. 22-21).

At a location adjacent to the keyhole incision, another incision is made just large enough to accommo-

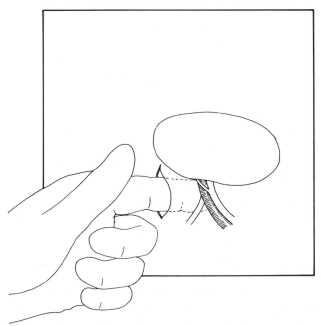

Fig. 22-20. *Schematic drawing of digital fixation of kidney. The index finger is used to hook hilar structures (renal vessels and ureter). Force is then applied to immobilize the kidney against the dorsolateral abdominal wall.*

date the biopsy needle. If a biopsy is being performed on the right kidney, the incision is usually cranial to the keyhole incision and may be located intercostally. Owing to the mobility of the left kidney, the incision for the needle placement can be cranial, caudal, or ventral to the keyhole incision, depending on the location of the kidney.

The biopsy needle is placed in the skin incision and is forced through the underlying tissue until contact is made with the renal capsule. The needle is then directed in such a fashion that the long axis is pointed away from the hilus and *only* cortical tissue is penetrated (see Fig. 22-13). (See the discussion on biopsy technique in the cat for technical aspects of operating the biopsy needle.)

When the biopsy needle has been withdrawn from the kidney, the biopsy site is compressed for 5 minutes, either directly by the index finger or indirectly by holding the kidney and biopsy site against the abdominal wall. Evidence of excessive hemorrhage at the keyhole incision warrants careful evaluation. If bleeding continues unabated, the keyhole incision may be enlarged to identify the source. Oxidized regenerated cellulose* may be placed on the renal capsule over the biopsy site. Closure of the keyhole incision requires 2 or 3 sutures in the abdominal muscle and skin.

Postoperative Care and Complications

Following the biopsy procedure, the animal should be confined to a cage for approximately 8 hours. Fluid

*Surgicel, Johnson & Johnson Products, Inc., New Brunswick, NJ 08903

therapy and diuretics are continued to maintain a mild diuresis. The patient should be evaluated periodically for bleeding. Strenuous physical activity should be limited for 7 to 10 days.

If proper technique is used, serious postoperative complications are rare. Bleeding is the most common complication following renal biopsy.[6] Insignificant, transient microscopic hematuria is routinely observed from 12 hours to 3 days postoperative. Gross hematuria is less frequent and may be significant, depending on the rate and volume of blood loss. Intra-abdominal and retroperitoneal hemorrhage are potentially the most serious forms of hemorrhage following biopsy, because large volumes of blood can be lost prior to detection of the disorder. Rest and transfusions (if indicated) control most such hemorrhaging. Surgical intervention is warranted for persistent bleeding when the patient is unable to maintain blood volume by transfusion.

Other complications reported in both human and veterinary literature[1,3,4,6,7] include: (1) hematoma formation (intrarenal, subcapsular, perinephric, retroperitoneal, and intra-abdominal); (2) excretory outflow obstruction (renal pelvis, ureter, and bladder) by clots; (3) intrarenal arteriovenous fistula; (4) infection (renal, perirenal, disseminated); (5) laceration or perforation of intra-abdominal organs and vessels; (6) pneumothorax; (7) failure to retrieve renal tissue; (8) biopsy of adjacent organs; (9) shock or hypotension; (10) hydronephrosis subsequent to outflow obstruction; (11) tumor seeding; (12) flank pain; (13) subcapsular and perirenal urinomas; and (14) pyelocutaneous fistula.

Tissue Handling

Once the renal biopsy has been performed, the tissue specimen is *gently* removed from the biopsy needle by teasing with a 25-gauge needle or by squirting with isotonic saline solution. Some have advocated obtaining a second biopsy if immediate inspection of the biopsy core with a hand lens or a dissecting microscope does not reveal glomerular tufts.

Fixation of the biopsy core for light-microscopic examination can be achieved with a 10% buffered neutral formalin solution. For those samples in which electron-microscopic study may be indicated, the dual fixative, Carson's fixative, allows both routine processing for histologic evaluation and processing for electron microscopy.[2]

Bacteriologic evaluation of the biopsy specimen is done by swirling the tip of the biopsy needle in an appropriate culture medium when the tissue core has been removed. The tissue core should be removed with a sterile 25-gauge needle because isotonic saline solution dilutes the residual bacterial population on the biopsy needle.

If fluorescent-microscopic examination is desired, the biopsy core should be kept moist with, but not immersed in, isotonic saline solution. The sample is then snap-frozen and is either sectioned or is stored at −70 C.

References and Suggested Readings

1. Almkuist, R. D., and Buckalew, V. M.: Techniques of renal biopsy. Urol. Clin. North Am., 6:503, 1979.
2. Carson, F. L., Martin, J. H., and Lynn, J. A.: Formalin fixation for electron microscopy; a re-evaluation. Am. J. Clin. Pathol., 59:365, 1973.
3. Kark, R. M.: Renal biopsy. JAMA, 205:80, 1968.
4. Lindeman, R. D.: Percutaneous renal biopsy. Kidney, 7:1, 1974.
5. Osborne, C. A., Finco, D. R., and Low, D. G.: Applied anatomy of the urinary system. In Canine and Feline Urology. Philadelphia, W. B. Saunders, 1972.
6. Osborne, C. A., Stevens, J. B., and Perman, V.: Kidney biopsy. Vet. Clin. North Am., 4:351, 1974.
7. Striker, G. E., Quadracci, L. J., and Cutler, R. D.: Use and Interpretation of Renal Biopsy. Philadelphia, W. B. Saunders, 1978.

Pyelolithotomy

by Clarence A. Rawlings

and Kenneth M. Greenwood

Renal calculi should be removed in order to treat an associated urinary tract infection effectively and to prevent pyelonephritis and hydronephrosis. When pyelonephritis or hydronephrosis has severely reduced renal function in a calculi-containing kidney, and when the opposite kidney is functional enough to support life, the nonfunctional kidney is removed by nephrectomy. When the calculi-containing kidney is worth salvaging, the calculi may be removed by either the traditional nephrolithotomy or a modified pyelolithotomy. Nephrolithotomy requires temporary obstruction of renal blood flow and an incision through the renal parenchyma, and it reduces the patient's postoperative glomerular filtration rate. These problems associated with nephrolithotomy can be avoided with the pyelolithotomy. This latter procedure can only be performed in those cases in which the calculi are large and fill an enlarged pelvis and proximal ureter.

Preoperative evaluation should include: (1) general renal function tests (blood urea nitrogen, creatinine, and urine specific gravity); (2) specific tests of renal function and anatomy, as demonstrated by intravenous excretory urography; and (3) characterization of any urinary tract infection by urinary sediment evaluation and bacterial culture. Uremic and azotemic patients should undergo diuresis preoperatively, and electrolyte imbalances should be corrected.

Once the animal has been successfully treated for uremia, the surgical procedure is performed while efforts are made to maintain renal perfusion. During the operation, the patient should be kept well hydrated, and its arterial pressure should be maintained within the normal range. The patient's urinary output should be monitored intra- and postoperatively, to identify incipient renal shutdown.

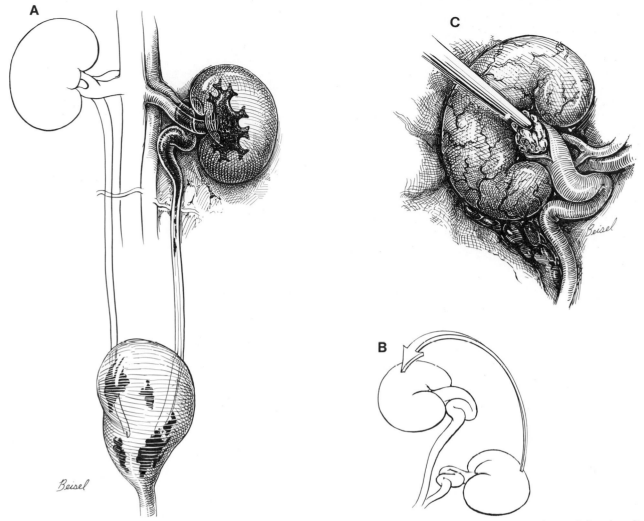

Fig. 22-22. A, *The urinary system is illustrated, with the right kidney being cranial to the left. The renal artery is cranial and medial to the ureter. B, The kidney is dissected along its greater curve from the retroperitoneal tissue. This illustration shows the left kidney being rotated medially from its retroperitoneal position. C, The dilated proximal ureter and pelvis of the left kidney is exposed. Care is taken to avoid the renal vessels. The ureter is incised longitudinally to expose the calculi. Calculi are removed with forceps, gentle manipulation, and flushing with sterile solution.*

Large calculi in both kidneys can usually be removed simultaneously by pyelolithotomy. This technique is less damaging to the kidneys than a nephrolithotomy because pyelolithotomy does not require renal artery occlusion.

Surgical Technique

A liberal midline celiotomy is performed to expose the kidneys and urinary bladder. The involved kidney is exposed by reflection of abdominal viscera and by dissection of the peritoneum and sublumbar fat from the lateral surface of the kidney (Fig. 22-22A). The kidney is reflected medially upon its hilus. Because the renal arteries are cranial and medial, and the renal vein is medial, to the ureters, the medial reflection exposes the ureters close to the renal pelvis (Fig. 22-22B). The calculi within the pelvis and proximal ureter should be palpated. If the proximal ureter is enlarged sufficiently to permit calculi removal, a longitudinal incision is made into the proximal ureter, and the calculi are gently removed (Fig. 22-22C). The renal pelvis is flushed and is explored for other calculi (Fig. 22-22D). A 3.5-French soft rubber catheter is passed through the ureter from the kidney to the bladder. If no resistance to catheter passage is met, and if cystic calculi are not present, the incision can be closed. If either cystic or ureteral calculi are present, a ventral cystotomy is performed to expose the ureteral orifices. Ureteral calculi are usually repulsed to the kidney by alternate flushing, manipulation, and perhaps, the use of a calculi basket catheter* (Fig. 22-22E). The incision into the proximal ureter is closed with a simple continuous 5-0 polypropylene suture, placed so as to minimize the amount of suture within the lumen (Fig. 22-22F).

*Dormia Ureteral Stone Dislodger, American V. Mueller, 6600 West Touhy Avenue, Chicago, IL 60648

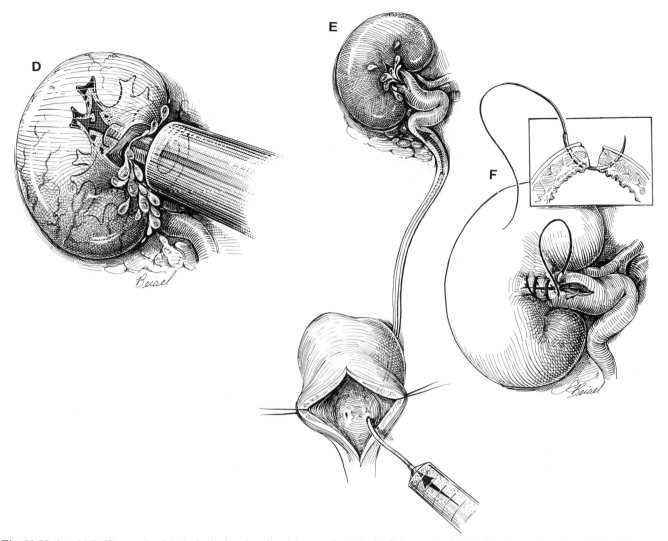

Fig. 22.22. (cont.) D, *The renal pelvis is flushed and explored for smaller calculi. Cultures should be taken from either the pelvis or the center of the calculi. E, If calculi are present in the ureter, a ventrocaudal cystotomy is performed to expose the ureters, which can be easily identified in the trigone. Calculi can be retropulsed to the kidney by flushing and manipulation. This incision can also remove cystic calculi. Even when only renal calculi appear to be present, the ureter should always be catheterized to ensure the absence of ureteral calculi. F, The pelvis and proximal ureter are closed with a simple continuous 5-0 polypropylene suture. The wall of the inflamed ureter is usually thick enough to permit splitting of the wall with the needle (inset). (Copyright University of Georgia.)*

Postoperative Management

Diuresis is maintained postoperatively, in order to aid in clot removal and to reduce the likelihood of azotemia or uremia. The calculi should be analyzed to aid in prevention of new calculi. If a urinary tract infection is present, vigorous antibiotic treatment and long-term medical management are required to prevent recurrence.

References and Suggested Readings

Gahring, D. R.: Comparative renal function studies of nephrotomy closure with and without sutures. J. Am. Vet. Med. Assoc., *171*:537, 1977.

Greenwood, K. M., and Rawlings, C. A.: Removal of renal calculi by pyelolithotomy. Vet. Surg., *10*:12, 1981.

Klausner, J. S., and Osborne, C. A.: Urinary tract infection and urolithiasis. Vet. Clin. North Am., *9*:701, 1979.

Osborne, C. A., Low, D. G., and Finco, D. R.: Canine and Feline Urology. Philadelphia, W. B. Saunders, 1972.

23 * Urinary Bladder and Ureter

Repair of the Traumatized Ureter

by CLARENCE A. RAWLINGS

Injury to the canine and feline ureter primarily occurs following penetrating trauma, usually due in dogs and cats to animal interactions and gunshots. Blunt trauma, which is much more frequent in dogs than penetrating trauma, seldom produces ureteral tears unless the kidney is severely displaced. Blunt ureteral injuries are usually close to the kidney or to the bladder. Injuries close to the bladder may be repaired by reimplantation of the ureter (see the next section of this chapter, on repair of ectopic ureter) or by the bladder-flap ureteroplasty described herein. Injuries close to the kidney require either direct repair of the ureter or nephrectomy.

Ureteral trauma in veterinary patients is usually diagnosed late. The early use of excretory urograms in humans, however, provides early diagnosis, repair, and improved success in managing ureteral trauma; unfortunately, these contrast procedures are usually delayed in veterinary hospitals because of their expense and the infrequent occurrence of ureteral trauma. Additionally, during emergency exploratory celiotomy, ureteral exploration is not usually performed because it produces further trauma and prolongs the operation.

When a leaking ureter is not diagnosed early, clinical signs develop slowly and insidiously during the first week after injury. Urine leakage can cause severe cellulitis and fistula formation. In penetrating trauma, this urine may both produce and sustain a fistula. In the absence of external drainage, urine-induced cellulitis produces a marked inflammatory response, fever, neutrophilia (with immature forms), anorexia, depression, abdominal pain, and occasionally a low-grade azotemia. If the opposite kidney is functional, the patient's blood urea nitrogen, ability to urinate, and urinalysis results may be normal. Because retroperitoneal urine leakage may not produce intraperitoneal collection of urine, diagnosis of the ureteral tear and its location requires an excretory urogram. This test also provides functional information about the opposite kidney if a nephrectomy is being considered.

Preoperative preparation of the patient should in-clude correction of fluid and electrolyte imbalances. Concurrent sepsis may be present, and concomitant treatment is necessary.

Surgical Technique

The urinary system is best explored through a midline celiotomy incision. If the ureteral damage is close to the kidney, primary repair is performed. The ends of the ureter are debrided and are spatulated. To decrease tension on the anastomotic site, the kidney may be freed from its retroperitoneal fossa and may be reflected caudally. The ureters are closed with a simple continuous pattern of 5-0 chromic catgut or polypropylene suture (see Fig. 23-1D). This closure should be watertight. In small ureters, a larger diameter may be gained with "Z" plasty than with spatulation, but "Z" plasty is technically more difficult. Ureteral tears of small longitude, especially those produced during the operation, may close better spontaneously and without sutures. A catheter stent may be responsible for ascending infection and fibrosis of the anastomosis and should not be placed unless complications, such as undue suture-line tension, obvious infection, ureteral infection, and adjacent pancreatic injury, are present.

An alternate urinary diversion technique is a nephrostomy tube. This tube is placed prior to anastomosis of a proximal ureteral transection by passing a hemostat from inside the pelvis to outside the kidney (Fig. 23-1A). The nephrostomy tube is withdrawn (Fig. 23-1B) and is left in the pelvis and proximal ureter (Fig. 23-1C). The ureteral surgical site should be wrapped with omentum, and a Penrose drain should be placed to permit exit of any urine leakage.

Ureteral transection close to the bladder may be repaired by reimplantation of the ureter into the bladder or by a bladder-flap ureteroplasty. This procedure is performed on the ventral floor of the bladder (Fig. 23-2A). The ureteral end is placed into this flap by a technique similar to that in the ureteral reimplantation procedure (Fig. 23-2B). The bladder flap is then closed by routine cystotomy closure techniques (Fig. 23-2C and D).

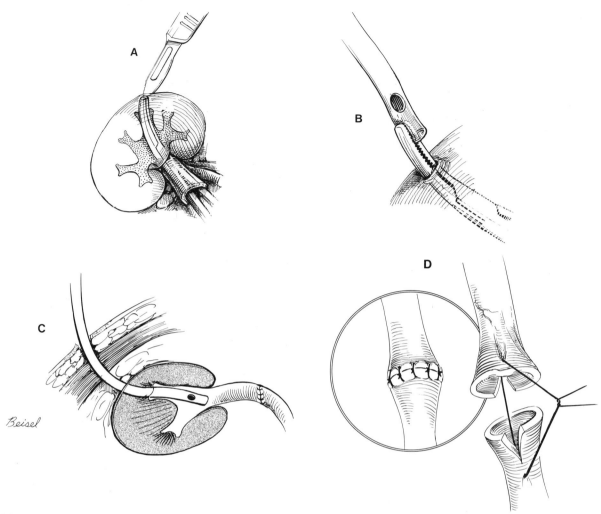

Fig. 23-1. A, *Passing a hemostat from inside the renal pelvis to outside the kidney in order to place a nephrostomy tube.* B, *Retraction of a nephrostomy tube.* C, *Proper placement of the nephrostomy tube in the renal pelvis and cranial ureter. Care is taken to avoid placing the catheter near the anastomosis site.* D, *Repair of a transected ureter, using spatulation and a simple continuous pattern. (Copyright University of Georgia.)*

Postoperative Management

Postoperative management must include: control of systemic sepsis and urinary tract infection, if present; maintenance of fluids, electrolytes, and calories; and constant surveillance for urine leakage. Urine leakage is evaluated by serial blood counts and by examination of the fluid coming from the Penrose drain. An excretory urogram is generally not done for several weeks after the surgical procedure.

References and Suggested Readings

Ambiavagar, R., and Nambiar, R.: Traumatic closed avulsion of the upper ureter. Injury, *11:*71, 1979.

Carlton, C. E.: Upper urinary tract trauma. *In* Urologic Surgery. 2nd Ed. Edited by J. F. Glenn. New York, Harper & Row, 1975.

Cass, A. S.: Immediate radiological evaluation and early surgical management of genitourinary injuries from external trauma. J. Urol., *122:*722, 1979.

Grayhack, J. T.: The urinary system. *In* Davis-Christopher Textbook of Surgery. 12th Ed. Edited by D. C. Sabiston. Philadelphia, W. B. Saunders, 1977.

Laberge, I., Homsy, Y. L., Dadour, G., and Beland, G.: Avulsion of ureter by blunt trauma. Urology, *13:*172, 1979.

Zamora-Munoz, S., et al.: A unified approach to management of genitourinary trauma. Ill. Med. J., *156:*165, 1979.

Repair of Ectopic Ureter

by CLARENCE A. RAWLINGS

Ectopic ureter is a surgically correctable congenital anomaly. Clinical signs include urinary incontinence and chronic vulvar dermatosis. The incontinence may be continual or intermittent; voiding of the urinary bladder may also be normal. Ectopic ureters are usually seen in bitches (female : male ratio of 25 : 1), particularly in Siberian huskies, West Highland white

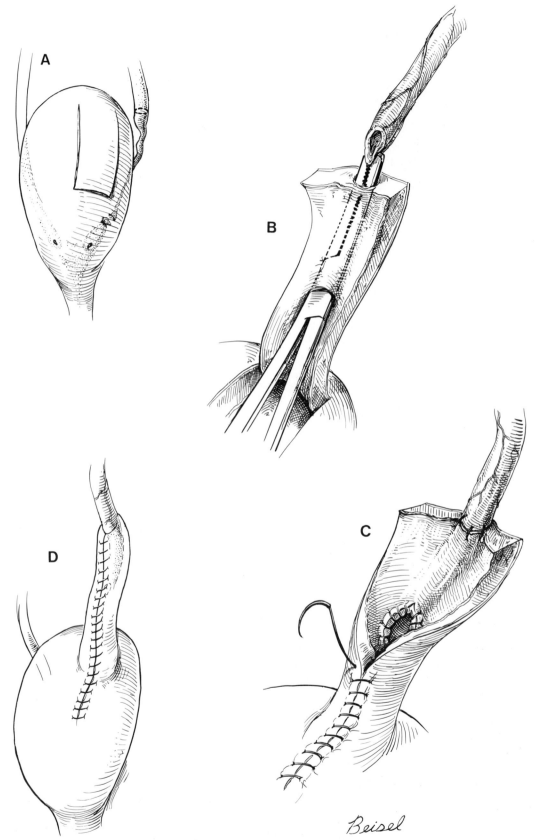

Beisel

Fig. 23-2. A, *Elevation of a bladder pedicle flap from the ventral bladder wall. This technique permits a bladder-flap ureteroplasty, to repair distal ureteral injuries. B, Implantation of the ureter into the bladder flap. C and D, Closure of the bladder defect and the bladder flap about the ureter entrance. (Copyright University of Georgia.)*

terriers, fox terriers, and poodles. The incidence of an anatomic ectopic ureter in the male dog is probably more frequent than its clinical incidence, because the ureteral entrance into the urethra may be closer to the bladder than to the tip of the penis. Urine in the urethra flows in the direction of least resistance and frequently accumulates in the bladder of these males dogs, rather than dribbling to the outside.

Preoperative diagnosis of ectopic ureter is by positive-contrast urinary radiography. An intravenous excretory urogram should be done routinely. These stud-ies frequently demonstrate the emptying of the ectopic ureter into the urethra, the uterus, or the vagina. Some diagnoses have been made either by a retrograde vaginogram or by endoscopic examination. Ectopic ureters frequently dilate (hydroureter, hydronephrosis) in response to an increased resistance to urine flow at the ureteral exit. The precise site of the ureteral termination may be difficult to identify on an excretory urogram. A dilated ureter and renal pelvis in an incontinent bitch are usually produced by an ectopic ureter, but they may also be produced by an upper urinary

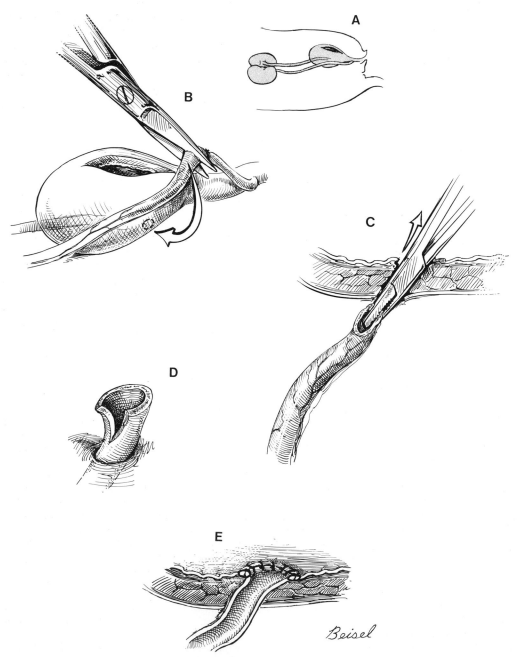

Fig. 23-3. A, *Caudal celiotomy and ventral cystotomy in order to expose the ureters and trigone. B, The ureter that bypasses the bladder caudally is ligated and transected. The end is passed through the dorsal cystic wall (circle). C, A mosquito hemostat is passed from inside to outside the bladder wall to withdraw the ureter into the bladder. D, The damaged portion of the ureter is excised, and the ureter is incised to provide a longer length for suturing. E, Simple interrupted sutures are placed between the ureteral wall and the cystic mucosa. (Copyright University of Georgia.)*

tract infection. These animals may require an exploratory ventral cystotomy, to determine the presence or absence of an anatomically correct ureteral termination.

Many patients with ectopic ureter also have urinary tract infections. These infections should be diagnosed by sediment examination and culture of urine obtained by cystocentesis. Antibiotic sensitivity determinations and treatment should be initiated prior to the surgical procedure. Renal function is usually normal, but should be confirmed by blood urea nitrogen and urine specific gravity measurements.

Surgical Techniques

A caudal midline celiotomy and a ventrocaudal cystotomy are performed to expose the ureters' entrance into the bladder (Fig. 23-3A). The entrance of both ureters into the trigone should be examined because ectopic ureters may be bilateral. If the ectopic ureter bypasses the bladder to enter caudal to the trigone, the ureter is cut and is reimplanted into the bladder. If the ectopic ureter enters the bladder serosa in the normal position to run caudally within the bladder wall, the ureter is left in place, and an appropriate entrance into the bladder is created directly from the ureter. A nephrectomy should be performed only on the large, nonfunctional hydronephrectic kidney and when the opposite kidney appears to be capable of sustaining normal life.

REIMPLANTATION

When the ureter bypasses the trigone, it is doubly ligated and is severed caudal to the trigone (Fig. 23-3B). By approaching it through a ventral cystotomy, a small circle of mucosa from the dorsal bladder wall is excised. A mosquito hemostat is passed through this excised area at an oblique angle from inside to outside the bladder (Fig. 23-3C). Other veterinary surgeons have recommended long submucosal tunneling of the ureter, to prevent vesicoureteral reflux. This long tunnel, in my experience, produces sufficient resistance to urine flow to cause hydroureter and hydronephrosis. The shorter tunnel can be situated such that urine leakage is not significant. Once inside the bladder, the ureter is transected and is incised 1 cm in the longitudinal direction (Fig. 23-3D). The ureter is sutured to the edges of the excised mucosa with interrupted 3-0 or 4-0 catgut suture (Fig. 23-3E). Care is taken to prevent twisting of the ureter and to preserve the ureteral blood supply. If an upper urinary tract infection is suspected, a 3.5-French soft rubber catheter is passed retrograde in the ureter to obtain a urine sample from the renal pelvis. The urinary bladder is closed, and omentum is placed over the cystotomy incision.

INTRAVESICULAR DIVERSION

Most ectopic ureters enter the serosa of the bladder dorsally in the normal position, but then course within the cystic and urethral wall before entering the lumen of the genitourinary tract outside the bladder. These anatomic features are documented by a ventral cystotomy and trigone exploration. These ureters can be dilated submucously by simultaneous caudal obstruction of the ureter and diuresis with fluids and furosemide.* To effect repair, the mucosa is incised into the ureter in order to permit urethral emptying directly into the bladder (Fig. 23-4A). The ureteral mucosa is then sutured to the cystic mucosa in a simple interrupted pattern with 3-0 or 4-0 catgut (Fig. 23-4C). A catheter is passed caudally through the ectopic ureter, to identify this anomaly. Several ligatures of a nonabsorbable suture (nylon or polypropylene) are placed to close the ureter, by entering and exiting of the suture through the serosa and by avoidance of the mucosa (Fig. 23-4B). At least one of these ligatures should be close to the caudal end of the new entrance of the ureter into the bladder. The bladder is closed, and omentum is placed over the cystotomy incision.

Postoperative Management

Medical management is as required for a routine cystotomy, and strict care is taken to treat urinary tract infections. Postsurgical problems have included persistent urinary tract infection, strictures, and calculi formation near the orifice of the ureteroneocystostomy. Many dogs with ectopic ureter continue to be incontinent after anatomic correction, probably because of neuromuscular dysplasia within the urethra as an associated congenital anomaly.

References and Suggested Readings

Bebko, R. L., Prier, J. E., and Biery, D. N.: Ectopic ureters in a male cat. J. Am. Vet. Med. Assoc., 171:738, 1977.

Biewenga, W. J., Rothuizen, J., and Voorhout, G.: Ectopic ureters in the cat—a report of two cases. J. Small Anim. Pract., 19:531, 1978.

Brodeur, G. Y.: Diagnosis of ectopic ureter. Canine Pract., 4:25, 1977.

Dingwall, J. S., Eger, C. E., and Owen, R. R.: Clinical experiences with the combined technique of ureterovesicular anastomosis for treatment of ectopic ureters. J. Am. Anim. Hosp. Assoc., 12:406, 1976.

Greene, J. A., Thornhill, J. A., and Blevins, W. E.: Hydronephrosis and hydroureter associated with a unilateral ectopic ureter in a spayed bitch. J. Am. Anim. Hosp. Assoc., 14:708, 1978.

Hare, W. C. D., and Bovee, K.: A chromosomal translocation in miniature poodles? Vet. Rec., 95:217, 1974.

Hayes, H. M., Jr.: Ectopic ureter in dogs: epidemiologic features. Teratology, 10:129, 1974.

Holt, P. E.: Ectopic ureter in the bitch. Vet. Rec., 98:299, 1976.

Johnson, T. C.: Surgical correction of ectopic ureter in the dog. J. Am. Vet. Med. Assoc., 169:316, 1976.

Johnston, G. R., Osborne, C. A., Wilson, J. W., and Yano, B. L.: Familial ureteral ectopia in the dog. J. Am. Anim. Hosp. Assoc., 13:168, 1977.

Lane, J. G.: Canine ectopic ureter—two further case reports. J. Small Anim. Pract., 14:555, 1973.

Lennox, J. S.: A case report of unilateral ectopic ureter in a male Siberian husky. J. Am. Anim. Hosp. Assoc., 14:331, 1978.

*Lasix, American Hoechst Corporation, Animal Health Division, Somerville, NJ 08876

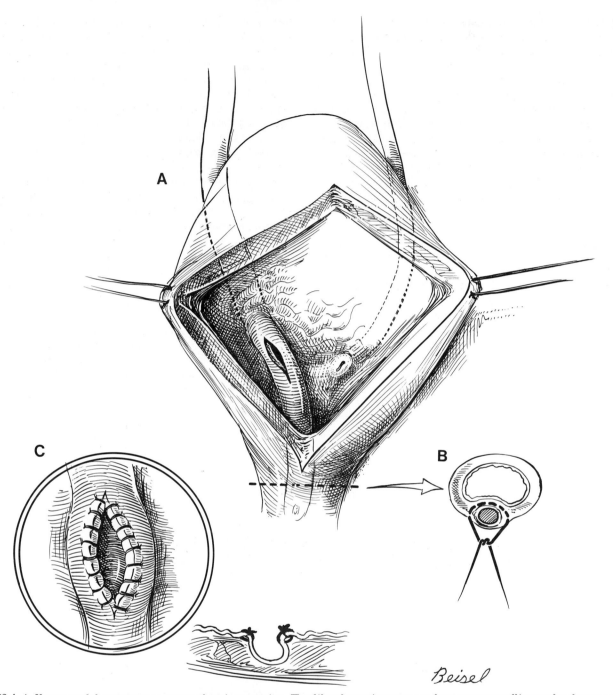

Fig. 23-4. A, *Ventrocaudal cystotomy to expose the trigone region. The dilated ectopic ureter can be seen as a swelling under the mucosa. It is incised. B, The ureter distal to this trigone incision is ligated by placing sutures through the outside and avoiding the cystic and urethral mucosa. Placing a catheter through this distal ureter can be helpful in identifying it for ligation. C, The edges of the incised ureter are sutured to the cystic mucosa in a simple interrupted pattern. (Copyright University of Georgia.)*

Osborne, C. A., Dieterich, H. F., Hanlon, G. F., and Anderson, L. D.: Urinary incontinence due to ectopic ureter in a male dog. J. Am. Vet. Med. Assoc., *166*:911, 1975.

Owen, R. R.: Canine ureteral ectopic—a review. 1. Embryology and aetiology. J. Small Anim. Pract., *14*:407, 1973.

Owen, R. R.: Canine ureteral ectopia—a review. 2. Incidence, diagnosis and treatment. J. Small Anim. Pract., *14*:419, 1973.

Seidenberg, L., and Knecht, C. D.: Ectopic ureter in the dog. J. Am. Vet. Med. Assoc., *159*:876, 1971.

Surgical Management of Canine Cystic and Urethral Calculi

by DEAN R. GAHRING

Patients with urinary calculi are commonly encountered in veterinary practice. Calculi most often occur in dogs between 3 and 7 years of age. Schnauzers, dachshunds, beagles, dalmations, terriers, pugs, bassets, corgis, and bulldogs seem to have a higher-than-normal incidence of urinary calculi, and calculi are seen frequently in poodles. Most calculi are radiopaque and are found in the urinary bladder or the urethra. Radiolucent calculi also occur.

The three main types of urinary calculi are (1) magnesium-ammonium-phosphate, with or without calcium; (2) cystine; and (3) ammonium urate. Calcium oxalate, calcium carbonate, xanthine, cholesterol, and silica calculi are uncommonly encountered. No predisposition exists for any type of calculi in any breed, except for a higher occurrence of urate calculi in dalmations. More than half the cases of urinary calculi have a positive urinary bacterial culture.

Clinical Features

The clinical signs of urolithiasis depend on the location of the stones, the duration of the problem, and any corresponding complicating factors, such as infection and azotemia. Dogs with cystic calculi usually have a history of increased frequency of urination, often with hematuria. Dogs with urethral calculi are presented to the veterinarian with a history of dysuria, dribbling of urine, stranguria, or anuria. When total urethral obstruction occurs, the patient soon develops azotemia

and uremia and becomes depressed, with a distended urinary bladder, and perhaps a history of vomiting. Calculi seldom lodge in the female urethra unless they are large, because the female urethra is distensible and more readily allows passage of a stone. Obstruction in the male urethra usually is seen at the level of the caudal os penis, but occasionally occurs in the perineal urethra.

Conservative Treatment

Azotemia and death result if urine flow is not reestablished. Smooth-muscle antispasmodic agents should be given, and then a urethral catheter should be passed. General anesthesia provides the best relaxation of the urethral musculature. If the obstruction is at the caudal os penis, repeated gentle passages of progressively smaller, semistiff polyethylene catheters may dislodge the calculi or may at least allow passage of a small catheter to the bladder. The catheter may also be passed to the point of obstruction and the tip of the penis may be occluded. Sterile saline solution may then be flushed with enough pressure to produce slight distension of the urethra in an effort to backflush the calculi into the bladder, in order to facilitate passage of the catheter (Fig. 23-5).

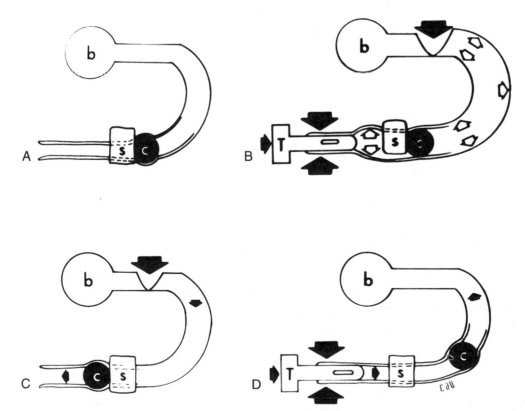

Fig. 23-5. *Schematic drawings illustrating removal of urethral calculi with the aid of fluid under pressure:* A, *Diagram of urethral calculus lodged behind os penis.* B, *Diagram illustrating dilatation of urethral lumen by injecting fluid under pressure. Pressure applied to the external urethral orifice and the pelvic urethra (large black arrows) has created a closed system.* C, *Diagram illustrating sudden release of digital pressure at the external urethral orifice and subsequent movement of fluid and calculus toward the external urethral orifice.* D, *Diagram illustrating sudden release of digital pressure at the pelvic urethra and subsequent movement of fluid and calculus toward the bladder.* b, *Urinary bladder;* s, *os penis;* c, *calculus;* T, *teat cannula (From Piermattei, D. L., and Osborne, C. A.: Nonsurgical removal of calculi from the urethra of small dogs. J. Am. Vet. Med. Assoc.,* 159: *1755, 1971.)*

Retrohydropulsion has also been a useful method for dislodging calculi in the male urethra. A finger is placed in the rectum to push down ventrally, to occlude the pelvic and perineal urethra. A teat-tube cannula or a large urethral catheter is inserted into the urethral meatus, which is held tightly closed around the cannula (Fig. 23-5). Fluid pressurization of the urethra by a syringe attached to the cannula results in distension of urethral lumen away from the calculi. At this point, the finger occlusion of the pelvic urethra is released to allow a sudden rush of fluid and small calculi toward the bladder.

These techniques establish urine flow in the majority of patients and thus give the veterinarian time to treat the medical complications before performing a definitive urolithectomy procedure. If the obstruction cannot be relieved by these "conservative" techniques, it must be decided whether to attempt a cystotomy and urethral lavage or to perform a urethrotomy. I prefer to avoid urethrotomies whenever possible because of the problems of postoperative hemorrhage and stricture formation. In the case of a critically azotemic patient, however, general anesthesia and an abdominal operation are not a prudent choice. Rather, a urethrotomy under light sedation and local anesthesia are preferred.

Surgical Techniques

CYSTOTOMY

Intravenous fluid therapy should be maintained during the surgical procedure. General anesthesia is induced, and the ventral abdomen is prepared and draped. A caudal midline abdominal incision from the umbilicus to near the cranial edge of the pubis is made in the female. In the male, a ventral midline abdominal skin incision is made from the umbilicus and is extended laterally to the cranial edge of the prepuce. The incision should extend far enough laterally to avoid the penile sheath. The caudal superficial epigastric vessels are ligated and are transected (Fig. 23-6A), the preputial ligament and superficial abdominal fascia are incised, the prepuce and penis are reflected laterally, and the incision is continued into the abdominal cavity by the linea alba.

The urinary bladder is exteriorized, is packed off with laparotomy pads, and is held at the apex by either a stay suture or Babcock forceps to facilitate manipulation (Fig. 23-6B). The cystotomy incision is made on the dorsal aspect of the bladder wall between major blood vessels and away from the ureters (Fig. 23-6C).

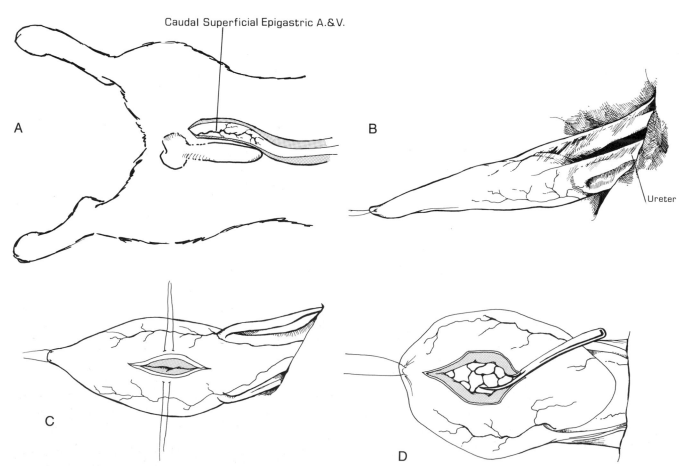

Fig. 23-6. A, *Ventral midline abdominal incision in male dog, extending lateral to the prepuce. B, The urinary bladder is exteriorized through a midline abdominal incision and held by a stay suture at the apex. C, The cystotomy incision is made on the dorsal aspect of the bladder between major blood vessels and between the ureters. D, Cystic calculi are removed from the urinary bladder with a smooth-edged spoon.*

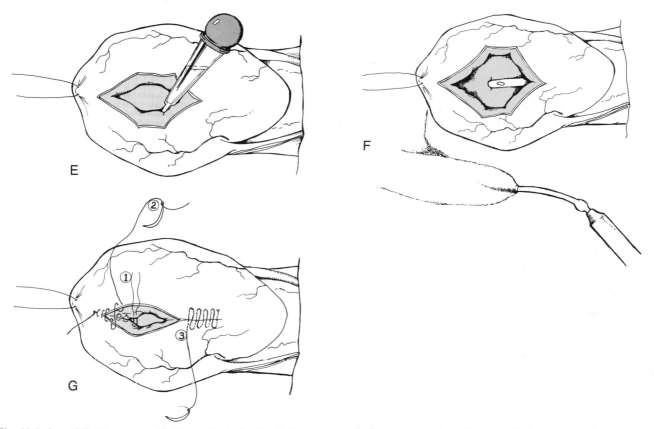

Fig. 23-6. *(cont.)* E, *The urinary bladder is flushed with a bulb syringe to flush out sand and small calculi. F, A urinary catheter is passed in both directions and flushed with saline solution, to flush calculi from the urethra. G, Cystotomy closure in three layers: the first layer is horizontal mattress everting sutures in the mucosa (1) with the knots outside the lumen. The second is a continuous Cushing suture (2), and the third is a continuous Lembert suture (3). The Lembert suture line is begun where the Cushing suture line ends and is tied to the long end of the initiating knot of the Cushing pattern.*

The cystotomy is preferred in the dorsal aspect because adhesions between it and the abdominal incision, which could interfere with future operations, do not form.

Following incision into the bladder, urine is removed with suction and cultures are taken directly from the bladder mucosa. The calculi are then removed with forceps or with a smooth-edged gallbladder spoon* and are saved for analysis (Fig. 23-6D) and possible culture of the center, especially in recurring cases. The mucosa is examined for any defects and is then flushed with a bulb syringe (Fig. 23-6E). A urinary catheter is also passed from the bladder into the urethra and is thoroughly flushed until all urethral stones have been removed and the catheter can be passed out freely. In the male, the catheter is also passed from the penis, and calculi are backflushed into the bladder, to be retrieved and removed (Fig. 23-6F).

The cystotomy incision is then closed in 3 layers with 3-0 or 4-0 catgut, sutures. Polyglycolic acid or polyglactin 910 suture material may also be used. The mucosa is closed with horizontal mattress everting sutures, tied so the knots do not lie in the bladder lumen. The tela submucosa and tunica muscularis are closed with 2 continuous inverting seromuscular suture lines

*American V. Mueller, 6600 West Touhy Avenue, Chicago, IL 60648

(Cushing, followed by Lembert); the end of the second layer is tied to the free end of the first (Fig. 23-6G).

The linea alba and subcutaneous closures are made with continuous or interrupted monofilament nylon, polyethylene, or polypropylene sutures. The preputial ligament should be properly reapposed, and the skin is closed with simple interrupted nonabsorbable sutures.

URETHROTOMY

If a temporary urethrotomy must be performed to remove calculi that cannot be flushed out with saline solution or grasped with forceps, a prepubic urethrotomy between the scrotum and caudal os penis is required (Fig. 23-7). A perineal urethrotomy should only be performed when it remains the sole remaining approach for removal of a stone lodged in the perineal urethra. The perineal urethra is more difficult to approach because of the bulbospongiosus muscles, and urine leakage can create severe cellulitis and postoperative strictures.

PREPUBIC. When a prepubic urethrotomy is to be performed, the patient is placed in dorsal recumbency and the groin is prepared for the procedure. A ventral midline incision is made in the prepuce and just caudal to the os penis to the base of the scrotum (Fig. 23-8A).

M. RETRACTOR PENIS

M. BULBOCAVERNOSUS

CORPUS CAVERNOSUM URETHRAE

CORPUS CAVERNOSUM PENIS

BULBUS GLANDIS

OS PENIS

PARS LONGA
GLANDIS

INCISION

INCISION

URETHRA

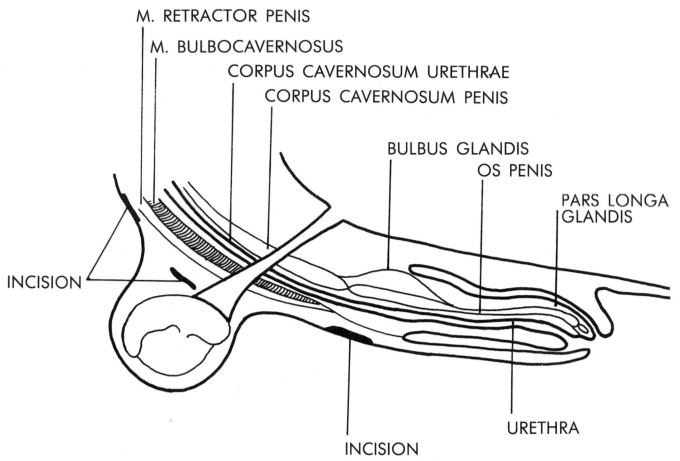

Fig. 23-7. *Sites of urethrotomies and urethrostomies and anatomic structures encountered.*

The subcutaneous tissue is dissected to expose the retractor penis muscle (Fig. 23-8B). This muscle is bluntly elevated from the corpus spongiosum penis and is retracted to the side (Fig. 23-8C). With a urethral catheter in place, and the penis stabilized in one hand, the corpus spongiosum penis is incised on its exact midline to the urethral lumen (Fig. 23-8D). This incision is extended to 1 or 2 cm in length.

PERINEAL. A perineal urethrotomy is performed with the patient sternally recumbent in the perineal position. The tail is secured over the patient's back. A pursestring suture is placed in the anus, and the area is prepared and draped for the surgical procedure. A midline perineal incision is made approximately halfway between the scrotum and the anus. The subcutaneous tissue is dissected to the level of the retractor penis muscle. This muscle is elevated and is retracted laterally to expose the bulbospongiosus muscles. The penis is stabilized, and the bulbospongiosus muscles are separated at their raphe to expose the corpus spongiosum penis. The corpus spongiosum penis is incised, over a previously placed urethral catheter, to the urethral lumen (Fig. 23-9A and B).

A urethrotomy may be either sutured closed (Fig. 23-9C) or left open to close on its own. In either case, complications are frequent. Fistulation and stricture

may occur; persistent hemorrhage may be expected when the incision is left unsutured, but edema and subcutaneous urine leakage can occur when the incision is sutured closed. I prefer to allow the prepubic urethrotomy to heal as an open wound and to allow the mucosa to re-establish continuity, to preclude the risk of stricture formation associated with suturing. All perineal urethrotomies should be sutured closed, however, because if left open, the problem of perineal and scrotal skin scalding may be severe. Using 4-0, 5-0, or 6-0 polyglycolic acid or polyglactin 910 sutures in simple interrupted pattern, the corpus spongiosum penis is closed. Sutures should be placed close to, but should not penetrate, the mucosa. When sutures penetrate the mucosa, resulting tears may exaggerate hemorrhage and may create avenues for scar tissue invasion. It is best to leave a small separation between the incised edges of urethral mucosa and to allow the mucosal epithelium to spread along the granulation base and cover the defect. The main cause of urethral stricture formation is excessive scar tissue production. All steps taken to minimize surgical trauma will in turn, help to minimize stricture formation. If the urethra is sutured closed, an indwelling catheter creates irritation, stimulates inflammation, and increases the risk of disruption of the suture line.

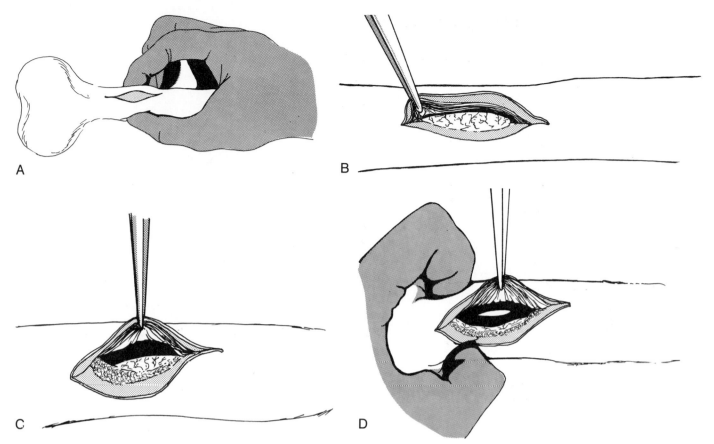

Fig. 23-8. A, *Prepubic urethrotomy incision.* B, *Retractor penis muscle identified (held by forceps).* C, *The retractor penis muscle is bluntly dissected and is retracted to expose the corpus spongiosum penis surrounding the urethra.* D, *Incision of the corpus spongiosum penis (over a previously placed urinary catheter) to the urethral lumen.*

URETHROSTOMY

A urethrostomy is the creation of a new and permanent urethral orifice. The three urethrostomy locations in the male dog are prepubic, scrotal, and perineal. The perineal region is by far the least desirable, both because of the problem of urine leakage and urine scald of the perineal skin and scrotum and because of the difficulty of suturing the deep urethra to the skin. If castration is not objectionable, scrotal urethrostomy is the most desirable, because of the large, distensible urethra in that region and the lack of problems with urine leakage or scald. Most calculi can be easily removed from this location without having to make the curve of the urethra at the area of the scrotum (Figs. 23-7 and 23-10). If castration cannot be performed, a prepubic urethrostomy is the alternative. Prepubic urethrostomies may be associated with the complication of urine scald of the scrotum, and the urethra is not as large in diameter as in the scrotal area.

INDICATIONS. A urethrostomy is indicated for the following: (1) recurrent stone formation that cannot adequately be treated and prevented by medical therapy; (2) strictures of the urethra that resulted from previous urethrotomy incisions or traumatic injuries; and (3) patients in which surgical management of recurrent calculi is preferred to medical management or in which

medical management may be harmful. At no time would a urethrostomy be elected in a dog that is to be kept for breeding.

TECHNIQUE. In the case of the prepubic and perineal urethrostomies, prepubic or perineal urethrotomies are first performed as described. In the case of the scrotal urethrostomy, the dog is placed in dorsal recumbency and is prepared and draped for the surgical procedure, including a complete shaving and scrubbing of the scrotum. The base of the scrotal sac is incised with a slightly elliptical incision, the tunica dartos is severed, and the skin is discarded. Care should be taken to leave enough skin so that suturing skin to urethral mucosa does not place the sutures under tension. The testes are then exposed, and castration is completed (Fig. 23-11A). The retractor penis muscle is exposed and is bluntly dissected from the corpus spongiosum penis. This muscle is retracted laterally, the penis is stabilized, and the urethra is incised over a previously placed urethral catheter, as described for prepubic urethrotomy (Fig. 23-8). The length of the urethrostomy should be at least 5 to 8 times the diameter of the urethral lumen, so that an adequate urethral orifice remains when the wound contracts.

Urethrostomies are first sutured by placing the 4 "corner" sutures at 45° angles. The lateral edges are

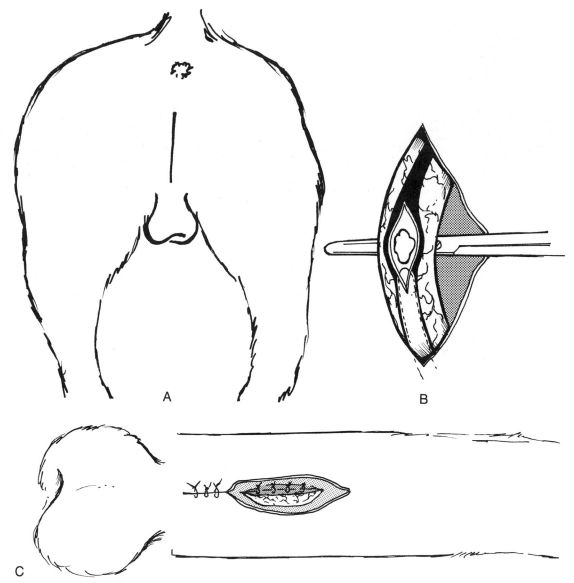

Fig. 23-9. A, *Site of incision for a perineal urethrotomy.* B, *The corpus spongiosum penis is incised (over a previously placed urinary catheter) to the urethral lumen.* C, *Closure of a urethrotomy in two layers: the first layer is simple interrupted closure of the corpus spongiosum penis, and the second is simple interrupted closure of the skin.*

then sequentially sutured with the corpus spongiosum penis apposed to the skin (Fig. 23-11*B*). Simple interrupted sutures of 4-0 or 5-0 monofilament nylon, polypropylene, or polyethylene, or 4-0 or 5-0 polyglycolic acid or polyglactin 910 sutures are used. These suture sizes and materials are the least irritating and the least inflammatory of available sutures. The skin is resected and is apposed as needed to create a tensionless, cosmetic closure (Fig. 23-11*C*). Tension leads to tearing of the tissue and thus leads to areas of excessive scar tissue production.

Elizabethan collars, muzzles, or body-neck braces may be required to prevent licking and automutilation of the urethrostomy by the patient. Any licking or automutilation increases the inflammatory response and ultimately leads to excessive scar tissue production.

Hemorrhage frequently occurs in the postoperative period when the dog becomes excited or urinates; the bleeding occurs from the suture tracts in the corpus spongiosum penis. Intermittent hemorrhage can be expected until the sutures are removed 7 to 14 days postoperatively. Episodes of intermittent bleeding usually do not last long, so efforts to control bleeding with topical hemostatic agents or tranquilization are not necessary or advisable unless bleeding is profuse.

Postoperative Care and Prevention of Recurrence

The removal of the calculi is only the beginning of treatment for urolithiasis. Calculi analysis, as well as direct bladder and urethral culture and sensitivity

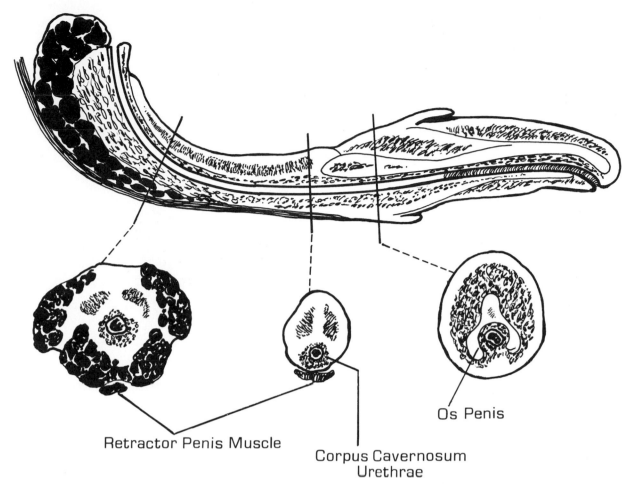

Retractor Penis Muscle

Corpus Cavernosum
Urethrae

Os Penis

Fig. 23-10. *Schematic illustration of cross sections of the urethra and penis at different levels. The urethra is larger in diameter and more distensible at the level of the scrotum than it is more cranially in the prepubic area. The urethra is essentially nondistensible at the level of the os penis.*

tests, must be obtained to provide the information necessary to treat rationally and to prescribe for nonrecurrence of calculi disease. Approximately two out of three cases of calculi are culture-positive, and approximately one out of three cases recurs.[3] For this reason, vigorous and prolonged therapy should be emphasized. Depending on the type of calculi found, more than one approach to therapy may be indicated.

Antibiotics found effective in the urinary tract include the following: (1) chloramphenicol (20 to 30 mg/kg tid orally); (2) nitrofurantoin (4 mg/kg orally with small amounts of food tid or qid); (3) penicillin G (40,000 U/kg tid orally); (4) trimethoprim, 20 mg and sulfadiazine 100 mg (one tablet/4 kg once or twice daily); (5) cephalexin (15 to 20 mg/kg tid orally); (6) sulfisoxazole (40 mg/kg tid orally); (7) penicillin VK, ampicillin, hetacillin (30 mg/kg tid orally); (8) amoxicillin (20 mg/kg tid orally); and (9) gentamicin (4 mg/kg subcutaneously bid).

Urinalyses and urine cultures should be checked at 2- to 4-week intervals, and therapy should be adjusted accordingly. Even if no bacteria are present, urinalyses should be checked regularly. In adition to antibiotics,

methylene blue (1/10 gr/4 kg orally tid) has been found effective in dissolving calculi and in preventing their recurrence in dogs.[4,7]

MAGNESIUM-AMMONIUM-PHOSPHATE CALCULI. These are the most common type of calculi to occur in dogs and are frequently associated with urinary tract infection. Because phosphate calculi form more readily in alkaline urine, attempts to acidify the urine, along with antibiotic therapy, may be helpful. The ability to maintain aciduria with chemotherapy is questionable, but ammonium chloride, ascorbic acid (vitamin C), and DL-methionine may be indicated in the early postoperative period.

Another reliable method of prophylaxis against urinary tract infection is to stimulate diuresis to dilute and urodynamically "flush out" bacteria. Liquids can be added to the food, and salt increases thirst and thus increases fluid intake.

CYSTINE CALCULI. High levels of the amino acid cystine may be excreted because of a hereditary metabolic defect of the renal tubules in certain male dogs. Cystine calculi form more readily in acid urine and are also associated with a high incidence of positive bacterial

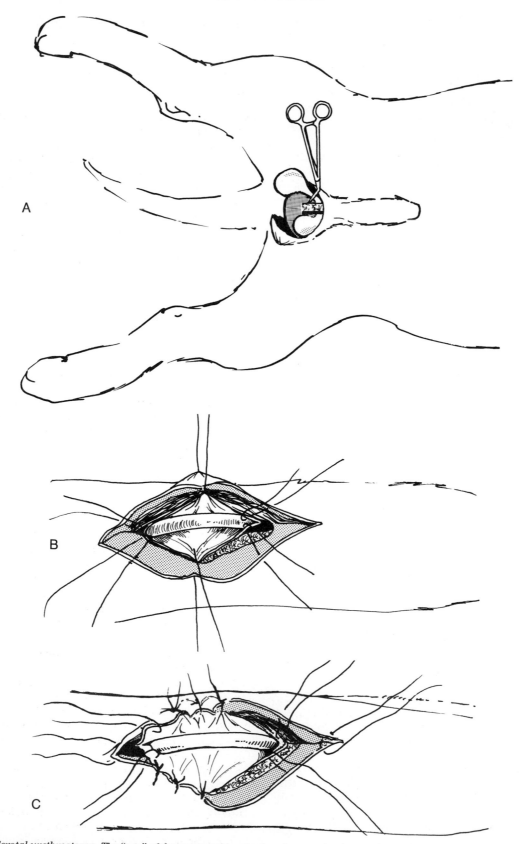

Fig. 23-11. A, *Scrotal urethrostomy. The "cap" of the scrotum is excised and castration is completed. One must be sure not to excise too much skin initially; excessive skin can be trimmed away later.* B, *Closure of urethrostomy. The "corner" sutures are placed first at 45° angles, apposing the corpus spongiosum penis to skin. No subcutaneous sutures are necessary. The caudal orifice should be where the perineal urethra curves to become the penile urethra.* C, *Closure of a urethrostomy. One should avoid using tension when suturing. One should trim excessive skin and suture to create a cosmetic closure.*

cultures. Urine alkalinization with sodium bicarbonate may be as difficult as attempts to acidify urine with chemotherapy. Stimulation of increased water intake and diuresis will help to reduce bacterial and cystine concentrations in the urine.

The drug D-penicillamine,* at a dose of 30 mg/kg divided bid, has been helpful in controlling recurring cystine calculi. The disadvantages of this drug are that it is expensive, can be toxic, and must be given for the rest of the dog's life. Nausea, vomiting, bone-marrow depression, and hypersensitivity may result from its use. If D-penicillamine is used, it should be used at the minimal effective, nontoxic dosage, and should be given with food; the dog should have pyridoxine added to the diet because D-penicillamine may increase the requirement for this vitamin. Consequently, owners often request that a urethrostomy be performed when the options are explained.

URATE CALCULI. Urate calculi occur primarily in the dalmatian breed of dog and have no sex predilection. Urate urolithiasis in the dalmatian is due to an inherited metabolic defect; a defective uricase system in the liver leads to incomplete breakdown of uric acid to allantoin and perhaps to a defective tissue transport system in the liver and kidney. This defect, in turn, increases the level of urates in the urine. The calculi consist primarily of ammonium urate, and unless they also contain some calcium, phosphate, or oxalate, they are radiolucent. Attempts to control the pH of the patient's urine have not satisfactorily prevented urate calculi recurrence. In cases of recurrence, urethrostomy may be recommended.

The drug allopurinol† is used successfully in preventing urate calculi recurrence. An effective recommended dose is 5 mg/kg orally bid indefinitely. Allopurinol inhibits xanthine oxidase from converting xanthine to uric acid in the liver. Side effects of the drug have been minimal, but the veterinarian should be aware of the possibility of xanthine calculi formation, which has been reported in man.

References and Suggested Readings

1. Bovee, K. C.: "Urinary Calculi in the Dog." In Current Veterinary Therapy V. Edited by R. W. Kirk. Philadelphia, W. B. Saunders, 1974.
2. Brown, N. O., Parks, J. L., and Greene, R. W.: Canine urolithiasis: retrospective analysis of 438 cases. J. Am. Vet. Med. Assoc., 170:414, 1977.
3. Brown, N. O., Parks, J. L., and Greene, R. W.: Recurrence of canine urolithiasis. J. Am. Vet. Med. Assoc., 170:419, 1977.
4. Donovan, C. A.: Clinical observations on use of methylene blue for urinary calculi and conception. VM SAC, 72:582, 1977.
5. Finco, D. R.: Current status of canine urolithiasis. J. Am. Vet. Med. Assoc., 158:327, 1971.
6. Peacock, E. E., and Van Winkle, W.: Wound Repair. 2nd Ed. Philadelphia, W. B. Saunders, 1976.
7. Schechter, R. D.: Personal communication, 1980.

*Caprimine, Merck, Sharp, & Dohme, West Point, PA 19486
†Zyloprim, Burroughs-Wellcome, Research Triangle Park, NC 27709

Diagnostic and Therapeutic Cystocentesis

by CARL A. OSBORNE, GEORGE E. LEES,

and GARY R. JOHNSTON

Cystocentesis is a form of paracentesis that consists of needle puncture of the urinary bladder for the purpose of removing a variable quantity of urine by aspiration. Although techniques and complications of cystocentesis have not been evaluated by controlled studies, clinical experience with many hundreds of canine and feline patients has revealed that properly performed cystocentesis is of great diagnostic and therapeutic value.[1,4] This procedure is associated with a much smaller risk of iatrogenic infection than catheterization and is better tolerated by most patients, especially cats and female dogs, than catheterization.

Diagnostic Indications

A resident population of bacteria normally is present in progressively increasing numbers from the midzone of the urethra to the distal urethra in humans and dogs and probably in cats. Resident bacteria are also present in the vagina and prepuce. In contrast, urine in the kidneys, ureters, and urinary bladder of normal animals typically is sterile. In addition to systemic natural defense mechanisms, the following local defense mechanisms are thought to prevent urinary tract infection in animals: normal micturition, normal anatomic features, mucosal defense barriers, antibacterial properties of urine, and renal defense mechanisms.[2]

Collection of urine during natural micturition is satisfactory for routine urinalyses performed to screen patients for abnormalities of the urinary tract and other body systems. Contamination of voluntarily voided urine with bacteria, cells, and other debris from the urethra, genital tract, and integument, however, sometimes makes it necessary to repeat analysis of urine collected by catheterization or cystocentesis. Urine samples obtained by catheterization may also be contaminated with resident urethral bacteria. In addition, catheterization, no matter how carefully executed, is always associated with the hazard of iatrogenic urinary tract infection caused by the transport of resident urethral bacteria into the bladder.[3] The risk of bacterial infection caused by catheterization depends on the integrity of systemic and local host defenses and is therefore higher in patients with: (1) pre-existing diseases of the urethra or urinary bladder; or (2) polysystemic diseases that alter host defenses, such as diabetes mellitus, hyperadrenocorticism, and primary renal failure. Potential problems associated with collection of urine samples by normal micturition, manual compression of the urinary bladder, and catheterization may be avoided by cystocentesis.

Diagnostic cystocentesis is indicated to: (1) prevent contamination of urine samples with bacteria, cells, and debris from the lower urogenital tract; (2) aid in

Table 23-1. *Comparison of Results of Urinalyses Performed on a Voluntarily Voided Urine Sample and a Sample Obtained by Cystocentesis*

	Method of Collection	
Factor	Voluntarily Voided	Cystocentesis
Color	Yellow	Yellow
Turbidity	Cloudy	Slightly cloudy
Specific Gravity	1.035	1.035
pH	7.5	7.5
Glucose	Negative	Negative
Bilirubin	Negative	Negative
Ketones	Negative	Negative
Occult Blood	4+	2+
Protein	3+	1+
RBC/HPF*	TNTC†	25–30
WBC/HPF*	TNTC†	50–60
Casts/LPF**	None	None
Epithelial cells	Many	Many
Crystals	Phosphate	Phosphate
Bacteria	Numerous rods	Occasional rods

*HPF, high power field = 450 × **LPF, low power field = 100×
†Too numerous to count

collection of urine for analysis prior to injection of solutions into the urethra to dislodge plugs or calculi; (3) aid in localization of hematuria, pyuria, and bacteriuria (Table 23-1); and (4) minimize iatrogenic urinary tract infection caused by catheterization, especially in patients with pre-existing diseases of the urethra or urinary bladder.

Therapeutic Indications

Therapeutic cystocentesis may be employed to provide temporary decompression of the excretory pathway of the urinary system when functional or mechanical urethral obstruction prevents normal micturition. It is frequently used in male cats when reverse flushing or other nonsurgical techniques have failed to dislodge urethral plugs. Following cystocentesis, attempts to dislodge urethral plugs by reverse flushing are frequently successful, perhaps because the patient has less discomfort and the skeletal muscle surrounding the distal urethra has relaxed.

Contraindications

The main contraindications to cystocentesis are an insufficient volume of urine in the urinary bladder and resistance of the patient to restraint and abdominal palpation. Blind cystocentesis performed without digital localization and immobilization of the urinary bladder is usually unsuccessful and may damage the bladder or adjacent structures.

In our experience, collection of urine by cystocentesis from patients with bacterial urinary tract infection has not been associated with detectable spread of infection outside the urinary tract. In fact, collection of a urine sample for bacterial culture that has not been contaminated by passage through the urethra and genital tract is a frequent reason for performing cystocentesis.

Iatrogenic loss of substantial quantities of urine through the needle tract in the bladder into the peritoneal cavity during or following properly performed cystocentesis is unlikely unless necrosis of the bladder wall is extensive. Transmural necrosis of the bladder wall is unlikely, but can occur following prolonged obstruction, especially with concomitant bacterial urinary tract infection, or traumatic infarction.

Equipment

We routinely use 22-gauge needles. Depending on the size of the patient and the distance of the ventral bladder wall from the ventral abdominal wall, 1.5-inch hypodermic or 3-inch spinal needles* may be selected.

We usually use small-capacity (2½- to 12-ml) syringes for diagnostic cystocentesis and larger-capacity (20- to 60-ml) syringes for therapeutic cystocentesis. Alternately, therapeutic cystocentesis may be performed with 6- to 12-ml syringes and a 2-way or 3-way valve.† If desirable, a 22-gauge needle may be transected midway between its tip and hub and reconnected with a section of flexible polyethylene tubing.‡

Site

Careful planning of the site and direction of needle puncture of the bladder wall is recommended. Although some clinicians recommend insertion of the needle into the dorsal wall of the bladder to minimize gravity-dependent leakage of urine into the peritoneal cavity following withdrawal of the needle (Fig. 23-12), we recommend that the needle be inserted in the ventral or ventrolateral wall of the bladder in order to minimize the chance of trauma to the ureters and major abdominal vessels (Figs. 23-12 and 23-13). If therapeutic cystocentesis is to be performed, we recommend insertion of the needle closer to the junction of the bladder with the urethra rather than the vertex of the bladder (Fig. 23-13). This maneuver permits removal of urine and decompression of the bladder without reinsertion of the needle into the bladder lumen (Fig. 23-13). If the needle is placed in or adjacent to the vertex of the bladder, it may not remain within the bladder lumen because the bladder progressively decreases in size following aspiration of urine.

We also recommend that the needle be directed through the bladder wall at approximately a 45° angle so that an oblique needle tract is created (Figs. 23-12 and 23-13). By directing the needle through the bladder wall in an oblique fashion, the elasticity of the vesical musculature and the interlacing arrangement of individual muscle fibers provide a better seal for the small pathway created by the needle when it is removed. In

*Yale spinal needle, Becton, Dickinson Co., Rutherford, NJ 07070
†Pharmaseal, Inc., Toa Alta, PR 00758
‡PE 60, Clay Adams, Inc., Parsippany, NJ 07054

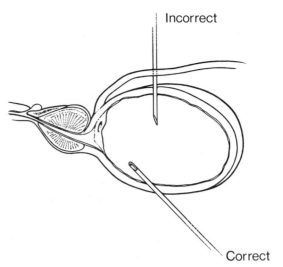

Fig. 23-12. *Schematic drawing illustrating correct and incorrect sites and angles of penetration of needle through the canine bladder wall. The needle should be directed through the bladder wall at approximately a 45° angle to create an oblique needle tract. By inserting the needle in the ventral or ventrolateral bladder wall, iatrogenic trauma to the ureters and major abdominal vessels is minimized.*

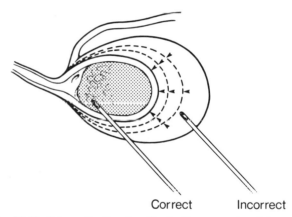

Fig. 23-13. *Schematic drawing illustrating correct and incorrect sites of insertion of a needle into the bladder for the purpose of evacuating urine. The needle should be inserted in the ventral or ventrolateral surface of the wall cranial to the junction of the bladder and the urethra rather than at the vertex of the bladder. This technique permits removal of urine and decompression of the bladder without need for reinsertion of the needle into the bladder lumen. (Illustration by Michael P. Schenk, College of Veterinary Medicine, University of Minnesota.)*

addition, subsequent distension of the bladder wall as the lumen refills with urine forces the walls of the needle tract into apposition in a fashion analogous to the flap valve of the ureterovesical junction.

Operative Considerations

Because insertion and withdrawal of a 22-gauge needle through the walls of the abdomen and bladder are associated with little discomfort, one rarely needs to administer tranquilization, general anesthesia, or local anesthesia for diagnostic or therapeutic cystocentesis.

If the urinary bladder does not contain a sufficient volume of urine to permit digital localization and immobilization, the patient may be given oral fluids or a diuretic. Although diuretics such as furosemide may be used to facilitate collection of urine samples by increasing urine formation, alteration of urine specific gravity and urine pH are notable drawbacks of this procedure. Even the quantity of bacteria per milliliter of urine may be reduced, altering the results of quantitative urine cultures. Use of diuretics to enhance urine collection by augmenting urine flow is therefore best suited for serial urine sample collections when information about urine specific gravity, urine pH, and semiquantitative evaluation of routine test components are not significant.

Surgical Technique

In order to perform cystocentesis without risk to the patient, adequate localization and immobilization of the urinary bladder, together with planning of the site and direction of needle puncture, are essential. The ventral abdominal skin penetrated by the needle should be cleansed with an antiseptic solution each time cystocentesis is performed. Excessive hair should be removed with a clipper if necessary. We usually drench the area with alcohol. Appropriate caution should be used to avoid iatrogenic trauma to or infection of the urinary bladder and surrounding structures.

In cats, it is usually easiest to perform the procedure with the patient in lateral or dorsal recumbency. In dogs, the procedure may also be performed when the patient is standing. In our experience, it is easier to palpate small urinary bladders while canine patients are standing, but more difficult to insert the needle into small bladders when such patients are standing. In this situation, we locate the bladders by palpation with the patients standing, and then place the animals in lateral recumbency without releasing the bladder. The needle is then directed into the bladder lumens. Abdominal palpation of the bladder may also be facilitated by an assistant who advances the bladder cranially by rectal palpation.

Following localization and immobilization of the urinary bladder, the needle should be inserted through the ventral abdominal wall and advanced to the caudoventral aspect of the bladder. The needle should be inserted through the bladder wall at an oblique angle. If a larger quantity of urine is to be aspirated, the needle should be directed to enter the bladder lumen cranial to the junction of the bladder with the urethra. If a small volume of urine is to be collected for analysis, any site along the ventrolateral or ventral surface of the bladder is satisfactory. While the needle and bladder are immobilized, urine should be gently aspirated into the syringe. If a large quantity of urine is to be evacuated from the bladder, a two-way or three-way valve may be used.

Excessive digital pressure should not be applied to the bladder wall while the needle is in its lumen, to prevent urine from being forced around the needle into

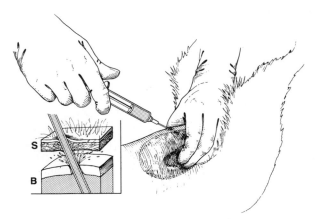

Fig. 23-14. *Schematic drawing illustrating escape of urine through the bladder wall adjacent to the needle tract as a result of excessive digital pressure used to localize and immobilize the bladder. Inset: S, skin of abdominal wall; B, wall of urinary bladder.*

the peritoneal cavity (Fig. 23-14). Use of a 3-inch spinal needle rather than a 1.5-inch hypodermic needle when the ventral surface of the bladder wall is more than 1 to 1.25 inches from the ventral abdominal wall permits immobilization of the urinary bladder without increasing intraluminal pressure by pulling it toward the ventral abdominal wall.

If disease of the bladder wall or virulence of urinary pathogens is a likely cause of complications associated with loss of urine into the peritoneal cavity, the bladder should be emptied as completely as is consistent with atraumatic technique. These potential complications have not been a problem in our patients.

Postoperative Care

The need for prophylactic antibacterial therapy following cystocentesis must be determined on the basis of the status of the patient and retrospective evaluation of technique. In most instances it is not required. In order to minimize contamination of the peritoneal cavity with urine, unnecessary digital pressure on the urinary bladder following cystocentesis should be avoided.

Complications

PATIENT

With the exception of occasional postcystocentesis hematuria, we have not observed significant antemortem or postmortem postoperative complications following use of cystocentesis in hundreds of dogs and cats in our clinical and experimental studies. Potential complications include damage to the bladder wall or adjacent structures with the needle, local or generalized peritonitis, vesicoperitoneal fistulas, and adhesion of adjacent structures to the bladder wall. These complications are most likely to occur if the technique is attempted in an uncooperative patient or in a patient with a small urinary bladder.

LABORATORY

We have encountered a few instances in which penetration of a loop of intestine by the needle resulted in false-positive significant bacteriuria. Varying degrees of microscopic hematuria might be expected for a short time following cystocentesis, but are of little consequence because samples for laboratory analysis are rarely collected at this time.

References and Suggested Readings

1. Osborne, C. A., Johnston, G. R., and Schenk, M. P.: Cystocentesis: indications, contraindications, technique, and complications. Minnesota Vet., *17*:9, 1977.
2. Osborne, C. A., Klausner, J. S., and Lees, G. E.: Urinary tract infections: normal and abnormal host defense mechanisms. Vet. Clin. North Am., *9*:587, 1979.
3. Osborne, C. A., and Schenk, M. P.: Techniques of urine collection. *In* Scientific Presentations and Seminar Synopses of the 44th Annual Meeting of the American Animal Hospital Association, South Bend, IN, 1977.
4. Osborne, C. A., and Stevens, J. B.: Handbook Of Canine And Feline Urinalysis. St. Louis, Ralston Purina, 1981.

24 * Urethra

Perineal Urethrostomy in the Cat

by GEORGE P. WILSON *and* JILL K. KUSBA

Obstruction of the male cat's distal urinary tract is common and represents all or part of the manifestations included in the feline urologic syndrome (FUS).[6] The clinical records of 501 male cats with FUS between January, 1975 through December, 1979 at The Ohio State University Veterinary Hospital were reviewed. The 97 intact males and 404 castrated males represented 8.0% of the total male cat population (6207) at that hospital. Affected cats ranged in age from 1 to 13 years, with 76% between 1 and 4 years old. Seven hundred and ninety-five obstructions were recorded in 501 male cats, with 1 to 7 recorded obstructions per cat. There were 450 domestic short- and long-haired cats, 36 Siamese cats, and 15 of other breeds. Six cats with postoperative complications seen at the University of Minnesota are included in these data.

The patient should be stabilized if possible; normal renal function should be restored before surgical intervention. If it is not possible to relieve the urethral obstruction, regardless of the cause, urethrostomy must be performed. A guarded prognosis is warranted in a cat with severely impaired kidney function due to prolonged urinary obstruction.

Surgical Anatomy

Knowledge of the anatomic features of the male cat's genitourinary tract is mandatory to perform the perineal urethrostomy.[2] The caudal scrotal arteries are paired vessels that arise from the perineal arteries; the cranial scrotal arteries, terminal branches of the external pudic artery, supply the prepuce, retractor scroti muscle, and dorsal artery of the penis. The corpus spongiosum penis is supplied by branches of the prostatic artery found on the lateral pelvic urethra coursing to the corpus spongiosum penis (Fig. 24-1). The veins of the penis drain through the left and right penile veins that lie on the ventral penis. These veins unite to form a single trunk through the bifid tendon of insertion of the ischiourethralis muscles. Because of the penile arterial and venous relationship, the blood supply of the penis is maintained following surgical urethrostomy (Fig.

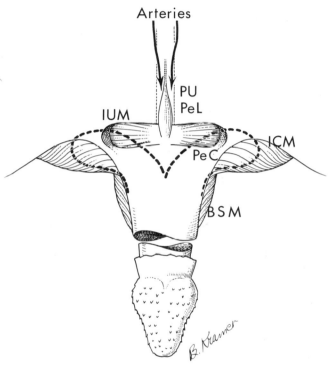

Fig. 24-1. *Relationship of the ischiocavernosus muscle, crura of penis, ischiourethralis muscle, and ligament of penis. The course of the penile artery on the sides of the pelvic urethra is indicated. PU, Pelvic urethra; PeL, ligament of penis; IUM, ischiourethralis muscle; ICM, ischiocavernosus muscle; PeC, crus of penis; BSM, bulbospongiosus muscle.*

24-1). The dorsal artery of the cat's penis is on the ventral surface of the cat penis, and this artery is the homologue of the dorsal artery of the penis of other domestic animals. In erection, the penis is directed ventrally, with its glans arched slightly forward; its dorsal and ventral surfaces are caudal and cranial, respectively.[5]

The penis is attached to the ischial arch by the paired ischiocavernosus muscles, the paired crura of the penis covered by the ischiocavernosus muscles, the paired ischiourethralis muscles, and the single midline penile ligament (Fig. 24-2). The penis and pelvic urethra have no other major pelvic attachments, except the genital folds attached on the lateral aspect of the pelvic urethra.

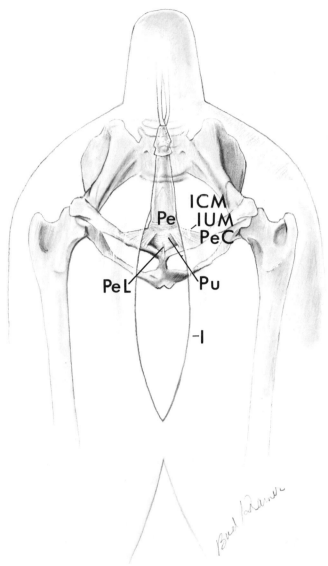

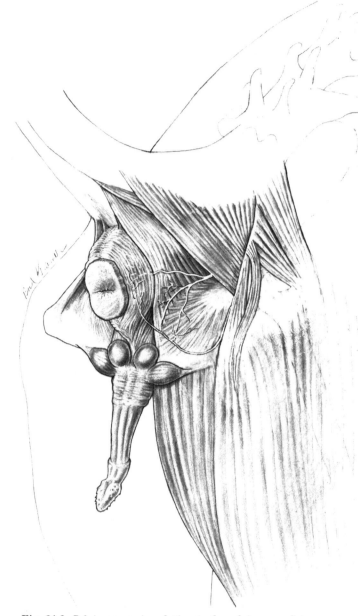

Fig. 24-2. *Pelvic attachments of the penis and pelvic urethra. ICM, Ischiocavernosus muscle; IUM, ischiourethralis muscle; PeC, crus of penis; Pe, penis; PeL, ligament of penis; Pu, pelvic urethra; I, skin incision. (From Wilson, G. P., and Harrison, J. W.: Perineal urethrostomy in cats. J. Am. Vet. Med. Assoc., 159:1789, 1971.)*

Fig. 24-3. *Pelvic nerves in relation to the pelvic musculature.*

The innervation to the pelvic viscera is complex and is not functionally well defined.[1,3,4] The ischiatic, the obturator, and the pudendal nerves are lateral to the levator ani muscle (Fig. 24-3); the autonomic pelvic plexus is medial to the levator ani muscle surrounding the colon, the rectum, and the pelvic urethra (Fig. 24-4). The control and coordination of urination and defecation depend on the continuity of the perineal ramus of the caudal cutaneous femoral nerve, the caudal rectal nerve, a branch of the pudendal nerve, and the pelvic nervous plexus. Any trauma, including surgical dissection, that disrupts these nerves produces fecal and urinary incontinence and rectal prolapse. Specifically, circumferential dissection of the pelvic urethra during perineal urethrostomy has the potential of disrupting the pelvic innervation producing incontinence, rectal prolapse, or both.

The retractor penis muscle is dorsal to the penile urethra, and this muscle is close to the penile urethra at the distal quarter of the penis. The retractor penis muscle runs toward and is part of the external anal sphincter and is covered dorsally by loose areolar tissue and the levator scroti muscle. The bulbospongiosus muscle is at the proximal quarter of the penile urethra, and the bulbourethral glands are at the caudal pelvic urethra. These two structures are the landmarks between the penile and pelvic urethra.

Preoperative Considerations

Gas anesthetic agents are the safest and the most effective for induction and maintenance of anesthesia in cats with urinary tract obstructions. Barbiturates should be avoided because these drugs are excreted by

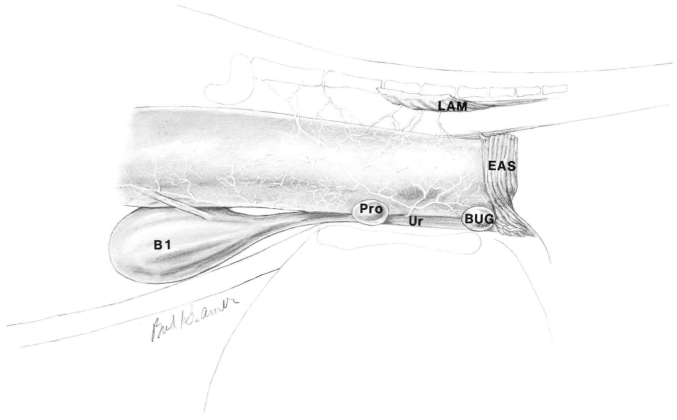

Fig. 24-4. *Autonomic pelvic plexus.*

the kidneys. To promote diuresis during the operation, the healthy patient is given a 10% dextrose solution intravenously. This solution causes diuresis and fills the urinary bladder during the surgical procedure, with no ill effects on the cat; the urinary bladder can be expressed manually immediately postoperatively to evaluate the urethrostomy and to clear debris in the urethra and bladder. Fluid administration must be carefully performed in cats with compromised renal function because of the many possible complications in kidney function resulting from acute urinary tract obstruction.

Surgical Technique

The hair on the perineum and the external genitalia is clipped, and the area is scrubbed. A pursestring suture is placed in the anus to eliminate fecal contamination of the surgical field. The patient is placed in ventral recumbency with the perineum elevated at approximately 30°. The tail is extended directly over the dorsal midline and is immobilized. (One should not place a towel clamp in the tail because the tail can be irreparably injured.)

An elliptical incision is made to excise the scrotum and prepuce (Fig. 24-5A). This maneuver exposes the testes in the intact male or a fat pad in a castrated male (Fig. 24-5B) and the levator scroti muscle dorsal to the retractor penis muscle. Castration should be performed at this time in an intact cat. The scrotal and

preputial blood vessels require ligation. The dorsal artery of the penis must be ligated.

The penis is reflected dorsolaterally at approximately 45°. The loose tissue surrounding the penis is dissected to the penile pelvic attachments on the ischial arch. The penile attachments (previously described) on the dissected side are severed from their ischial origins (Fig. 24-5C). If this procedure is done carefully, it is possible to avoid incising the crus of the penis, which is covered by the ischiocavernosus muscle, and thereby to eliminate a source of hemorrhage. The penis is reflected to the opposite side; the dissection and incision of the contralateral penile attachments are performed. One should keep the scissors parallel to the bony pelvis to avoid lacerating the pelvic urethra during the dissection of the penile pelvic attachments. The penis is directed on the dorsal midline, and the penile ligament of the penis is incised (Fig. 24-5D). All the major attachments of the penis are cut; the penis and pelvic urethra are freed from the pelvic floor by blunt digital dissection.

The penis is reflected ventrally, and the levator scroti muscle and the loose areolar tissue on the dorsal aspect of the penis are excised, exposing the retractor penis muscle lying dorsal to the penile urethra (Fig. 24-5E). A fine probe is inserted in the penile urethra, and the retractor penis muscle is carefully removed from the dorsal aspect of the penis to expose the urethral cavernous body surrounding the penile urethra (Fig. 24-5F). The bulbospongiosus muscle is exposed

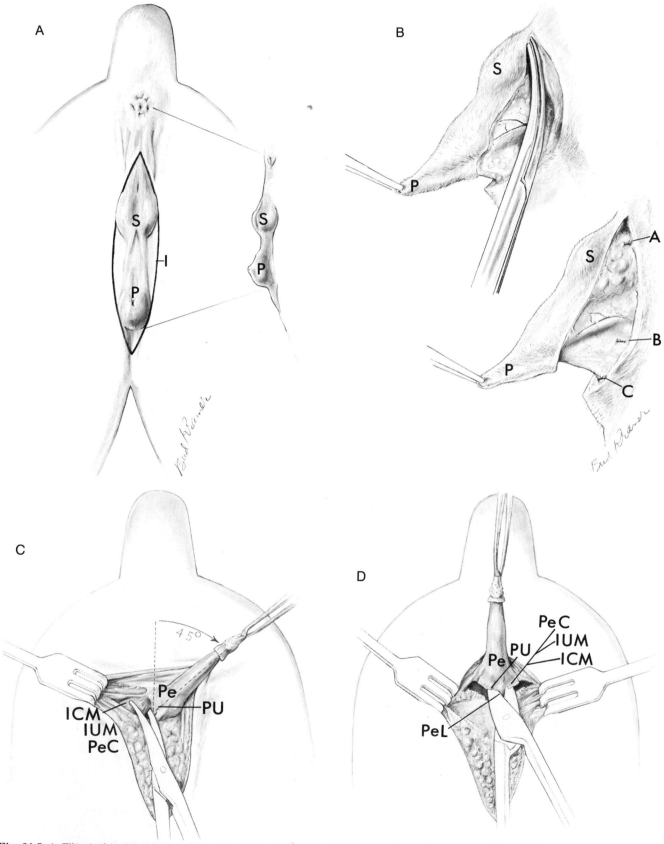

Fig. 24-5. A, *Elliptical incision incorporating the scrotum and prepuce. S, Scrotum; P, prepuce; I, skin incision. B, Removal of prepuce and scrotum. S, Scrotum; P, prepuce; A, caudal scrotal artery; B, cranial scrotal artery; C, dorsal artery and vein of penis, prostatic artery. C, Dissection of penis from surrounding tissue to its pelvic attachments on the ischium. ICM, Ischiocavernosus muscle; IUM, ischiourethralis muscle; PeC, crus of penis; Pe, penis; PU, pelvic urethra. D, Incision of ligament of penis. PeC, Crus of penis; IUM, ischiourethralis muscle; ICM, ischiocavernosus muscle; PU, pelvic urethra; Pe, penis; PeL, ligament of penis.*

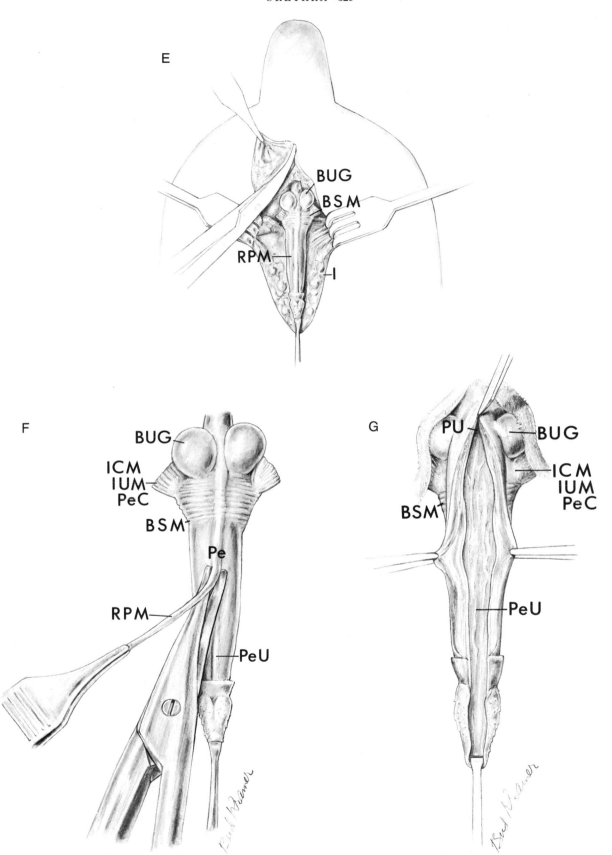

Fig. 24-5. *(cont.)* E, *Exposure of the retractor penis muscle. BUG, Bulbourethral glands; BSM, bulbospongiosus muscle; RPM, retractor muscle of penis; I, skin incision. F, Insertion of probe into penile urethra. BUG, Bulbourethral gland; ICM, ischiocavernosus muscle; IUM, ischiourethralis muscle; PeC, crus of penis; BSM, bulbospongiosus muscle; Pe, penis; RPM, retractor muscle of penis; PeU, penile urethra. G, Incision of the penile urethra through the glans penis to the pelvic urethra. PU, Pelvic urethra; BUG, bulbourethral gland; ICM, ischiocavernosus muscle; IUM, ischiourethralis muscle; PeC, crus of penis; PeU, penile urethra; BSM, bulbospongiosus muscle.*

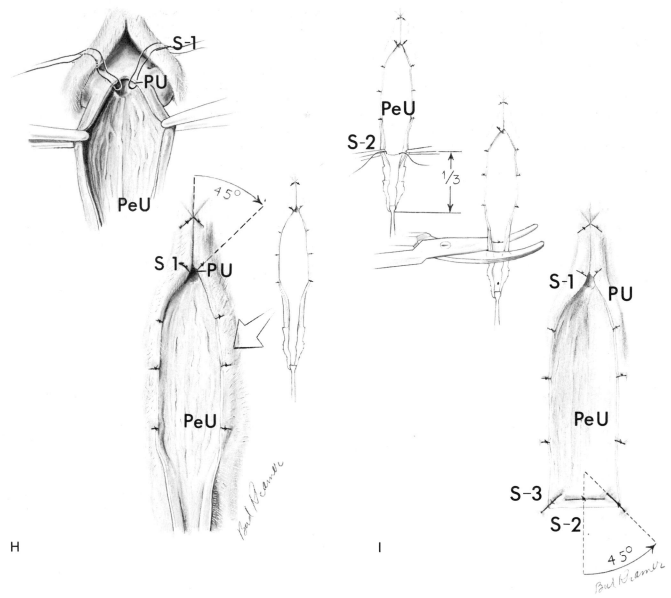

Fig. 24-5. (cont.) H, *Suture of the pelvic and penile urethral mucosa to the perineal skin. S-1, Initial sutures; PU, pelvic urethra; PeU, penile urethra. I, Placement of through-and-through suture through body of penis. PeU, Penile urethra; S-2, through-and-through mattress suture; S-1, initial sutures; PU, pelvic urethra; S-3, mucosa-to-skin sutures. (From Wilson, G. P., and Harrison, J. W.: Perineal urethrostomy in cats. J. Am. Vet. Med. Assoc. 159:1789, 1971.)*

at the proximal penile urethra. The bulbourethral glands are atrophic in the castrated male, in contrast to those of the intact male, in which the glands may be large. Removal of the bulbourethral glands is not necessary.

The penile urethra is incised dorsally and longitudinally through the glans penis to the pelvic urethra with small, sharp-sharp tenotomy scissors (Fig. 24-5G). The penile urethral incision must extend into the pelvic urethra. The pelvic urethra varies in size up to 4.5 mm in diameter. The opening of the pelvic urethra may be identified by a distinct feeling of cutting dense tissue; it is the fascia of the bulbospongiosus muscle. The narrow penile urethra is not completely incised if the urethral incision is not carried to the pelvic urethra and the penile urethra continues to serve as a site of ob-

struction. A blunt instrument, such as closed Rochester Pean forceps,* introduced carefully into the pelvic urethra, ascertains that the incision is adequate.

The pelvic and penile urethral mucosa are carefully identified and are sutured to the perineal skin with 4-0 suture (Fig. 24-5H). Excessive tissue incorporated into the sutures causes postoperative problems. It is possible to suture the pelvic urethra closed if the urethral mucosa is not carefully identified. The dorsolateral pelvic urethra is sutured to the perineal skin with sutures placed bilaterally at approximately 45° to the midline. These sutures pull the pelvic urethra caudally and widen the urethrostomy. Two-thirds of the penile urethra is sutured to the perineal skin.

*Rochester–Pean hysterectomy forceps, American V. Mueller, 6600 West Touhy Avenue, Chicago, Il 60648

A through-and-through mattress suture of 4-0 chromic catgut is placed through the body of the penis to arrest bleeding from the distal cavernous body. The penis distal to the mattress suture is amputated, the remaining penile urethral mucosa is sutured to the skin. The last 2 urethral mucosal sutures are placed at 45° to the midline at the ventral end of the flap to widen the urethrostomy mucosal flap (Fig. 24-5*I*). A few skin sutures may be necessary to close the skin incision. The bladder is expressed to demonstrate the patency of the urethrostomy and to clear debris that can be present in the bladder and urethra.

Postoperative Care

The pursestring suture in the anus is removed. The cat does not usually mutilate the urethrostomy site, and sutures may be removed in 7 to 10 days following the operation. We recommend the use of shredded paper in the litter box to eliminate irritation from litter sticking to the urethrostomy. One should not probe or manipulate the urethrostomy before suture removal because this maneuver may result in laceration of the urethra. Urine will infiltrate the subcutis and muscle of the posterior thigh regions and will cause severe inflammation or muscle necrosis if the pelvic urethra is lacerated caudal to the levator ani muscle. Urethral lacerations cranial to the levator ani muscle cause urine to fill the peritoneal cavity. The urethra, if lacerated, can be stented with an indwelling catheter for several days to direct urine flow while the lacerated tissue heals.

Complications

The perineal urethrostomy technique[7] was performed on 204 male cats, 175 castrated and 29 intact. During the 5-year period, 37 cats developed 38 postsurgical complications. Eight of the 37 cats were referred to the Ohio State University Veterinary Hospital, and 6 cats were referred to the University of Minnesota Veterinary Clinic for similar postoperative complications; all these cats' postoperative problems resulted from an incomplete surgical dissection of the penile pelvic attachments or failure to incise the penile urethra to the pelvic urethra.

Twenty-nine cats treated at The Ohio State University Veterinary Hospital had postoperative complications: 1 cat developed a mucosal flap across the urethrostomy site, and 23 postoperative strictures occurred in 22 cats. The pelvic urethra was ruptured in 7 cats before or during the surgical procedure, and consequently urine ran into the caudal thighs or peritoneal cavity. Four male cats had rectal prolapse and fecal and urinary incontinence postoperatively: 3 of these cats also had fractures of the pelvis or sacrum, and the fourth cat had a circumferential dissection of the pelvic urethra as part of the perineal urethrostomy technique. Ulceration of exposed penile urethral mucosa did not occur in the 204 perineal urethrostomies reviewed. Recurrent hematuria and obstruction from calculus

occurred, and 3 male cats with perineal urethrostomies and bladder diverticula had unremitting hematuria.

The following is a list of the postoperative complications identified at Ohio State and Minnesota:

1. Inaccurate surgical technique is the most common complication in patients referred to the veterinary hospitals of the University of Minnesota and Ohio State University. If the ischial pelvic attachments of the penile and pelvic urethra are not freed adequately, and if the penile urethra is not incised completely, failure is sure.

2. Excessive circumferential dissection of the pelvic urethra, especially the dorsal pelvic urethra, has denervated the pelvic viscera and has caused postoperative incontinence and rectal prolapse.

3. Indiscriminate and inaccurate suturing of the urethrostomy, such as by using suture material that is too large or by applying too much tension, has caused tissue necrosis and wound disruption.

4. Laceration of the pelvic urethra before or during the surgical procedure has caused urine infiltration of the caudal thighs or peritoneal cavity. Severe inflammation, tissue necrosis, and sloughing of the caudal thighs has resulted, or the urine has filled the peritoneal cavity.

5. In some long-haired cats, the perineal hair mats over the urethrostomy site and obstructs the urethrostomy.

6. During incision of the penile urethra, the urethral cavernous body is incised, leaving the tubular penile urethral mucosa intact; this complication occurs when the distal penile urethra is traumatized excessively by long term catheterization.

7. The penile urethra must be accurately incised on the dorsal midline; if the penile urethra is not incised carefully, inaccurate closure occurs, and the potential for stricture is increased.

8. Following urinary tract obstruction, some cats have manifested a nonregenerative anemia. The cause of this anemia is unknown; it is most likely that the bone-marrow suppression is related to the uremia of FUS.

9. Some cats have chronic struvite calculi formation. It is possible to fill the urethra and bladder with these fine calculi. In such a case, a cystotomy is performed, and the bladder and urethra are flushed free of the calculi.

SURGICAL TECHNIQUE FOR POSTOPERATIVE
STRICTURE OF THE PERINEAL URETHROSTOMY

The cat with a stenotic urethrostomy acts as it did during the initial obstruction; the animal strains to urinate and is able to produce urine only in a fine stream or in drops. The urethrostomy should be examined carefully for occluding urinary calculus (struvite). The strictured urethrostomy usually does not allow the passage of a urinary catheter.

The cat is treated medically in the same manner as for the original urinary tract obstruction. The site of the

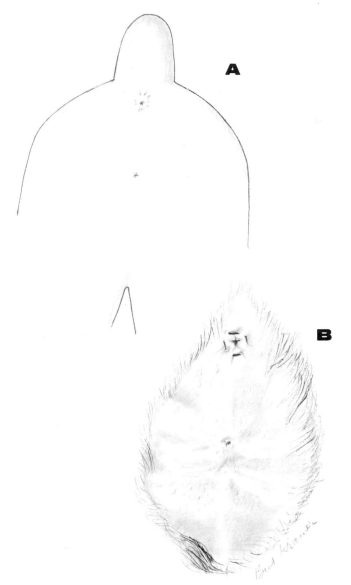

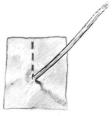

Fig. 24-7. *Strictured distal pelvic urethra with a fine probe inserted.*

urethrostomy is examined closely, and a drop of urine is usually seen forming at the strictured end of the pelvic urethra (Figs. 24-6 and 24-7). The stenotic urethral site is incised carefully circumferentially and is carefully freed from the surrounding tissues (Fig. 24-8 *A*, *B*, and *C*); little dissection is necessary. An incision is made on the dorsal side of the freed tissues (Fig. 24-8*D*); this dorsal incision usually opens the stenotic distal urethra (Fig. 24-8*E*). The urethral mucosa is distinguished readily by its characteristic pink color, and the bladder empties with a full stream of urine.

The skin edges attached to the urethral mucosa are carefully removed (Fig. 24-8 *F*, *G*, and *H*), and the free urethral mucosal margins are sutured to the skin 45° to the midsagittal line of the urethra (Fig. 24-8*I*). This procedure is all that is needed to alleviate the strictured distal pelvic urethra, unless other complications can be identified.

References and Suggested Readings

1. Martin, W. D., Fletcher, T. F., and Bradley, W. E.: Innervation of feline perineal musculature. Anat. Rec., *180:*15, 1974.
2. Martin, W. D., Fletcher, T. F., and Bradley, W. E.: Perineal musculature in the cat. Anat. Rec., *180:*3, 1974.
3. Oliver, J., Bradley, W., and Fletcher, T.: Spinal cord distribution of the somatic innervation of the external urethral spincter of the cat. J. Neurol. Sci., *10:*11, 1970.
4. Oliver, J. E., Bradley, W. E., and Fletcher, T. F.: Spinal cord representation of the micturition reflex. J. Comp. Neurol., *137:*329, 1969.

Fig. 24-6. A *and* B, *Two views of stricture of the distal pelvic urethra, perineum of cat with distal urethral stricture, and strictured distal urethra with scarring resulting from excessive suturing.*

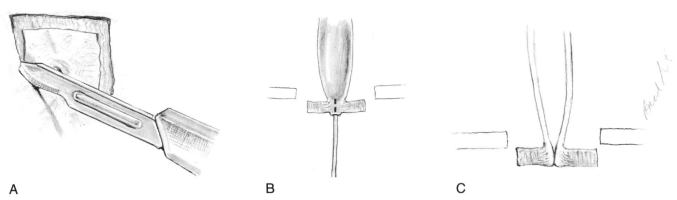

A   B   C

Fig. 24-8. A, *The strictured distal urethra is circumferentially freed from the perineum with attached perineal skin.* B, *Dorsal schematic view of strictured distal pelvic urethra attached to perineal skin.* C, *Sagittal section through distal strictured pelvic urethra and attached perineal skin.*

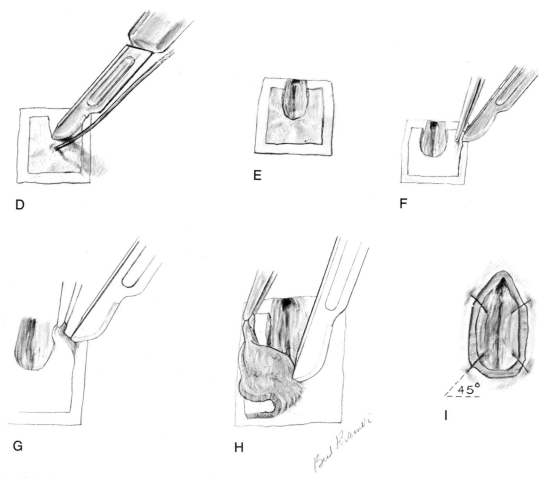

Fig. 24-8. (cont.) D, *Incision demonstrated through perineal skin dorsal to strictured pelvic urethra. This incision should open the strictured pelvic urethra. E, Strictured pelvic urethra opened with perineal skin attached. F, G, and H, Dissection of perineal skin from the strictured pelvic urethra. The removal of this perineal skin is essential to avoid another stricture resulting from wound contracture. I, The distal pelvic urethral mucosa is sutured to the perineal skin. These sutures should be placed through the urethral mucosa and skin only.*

5. Redich, G.: Das Corpus penis des Katern und seine Erektions Veranderung, eine functionellanatomische Stude. Gegenbaurs Morphol. Jahrb., *104*:561, 1963.
6. Willeberg, P.: A case-control study of some fundamental determi-

nants in the epidemiology of the feline urologic syndrome. Nord Vet. Med., *27*:1, 1975.
7. Wilson, G. P., and Harrison, J. W.: Perineal urethrostomy in cats. J. Am. Vet. Med. Assoc., *159*:1789, 1971.

25 * Uterus

Ovariohysterectomy in the Dog and Cat

by GEORGE P. WILSON *and*

HOWARD M. HAYES, JR.

Ovariohysterectomy is the most common abdominal surgical procedure performed in veterinary medicine. The primary indication for this procedure is elective sterilization. Ovariohysterectomy is also indicated in many cases of reproductive tract disease.

At the Veterinary Hospital of The Ohio State University from January of 1975 through June of 1979, 1712 ovariohysterectomies were performed on dogs; of these, 1409 were for sterilization, 313 for reproductive tract disease, 122 for mammary neoplasia, 100 for pyometra, 14 for endometrial hyperplasia, 8 for vaginitis, and 79 for miscellaneous diseases of the genital tract.

Surgical Anatomy

The reproductive tract of the female dog or cat is approachable through the flank (laparotomy) or the ventral abdominal wall (celiotomy); the latter technique is more common. The flank approach for ovariohysterectomy in a dog or cat with a diseased reproductive tract can be a difficult surgical procedure.

Removal of the ovaries is of primary concern for sterilization. Anatomically, the ovaries are located dorsal and cranial to the umbilicus. For the best surgical exposure of the ovaries and for oophorectomy, the abdominal wall incision is extended cranially through the umbilicus. This incision provides adequate exposure of the ovaries, and less effort is required to isolate the ovarian and uterine ligaments. A long incision is required to perform the ovariohysterectomy in patients with pyometra. The length of the abdominal wall incision for an ovariohysterectomy should be long enough to gain adequate exposure of the ovaries and uterus, to obviate intraoperative and postoperative complications.

Partial removal of the falciform ligament during an ovariohysterectomy is not necessary to effect better exposure of abdominal viscera and closure of the abdominal wall. The falciform ligament does not anatomically interefere with closure of the abdominal wound, if the linea alba or the abdominal fascial sheaths are used for this closure.[4]

When the patient is placed on the operating table in dorsal recumbency, the ovaries and uterine horns fall into the right and left lumbar gutters caudal to their respective kidneys. The left ovary and uterine horn are more caudal and are more readily accessible than the right ovary and uterine horn. For convenience, the left ovary and uterine horn are removed from the abdominal cavity first.

Three techniques are used to identify and to remove the ovary and uterine horn from the peritoneal cavity: one is to visualize the uterine horn and its ligamentation; the second is to use an ovariohysterectomy hook; and the third is to use the right or left index finger as a tissue hook. The structures commonly delivered into the surgical wound by these maneuvers are the round and broad ligaments. The round ligament originates cranially at the ovarian bursa and serves as a means to identify the ovary. In any female dog or cat, it is possible to push the uterine horn across the midline; such displacement necessitates moving the abdominal viscera to the cranial abdomen to identify the left or right uterine horn. The first-isolated uterine horn (cornu) is used to identify the opposite uterine horn by following the horn caudally to the uterine body.

The blood supply to the reproductive tracts of the female dog and cat is complex but constant, regardless of the stage of estrus or disease (Fig. 25-1). From cranial to caudal, both left and right, multiple arteries are found, with their satellite veins. Beginning with the suspensory ligaments, arteries in these ligaments originate from the phrenicoabdominal artery or the renal arterial complex. These arteries have companion veins that drain into the phrenicoabdominal veins, the renal veins, or the adrenal venous complex. This complex of blood vessels associated with the suspensory ligament can maintain the blood supply to a kidney that has slowly lost its renal arterial blood supply.[1,2]

The ovarian arteries and veins are caudal to the vessels of the ovarian suspensory ligament. This ovarian arteriovenous (AV) complex is a distinct, tube-like structure on the medial side of the broad ligament, coursing from the aorta to the ovary. The ovarian ar-

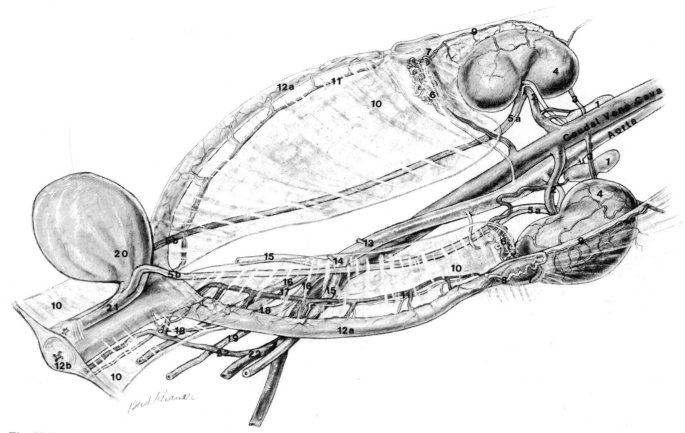

Fig. 25-1. *Schematic drawing of the female canine reproductive tract demonstrating the blood supply to the reproductive tract and the relation of other abdominal organs to the reproductive tract. (Species variations are found in the female cat.) 1, Adrenal gland; 2, renal artery and vein; 3, phrenicoabdominal vessels; 4, kidneys; 5 a and b, ureters and ureteral vessels; 6, ovarian arteriovenous complex; 7, ovarian bursa containing ovaries; 8, uterine tube (fallopian tube); 9, suspensory ligament of ovary and broad ligament of uterus; 10, broad ligament (medial aspect), ligament of uterine body; 11, uterine arteriovenous complex branches or tributaries of the vaginal vessels; 12, uterine cornua (a) and body (b); 13, caudal mesenteric artery; 14, umbilical artery; 15, external iliac arteries; 16, internal iliac arteries; 17, middle caudal artery; 18, vaginal artery; 19, internal pudendal artery; 20, urinary bladder*; 21, urethra; 22, vaginal vein; 23, pudendal vein.*

teries originate from the aorta caudal to the renal arteries. The left ovarian vein drains into the left renal vein, and the right ovarian vein drains into the caudal vena cava.[4] The distal two-thirds of the ovarian AV complex are convoluted, similar to the pampiniform plexus of the testes. The ovarian arteries and veins separate during the proximal and distal third of their courses and are juxtaposed at this point to the right and left ureters. This relationship between the ureters and the ovarian AV complex accounts for the ease with which the ureters can be ligated at the kidney during ovariohysterectomy. It is also possible to ligate the ureters in the area of the bladder because of the close anatomic relationship of the neck of the bladder with the uterine body.

Just caudal to the left ovarian AV complex, a large artery and vein course caudally through the left broad ligament. This large branch of the ovarian vessels can be easily overlooked when the ovarian AV complex is

---

*The urinary bladder venous drainage does not have the usual pattern of venous drainage of most organs. The veins of the urinary bladder drain into the caudal vena cava through the pelvic venous plexus.

ligated; such an oversight thus causes serious blood loss.

The uterine broad and round ligaments do not contain any distinctly large blood vessels, with the exception of the uterine AV complex parallel to the uterine horn that is the continuation of the vaginal vessels. If broad and round ligaments are cut or torn without ligation, hemorrhage issues from these lacerated ligaments in their respective lumbar gutters.

The vaginal arteries are terminal branches of the internal pudendal arteries. The vaginal artery divides at the uterine body; one branch runs parallel to the uterine body in the dorsolateral ligaments of the uterine body, and another branch penetrates the uterine body and sends several dorsal and ventral communicating loops around the uterine body (Fig. 25-2). The convoluted, looping vessels in the uterine body wall continue cranially in their respective dorsolateral uterine horn walls. These convoluted intramural vessels of the uterine body and uterine horns become straight as a result of any phenomenon that enlarges the uterus, such as pregnancy or pyometra (Fig. 25-3).

The AV complex that courses in the ligaments paral-

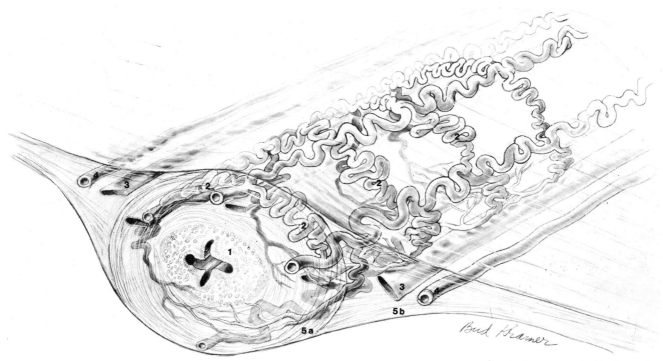

Fig. 25-2. *Schematic drawing of a transverse section of the anestrus uterine body of the female dog. 1, Endometrium; 2, blood vessels of contracted uterine body; 3, vaginal vein in lateral ligaments; 4, vaginal artery of uterine body; 5, myometrium: layer adjacent to endometrium (a) and layer of muscle extending into lateral uterine body ligament (b).*

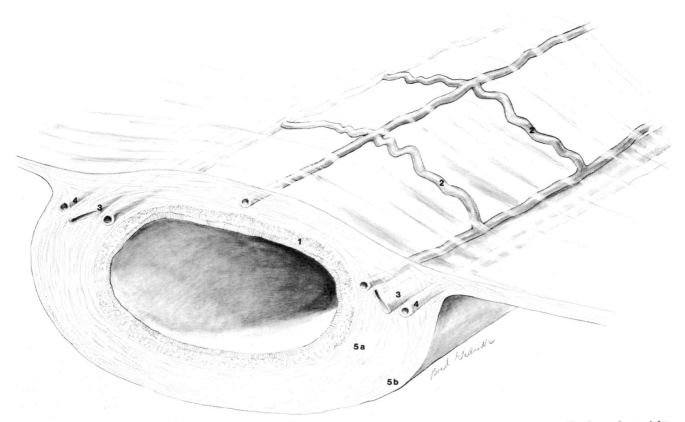

Fig. 25-3. *Schematic drawing of a transverse section of a gravid or disease-distended uterine body. The tortuous blood vessels straighten when the reproductive tract distends. 1, Endometrium; 2, Blood vessels of contracted uterine body; 3, vaginal vein in lateral ligaments; 4, vaginal artery of uterine body; 5, myometrium: layer adjacent to endometrium (a) and layer of muscle extending into lateral uterine body ligament (b).*

lel to the uterine body continues cranially in the broad ligament parallel to the uterine horn toward the ovary. From the uterine body to the proximal uterine horn, six to eight AV branches lead to the uterine body (see Fig. 25-1). Contrary to previous reports, limited anastomoses exist between the uterine and ovarian blood vessels in the female dog.[3] The venous drainage of the uterine body is through the pelvic plexus to the caudal vena cava. Increased intra-abdominal pressure may shunt venous blood from the pelvic plexus into the vertebral sinuses and may bypass the caudal vena cava.

Surgical Technique

The left ovary and the left uterine horn are most easily isolated; these structures are removed first, regardless of the reason for ovariohysterectomy. Constant digital contact must be maintained with the ovary so that the ovary is surgically removed. Intraoperative problems may occur, especially in dogs and cats with reproductive tract disease. The previously described three-forceps technique[5] has been modified to eliminate the complications resulting from mass ligation of the torn suspensory ligament and ovarian AV complex.

An avascular site is perforated in the broad ligament between the suspensory ligament and the cranial edge of the ovarian AV complex. The isolated suspensory ligament is cross-clamped, cut, and ligated. The ligated suspensory ligament and its blood vessels are returned to the abdominal cavity lateral to the kidney. This maneuver frees the left ovarian AV complex to a greater degree than does tearing the ovarian suspensory ligament. The ovarian AV complex can be specifically and safely ligated. This technique accomplishes two things: first, it eliminates the mass ligation of the suspensory ligament and the ovarian complex; and second and most important, it reduces the possibility of "dropping" the ovarian AV complex.

The broad ligament is first stretched over the fingers to identify the ovarian AV complex and then is perforated with forceps at an avascular site caudal to the ovarian AV complex. Two forceps are placed proximal to the ovary on the ovarian AV complex; a third forcep is placed between the ovary and the uterine horn. The ovarian AV complex is incised between the two proximal clamps and the ovary; the excised ovary and the uterine body are reflected caudally. The ovarian AV complex is ligated proximal to the proximal most clamp. This clamp is loosened after the first throw of the ligature, so that the blood vessels distorted by the hemostatic clamp may return to a normal configuration. This step of releasing the hemostatic clamp is essential for the ligature to hold in the ligamentous tissues. If the clamp is not loosened or released, the ligation will be loose and very likely will fall off the blood vessels; hemorrhage results. If the tissues of the ovarian AV complex are correctly handled, a square-knot ligation will suffice.

The broad and round ligaments are cross-clamped and ligated, rather than being torn or incised. This ligation may appear to be superfluous, but if the lumbar gutter is examined after tearing the round and broad uterine ligaments, hemorrhage will be observed.

The left uterine horn is followed to the uterine body to identify the right side of the reproductive tract. The right uterine horn is followed cranially to identify the right ovary and the suspensory ligament. The surgical techniques previously described are repeated for removal of the right ovary and uterine horn.

The next step is evaluation of the ligatures placed on the suspensory ligament, the broad ligament, and the ovarian AV complex. The ligated suspensory ligament pedicles are found lateral to their respective kidneys, the ligated ovarian AV complex is at the caudal pole of its respective kidney, and the ligated broad and round ligaments are at the inguinal canal and the pelvic inlet.

Hemostatic clamps are not used on the uterine body because the uterine body is distorted, is sometimes cut, and is not crushed by these clamps. The myometrium is resilient or elastic, and the uterine body arteries are thick-walled and elastic. The myometrium distorts, the elastic arteries retract out of the hemostatic clamps, and severe hemorrhage results. This hemorrhage may not be apparent during the operation because of the distortion of the uterine body tissues. Significant hemorrhage begins when the uterine body is returned to its normal location between the ventral colon and the dorsal urinary bladder. Therefore, we prefer a technique using suture ligature of the uterine body and its blood vessels.

In young female dogs or cats, a suture ligature is placed through the uterine body and around the uterine blood vessels. In older female dogs or cats or in animals with diseased reproductive tracts, the blood vessels in the ligament of the uterine body and in the uterine body are ligated individually. First, the blood vessels in the ligaments (see Fig. 25-2) parallel to the uterine body are ligated and the suture tags are cut long. These uterine body vessels are clamped proximal to the ligatures and then are incised, leaving only the uterine body to ligate. A suture ligature is placed through and around the uterine body, and the suture tags are again left long. The uterine body is incised proximal to the body ligature. The uterine body stump and the ligated vessels are returned to their normal location with the long suture tags; if hemorrhage is seen, the stump is retrieved, and hemostasis is performed. If no hemorrhage occurs when the uterine body remains in its normal location, the individual suture tags are cut.

In pyometra, the ligation technique is performed as described, with the following modification: two suture ligatures are placed in the uterine body, and the uterus is removed by incising between these two ligatures. Cross-clamping the uterine body can rupture the pus-filled uterus of a female dog or cat and may thereby fill the peritoneal cavity with pus and other uterine contents. In animals with pyometra, it is recommended that the uterine body stumps be inverted into the vaginal canal. If the uterine body is ligated during ovariohysterectomy, inverting the uterine stump into the vagina is not possible. Most important, if the uterine stump and its blood vessels are inverted into the vagina and the intramural blood vessels of the uterus are not ligated, severe hemorrhage results.

Complications

1. Hemorrhage from many unligated blood vessels into the abdominal cavity is a common complication, especially hemorrhage of the blood vessels of the uterine body and its ligaments.

2. Hollow viscus such as bladder and small bowel may be trapped between commonly ligated uterine horns.

3. Ureters can be clamped, crushed, and ligated, usually following the loss of the unligated ovarian AV complex and the indiscriminate clamping of hemorrhaging reproductive tract tissues in the lumbar gutter area.

4. Excessive inflammation of the uterine body ("stump granuloma") following surgical manipulation can cause adhesions to the bladder, colon, or both. If the ovaries are removed, endometrial hyperplasia will not occur, and this complication is usually the result of excessive trauma.

5. Fistulas in the flank, ventral abdominal wall, or medial thigh can result from contaminated suture material used to ligate the reproductive tract and its vessels.

6. If an angiotribe is used to perform an ovariohysterectomy, this instrument can cut tissues, rather than crush them, the lacerated blood vessels fall into the abdomen, and hemorrhage occurs.

7. It is possible to incise an engorged spleen or a full urinary bladder while opening the abdominal cavity in female dogs and cats. The spleen normally enlarges following barbiturate anesthesia and is found in the cranial abdomen at the umbilicus.

8. Ovaries can be left behind in the ovarian bursa at the completion of an ovariohysterectomy. Before abdominal closure, the tissues excised during ovariohysterectomy should be carefully examined to ensure that the ovaries have been removed.

9. When ovariohysterectomy is performed late in pregnancy, parts of fetuses can be left in the vaginal canal, especially if hemostatic clamps are used to clamp the uterine body.

10. Surgical sponges can be left in the abdominal cavity. The severe consequences of this problem are avoided by performing a sponge count both at the beginning of the procedure and before abdominal closure.

References and Selected Readings

1. Abrams, H. L., and Cornell, S. H.: Patterns of collateral flow in renal ischemia. Radiology, 84:1001, 1965.
2. Christie, B. A.: Collateral arterial blood supply to the normal and ischemic kidney: Am. J. Vet. Res., 41:1519, 1980.
3. Del Campo, C. H., and Ginther, O. J.: Arteries and veins of uterus and ovaries in dogs and cats. Am. J. Vet. Res., 35:409, 1974.
4. Evans, H. E., and Christensen, G. C.: Miller's Anatomy of the Dog. 2nd ed. Philadelphia, W. B. Saunders, 1979.
5. Archibald, J. (ed.): Canine Surgery. 2nd Ed. Santa Barbara, CA, American Veterinary Publications, 1974.

Diagnosis and Management of Dystocia in the Bitch and Queen

by Victor M. Shille

The time of parturition is one of the most critical stages in the life of an animal. Iatrogenic mismanagement of parturition can result in death or injury to the fetus and dam and can reduce the future fertility of the dam. This period is of great concern to the breeder who has a considerable economic investment in the animals, as well as to the pet owner whose anxiety is based on emotional grounds.

Etiology

Dystocia has classically been regarded as being either maternal or fetal in origin. More realistically, however, dystocia should be considered in relation to a failure of the three components of the process of parturition: the expulsive forces, the birth canal, and the fetus. Difficult birth occurs when the expulsive forces are insufficient, when the birth canal is constricted, or when the presenting diameter of the fetus is too large for the birth canal. A diagrammatic representation of the interrelationships of these three components may be seen in Figure 25-4.

The immediate causes of difficult birth as outlined in Figure 25-4 are easily recognized and permit the application of appropriate, timely treatment. The veterinarian should recognize the fundamental causes of dystocia, however, in order to prevent its occurrence. These causes may be loosely grouped into genetic factors, endogenous chemical factors, and environmental influences.

When a certain type of dystocia has a high incidence in a particular breed, it is probably due to genetic factors. For example, primary uterine inertia frequently occurs in Scottish and Aberdeen terriers and miniature dachshunds, whereas the corgi shows variations in the size of the fetus that predispose the breed to dystocia from absolute or relative fetal oversize.[2] Brachycephalic breeds and Sealyham and Scottish terriers are prone to obstructive dystocias because the fetuses have comparatively large heads and the dams have shallow (flattened) pelvises. Fetal oversize is common in breeds that have small litters, which cause obstructive dystocias; liberal uterine nutrition of the individual fetus allows it to grow to a disproportionate size and thereby to cause difficult delivery.

Litter size may be important in endocrine triggering of the onset of parturition. The gestation period is often increased in bitches with a single fetus and is decreased in those carrying many fetuses. Irregularities

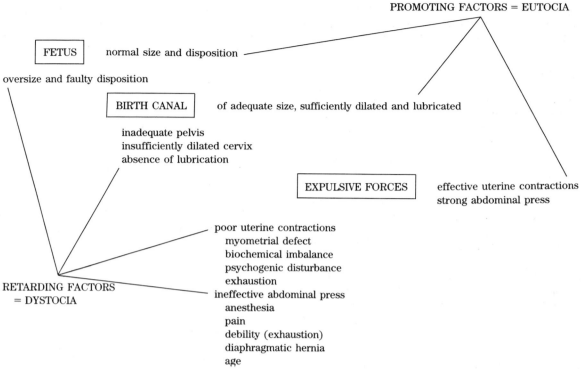

Fig. 25-4. *Diagrammatic representation of the factors operative during parturition.*

in the biochemical environment of the uterus, such as the failure of the appropriate reversal of the estrogen-progesterone ratio or the lack of adequate levels of calcium, can cause myometrial insufficiency and primary incrtia. Studies in the cow have suggested that limb posture of the calf at parturition can be affected by prepartum hormone imbalance.[6] This hypothesis has not been investigated in the bitch.

The entry of the fetus into the cranial vagina initiates a neuroendocrine reflex (Ferguson reflex) that releases oxytocin and triggers the onset of the propulsive stage of labor. Postponement of the first stage of labor by a bitch or queen that is disturbed by an inappropriate or strange environment appears to affect the early onset of the propulsive stage and may result in primary uterine inertia.

Secondary uterine inertia is essentially due to exhaustion and is in this sense more a result than a cause of dystocia. It is frequently followed by retention of fetal membranes and retarded involution of the uterus. These factors predispose the dam to puerperal metritis. Generally speaking, secondary inertia is a preventable condition, depending on early recognition of nonproductive labor. In some individuals, secondary inertia may intervene before any great expenditure of effort is clinically recognized.

In the cat, the overall incidence of dystocia is lower than in the special canine breeds mentioned earlier, but certain cat breeds such as the Persian and some particular family lines in all breeds have been observed to have frequent dystocias. Other common causes of dystocia in the cat are pelvic deformities from trauma or secondary hyperparathyroidism and sacroiliac ankylosis and pelvic exostoses from vitamin A overdose. Queening complications arising from uterine inertia are not rare and can be anticipated in the primigravid cat over 5 years old and in the multiparous queen over 8 years of age.[7]

Normal Parturition (Eutocia)

A thorough knowledge of the normal sequence of events in parturition is essential for the recognition of the abnormal when it occurs. The first stage of parturition is characterized by the onset of regular, peristaltic, myometrial contractions and cervical relaxation. The duration of this stage varies from 6 to 12 hours, but may be as long as 36 hours. The externally visible signs include anorexia, restlessness, and preparation of the nest by the dam. Physical examination shows relaxation of the pelvic and perineal musculature and swelling and softening of the vulva. Clear mucus is visible in the vagina and the vestibule. Rectal temperature declines to less than 37° C (99° F).

Entry of the head of the fetus into the pelvic cavity causes distension of the birth canal and elicits reflex contractions of the abdominal musculature. The chorioallantoic sac ("water bag") ruptures as a consequence of the straining, and a gush of fluid escapes from the vagina. The rupture of the chorioallantois is easily recognized by the layman and can be used to time the onset of the second or propulsive stage of labor in the bitch and queen. The time interval from the rupture of the chorioallantois to the delivery of the first fetus varies from 20 to 60 minutes, but it should not be allowed to exceed 1.5 to 2 hours without examination to determine the cause of the delay.

The period between successive deliveries allows for expulsion of fetal membranes and resting of the dam, but involution of the uterus does not begin in polytocous species until after the delivery of the last fetus. The bitch or queen may take as long as 6 hours to deliver successive fetuses, and uncomplicated delivery of a litter has, on rare occasion, taken as long as 24 hours.

The three-dimensional relation of the fetus to the birth canal is described by presentation, position, and posture. Presentation describes the orientation of the long axis of the fetus to the vagina; it may be longitudinal or transverse. Depending on the portion of the fetal body presented to the veterinarian, presentation may also be defined as cranial or caudal and dorsal or ventral. The relation of the fetal vertebral column to the dam's pelvis is indicated by its position; it may be dorsosacral, dorsopubic, or left or right dorsoilial. Posture refers to the disposition of the fetal limbs and head and involves flexion and retention at the various joints. Because fetal limbs are short and flexible, postural abnormalities that result in dystocia are infrequent in the bitch and queen.

Role of The Client

The initial management of parturition in the bitch and queen is affected by the degree of communication between the veterinarian and the owner. If the owner is a complete novice, the practitioner should have prepared the way by a preparturient examination and a discussion of the practical aspects of parturition and care of the neonate. An overanxious owner should be urged to avoid disturbing the bitch or queen because extensive intrusion may cause a voluntary delay of the second stage of labor by the dam that could result in primary uterine inertia.

In the case of the experienced breeder, the relationship between practitioner and client may become more delicate, because breeders vary in their ability to observe the progress of labor and to judge when assistance is needed. In many cases, it is to the practitioner's advantage to instruct the breeder carefully in the basics of good hygiene and obstetric manipulation, rather than to forbid all interference and to run the risk of covert manipulations with dirty fingers or instruments. The use of ecbolic agents by the breeder before a correct diagnosis is established is to be strongly discouraged.

The owner should advise the veterinarian of the expected delivery date, so that appropriate arrangements for emergency help may be made in advance. The client may be asked to telephone during the onset of the first stage of labor (panting, restlessness, digging of the nest), and again when the chorioallantois ruptures and straining first becomes visible (onset of second stage of labor). The call for actual help should come if the bitch or queen fails to produce a neonate within an hour after the rupture of the chorioallantois.

Data Base

It is important to establish as accurately as possible the parity of the bitch and queen, the course of prior deliveries, and the breeding date(s), as well as the duration of the first and second stages of labor in the present delivery. The time of rupture of the chorioallantois (onset of second stage of labor) is useful in deciding whether the patient may be allowed to continue labor at home undisturbed or whether the patient should be examined in the veterinarian's office.

To assess the status of the patient at presentation, the initial work-up should include determination of the hematocrit, total protein, and blood urea nitrogen. Abdominal palpation yields information about the approximate number of fetuses, the amount of fetal fluids, and possibly fetal movements (viability). A vaginal examination should only be made after scrubbing the patient's perineum and vulva and the veterinarian's hands. A sterile glove should be put on the hand, and the index and middle fingers used for intravaginal manipulation should be well lubricated. The opposite hand provides abdominal counterpressure and manipulation (Fig. 25-5).

Visual examination of the vagina may be made with a sterile, lubricated vaginoscope with a minimal length of 25 cm. Such an examination provides further information about the condition of the birth canal, particularly the presence and degree of injury caused by any prior assistance. The degree of dilation and relaxation of the vagina and cervix should be assessed. The cervix may be too far cranial to examine in larger breeds. The condition of the birth canal allows a rough estimate of the time spent in unproductive labor. A dry, sticky fetus surrounded by a dry vaginal wall indicates that the chorioallantoic sac ruptured some time ago. The force of the labor contractions may be appraised by pressing upwards against the roof of the vagina ("feathering"). This maneuver elicits the abdominal press and uterine contractions, in response to the neuroendocrine reflex mediated by the pelvic nerves. If the examining finger contacts membranes filled with fluid only, and if this finding correlates with the information supplied by the owner, it may be assumed that rupture of the chorioallantois has not occurred and second stage of labor either has not begun or has begun only a short time ago. When membranes that contain the fetus are palpated, it is impossible to distinguish between the chorioallantois and the amnion, and the timing of the rupture of the chorioallantois must be estimated from subjective information.

Diagnosis of disposition, size, and viability of the fetus may be made by identifying anatomic landmarks and responses of the fetus and by estimating the degree of fetal advancement through the birth canal. In the normal cranial presentation, the blunt nose of the fetus is contacted. The membranes are ruptured, so that a finger may be inserted into the mouth of the fetus to identify its position by landmarks such as the ridges on the hard palate, the soft tongue, and the hard edges of the mandibles. The presence of the forelimbs should be

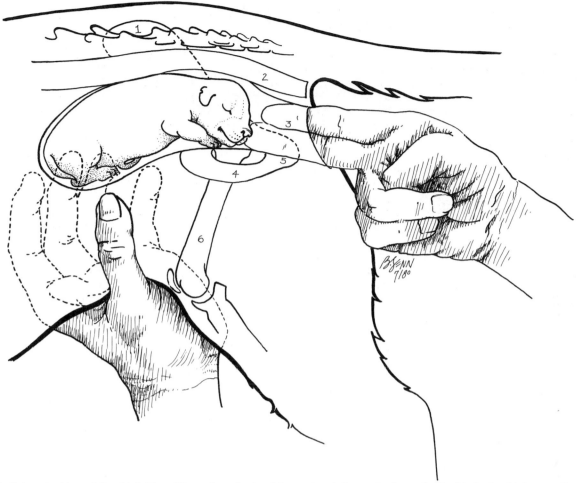

Fig. 25-5. *Determination of the fetal disposition when the head has entered the vaginal canal. The bitch should be standing for this procedure. 1, Right wing of ilium; 2, rectum; 3, lumen of vaginal vestibule; 4, right half of pubic symphysis; 5, right wing of ischium; and 6, right femur.*

ascertained, because their retention may cause relative oversize of the fetus at the shoulders and the inability to deliver vaginally. In the vertex posture, the forelimbs are retained at the shoulder, and only the crown of the head is presented; this posture may be identified by palpation of the crown, the nape of the neck, and the ears.

The presence of a single forelimb in the vagina indicates that lateral neck flexion has occurred and results in the presentation of the foreleg on the side away from which the head is turned. To verify the diagnosis, and to determine to which side the head is deviated, the fetus must be repelled with obstetric forceps,* usually in stages, and the finger is directed laterally toward each iliac shaft in turn, to detect the occiput and ears. This procedure is usually impossible in bitches of larger breeds, and a cesarean section is indicated.

Caudal presentation unaccompanied by dystocia occurs with such frequency in the dog and cat that it is considered normal. One or both hind feet may be retained, leaving the tail as the only recognizable structure to be palpated in the birth canal. Retention of the

hindlimbs in caudal presentation is not normal and frequently results in dystocia. A caudal presentation with retention of both hind feet is commonly known as a "true breech."

The viability of the fetus in cranial presentation may be assessed by sucking movements when the examiner places his fingertip in the fetus's mouth, although a fetus weakened by prolonged compression against the pelvic brim may not respond to this stimulus and may yet be alive. In caudal presentation, the tail and hindlimbs seldom respond to pinching and pulling, and the viability of the fetus is difficult to determine.

Fetal size may be estimated by observing whether progress through the birth canal can be achieved after judicious and gentle use of traction. If delivery with the aid of instruments and with minimal application of force is unsuccessful within 25 to 30 minutes, a cesarean section is recommended.

Biplane, abdominal radiographic studies of the bitch may be useful to demonstrate the position, the size, and the number of fetuses to be delivered and the disposition of the fetus presented in the birth canal. Fetal death may be indicated by inequality in skeletal mineralization, intrafetal or intrauterine gas accumulations,

*American V. Mueller, 6600 West Touhy Avenue, Chicago IL 60648

or obvious crenation. It is important to distinguish between fetuses in the uterus and those in the stomach from the animal's eating her own newborn.

Treatment of Dystocia

Diagnosis of the immediate cause of dystocia determines, to a large extent, the mode of treatment to be used. Findings compatible with primary or secondary uterine inertia suggest the use of ecbolic agents if the birth canal is dilated. Diagnosis of obstructive dystocia precludes the use of oxytocic drugs until the obstruction is relieved. The drug commonly used to promote uterine contractions at parturition is the extract of the posterior pituitary or synthetic oxytocin injected intramuscularly at 5 to 20 U.S.P. units in the bitch or 2.5 to 10 U.S.P. units in the queen. These drugs have a short duration of action and may be repeated to stimulate delivery of subsequent fetuses, if necessary. If the initial injection fails to cause uterine contractions, the dose may be repeated in 40 to 60 minutes and may be preceded by an intravenous injection of calcium gluconate (1 to 2 ml of 10% solution). Lack of response to this treatment indicates the need for a cesarean section.

The use of oxytocin before the onset of the propulsive stage of labor with the first or any subsequent fetus may result in premature separation of the placentas and in death of fetuses from hypoxia in utero. Ergot drugs cause powerful, sustained contractions of the uterine musculature, are recommended to promote involution of the uterus post partum, and are useful in the aftercare of the patient with dystocia. Ergot drugs are generally not suitable for use in the immediate treatment of dystocia. Estrogen compounds have been previously recommended for use with ecbolic agents, to sensitize the uterus to the action of oxytocin and to relax the cervix. The evidence for efficacy of these drugs when used for this purpose is equivocal. In my opinion, they cannot be recommended. Supportive treatment with calcium gluconate and glucose is indicated in cases of primary uterine inertia due to hypocalcemia and hypoglycemia. Other supportive treatments are dictated by the status of the dam.

Sedation is usually contraindicated in vaginal delivery because it is not desirable to depress the fetuses and to retard the subsequent course of parturition. A patient that is either sensitive to pain or aggressive is best restrained manually, preferably not by the owner. In the bitch, a comfortable muzzle applied in a way that permits panting is sufficient. In the queen, the forepaws may have to be taped to prevent scratching. A cesarean section should be considered if the patient continues to be difficult to manage.

Manipulative vaginal delivery should be considered whenever examination of the dam suggests that delivery of the fetus can be accomplished within 20 to 30 minutes and subsequent parturition will proceed normally. This situation is exemplified by the dystocia of a few hours duration that is caused by relative oversize in cranial or caudal presentation or by an easily cor-

rectable vertex or full-breech presentation. An early cesarean section is indicated when dystocia is due to primary uterine inertia, when secondary inertia has supervened in protracted cases of over 24 hours' duration, when the fetus is grossly oversized, or when the removal of the obstructed fetus is not likely to alter the ultimate outcome of the dystocia.

Attempts to deliver a dead and putrifying fetus often result in its breaking apart, and piecemeal removal is a difficult and dangerous procedure, particularly because the uterus becomes fragile and is readily punctured under these conditions.

It has been recommended by Arthur[2] that, in some cases, the grossly contaminated fetus impacted in the pelvis should be removed vaginally with forceps prior to commencing the abdominal procedure. The rationale is to prevent contamination from the opened uterus. I feel that this procedure subjects the dam to additional manipulations that may jeopardize her capacity to withstand the necessary hysterotomy. Because of this consideration, removal of the presented fetus through the hysterotomy incision is usually preferable. It is imperative, however, to observe careful procedure during the operation and to isolate the exteriorized uterus by packing it off to prevent leakage of the septic contents into the abdominal wound.

The fetus in the vagina rarely lives beyond 6 to 8 hours after the onset of second stage labor because, by that time, the placenta has completely separated. The fetuses remaining in utero, however, may remain viable for as long as 36 and in some cases 48 hours. As a general rule, a simple cesarean section without hysterectomy may be safely performed within the first 12 to 24 hours after the onset of the propulsive stage of labor. In hysterotomies performed more than 24 hours after the onset of the propulsive stage of labor, one is likely to find dead fetuses and a septic uterus. In these cases, a combined hysterotomy and hysterectomy is recommended. Amputation of the uterine body is made in the vagina just caudal to the cervix to reduce abdominal contamination.

OBSTETRIC TECHNIQUES

Before delivery is attempted with the aid of instruments, digital manipulation should be attempted. The birth canal should be thoroughly lubricated with a sterile, water-soluble jelly. Lubricant may be injected with a syringe around and proximal to the fetus through a sterile disposable urethral catheter. Soaps and detergents are contraindicated.

In the cranial presentations, it may be possible to introduce the index and middle fingers along and behind the sides of the mandible of the fetus and to apply traction and guidance to the head (Fig. 25-6). In the vertex posture, the index finger must be first inserted beneath the fetal chin to direct the muzzle upward into the birth canal. The limbs may be left uncorrected in most cases because they fold along the trunk and present little trouble. Once the head posture is corrected, delivery can proceed as shown in Figure 25-6.

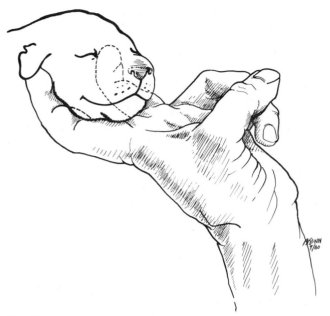

Fig. 25-6. *The index and middle fingers are used to guide the head and exert moderate traction in a cranial presentation.*

In the caudal presentations, the index, middle, and ring fingers may be used to grasp the hind legs proximal to the hocks (Fig. 25-7). If the legs are retained, as in breech presentation, it may be possible to hook the index finger around the retained limbs and to draw them upward and backward into the opening of the birth canal. Then they may be grasped, and traction may be applied to help delivery.

Once the fetus has reached the vestibule, traction is directed ventrally toward the hocks of the dam. The perineum may be lifted and pushed proximally to allow easier exit of the presenting part of the fetus through the vulva.

Instruments should never be used unless the disposition of the fetus is determined and the parts to be grasped can be reached with the finger to guide the instrument. Forceful, impatient, or blind use of instruments is likely to injure the fetus. Injury to the dam can be avoided by the liberal use of lubricants, gentle manipulation, and adherence to the rule that traction is never applied until the forceps grip has been checked to ensure that no maternal tissue is included. Specific manipulations in dystocias are as follows: In the cra-

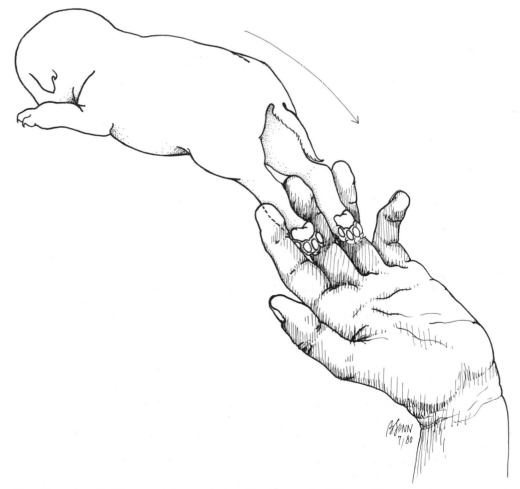

Fig. 25-7. *Manual traction as applied in a caudal presentation. The fingers should be positioned proximal to the hocks for best results.*

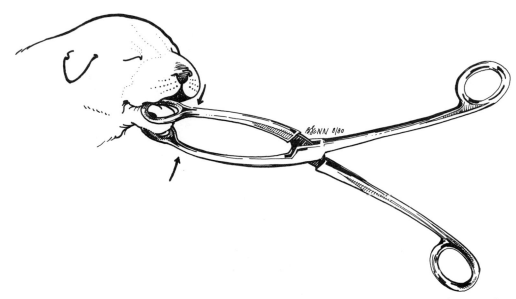

Fig. 25-8. *Hobday's obstetric forceps applied to the lower jaw to guide the head during delivery. Lifting the jaw must be avoided to prevent fracture.*

nial presentation, the veterinarian uses his index finger as a guide to apply forceps lightly to the upper jaw, the lower jaw, or the whole snout. Application to the lower jaw (Fig. 25-8) is easier in fetuses that are difficult to reach, but this grip carries the risk of cutting the tongue or fracturing the jaw if lifting traction is applied too vigorously. Advantage is taken of each straining effort of the dam, and rest is allowed after each contraction. Once the fetus is brought far enough for the fingers to reach behind the head, the instrument should be relinquished, and delivery should be continued by means of fingers, as discussed earlier (see Fig. 25-6).

Assistance for the initial alignment, but not traction, in small breeds of dogs or in the cat may be provided by the use of an ovariectomy hook[4] applied to the lower jaw inside the mouth while the index finger of the same hand is pressed against the hook from below (Fig. 25-9). This procedure should not be used to apply traction, but merely to guide the head during the propulsive efforts of the dam.

In the caudally presented fetus, one should apply the forceps to the lateral and medial aspects of the hock (Fig. 25-10). Two pairs of obstetric forceps, one on each hock, may be used with the ratchets closed on the first step. Traction should be straight at first, until the ribs are felt to engage the pelvic opening; then traction should be applied to one side until the rib cage enters the pelvic cavity. The direction of the pull is then changed to the opposite side. A similar maneuver is made to bring the shoulders into the birth canal. The entry of the fetal occiput into the pelvis causes the next point of resistance, which is alleviated by slight rotation to an oblique position. The forceps should be removed, and fingers should be used for traction and manipulation as soon as possible.

In the full-breech posture, it has been recommended to lift the fetus by the tail to deliver the retained limbs into the pelvic cavity. In my experience, this maneuver frequently results in amputation of the tail, and therefore a hysterotomy is recommended in these cases.

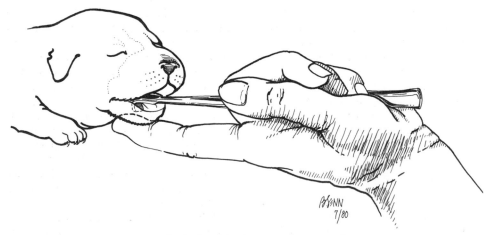

Fig. 25-9. *The Snook ovariectomy hook used to guide the head in the cranial presentation.*

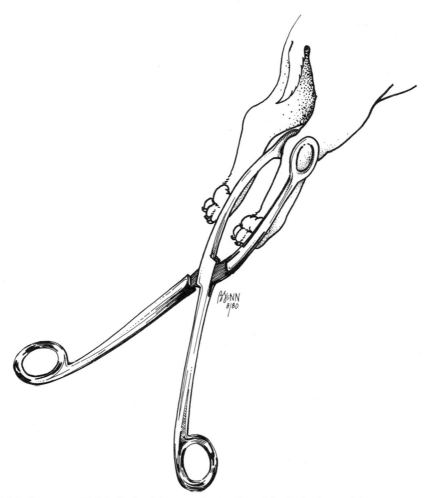

Fig. 25-10. *Hobday's obstetric forceps applied to the hock to prevent retention of the limbs in caudal presentation. Alternating traction on the left and right leg aids in expulsion of the fetus.*

Immediate Care of the Neonate

The newborn puppy or kitten requires considerable attention at birth, particularily when stressed by a prolonged delivery. It is essential that a patent airway be ensured immediately upon presentation, by removal of the amniotic membrane and by clearing of mucus from the mouth and nose; the latter may be accomplished with a rubber bulb syringe. After delivery, neonatal respiration and cardiovascular function may be stimulated by brisk rubbing with a coarse towel. Hypothermia must be prevented by maintaining the ambient temperature at 30 to 33° C (86 to 92° F) while the neonates are not under the dam's care. Nursing should be encouraged immediately, to ensure adequate hydration and intake of colostrum. If nursing is not possible, dehydration must be prevented by administering a 5% glucose solution (0.25 ml/30 g body weight) orally.

Aftercare of the Dam

The postparturient phase is important in restoring the reproductive organs to their prepregnant condition. The puerperal uterus contains a fluid mixture of fetal fluids, blood, mucus, and tissue detritus collectively known as lochia. The lochia is expelled, and the uterine horns regress gradually to their prepregnancy size during the first 4 weeks following parturition in the bitch.[2] Histologic evidence of completed healing of placental attachment sites was found in several healthy beagle bitches to take as long as 150 days after breeding, or 90 days after parturition.[1] The immediate postpartum discharge is dark green in the bitch and queen, but it changes within 12 hours to a blood-tinged (reddish brown) mucoid fluid that may continue to be discharged until the placental attachment sites are healed.

When parturition is thought to be completed, the general status of the dam should be assessed, and the mammary glands should be checked for an adequate supply of milk and the functional patency of the nipples. The dam should be thoroughly examined for the presence of any remaining fetuses, particularly large breeds of dogs in which the last 1 or 2 fetuses may be retained in the tips of the uterine horns. A radiograph should be taken if any doubt exists as to whether the uterus has been emptied.

Retention of fetal membranes is rare in the bitch and queen. In the bitch, it is usually limited to retention of 1 or 2 placentas in the tips of the uterine horns after a long delivery in toy breeds. If the dark green discharge is seen to persist for longer than 12 hours post partum, retention of membranes should be suspected.[2] If the placentas are not expelled spontaneously or after treatment, fatal necrotic perforation of the uterine wall at the placental attachment sites may result. To ensure delivery of placentas, to empty the uterus of lochia, and to aid in the healing of placental attachment sites, it is recommended to administer an appropriate dose of oxytocin routinely 24 to 48 hours after completion of delivery. The routine postpartum use of antibiotics is contraindicated and may cause gastrointestinal disturbances in the neonate from ingestion of the compound secreted in the dam's milk. On the other hand, if delivery was prolonged for more than 24 hours, or if manipulative ingression caused trauma and introduced contamination, broad-spectrum antibiotic therapy may be necessary. The use of compounds containing chloramphenicol, ampicillin, gentamicin, and kanamycin has been recommended. The neonates must be prevented from nursing during the period of treatment. In these cases, it may be desirable to hasten the involution of an unhealthy uterus by administering ergot derivatives. In the bitch, ergotamine maleate may be given by mouth for a period of 3 to 5 days post partum (0.2 mg tablet every 8 or 12 hours).

Acknowledgment

I gratefully acknowledge the talented efforts of Beth Senn, who prepared the illustrations.

References and Suggested Readings

1. Anderson, A. C., and Simpson, M. E.: The Ovary and Reproductive Cycle of the Dog (Beagle). Los Altos, CA, Geron-X, 1973.
2. Arthur, G. H.: Veterinary Reproduction and Obstetrics. 5th Ed. London, Bailliere, Tindall, 1982.
3. Bennett, D.: Normal and abnormal parturition. In Current Therapy in Theriogenology. Edited by D. A. Morrow. Philadelphia, W. B. Saunders, 1980.
4. Collins, D. R.: A simple obstetrical technique for assisting with fetal delivery. Vet. Med./Small Anim. Clin., 61:455, 1966.
5. Freak, M. J.: Abnormal conditions associated with pregnancy and parturition in the bitch. Vet. Rec., 74:1323, 1962.
6. Jöchle, W., Esparza, T., Gimenez, T., and Hidalgo, M. A.: Inhibition of corticoid-induced parturition by progesterone in cattle: effect on delivery and calf viability, J. Reprod. Fertil., 28:407, 1972.
7. Stein, B. S.: The genital system. In Feline Medicine and Surgery. 2nd Ed. Edited by E. J. Catcott. Santa Barbara, CA, American Veterinary Publications, 1975.

Cesarean Section in the Dog and Cat: Anesthetic and Surgical Techniques

by CURTIS W. PROBST *and* A. I. Webb

Cesarean section is normally an emergency procedure because the delay in resolution of dystocia risks the life of the mother or neonate. When dystocia can be predicted owing to preexisting injuries or abnormalities that compromise the birth canal, the surgical procedure can be planned and performed before the onset of active parturition. The diagnosis and nonoperative management of dystocia, as well as indications for cesarean section, are discussed in the previous section of this chapter.

Surgical Anatomy

The gravid uterus lies on the abdominal floor during the last half of pregnancy. Unlike the divergent uterine horns in the nonpregnant state, the heavily gravid horns are parallel and in contact with each other. As the horns enlarge, they also flex and bend the uterus cranially and ventrally upon itself. It is important to appreciate that when making the abdominal incision during a cesarean section, the uterus is close to the thin, distended abdominal wall.

The uterus is composed of three layers: tunica serosa, or perimetrium, tunica muscularis, or myometrium and tunica mucosa or endometrium. The tunica serosa is a layer of peritoneum that covers the entire uterus and is continuous with the mesometrium (broad ligaments). The muscular layer consists of a thin longitudinal outer muscle layer and a thick inner layer. The deeper myometrium contains blood vessels, nerves, and circular and oblique muscle fibers. The tunica muscularis is also the layer of greatest tensile strength. The tunica mucosa is the thickest of the three layers.

The uterus is well supplied with arterial blood. The reader is referred to the earlier section of this chapter on ovariohysterectomy for a discussion of the blood supply to the female reproductive tract. During gestation, the uterine vessels enlarge greatly and potentially complicate an ovariohysterectomy performed in conjunction with a cesarean section. Lymphatic drainage of the uterus is through the internal iliac and lumbar lymph nodes. Autonomic nervous innervation is through the hypogastric and pelvic plexuses.

Preoperative Preparations

Animals considered for cesarean section are often in poor physiologic condition at the time of presentation and should be carefully examined. Clinical tests are often limited to measurement of the patient's hematocrit, total plasma protein, blood urea nitrogen, and urine specific gravity. These tests assist in evaluating the need for corrective fluid therapy or cross-matching of potential blood donors. Before any anesthesia is given, an intravenous fluid drip should be established. The fluid of choice is a balanced electrolyte solution such as lactated Ringer's solution. If the patient has not eaten, a solution of 2.5% dextrose and half-strength lactated Ringer's may be more appropriate if hypoglycemia is likely. A base-line administration rate of 10 ml/kg/hour may be increased as indicated by individual clinical needs. All volume deficits should, if possible, be corrected prior to commencing the surgical procedure. If the fetuses are known to be dead and decomposing, or if uterine infection is established, intravenous antibiotic therapy (ampicillin sodium 20 mg/kg IV over 30 minutes) should be instituted at this time.

Before the operation, the veterinarian and the client should discuss the nature of the surgical procedure, its potential complications, and the issue of simultaneous ovariohysterectomy. We feel that the advisability of an additional surgical procedure should be carefully considered and that ovariohysterectomy may be better postponed until the litter is weaned.

Anesthetic Technique

The physiologic changes that take place in late pregnancy in the bitch and queen have not been documented; therefore, the following is based on studies of pregnant women.

Blood volume that increases by up to one-third at term is largely a plasma volume increase. Blood coagulability also increases because of reduced fibrinolytic activity. Cardiac output and pulse rates are increased 30 to 50%. Because the gravid uterus increases abdominal pressure on the diaphragm, pulmonary functional residual capacity (FRC) is reduced. At the same time, the tidal volume is increased. These changes mean that alveolar gas tensions may change more rapidly than normal and result in a more rapid uptake of inhalation anesthetic agents. The risks of hypoxia are also increased because there is less pulmonary reserve capacity.

Although the dog and cat have uterine mucosal vessel endothelium in addition to the chorion, mesenchyme, and endothelium of the fetal tissues (four structures) separating the maternal and fetal blood, all anesthetic drugs cross the placenta and may be detected in neonates after delivery. Because of differing placental morphologic features, however, drug transmission studies in man cannot be extrapolated to other species. For example, carnivores with their endotheliochorial placenta have an additional cell layer through which these drugs must diffuse. Additionally, the maternal endothelium of the pregnant bitch is strikingly hypertrophied.

Once a drug has crossed into the fetal bloodstream, its activity depends upon how much is in the "bound" versus the "available" form. The unbound un-ionized form of a drug crosses the placenta. Another factor affecting fetal depression is the sensitivity of the fetus to the drug. This latter aspect is not well known, except neonates appear more sensitive to barbiturates and nondepolarizing muscle relaxants than juvenile or adult animals.

A variety of anesthetic techniques are advocated for cesarean section in dogs and cats, but the two most popular techniques are regional analgesia (epidural) and general anesthesia. Each of these techniques has its own indications and disadvantages. A familiar and simple technique usually provides the most consistent results.

When the epidural method is used in humans, the neonate is born in superior condition, and the risk of maternal vomiting and aspiration is less. In dogs and cats, however, preoperative sedation is usually required to provide calming restraint for the lumbosacral injection and to prevent excessive struggling and movement once the patient is placed in dorsal recumbency. Neuroleptanalgesia combinations such as fentanyl and droperidol (1 ml/10 to 15 kg IV) or oxymorphone and acepromazine (0.1 to 0.2 mg/kg and 0.05 to 0.1 mg/kg IV) are useful in dogs. Ketamine, at 2 to 5 mg/kg IV, can be used in cats, but epidural anesthesia is not favored in this species because of the technical difficulties in administering the injection.

Analgesia is produced by the epidural injection of local anesthetic at the lumbosacral space with a spinal needle. A dose of 1 ml/4 kg body weight of 2% plain lidocaine provides analgesia to just above the umbilicus. This technique is usually easy and rapid; however, technical problems may arise in large or obese animals. Hypotension, a common complication of epidural anesthesia, may result from sympathetic blockade above the level of anesthesia. If hypotension occurs, fluid loading, or perhaps administration of vasoconstrictor agents such as phenylephrine or ephedrine (if response to fluid therapy is insufficient), is indicated. Oxygen should also be administered to assist adequate maternal and fetal oxygenation during the hypotensive period. When general anesthesia, also a popular anesthetic technique, is used for cesarean section, neonates may be delivered in a condition only slightly more depressed than when unsedated epidural methods are used. Regardless of the general anesthesia technique elected, the patient should be well oxygenated by mask or induction chamber preoperatively. Such treatment ensures optimal maternal and fetal oxygenation for induction and hastens denitrogenation prior to the use of nitrous oxide.

The general anesthetic technique we prefer is a balance of narcosis produced by ultrashort-acting barbiturates and nitrous oxide, with relaxation from muscle relaxants. Additional analgesia can be obtained by the use of narcotic analgesics in low doses, when necessary. Other methods include masking with inhalation agents and the administration of intravenous narcotics.

Premedication is usually omitted because it increases neonatal depression. An exception is when succinylcholine is to be administered to cats; atropine (0.3 mg) is given subcutaneously to prevent the bradycardia that occurs in that species.

An intravenous dose of 6 to 8 mg/kg thiamylal (2 to 4 mg/kg methohexital for greyhounds), followed by 0.3 mg/kg succinylcholine is suggested for induction of anesthesia. Thiobarbiturates such as thiamylal enter the fetal circulation rapidly and reach their peak concentrations in 2 to 3 minutes. This delay in equilibration means that the peak fetal concentration is only a fraction of that in the maternal blood, which occurred immediately after injection; the barbiturate's fetal depressive potential is thus limited. Controlled ventilation using a cuffed endotracheal tube is mandatory because succinylcholine provides 15 to 30 minutes of muscle

26 * Vagina and Vulva

Masses of the Vagina and Vulva

by GHERY D. PETTIT

In the bitch, physiologic enlargement of the vulvar labia during proestrus and estrus is a normal estrogenic response. It may be mimicked or exaggerated by masses within the vestibule of the vulva or the vagina that cause the labia to protrude. Such masses include hyperplasia of the vaginal floor, vaginal prolapse, and vestibular or vaginal tumors. These masses usually become apparent to an animal's owner when they visibly protrude through the vulva, although subtle perineal bulges may be detected. Rarely, dysuria is the presenting complaint.

Inspection and vaginal or rectal digital palpation provide adequate identification of most vaginal lesions. In at least one instance, an intraluminal vaginal tumor was diagnosed by pneumovaginography. Surgical treatment of these lesions is facilitated by episiotomy.

Hyperplasia of the Vaginal Floor

During proestrus and estrus, the vestibular and vaginal mucosae normally become swollen, thickened, and turgid. Exaggeration of this estrogenic response occasionally leads to the development of a transverse mucosal fold on the floor of the vagina just cranial to the external urethral orifice. If it becomes large enough, the redundant fold protrudes between the labia of the vulva as a red, fleshy mass (Fig. 26-1A). The condition is seen most often during a bitch's first estrus and seems to occur most often in brachycephalic breeds, such as boxers and English bulldogs. Spontaneous regression occurs during metestrus, but recurrence is common at the next estrus. The protrusion is vulnerable to trauma, ulceration, and inflammation. The mass mechanically interferes with mating and is esthetically objectionable. For these reasons, amputation is the treatment of choice.

Recurrence after surgical excision is rare, and natural mating is possible at subsequent estrous periods. Although it is not usually recommended, surgical excision of the mass and artificial insemination can be performed during the same estrus. With or without surgical excision, oophrectomy provides permanent relief of the condition.

SURGICAL TREATMENT

The patient is prepared and is positioned for episiotomy, which is performed as described in a later section of this chapter. Elevating the margins of the episiotomy incision exposes the vaginal lumen. The hyperplastic protrusion must be elevated for catheterization of the urethra, to identify and protect that structure (Fig. 26-1B and C). The mass is amputated by making connecting, curved, transverse incisions through its base. One incision is made on the dorsal surface of the mass (the cranial aspect of its base), and the other on its ventral surface cranial to the external urethral orifice (the caudal surface of the base of the mass). The incisions should be made no deeper than necessary to dissect the mass. Closure is accomplished with a simple continuous transverse suture of 2-0 chromic catgut (Fig. 26-1D). The catheter is removed, and the episiotomy incision is closed (Fig. 26-1E). If bleeding persists, a vaginal tampon may be left in place for 12 hours following the operation.

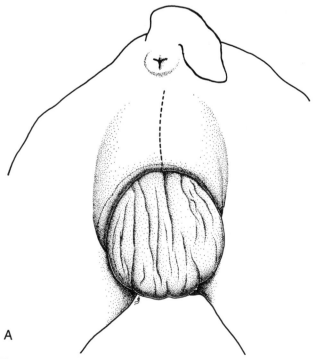

A

Fig. 26-1. *Legend is on opposite page.*

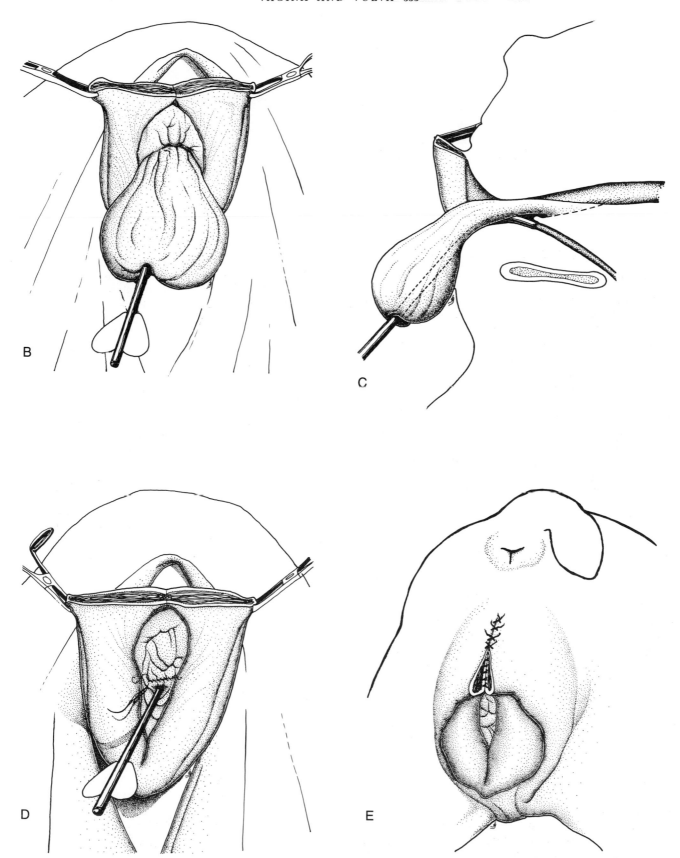

Fig. 26-1. *Hyperplasia of the vaginal floor. A, The broken line indicates the site of the episiotomy incision. B, The vestibule has been opened by performing an episiotomy and a urethral catheter has been inserted. C, Lateral view. Episiotomy and urethral catheterization have been performed. The broken line on the floor of the vagina indicates the incision site for amputation of the redundant mucosal mass. D, The mass has been amputated and the mucosal incision closed with a simple continuous suture. E, Postoperative view. The catheter has been removed and the episiotomy incision is being closed.*

Vaginal Prolapse

Much rarer than hyperplasia of the vaginal floor is a cylindrical prolapse of the vaginal wall. In this condition, which also occurs during estrus, a doughnut-shaped eversion of the entire vaginal circumference protrudes from the vulva (Fig. 26-2). Vaginal prolapse has been said to occur after forcible separation of the male and female before coitus is terminated. As in hyperplasia of the vaginal floor, the external urethral orifice is ventral to the entire mass, but access to the vaginal canal is through the center of the protrusion rather than dorsal to it.

Complete vaginal prolapse may also occur during parturition or advanced pregnancy, as a prelude to prolapse of the cervix, uterine body, and one or both uterine horns. It results from excessive straining while the supportive tissues are relaxed. The everted organs are usually discolored from venous congestion, are soiled, and are traumatized.

It may be possible to reduce a recent prolapse, but recurrence is likely. Recurrence, hemorrhage, infection, and necrosis make amputation necessary. Shock and dehydration are common complications that must be treated appropriately.

SURGICAL TREATMENT

With the patient under general anesthesia, the protruding structures are washed gently with warm saline solution or a mild detergent; additional trauma is avoided. The mass is compressed manually to reduce edema, and reduction is attempted. Sprinkling the mucosal surface with table sugar may further reduce the swelling, and episiotomy may make reduction of the mass easier. Once accomplished, reduction is maintained by placing heavy nonabsorbable sutures across the vulvar labia.

Reduction of vaginal prolapse may be assisted by traction on the uterus through a ventral abdominal incision. If this technique is used, protection against recurrence can be gained by hysteropexy, that is, suturing the uterine body or horns to the abdominal wall.

If reduction is impossible or inadvisable, the protruding tissue must be amputated. Paying careful attention to the distorted anatomic features minimizes errors. With a catheter in place to identify and protect the urethra, a circumferential incision is made in stages through the vaginal wall. The outer, everted mucosa is incised first, and the incision is deepened to penetrate all layers of prolapsed vaginal tissue until the inner, noneverted mucosa is reached. Hemostasis is maintained by ligation or by electrocautery, and the proximal mucosal margins are united with horizontal mattress sutures. The incision is extended for another short distance, the exposed segment is sutured, and the process is repeated until the amputation is complete.

Tumors of the Vulva and Vagina

Any tumor of skin and adnexal tissue may occur on the labia of the vulva, although this site is unusual. The most common tumors of the vulva and vagina include leiomyoma, fibroma, lipoma, and in some geographic areas, transmissible venereal tumor. Mast-cell tumors, sebaceous adenomas, and epidermoid carcinomas have been reported. Malignant tumors are rare.

Leiomyomas and fibromas are often grossly indistinguishable. They form smooth, firm, spherical masses that are often pedunculated and protrude into the vestibular or vaginal lumen. They may protrude from the vulva and may resemble an early hyperplasia of the vaginal floor. Lipomas occur as a gradually enlarging mass under the intact mucosa; they may protrude into the lumen or may become apparent under the perineal skin adjacent to the vulva. In the female, transmissible venereal tumors appear as single or multiple projecting masses with roughened or reddened, ulcerated surfaces.

SURGICAL TREATMENT

Episiotomy is performed for better exposure. Pedunculated intraluminal tumors can be amputated, but encapsulated extraluminal tumors are removed by submucosal resection (Fig. 26-3). An incision is made through the mucosa, and the tumor is bluntly peeled out. The mucosal incision is closed with absorbable sutures. Submucosal resection is especially useful for large or multiple tumors.

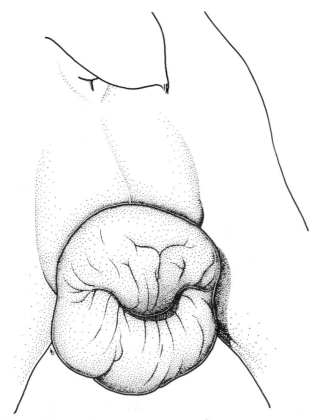

Fig. 26-2. *Vaginal prolapse. The entire circumference of the vaginal wall has everted.*

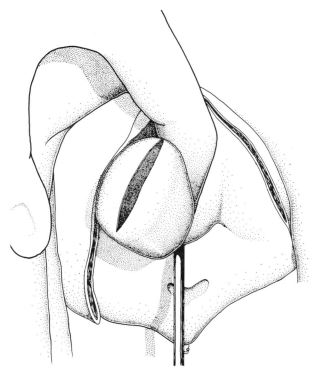

Fig. 26-3. *Vestibular leiomyoma. Episiotomy has been performed and a mucosal incision has been made to facilitate submucosal resection of the tumor.*

References and Suggested Readings

Adams, W. M., Biery, D. N., and Millar, H. C.: Pneumovaginography in the dog: a case report. J. Am. Vet. Radiol. Soc., *19*:80, 1978.

Alexander, J. E., and Lennox, W. J.: Vaginal prolapse in a bitch. Can. Vet. J., *2*:428, 1961.

Blakely, C. L.: Prolapse of the vagina. *In* Current Veterinary Therapy II. Edited by R. Kirk. Philadelphia, W. B. Saunders, 1966.

Brodey, R. S., and Roszel, J. F.: Neoplasms of the canine uterus, vagina, and vulva: a clinicopathologic survey of 90 cases. J. Am. Vet. Med. Assoc., *151*:1294, 1967.

Gilmore, C. E.: Tumors of the female reproductive tract. Calif. Vet., *19*:12, 1965.

Schutte, A. P.: Vaginal prolapse in the bitch. J. S. Afr. Vet. Med. Assoc., *38*:197, 1967.

Theilen, G. H., and Madewell, B. R.: Veterinary Cancer Medicine. Philadelphia, Lea & Febiger, 1979.

Episioplasty

by Jerry A. Greene

Episioplasty is defined as a reconstructive procedure used to correct a defect in the perineum or the vulva. In veterinary medicine, it usually refers to the specific technique used in the treatment of perivulvar pyoderma. Perivulvar pyoderma is usually seen in obese, older bitches with an immature vulva in which redundant skin folds develop both dorsally and laterally and give the vulva a recessed appearance. Surgical correction is aimed at removing the redundant skin folds that predispose the area to moisture, irritation, and infection.

The pyoderma is treated with cleansing and drying agents preoperatively to reduce inflammation. In severe infections, culture and sensitivity tests and antibiotic therapy should be commenced prior to the surgical procedure.

Surgical Technique

The surgical procedure may be performed either under general (preferred) or epidural anesthesia. The patient and operative site are prepared for the procedure in a routine manner. A pursestring suture is placed around the anus to prevent fecal contamination. The patient is positioned in ventral recumbency, with the rear quarters elevated to a comfortable operating height for the veterinary surgeon. Care is taken to prevent unnecessary pressure on the diaphragm caused by tilting the patient too far forward.

A sufficient amount of skin must be removed to prevent recurrence of the condition. By grasping the skin around the vulva, the amount of tissue requiring excision may be approximated (Fig. 26-4A). A sterile skin marker can be used to mark off the area to be removed.

With a scalpel, a crescent-shaped, bilaterally symmetrical piece of skin is outlined dorsal and lateral to the vulva. The first incision begins lateral to the ventral commissure of the vulva, proceeds dorsally to the juncture of the labia and the skin around the vulva, and continues to the opposite side (Fig. 26-4B). The second incision starts at the same point as the first, but extends in a wider arc outlining the skin to be removed. If necessary, the second incision may be made narrower initially and widened later. The underlying subcutaneous fat is removed with scissors (Fig. 26-4C). Hemorrhage is controlled with hemostats and ligature or pinpoint electrocoagulation. Sufficient subcutaneous fat must be removed to ensure that the vulva does not invert into a recess.

Skin closure is begun by placing simple interrupted skin sutures of monofilament nylon or stainless steel at the 9-, 12-, and 3-o'clock positions to ascertain whether sufficient tissue has been removed (Fig. 26-4D). If sufficient tissue has not been excised, these sutures are removed, and an additional excision is made. Once sufficient tissue has been excised, interrupted subcutaneous sutures of 3-0 or 4-0 absorbable material are placed to relieve skin tension. Closure of the skin incision is completed by placing additional monofilament nonabsorbable sutures alternately between the previous 3 sutures (Fig. 26-4E). The pursestring suture is removed at the conclusion of the operation.

Postoperative Care

An Elizabethan collar or a side brace is applied to prevent self-mutilation. Antibiotics are administered postoperatively if indicated.

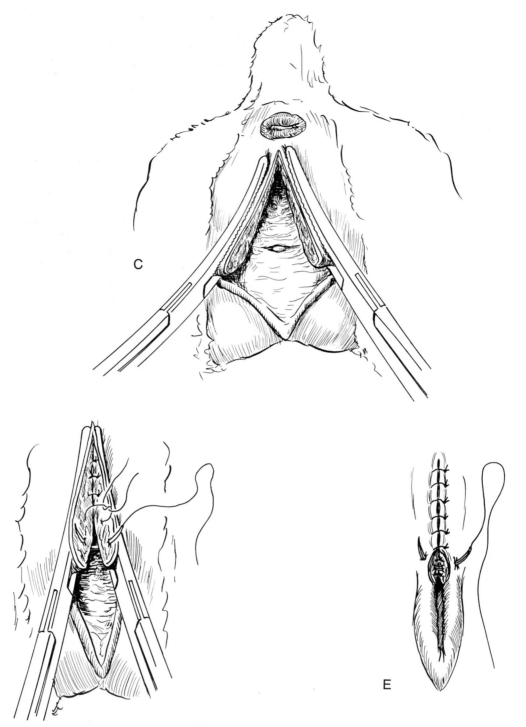

Fig. 26-5. *(cont.)* C, *Completed incision showing exposure of vagina.* D, *The mucosa is sutured with absorbable sutures.* E, *The skin is apposed with nonabsorbable sutures in a simple interrupted pattern. (A and C to E, From Annis, J. R., and Allen, A. R.: An Atlas of Canine Surgery. Philadelphia, Lea & Febiger, 1967.)*

necrosis may be induced. The episiotomy is completed with scissors.

The skin incision is made with a scalpel from the dorsal commissure of the lips of the vulva to a point opposite the dorsal wall of the horizontal vaginal canal (Fig. 26-5B). One blade of the scissors is placed in the vestibulovaginal cavity, and the other is placed externally, and the incision is completed. Hemorrhage is

controlled with hemostats and ligature or electrocoagulation.

Following completion of the procedure (Fig. 26-5C), the vaginal wall is reconstructed. The mucosa is apposed with simple interrupted 3-0 absorbable sutures (Fig. 26-5D). In heavily muscled or obese animals, it may be necessary to close the musculature separately with absorbable sutures. The skin is apposed with non-

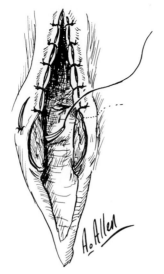

Fig. 26-6. *In episiostomy, the vulvar mucosa is sutured to the skin. (From Annis, J. R., and Allen, A. R.: An Atlas of Canine Surgery. Philadelphia, Lea & Febiger, 1967.)*

absorbable suture material in a simple interrupted pattern (Fig. 26-5*E*).

In episiostomy, the mucocutaneous tissue on each side (Fig. 26-6) is sutured, to enlarge the vestibulo-vaginal opening permanently. A simple interrupted suture pattern of either 3-0 or 4-0 nonabsorbable material is preferred.

Postoperative Care

Antibiotics are usually not administered postoperatively. An Elizabethan collar or a side brace may be indicated to prevent self-mutilation in the immediate postoperative period.

Pain or discomfort following the episiotomy is usually associated with poor technique in the repair of the incision, such as poor suture placement, excessive tension, and closure with a through-and-through suture pattern. Surgical correction may be indicated. Skin sutures are removed in 7 to 10 days postoperatively, once healing is ensured.

27 * Prostate Gland and Testes

Prostate

by THOMAS R. CHRISTIE

The canine prostate gland is a dynamic organ that functions at rest as well as during ejaculation. Its function is mediated by complex neurologic, hormonal, and anatomic influences. Disease processes in the prostate are common. An increase in disease is seen with age. For simplicity, the prostatic diseases have been classified into five categories (Table 27-1). In this discussion of surgical techniques that may be applied to the prostate gland, I refer to these disease classifications. It is wise to keep in mind, however, that more than one of these diseases may be present in the same gland concurrently. The following pathophysiologic sequence has been suggested:

prostatic hypertrophy → ductile blockage →
prostatic fluid stasis → prostatic cyst formation
+ infection → prostatitis → prostatic abscessation →
END-STAGE PROSTATE DISEASE

It is not within the scope of this text to discuss non-surgical prostatic disease treatment, except to say that the complex interaction of hormonal influences on the prostate can make hormonal therapy difficult,[11] and a "prostatic barrier" has been described that makes penetration of many antibiotics into the gland parenchyma difficult.[3,18,24-26] For these reasons and others, nonsurgical treatments of prostatic diseases are often unre-

Table 27-1. *Prostatic Diseases*

1. Prostatic hypertrophy
2. Prostatic cysts
   glandular
   paraprostatic
3. Prostatitis
   acute
   chronic
4. Prostatic abscess
5. Prostatic neoplasia

warding. Prostatic surgical techniques are discussed in order of increasing complexity. Surgical intervention in prostatic diseases can offer rapid resolution of clinical signs in selected cases if properly applied.

The influence of testicular secretions on the prostate is profound. When the androgen-estrogen balance is upset by testicular dysfunction, prostatic disease often results. Either excessive androgen or excessive estrogen can enlarge the prostate. Although the cell populations of two enlargements may differ, the end result is a predisposition to prostatic disease.[20,21]

Prostatic hypertrophy and cysts often resolve when castration alone is used as a treatment. Thus, *castration is an important adjunct to all prostatic surgical procedures.* Only in the valuable breeding male should castration not be advised as the first and most necessary step in the treatment of prostatic disease. Demonstrable involution of prostatic parenchyma is seen as soon as 2 weeks following surgical castration. The technique for castration is described in the following section of this chapter.

Surgical Techniques

KEYHOLE NEEDLE BIOPSY

Many prostatic biopsy techniques have been described.[9] The prostate gland is not visualized during most of these procedures, and major disadvantages exist with such "blind" procedures. The diseased portion of the prostate may not be included in a biopsy specimen, thus, the sample is not representative of the prostatic condition. Considerable expertise must be developed, especially with the perineal and transrectal techniques, to avoid iatrogenic injury to a nearby anatomic structure. Dissemination of disease, such as infection in the case of prostatic abscess, may also result from indiscriminate needle biopsy into an infected area.

For these reasons, actual visualization of the prostate gland by celiotomy prior to biopsy selection is the preferred method of obtaining a representative sample. At times, extenuating circumstances such as anesthetic risk, financial restrictions, or concurrent diseases make visual incisional biopsy impossible. Of the "blind techniques" available, the keyhole needle biopsy technique appears to be the most practical and is described here. The procedure can usually be performed with sedation (acepromazine, .3 mg/kg, intramuscularly), although certain patients may require general anesthesia.

An area of several square centimeters is surgically prepared in the lateral prepubic area of the ventral abdomen. Generally, the prostate becomes more and more abdominal as it enlarges. Selection of the site depends upon distribution of the palpable prostatic lesion. Asymmetry in one lobe or the other may alter the site of entry.

The skin and abdominal musculature are anesthetized with 2% lidocaine* at the proposed biopsy site. An assistant stabilizes the prostate gland by abdominal or rectal manipulation or a combination of both. The gland is held firmly against the abdominal wall. An incision about an inch in length is made through the skin directly over the immobilized prostate. The musculature is separated by blunt dissection to the caudal abdominal peritoneum, which is thin and is easily divided.

The veterinary surgeon's index finger is introduced into the abdomen to palpate the immobilized gland and to ensure that no unwanted tissue obstructs the needle's path to the gland (Fig. 27-1).

The direction of the biopsy needle should be determined with care to avoid penetration of the prostatic urethra, which passes centrally through the gland between the prostatic lobes. A Franklin-modified Vim-

Silverman biopsy needle* is an efficient instrument for this procedure[19] (Fig. 27-2). First, the needle, with the stylet and outer cannula, is advanced into the prostatic capsule (Fig. 27-3). The stylet is then removed, and the cutting prongs are inserted. These prongs are then advanced into the gland parenchyma beyond the tip of the outer cannula. The halves of the cutting prongs splay out to encompass a portion of the glandular tissue. The outer cannula is then advanced as a sheath over the cutting prongs and causes the filled tip of the cutting prongs to sever and to retain a piece of prostatic tissue. The components of the system are then withdrawn as a unit, and the biopsy specimen is harvested from the needle into a preservative solution. Digital pressure for 5 minutes on the biopsy needle hole results in adequate hemostasis.

The muscular fascia is closed with a continuous catgut suture, and the skin is closed using a simple interrupted pattern of nonabsorbable suture material.

MARSUPIALIZATION OF THE PROSTATE GLAND

Marsupialization of the prostate gland is the treatment of choice for large, fluid-filled prostatic cysts, paraprostatic cysts, and abscesses. A major criterion in electing to marsupialize such a lesion is that the fluid-filled structure must be large enough to make contact with the ventral abdominal wall at rest. Marsupialization then provides for ventral drainage until the causative factors are eliminated. Concurrent castration and appropriate antibiotic therapy, if needed, provide permanent resolution of the prostatic problem in a number of cases. The clinical signs caused by the

*Xylocaine, Astra Pharmaceutical Products, Inc., Worcester, MA

*Available from American V. Mueller, 6600 West Touhy Avenue, Chicago, IL 60648

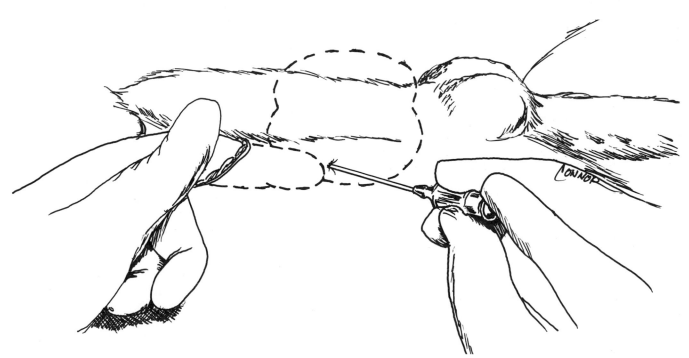

Fig. 27-1. *Index finger of the veterinary surgeon guides the biopsy needle into the prostate gland through a keyhole abdominal incision.*

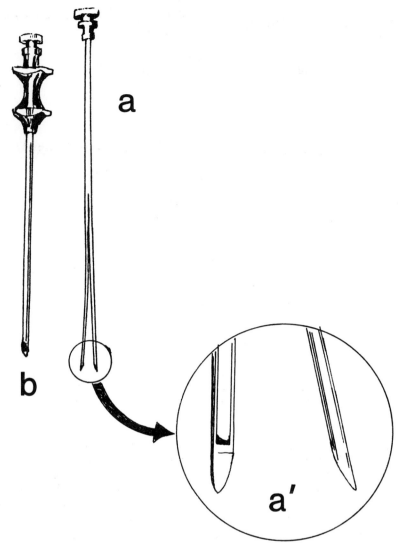

Fig. 27-2. A, *Franklin-modified Vim Silverman biopsy needle; inset, filled-in tip of the cutting prongs, which severs a piece of prostatic tissue when the outer needle sheath is advanced around it.* B, *Needle cannula with inner stylet.*

space-occupying nature of large, fluid-filled prostatic structures are immediately alleviated. A fistula is surgically created to allow for necessary drainage.

The dog is placed in dorsal recumbency, and a caudoventral abdominal midline incision is made. The skin incision extends from the umbilicus to a point 1 cm cranial to the prepuce. It then turns to course caudally, lateral to the prepuce, to the level of the inguinal nipple (Fig. 27-4A). The prepuce is reflected to one side, and the celiotomy incision is made through the linea alba to the prepubic tendon. The prostate is visualized to determine the extent of disease. One should choose an incision site in the cyst or abscess that is near the abdominal wall. This region is isolated from the rest of the abdomen using laparotomy pads moistened with saline solution. A stab incision is made into the cystic area, and all cystic fluid or pus is removed by suction. Cultures and fluid samples are obtained at this time. The cystic cavity is repeatedly flushed using Ringers solution and an appropriate antibiotic, if necessary.

A two- to three-inch incision is made in the skin directly over the planned site of drainage, but lateral to the prepuce. If possible, the marsupialization should be on the opposite side of the parapreputial incision used during the abdominal approach. Blunt dissection is continued through the abdominal musculature, and a stab incision is made through the peritoneum directly over the cystic area. The wall of the cyst or abscess is exteriorized through the abdominal incision and is sutured directly to the skin using a simple interrupted suture pattern (Fig. 27-4*B*). Size 2-0 monofilament nylon is the suture material of choice. The sutures should pass well away from the incised margin of the cyst, so that the cyst wall adequately folds over the skin margin to which it is sutured.

The midline abdominal incision is then closed in routine fashion. A Foley catheter or a large Brunswick feeding tube is sutured into place within the cavity to provide maximum drainage for the first 48 hours postoperatively. Sutures are removed in 10 days, and the

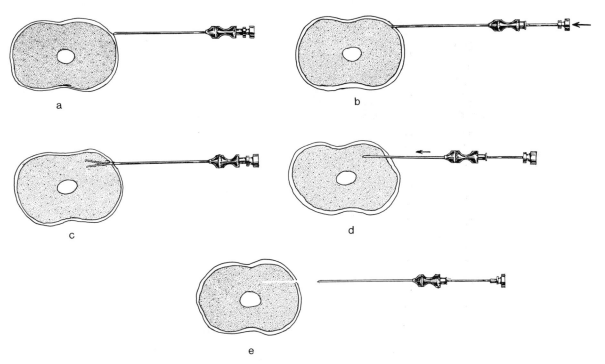

Fig. 27-3. *Prostatic biopsy technique with a Franklin-modified Vim Silverman biopsy needle. A, Needle with stylet is advanced to the prostatic capsule. B, The stylet is removed and the cutting prongs are introduced through the needle cannula to the tip of the needle. C, The cutting prongs are plunged into the prostatic parenchyma. D, The needle cannula is advanced to the tip of the cutting prongs causing a piece of prostatic tissue to be cut off and compressed into the cutting prongs. E, The entire assembly is withdrawn from the prostate, and the biopsy specimen is harvested.*

fistula usually seals completely within a month postoperatively. If fluid accumulates, frequent probing of the opening will ensure a patent fistula.

When anesthesia risk is a significant factor, the marsupialization procedure can be performed without a large abdominal midline incision, but rather through a more limited paramedian approach. The disadvantage of this approach is that it does not allow visualization of the entire prostate for complete assessment of the disease process. The location chosen for the paramedian incision should provide adequate ventral drainage. A skin incision an inch and a half to three inches long is made, and the abdominal musculature is bluntly dissected to expose peritoneum. An incision is carefully made through the peritoneum to expose the cyst wall. Care should be taken to identify the cystic structure, so

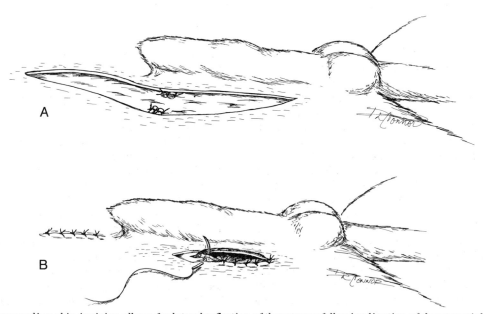

Fig. 27-4. A, *The paramedian skin incision allows for lateral reflection of the prepuce following ligation of the preputial artery and vein. B, The cyst or abscess wall is sutured to the skin with a simple interrupted pattern.*

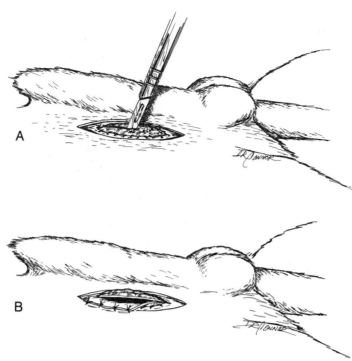

Fig. 27-5. A, *The cyst wall is sutured in a continuous pattern to the internal and external rectus fascia and the peritoneum. The cyst is then lanced and flushed.* B, *The margin of the cyst is then sutured directly to the skin.*

that the urinary bladder is not mistaken for a cyst wall. The circumference of the cyst wall is then sutured to the external rectus fascia, the internal fascia, and the peritoneum using a simple continuous pattern of 2-0 chromic catgut (Fig. 27-5A). The cyst wall is then lanced, is drained, and is flushed. The margin of the cyst wall is then sutured directly to the skin using a simple interrupted suture pattern with 2-0 monofilament nylon (Fig. 27-5B). A large Brunswick catheter or a Foley catheter is sutured in place to ensure maximum ventral drainage.

DRAINAGE OF PROSTATIC ABSCESSES

This technique should be considered when a prostatic abscess or multiple prostatic abscesses are either too small or too numerous to allow marsupialization.[27,28] The prostate gland is exposed along the ventral midline as previously described for marsupialization (see Fig. 27-4A). Using No. 1 chromic stay sutures, cranial traction is applied to the urinary bladder. Prostatic fat is incised along the midline of the gland ventrally between the parenchymal lobes (Fig. 27-6A). The fat is then gently reflected laterally and dorsally to allow exposure of the entire gland. The fat must not be excised or traumatized because small autonomic nerves are present in the peritoneum covering the fat. The prostatic abscess is located, and laparotomy pads moistened with saline solution are placed around the area to confine and to collect any leakage of exudate. The abscess is aspirated with a needle, and a specimen is saved for culture. The abscessed area is lanced and is drained with a stab incision ventrally and then is drained further with surgical suction (Fig. 27-6B). Next,

the initial incision is enlarged to permit digital entry into the abscess cavity for exploration of abscessed glandular tissue, fibrous adhesions, and any nearby loculi that may be present. The abscess is then flushed repeatedly with Ringers solution, sterile saline solution, or a 10% povidone-iodine* solution. It is important that the flushing be vigorous, with a large volume of warmed solution. When the entire cavity has been flushed repeatedly, the procedure is repeated in other abscessed areas.

Finally, the abscess cavity is incised dorsally to allow two to four Penrose drains half an inch to an inch in diameter to be inserted into the abscess cavity from ventral to dorsal (Fig. 27-6C). These drains are sutured in place dorsally with one 4-0 chromic catgut suture through the glandular capsule. The drains are then exteriorized to one side of the abdomen through a single ventral opening. Two to four additional drains are then placed into the peritoneal cavity near the abscessed area and are exteriorized through another incision in the opposite side of the abdomen. The entire area is flushed thoroughly again. The ventral midline is then closed using 2-0 monofilament stainless steel wire or 2-0 monofilament nylon suture in an interrupted pattern. Subcutaneous 2-0 catgut sutures realign the prepuce, and a simple interrupted skin closure completes the procedure.

Castration is performed as a routine therapeutic adjunct. Vigorous systemic antibiotic therapy follows postoperatively, based on culture and sensitivity test results. The intraprostatic drains are removed first, in 3 to 5 days, and the peritoneal drains are removed 2 days later.

*Betadine, Purdue Frederick Company, Norwalk, CT

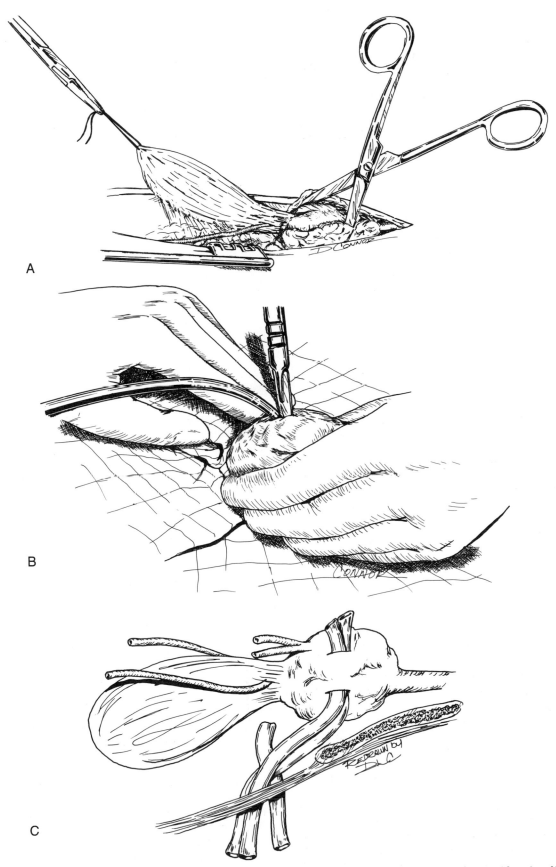

Fig. 27-6. A, *Cranial traction of the urinary bladder and midline incision and reflection of the prostatic fat provides visualization of the diseased prostate.* B, *A stab incision is made into the immobilized prostate gland and the abscess cavity is drained using surgical suction.* C, *Penrose drains are installed into the glandular cavity.*

This technique has the advantages of allowing the veterinarian to deal with prostatic abscesses quickly and to avoid the lengthy and difficult dissections associated with total prostatectomy. Contamination of the abdomen is inevitable, but is well managed with vigorous, liberal flushing and extensive drainage. In cases of extreme contamination, peritoneal lavage may be considered postoperatively.

SUBTOTAL PROSTATECTOMY—"FILLET TECHNIQUE"

Subtotal prostatectomy[10,15] is indicated when the risk of total prostatectomy is not warranted, or for the removal of localized prostatic neoplasia or infection. This procedure may also be indicated for the removal of a large portion of an infected gland that has proved to be untreatable by other means.

Subtotal prostatectomy has the advantages over total prostatectomy of shortened operative time and fewer potential postoperative complications, and it usually does not result in surgical interruption of the vas deferens. The major disadvantage of this procedure is that neither the entire gland nor any diseased portion of the prostatic urethra is removed.

Before beginning the surgical procedure, it is necessary to review the anatomic blood supply to the prostate gland, to facilitate proper hemostasis. The prostatic arteries branch off directly from the paired urogenital arteries (Fig. 27-7). The urogenital arteries then continue as the caudal vesicular arteries to supply the urinary bladder. This bifurcation is an important surgical landmark.

With the dog in dorsal recumbency, the prostate gland is identified and is approached along the ventral midline as previously described. Cranial traction is applied to the apex of the urinary bladder. Periprostatic fat is reflected dorsally to either side of the gland to expose the vasculature on the dorsolateral surface of the gland (see Fig. 27-6A). By rolling the isolated gland to one side, the bifurcation of the urogenital artery can easily be seen (Fig. 27-8A). The prostatic vessels are then doubly ligated with nonabsorbable suture material or metal clips. Care is taken to preserve the caudal vesicular artery as it courses cranially to supply the trigone area of the urinary bladder. By rolling the prostate gland to the other side, ligations are repeated on the remaining prostatic vessels at the contralateral urogenital arterial bifurcation.

Once the prostatic vessels have been ligated, the diseased portion of the prostate can be excised (Fig. 27-8B). A urinary catheter should be in place during the "fillet" maneuver, which is performed by successive passes with a scalpel or electrosurgical equipment. Care should be taken to note any large communication between excised parenchyma and the prostatic urethra.

Large iatrogenic rents or pre-existing fistulas into the prostatic urethra should be closed with 4-0 chromic

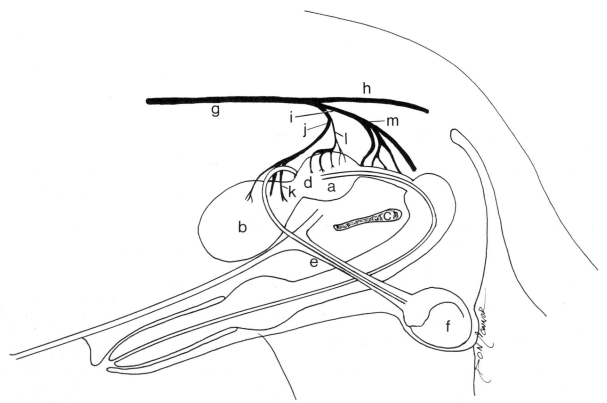

Fig. 27-7. *Illustration of the prostatic blood supply: a, prostate gland; b, urinary bladder; c, os pubis; d, ampulla of vas deferens; e, vas deferens; f, testes; g, aorta; h, parietal branch of internal illiac artery; i, visceral branch of internal illiac artery; j, urogenital artery; k, caudal vesicular artery; l, prostatic arteries; m, internal pudendal artery.*

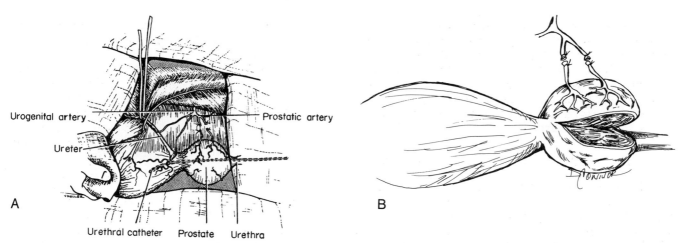

Urogenital artery — Prostatic artery

Ureter

Urethral catheter   Prostate   Urethra

A

B

Fig. 27-8. A, *With cranial pressure on the bladder and paraprostatic fat reflected dorsally, the prostate can be rolled to one side exposing the bifurcation of the urogenital artery. The prostatic vessels are shown doubly ligated. B, When the prostatic vessels have been ligated, selective excision of a portion of the prostate can be accomplished.*

catgut suture in a simple interrupted pattern if enough viable urethral tissue exists to suture. Smaller communications need not be sutured. If any significant communication exists with the prostatic urethra, a large, indwelling Foley catheter or Brunswick feeding tube should be left in place postoperatively to divert urine while urethral epithelium heals. Installation of a large catheter may necessitate a temporary perineal urethrotomy to bypass the restrictions of the os penis. This catheter should be left in place for 5 to 10 days postoperatively, depending on the size of prostatic urethral defect.

Following the resection of a portion of the prostate, Gelfoam* or Surgical† should be used along with firm pressure to control hemorrhage from the remaining glandular tissue. If infection in the gland is present at the site of resection, the entire area should be well flushed with sterile saline solution and an appropriate antibiotic. Local abdominal drainage with two double-lumen Penrose-Brunswick drains is advised following this procedure. These drains serve not only to drain the area, but are also useful in the early detection of prostatic urethral leakage and postoperative bleeding.

TOTAL PROSTATECTOMY

Total prostatectomy should be reserved only for patients with "end-stage" prostate disease. Extensive, saccular abscessation and advanced but operable prostatic neoplasia are the most common indications. Total transurethral prostatectomy is technically difficult and often causes significant surgical stress to the patient. Complications are not uncommon. This technique, however, is the only way to remove completely the diseased prostatic urethra along with diseased glandular elements.

Before the total prostatectomy procedure is begun, a jugular catheter is installed to allow continuous fluid replacement and shock therapy if needed during the

*Upjohn Company, Kalamazoo, MI
†Surgikos Company, New Brunswick, NJ

operation. Whole blood should be available in case of severe blood loss. The largest urinary catheter that will fit is introduced into the patient's urinary bladder. As previously described, a ventral midline abdominal incision is made from the umbilicus to the pubis, following lateral reflection of the prepuce. The prepubic tendon is severed at the cranial rim of the pubis to allow maximum exposure of the prostate (Fig. 27-9A). A Balfour abdominal retractor is useful to provide wide exposure.

It is not necessary to split the pelvic symphysis to perform a total prostatectomy because the enlarged gland is in the abdominal cavity. The prostatic fat is incised ventrally directly over the prostate and is reflected laterally; one must take care to protect small wispy nerves in the loose tissue surrounding the fat. The prostate is rotated to one side, and the prostatic arteries and veins are located and are doubly ligated (see Fig. 27-8A). The vessels are similarly ligated on the other side. Using gauze sponges and blunt dissection, the prostate gland parenchyma is gently teased caudally from the ventral bladder neck and proximal urethra (Fig. 27-9B). This blunt dissection is continued caudally onto the prostatic urethra to the level of the ampulla of the vas deferens. Careful reflection of the gland to this level ensures preservation of the dog's ability to avoid indiscriminate urination postoperatively. The vas deferens is then doubly ligated and severed. A strip of umbilical tape or a Penrose drain is then placed around the urethra just cranial to the ampulla of the vas deferens. Two "stay" sutures are placed through the urethral wall just caudal to the prostate gland. These sutures help to control the distal urethral segment when the urethra is severed and may be incorporated into the urethral anastomosis.

The urethra is then transected at the level of the ampulla of the vas deferens and again at the caudal border of the prostate (Fig. 27-9C). The entire prostate with prostatic urethra intact is then lifted from the catheter and out of the abdomen. The tip of the catheter is replaced into the bladder, and the urethral sur-

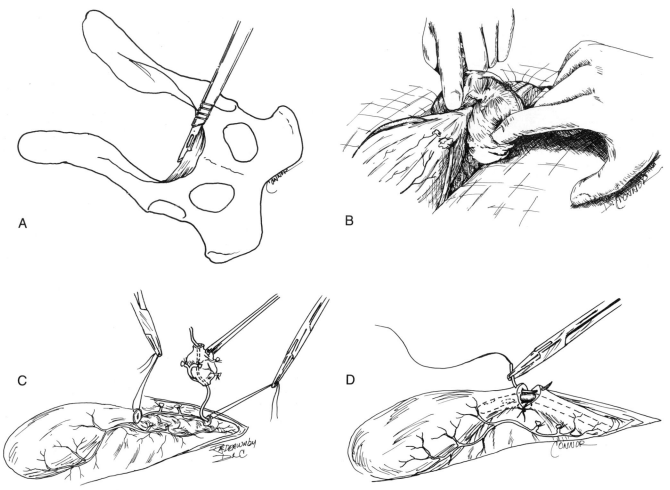

Fig. 27-9. A, *The prepubic tendon is severed to allow maximum exposure in performing a prostatectomy.* B, *The gland is teased off the prostatic urethra using blunt dissection caudally to the ampulla of the vas.* C, *The prostatic urethra is transected proximally and distally to the gland and the entire prostatic segment is lifted out of the abdomen.* D, *Urethral anastomosis. A simple interrupted suture pattern reunites the urethra.*

faces are apposed. These urethral segments are then anastomosed using full-thickness 2-0 monofilament nylon suture in a simple interrupted pattern (Fig. 27-9D). Eight equally spaced sutures are usually adequate to provide a tight seal of the entire urethral circumference. The caudal abdomen is flushed vigorously with Ringers flush solution. Two Penrose-over-Brunswick tube drains may be installed, and the abdomen is closed in routine fashion.

Postoperatively, an attempt should be made to keep the urinary catheter in place for at least 7 days, by suturing the catheter to the prepuce and by applying an Elizabethan collar or a head-bucket type of restraint as soon as the dog is awake. The catheter serves to decrease intraluminal urethral pressure and provides an adequate conduit for the urine.

The most common complications of total prostatectomy are urethral anastomosis leakage and urinary incontinence. Anastomosis leakage usually occurs from 2 to 7 days postoperatively and is generally due to premature removal of the urethral catheter, lack of adequate urethral blood supply, or an error in suture tech-

nique. Signs of leakage are fever, caudal abdominal pain, and decreased urine output. A positive contrast urethrogram may be useful in detecting anastomosis leakage, but care must be taken to introduce the contrast at low pressure, so that further suture line disturbance does not result.

Small urethral leaks can be treated conservatively. A Foley catheter should be placed into the urinary bladder. In some cases, a temporary urethrotomy may have to be performed to facilitate placement because of the restrictive nature of the os penis. With the cuff on the Foley catheter well inflated, the catheter acts to shunt nearly all of the urine past the urethral suture line. Small leaks heal in 3 to 4 days following placement of such a catheter. If the leak is large, or if a catheter cannot be placed, the area must be re-explored surgically, and the leaking areas must be resutured. A large Brunswick catheter or a Foley catheter should be placed following such a repair. Abdominal lavage is advised following resuturing, to provide for treatment of the urine peritonitis until the dog's condition stabilizes.

Short-term urinary incontinence is often present postoperatively. This incontinence is usually neurogenic and is caused by trauma and irritation to the nerves of the pelvic plexus, which supply the bladder syncytium. Full urinary continence usually returns within 2 weeks. If incontinence persists beyond a month, Enuretrol* may help to speed return of control. Occasionally, the incontinence persists permanently. Reasons for this permanent condition may be twofold: If the urethra is transected cranial to the ampulla of the vas deferens, a portion of the muscular syncytium at the neck of the bladder is also removed. Iatrogenic damage to the nervous or blood supply to the bladder neck may also result in permanent incontinence. A bladder-neck fascial sling operation may offer a solution to such postoperative incontinence.

In most cases, castration should be performed as an adjunct to total prostatectomy. It is possible, with meticulous dissection and beveling of the proximal urethral transection, to preserve the ampulla of the vas deferens. If this preservation is successful, sexual potency can be retained. Owing to the technical difficulty of performing such a prostatectomy, however, this procedure is not advised unless extreme circumstances require that the dog be used for breeding purposes postoperatively.

References and Suggested Readings

1. Annis, J., and Allen, A.: An Atlas of Canine Surgery. Philadelphia, Lea & Febiger, 1967.
2. Archibald, J. (ed.): Canine Surgery. 2nd Ed. Santa Barbara, CA, American Veterinary Publications, 1974.
3. Barsanti, J. A., and Finco, D. R.: Canine bacterial prostatitis. Vet. Clin. North Am., 4:679, 1979.
4. Barsanti, J. A., Shotts, E. B., Prasse, K., and Crowell, W.: Evaluation of diagnostic techniques for canine prostatic diseases. J. Am. Vet. Med. Assoc., 177:160, 1980.
5. Buckner, R. G.: The genital system. In Canine Medicine. 4th Ed., Vol. 1. Edited by E. J. Catcott. Santa Barbara, CA, American Veterinary Publications, 1979.
6. Bushby, P. A., and Hankes, G. H.: Sling urethroplasty for the correction of urethral dilatation and urinary incontinence. J. Am. Anim. Hosp. Assoc., 16:115, 1980.
7. Christie, T. R.: The prostate. In Pathophysiology of Small Animal Surgery. Edited by M. J. Bojrab. Philadelphia, Lea & Febiger, 1981.
8. Evans, H. E., and Christensen, G. C.: Miller's Anatomy of the Dog. 2nd Ed. Philadelphia, W. B. Saunders, 1979.
9. Finco, D.: Prostate gland biopsy. Vet. Clin. North Am., 4:367, 1974.
10. Gahring, D. R.: Surgical Management of Prostatic Diseases. Sixth American College of Veterinary Surgeons Forum, Chicago, 1978.
11. Greiner, T. P., and Betts, C. W.: Diseases of the prostate gland. In Textbook of Veterinary Internal Medicine: Diseases of the Dog and Cat. Edited by S. J. Ettinger. Philadelphia, W. B. Saunders, 1975.
12. Howard, D. R.: The prostate gland. In Current Techniques in Small Animal Surgery. Edited by M. J. Bojrab. Philadelphia, Lea & Febiger, 1975.
13. Howard, D. R.: Surgical Approach to the Canine Prostate. J. Am. Vet. Med. Assoc., 155:2026, 1969.
14. Knecht, C. D.: Diseases of the canine prostate gland (part 1). Compend. Contin. Ed. Small Anim. Pract., 1:385, 1979.
15. Knecht, C. D.: Diseases of the canine prostate gland (part II). Compend. Contin. Ed. Small Anim. Pract., 1:427, 1979.
16. Kopp, H., and Stockton, N.: Ligation of blood supply in the treatment of canine prostatic hyperplasia. J. Am. Vet. Med. Assoc., 136:327, 1960.
17. Leeds, E. B., and Leav, I.: Perineal punch biopsy of the canine prostate gland. J. Am. Vet. Med Assoc., 154:925, 1969.
18. Madsen, P. O., Wolf, H., Barquin, O., and Rhodes, P.: The nitrofurantoin concentration in prostatic fluid of humans and dogs. J. Urol., 100:54, 1968.
19. Osborne, C. A., Stevens, J. B., and Perman, V.: Kidney biopsy. Vet. Clin. North Am., 4:351, 1974.
20. O'Shea, J. D.: Squamous metaplasia of the canine prostate gland. Res. Vet. Sci., 4:431, 1963.
21. O'Shea, J. D.: Studies on the canine prostate gland. J. Comp. Pathol., 73:244, 1962.
22. Pettit, G.: A clinical evaluation of prostatectomy in the dog. J. Am. Vet. Med. Assoc., 136:486, 1960.
23. Smith, C. W.: Marsupialization of the prostate gland. In Current Techniques in Small Animal Surgery. Edited by M. J. Bojrab. Philadelphia, Lea & Febiger, 1975.
24. Stamey, T. A., and Meares, E. M., Winningham, D. G.: Chronic bacterial prostatitis and the diffusion of drugs into prostatic fluid. J. Urol., 103:187, 1970.
25. Winningham, D. G., and Stamey, T. A.: Diffusion of sulfonamides from plasma into prostatic fluids. J. Urol., 104:559, 1970.
26. Wolf, H., Madsen, P., and Rhodes, P.: The ampicillin concentration in prostatic tissue and prostatic fluid. Urol. Int., 22:453, 1967.
27. Zolton, G. M.: Surgical techniques for the prostate. Vet. Clin. North Am., 9:349, 1979.
28. Zolton, G. M., and Greiner, T. P.: Prostatic abscesses: a surgical approach. J. Am. Anim. Hosp. Assoc., 14:697, 1978.

*Berlex Laboratories, Inc., Cedar Knolls, NJ 07927

Orchiectomy of Descended and Retained Testes in the Dog and Cat and Biopsy of the Testis

by STEPHEN W. CRANE, JAMES E. SMALLWOOD, *and* CORNELIS J. G. WENSING

Castration (orchiectomy) is one of the more frequently performed surgical procedures in veterinary practice. The usual reasons for removal of the male gonads are to effect sexual sterilization and to modify or eliminate certain behavior patterns characteristic of intact males. Castration is also used as adjunct therapy in reducing aggressive behavior. Neoplasia, severe blunt or penetrating traumatic injury, torsion, orchitis, and epididymitis represent primary medical indications for orchiectomy. Castration may also be employed to remove the source of androgenic and estrogenic hormones, which may be mediators in other conditions such as benign prostatic hypertrophy, perianal adenoma, and perineal hernia. In addition, castration, coupled with scrotal ablation, is the initial surgical step in the perineal urethrostomy of the cat and in the permanent urethrostomy for chronically recurring urinary calculi in the dog. These urethrostomy procedures are covered in detail in Chapters 23 and 24.

Surgical Anatomy

The thin and sensitive skin of the scrotum can be easily irritated by surgical soap and other surgical preparations. If incised, the scrotum typically bleeds heavily and swells postoperatively. Because of these difficulties in preparing for asepsis and the local responses to injury, routine castration of the dog is performed through a single median incision cranial to the scrotum. Exceptions are those cases in which scrotal ablation is to be accomplished. In orchiectomy of the cat, a sagittal incision is made on each side of the scrotum.

Intimately associated with the deep surface of the scrotal skin is the tunica dartos, which consists of smooth muscle bundles and connective tissue. Deep to the tunica dartos is the spermatic fascia, which loosely attaches the scrotal wall to the parietal layer of the vaginal tunic (Fig. 27-10). The vaginal tunic is the peritoneal evagination that envelopes the spermatic cord, the testis, and the epididymis (Fig. 27-11).

The spermatic cord requires transection in any castration procedure. This structure originates near the vaginal ring as its individual components converse to exit the abdominal cavity. The spermatic cord consists of the testicular artery, the testicular vein (which forms the pampiniform plexus), the lymphatic vessels, the smooth muscle bundles, the ductus deferens with its associated vessels, and the testicular plexus of autonomic nerves.

The cremaster muscle, a fascicular division of the internal abdominal oblique muscle, is closely associated with the external surface of the parietal layer of the vaginal tunic, which surrounds the spermatic cord. Between the superficial inguinal ring and its entrance into the scrotum, the spermatic cord, surrounded by the vaginal tunic and a variable amount of fat, passes ventral to the pelvis in a subcutaneous position. Within the abdominal cavity, the ductus deferens courses from the vaginal ring to its termination at the prostate gland by looping caudally and medially around each ureter (Fig. 27-12).

Orchiectomy of the dog is generally performed under ultrashort intravenous anesthesia. In all cases of general anesthesia, the patency of the patient's airway should be protected by an endotracheal tube. In the cat, dissociative anesthesia by ketamine, with or without supplemental preoperative tranquilization, is commonly used. Ultrashort intravenous anesthetic agents are also popular, and perhaps preferable, whenever procedures such as declawing are to be combined with castration. Because the surgical approaches differ considerably between the dog and cat, they are described separately.

Castration of the Dog

SURGICAL TECHNIQUE

In the dog, the patient is positioned in dorsal recumbency, with retention of the pelvic limbs to the operating table. The hair from the surgical field, including the medial thigh areas, is clipped, and the entire region is scrubbed thoroughly with water and a mild soap. The prescrotal area, but not the scrotum, is next prepared for an aseptic surgical approach with scrub soap and skin-preparation solution. Contact of the scrotum with surgical antiseptics, especially the iodinated compounds, often incites scrotal dermatitis and results in increased postsurgical licking of the area by the patient. Because the scrotum has not received surgical preparation, the operative field is quadrant-toweled to cover the scrotum fully. A fenestrated drape is positioned over the surgical site. All further manipulations of the scrotum are performed through the sterile fabric of the towels and the fenestrated overdrape.

A median skin incision is made cranial to the scrotum and is carefully extended through the subcutaneous tissue layers. This incision should extend from the base of the scrotum a sufficient length cranially to allow expression of each testis through it. Next, one testis is manipulated toward the incision by digital pressure on the scrotum through the drape and towel

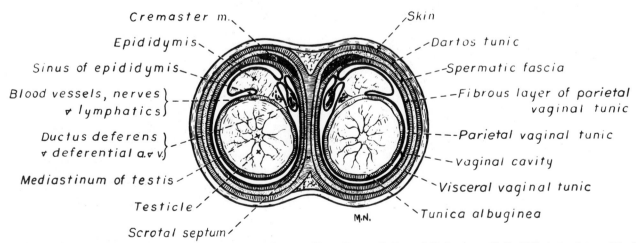

Fig. 27-10. *Schematic cross-section through the scrotum and testes. (From Evans, H. E., and Christensen, G. C.: Miller's Anatomy of the Dog. 2nd Ed. Philadelphia, W. B. Saunders, 1979.)*

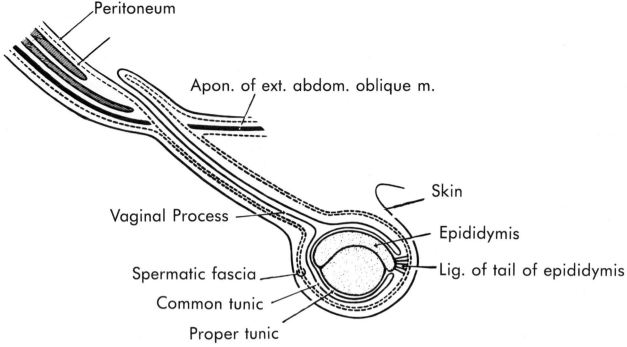

Fig. 27-11. *Schematic sagittal section of the inguinal canal showing the relationship of the peritoneum to the testis and the spermatic cord. (From Evans, H. E., and Christensen, G. C.: Miller's Anatomy of the Dog. 2nd Ed. Philadelphia, W. B. Saunders, 1979.)*

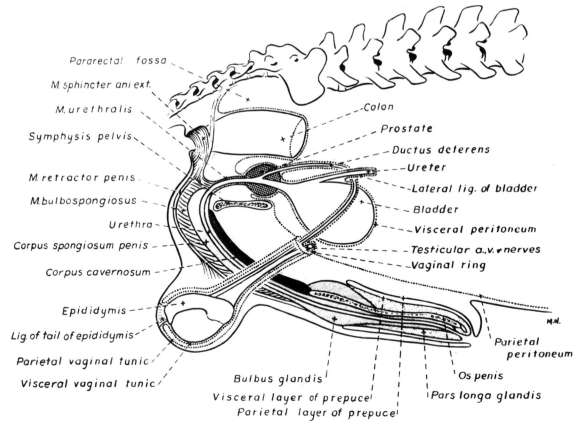

Fig. 27-12. *Schematic diagram of peritoneal reflections and the male genitalia. Note the looping of the ductus deferens caudally and medially around the ureters. (From Evans, H. E., and Christensen, G. C.: Miller's Anatomy of the Dog. 2nd Ed. Philadelphia, W. B. Saunders, 1979.)*

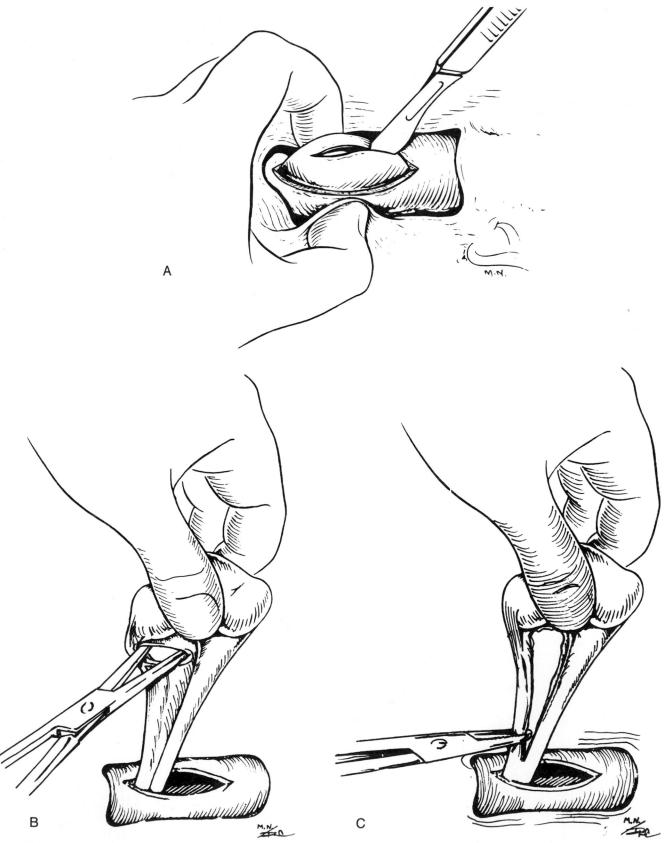

Fig. 27-13. A, *One testis is forced cranially to the incision and the spermatic fascia is carefully incised down to the parietal layer of the vaginal tunic. (From Leonard, E. P.: Fundamentals of Small Animal Surgery. Philadelphia, W. B. Saunders, 1968.) B, The testis is delivered with an intact parietal vaginal tunic through the incision. C, The condensation of the scrotal fascia between the scrotal wall and the parietal layer of the vaginal tunic is either crushed with a tissue clamp or ligated prior to transection to effect hemostasis.*

(Fig. 27-13*A*). The tissue that limits extrusion of the testis at this point is the spermatic fascia, which must be carefully incised down to the parietal layer of the vaginal tunic. The latter structure is recognized as a distinct, white, glistening layer that surrounds the testis. Once the spermatic fascia has been divided and the incision is long enough, the tunic-covered testis is delivered through the skin incision. Shortly after the testis appears, its outward progress is resisted by additional attachments of the spermatic fascia. A natural cleavage plane between the parietal layer of the vaginal tunic around the spermatic cord and the spermatic fascia can be developed. The spermatic fascia is fenestrated with the tips of hemostatic forceps to isolate the tunic-covered spermatic cord (Fig. 27-13*B*). Because some of the vessels of the spermatic fascia are concentrated in the remaining fascial attachment, hemostatic forceps are briefly clamped across the fascial condensation to effect hemostasis (Fig. 27-13*C*). In the case of testicular neoplasia or orchitis, the vessels are ligated

to preclude the troublesome and unnecessary complication of scrotal hematoma.

Following clamping and ligation, severance of the remaining connections between the fascia and the parietal layer of the vaginal tunic releases the invagination of the scrotal skin and allows free manipulation of the testis. Caudal and outward traction is then applied to the tunic-covered spermatic cord to break down the remaining loose connective tissue attachment. Any fat surrounding the parietal layer of the vaginal tunic is gently stripped proximally with a dry surgical sponge. At this stage, the testis and a considerable portion of the intact parietal layer of the vaginal tunic are exteriorized, and the cremaster muscle should be visible on the external surface of the vaginal tunic. The tunic-covered spermatic cord must next be severed to remove the testis and epididymis, to complete the operation; our technique depends on the patient's size.

"Closed" Castration. In patients under 35 kg, a "closed" castration technique is employed. Triple he-

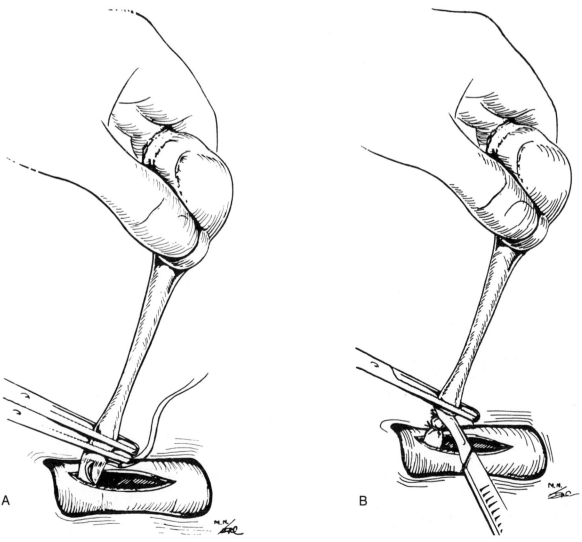

A

B

Fig. 27-14. A, *The "closed" castration technique begins with the application of three Carmalt hemostatic forceps and then the removal of the one closest to the patient.* B, *The intact vaginal tunic and enclosed spermatic cord are severed along the proximal edge of the distal clamp.*

mostatic forceps, such as Carmalt forceps, are applied across the tunic-covered spermatic cord. The most proximal clamp is removed, and synthetic absorbable or nonabsorbable suture material is used to create a transfixation ligature through the parietal layer of the vaginal tunic and cremaster muscle and around the spermatic cord at the level of the crush mark (Fig. 27-14A). The first loop of the triple square knot is tied tightly. The transfixation method of securing the ligature prevents a potential complication of the closed castration method. This complication is internal retraction of the testicular artery within the ligature that results in intra-abdominal or subcutaneous hemorrhage. The middle clamp is next removed, and another ligature is placed in the crush mark. The intact vaginal tunic and enclosed spermatic cord are then severed along the proximal edge of the distal clamp, and the testis, epididymis, and associated spermatic cord are removed (Fig. 27-14B).

"OPEN" CASTRATION. Large and giant breeds of dogs are castrated by the "open" method; the parietal layer of the vaginal tunic is incised and is opened longitudinally with scissors or a scalpel to expose the vascular structures of the spermatic cord (Fig. 27-15). Proximal to the pampiniform plexus, the testicular artery and vein and the ductus deferens are collectively ligated with nonabsorbable suture material. The advantage of the open method is that the vascular ligations are more secure. The disadvantages include the opening of the cavity of the vaginal tunic, which communicates proximally with the main peritoneal cavity. It is also necessary to resect the excessive portions of the vaginal tunic and cremaster muscle as an additional and separate step after the testicular amputation.

With either method, the proximal stump of the spermatic cord is held with a thumb forceps and is examined for complete hemostasis. The cord is released under direct thumb forceps control so that it may be retrieved and re-examined if bleeding begins when the vessels shorten and dilate. The structure is then allowed to retract into the subcutaneous tissue toward the superficial inguinal ring.

Following the first half of the procedure, the remaining testis is produced through an incision in the contralateral spermatic fascia and is removed in the same manner to complete the castration. At no time is it necessary to invade the scrotal septum. To do so is to invite the complication of scrotal hematoma. Following inspection for the complete arrest of bleeding, the deep and superficial subcutaneous layers are closed with synthetic absorbable sutures in the simple interrupted pattern. The skin is carefully closed with a fine nonabsorbable material in an intracuticular or a simple interrupted pattern. Skin sutures that are placed carelessly or too tightly invite the interest of the patient and perhaps encourage automutilation. Such patients require restraint devices, tranquilization, and removal and replacement of the sutures, or a combination of the methods, to prevent licking or chewing the sutures or incision.

An alternate method for canine orchiectomy has

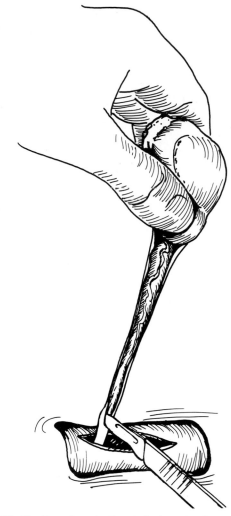

Fig. 27-15. *The "open" castration technique involves opening the parietal vaginal tunic longitudinally after its exteriorization. After clamping and ligation of the vessels, the testis is amputated.*

been described for those situations in which the patient has been positioned in sternal recumbency on a perineal stand for perineal herniorrhaphy or removal of perianal adenomas. An incision is made caudodorsal to the scrotum at the perineal junction. The spermatic fascia is incised, and the testes are delivered dorsocaudally into the operative field (Fig. 27-16). The remainder of the operation is performed as previously described.

POSTOPERATIVE COMPLICATIONS

Serious postsurgical complications include automutilation, scrotal hematoma, and local cellulitis or abscessation. These major complications are best handled by scrotal ablation with primary closure. In fact, some veterinary surgeons perform scrotal removals on all large (over 25 kg) dogs they castrate. Closure over drains may or may not be indicated. Another technique is to delay primary closure of the wound until infection has cleared and a bed of healthy granulation tissue has been established.

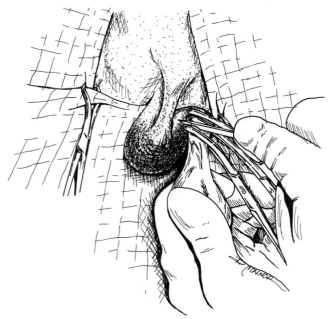

Fig. 27-16. *An alternative technique for orchiectomy from the perineum requires a dorsal, caudal, and lateral surgical approach when the patient is already suitably positioned. (Redrawn from Knecht.)*

Castration of the Cat

It is generally accepted that male cats make superior pets if sexually neutered at or before sexual maturity. The typical intact tom cat cannot usually be tolerated as an exclusively indoor companion animal because of its marking and spraying of odoriferous urine. Nocturnal fighting and roaming are also behavior patterns of male cats that are often successfully controlled by orchiectomy. Because the feline scrotum is located in the nondependent perineal position (Fig. 27-17), the surgical technique is different from that used for the dog.

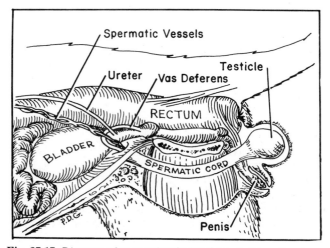

Fig. 27-17. *Diagram of anatomic relationships in the male cat genital tract.*

SURGICAL TECHNIQUE

The cat is anesthetized and is placed in dorsal recumbency. The perineal area can be conveniently exposed by bringing the patient's hindquarters to the edge of the table and by allowing its tail to fall toward the floor. The patient's pelvic limbs are secured in an abducted position, and the fine hair covering the scrotum is plucked with the fingers (Fig. 27-18A) or is clipped with a No. 40 clipper blade. The scrotal area is prepared with surgical soap and scrub solutions, and an overdrape is applied to the area. Such drapes limit the inherent contamination associated with the perineal area, especially when most of the hair is still present. The drapes used for this purpose are easily made from surgical muslin or paper draping material and should be about the size of a large handkerchief, with a presewn fenestration about 20 mm in length. The prepared scrotum is then expressed through the fenestration to create an acceptably draped surgical area.

Each side of the scrotum is carefully opened with a hand-held No. 10 scalpel blade. Both the length and the depth of the initial incisions are important. The length should fully scribe the scrotum from the dorsal to the ventral aspect to allow ample postoperative drainage. The depth should be sufficient to completely divide the skin and spermatic fascia, but not the underlying parietal layer of the vaginal tunic (Fig. 27-18B). With a gentle pinching maneuver, the testis, still enclosed in the vaginal tunic, is "popped" out of the incision. The testis is pulled caudally or caudoventrally with firm traction until considerable exposure of the tunic-covered spermatic cord is obtained and resistance to further traction is met. Fat is stripped from the vaginal tunic with a dry sponge. Two Halstead mosquito forceps are then placed across the spermatic cord, which is subsequently transected caudal to the forceps (Fig. 27-18C). One ligature of plain or chromic catgut suture is placed in the crushmark of the cranial forceps and is tightly tied. The testis is then amputated, and the cranial spermatic cord is released under direct forcep control so that it may be retrieved if bleeding commences. The tunic-covered spermatic cord is then released into the subcutaneous tissues. After removing the other testis, both incisions are dilated by spreading the tips of the mosquito forceps between the wound edges (Fig. 27-18D). The purpose of this last step is to reduce the likelihood of an early fibrin seal across the incision that might prevent drainage. Topical ointments or powders and systemic antibiotics are unnecessary. Proper ligature technique and avoidance of the scrotal septum preclude postoperative hemorrhage.

An open method of feline castration has been described wherein the ductus deferens is separated from the testicular vessels, and these two components of the spermatic cord are tied into a square knot (Fig. 27-19). An alternate method involves placing one throw of an overhand knot into the spermatic cord and cinching down the throw to occlude the testicular artery. Excessive portions of the proximal parietal vaginal tunic are then excised. These procedures have the advantages of

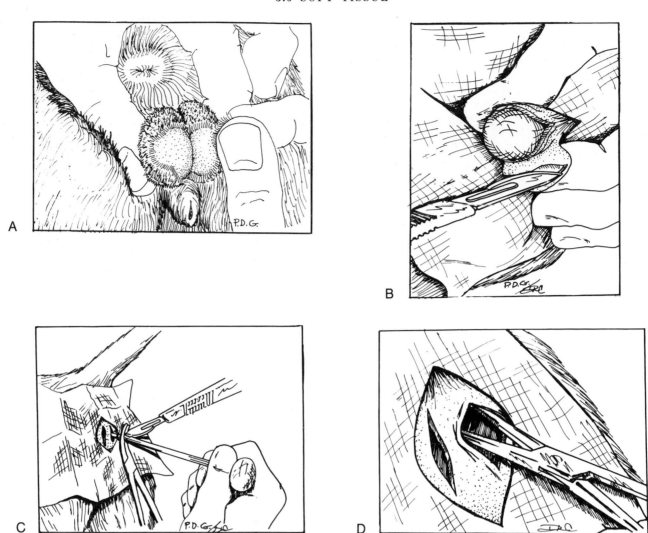

Fig. 27-18. A, *The fine hair covering the scrotum is plucked.* B, *The initial incision in a "closed" feline orchiectomy should divide the skin and spermatic fascia but not enter the parietal vaginal tunic.* C, *Two Halstead mosquito forceps are placed across the spermatic cord and a ligature of absorbable suture material is placed in the crush mark of the removed proximal clamp.* D, *The scrotal incisions are spread apart as the final step in the procedure.*

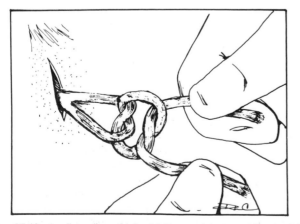

Fig. 27-19. *An "open" method of feline orchiectomy. See text for details.*

using no suture material and of being rapidly performed with practice. The vascular ligation is probably less secure than with direct closed ligation of the spermatic cord, however, and the latter method is our choice.

The patient is discharged the same day, with the recommendation that shredded newspapers be used to replace clay cat litter for 5 days.

Alternate procedures for castration of the cat have been described or are a part of veterinary historical lore. Included are techniques to accomplish neutering without analgesia and the practice of traction avulsion of the spermatic cord. The traction avulsion technique has been associated with a substantial risk of postoperative intra-abdominal hemorrhage and is inconsistent with accepted surgical principles.

Cryptorchidism

Unilateral or bilateral cryptorchidism, especially in the dog, is frequently encountered in small animal practice. Current understandings relating to canine cryptorchidism include the following:

1. The condition is genetically carried and is transmitted in a single autosomal recessive manner.

2. Unilaterally cryptorchid males are typically fertile and usually possess normal libido. Thus, a wide dissemination of the trait is theoretically possible and has apparently occurred. The prevalence rate of cryptorchidism is 13/1000.

3. The condition occurs most frequently in small or purebred dogs, with a right-to-left ratio of 2.3 : 1.

4. Testicular descent should be complete shortly after birth. Testes not located within the scrotum by 2 months of age should be considered permanently retained. Figure 27-20 depicts the descent of the canine testis in prenatal and postnatal life.

5. Medical therapy using luteinizing hormone releasing factor or human chorionic gonadotropin is useless, because increasing the size of the interstitial cells does not stimulate testicular migration when the gubernaculum testis has regressed. Orchiopexy or prosthetic testicular implants are of no psychologic benefit to the patient, represent unjustified operative risks, and are illegal and unethical for show purposes. Such procedures may also contribute to the perpetuation of cryptorchidism.

6. Testes retained in an inguinal or abdominal position are predisposed to malignant changes (seminoma and Sertoli cell tumor) in later life.

These observations justify that the veterinarian should strongly recommend complete castration of cryptorchid animals.

Testicular Descent in the Dog

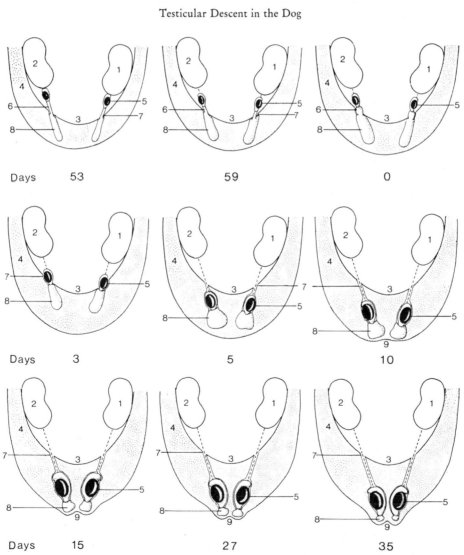

Days 53   59   0

Days 3   5   10

Days 15   27   35

Fig. 27-20. *Schematic diagram of the maturation and descent of the canine testis at various intervals in development, from the fifty-third day after conception to the thirty-fifth day after birth. 1, Left kidney; 2, right kidney; 3, abdominal wall; 4, subcutis; 5, testis; 6, gubernaculum (intra-abdominal); 7, inguinal canal; 8, gubernaculum (extra-abdominal); 9, scrotum. (From Baumans, V., Dijkstra, G., and Wensing, C. J. G.: Testicular descent in the dog. Zentralbl. Veterinaermed. [C], 10:97, 1981.)*

PHYSICAL DIAGNOSIS

The palpable absence of one or both testes during multiple examinations confirms the diagnosis of cryptorchidism. The veterinarian should be aware that cremaster muscle spasm may cause an artifactual retention of the testis to an elevated position in some young puppies.

Once a diagnosis of cryptorchidism has been established, it remains to be determined at what point along the normal path of descent testicular migration became arrested.

During embryonic development, the gonad develops in the urogenital ridge in the dorsal wall of the abdomen. When descent begins, the gonad is located caudal to the kidney. Migration of the testis to the vaginal ring normally takes place near the time of birth and is totally dependent on the proper development and enlargement of the gubernaculum testis (Fig. 27-20). Any substantive error in the segmental enlargement of the gubernaculum testis can result in failure of the descent mechanism and thus, intra-abdominal cryptorchidism. Although the specific mediator of this critical enlargement process is still under investigation, cryptorchidism is a direct result of the dysplasia in gubernacular development. Once near or in the inguinal canal, the final stage of testicular descent depends on regression of the extra-abdominal part of the gubernaculum testis, which guides the testis to the scrotum.

Thus, the undescended testis may be located anywhere along the path between kidney and scrotum. In the dog, the most common location for retention is intra-abdominal. Although this location is also the most frequent in feline cryptorchidism, the cat has a higher percentage of retained testes in the superficial inguinal of prescrotal areas. Careful palpation of the patient in dorsal recumbency sometimes allows the presurgical identification of the gonad if it is in the extra-abdominal position. If the gonad is not identified by palpation, abdominal exploration is necessary to locate and to remove the retained testis. Other diagnostic techniques include pneumoperitonography, laparoscopy, and ultrasonography.

SURGICAL TECHNIQUE

Because most retained canine testes are located within the abdominal cavity, exploratory celiotomy is required for their removal. With the patient under general anesthesia, the ventral abdominal wall is clipped and is prepared for an aseptic surgical procedure; the preputial cavity is lavaged with surgical scrub solution and is then irrigated with sterile saline solution to reduce subsequent contamination of the operative field. The patient is positioned in dorsal recumbency, and towels and a large fenestrated drape are arranged so as to expose the ventral abdominal wall. It is almost always possible to locate, to exteriorize, and to remove the intra-abdominal testis through an incision located between the umbilicus and the prepuce. The median skin and subcutaneous tissue incision should extend from just cranial to the umbilicus to near the prepuce. A midline celiotomy is performed through the linea alba.

Frequently, the testes are located in the midabdominal region as a movable, tan or gray gonad of about half the normal size. Arterial supply from the testicular artery (a direct branch of the aorta) and a small artery in the gubernacular remnant or the deferential fold of the peritoneum are typically visualized. A small epididymis and ductus deferens are seen to course toward the caudal aspect of the abdomen.

If the testis cannot be located in the midabdominal area, one should examine the area of the vaginal ring. When the testicular descent is arrested at this location, it is usually possible to palpate the testis by moving the index or middle finger caudolaterally along the abdominal wall toward the vaginal ring. If the testis cannot be located on cursory inspection, the prostate gland should be palpated or visualized to locate the termination of the ductus deferens. Once identified, the ductus deferens can be traced proximally to the testis. Careful traction on the ductus deferens aids in bringing the testis and the testicular vessels into view. The testicular vessels are isolated, are triple-clamped, then are double-ligated with nonabsorbable suture material, and finally are divided. Triple Halstead hemostatic forceps are applied to the ductus deferens well past the epididymis. The ductus deferens and its associate vessels are double-ligated and are divided distal to the ligatures. The abdominal cavity is checked carefully for bleeding, and the celiotomy is closed.

PRESCROTAL TESTIS. If the testis is descended through the inguinal canal, but is located in the prescrotal position, removal is accomplished by making a skin incision just cranial to the scrotum and manipulating the testis by digital pressure into the incision. The spermatic fascia and spermatic cord are then managed as in routine orchiectomy.

Biopsy of the Testis

In some cases, it may be necessary to confirm a clinical diagnosis of impaired fertility or other testicular disorder by histopathologic means. It should be recognized that significant complications may occur following biopsy, including hemorrhage and even further impairment of fertility. An open incisional biopsy of the testis, however, is considered superior to needle biopsy when histopathologic diagnosis is required. The advantages of an open method include direct assessment of the testis and precise harvesting of representative tissue. Open biopsy also provides the most atraumatic technique because all major steps in the procedure can be done gently and under direct visual control. Because postoperative hemorrhage is a potential complication the ability to observe the testis after biopsy to ensure hemostasis is another significant advantage.

The patient is placed under general anesthesia or is given a tranquilizer and an epidural infusion of 2% lidocaine. The abdominal and inguinal areas are prepared

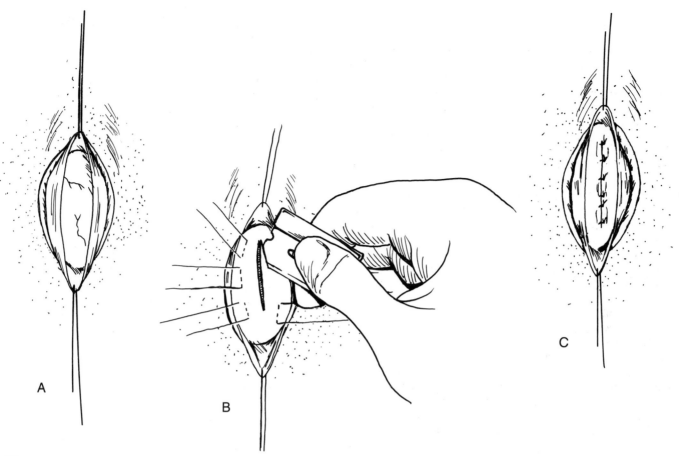

Fig. 27-21. *A, Biopsy of the testis is accomplished by the same initial approach as for orchiectomy. The cut edges of the tunic are temporarily secured by stay sutures. B, Two rows of fine, synthetic absorbable suture material are preplaced into the visceral vaginal tunic and tunica albuginea. A wafer-thin wedge biopsy is harvested with a sterile, new single-edge razor blade. C, Following biopsy the preplaced sutures are quickly tied to oppose the edges of the testicular wound gently. Closure of the wound is as for orchiectomy.*

and are draped as for orchiectomy. The testis is approached as for castration by a median skin incision just cranial to the scrotum. The parietal vaginal tunic, once identified, is brought into the incision with fine-toothed forceps and is secured with traction from an assistant. Countertraction is provided by the spermatic fascia.

The parietal tunic is incised to expose the extreme distal spermatic cord and testis. The cut edges of the tunic are retracted with temporary stay sutures (Fig. 27-21A). The testis is carefully examined, and the biopsy site is chosen. Two rows of interrupted horizontal mattress sutures of synthetic absorbable material (size 4-0 to 6-0, swaged onto a fine half- or ⅝-circle tapered needle) are preplaced through the visceral vaginal tunic and tunica albuginea. The suture "bites" are placed parallel to the proposed biopsy site (Fig. 27-21B). A thin-wedge testicular biopsy is taken by sharp dissection with a new, sterile, single-edged razor blade. A depth halfway to the center of the testis should be an adequate sample. One should work to complete the biopsy atraumatically and rapidly. The harvested tissue is briefly set aside, and the preplaced sutures are tied by hand to appose tissue edges gently but completely (Fig. 27-21C). Immediate postoperative hemorrhage

usually abates with direct pressure. Specimens for exfoliative cytologic study and bacterial culture are taken from the biopsy specimen when hemostasis from the sutured testis is being confirmed. The sample is then added to Bouin's fixative.

The testis is checked a final time for control of bleeding, and the parietal layer of the vaginal tunic is closed with fine synthetic absorbable suture material. The subcutaneous layers are reapposed, and the skin is closed with simple interrupted sutures.

References and Suggested Readings

Baumans, V., Dijkstra, G., and Hensing, C. J. G.: Testicular descent in the dog. Zentralbl. Veterinaermed. [A], *10*:97, 1981.

Burke, T. J.: Sterility in the male. *In* Pathophysiology in Small Animal Surgery. Edited by M. J. Bojrab. Philadelphia, Lea & Febiger, 1981.

Burke, T. J., and Reynolds, H. A.: The testis. *In* Pathophysiology in Small Animal Surgery. Edited by M. J. Bojrab. Philadelphia, Lea & Febiger, 1981.

Evans, H. E., and Christensen, G. C.: Miller's Anatomy of the Dog. 2nd Ed. Philadelphia, W. B. Saunders, 1979.

Knecht, C. D.: An alternative approach for castration of the dog. VM SAC, *71*:469, 1976.

Reif, J. S., Moquiri, T. G., and Kenney, R. S.: A Comort study of canine testicular neoplasia. J. Am. Vet. Med. Assoc., *175*:719, 1979.

28 * Penis

Surgical Procedures of the Penis

by H. PHIL HOBSON

Amputation Techniques

Partial or "complete" amputation of the penis may be indicated in certain congenital, traumatic, or neoplastic conditions. The most common neoplasm of this area, transmissible venereal tumor, is responsive to radiotherapy in most cases. Thus, amputation of the penis should be considered rarely, if ever, as a corrective measure for this condition.

PARTIAL AMPUTATION

The exact location of the amputation is determined by the site of the lesion. In most cases, the penis can be extruded, (Fig. 28-1*A*) and it may be held in the extruded position by clamping the preputial orifice with a towel clamp just caudal to the bulbus glandis. The sheath may be opened full thickness, when necessary, to expose the penis. A Penrose drain tube works well as a tourniquet around the base of the penis.

Amputation of the tip of the penis may be necessary in chronic or recurrent prolapse of the urethra (Fig. 28-1). It is advantageous to place a catheter in the urethra in order to identify the limits of the lumen. One should make the incision partway across the tip, place a stay suture to unite the mucosa of the urethra with the mucosa of the penis, and then complete the excision of the tip of the penis (Fig. 28-1*B*). The triangulation technique (Fig. 28-1*C* and *D*) conserves a patent lumen to the tip of the urethra. Careful apposition of the cut mucosal edges to the penile tunic helps to avoid excessive scar-tissue proliferation and stricture. A continuous suture pattern helps to control seepage from the cavernous erectile tissue. Synthetic absorbable suture is used for the mucosal closure.

An Elizabethan collar or a side bar restraint device should always be used to prevent the patient from licking the wound (see Chap. 3). Castration or careful hormone therapy may be indicated to help to prevent erection during healing.

Amputations of the main body of the penis require the severing of the os penis, as well as the salvaging of

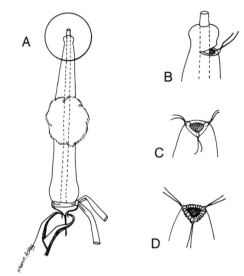

Fig. 28-1. A, *Amputation of the tip of the penis.* B, *Securing the urethral mucosa to the penile mucosa.* C, *Triangulating the urethral orifice with stay sutures.* D, *Placement of a simple continuous suture pattern between the stay sutures with the orifice in maximal dilatation.*

enough urethra distal to the severed os penis to create a urethral flap to anastomose to the penile mucosa. A catheter is placed within the lumen of the urethra, and the soft tissue is reflected in a flap-like fashion distally from the urethra and os penis for a distance of 1 cm. The os penis and urethra are severed with bone-cutting forceps and a scalpel. The urethra is isolated subperiosteally from the groove of the os penis with a small dental chisel. The urethra is split, flared, trimmed, and sutured to the infolded tunica albuginea, as shown in Figure 28-2. Care should be taken to appose the mucosal surfaces carefully. It is perhaps easier to achieve excellent apposition with fine, closely placed interrupted sutures, but a continuous pattern is more likely to control bleeding. Some bleeding, especially at the end of urination, is common, even for a period of several days following the operation. It is difficult to identify and to ligate individual vessels in this area. Releasing the tourniquet while the wound is open, in an effort to identify and to ligate the vessels within the corpus spongiosum penis, may prove unrewarding.

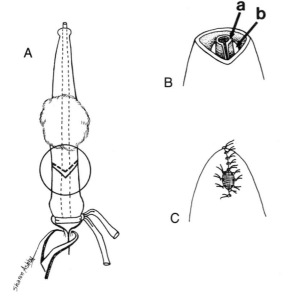

Fig. 28-2. *A, Amputation of the penis proximal to a lesion. The corpus spongiosum penis is incised at a 45° angle. The os penis and urethra are incised 1 cm further distal than the corpus spongiosum penis. B, The urethra (1) is elevated subperiosteally from the groove in the os penis. The os penis (2) is trimmed away with a rongeur to the level of the corpus spongiosum penis. C, The urethra is sutured to the penile mucosa, and the remainder of the penile stump is closed.*

PREPUTIAL AMPUTATION

When pooling of urine within the prepuce becomes a concern following partial amputation of the penis, shortening of the entire prepuce may be desirable. For the best cosmetic results, a full-thickness section of the prepuce may be removed (Fig. 28-3). The length of pre-puce to be removed should be the same as the length of the penile resection. In cases of congenital micropenis, the tip of the prepuce should cover the tip of the penis by approximately 1 cm. The cranial transverse incision is made 2 cm caudal to the cranial junction of the pre-puce and to the body wall, in order to allow adequate circulation to the cranial end of the prepuce. The location of the caudal transverse incision is determined by the length of the penis. The two incisions are extended laterally in an elliptical fashion to facilitate a smooth closure of the skin.

Next, the dorsal aspect of the section of prepuce to be removed is dissected free from the body wall with scissors. With careful dissection, most of the preputial vessels, which lie immediately subcutaneously on ei-ther side of the sheath, can be identified and preserved. To close the amputation, the preputial mucosa is ap-posed with 4-0 chromic catgut suture, using a sub-mucosal pattern. If a continuous pattern is used around the circumference of the prepuce, care should be taken to avoid a pursestring effect, which would limit the movement of the penis. The veterinarian may find it easier to close the dorsal mucosa if the penis is allowed to protrude through the incision site during this phase of closure.

COMPLETE AMPUTATION

The initial skin incision is made in an elliptical fash-ion around the entire external genitalia (Fig. 28-4A). The preputial vessels are ligated, as well as any addi-tional branches of the caudal superficial epigastric ves-sels that may cross the incision line. The spermatic cords are isolated, ligated, and severed. Care must be taken to place the ligatures tightly enough to prevent retraction of the severed spermatic artery if the tunics

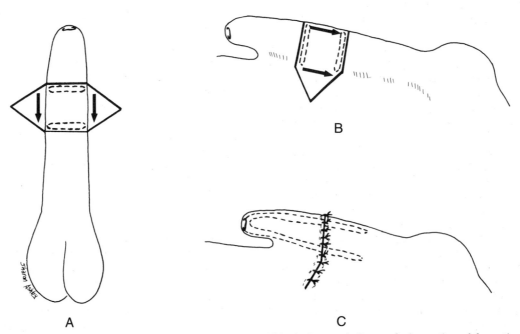

Fig. 28-3. *Shortening of the prepuce in cases of pooling of the urine within its lumen. A, Removal of a section of the entire prepuce. B and C, Reapposition of the mucosa and skin.*

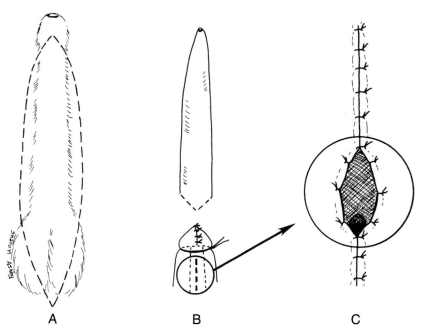

Fig. 28-4. *Ablation of the external male genitalia. A, The skin incision extends from cranial to the prepuce to caudal to the scrotum. B, Amputation of the shaft of the penis in the area of the scrotum. The penis is ligated, incised, and sutured. C, The urethrostomy is established by careful apposition of the urethral mucosa to the edge of the skin.*

are incorporated in the ligature. When the penis and the prepuce have been stripped from the body wall in a caudal direction, the dorsal penile vessels are identified and are ligated just caudal to the level of the desired penile amputation site. The retractor penis muscle is reflected from the urethra, and with a catheter in place, a midline incision is made into the urethral lumen at the desired urethrostomy site. A 1-0 chromic ligature, which circumscribes the penis, is placed just caudal to the amputation site and just cranial to the urethrostomy site (Fig. 28-4*B*). The shaft of the penis is amputated in a wedge fashion, and the tunica albuginea is apposed over the amputation stump.

The urethrostomy should be located in the scrotal area whenever possible. Careful apposition of penile urethra and skin edge, as the urethrostomy is completed, minimizes postoperative bleeding and scar-tissue formation (Fig. 28-4*C*). Although suture patterns and materials are a matter of choice, a continuous pattern aids in controlling hemorrhage from any incised erectile tissue. The use of a synthetic absorbable suture eliminates the need for suture removal.

Particular care should be taken to obliterate "dead space," especially cranial to the stump of the amputated penis, when closing the subcutaneous tissue. The use of a restraint device, to prevent licking of the surgery site by the patient, is imperative.

Hypospadias

Hypospadias is a congenital anomaly of the external genitalia in which the penile urethra terminates ventrally and caudally to its normal opening. The urethra may terminate at any level from the perineum to the tip of the penis (Fig. 28-5) because the urethral folds fail to

fuse (see Fig. 28-9). In severe cases, the two halves of the scrotum may fail to fuse, the penis fails to develop normally, and the urethra fails to close in the perineal area (Fig. 28-6). Frequently, the analogue of the urethra may be present as a fibrous cord that runs from the

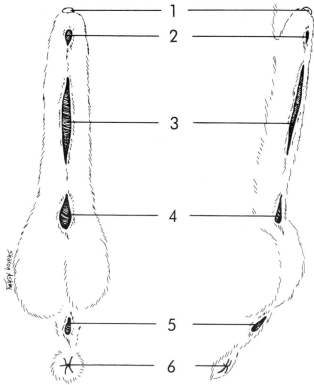

Fig. 28-5. *Normal urethral meatus (1) and types of hypospadias: glandular (2); penile (3); scrotal (4); perineal (5); and anal (6).*

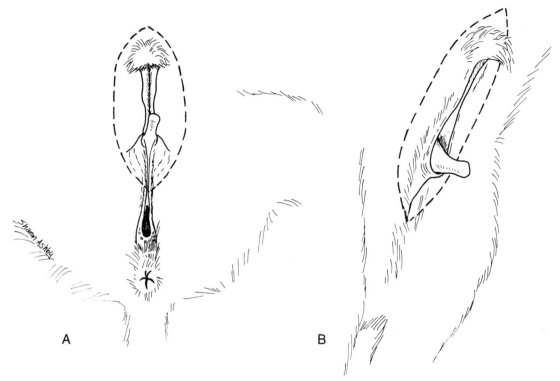

Fig. 28-6. A *and* B, *Severe hypospadias with concurrent defects of penile and preputial development. Excision of the entire external genitalia is the approach of choice.*

glans penis to the urethral opening and pulls the penis into a deforming ventral curvature (chordae) (Fig. 28-6).

Minimal defects may require no urethral surgery. The constant extrusion of the tip of the glans penis can often be relieved by closing the prepuce to its normal extent (Figs. 28-7 and 28-8) on its caudoventral aspect. Should the resulting orifice be too small to allow extension of the penis, the opening may be increased to the desired diameter by enlarging the lumen on the craniodorsal aspect. Simply leaving the orifice larger by not closing the caudoventral defect to its fullest extent may well result in the tip of the penis continuing to droop from the prepuce and may thus subject it to continual drying, licking, and trauma.

Caudoventral closure is accomplished by excising the mucocutaneous junction, separating the mucosa from the skin, and closing the two layers individually (Fig. 28-8A). Sutures of 4-0 to 6-0 absorbable synthetic material are preferred. Should the orifice need to be enlarged dorsally, one scissor jaw is inserted into the lumen of the prepuce, and the orifice is cut to the needed extent. With a minimum of undermining, the cut mucosal and skin edge can be apposed (Fig. 28-8 B). Failure to appose the skin and mucosal edges adequately may result in closure by granulation, and should the patient be allowed to lick out the sutures, the same is likely to occur.

Small urethral defects can be closed successfully with a two-layer closure (Fig. 28-9). A catheter is in-

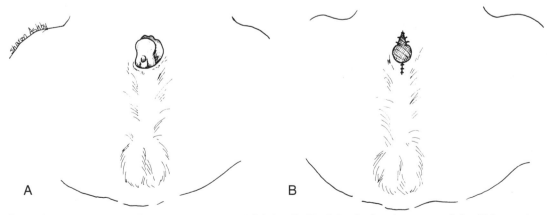

Fig. 28-7. A, *Glandular hypospadias with a concurrent preputial defect.* B, *The defect is closed ventrocaudally. If the resulting orifice is too small, it is enlarged by incising the prepuce dorsocranially. The preputial mucosa is sutured to the skin edge.*

29 * Endocrine

Adrenalectomy in the Dog

by DUDLEY E. JOHNSTON

Adrenalectomy has been performed in the dog for treatment of hyperadrenocorticism, or Cushing's syndrome. This syndrome can be caused by bilateral adrenocortical hyperplasia or by neoplasia of the adrenal cortex. The adrenocortical hyperplasia may, in turn, be the result of tumor growth in the pituitary gland. The standard treatment for adrenocortical hyperplasia is the use of ortho, para prime-DDD (O, p[1]-DDD), an adrenocorticolytic drug. Currently, adrenalectomy is used in veterinary surgery to treat adrenocortical hyperplasia when pharmacologic intervention is not successful and to remove adrenal tumors.

One surgical approach is bilateral paracostal laparotomy.[3,4] A ventral midline celiotomy gives excellent exposure of both adrenal glands; however, problems are associated with wound healing in the presence of high levels of corticosteroids, and therefore, a ventral weight-bearing incision should be avoided. A retroperitoneal approach to adrenalectomy gives adequate exposure of the adrenal glands and avoids the problems associated with delayed wound healing.[1]

Surgical Considerations

Prevention of bleeding from adrenal vessels is a major part of the surgical procedure. The adrenal gland develops in a highly vascular area and can receive branches from the aorta as well as from the caudal phrenic, cranial abdominal, renal, celiac, and lumbar arteries. Hypervascularity associated with pathologic processes aggravates this situation. Hemostatic clips* are used as the sole means of achieving hemostasis in the adrenal vessels.

Hormonal therapy and fluid and electrolyte balance are extremely important before, during, and after adrenalectomy. The recommendations of Siegel can be followed.[2] In bilateral adrenalectomy, 1 to 2 mg desoxycorticosterone acetate (DOCA) is given once daily, and 25 to 50 mg cortisone acetate are given twice daily for 2 days prior to and on the morning of the operation. Hydrocortisone sodium succinate, 10 to 20 mg/kg, in electrolyte solution is infused slowly during the operation until the second adrenal gland is ligated, when the flow rate is increased. Additional hydrocortisone sodium succinate is given later in the same day. DOCA pellets for implantation, as recommended by Siegel, are no longer available, and therefore a substitute for this convenient long-term therapy is used. Dogs are usually maintained on oral doses of prednisolone and Fludrocortisone acetate. Salt is given in the food.

Surgical Approaches

For right adrenalectomy, the dog is placed in left lateral recumbency. When the right gland has been removed, all instruments are replaced, and the procedure is repeated on the left side.

The external landmarks for the surgical approach are readily determined. Dorsally, the epaxial muscles are palpated as a round mass extending longitudinally above the transverse processes of the lumbar vertebrae. Cranially, the thirteenth rib is palpated up to where it passes ventral to the epaxial muscles. The surgical approach is in the angle between the thirteenth rib and the epaxial muscles (Fig. 29-1).

An 8- to 10-cm skin incision is made parallel and 1 cm caudal to the thirteenth rib. The external abdominal oblique muscle and the underlying internal abdominal oblique muscle are split in the direction of their fibers. When the cranial abdominal artery is encountered, it is ligated and divided.

To enter the retroperitoneal space, a finger is inserted through the opening in the oblique muscles, in a slightly cranial and dorsal direction, in the angle between the thirteenth rib and the epaxial muscles. Only fatty tissue is encountered until the deeply lying transverse abdominal muscle is felt near its origin at the transverse processes of the lumbar vertebrae and the deepest division of the thoracolumbar fascia (Fig. 29-2). An opening is made bluntly in the transverse abdominal muscle; through this opening, the soft fatty tissue around the kidney is felt, and the adrenal gland is detected as a firm body in the mass of fatty tissue.

Soft, moistened abdominal sponges are inserted into the opening under the blades of malleable hand-held

*Hemoclips, Edward Weck & Co., Inc., Research Triangle Park, NC

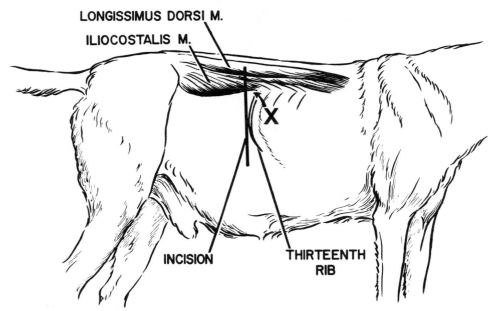

Fig. 29-1. *Site of the skin incision for adrenalectomy. The site for entry into the retroperitoneal space is indicated (X). (From Johnston, D.: Adrenalectomy via retroperitoneum in dogs. J. Am. Vet. Med. Assoc., 170:1092, 1977.)*

retractors. The width of the retractors varies with the size of the dog; however, they are either 2.5 or 5 cm wide. Three retractors are inserted: the first is placed in the craniodorsal angle, the second in the caudodorsal angle, and the third is ventral in position. The shape of the retractor blade is determined carefully, with particular emphasis on the size of the angle at the bend in the retractor and the length of the blade in the wound. It is necessary to ensure that the retractor blade extends to the depth of the adrenal gland, so that the fatty tissue is kept away from the adrenal gland. In addition, the ventral retractor forces the kidney ventrocaudally, so that the kidney and adrenal gland are drawn caudally and out from under the costal margin. The desired result of the retraction is the formation of a funnel, the base of which is a large opening at the level of the skin and the apex of which is a flat surface approximately 5 cm in diameter, with the adrenal gland in the center of the flat surface.

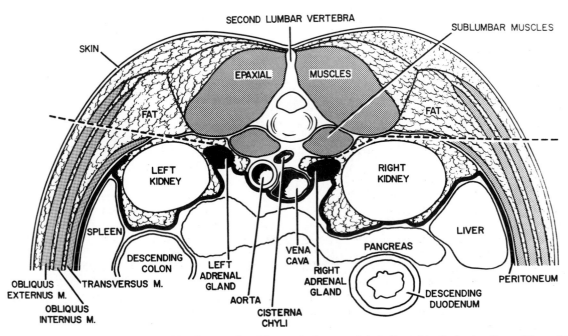

Fig. 29-2. *Cross-section of the dog at the second lumbar vertebra. The surgical approach is indicated by the broken lines. (From Johnston, D.: Adrenalectomy via retroperitoneum in dogs. J. Am. Vet. Med. Assoc., 170:1092, 1977.)*

RIGHT ADRENALECTOMY

From the veterinary surgeon's viewpoint, the right adrenal gland lies on top of the vena cava; the caudal phrenic vein, approximately 3 mm in diameter, lies in its upper surface in a cranioventral direction (Fig. 29-3).

Removal of the adrenal gland commences at the caudal pole. Using long scissors and forceps, the veterinarian separates the gland bluntly from the underlying vena cava. Tissue that cannot be separated bluntly is isolated into a pedicle; a small or medium-sized hemostatic clip is placed on the pedicle, which is divided between the clip and the gland. This dissection proceeds cranially while the adrenal gland is gently elevated, either with one blade of Tuttle's forceps used as a spoon, or by grasping the loose areolar tissue attached to the gland.

The caudal phrenic vein is isolated dorsal to the adrenal gland, that is, on the edge of the gland farthest from the vena cava. Two clips are applied to the vein, which is then divided between the clips (Fig. 29-4A). Dissection continues by blunt separation and by applying clips to pedicles until the junction of the caudal phrenic vein and vena cava is reached. Two clips are placed on the vein near the vena cava, and the vein is divided between the clips (Fig. 29-4B). The cranial pole of the gland is dissected from surrounding tissue. In most instances, a small opening is made in the peritoneum when the cranial pole of the gland is dissected free. If omentum protrudes through this opening before the dissection is completed, the opening is packed with a portion of gauze sponge soaked in saline solution.

LEFT ADRENALECTOMY

The left gland is removed in a similar manner. The dissection of this gland is easier than that of the right, inasmuch as the gland is situated more caudally and is not immediately adjacent to the vena cava. The method of blunt separation and application of hemostatic clips to pedicles is used.

References and Suggested Readings

1. Johnston, D. E.: Adrenalectomy via retroperitoneal approach in dogs. J. Am. Vet. Med. Assoc., *170*:1092, 1977.
2. Siegel, E. T.: Endocrine Diseases of the Dog. Philadelphia, Lea & Febiger, 1977.
3. Siegel, E. T., Kelly, D. E., and Berg, P.: Cushing's syndrome in the dog. J. Am. Vet. Med. Assoc., *157*:2081, 1970.
4. Usenik, E. A., and Arnold, J. P.: Bilateral adrenalectomy in the equine species. J. Am. Vet. Med. Assoc., *136*:19, 1960.

Thyroid Biopsy and Thyroidectomy

by ANTHONY P. BLACK *and* MARK E. PETERSON

Biopsy or surgical removal of the thyroid gland is indicated when a goiter, or enlargement of the thyroid, is detected during physical examination. Most goiters in

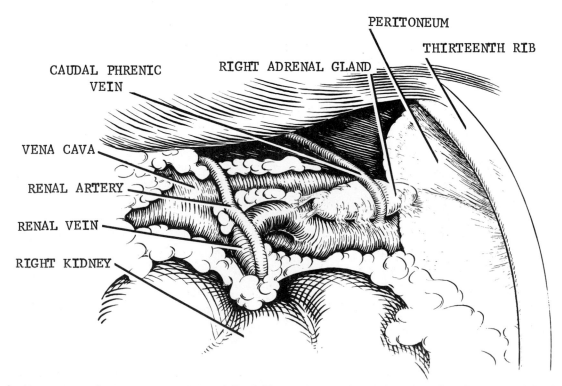

Fig. 29-3. *Veterinary surgeon's view of the right adrenal gland. The retractors and some fatty tissue have been omitted for clarity. (From Johnston, D.: Adrenalectomy via retroperitoneum in dogs. J. Am. Vet. Med. Assoc., 170:1092, 1977.)*

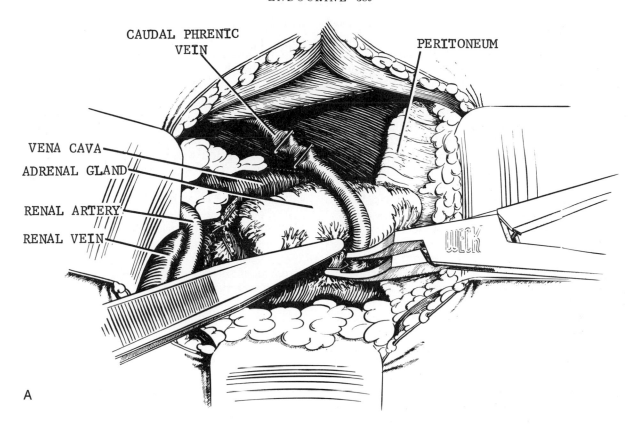

A

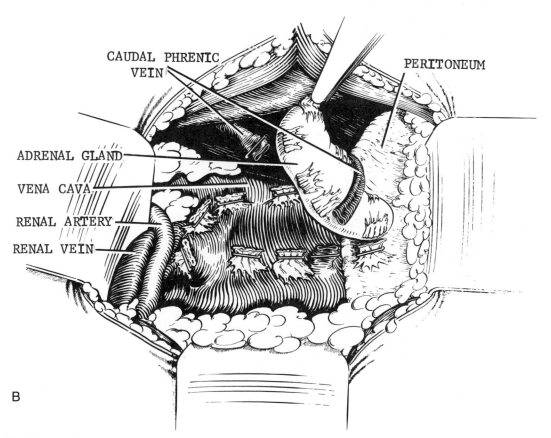

B

Fig. 29-4. A, *Clip being applied to a pedicle. The caudal phrenic vein is to be divided between the top two clips. Cloths under the retractor blades have been omitted for clarity. B, The adrenal gland is separated at the cranial pole by removing a small section of peritoneum. (From Johnston, D.: Adrenalectomy via retroperitoneum in dogs. J. Am. Vet. Med. Assoc., 170:1092, 1977.)*

veterinary practice are unilateral or bilateral thyroid neoplasms. Thyroid biopsy has also been advocated as a means of diagnosing canine hypothyroidism and of distinguishing between primary and secondary causes of thyroid hypofunction.

In the dog, most benign tumors of the thyroid are small and are unassociated with obvious clinical signs. They are not usually detected during life. Fifty to 80% of canine thyroid neoplasms are malignant.[4,6] Thyroid adenocarcinomas are characteristically large, locally invasive, rapidly growing tumors; distant metastasis occurs frequently. In advanced cases, dysphagia and respiratory distress may result from compression of the esophagus and the trachea. In approximately 20% of dogs with thyroid carcinoma, hypersecretion of thyroid hormones leads to signs of hyperthyroidism. Polydipsia and polyuria are the most frequent signs of hyperthyroidism in the dog. Weight loss, polyphagia, nervousness, weakness, and panting are also common clinical signs.

In the cat, most thyroid adenomas are small, are difficult to palpate, and are usually associated with signs of hyperthyroidism. Feline thyroid carcinomas, although rare, may also lead to hypersecretion of thyroid hormones. Weight loss is the most common sign of feline hyperthyroidism, followed by hyperexcitability, polyphagia, and tachycardia. In some cats, gastrointestinal disturbances, such as frequent defecation with the production of voluminous stools or frank diarrhea, may also occur. Polyuria and polydipsia are seen in only one-third of cats with hyperthyroidism.

Other thyroid tumors, such as medullary (C-cell) carcinomas and miscellaneous mesenchymal tumors, are extremely rare in the dog and have not been described in the cat.

Under normal circumstances, the thyroid gland is not palpable in the dog or cat. When attempting to palpate the canine or feline thyroid, the animal's neck should be slightly extended with the head tilted backward. Careful inspection using the thumb and index finger should be performed. One starts at the laryngeal area and progresses ventrally along both sides of the trachea to the thoracic inlet. Because the thyroid lobes in both the dog and cat are loosely attached to the trachea, the diseased lobe(s) frequently descends ventrally from its normal location adjacent to the larynx.

Thyroid surgical procedures are being performed more commonly in the dog and cat as a result of advances in the recognition and diagnosis of feline hyperthyroidism. Adjuvant therapy following operations for thyroid carcinoma is also feasible.

In this chapter, the basic principles and techniques of thyroid biopsy in the dog and cat and thyroidectomy in the cat are presented.

Thyroid Biopsy

Thyroid biopsy is indicated to confirm that a cervical mass is of thyroidal origin and to differentiate among thyroid adenoma, thyroid adenocarcinoma, medullary C-cell carcinoma, and colloid goiter. It is also indicated to confirm hypothyroidism in the dog and to distinguish between primary and secondary causes of thyroid hypofunction. Results of histopathologic examination allow the clinician to institute more definitive therapy with chemotherapeutic agents or radioactive iodine and to give a more accurate prognosis to the owner.

Two general methods are used in thyroid biopsy—open and closed. Closed thyroid biopsy is less invasive and is performed when the enlarged thyroid is easily immobilized. The highly vascular nature of most canine thyroid adenocarcinomas dictates that the closed rather than the open biopsy technique be used.

An open operation becomes necessary when the thyroid cannot be firmly grasped or when a closed biopsy fails to yield adequate tissue for cytologic or histologic analysis. An open biopsy is also performed if complete removal of the involved thyroid lobe is not possible during neck exploration.

In the cat, open biopsy is most commonly performed during surgical exploration of the thyroid for hyperthyroidism. If one thyroid lobe is definitely enlarged while the other lobe is equivocally abnormal in size, color, or location, hemithyroidectomy of the obviously abnormal lobe and biopsy of the suspicious lobe should be performed. Because biopsy results may demonstrate that no abnormalities are present, the procedure may prevent the necessity of lifelong thyroid hormone replacement therapy and reduces the incidence of hypoparathyroidism.

CLOSED BIOPSY TECHNIQUE

Three biopsy needles can be used to perform a closed thyroid biopsy: (1) fine needle, (2) Franklin-modified Vim-Silverman,* and (3) Vim Tru-Cut.†

The main advantage of fine-needle aspiration is its simplicity. Anesthesia is usually not required. The only instrumentation needed is a 20- to 22-gauge needle attached to a 12-ml syringe. With this technique, the needle is introduced into the thyroid mass, and the plunger is retracted to create a vacuum in the syringe. Repeated, vigorous suction of short duration is applied while the needle is moved back and forth in different directions. When the plunger has been released to eliminate the vacuum, the needle is withdrawn from the thyroid, and the aspirate is spread on glass slides with the same technique as for standard blood films. The smear is air-dried and is stained for cytologic examination. The main disadvantage of fine-needle aspiration is that it provides essentially no information concerning the structural architecture of tissues. Therefore, it may be difficult using this technique to distinguish between benign and malignant tumors.

The technique for performing a closed thyroid biopsy with either a Franklin-modified Vim-Silverman or a Vim Tru-Cut needle is basically the same, but it requires general anesthesia or heavy tranquilization. An area over the mass is surgically prepared and is draped,

*American V. Mueller, 6600 Touhy Avenue, Chicago, IL 60648
†Baxter Laboratories, Morton Grove, IL

and a small skin nick is made on the ventrolateral margin of enlargement. The Franklin-modified Vim-Silverman biopsy needle, with the stylet in place, is inserted through the skin incision into the thyroid mass in a direction parallel to the lateral side of the trachea. The stylet is then withdrawn and is replaced with the cutting prongs, which are advanced into the thyroid mass. The outer cannula of the Franklin-modified Vim-Silverman needle is then moved forward so as to cut the tissue next to the cutting prongs. A core of tissue suitable for examination should be obtained as the cutting prongs and outer cannula are withdrawn as a unit. Additional plugs of tissue may be obtained if needed. Firm digital pressure is immediately applied over the biopsy site until hemostasis is achieved. The small skin incision is closed with one suture.

When using the Vim Tru-Cut biopsy needle, the needle unit is advanced into the cervical mass, with the obturator specimen rod retracted within the outer cannula of the needle. The obturator specimen rod is then advanced into the mass without moving the outer cannula. While keeping the obturator specimen rod stationary, the outer cannula is next advanced over the specimen rod, and the biopsy is withdrawn.

The major advantage of the Franklin-modified Vim-Silverman or the Vim Tru-Cut needle is that the piece of tissue obtained from the thyroid parenchyma is suitable for histologic examination, as opposed to fine-needle aspiration, in which a smear is made of the aspirate for cytologic examination only. Therefore, more information is gained from the large-bore, closed-needle biopsy.

OPEN BIOPSY TECHNIQUE

The two thyroid lobes of the dog and cat are located on either side of the trachea. They extend from just below the level of the cricoid cartilage to the fifth or sixth tracheal ring. In dogs with hypothyroidism, the thyroid gland lies in the normal location, but it is reduced in size. In the dog with thyroid neoplasia, the affected lobe or lobes are enlarged and may have descended caudoventrally from their normal location.

In the dog, the thyroid lobes are bounded dorsolaterally by the common carotid artery and the vagosympathetic trunk. The right recurrent laryngeal nerve passes along the dorsal aspect of the right thyroid lobe. The sternocephalicus and sternohyoideus muscles are located immediately lateral to each lobe while the sternothyroideus covers each lobe on its ventral surface. The major blood vessels that supply the canine thyroid gland are the cranial and caudal thyroid arteries and veins.

Two parathyroid glands are usually associated with each thyroid lobe. The "external" parathyroid gland normally lies on the cranial, dorsolateral surface of the thyroid and is superficial to the capsule of the lobe. This parathyroid gland is readily visible. In most dogs, the "internal" parathyroid glands are situated within the thyroid parenchyma and therefore cannot usually be visualized during surgical procedures.

To perform an open thyroid biopsy, the dog is anesthetized, an endotracheal tube is placed, and the dog is positioned in dorsal recumbency. A ventral midline skin incision is extended from the cranial larynx to a midpoint between the larynx and the thoracic inlet. The trachea is exposed by midline dissection between the sternohyoideus muscles. The sternothyroideus muscles should next be located by lateral retraction of the sternohyoideus muscles. The dorsomedial surface of the sternothyroideus muscle is exposed by gentle retraction and reveals the thyroid lobes. The use of self-retaining or hand-held retractors facilitates further dissection. Care must be taken not to injure the carotid sheath, the esophagus, the recurrent laryngeal nerves, or other vital structures by faulty positioning of retractor blades.

The biopsy specimen should be taken from the caudal aspect of the gland. This region of the gland is the least vascular and preserves the external parathyroid gland. The caudal thyroid artery and vein, which exit from the caudal pole of the lobe, are identified, are ligated, and are transected. If the lobe is small, gentle blunt dissection around the caudal pole of the lobe enables a suture of polyglycolic acid,[*] polyglactin 910,[†] or silk to be placed around its caudal tip. Tightening of this cutting suture partially amputates the gland, achieves hemostasis, and allows the biopsy tissue to be removed with a scalpel blade (Fig. 29-5).

If the cutting suture is unsuccessful, or if the thyroid capsule is grossly thickened, a wedge biopsy of the same area can be performed. Hemorrhage is controlled either with digital pressure or with a deep, horizontal mattress suture. The fascia of the sternohyoideus muscles and the subcutaneous tissue are approximated with absorbable suture material in a simple interrupted or a continuous pattern. The skin is closed routinely.

In the cat, the general technique for open biopsy of the thyroid is similar to that in the dog. Biopsy of a suspicious thyroid lobe in the cat is usually performed in conjunction with surgical removal of the opposite lobe, which is greatly enlarged as a result of tumor. The surgical anatomy of the feline thyroid gland is described in the discussion of the technique for thyroidectomy.

Thyroidectomy in the Dog and Cat

Complete surgical removal of the affected thyroid lobe or lobes is the treatment of choice in most animals with thyroid tumors. If an enlarged thyroid gland is palpated, thyroid hormone levels should be determined to ascertain the thyroid status of the animal. Dogs with thyroid tumors may have normal, elevated, or decreased levels of thyroxine. Hypothyroidism usually results from extensive infiltration of normal thyroid tissue with nonfunctional tumor. Almost all cats with detectable thyroid tumors have elevated thyroid hormone levels. If hypothyroidism or hyperthyroidism is present,

*Dexon, Davis & Geck, Inc., Manati, PR 00701
†Vicryl, Ethicon, Inc., Somerville, NJ 08876

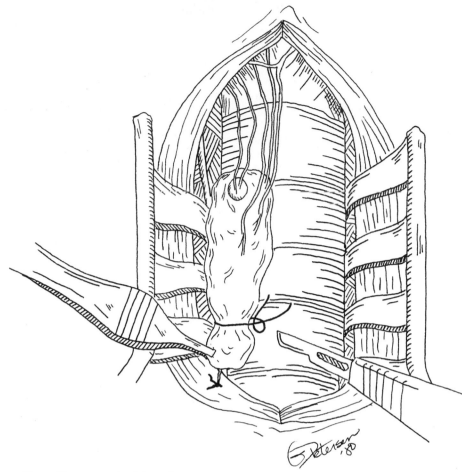

Fig. 29-5. *Open biopsy. The cutting suture is tightened around the caudal aspect of the gland. The partially amputated biopsy tissue is incised caudal to the ligature.*

it is prudent to return the animal to a euthyroid state before thyroidectomy is attempted.

In the cat, thyroidectomy is usually accomplished with ease. Total resection of most canine thyroid neoplasms is difficult, however, owing to their highly malignant and locally invasive behavior. If the canine thyroid carcinoma cannot be completely surgically removed, chemotherapy or radioactive iodine therapy may be instituted, but most dogs either die or are subject to euthanasia as a result of the disease. Therefore, only the technique for thyroidectomy in the cat is discussed here.

SURGICAL TECHNIQUE IN THE CAT

Preoperative Treatment

Most cats requiring hemi- or total thyroidectomy are hyperthyroid as a result of either a benign functional thyroid tumor or adenomatous hyperplasia. Surgical removal of one or both thyroid lobes effectively corrects the hyperthyroid state in these cats. Although the procedure for correcting it is simple, hyperthyroidism is a systemic illness with a profound effect on several body systems. Cardiovascular, gastrointestinal, he-

patic, and neuromuscular functions may all be seriously compromised.

To prepare cats with hyperthyroidism for surgical procedures, we prefer to administer propranolol,* and a saturated solution of potassium iodide, or propylthiouracil to mitigate the metabolic and cardiovascular complications associated with hyperthyroidism. Propranolol may be administered in doses of 2.5 mg tid for 7 to 14 days prior to operation. The elevated thyroid hormone levels remain unchanged while the cat is being treated with propranolol, but the drug acts to block the peripheral effects of toxic levels of circulating thyroid hormones. The result is an attenuation of the tachycardia and hyperexcitability commonly observed in hyperthyroid cats. This potent myocardial depressant should be used with extreme caution if cardiac failure is present. Congestive heart failure should be controlled with digitalis and furosemide in conjunction with propranolol. The apparent ineffectiveness of propranolol in some cats is probably related to the highly variable circulating propranolol levels observed in hyperthyroidism. Plasma propranolol levels are decreased in humans with hyperthyroidism; thus, dosage

* Inderal, Ayerst Laboratories, 685 Third Avenue, New York, NY 10017

schedules based on observations in euthyroid animals may not be applicable to some hyperthyroid cats.[10]

A saturated solution of potassium iodide may also be used alone or in combination with propranolol. Administration of this potassium iodide solution should begin 7 to 14 days preoperatively in doses of 2 to 3 drops per day. This solution acts to block the release of thyroid hormone from the thyroid gland. In most cats, the administration of saturated solution of potassium iodide causes thyroid hormone levels to decrease within a 2-week period. The major disadvantage of this agent is the unpleasant, brassy taste of iodine, which results in excessive salivation and partial-to-complete anorexia in some cats.

Propylthiouracil is a valuable and effective pharmocologic agent in the preoperative preparation of a hyperthyroid cat. This agent acts to block thyroid hormone synthesis and thereby lowers thyroid hormone concentrations. By administering propylthiouracil in doses of 50 mg tid, most hyperthyroid cats return to a euthyroid state within 1 to 2 weeks. Most systemic problems are resolved in 2 to 4 weeks, and intraoperative complications are thus minimized.

Anesthesia

It is extremely important to recognize that cats with hyperthyroidism have an increased metabolic rate. Therefore, the absorption, distribution, tissue uptake, and metabolism of an anesthetic agent may be more rapid than normal. In addition, most cats with hyperthyroidism have moderate-to-severe weight loss. All cats should be weighed before a surgical procedure, so that accurate drug dosages can be precalculated. It is also imperative to titrate carefully the doses of all drugs used.

Many anesthetic regimens are successful. Premedication with acepromazine, given intramuscularly in a dose of 0.1 mg/kg, reduces the autonomic manifestations of hyperthyroidism, in addition to causing sedation. Anticholinergic agents such as atropine are usually omitted because they cause sinus tachycardia and are known to enhance anesthetic-induced cardiac arrhythmias. Ketamine hydrochloride, given intramuscularly in a dose of 5 mg/kg, is both safe and effective in inducing anesthesia in cats, although barbiturates such as thiamylal sodium can be used for induction of anesthesia. After induction with either thiamylal sodium or ketamine, an endotracheal tube should be placed, and anesthesia maintained with nitrous oxide and oxygen. Halothane or methoxyflurane may also be administered, if required, to maintain an adequate plane of anesthesia.

Whatever anesthetic regimen is used, the cat must be carefully monitored. In addition to an esophageal stethoscope, an electrocardiogram is mandatory because many cats with hyperthyroidism have cardiac disease associated with arrhythmias. The most common cause of surgical mortality during thyroidectomy is cardiac dysrhythmias.

Surgical Anatomy

The normal thyroid lobes in the cat are approximately 2 cm long, 0.5 cm thick, and 0.3 cm wide. They are light brownish yellow in color and are usually oval in shape. A fibrous capsule surrounds each lobe, which lies within the cervical fascia between the sternothyroideus muscle and the trachea. Dorsally, the lobes are in close proximity to the carotid sheath and the vagosympathetic trunk. The right recurrent laryngeal nerve is medial to the gland and courses along the trachea's right dorsolateral surface. The left recurrent laryngeal nerve lies between the trachea and the esophagus.

The caudal thyroid vein leaves the caudal pole of the gland as a single vessel; the caudal thyroid artery is usually not present in the cat.[7] The cranial thyroid artery and vein form multiple branches at the cranial pole of each lobe. The external parathyroid glands are located near the cranial pole of each thyroid lobe external to the thyroid capsule. They are pink, approximately spherical, and vary in size from 3 to 7 mm. The branching cranial thyroid vessels lie along the dorsal aspect of the glands. The internal parathyroid glands are more variable in location, although they commonly lie within the parenchyma of the caudal pole of each lobe. They arc rarely visible at the time of operation. Accessory thyroid and parathyroid tissue and embryonic remnants may also be found in the neck and the thorax.[7]

Unilateral Thyroidectomy and Parathyroidectomy

Using the previously described approach, the mobile, enlarged thyroid lobe is moved to the center of the incision. The cranial and caudal thyroid vessels are ligated and are transected (Fig. 29-6). Dissection through the loose cervical fascia surrounding the gland with fine Metzenbaum scissors allows for removal of the mass. The fascia of the sternohyoideus muscles and the subcutaneous tissue are closed separately using 3-0 absorbable suture material in a simple interrupted or a continuous pattern. The skin is closed routinely.

Bilateral Thyroidectomy

This procedure is indicated when both thyroid lobes are palpably enlarged or are obviously abnormal at surgical exploration. If one lobe is unquestionably enlarged while the other lobe is equivocally abnormal, the definitely abnormal and enlarged lobe should be removed by intracapsular dissection, and the external parathyroid gland should be preserved. The questionable lobe may be removed in a similar manner, or a biopsy may be performed on it, as described in our discussion of the open biopsy technique.

The surgical approach is the same as for unilateral thyroidectomy and parathyroidectomy. After exposure and inspection of both thyroid lobes, the external parathyroid gland of each lobe is identified. It is imperative that hemostasis be maintained throughout the proce-

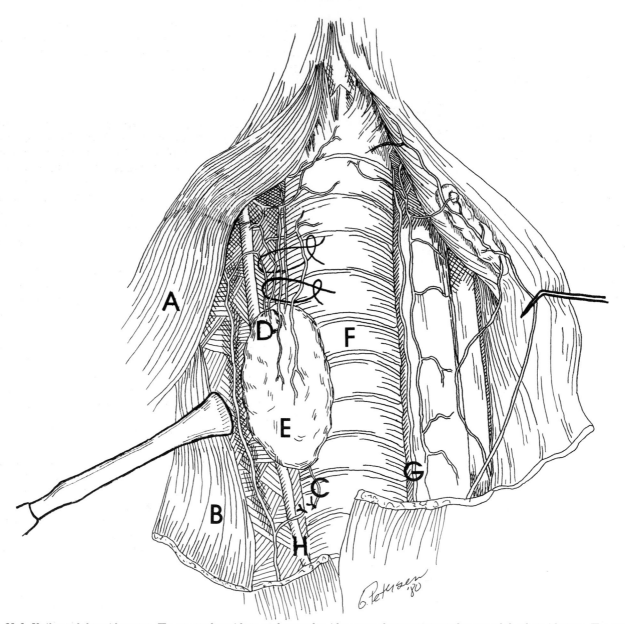

Fig. 29-6. *Unilateral thyroidectomy. The sternothyroideus and sternohyoideus muscles are retracted to reveal the thyroid mass. The cranial and caudal vessels are ligated and transected between ligatures. A, Sternohyoideus muscle; B, sternothyroideus muscle; C, caudal thyroid vein; D, external parathyroid gland; E, thyroid gland; F, trachea; G, recurrent laryngeal nerve; H, external carotid artery.*

dure to ensure continuous visualization of the external parathyroid glands. If extensive hemorrhage occurs within the fascia of the cranial pole of the thyroid lobe, identification of the external parathyroids will be difficult. Care is also taken to visualize and to avoid the recurrent laryngeal nerves.

The caudal thyroid vein of one lobe is ligated and transected as it leaves the lobe. The least vascular area of the thyroid capsule near the caudal portion of the lobe is incised with a scalpel. The incision is enlarged with fine scissors, and the parenchyma is bluntly dissected away from the capsule wall (Fig. 29-7A). A sterile, cotton-tipped applicator may be used to move the parenchyma away from the capsule (Fig. 29-7B). This

dissection avoids traumatizing the parenchyma. When the caudal pole has been dissected free, one moves cranially using the cotton applicator to separate the capsule and the external parathyroid gland from the thyroid gland. The glandular tissue is then removed, leaving the external parathyroid gland and thyroid capsule in situ with the cranial thyroid vessels intact. Occasionally, a portion of the thyroid parenchyma breaks free and causes minor hemorrhage. This bleeding is controlled by digital pressure. The procedure is repeated for the opposite lobe.

If the external parathyroid glands are visualized, but cannot be preserved on a vascular pedicle during dissection, an attempt may be made to dissect them free

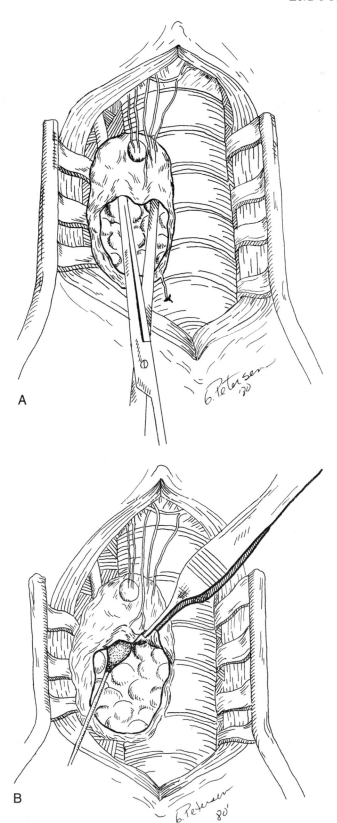

Fig. 29-7. *Bilateral thyroidectomy. A, The thyroid capsule has been incised, and fine Metzenbaum scissors are used to further dissect the parenchyma from the capsule. The caudal thyroid vein is ligated. B, The use of a cotton-tipped applicator facilitates blunt dissection of the parenchyma from the capsule.*

and to transplant them into a muscular pouch. This technique has been successful in the prevention of postoperative hypocalcemia in the dog.[12] Closure is as previously described.

Postoperative Care

Our feline patients have become euthyroid within 48 hours postoperatively if removal of all involved tissue has been complete. If a total thyroidectomy has been performed, replacement therapy, using thyroxine at a dose of 0.1 mg bid, should be instituted. If a hemithyroidectomy has been performed, most cats do not require thyroxine supplementation, although the majority have thyroid hormone levels in the hypothyroid range for 2 to 3 months postoperatively. If severe lethargy, anorexia, or weakness develops soon after the removal of one thyroid lobe, thyroxine therapy should be initiated and should be continued for 2 to 3 months.

Potential complications following thyroidectomy include hypoparathyroidism, Horner's syndrome, vocal cord paralysis, and wound infection. The most serious complication is profound hypolcalcemia, which occurs secondarily to a loss of parathormone if the glandular tissue has been devascularized or inadvertently removed in the course of thyroidectomy. After total thyroidectomy, the patient's serum calcium level should be monitored on a daily basis, because mild hypocalcemia is common after removal of both thyroid lobes. Although mild hypocalcemia does not itself require therapy, overt hypoparathyroidism and severe hypocalcemia cause severe depression that progresses to tetany or convulsions. Sudden signs of hypocalcemia require immediate administration of calcium (1½ ml/kg body weight of 10% calcium gluconate) by slow intravenous injection. Subsequent calcium administration should be both oral and by slow, intravenous infusion of calcium gluconate in saline solution. Vitamin D (calciferol) or dihydrotachysterol may also be added to the patient's food if oral calcium alone is not sufficient to maintain normal serum calcium values. Some cats require calcium and vitamin D supplementation for a few days only, whereas others may require it for several weeks. In most cases, the vitamin D and calcium supplementation is ultimately stopped.

Cats in which only one lobe is removed should have thyroid hormone values determined at 6-month intervals, to ensure that the remaining lobe is functionally normal and that hyperthyroidism does not recur.

References and Suggested Readings

1. Edis, A. J.: Prevention and management of complications associated with thyroid and parathyroid surgery. Surg. Clin. North Am., *59*:83, 1979.
2. Feek, C. M., et al.: Combination of potassium iodide and propranolol in preparation of patients with Grave's disease for thyroid surgery. N. Engl. J. Med., *302*:883, 1980.
3. Holzworth, J., et al.: Hyperthyroidism in the cat: ten cases. J. Am. Vet. Med. Assoc., *176*:345, 1980.

4. Leav, I., et al.: Adenomas and carcinomas of the canine and feline thyroid. Am. J. Pathol., *83:*61, 1976.

5. Lowhagen, T., et al.: Aspiration biopsy cytology (ABC) in nodules of the thyroid gland suspected to be malignant. Surg. Clin. North Am., *59:*3, 1979.

6. Mitchell, M., Hurov, L. I., and Troy, G. C.: Canine thyroid carinomas: clinical occurrence staging by means of scintiscans, and therapy of 15 cases. Vet. Surg., *8:*112, 1979.

7. Nicholas, J. S., and Swingle, W. W.: An experimental and morphological study of the parathyroid glands of the cat. Am. J. Anat., *34:*469, 1933.

8. Osborne, C. A.: General principles of biopsy. Vet. Clin. North Am., *4:*213, 1974.

9. Peterson, M. E., et al.: Spontaneous feline hyperthyroidism. *In* Program of the 62nd Annual Meeting of the Endocrine Society, June 1980.

10. Rubenfeld, S., et al.: Variable plasma propranolol levels in thyrotoxicosis. N. Engl. J. Med., *300:*353, 1979.

11. Stenling, L. C.: Anesthetic management of the patient with hyperthyroidism. Anesthesiology, *41:*585, 1974.

12. Wells, S. A., et al.: Transplantation of the parathyroid glands in dogs. Transplantation, *15:*179, 1973.

30 * Hernias

Umbilical Hernia

by M. Joseph Bojrab

and William J. Taylor

Etiopathogenesis

Umbilical hernias, while they usually occur randomly, may show a breed and familial risk.[1,3,4] The incidence of occurrence is low in the domestic cat, but a high incidence of the disorder has been reported in a family of Cornish rex cats.[4] The incidence is sporadic, with occasional concentration, in other feline families. The breeds of dogs showing a high risk of umbilical herniation include the Airedale terrier, basenji, Pekingese, pointer, and weimaraner.[3] The explanations put forward include single or multiple, dominant or recessive genetic traits, and in one study, mutation in the germinal tract was cited.[4] The degree of sex predilection varies from study to study: in one study, males and females were equally affected; in another, 20 males were affected to each female; and in another study, twice as many females as males were affected.[1,3]

Congenital umbilical hernias result from a failure of proper closure of the umbilical ring or from maldevelopment or hypoplasia of the abdominal rectus abdominis muscle and the aponeurosis of the two abdominal oblique muscles. Both causes allow for an opening in the musculature and fascia of the abdominal wall with an outpouching of the peritoneum. The acquired umbilical hernia may occur following the incision of the umbilical cord too close to the abdominal wall either by the bitch, the owner, or the veterinarian. This hernia may result in evisceration of the abdominal contents.

Clinical Signs

An umbilical hernia consists of the protrusion of abdominal contents through the open umbilicus. This protrusion may contain omentum, falciform fat, or any abdominal organ. The abdominal viscera are usually contained within a peritoneal sac. The layers of an umbilical hernia are usually skin, subcutaneous tissue, and peritoneum; however, in the case of an umbilical cord hernia, as described, the viscera pass through the abdominal wall without being covered by peritoneum.

Although an umbilical hernia is easier to diagnose than a ventral abdominal hernia, it must be differentiated from an abscess, from cellulitis, and from a subcutaneous or a dermal mass because of its location. The contents of the hernial sac may resist reduction, but if reduction can be accomplished, identification of the edges of the hernial ring is possible. The palpation of a small, firm mass is consistent with the presence of omentum or faliciform ligament and fat. A larger mass may be indicative of small intestine; if incarcerated, the gut will be swollen, painful, and often irreducible.

Ancillary tests may be performed to substantiate the diagnosis of an umbilical hernia. These tests are often unnecessary because the location and physical characteristics of the ring and contents are diagnostic.

Surgical Treatment

Although a surgical procedure is the most common method of treatment, spontaneous correction may occur. A small, open umbilical ring may contract in size as the animal grows and may remain as a small imperfection of the abdominal wall. In the female, a persistent small umbilical hernia may be left until an ovariohysterectomy is performed, when the hernia is also corrected.

Prompt surgical correction is necessary for a large hernia, particularly if a loop of incarcerated bowel is present in the hernial sac, or when the abdominal wall is imperfect in its development as with hypoplastic muscular and fascial development.

The size of the hernial sac determines the type of skin incision made. A single incision over the hernial sac or ring, extending slightly beyond its cranial and caudal edges, is used for the small umbilical hernia. When the hernial sac is large and excessive skin is present, an elliptical incision is made on either side of the sac (Fig. 30-1A). The incisions should be of sufficient length to allow for a length-to-width incision ratio of 4:1, thus allowing proper cosmetic skin closure.

When the animal is in dorsal recumbency, the hernial sac may reduce itself, and thus the peritoneal sac may

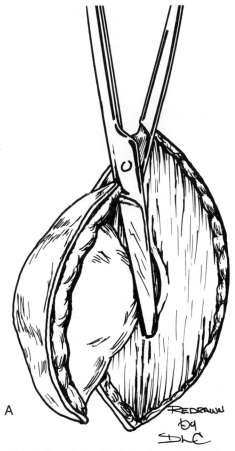

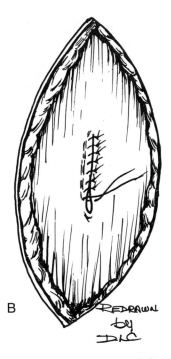

Fig. 30-1. A, *An elliptical incision for repair of a large umbilical hernia. The redundant skin overlying the hernial sac is removed along with the hernial sac.* B, *Closure of abdominal wall after hernial sac removal. (Redrawn from Archibald, J., and Sumner-Smith, G.: Abdomen.* In *Canine Surgery. 2nd Ed. Edited by J. Archibald. Santa Barbara, CA, American Veterinary Publications, 1974.)*

be invaginated and may not be apparent. In this case, the hernial ring can be closed without entering the peritoneal cavity. A large hernia may have attachments from the peritoneum to the subcutaneous tissue and skin, as well as internally from the peritoneum to the abdominal viscera. In these cases, it is necessary to isolate the peritoneum from its attachments. If this isolation is done, an "open reduction" is performed by removing the peritoneal tissue making up the hernial sac.

Closure of the open repair is performed with size 2-0 or 3-0 synthetic absorbable in a simple interrupted suture pattern (Fig. 30-1B).

It is rarely necessary to imbricate or to use a synthetic implant in closure of umbilical hernias. Correction of a large hernia in a medium-to-giant breed of animal may require stainless steel sutures. Congenital hypoplasia of abdominal fascia and muscle may require the use of a mesh implant to provide support and a framework for healing (Fig. 30-2).

When apposed, the large hernial ring may place excessive tension on the suture line. In such a case, two procedures may be performed. The first is bilateral release by incision of the fascia of the rectus abdominis muscle (Fig. 30-3). It is important to incise only the rectus fascia and not the deeper muscle and fascia, in order to avoid an iatrogenic hernia.[2] The second method involves placement of several large mattress tension sutures through abdominal muscle fascia several centimeters lateral to the suture line, using synthetic absorbable suture material.

Postoperative Care

It is best to restrict the movement of the patient for a week postoperatively. This period may be extended, depending upon the size and the extent of hernial repair. Education of the client is important in the early detection of dehiscence, recurrence, or infection.

References and Suggested Readings

1. Angus, K., and Young, G. B.: A note on the genetics of umbilical hernia. Vet. Rec., *90*:245, 1972.
2. Archibald, J., and Sumner-Smith, G.: Abdomen. *In* Canine Surgery. 2nd Ed. Edited by J. Archibald. Santa Barbara, CA, American Veterinary Publications, 1974.

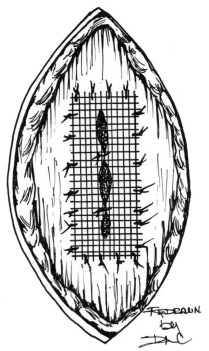

Fig. 30-2. *Mesh implant helps to provide support and a framework for healing in congenital hypoplastic hernia. (Redrawn from Archibald, J., and Sumner-Smith, G.: Abdomen. In Canine Surgery. 2nd Ed. Edited by J. Archibald. Santa Barbara, CA, American Veterinary Publications, 1974.)*

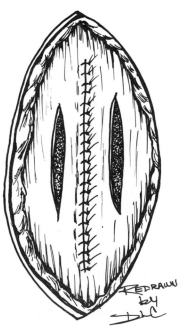

Fig. 30-3. *Relieving incisions in the rectal fascia help to decrease suture line tension in large umbilical hernia repairs. (Redrawn from Archibald, J., and Sumner-Smith, G.: Abdomen. In Canine Surgery. 2nd Ed. Edited by J. Archibald. Santa Barbara, CA, American Veterinary Publications, 1974.)*

3. Hayes, H. M.: Congenital umbilical and inguinal hernias in cattle, horses, swine, dogs and cats: risk by breed and sex among hospital patients. Am. J. Vet. Res., *35*:839, 1974.
4. Robinson, R.: Genetic aspects of umbilical hernia incidence in cats and dogs. Vet. Rec., *100*:9, 1977.

Inguinal Hernias

by M. JOSEPH BOJRAB

Etiology

Herniation in the inguinal region is a common condition in the bitch, but has been reported only rarely in cats and male dogs.[1,3,4] When present in the male, it may progress to an inguinoscrotal hernia. Most afflicted animals probably have a structural predisposition and possibly a hereditary basis for the disease.[1,2,4]

Inguinal hernias are classified anatomically as either direct or indirect. Direct herniation is a separate outpocketing of peritoneum through the inguinal canal not involving the vaginal process. Indirect herniation is a protrusion of abdominal contents into the vaginal process and is the most common type found in domestic animals.[2,3]

Over a period of time, small hernias may be enlarged by various stresses such as pregnancy, obesity, mammary tumors, and occasionally trauma.[1,5] Increased abdominal pressure may account for the higher incidence of this disorder in pregnant bitches.

Anatomic Considerations

Structural defects in the inguinal region tend to predispose an animal to herniation. Although the size of the external inguinal ring varies little from animal to animal, the size of the internal inguinal ring may be different, depending on the caudal extent of the internal abdominal oblique muscle. In those animals in which the caudal edge of the muscle does not extend past the cranial edge of the external inguinal ring, the inguinal canal is virtually nonexistent. This leaves a defect in the abdominal floor directly over the external inguinal ring.[2]

The vaginal process, which, other than the external pudendal vessels and genital nerve, is the major structure to traverse the inguinal canal, is an evagination of the peritoneum containing spermatic cord in the male and round ligament of the uterus in the female. In the male, the vaginal process continues caudally on each side to the scrotum ending with the testes. In the female, it may extend as far caudally as the vulva.

The vaginal cavity, the space between the peritoneal covering of the process and its contents, communicates with the peritoneal cavity by a slit-like orifice at the origin of the vaginal process. In an indirect herniation, the viscera enter the cavity of the vaginal process through this orifice. The round ligament is probably responsible for directing the uterine horn or the uterus into the vaginal process during herniation. The vaginal

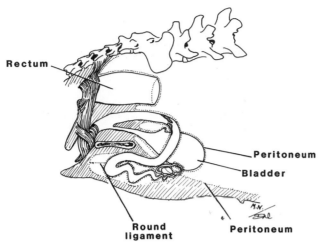

Fig. 30-4. *Diagram of uterus and ovary in an inguinal hernia. (Modified from Evans, H. E., and Christensen, G. C.: Miller's Anatomy of the Dog. 2nd Ed. Philadelphia, W. B. Saunders, 1979.)*

process forms the hernial sac with the viscera lying alongside the round ligament or spermatic cord (Fig. 30-4). Enlargement of the vaginal orifice is probably an important predisposing factor in herniation.[2,5]

Diagnosis

The majority of inguinal hernias are soft, doughy, unilateral swellings that are painless on palpation. Although most are located in the inguinal region, it is possible for the contents to migrate caudally and to lie lateral to the vulva, thereby resembling a perineal hernia.[1] Careful palpation may reveal bilateral involvement.

The size and consistency of the swelling depend on the hernial contents and the length of time the hernia has been present. A gravid or diseased uterus is a common finding, but intestine, omentum, or bladder may also be involved.[1,3,5] The uterus usually herniates during the progestational phase of estrus because of increased laxity of the support structures of the genital tract at that time. In some animals, the swelling may be so minor as to be obscured by the caudal mammary glands.

If easily reducible, the hernial ring may be palpated, and diagnosis may be simplified. Reducing pressure in the caudal abdomen by elevating the hind quarters while the animal is in dorsal recumbency may aid in identification. Irreducible hernias may be caused by strangulation of an organ, retention of urine in the bladder, or growth of fetuses in the uterus after herniation. In these instances, diagnosis becomes more difficult, and the swelling must be differentiated from a mammary tumor, an abscess, or a hematoma. An irreducible swelling may also be due to the deposition of fat around the round ligament that enlarges the vaginal process in the absence of herniation.

When the diagnosis is in question, radiography may be helpful. A gravid uterus appears as a lobulated fluid density, with fetal skeletons if gestation is of sufficient

duration. Contrast studies of the gastrointestinal or urinary systems are useful in some cases.

Surgical Correction

A ventral midline incision can be used for all inguinal hernias. This approach allows visualization of both inguinal rings and repair of bilateral herniation through a single incision. It also permits extension of the incision cranially, when necessary, without invasion of mammary tissue or its blood supply.[4]

The surgical incision extends from the cranial brim of the pelvis cranially as far as necessary to allow exposure of the hernial sac (Fig. 30-5A). This incision is continued through the subcutaneous tissue down to the ventral rectus sheath. The mammary tissue is undermined and is retracted laterally to expose the inguinal ring and hernial sac; this sac is bluntly dissected from the subcutaneous tissue (Fig. 30-5B). The hernial sac is then opened, and its contents are inspected. Any adhesions between the sac and the viscera are broken down, and the contents are then returned to the abdominal cavity (Fig. 30-5C).

In some cases, it may be necessary to enlarge the hernial ring cranially to facilitate reduction of the hernia. If the urinary bladder is included in the hernia, aspiration of urine simplifies reduction. When one or both horns of the uterus are included and ovariohysterectomy is necessary or desired, the incision may need to be extended in a cranial and medial direction as far as necessary to complete the procedure.[1,4]

On replacement of viscera to the abdomen, the redundant sac is trimmed at the margins of the inguinal ring, and the hernial ring is sutured with simple interrupted sutures of 2-0 stainless steel (Fig. 30-5D). Care must be taken during closure to avoid the external pudendal vessels and nerves, which exit from the caudomedial aspect of the ring.

The inguinal ring on the other side is inspected, the vaginal process is removed, and the ring is sutured closed. The mammary tissue is then drawn back to the midline, and a Penrose drain is positioned. The skin is closed in a routine manner.

Postoperative Care

The caudal abdomen is bandaged immediately after the procedure; one must allow space for drainage. Bandaging helps to eliminate dead space and increases the comfort of the patient. The Penrose drains are removed 3 to 5 days postsurgically, prior to the patient's discharge from the hospital.

References and Suggested Readings

1. Archibald, J., and Sumner-Smith, G.: Hernia. *In* Canine Surgery. 2nd Ed. Edited by J. Archibald. Santa Barbara, CA, American Veterinary Publications, 1974.
2. Ashdown, R. R.: The anatomy of the inguinal canal in the domesticated mammals. Vet. Rec., 75:1345, 1963.

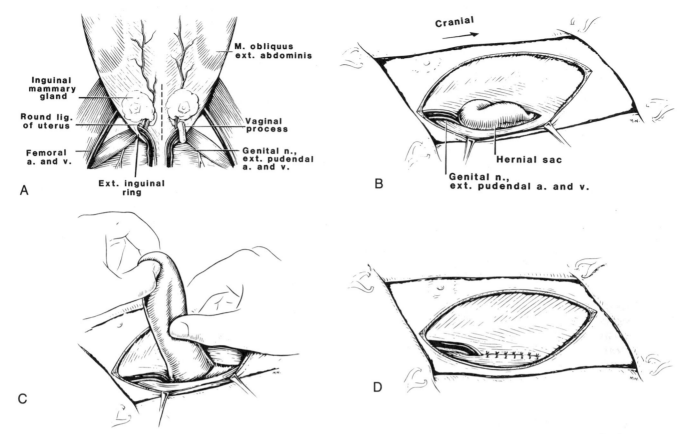

Fig. 30-5. A, *Diagram of vaginal process through inguinal ring. Dashed line indicates midline incision site for inguinal hernia repair.* B, *Exposed inguinal area showing vaginal process containing hernial contents. Note pudendal vessels and nerve.* C, *Vaginal process is dissected and freed.* D, *The inguinal ring is sutured. (From Leonard, E. P.: Fundamentals of Small Animal Surgery. Philadelphia, W. B. Saunders, 1968.)*

3. Grier, R. L., Hoskin, J. D., and Whalstrom, J. D.: Inguinal hernia and Richter's hernia in a dog. J. Am. Vet. Med. Assoc., *159*:181, 1971.
4. Worth, A. F.: A new surgical approach to inguinal hernia in the dog. Cornell Vet., *49*:379, 1959.
5. Wright, J. G.: The surgery of the inguinal canal in animals. Vet. Rec., 75:1352, 1963.

Perineal Hernia

by M. Joseph Bojrab

and Amelia A. Toomey

Perineal hernia has long been recognized as a disease of older intact male dogs. The peak incidence is approximately 8 years of age.

Etiology

Many factors have been incriminated in the etiopathogenesis of this disease. Suggested theories include congenital predisposition, structural weakness of the pelvic diaphragm, hormonal imbalance, and chronic constipation. Because firm evidence to support any one of these theories does not exist, the origin of this disorder probably involves a combination of contributing factors.

Most authors agree that the exceptionally strong predisposition among sexually intact males suggests that hormonal influences play an important role in the development of this condition. Several theories have been advanced to explain this role, but as yet no evidence conclusively links hormonal factors to maintenance of pelvic diaphragm integrity.

Several authors have suggested an association between prostatic enlargement and the development of perineal hernias.[1,9] Prostatic enlargement secondary to an imbalance of sexual hormones is a common finding in adult male dogs. It is theorized that a relative increase in estrogen or androgen levels, owing to an increased or decreased production of either hormone, may lead to benign prostatic hyperplasia.[5] Increased androgen stimulation leads to hyperplasia of glandular structures, whereas increased estrogen influence causes squamous metaplasia of glandular epithelium, proliferation of the fibromuscular stroma, and cyst formation. Enlargement due to androgen stimulation is seen more commonly, but the type of enlargement associated with perineal hernias is more characteristic of excessive estrogen stimulation.[5]

Constipation and tenesmus are the most common clinical features seen in animals affected with prostatic enlargement.[5] It is felt that chronic straining to defecate may weaken the pelvic diaphragm and may predispose the animals to perineal herniation. The actual percentage of animals with perineal hernias who also have prostatic enlargement has not been established.

Further evidence of hormonal interactions in the genesis of perineal hernias is provided by the beneficial effect that castration has on animals afflicted with this condition. Although several authors have disputed the benefit of castration at the time of initial herniorrhaphy,[2,7,11,12] sufficient evidence exists to support the claim that castration has a significant sparing effect on the recurrence of perineal hernias following surgical repair.[8,9] In a retrospective study of surgical cases from 14 North American veterinary teaching hospitals, it was found that the risk of recurrence among noncastrated patients was 2.7 times greater than that for castrated males.[8] It is not known, however, how the removal of testicular hormones provides this sparing effect.

Whatever the inciting cause or causes, once the pelvic diaphragm is sufficiently weakened, herniation of a rectal dilatation or abdominal organ soon occurs. Accumulation of feces in this dilatation or strangulation of an organ leads to the development of clinical signs.

Clinical Signs and Diagnosis

Straining to defecate and perineal swelling are the most consistent clinical features.[1,2,14] Approximately 75 to 80% of animals are presented to the veterinarian with the complaint of straining at defecation.[2] Flatulence, pain on defecation, and irregular bowel movements are also commonly reported.[2,4]

The swelling in the perineal region is usually obvious and may be either unilateral or bilateral. Unilateral hernias are seen in about two-thirds of cases, with over 80% of these on the right side.[2,6,14] Careful palpation of the opposite side often reveals a weakness of the musculature there also.

The herniated mass is usually soft and fluctuant and can often be replaced into its normal position by applying digital pressure in a cranial direction. A firm, painful swelling is seen with a strangulated hernia, which most commonly contains urinary bladder/or prostate gland. The skin covering the perineal region may be red, edematous, or ulcerated from pressure exerted by the herniated mass.

Digital examination of the rectum helps to establish the contents of the hernia. Impaction of feces in a laterally deviated rectal dilatation is often found. Removal of these fecaliths allows a more thorough examination. With an index finger in the rectum and a thumb on the skin lateral to the anus, the extent and contents of the hernia can be determined. Over 90% of these hernias contain a rectal dilatation.[2] Approximately 20% contain urinary bladder or prostate.[2] Other organs are rarely found. Hernias containing only fluid or retroperitoneal fat are seen in a few patients.

Patients with perineal hernias presented to the veterinarian are rarely emergency cases. If strangulation of the urinary bladder has occurred and the animal is unable to urinate, then immediate therapy must be initiated. An attempt should be made to catheterize and to empty the bladder. If this is not successful, paracentesis with a small-bore needle is adequate. Once the bladder is emptied, the hernia is manually reduced, if possible. Biochemical evaluation often reveals a uremic patient, owing to the postrenal obstruction. Fluid diuresis and maintenance of the urinary outflow tract is begun prior to a surgical procedure. Surgical repair should follow as soon as possible.

In patients without such complications, surgical treatment is an elective procedure. If the skin overlying the hernial mass is edematous or ulcerated, the operation should be delayed a few days, medical therapy should be begun to return the skin to normal.[4] When the surgical procedure is delayed, fecal impactions should be removed, and a low-residue diet should be fed until the day of operation.

Because patients undergoing repair of perineal hernias are usually old, laboratory evaluation should include a minimum of a complete blood count, biochemical profile, and urinalysis. Any abnormalities should be further investigated and corrected, if possible, prior to the operation.

The day before the surgical procedure the animal is fasted. That evening, any fecal concretions are manually removed, and the animal is given one or more warm, soapy water enemas to empty the digestive tract. The surgical area is liberally clipped to include the perineal and groin regions, the caudal aspect of the rear legs, and the base of the tail.

After anesthetizing the animal, the anal sacs are expressed, and a pursestring suture is placed to close the anal opening. A preliminary scrub is applied to remove any gross contamination, and the animal is positioned for the procedure.

The patient is placed in sternal recumbency with its rear legs over the end of the table. The patient's hindquarters are elevated by tilting the operating table or by using a rectal stand. If these means are not available, sandbags or other forms of padding sufficient to elevate the hindquarters may be used. Care must be taken so that the animal is not elevated steeply enough to compromise respiratory function. Adequate padding between the patient and the edge of the operating table or rectal stand is important to prevent femoral nerve damage due to stretching or pressure in this region.[4]

The hindlegs are gently pulled forward and are tied to the operating table. The tail is pulled in a craniodorsal direction and is secured in this position, with adhesive tape extending from a point several inches above the base of the tail to each side of the table. Once the patient is positioned, the final surgical scrub is applied.

Surgical Correction

The surgical site is isolated using a four-drape method. The side of the perineal region to be operated and the anus are left exposed to the veterinary surgeon. Another drape is placed medially and is clamped to the skin, to cover the anus. A fenestrated, water-

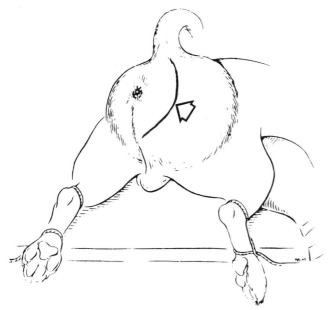

Fig. 30-6. *Schematic diagram of a dog positioned for perineal herniorraphy. A half-circle skin incision site (arrow) is identified. Note pursestring suture in anus. (Redrawn from Leonard, E. P.: Fundamentals of Small Animal Surgery. Philadelphia, W. B. Saunders, 1968.)*

proof drape, with an opening large enough to include the entire surgical site, is then placed over these drapes.

A half-circle skin incision (Fig. 30-6) is made over the hernia in a dorsoventral direction, beginning near the base of the tail and extending ventrally to a point below the hernial mass. This incision is curved slightly in a lateral direction. Care must be taken not to incise too deeply and inadvertently damage the hernial contents.

Blunt dissection is used to enter the hernial sac and to expose its contents. Serous fluid escapes once the sac is opened. Nodules of necrotic retroperitoneal and paraprostatic fat are often encountered. These firm, yellow to brownish masses should be excised and removed. The herniated organs are then replaced into the pelvic or abdominal cavity by gentle but firm pressure in a cranial direction, through the muscular defect.

Following reduction, the outline of the muscular defect and landmarks for surgical closure can be identified. The medial side of the defect is bordered by the rectum ending with the external anal sphincter caudally. The sphincter is the only tissue available for closure on the medial side and must be well visualized because placement of sutures into the rectum may lead to postoperative problems.

Dorsolaterally are the coccygeus and levator ani muscles. Frequently, the fibers of the levator ani muscle and, sometimes, portions of the coccygeus muscle are atrophied and are unsuitable for use in the closure.[4,8] The sacrotuberous ligament can then be used as the lateral landmark for repair. This ligament is a broad, fibrous cord extending from the sacrum to the

ischiatic tuberosity. It can be identified by running a finger along the medial wall of the rectum and hooking it backwards until a hard band of tissue is felt.

The ventral boundary of the hernia is the internal obturator muscle, which lies on the floor of the pelvis. Overlying this muscle is a band of tissue coursing in a caudomedial direction that contains the pudendal nerve and internal pudendal vessels. It is important to identify and to avoid these structures because they supply the external anal sphincter, and damage to them may lead to fecal incontinence. This factor is more critical in bilateral repair because unilateral injury to the pudendal nerve may only lead to temporary incontinence. Within weeks, reinnervation from the opposite side usually occurs.[1]

Suture placement is begun in the dorsalmost aspect of the defect. The first suture includes fibers of the coccygeus muscle dorsolaterally, near the base of the tail, and the external anal sphincter medially (Fig. 30-7). Ventral to this, two sutures are placed between the sacrotuberous ligament and the external anal sphincter. The more dorsal suture of these should also include a portion of the coccygeus muscle. Extreme care must be taken when placing the lateral suture bite to avoid damage to or inclusion of the caudal gluteal vessels and sciatic nerve, which lie just cranial to the sacrotuberous ligament (Fig. 30-8).

The last suture is inserted from the internal obturator muscle ventrally, to the ventral surface of the external anal sphincter. Placement of this suture is difficult because the structures lie deeply within the pelvis and, as mentioned previously, care must be taken in this area to avoid the pudendal nerve. These four sutures are usually sufficient to obtain adequate closure of the defect, but additional sutures may be required in larger animals.

Following closure of the initial suture line, a second row of sutures of 1-0 chromic catgut is placed. The perineal fascia, which has usually retracted laterally, is located and is grasped with Allis tissue forceps. Dissecting this fascia from the overlying skin creates a flap

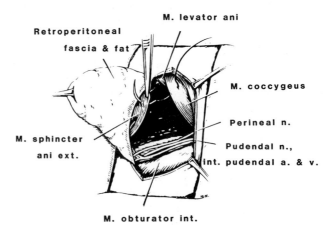

Fig. 30-7. *Placement of the first reconstruction suture. Note pertinent anatomic features. (From Leonard, E. P.: Fundamentals of Small Animal Surgery. Philadelphia, W. B. Saunders, 1968.)*

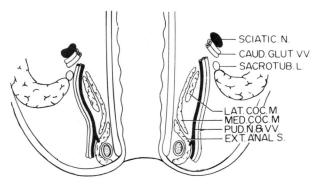

Fig. 30-8. *Cross-section through the normal anus and rectum showing the relationships of structures pertinent to perineal hernia repair. (From Borrows, C. F., and Harvey, C. E.: Perineal hernia in the dog. J. Small Anim. Pract., 14:315, 1973.)*

that is then sutured to the caudal portion of the external anal sphincter. Chromic catgut is used here to initiate a greater inflammatory response.

The subcutaneous tissue and skin are closed in a routine manner. When an excess of redundant skin is present, this should be trimmed before closure to ensure a cosmetic result. If a considerable amount of dead space is present or if contamination is suspected, a Penrose drain should be placed prior to closure.

Repair of a perineal hernia consists of reconstruction of the pelvic diaphragm and castration. Size 2-0 stainless steel wire with a swaged-on, half-circle, taper-point needle is used in the pelvic reconstruction.

If bilateral hernias are present, both sides should not be operated at the same time because bilateral repair puts extreme stress on the external anal sphincter. I prefer to wait 4 to 6 weeks before repairing the second hernia.

Once the hernia operation is completed, the animal is repositioned in dorsal recumbency, and the area cranial to the scrotum is surgically prepared. A castration is then performed. Following this procedure, the purse-string suture is removed, and the animal recovers from anesthesia.

Postoperative Care and Complications

Prophylactic antibiotics are administered postoperatively because of the high incidence of postoperative infection in this area. A low-residue diet and a stool softener* are fed for several days to help eliminate straining and to prevent wound disruption. If the animal continues to strain, narcotics may be administered to help alleviate this problem. An Elizabethan collar, side braces, or a plastic bucket around the neck may be placed on the animal if it licks or chews the incision line (see Chap. 3). Sutures are removed in 10 to 14 days.

The list of postoperative complications from this procedure is long, but fortunately, several are temporary and respond to therapy, whereas others are of an

* Metamucil, Searle Consumer Products, Box 5110, Chicago, IL 60680

iatrogenic origin and can be avoided if proper precautions are taken. The immediate postoperative complications include wound breakdown or infection, fecal incontinence, sciatic nerve paralysis, urinary abnormalities, excessive straining, and prolapse of the rectum.[2,4]

The incidence of wound infection following surgical procedures of the anal region is understandably high. As discussed earlier, drainage should be established at the time of the operation if contamination is suspected, and antibiotic therapy should accompany all perineal hernia repairs. When infection does not become evident until later, Penrose drains should be placed into the purulent area; these drains should exit from the ventral aspect of the wound and should be sutured in place. The exudate is cultured, and the wound is flushed around the drains with antibacterial solution until the drainage is minimal and the infection is eliminated.

The problem of fecal incontinence was mentioned earlier. This problem is often only temporary in unilateral hernia repair, but bilateral damage to the pudendal nerves leads to permanent fecal incontinence.[1] Damage to the sciatic nerve is much more devastating and is evident immediately following anesthetic recovery. If the nerve is impinged by the suture material, the animal will be in extreme pain, and a sciatic palsy will be present in the affected limb.[4] Immediate surgical intervention to remove the offending suture is indicated. This procedure may be performed through the original surgical incision or through a caudolateral approach to the hip or the affected side. The latter approach allows visualization of the sciatic nerve and an assessment of the degree of damage.[4]

Urinary problems postsurgically are manifested by anuria, following retroflexion of the bladder into the hernia. This complication is probably due to damage to the nerve or blood supply of the bladder or to prolonged stretching of the bladder musculature. The atony is usually temporary, and bladder function is regained in several days.[2] Catheterization or manual expression of the bladder must be instituted until function returns.

Excessive straining is a common problem and is most often due to postsurgical pain.[2,4a] Digital rectal examination should be performed to rule out the placement of a suture in the rectal mucosa. If this error has occurred, it will usually resolve itself with time and supportive care, but abscess formation may be a problem.[4] Administration of narcotics helps to alleviate the pain and thus decreases straining. In some patients, this straining, along with the tension on the external anal sphincter, results in a minor rectal prolapse. Such a prolapse is usually temporary and regresses spontaneously when the straining ceases, but cases requiring resection have been reported.[2]

Any of these postsurgical complications may persist to become permanent afflictions. The most common long-term complications include straining to defecate, flatulence, and pain on defecation.[2] Although these problems are similar to those experienced by most animals presurgically, improvement with surgical intervention is generally considerable. The percentage of animals affected postsurgically is reduced, and the severity and frequency of signs are diminished.[2] Medical management may further alleviate the animal's discomfort.

Recurrence

Factors which have been shown to affect recurrence rates include sexual status of the animal, experience of the surgeon, and type of suture material used in the repair. Despite controversy surrounding the influence of castration on perineal hernias,[1,2,7,8,11,13] I feel that existing evidence supports the claim that castration reduces the risk of recurrence and therefore recommend this procedure with all perineal hernia repairs. Since castration can also spare the animal from testicular or perianal gland neoplasm later[8] it is hard to argue against this recommendation.

References and Suggested Readings

1. Blakely, C. L.: Perineal hernia. *In* Canine Surgery. Edited by K. Mayer, J. V. Lacroix, and H. P. Hoskins. Santa Barbara, CA, American Veterinary Publication, 1959.

1a. Bojrab, M. J., and Toomey, A.: Perineal hernia. Compend. Contin. Ed. Small Anim. Pract., *3*:8, 1981.

2. Burrows, C. F. and Harvey, C. E.: Perineal hernia in the dog. J. Small Anim. Pract., *14*:315, 1973.

3. DeVita, J.: Factors responsible for perineal hernias in male dogs. *In* Canine Surgery. 4th Ed. Edited by K. Mayer, J. V. Lacroix, and H. P. Hoskins. Santa Barbara, CA, American Veterinary Publications, 1959.

4. Dietrich, H. F.: Perineal hernia repair in the canine. Vet. Clin. North Am., *5*:383, 1975.

5. Greiner, T. P., and Betts, C. W.: Diseases of the prostate gland: benign prostatic hyperplasia. *In* Textbook of Veterinary Internal Medicine: Diseases of the Dog and Cat. Edited by S. G. Ettinger. Philadelphia, W. B. Saunders, 1975.

6. Harvey, C. E.: Anal splitting in dogs with perineal hernia: technique and results. J. Am. Anim. Hosp. Assoc., *14*:243, 1978.

7. Harvey, C. E.: Treatment of perineal hernia in the dog—a reassessment. J. Small Anim. Pract., *18*:505, 1977.

8. Hayes, H. M., Wilson, G. P., and Tarone, R. E.: The epidemiologic feature of perineal hernias in 771 dogs. J. Am. Anim. Hosp. Assoc., *14*:703, 1978.

9. Holmes, J. R.: Perineal hernia in the dog. Vet. Rec., *76*:1250, 1964.

10. Larsen, J. S.: Perineal Herniorrhaphy in dogs. J. Am. Vet. Med. Assoc., *149*:277, 1966.

11. Lawson, D. D., and Campbell, J. R.: Perineal hernia in the dog. Vet. Rec., *76*:1522, 1964.

12. Leighton, R.L.: Surgical procedures for the routine small animal practice. Perineal herniorrhaphy. Vet. Med., *55*:33, 1960.

13. Moltzen-Nielsen, H.: Perineal hernia. *In* Proceedings of the Fifteenth International Veterinary Congress. Vol. I. Stockholm, 1953.

14. Pettit, G. D.: Perineal hernia in the dog. Cornell Vet., *52*:261, 1962.

15. Schnelle, G. B.: Perineal hernia. *In* Proceedings of the Fifteenth International Veterinary Congress. Vol. I. Stockholm, 1953.

16. Wainman, P., and Shipounoff, G. C.: The effects of castration and testosterone propionate on the striated perineal musculature in the rat. J. Endocrinol., *29*:975, 1941.

Perineal Hernia in the Dog: An Alternative Method of Correction

by THOMAS D. EARLEY

and RONALD J. KOLATA

The traditional method of repairing a perineal hernia involves reconstruction of the pelvic diaphragm by suturing the external anal sphincter to the internal obturator muscle ventrally and the sacrotuberous ligament laterally and dorsally.[1,3] This repair has a reported recurrence rate of between 22 and 48%.[1,2] Multiple factors may contribute to recurrence of the hernia; one of these may be the great amount of tension that must sometimes be applied to the sutures used to appose the components of the pelvic diaphragm. Our method for repairing perineal hernias reduces tension on the sutures approximating the reconstructed pelvic diaphragm and thereby decreases the likelihood of their cutting through tissues. This method brings muscular tissue bulk and an additional blood supply into the area that may also foster secure healing.

Surgical Procedure

The approach to the hernia is the same as in the traditional technique. Once exposed, the herniated structures are reduced into the abdomen, and redundant fat is excised. Care is taken to identify and to preserve the pudendal artery, vein, and nerve (Fig. 30-9*A*).

Once the external anal sphincter, and sacrotuberous ligament, and the internal obturator muscle are identified, the caudal border of the origin of the internal obturator muscle is incised, and a periosteal elevator is used to elevate it from the ischiatic table (Fig. 30-9*B* and *C*). Elevation should not proceed beyond the caudal edge of the obturator foramen because the obturator nerve and the artery supplying the internal obturator muscle may be injured. The tendon of the internal obturator muscle is severed at the point at which it condenses and begins to pass laterally over the body of the ischium (Fig. 30-9*D*). Care is taken to sever the tendon medial to the ischium as the ischiatic (sciatic) nerve crosses the tendon just lateral to the ischium (see Fig. 30-9*B*). Once the caudal portion of the internal obturator muscle is elevated and its tendon is severed, it is brought dorsally to fill the hernial defect (Fig. 30-9*E*). The lateral aspect of the external anal sphincter is freed of as much connective tissue as possible in order to create a surface that will adhere to the internal obturator muscle. An initial suture is placed between the external anal sphincter and the sacrotuberous ligament and gluteal fascia as far dorsal as possible to create a point to which the apex of the internal obturator muscle is sutured. The caudolateral border of the internal obturator muscle is sutured to the caudomedial edge of the sacrotuberous ligament using 4 to 6 cruciate sutures of 1-0 nylon (Fig. 30-9*F*). *Care must be*

den increase in intra-abdominal pressure due to blunt trauma from any source is presumed responsible for creating a diaphragmatic tear, usually in the muscular diaphragm. During herniorrhaphy of a recently induced diaphragmatic hernia, a hematoma is often identified in the abdominal wall; this phenomenon lends evidence to the hypothesis that blunt abdominal trauma increases intra-abdominal pressure.[4]

Trauma is recorded as the cause of diaphragmatic hernia in 93% of cases; developmental hernias occurred in 6% of cases in dogs and cats. These data are similar to those reported previously.[4]

The tear or tears in the diaphragm are intramuscular, ventral to the esophageal hiatus, and many tears include the diaphragmatic costal origins. The diaphragmatic tear locations and size determine which viscera migrate into the chest. The visceral organs migrate freely or become incarcerated and partially strangled. The organs in the chest at the time of radiographic examination are not necessarily the same as those found at herniorrhaphy. This difference is attributable to the free movement of abdominal organs between the pleural and peritoneal cavities. Most frequently seen in the thoracic cavities of patients undergoing operations to repair diaphragmatic hernias are liver, small bowel, stomach, spleen, and fluid.[4] Abdominal organs that cross the diaphragm and become incarcerated have some degree of venous obstruction and congestion. The liver can produce large quantities of fluid that is exuded through the liver capsule.[2] The fluid produced by the strangled liver has the characteristics of a transudate, similar to normal extracellular fluid. Twenty-eight patients (24%) of the total population with partially strangulated liver lobes had accumulated large quantities of fluid in their thoracic or abdominal cavities. Removal of this fluid temporarily relieves the patient's dyspnea; only hernia reduction and herniorrhaphy correct the fluid production and accumulation.

The clinical records of 191 animals from 1970 through 1979 were reviewed to characterize the population of animals with diaphragmatic hernias. Sixty percent of these patients were male, and 40% were female dogs. The dogs with diaphragmatic hernias ranged in age from less than 6 months to 12 years; 70% were 3 years old or younger. Mixed-breed dogs represented 40% of the population with traumatic diaphragmatic hernias. Poodles, Irish setters, beagles, and German shepherd dogs represented 27% of the population; 28 other breeds made up the remainder.

Diagnosis

A number of clinical signs have been described as classic for a patient with diaphragmatic hernia but these signs are unreliable and include "tucked-up" abdomen, intestinal sounds in the chest, and muffled heart and lung sounds. The movement of viscera between the abdomen and the thorax is in part responsible for the unreliability of these "classic" clinical signs of diaphragmatic hernia. Many hernia patients assume postures that accommodate their reduced tidal volume; many are reluctant to lie down. The only consistent clinical sign is compromised respiratory function exaggerated by stress.

After a thorough physical examination, a radiographic examination of the chest is imperative. The diaphragmatic silhouette is incomplete in most diaphragmatic hernias. Other diseases, such as hydrothorax, can also produce a loss of diaphragmatic silhouette. Thoracentesis and fluid removal define the quantity and, possibly, the character of the fluid and the cause of the existing fluid accumulation.

Anesthesia

The surgical repair of acute or chronic diaphragmatic hernia presents important anesthetic problems. The presence of broken ribs, pneumothorax, or abdominal viscera within the thoracic cavity predisposes a patient to the sudden onset of respiratory distress and hypoxemia. The administration of potent respiratory depressant drugs for preanesthetic medication or for the maintenance of general anesthesia predisposes a patient to respiratory embarrassment prior to, during, or for several hours following diaphragmatic herniorrhaphy. The intraoperative mismanagement of spontaneous or controlled ventilation can result in respiratory acidosis, hypoxemia, and hypotension.

Prior to the administration of preanesthetic medication, the patient should be thoroughly evaluated, with special emphasis on the animal's heart and respiratory rates, the color of mucous membranes, perfusion time, and the intensity of lung and heart sounds. Animals with diaphragmatic hernia can demonstrate dyspnea, tachypnea, tachycardia, cyanosis, and muffled or absent heart and lung sounds. These clinical signs result from the presence of air, fluid, or abdominal viscera in the thoracic cavity, all of which contribute to respiratory insufficiency. Patients with diaphragmatic hernia demonstrating cyanosis and respiratory distress must be handled carefully, with minimal physical restraint, to avoid an exacerbation of their condition. Drugs used prior to the induction of anesthesia should have minimal respiratory depressant effects. Diazepam and low doses of phenothiazine tranquilizers or narcotics are preferred to large doses of narcotics, xylazine, or an intravenous infusion of fentanyl and droperidol. The patient should be administered oxygen by face mask prior to and during the anesthetic induction period if respiratory distress or cyanosis is obvious.

The intravenous administration of low doses of ultrashort-acting barbiturates such as thiamylal, thiopental, and methohexital are preferred to combinations of intravenous narcotics and tranquilizers and to mask or chamber anesthetic induction techniques. The reasons for using ultrashort-acting barbiturates include: (1) rapid induction of anesthesia allowing rapid endotracheal intubation and ventilatory control; (2) minimum of physical restraint; and (3) rapid redistribution of the ultrashort-acting barbiturates minimizing prolonged respiratory depressant effects. General anesthesia is maintained using inhalation anesthetics that can be easily controlled and rapidly eliminated. Halothane, enflurane, or isoflurane are the preferred inhalant drugs. Methoxyflurane can be used, but because of its high blood solubility and respiratory depressant effects, its use prolongs recovery from anesthesia and may cause marked hypoventilation.

Nitrous oxide may be contraindicated as an adjunct to anesthesia. Nitrous oxide hastens the rate of uptake of the primary inhalation anesthetic (second gas effect)[3] and reduces the amount of more potent and potentially more dangerous drugs, such as halothane and enflurane, used to maintain general anesthesia. The use of nitrous oxide during induction of anesthesia or after diaphragmatic herniorrhaphy can result in respiratory embarrassment. Nitrous oxide is comparatively less soluble in blood than inhalation anesthetic drugs, but it is approximately 34 times more soluble in blood than nitrogen. Because of the greater blood solubility of nitrous oxide as compared to nitrogen, greater quantities of nitrous oxide are carried into closed gas spaces[4] (thoracic cavity) than quantities of nitrogen are carried away. The entrance of nitrous oxide into any compliant space, such as air embolism, pneumoperitoneum, pneumothorax, and obstructed bowel, causes the gas space to expand or the pressure to increase. It has been demonstrated in dogs that inspiration of 75% nitrous oxide and 25% oxygen doubled a 300-ml pneumothorax in 10 minutes and tripled it in 45 minutes. This effect could cause severe respiratory embarrassment in dogs having a diaphragmatic herniorraphy and closed pneumothorax.

Nitrous oxide should be avoided in diaphragmatic hernia patients because of the potential development of diffusion hypoxia. Following general anesthesia, when the patient is allowed to breathe room air, nitrous oxide rapidly leaves the blood and dilutes the alveolar oxygen and carbon dioxide. This dilution effect is the result of the lower solubility of nitrous oxide in the blood, as compared with oxygen. The resulting dilution of lung alveolar oxygen and carbon dioxide causes hypoxemia and respiratory depression. The maximum duration of diffusion hypoxemia in normal patients is generally 3 to 5 minutes, but if ventilation is compromised, such as by pain, broken ribs, or pulmonary distress, or if ventilation-perfusion inequalities are present, the arterial hypoxemia can last much longer.

During recovery from anesthesia the patient should be placed in an oxygen enriched (40%) environment. Intermittent respiratory support (mechanical ventilator) may be required during the early postoperative period. Careful and frequent monitoring of mucous membrane color and perfusion, heart rate, and respiratory rate are essential. If narcotics (oxymorphone, fentanyl) were used to maintain anesthesia and respiratory depression is apparent, the use of narcotic antagonists (naloxone nallorphine, levallorphan) should be considered. Local anesthetic agents (lidocaine) can be given if severe pain occurs and predisposes to respiratory distress. Restrictive thoracic bandages should be avoided.

Surgical Correction

Data were available on 115 dogs from the time between the initial trauma causing the hernia and diaphragmatic herniorrhaphy. Eighty percent of these animals had a herniorrhaphy 54 days ± 14 days after trauma, and 20% had herniorrhaphy 283 days ± 43 days after trauma. The postoperative mortality rate was significantly greater (p < 0.01) the longer the traumatic hernia persisted. In this group of patients, survival following diaphragmatic herniorrhaphy was due to several factors. A major consideration was the extent of the trauma other than the diaphragmatic tear. The time required to repair the diaphragmatic defect successfully in the immediately repaired hernias was an important factor in the patient's surviving the herniorrhaphy and the immediate postoperative period.

Generally, the earlier the herniorrhaphy is performed, the better the outcome, but clinical judgment and evaluation of the patient's ability to withstand anesthesia and operation are important. The condition of the suddenly traumatized patient may sometimes be stabilized before the surgical procedure. In other instances, because of a life-threatening intercurrent problem, the herniorrhaphy is performed in an unsta-

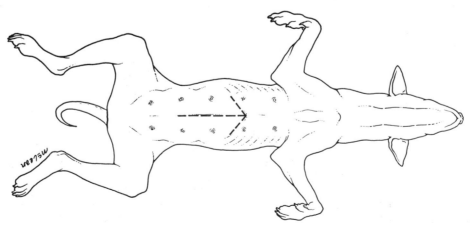

Fig. 30-10. *Paracostal extension of the midabdominal incision.*

ble patient, in which the prognosis is guarded. The animal with a chronic hernia is stable, but is prone to develop problems from abnormal visceral changes resulting from the long-standing hernia.

The midline abdominal approach is preferred because it allows accessibility to the entire diaphragm, in spite of the disadvantage of dealing with the abdominal viscera. The abdominal exposure can be enlarged by extending the incision paracostally from the cranial midline or cranially through the sternal midline (Fig. 30-10). The paracostal incision transects the rectus abdominis muscle and the cranial deep and superficial epigastric arteries and veins. The closure of this paracostal wound is not difficult if done anatomically.

The abdominal wall should be explored for other traumatic effects, including hematomas and other hernias. The oblique and transverse abdominal muscles are sometimes torn from the costal arch, and the abdominal viscera therefore spill into the subcutaneous tissues. This paracostal hernia is closed when the diaphragm is repaired. The abdominal cavity is explored, and all organs, especially those that have traversed the diaphragm, should be examined to determine the extent of injury. The herniated, strangled liver lobes can appear severely diseased, but the liver lobes resume their normal state when returned to their anatomic location and when the vascular obstruction is removed.

The size and location of the diaphragmatic tear determine which viscera enter the thorax and whether the organs are freely movable or incarcerated. It is sometimes necessary to enlarge the diaphragmatic defect in order to facilitate hernia reduction and to eliminate the risk of damage to herniated organs in the chest. Fluid and debris are evacuated as completely as possible from the body cavities after hernia reduction and before herniorrhaphy.

The diaphragmatic wound margins are carefully evaluated; if the wound is recent, sutures must be placed in tissues that will hold the sutures, to avoid reherniation. The wound margins have more tensile strength if the hernia is long standing because of the increased collagen in the healing wound margin. The diaphragm is returned to a normal location, although this maneuver is not always possible, owing to muscular contraction and scar contracture. The liver as well as muscle flaps from the abdominal wall have been used to close diaphragmatic defects.

The closure of the diaphragmatic tear begins at the most remote site and progresses to the most accessible site. Preplacement of sutures in the diaphragmatic wound edges facilitates closure; long suture ends can be used for traction. Nonabsorbable suture material is preferable for herniorrhaphy because of its longer-lasting tensile strength. Suture pattern is a matter of personal preference. An interrupted suture pattern is safer than a continuous suture pattern because one untied knot or torn suture does not totally disrupt the hernia repair. Closure of the diaphragm should be secure and as airtight as possible. When the diaphragm is torn from its costal insertions, paracostal sutures are necessary to reattach the diaphragmatic costal insertions.

The abdominal incision is closed. In a long-standing hernia, the abdominal organs may not fit comfortably in the abdominal cavity, and care must be exercised to avoid injury to the abdominal organs during the abdominal wall closure. The abdominal musculature, in time, relaxes to accommodate the returned visceral organs.

Residual air should be evacuated from the patient's chest. One method of removing this air is to expand the lungs to a positive pressure of approximately 20 cm water. While the lungs are expanded, the intrathoracic air is allowed to escape by opening a space in the diaphragmatic wound closure with a hemostatic forcep. When the abdominal wound is closed, one should place the patient in lateral recumbency and aspirate the nondependent pleural space with a hypodermic needle, a 2-way valve, and a large syringe; this procedure removes more air. Needle aspiration carries the risk of lacerating the lung. Chest drains can be placed during herniorrhaphy, but constant postoperative surveillance is necessary to avoid pneumothorax. A rapid return to normal negative thoracic pressure and normal tidal volume is most desirable.

PERICARDIAL (DEVELOPMENTAL) DIAPHRAGMATIC HERNIA

In a previous study, pericardial (pleuroperitoneal) diaphragmatic hernia was found in 1 of 10 patients with diaphragmatic hernias. In a more current review, only 6% of the population has this type of hernia. Communication exists between the peritoneal cavity and the pericardial sac. The pericardial sac is greatly distended by small bowel, liver, and omentum. This hernia represents a developmental defect in the muscular portion of the diaphragm that is derived from the fetal body wall. About half the patients with this hernia have large ventral abdominal defects cranial to the umbilicus. The defect can include the caudal sternum. Some hernias are clinically silent and are only identified because thoracic radiographs are taken for reasons such as heart disease, muffled heart sounds, pneumonia, neoplasia, and gastroenteritis. The diagnosis of developmental hernia is made in most affected animals when they are under 2 years of age, but this hernia can go undetected for several years. No specific clinical signs exist.

Even though the pleural cavity is not entered, positive-pressure ventilation is required during herniorrhaphy because the dilated pericardial sac interferes with respiratory function. A ventral abdominal midline approach is best; if the ventral body wall is defective, only the skin and falciform ligament are incised to open the peritoneal cavity. The abdominal organs in the pericardial sac are replaced in the abdomen. The hernial ring and fibrous margin do not usually exceed 6.0 cm in diameter. The hernial ring may have to be incised and enlarged to reduce the herniated abdominal organs. Closure is accomplished with nonabsorbable interrupted mattress sutures along the length of the defect; the first layer is oversewn with simple interrupted sutures. If the abdominal wall is normal, it is closed; if a belly wall defect exists, the widely separated internal and external sheaths of the rectus abdominis muscle are closed. This abdominal wall separation is predisposed to considerable tension during wound closure and may need reinforcement.

The dilated pericardial sac is filled with air after herniorrhaphy. The air in the pericardial sac is difficult to remove, but it is absorbed by the serosal surface of the pericardial sac in a short time. Based on evaluation of up to 5-year follow-ups, no deleterious cardiac effect results from leaving the chronically dilated pericardial sac intact. Postoperative thoracic radiographs of animals with pericardial diaphragmatic hernias demonstrate that the pericardial sac contracts to normal size surrounding the heart within 3 weeks.

References and Suggested Readings

1. Eger, E. I., III, and Saidman, J. J.: Hazards of nitrous oxide anesthesia in bowel obstruction and pneumothorax. Anesthesiology, 26:61, 1965.
2. Sodeman, W. A., and Sodeman, T. M.: Sodeman's Pathologic Physiology. 6th Ed. Philadelphia, W. B. Saunders, 1979.
3. Stoelting, R. K., and Eger, E. I., III: An additional explanation for the second gas effect. A concentrating effect. Anesthesiology, 30:273, 1969.
4. Wilson, G. P., Newton, C. D., and Burt, J. K.: A review of 116 diaphragmatic hernias in dog and cats. J. Am. Vet. Med. Assoc., 159:1142, 1971.

31 * Mammary Glands

Mammary Glands

by GEORGE P. WILSON

and HOWARD M. HAYES, JR.

Mammary Tumors

Mammary cancer is the most frequently occurring neoplasm in the female dog, and mammary gland neoplasms are the third most frequently found tumors in the female cat.[7]

Mammary gland neoplasms occur in the intact and spayed female dog or cat that has had multiple estrous cycles. It is not unusual for the spayed female dog with a history of pyometra or pseudocyesis to develop mammary gland tumors. There is little doubt that ovaries play a role in the development of canine and feline mammary neoplasia. The long ovarian luteal phase of the canine estrous cycle makes a major contribution to the development of mammary tumors;[3,9] the ovarian role in mammary neoplasia needs further clarification in the cat.

A review of 132 cats with mammary neoplasia indicates that the biologic behavior of feline mammary neoplasia differs from that of the dog.[5] This behavioral difference can be attributed, in part, to the distinctions between the cyclic estrus of the dog and the continuous estrus of the cat. The prolonged progestational (luteal) period of the canine estrous cycle does not occur in the continuous estrus of the cat. Mammary neoplasia has been produced in the female dog by prolonged administration of high doses of progestational contraceptive drugs.[3]

Many reports indicate that the most common sites for the occurrence of mammary tumors are the caudal abdominal and inguinal mammary glands. Careful palpation and examination of excised mammary chains demonstrate that solitary mammary nodules or tumors are uncommon;[4] multiple nodules or tumors are present throughout the length of the mammary chain. Eighteen percent of these mammary tumors examined histologically are reported to be malignant neoplasms.[2]

Nodules in the mammary glands on occasion appear to enlarge during estrus and to decrease in size at anestrus. This fluctuation can happen several times, but at some point the tumors continue to enlarge after estrus. This continued enlargement reflects three possible changes: loss of hormone dependency,[2] malignant transformation, or both. Tumor size has been used as a criterion to determine the necessity of surgical treatment. Widespread metastases may be present even though the size of a mammary tumor appears static. A tumor of the mammary glands should be considered malignant regardless of its size.

The mixed mammary tumor is the most commonly reported neoplasm in the dog; malignant tumors frequently arise from these benign masses. About 70% of dogs with mammary neoplasms have mixed-type tumors, and 50% of these have coexisting malignant neoplasms of a different type. A study at the Ohio State University revealed multiple mammary tumors with as many as four malignant histologic types identified in one individual.[4] To date, surgical excision at the earliest opportunity is the most effective therapy for any neoplasm; excision must be complete to control the disease.

Surgical Anatomy

A thorough knowledge of the anatomy of the mammary glands, including their vascular and lymphatic systems, augments evaluation of the patient and surgical excision. The glandular tissue extends bilaterally from the cranial pectoral region to the lateral vulva; no cranial-to-caudal anatomic glandular demarcation is present, with the exception of the nipples. The right and left chains are clearly separated from each other on the ventral midline; the stage of estrus or lactation determines the size of the glandular chain. The removal of the canine or feline ovaries causes normal gland atrophy.

It is customary to number the mammary nipples of the cat and dog cranially to caudally. Careful observation of the mammary chains demonstrates that an unequal number of nipples (4.85 per side) and mammary glands exist;[2,6] the most commonly missing gland is the right or left cranial abdominal gland. This anatomic observation affects the results of segmental mastectomy based on lymphatic drainage. Because of this characteristic glandular distribution, the glands are more accurately named cranial and caudal thoracic, cranial and caudal abdominal, and inguinal.

The mammary glands are modified skin glands attached to the ventral thoracic and abdominal wall. The thoracic mammary glands are closely adherent to the pectoral muscles, whereas the abdominal and inguinal glands are loose and pendulous, especially after estrus or lactation. The glandular tissue is between the skin and cutaneous musculature, the suspensory apparatus of the mammary glands. The cutaneus trunci muscle in the subcutaneous tissues provides a discrete plane, in the lateral thorax and the abdomen, to define the lateral margin of the mammary tissue. This line of demar-

cation is important for complete excision of mammary gland tissue. Mammary tissue left in the surgical margins following mastectomy has been the site of mammary neoplasms.

BLOOD SUPPLY (ARTERIAL, VENOUS, LYMPHATIC) (FIG. 31-1). The branches of the lateral thoracic artery from the axilla and contributions of the intercostal vessels supply the thoracic mammary glands and the lateral rib cage. The deep mammary tissue of the thoracic mammary glands is supplied by perforating branches of the internal thoracic artery. At the margin of the caudal rib cage, the internal thoracic vessels divide to form the cranial deep and superficial epigastric arteries. The superficial epigastric artery penetrates the mammary

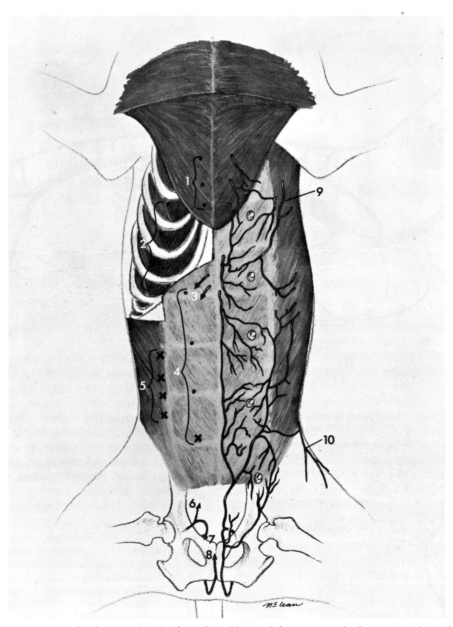

Fig. 31-1. *Blood supply to mammary glands: 1, perforating branches of internal thoracic vessels; 2, intercostal vessels; 3, cranial superficial epigastric vessel; 4, perforating branches of the cranial deep epigastric vessel; 5, segmental lateral abdominal and circumflex iliac vessels; 6, anterior branch of the caudal superficial epigastric vessel; 7, posterior branch of the caudal superficial epigastric vessel; 8, labial vessels; 9, lateral thoracic vessels; and 10, circumflex iliac vessels.*

33 * Skin

Plastic and Reconstructive Surgery in the Dog and Cat

by Michael M. Pavletic

and Llewellyn C. Peyton

Skin wounds are among the most common injuries seen by the veterinarian. Despite their frequency, even minor skin wounds are potentially dangerous, and individualized evaluation and treatment are indicated.

Most skin injuries are handled by primary closure, delayed closure, or healing by contraction and epithelialization. The method chosen depends upon the size, the location, and the condition of the wound.

Preoperative Considerations

The initial treatment for contaminated wounds is considered in Chapter 40. Many cutaneous defects can be closed by simple debridement and direct closure, allowing the wound to heal by primary closure. (Fig. 33-1). Local lines of tension should be determined prior to debridement of devitalized skin by manually pushing the peripheral skin toward the center of the area to be excised. An incision made perpendicular to skin tension lines gapes widely. An incision and a closure made along tension lines separate minimally and heal optimally. Skin incision and closure should therefore be oriented to the line of least tension to facilitate closure, to minimize the risk of dehiscence and tissue necrosis,

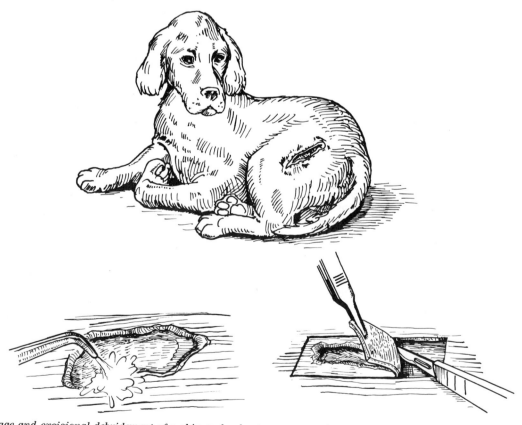

Fig. 33-1. *Lavage and excisional debridement of a skin and subcutaneous wound.*

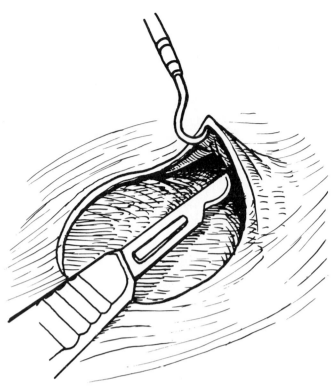

Fig. 33-2. *A scalpel blade or Metzenbaum scissors may be used to undermine the skin.*

and to minimize scarring. Subcutaneous undermining is usually performed in order to allow accurate apposition of skin edges (Fig. 33-2).

Tension relief to local wound excisions or defect reconstruction should be carefully considered. Preplanning for local tension relief maneuvers should be a standard consideration for any surgical procedure requiring removal of skin (Fig. 33-3 and see Figs. 33-18 to 33-20 and 33-24 and 33-25).

Development of skin flaps or skin grafting may be necessary to achieve skin closure in some instances. This section discusses basic reconstructive techniques employed in veterinary medicine.

Suture Materials and Patterns

Many suture materials can be used effectively for wound closure. In general, fine, nonreactive, monofilament suture material on a swaged-on reverse cutting

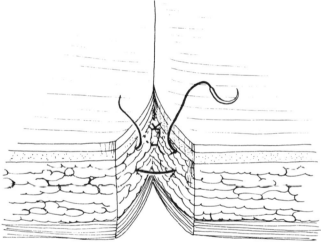

Fig. 33-4. *Interrupted subcuticular pattern. This useful pattern allows accurate skin alignment. In addition, it can be used to relieve wound tension, permitting more accurate apposition with fine simple interrupted sutures.*

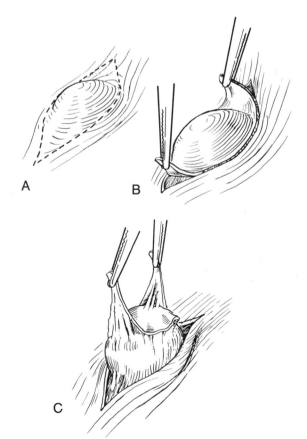

Fig. 33-3. A to C, *Local excisions of tumors or blemishes are planned so that lines of least tension will parallel the intended incisions. Such consideration reduces the tension on closure.*

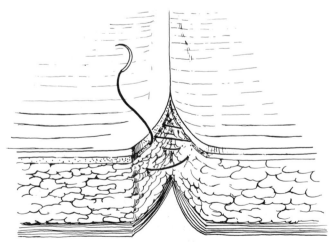

Fig. 33-5. *Continuous subcuticular pattern. Generally used for longer incisions, this pattern has applications similar to the interrupted subcuticular pattern.*

needle passes through skin with minimal friction and trauma. Suture material of 3-0 and 4-0 monofilament nylon* or polypropylene† meets these criteria for most companion animals, although finer suture material may be used for more delicate tissues. Subcutaneous sutures are generally needed to appose skin edges accurately prior to skin closure (Figs. 33-4 and 33-5). The suture pattern for the skin should accurately approximate the wound edges without restricting local circulation. Sutures should be placed at least 5 mm from the wound's edge and 5 to 10 mm apart. Of the numerous suture patterns available, the simple interrupted, the vertical mattress, the far-near-near-far, and the subcuticular suture patterns are strong, cause minimal circulatory interference, and can be used effectively in most skin closures (Figs. 33-6 to 33-8).

*Dermalon, Ethicon, Inc., Somerville, NJ 08876
†Prolene, Ethicon, Inc., Somerville NJ 08876

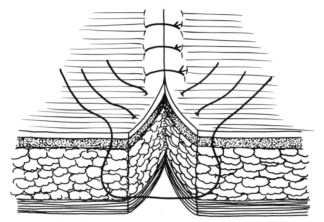

Fig. 33-6. *Simple interrupted suture pattern. The needle should pass principally through the dermis, with minimal subcutaneous tissue. The knot should be offset to avoid placement over the incision.*

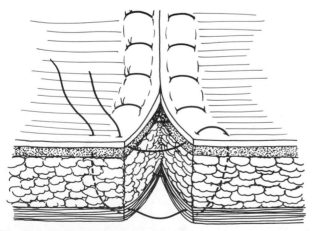

Fig. 33-7. *Vertical mattress suture pattern. This pattern provides accurate apposition with slight eversion. It is often employed where skin is mobile, poorly supported, and has a tendency to invert. Vertical mattress and simple interrupted sutures can be alternated if necessary. The vertical mattress pattern causes minimal circulatory impedance to the skin's edge, unlike the horizontal mattress pattern.*

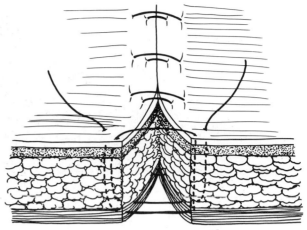

Fig. 33-8. *Far-near-near-far "pulley" suture pattern. This pattern is commonly employed in areas subject to mild tension. The "far" component of the pattern relives tension while the "near" component provides apposition. Excessive tightening should be avoided. The far component should be started first, to avoid placing the knot over the incision line.*

Surgical Anatomy

The survival of skin or a skin flap is dependent upon the preservation of its blood circulation. It is important to understand the cutaneous circulation in order to construct pedicle grafts with consistent success.

The cutaneous circulation is divided into three plexuses: the deep or subdermal plexus, the middle or cutaneous plexus, and the superficial or subpapillary plexus (Fig. 33-9). The subdermal plexus is the major blood supply to the skin. Its preservation is essential for the survival of a skin flap. The subdermal plexus lies in the subcutaneous fatty and areolar tissues along the deep face of the dermis (Fig. 33-9D). It is important to undermine skin in the subcutaneous tissue below this level to avoid deep plexus injury. In areas where a panniculus muscle is closely associated with the overlying skin, the subdermal plexus lies both superficial and deep to it. In such a case, one should undermine beneath the panniculus muscle to preserve the subdermal vasculature. Bleeding cutaneous vessels commonly seen during a surgical procedure generally originate from the subdermal plexus.

Branches from the deep plexus next ascend into the dermis and arborize to form the middle plexus. The middle plexus supplies blood to the adjacent cutaneous adnexa. Branches from the middle plexus ascend to form the superficial or subpapillary plexus. The superficial plexus lies below the epidermis to supply circulation to the adjacent stratum basale (Fig. 33-9).

Arteries supplying the skin in the dog and cat approach and course beneath the skin in parallel fashion. These vessels are termed direct cutaneous arteries and are the predominant blood supply to the canine skin (Figs. 33-10 and 33-11). Veins are generally parallel to these arteries. Direct cutaneous arteries arborize to

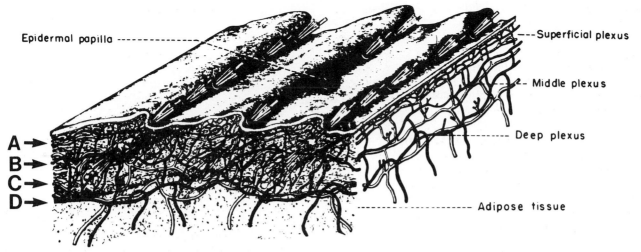

Epidermal papilla

Superficial plexus

Middle plexus

Deep plexus

A
B
C
D

Adipose tissue

Fig. 33-9. *Cutaneous vasculature of the dog demonstrating the three cutaneous plexuses. The arrows illustrate various free-graft thicknesses in relation to the dermis and cutaneous plexuses: (A) thin split-thickness graft, (B) intermediate or medium split-thickness graft, (C) thick split-thickness graft, and (D) full-thickness graft. (Adapted from Evans, H. E., and Christensen, G. C.: Miller's Anatomy of the Dog. 2nd Ed. Philadelphia, W. B. Saunders, 1979.)*

form and supply the subdermal plexus. Although man has direct cutaneous vessels supplying the skin, the predominant blood supply is from numerous musculocutaneous vessels running perpendicular to the skin. Therefore, human grafting techniques must be reviewed with caution because of the distinct anatomic differences between man and the dog and cat.

Surgical Techniques

PEDICLE GRAFTS (SKIN FLAPS)

A pedicle graft is a portion of skin and underlying subcutaneous tissue attached to the body by means of a vascular pedicle (base). Graft survival depends upon maintaining an adequate perfusion pressure from the pedicle until neovascularization establishes a secondary blood supply from the recipient bed.

Local skin flaps are the most practical method in veterinary surgery to close cutaneous defects unamenable to simple closure techniques. Their effective use, however, requires the availability of adjacent loose or elastic skin. Extensive skin losses in areas with minimal loose skin, such as the distal extremities, necessitates a distant graft or a free graft, both of which require greater surgical time and postoperative care.

Local flaps are capable of (1) rapidly restoring the anatomic and functional continuity to an area, (2) covering a recipient bed poorly suited for a free graft, (3) providing a durable surface over bony prominences, and (4) covering body structures that poorly tolerate exposure, such as tendons, blood vessels, and nerves. Local flaps can be classified according to their blood supply and design.

Flap Classification Based upon Blood Supply

Flaps dependent upon the deep or subdermal plexus may be termed subdermal plexus flaps. Flaps incorpo-

rating a direct cutaneous artery and vein into the flap pedicle are termed axial pattern flaps (direct cutaneous arterial pedicle grafts). An "island" of skin connected to the body by a direct cutaneous artery and vein is called an island arterial flap.

SUBDERMAL PLEXUS FLAP. This flap is the most common pedicle graft in veterinary medicine. Its survival is dependent upon adequate perfusion through the pedicle's subdermal plexus. No generalized length-to-width flap ratio can be used for safe flap dimensions in all areas of the body because the cutaneous circulation differs in various areas of the dog. More important, flaps based over a similar blood supply survive to the same length *regardless of the flap's width.* The only advantage of widening a subdermal plexus flap would be to incorporate a direct cutaneous artery and vein into the pedicle to form an axial pattern flap (see Fig. 33-10B).

Long subdermal plexus flaps require time to elapse after their creation to improve their circulation prior to transfer to the recipient bed. A 3-week delay is common, but the optimal time of transfer varies with individual dogs. The considerable time, cost, and potential complications associated with delayed procedures can be avoided with axial pattern flaps. Whenever possible, the subdermal plexus flap pedicle should be oriented toward a known direct cutaneous artery arborizing in the general vicinity of the wound (see Fig. 33-11). This orientation helps to ensure an adequate perfusion pressure to the flap.

AXIAL PATTERN FLAPS. A direct cutaneous artery and vein are incorporated into axial pattern flaps to help ensure an adequate perfusion pressure to the graft. Axial pattern flaps of considerable dimension may be developed and transferred in a single stage because of their excellent blood supply.

Anatomic landmarks are required to locate predictably the direct cutaneous vessels for axial pattern flap development. Four major direct cutaneous arteries

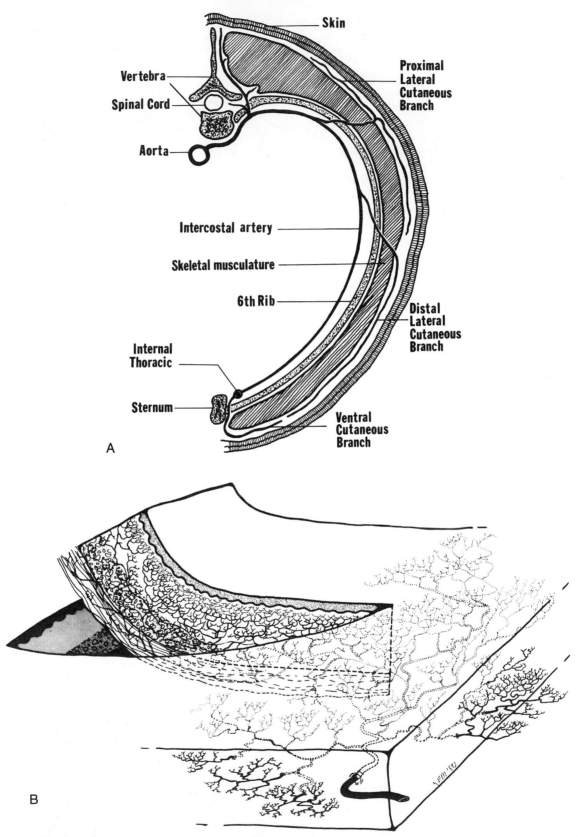

Fig. 33-10. A, *Cross-section of the thoracic wall illustrating the proximal and distal lateral cutaneous branches of the intercostal arteries. Note the parallel relationship of the direct cutaneous arteries (and veins) with the overlying skin. B, Schematic diagram of the subdermal plexus flap. Terminal branches of a direct cutaneous artery form and supply the subdermal plexus. Note the panniculus muscle associated with the subdermal (deep) plexus and the overlying skin. (From Pavletic, M. M.: Canine axial pattern flaps using the omocervical, thoracodorsal and deep circumflex iliac direct cutaneous arteries. Am. J. Vet. Res. 42:391, 1981.)*

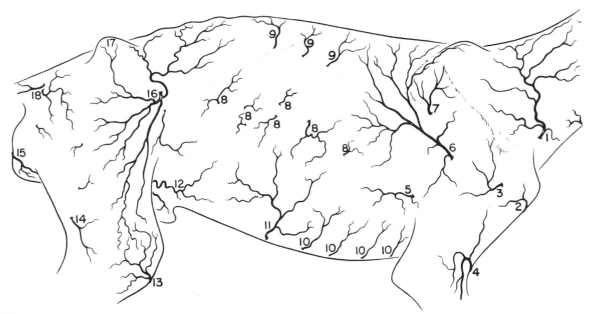

Fig. 33-11. *Superficial arteries of the canine trunk: 1, superficial cervical branch of the omocervical; 2, cranial circumflex humeral; 3, caudal circumflex humeral; 4, proximal collateral radial; 5, lateral thoracic; 6, cutaneous branch of thoracodorsal; 7, cutaneous branch of subscapular; 8, distal lateral cutaneous branches of intercostals; 9, proximal lateral cutaneous branches of intercostals; 10, ventral cutaneous branches of internal thoracic; 11, cranial superficial epigastric; 12, caudal superficial epigastric; 13, medial genicular; 14, cutaneous branch of caudal femoral; 15, perineal; 16, deep circumflex iliac; 17, tubera coxae; 18, cutaneous branches of superficial lateral coccygeal. (From Evans, H. E. and Christensen, G. C.: Miller's Anatomy of the Dog. 2nd Ed. Philadelphia, W. B. Saunders, 1979.)*

have been mapped in the dog: the caudal superficial epigastric artery, the cervical cutaneous branch of the omocervical artery, the thoracodorsal artery, and the deep circumflex iliac artery (Fig. 33-12). The skin to be incorporated into the flap must be in a natural, undis-

torted position in relation to the landmarks, to ensure that the direct cutaneous vessels are included in the flap. Flap boundaries should then be sketched onto the skin with ink before the animal is positioned for the surgical procedure (Figs. 33-13 to 33-15).

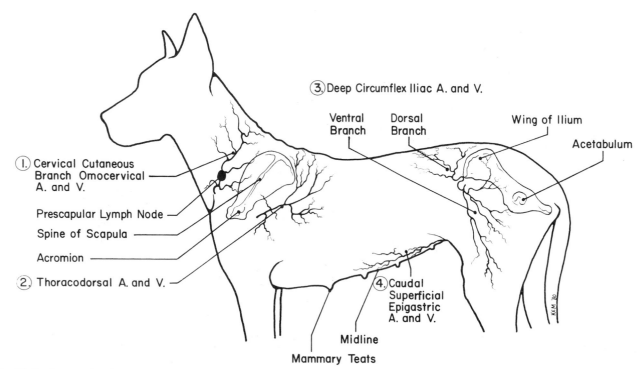

Fig. 33-12. *Four major direct cutaneous arteries are illustrated in relation to their anatomic landmarks. (From Pavletic, M. M.: Canine axial pattern flaps using the omocervical, thoracodorsal, and deep circumflex iliac direct cutaneous arteries. Am. J. Vet. Res., 42:391, 1981.)*

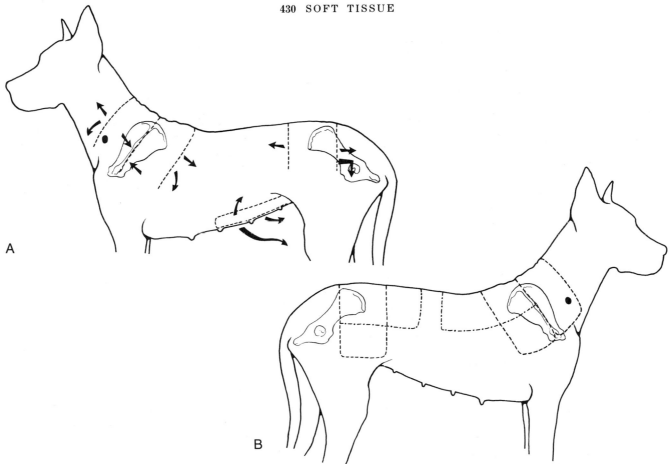

Fig. 33-13. A *and* B, *Reference lines for the omocervical, thoracodorsal, deep circumflex iliac, and caudal superficial epigastric axial pattern flaps. Flaps may be created in the standard peninsula (dashed lines) or "L" or Hockey-stick (dashed and dotted lines) configuration. (From Pavletic, M. M.: Canine axial pattern flaps using the omocervical, thoracodorsal, and deep circumflex iliac direct cutaneous arteries. Am. J. Vet. Res., 42:391, 1981.)*

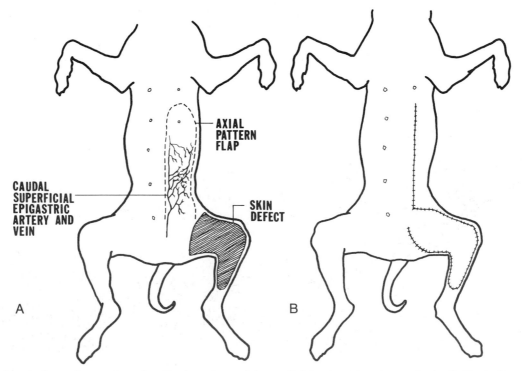

Fig. 33-14. A, *Extent of vascular supply to the skin from the caudal superficial epigastric artery and vein.* B, *illustration of one potential application of such an axial pattern flap. The flap can be transplanted within 180° as long as care is taken to avoid twisting or kinking the direct cutaneous artery and vein.*

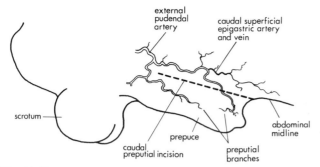

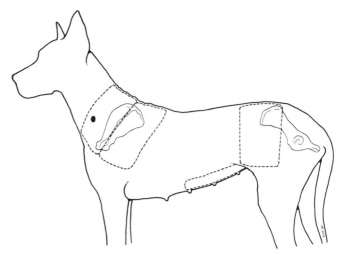

Fig. 33-15. *In the male, care must be taken to avoid transection of the caudal superficial epigastric artery and vein by including the base of the prepuce in the medial incision.*

Fig. 33-17. *General reference lines for island arterial flaps. Larger island arterial flaps may be created. (From Pavletic, M. M.: Canine axial pattern flaps utilizing the omocervical, thoracodorsal and deep circumflex iliac direct cutaneous arteries. Am. J. Vet. Res., 42:391, 1981.)*

ISLAND ARTERIAL FLAPS. These are axial pattern flaps in which the cutaneous pedicle is severed. Thus, the direct cutaneous artery and vein are the only source of circulation to the flap (Fig. 33-16). The direct cutaneous artery and vein are capable of supporting island flaps of considerable dimension (Fig. 33-17). These dimensions are comparable to axial pattern flaps even without the additional circulation from a cutaneous pedicle. Another advantage to island flaps is greater mobility, as compared with axial pattern flaps.

It is possible to sever an island arterial flap's direct cutaneous vessels and anastomose them, through the use of microvascular surgical techniques, to a donor artery and vein at or near the recipient site. Microvascular graft transfer has limited clinical application in the dog at the present time, however.

Local Pedicle Grafts (Flaps)

Local pedicle grafts can be either advanced forward or rotated into the recipient bed.

ADVANCEMENT FLAPS. The single square or rectangular pedicle advancement flap is one of the more common local flaps and is advanced forward into the defect

(Fig. 33-18). In addition, two opposing single pedicle advancement flaps can be used to close large recipient beds. This form of closure is called "H" plasty (Fig. 33-19). In man, Burow's triangles have been employed at the base of the flap, to facilitate flap advancement and to eliminate corner "kinks" or "dog-ears." They are rarely, if ever, required in companion animals because of the elastic nature of the skin of companion animals.

"V-Y" advancement is a "lengthening procedure" occasionally used to relieve excessive tension to an area. Conversely, "Y-V" closure can be used to increase local tension to an area. A "V" incision is made, and the edges are undermined if necessary. Closure of the outer incision edges at the point of the "V" pushes the inner triangular flap forward to relieve local tension (Fig. 33-20).

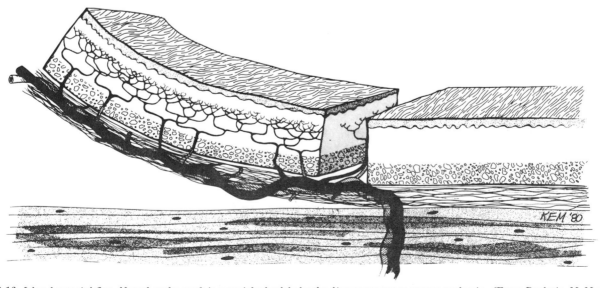

Fig. 33-16. *Island arterial flap. Note that the graft is nourished solely by the direct cutaneous artery and vein. (From Pavletic, M. M.: Canine axial pattern flaps using the omocervical thoracodorsal, and deep circumflex iliac direct cutaneous arteries. Am. J. Vet. Res., 42:391, 1981.)*

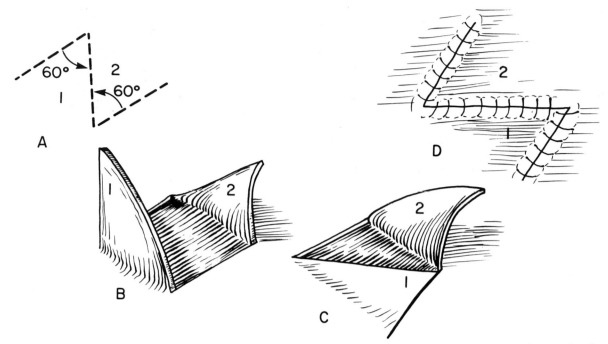

Fig. 33-24. *"Z" plasty. A, A "central" incision is made over the restrictive scar or parallel to the lines of tension when employed to relieve excessive tension on a suture line. Local restrictive scar tissue may be excised or divided to facilitate scar lengthening. Two incisions are made 60° to the central incisions. All three incisions are equal in length to form two equilateral triangular flaps. B, Both flaps are undermined. C, Both flaps are rotated to their opposing donor beds. D, The flaps are sutured into place; the result is a net lengthening of approximately 75%.*

Distant Pedicle Grafts (Flaps)

Distant pedicle grafts are used when insufficient loose skin is available to develop a local flap for wound closure. This situation is most common with large skin losses involving the distal extremities.

Distant flaps can be *transferred directly* or *indirectly*. Direct transfer involves elevation of the affected limb beneath a lateral thoracic or abdominal flap (hinge flap[6]) or placement beneath a bipedicle flap (tunnel or pouch flap[21]). Indirect transfer involves tubed flap development and movement to the recipient

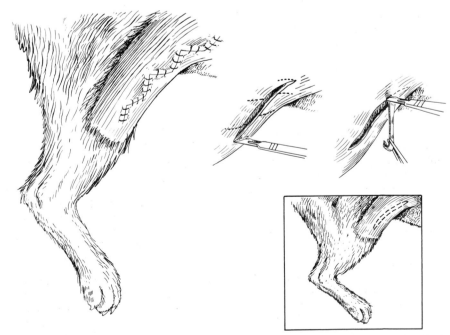

Fig. 33-25. *Multiple "Z" plasties. Multiple "Z"s have a cumulative lengthening effect which can be employed effectively in areas where a single "Z" plasty procedure is impossible or unadvisable.*

bed. All distant flaps must be carefully planned for consistent success. Distant flaps transferred in direct fashion must be adequately immobilized to the trunk to prevent movement of the flap and tension on the flap pedicle for 10 to 14 days. The pedicle(s) should be divided in stages (one-third to half the pedicle(s) every 2 to 3 days) to prevent sudden vascular compromise to the flap.

Tube flaps based upon the subdermal plexus require a delay of 2 to 3 weeks to enhance the blood supply prior to severing one pedicle and transferring the flap. Care must be taken to avoid kinking or twisting the transfer pedicle. In general, 2 weeks more are required before this pedicle can be severed (in stages) to complete the transfer. Although distant flaps can provide full-thickness skin coverage to an area, considerable time and money are required with inherent risks of flap necrosis during their development and transfer. Free skin grafts are an alternate method of skin coverage for extensive distal extremity defects.

FREE SKIN GRAFTS

Free skin grafts lack a vascular attachment upon transfer to the recipient graft bed. These grafts must survive the initial transfer by absorbing tissue fluid from the recipient bed by capillary action during the initial 48 hours after transplantation. During this period, capillaries from the recipient bed unite with the exposed graft plexuses to reestablish vital circulation. New capillaries later grow into the graft, and the vascular channels remodel. In addition, fibrous connective tissue forms to hold the graft securely in place. Grafts assume a pink color in 48 hours if circulation is adequate. Grafts with venous obstruction have a cyanotic hue until circulation improves.

An accumulation of materials such as pus, serum, blood, hematoma, or foreign matter between the graft and recipient bed delays or prevents graft revascularization. This delay often results in graft necrosis. Motion between the graft and the recipient bed has a similar effect. Fibrinolysis secondary to bacterial infection destroys the early fibrin "glue" between the graft and the bed, resulting in motion and graft necrosis. Improper contact between the graft and the recipient bed prevents proper surface-to-surface interdigitation and poor graft revascularization. This improper contact may occur if the graft is stretched over the bed like a "drum skin" or if an excessively large graft is applied to form graft folds that lack proper recipient-bed contact.

Although grafts require a vascularized recipient bed for survival, granulation tissue is not necessary before a graft is applied. Healthy pink granulation tissue, however, is an excellent recipient bed for skin grafts. Chronic granulation tissue has a poor vascular supply and should be excised to promote formation of healthy granulation tissue. Contamination and infection should be controlled, and the granulation surface must be free of any "epithelial cover" prior to graft application.

Free grafts can be classified according to the source of the graft, the graft thickness, and the graft shape or

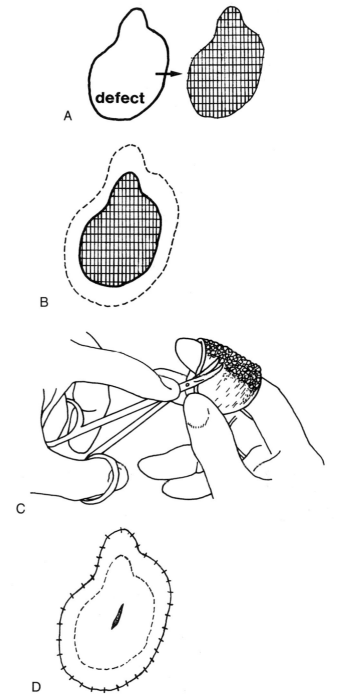

Fig. 33-26. *Free full-thickness graft. A, The recipient bed has been prepared for operation. Any epithelialized areas have been excised to accept full graft coverage. A sterile gauze or paper template is made of the recipient bed. B, The template is transferred to the prepared donor site. A sterile ink applicator is used to outline the template on the donor site 1 cm outside its border. C, The graft is removed, and the donor bed is closed. The graft is "defatted" by trimming away all subcutaneous tissue. The resultant graft appears opaque when held to a light source. The graft must be kept moist at all times. D, The graft is laid over the wound. Stab incisions may be used to prevent fluid accumulation beneath the graft. The graft overlaps the recipient bed and is sutured into place with a simple interrupted or continuous pattern. (The overlapped border eventually sloughs, leaving complete graft coverage over the recipient bed.) The graft is dressed and bandaged postsurgically.*

design. Whereas autogenous grafts are used for permanent free graft coverage in the dog, allografts (homografts) and xenografts (heterografts) are used as a temporary biologic dressing until an autogenous graft can be successfully applied. Free grafts can be harvested as full-thickness or split-thickness skin grafts. Split-thickness grafts are harvested with razor blades, graft knives, or a dermatome. Graft thickness varies according to the amount of dermis included with the overlying epidermis (see Fig. 33-9). The donor bed of a split-thickness graft bed can be excised and closed, or it may be left to heal by adnexal regeneration and epithelialization.

Thin split-thickness grafts "take" more readily than full-thickness grafts, but they lack durability and proper hair growth, and they are more susceptible to secondary graft contraction. Full-thickness grafts are preferred by many veterinarians for these reasons. (See the next section of this chapter, "split-thickness skin grafting.") Free grafts can be applied as a "sheet" over the entire recipient bed (Fig. 33-26), or they may be divided into various shapes or patterns. Pinch grafts,[1,7] strip grafts, stamp grafts, and mesh grafts[8] are commonly used as partial-coverage grafts to increase the total recipient surface area that a small graft harvest can cover (Figs. 33-27 to 33-30).

Open spaces between the graft perimeters also allow for drainage until the granulation tissue bed is covered by the advancing sheet of epithelial cells originating from the graft. As a result, partial-coverage grafts are useful for recipient beds with low-grade infections. Small grafts also conform to irregular recipient beds, are simple to apply, and are economical to perform. Unfortunately, the resultant epithelialized surface lacks the functional and cosmetic results achieved with full-thickness graft coverage.

Postoperative Care

Proper protection is essential for survival of a skin graft. The animal should be confined to a cage, and sedatives should be administered if the patient is excita-

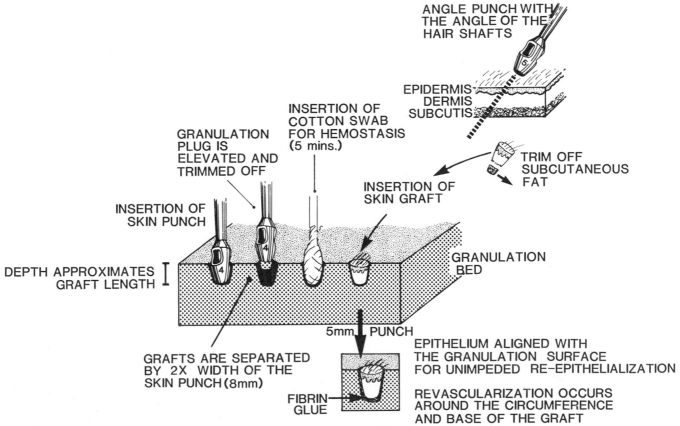

Fig. 33-27. *Punch graft technique (pinch grafts). A sharp 5- or 6-mm biopsy punch is used to harvest the graft plugs from a suitable donor site. The donor area is clipped, leaving the hair shafts exposed. Subcutaneous fat is trimmed off the graft base. A single stitch is used to close the donor bed. The grafts are placed between 2 moistened saline pads until needed. A 4-mm biopsy punch is used to remove cores of granulation tissue. Holes are spaced 8 mm apart (twice the width of the biopsy punch). Fine scissors are required to remove the granulation core. A sterile cotton swab is inserted into each hole for 5 minutes. The graft plugs are then inserted in the direction of natural hair growth. A firm dressing is applied postsurgically to maintain the position of the grafts. The following advantages may be noted with this procedure: (1) 4-mm granulation holes compensate for graft shrinkage and allow the grafts to fit more snugly; (2) the epithelial surface of the graft is level with the granulation bed, and re-epithelialization is unimpeded; (3) as many hair follicles as possible are included into each graft to promote hair growth; (4) re-epithelialization is possible despite partial graft necrosis from surviving hair follicles and skin adnexa deep in the graft; and (5) graft revascularization occurs around the circumference as well as through the base of the graft plug, a comparatively large surface area.*

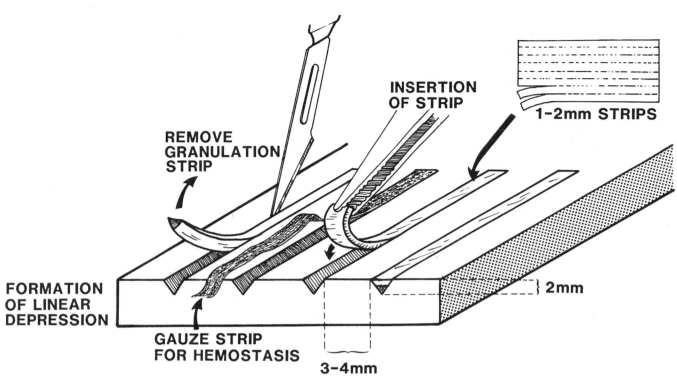

Fig. 33-28. *Strip grafts. Application of strip grafts is similar to that of punch grafts. Linear strips of skin are laid in granulation troughs cut with a scalpel blade. Granulation tissue between the strips is eventually re-epithelialized from the graft.*

ble. The type of bandage, the dressing, and the sequence of bandage changes may vary. We prefer covering grafts postoperatively with an Adaptic* pad and a bland antimicrobial ointment followed by an even layer of gauze pads. Alternate layers of adherent gauze and cotton are applied. A layer of elastic tape is applied to complete the bandage. Such bandages are bulky and restrict motion to the graft. Additional external support, such as with splints, casts, slings, and reinforcement rods, is used if necessary.

The bandage is changed 4 to 5 days postsurgically with the patient under light anesthesia. Earlier bandage changes risk graft motion during the critical 48-hour-

*Adaptic Nonadherent Dressing, Johnson & Johnson, Products, Inc., New Brunswick, NJ 08903

period of graft revascularization. The veterinarian must resist the tremendous temptation to "check" the graft in the early stages. To remove the bandage, the outer layers are cut away, but the Adaptic pad is left in place. Any bandage materials sticking to the graft should be left alone because "graft picking" and "scab pulling" may move or remove the graft. At 4 to 5 days postoper-

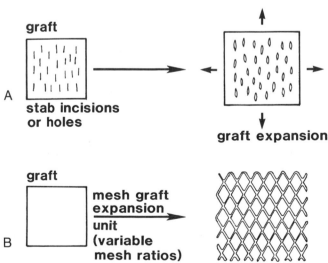

Fig. 33-30. *Mesh grafts. Both full-thickness and split-thickness grafts may be used. A, Multiple stab incisions or holes are cut into the graft to allow the graft to expand and to provide adequate drainage. The graft is sutured at the periphery. B, Mesh-graft expansion units have been developed to expand the graft into a uniform mesh. A graft can be expanded 1.5 to 9 times its original surface area to cover extensive skin defects.*

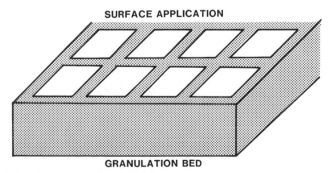

Fig. 33-29. *Stamp grafts. Full-thickness or split-thickness grafts are harvested and are divided into squares. Size can vary up to the size of postage stamps. Grafts are laid over the recipient bed a few to several millimeters apart. Square depressions may be cut into a granulation bed if necessary to improve graft immobilization.*

atively, the graft is inspected, if visible, for signs of infection, necrosis, or elevation from the graft bed. Cultures are taken if necessary. Early signs of graft necrosis are discouraging, but not always catastrophic, because hair follicles and cutaneous adnexa in the deep portion of the graft may survive and may serve as a source for wound epithelialization. Subsequent bandage changes are repeated in similar fashion every 2 to 4 days, depending on the condition of the graft. This routine is continued for approximately 2 weeks, followed by application of a lighter bandage for an additional 10 to 14 days.

One must also keep in mind the potential adverse effects of bandages. Excessive pressure or application of wrinkled bandage material over the graft can result in graft necrosis. In addition, bandage materials can act as an abrasive on the graft if immobilization of the affected area is inadequate.

Comments

Flap necrosis is usually attributed to insufficient vascular perfusion. Poor planning and rough technique also contribute to flap failure. Thus, flaps should be planned with the blood supply as a primary consideration, and the technique should be the simplest and gentlest possible to safely restore the anatomic and functional continuity of the affected area. The direction of hair growth from the flap is also considered if other surgical factors are considered to be equal.

Atraumatic surgical technique is essential for consistent success in skin grafting. Tissue trauma (1) compromises vascular channels in the flap, (2) damages and destroys cells that may then serve as a bacterial growth medium, (3) prolongs wound healing, and (4) further compromises the ability of the flap to resist infection. Sharp surgical blades should be used to cut skin. Scissors crush skin and should be avoided. Skin hooks and Brown-Adson forceps should be used to manipulate the flap. Allis tissue forceps and other crushing forceps should not be used on any epithelial surface.

The skin of the dog and cat is loosely attached, pliable, and elastic and often "molds" to skin closures that would cause skin "puckers" or "dog ears" in man. Consequently, the use of Burow's triangles and other methods to minimize "dog ears" (Fig. 33-31) and to facilitate flap rotation or advancement are usually unnecessary. Skin grafting in the dog and cat can be kept on a simple surgical level in most cases with gratifying results.

References and Suggested Readings

1. Alexander, J. W., and Hoffer, R. E.: Pinch grafting in the dog. Canine Pract., *3*:27, 1976.
2. Converse, J. M.: Reconstructive Plastic Surgery. Vol I. Philadelphia, W. B. Saunders, 1977.
3. Evans, H. E., and Christensen, G. C.: Miller's Anatomy of the Dog. 2nd Ed. Philadelphia, W. B. Saunders, 1979.
4. Finseth, F. J.: Anatomy and design of flaps. *In* Symposium on Basic Science in Plastic Surgery. Edited by T. J. Krizek and J. G. Hoopes. St. Louis, C. V. Mosby, 1976.
5. Grabb, W. C., and Myers, M. B.: Skin Flaps. Boston, Little, Brown, 1975.
6. Grabb, W. C., and Smith, J. W.: Plastic Surgery. Boston, Little, Brown, 1973.
7. Hanselka, D. V., and Boyd, C. L.: Use of mesh grafts in dogs and horses. J. Am. Anim. Hosp. Assoc., *12*:650, 1976.
8. Hoffer, H. E., and Alexander, J. W.: Pinch grafting. J. Am. Anim. Hosp. Assoc., *12*:664, 1976.
9. Hoffmeister, F. S.: Studies on timing of tissue transfer in reconstructive surgery. Plast. Reconstr. Surg., *19*:283, 1957.
10. Jensen, E. C.: Canine autogenous skin grafting. Am. J. Vet. Res., *20*:898, 1959.
11. Jensen, E. C.: Skin grafting in the dog. Iowa State Coll. Vet., *3*:163, 1957.
12. Keefe, F.: Skin grafting in a cat. J. Am. Vet. Med. Assoc., *108*:43, 1946.
13. Milton, S. H.: Experimental studies of island flaps. I. The surviving length. Plast. Reconstr. Surg., *48*:574, 1971.
14. Milton, S. H.: Pedicled skin flaps: the fallacy of the length:width ratio. Br. J. Surg., *57*:502, 1970.

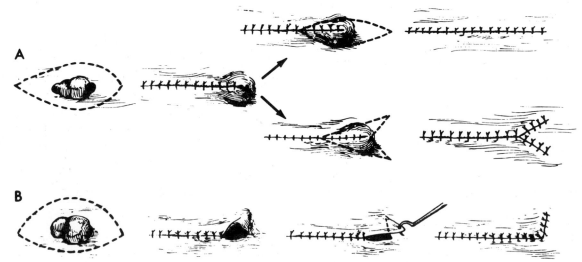

Fig. 33-31. A, *Two methods of removing a dog ear caused by an elliptical excision that is too short.* B, *A method of removing a dog ear caused when one side of the ellipse is longer than the other. (From Grabb, W. C., and Smith, J. W.: Plastic Surgery. Boston, Little, Brown, 1973.)*

15. Myer, M. B.: Anatomy and design of flaps. *In* Symposium on Basic Science in Plastic Surgery. Edited by T. J. Kirzek and J. E. Hoopes. St. Louis, C. V. Mosby, 1976.

16. Nathanson, S. E., and Jackson, R. J.: Blood flow measurements in skin flaps. Arch. Otolaryngol., *101*:354, 1975.

17. Orentreich, N.: Hair transplantation: the punch graft technique. Surg. Clin. North Am., *51*:511, 1971.

18. Pavletic, M. M.: Canine axial pattern flaps utilizing the omocervical thoracodorsal and deep circumflex iliac direct cutaneous arteries. Am. J. Vet. Res., *42*:391, 1981.

19. Pavletic, M. M.: Caudal superficial epigastric arterial pedicle grafts in the dog. Vet. Surg., *9*:103, 1980.

20. Pavletic, M. M.: Vascular supply to the skin of the dog: a review. Vet. Surg., *9*:77, 1980.

21. Pullen, C. M.: Reconstruction of the skin. *In* Current Techniques in Small Animal Surgery. Edited by M. J. Bojrab. Philadelphia, Lea & Febiger, 1975.

22. Ross, G. E.: Clinical canine skin grafting. J. Am. Vet. Med. Assoc., *153*:1759, 1968.

23. Self, R. A.: Skin grafting in canine practice. J. Am. Vet. Med. Assoc., *82*:163, 1934.

24. Swaim, S. F.: Surgery of Traumatized Skin: Management and Reconstruction in the Dog and Cat. Philadelphia, W. B. Saunders, 1980.

25. Vallis, C. P.: Hair transplantation for male pattern baldness. Surg. Clin. North Am., *51*:519, 1971.

26. Wallace, A. B., Spruell, J. S. A., and Hamilton, H. A.: The use of autogenous free full thickness skin graft in the treatment of a chronic inflammatory lesion in a dog. Vet. Rec. *74*:286, 1962.

27. Zoltan, J.: Techniques for Ideal Wound Healing. Cicatrix Optima. Baltimore, University Park Press, 1977.

Split-Thickness Skin Grafting

by Curtis W. Probst

and Llewellyn C. Peyton

Split-thickness skin grafts are used extensively to treat a variety of cutaneous injuries in man. Split-thickness skin grafting in the dog has had limited use; however, skin grafting should be considered in certain cases for reconstruction of cutaneous defects. In man, one of the major indications for the use of split-thickness skin grafts is in the repair of burn wounds. In dogs, split-thickness skin grafts can be used to treat massive wounds, wounds of the face and extremities and to cover secondary defects created by full-thickness grafts or pedicle flaps.

Surgical Anatomy

The canine skin is composed of two main layers: the epidermis and the dermis. The thickness of these layers and the hair density vary on different parts of the body; the skin is thickest over the dorsum and neck and thinnest over the abdominal, sternal, axillary, and inguinal regions.

The epidermis lacks blood vessels and receives nourishment from fluid that penetrates from the deeper layers and from dermal capillaries. The dermis, which is vascular and usually much thicker than the epidermis, contains blood and lymph vessels, nerves, hair follicles, glands and their ducts, and smooth muscle fibers.

The arteries supplying the skin form three vascular plexuses: (1) the subcutaneous plexus, (2) the cutaneous plexus, and (3) the superficial plexus. These vascular plexuses are important in gauging the thickness of a split-thickness skin graft. A thin graft leaves many small, superficial bleeding vessels, whereas a thick graft leaves a donor site with fewer but larger bleeding vessels.

Split-thickness skin grafts contain epidermis and a variable quantity of dermis, in contrast to full-thickness grafts, which include the entire thickness of dermis. Split-thickness grafts may be classified as thin (less than .008 inch thick), intermediate (.010 to .015 inch thick), or thick (.015 to .025 inch thick), depending on the amount of dermis included in the graft (Fig. 33-32).

Advantages and Disadvantages

Some of the advantages of split-thickness skin grafts are as follows: (1) free split-thickness skin grafts take more readily than full-thickness free grafts; (2) split-thickness grafts leave adnexal remnants, and therefore, donor sites heal spontaneously; (3) multiple crops of split-thickness skin can be harvested from areas of thick skin; and (4) split-thickness skin grafts can cover wounds with only one surgical procedure.

The disadvantages of split-thickness skin grafting include the following: (1) split-thickness grafts may lack hair growth; (2) the grafts may have a scaly appearance and may lack sebaceous and sweat secretions; (3) split-thickness skin grafts tend to contract; (4) split-thickness grafts are less durable than full-thickness grafts; and (5) the donor sites may heal with little or no hair growth.

Many of the disadvantages of split-thickness grafts

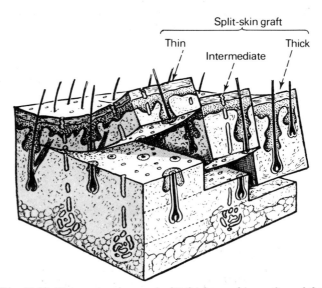

Fig. 33-32. *The varying degree of split-thickness skin grafts and the constituents of each is shown. (From McGregor, I. A.: Fundamental Techniques of Plastic Surgery. 7th ed. Edinburgh, Churchill Livingstone, 1980.*

are a result of the graft's thickness. Thick split-thickness skin grafts grow hair, contract less, and may have sebaceous and sweat secretions. If a graft is cut thickly enough to grow hair, however, the donor site will heal slowly and may lack hair growth. In such instances, the donor site can be excised and closed by direct suture, provided enough loose skin is available. Intermediate and thick split-thickness grafts usually withstand the stresses placed on them by active dogs.

Grafting Techniques

AREAS THAT ACCEPT SKIN GRAFTS. A skin graft can be placed either on a healthy granulation bed or on a fresh, surgically clean wound. As a general rule, a free skin graft is accepted by any site that, left ungrafted, would rapidly develop granulations. Soft tissues such as muscle and fascia usually accept grafts readily. Cartilage covered with perichondrium, bone covered with periosteum, and tendon covered with paratenon all accept grafts; however, bare cartilage, bone, or tendon cannot be relied on to take a graft. Grafts may survive laterally for a distance of about 1 cm from their underlying blood supply. Because of this ability, grafts may survive over areas of bare bone, cartilage, or tendon, provided the area is small.

DONOR SITE SELECTION. Factors to consider when choosing a donor site include the amount of skin required, the amount of skin available, local convenience, whether a good color and texture match is needed, the necessity of having hair on the graft, and the cutting instrument available. The thorax, the lateral thigh, and the neck are the most common donor sites, but virtually any area of the body can be used.

GRAFT-CUTTING INSTRUMENTS. The various instruments used to harvest split-thickness skin grafts fall into one of three categories: (1) freehand instruments, (2) drum dermatomes, and (3) electric or pneumatic dermatomes.

Several skin graft knives with depth control devices are available (Fig. 33-33). Split-thickness skin grafts

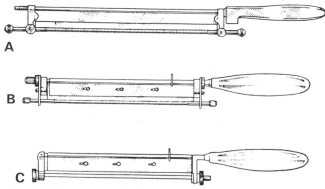

Fig. 33-33. *Several hand-held graft knives with a depth control device are shown. A, Humby knife (Bodenham modification); B, Humby knife (Braithewaite pattern); and C, Humby knife (Watson modification). (From McGregor, I. A.: Fundamental Techniques of Plastic Surgery. 7th ed. Edinburgh, Churchill Livingstone, 1980.)*

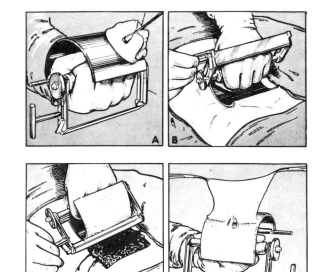

Fig. 33-34. *The use of the Padgett-Hood dermatome is shown. A, The adhesive compound is applied to the drum. B, The drum is secured to the skin. C, The graft is cut to the desired thickness. D, The graft is removed from the drum prior to placing it on the wound. (From McGregor, I. A.: Fundamental Techniques of Plastic Surgery. 7th ed. Edinburgh, Churchill Livingstone, 1980.)*

can also be harvested with safety or injector razors and a scalpel.

The Padgett-Hood* and Reese† dermatomes are drum dermatomes. The skin is secured to the drum either by rubber cement (Padgett-Hood) or with a special tape (Reese) and then cut to a predetermined thickness with an oscillating blade (Fig. 33-34). These dermatomes cut a uniform thickness of graft, but the length and width of the graft are limited by the size of the drum.

The electric or pneumatic dermatome (Brown dermatome‡) has a rapidly oscillating blade that can cut long strips of split-thickness skin without the use of adhesives (Fig. 33-35). The skin can be cut to a variety of depths and widths by calibrating the instrument. With the Brown dermatome, one may cut skin from almost any part of the body.

HARVESTING THE GRAFT. Once the wound is deemed ready for grafting, the patient is anesthetized in a standard manner. The donor site and the skin surrounding the wound are routinely clipped and are aseptically prepared. Strong antiseptic solutions should not be applied directly on granulating wounds. Rinsing the wound with sterile saline solution is usually sufficient preparation of the recipient site.

The recipient site should be prepared first in order to achieve maximum hemostasis prior to the application of the graft. Generally, grafts take more completely if the surface of the granulation is removed. Because

*Kansas City Assemblage Co., 3953 Broadway, Kansas City, MO 64111
†Bard-Parker Co., Danbury, CT 06810
‡Zimmer Manufacturing, Warsaw, IN 46580

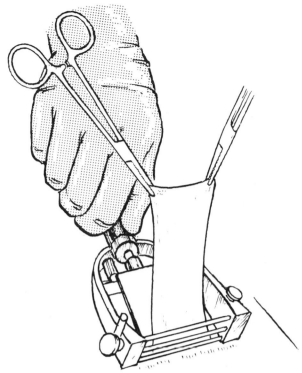

Fig. 33-35. *The use of the Brown pneumatic dermatome is shown. The dermatome is pressed firmly against the skin and is slowly advanced as the oscillating blade cuts the graft. (From McGregor, I. A.: Fundamental Techniques of Plastic Surgery. 7th ed. Edinburgh, Churchill Livingstone, 1980.)*

scraping interferes with the graft's success, granulations should never be scraped, but should be cleanly sliced off with an old graft knife or scalpel blade. The superficial, .5- to 2-mm layer of granulation is all that needs to be removed. Care should be exercised to avoid undue contamination of the underlying recipient bed or damage to important underlying tissues. When removing surface granulations, the underlying bed should be as level as possible, to avoid irregularities that may cause tenting of the graft across the hollows. Tenting causes the graft to fail because the graft must maintain constant contact with the recipient bed in order to take successfully.

After removal of surface granulations, the resulting hemorrhage must be controlled because hematoma formation is a major cause of graft failure. Applying gauze sponges soaked in a 1:200,000 dilution of epinephrine to the recipient site is effective in controlling most hemorrhage. Vessels that continue to bleed may be ligated, or electrocoagulation may be performed; however, care must be taken to cause only minimal tissue necrosis. If hemorrhage cannot be controlled, a firm dressing is applied over the wound and is left in place for 24 to 48 hours. Grafts placed in the dry bed of a 24-hour-old recipient site can be expected to take without difficulty.

After preparation of the recipient site, the graft can be harvested. If the Padgett-Hood dermatome is used, the skin and drum are painted with an adhesive com-

pound; if the Reese dermatome is used, Dermtape* is applied. Where the drum is pressed against the skin, the two surfaces adhere, and the skin can be lifted with the drum for cutting by the knife blade, which is moved to and fro (see Fig. 33-34).

The use of the Brown dermatome and freehand graft knives requires a flat skin surface for best results. The dog has few naturally flat skin surfaces; however, the lateral thorax provides an adequate donor site. Sterile saline solution is injected subcutaneously to elevate the skin over the ribs and thereby to make the entire thorax an acceptable donor site. Once a flat surface has been obtained, the skin is lubricated with sterile mineral oil or water-soluble jelly. The skin is held taut by an assistant, and the graft is cut to the desired specifications. The Brown dermatome can be set to cut a graft of uniform depth and width. Downward pressure must be applied to the Brown dermatome while cutting in order to obtain an adequate graft (Fig. 33-35). If a hand-held graft knife is used, the blade is held parallel to the surface of the skin, and the knife is rapidly moved to and fro. The knife is advanced while maintaining this oscillating movement to cut the graft (Fig. 33-36). One should avoid putting excessive downward force on the knife so as not to cut the graft thicker than desired. Judging the depth of the cut with a freehand knife requires experience. When the depth is correct, the knife blade can just be seen through the graft, and the dermis presents a definite resistance to cutting.

Once harvested, the graft is applied to the recipient site with the dermal side down. The direction of hair growth on the graft should match that of the surrounding skin as closely as possible because a thick split-thickness graft grows hair. The edges of the graft should overlap the edges of the defect by 2 to 4 mm (Fig. 33-37). If one attempts to suture the graft-skin margin accurately edge to edge, the graft is apt to roll inward resulting in a poor scar. The edges of the graft are then secured to the skin with fine (3-0 to 4-0) suture material. The use of absorbable suture material eliminates the need for suture removal. If the wound cannot

*Bard-Parker Co., Danbury, CT 06810

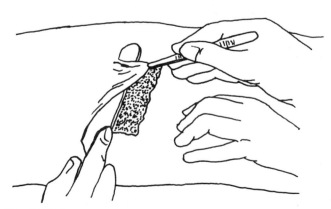

Fig. 33-36. *The use of a hand-held graft knife is shown. The skin is held taut. The knife blade is held parallel to the skin surface and is moved rapidly in a to-and-fro fashion to harvest the graft.*

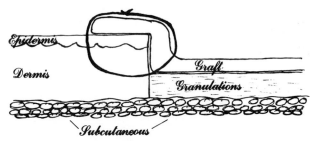

Fig. 33-37. *A correctly sutured split-thickness skin graft is shown. The edge of the graft overlaps the edge of the wound. The sutures are placed in such a manner as to provide maximum contact between the graft and its bed.*

be covered with one graft, multiple grafts should be sutured to one another and tacked down to the granulating bed. Before placing the last few sutures, any air bubbles or accumulated serum should be removed from under the graft by rolling a moistened, cotton-tipped applicator over the graft toward the unsutured opening. The graft only takes to the edges of the wound, and the overlapping skin may be trimmed during subsequent dressing changes.

Postoperative Management

The requirement for a successful graft (given a suitable bed) is close and immobile contact between the graft and its bed. Grafts are lost when a hematoma separates the graft from its bed and when shearing movements prevent adhesion and capillary linkup between the graft and its bed.

Pressure bandages provide close contact between the graft and the recipient bed. These bandages can be applied as tie-over bolus dressings or as diffuse-pressure dressings that provide not only pressure, but immobilization as well. A tie-over bolus dressing is reserved for clean wounds with a concave surface. When suturing the graft to the wound, the ends of the suture are left long. Petrolatum-impregnated gauze is placed directly on the graft. A cotton bolus is then placed over the gauze and the ends of the sutures are tied to one another over the cotton (Fig. 33-38). The diffuse-pressure dressing is particularly useful when grafts have been applied on the distal extremities. Petrolatum-impregnated gauze is placed directly over the graft, which is then covered with roll cotton (cast padding). The roll cotton is covered with a layer of stretch gauze, followed by a layer of elastic tape. Casts and splints can be used in conjunction with pressure dressings to aid in graft immobilization.

The bandages should be changed 48 hours postoperatively. During bandage changes, the primary concern is not to disturb the graft. In 48 hours, graft adherence is usually sufficient that the graft will not be disturbed. If available, early graft inspection allows one to drain seromas and thereby to save a graft that might otherwise fail. Seromas can be drained by lancing them with a No. 11 scalpel blade at the ventralmost aspect and by rolling the serum out with a cotton-tipped applicator.

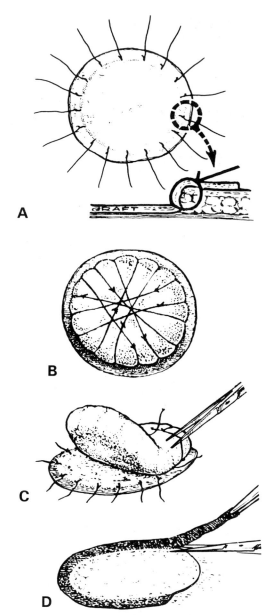

Fig. 33-38. *The use of a tie-over bolus dressing is shown. A, The ends of the sutures are left long in order to tie them over the bolus. B, The bolus is shown in place. C, The bolus is removed in 10 to 14 days, and D, the overlapped edge of the graft is trimmed away. (From McGregor, I. A.: Fundamental Techniques of Plastic Surgery. 7th ed. Edinburgh, Churchill Livingstone, 1980.)*

Subsequent dressing changes depend upon the cooperation of the patient. The dressing is not to be disturbed as long as it is clean, dry, and in place. The dressing can be removed in 10 to 14 days. If a tie-over dressing is used, it should be left in place for 10 to 14 days.

Donor sites left exposed to the air form a thin protective crust that loosens spontaneously as complete epithelialization takes place underneath. The donor area can be covered with a light dressing immediately after harvesting the graft. A single layer of Scarlet Red Ointment Dressing* or a sterile gauze sponge is placed

*Cheesebrough-Ponds, Inc., Hospital Products Division, Greenwich, CT 06830

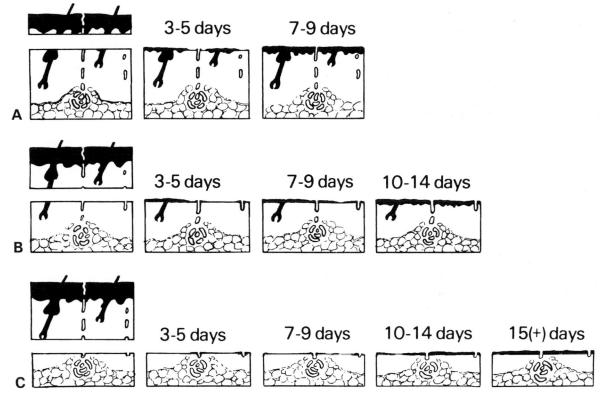

Fig. 33-39. *The healing of various thicknesses of split-thickness skin grafts is shown: A, thin; B, intermediate; and C, thick. Epithelial regeneration occurs from the pilosebaceous apparatus, sweat glands, and the skin edge. (From McGregor, I. A.: Fundamental Techniques of Plastic Surgery. 7th ed. Edinburgh, Churchill Livingstone, 1980.)*

directly on the wound immediately after the graft is harvested. This dressing is covered with a light bandage, which can be removed in 24 to 48 hours. An Elizabethan collar should be kept on the dog to prevent it from disturbing the donor site. The dressing immediately covering the donor site usually adheres and is left in place until it loosens as epithelialization becomes complete. If the dressing does not adhere, the donor site can be left exposed to the air once the protective crust forms.

DONOR SITE HEALING. The donor sites heal by re-epithelialization from the pilosebaceous apparatus. Time for healing of donor sites varies between 7 and 14 days, depending on the thickness of the grafts (Fig. 33-39). Hair regrowth is complete with thin or intermediate thickness grafts, but may be sparse with thicker grafts.

SKIN GRAFT HEALING. The graft initially adheres to its new bed by means of fibrin and survives on "plasmatic circulation." Circulation is rapidly re-established through the vessels transferred with the graft. Color changes take place in the graft during vascular linkup. During the first few days, the graft has a bluish tinge with a faint reddish color. The reddish tint becomes more vivid as the graft "takes." A white or black color indicates graft failure. Concomitantly with the vascular linkup, the fibrin is infiltrated by fibroblasts that secrete collagen and by ground substance that increases the tensile strength and attachment of the graft. The connection between the graft and bed is firm and complete within the first 10 days.

References and Suggested Readings

Brown, J. B., and McDowell, F.: Skin Grafting. 3rd Ed. Philadelphia, J. B. Lippincott, 1958.

Converse, J. M.: Plastic surgery and transplantation of skin. In Skin Surgery. 4th Ed. Edited by E. Epstein and E. Epstein, Jr. Springfield, IL, Charles C Thomas, 1977.

Dingman, R.: General principles of skin surgery. In Skin Surgery. 4th Ed. Edited by E. Epstein and E. Epstein, Jr. Springfield, IL, Charles C Thomas, 1977.

McGregor, I. A.: Fundamental Techniques of Plastic Surgery. 7th Ed. New York, Churchill Livingstone, 1980.

McKeever, P. J., and Braden, T. D.: Comparison of full- and partial-thickness autogenous skin transplantation in dogs: a pilot study. Am. J. Vet. Res., *39*:1706, 1978.

Polk, H. C.: Adherence of skin grafts. Surg. Forum, *17*:487, 1966.

Swaim, S. F.: Surgery of Traumatized Skin: Management and Reconstruction in the Dog and Cat. Philadelphia, W. B. Saunders, 1980.

Hygroma of the Elbow

by AMELIA A. TOOMEY

and M. JOSEPH BOJRAB

The development of hygromas in immature dogs of the large and giant breeds is not an uncommon finding for the veterinary practitioner. Most hygromas are painless swellings that develop between 6 to 18 months of age.[5] Although these fluid-filled structures may be found over any bony prominence, including the greater trochanter of the femur, tuber calcanei, ischial tuberosity, and occipital protuberance, most hygromas occur on the lateral aspect of the elbow, overlying the olecranon.[1-5] Their formation is related to trauma of the soft tissues covering these prominences, usually incurred when the animal is sitting or lying down on hard surfaces.[5] In the case of occipital hygromas, this trauma may be induced by confinement in a cage small enough to allow the animal to strike its head repeatedly against the top of the cage.

In most dogs, as they mature, minor repeated trauma over these bony prominences leads to the development of a skin callus that protects against the formation of hygromas. When excessive trauma occurs before this callus has formed, an inflammatory response develops in the overlying soft tissues. The pressure exerted from hard surfaces is transmitted to the bone, compresses the intervening soft tissue structures, and compromises blood flow to the area. This obstruction to blood flow leads to edema formation, local ischemia, and cellular death.[6] The tissue destruction is accompanied by seroma formation in the subcutaneous tissue, and because the surrounding tissues are also damaged, this fluid is not absorbed.[1] A dense, connective wall forms to enclose the fluid.

The wall of the hygroma consists of varying stages of granulation tissue with a high collagen content.[5] The lining is irregular, owing to villous projections of fibrinous tissue into the lumen. Because the lining is not secretory, the cavity is not a true cyst. The edema fluid is yellow to red in color, mucinous and is less viscid than synovial fluid.[5]

Surgical Treatment

The optimal treatment of elbow hygromas is prevention of their formation. Inflammation and edema of the skin over the olecranon, without cavitation, are the first indications that a hygroma is developing.[1] At this stage, if the elbow is protected, the tissues heal without surgical intervention. Protection is provided by covering the elbow with a loose padded bandage for 2 to 3 weeks and covering the floor of the animal's resting area with soft bedding or straw. With time, a protective callus forms.

If cavitation has already occurred, conservative management may be successful if the hygroma is small and the wall is not yet thick and rigid.[1] Some small hygromas may be present for the life of the animal without causing any problems and, therefore, need not be treated. If desired, treatment by aspiration may be attempted. One must pay strict attention to aseptic technique. Protective padding is applied to the elbow. Corticosteroid preparations should not be injected into the hygroma. These drugs have not been shown to be helpful and may actually impede the healing process.[1-3] Weekly aspirations may be necessary, but if fluid is still present after several treatments, success by this method is unlikely.[1]

Surgical intervention is recommended for small,

thick-walled hygromas and all large hygromas.[1] The objective of surgical treatment is to obliterate the cystic cavity by establishing drainage for the encapsulated fluid. This treatment allows apposition of the two granulating surfaces of the inner wall of the hygroma, so that permanent bridging between the two may take place.

Following aseptic surgical preparation, stab incisions are made into the cavity of the hygroma at its most proximal and distal aspects. By inserting a finger into these openings, any loculi or fibrin masses that are present can be broken down and removed. A Penrose drain one-quarter inch in diameter is placed through the cavity and is sutured to the skin above and below the hygroma (Fig. 33-40A). A Telfa Wet-Pruf* pad is placed over the drains, and a Robert Jones' bandage is applied over the elbow and is changed at weekly intervals. The Penrose drain is removed in 2 to 3 weeks, once the cavity of the hygroma is obliterated, and a bulky padded bandage is reapplied for another 1 to 2 weeks.[1-3]

Once the elbow is healed, some excess skin may be present if the hygroma was large. Over a period of several months, this skin contracts, but some redundant skin may be present for the life of the animal.[1] It is important to provide soft bedding for the animal and to monitor the area for any redness or swelling until a protective callus has formed. Recurrence of the hygroma is uncommon.

Infected hygromas may be handled in the same manner if extensive ulceration of the overlying skin has not occurred. An infected hygroma is painful, the overlying skin is inflamed, and sinus openings are often present. Although hematogenous spread of bacteria to the hygroma is possible, most infections are due to the introduction of organisms from needles or medications.[3,5] Along with surgical drainage, culture of the infected material and antibiotic therapy are indicated.

More complex surgical techniques, which require partial or total excision of the hygroma, are usually not indicated and often provide less satisfactory results. Owing to the lack of loose skin in this area, when tissue is excised, considerable tension is applied to the suture line whenever the elbow is flexed. Because the elbow area is difficult to protect postoperatively, wound dehiscence is common.[3] Excision of the hygroma also removes any protective callus that has already formed in the overlying skin. This callus provides protection against recurrence of the hygroma and should be left intact. In certain instances, however, total surgical excision of the hygroma and overlying skin is necessary. Some advanced hygromas have large areas of ulceration and scar tissue over the olecranon. These ulcerated areas are a result of wound dehiscence following previous surgical procedures, necrosis secondary to repeated trauma, or advanced infection that has broken through the skin.[4] Because these wounds heal with extreme difficulty, owing to continual trauma to the

---

*Kendall Veterinary Products Division, One Federal Street, Boston, MA 02101

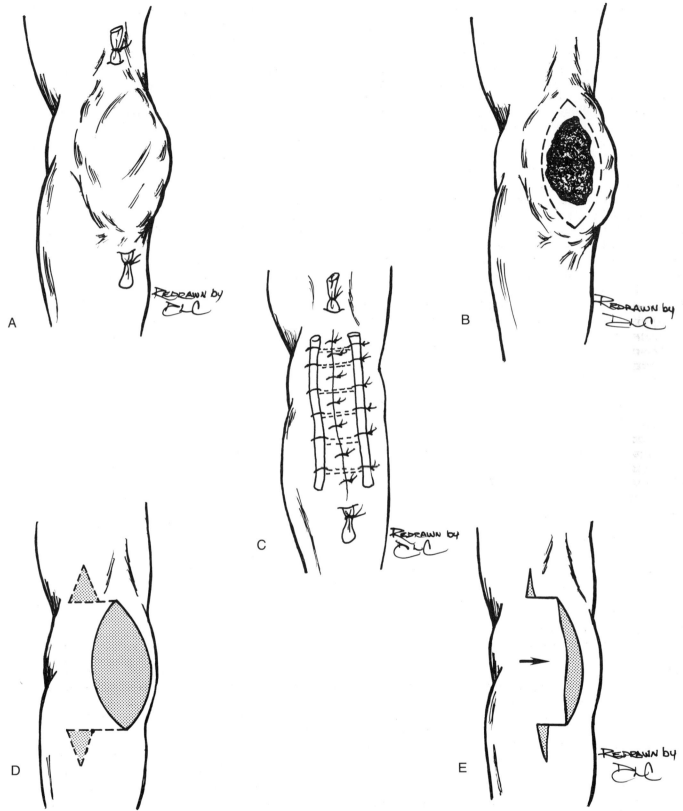

Fig. 33-40. A, *Drained hygroma with Penrose drain sutured in place.* B, *An elliptical incision is made around the area of ulceration.* C, *With the Penrose drain in place, vertical mattress sutures are placed around rubber or gauze stents to relieve tension from the primary suture line. Simple interrupted sutures are used to close the surgical wound.* D, *Burows triangles are made in the loose skin above and below the elbow to allow formation of an advancement flap.* E, *After undermining the skin lateral and medial to the wound, the flap is advanced into place and sutured.* (C and E, redrawn from D. J. Krahwinkel. In *Surgery of Traumatized Skin.* Edited by S. F. Swaim. Philadelphia, W. B. Saunders, 1980.)

area, complete resection of the affected tissue is indicated.[1]

Several days before the surgical procedure, the wound is cleaned, and an aqueous antibiotic dressing is applied. The area is cultured, and systemic antibiotics are administered. Following surgical preparation, an elliptical incision is made around the entire ulcerated area; one must be careful to preserve as much healthy tissue as possible for closure (Fig. 33-40B). The ulcerated tissue is excised, and the surrounding skin is undermined. To relieve the tension on the primary suture line, a row of interrupted vertical mattress sutures is placed over soft rubber or gauze stents.[1] A Penrose drain one-quarter inch in diameter is inserted to allow drainage of the undermined area postsurgically. The skin edges are sutured in a simple interrupted pattern (Fig. 33-40C). When a large amount of tissue has been removed, construction of an advancement flap (Fig. 33-40D and E) may be helpful in mobilizing more skin for closure.[4]

The limb must be immobilized postsurgically to prevent stress on the suture line. The elbow is covered with a Telfa Wet-Pruf pad and loosely bandaged. The leg is then placed in a Schroeder-Thomas splint or Robert Jones' bandage. The drains are removed in 5 days, and the stent sutures are removed in a week. Healing of the primary suture line usually occurs in 10 to 14 days, when the skin sutures and splint are removed.[1,4] The elbow is bandaged for another 2 weeks following splint removal. As emphasized before, careful monitoring of the elbow and protective measures must be instituted until sufficient callus has formed to protect against recurrence.

References and Suggested Readings

1. Johnston, D. E.: Hygroma of the elbow in dogs. Compend. Contin. Ed. Vet. Pract., 1:157, 1979.
2. Johnston, D. E.: Hygroma of the elbow in dogs. In Current Techniques in Small Animal Surgery. Edited by M. J. Bojrab. Philadelphia, Lea & Febiger, 1975.
3. Johnston, D. E.: Hygroma of the elbow in dogs. J. Am. Vet. Med. Assoc., 167:213, 1975.
4. Krahwinkel, D. J.: Elbow hygroma. In Surgery of Traumatized Skin. Edited by S. F. Swaim. Philadelphia, W. B. Saunders, 1980.
5. Newton, C. D., Wilson, G. P., Allen, H. L., and Swenberg, J. A.: Surgical closure of elbow hygromas in the dog. J. Am. Vet. Med. Assoc., 164:147, 1974.
6. Shea, J. D.: Pressure sores: classification and management. Clin. Orthop., 112:89, 1975.

Cheiloplasty

by STEVEN G. STOLL

In small animals, cheiloplasty is primarily concerned with function rather than cosmetics, although a pleasing cosmetic result is always desirable.

Certain anatomic features of small animals are advantageous to the veterinary surgeon contemplating a surgical procedure of the lips. For example, the blood supply to the lips and the entire head region is abundant. This feature promotes rapid healing and provides resistance to infection as long as proper general surgical techniques are followed. Furthermore, in most breeds of dogs, the lips themselves have considerable redundant skin. This extra skin makes resection of a substantial amount of lip possible without the need for complicated plastic surgical procedures, and primary closure is accomplished without undue tension at the incision site.

Basically, the lips are divided into an outer cutaneous lining, a layer of muscle fibers, called the media, and an inner lining of mucous membranes, called the buccal surface, which becomes continuous with the gums. The continuity of the mucocutaneous border must be maintained when cheiloplasty involves this margin. The point at which the upper lip joins the lower lip caudally is known as the commissure of the lip; its preservation is important when lesions involve this area.

Problems requiring surgical procedures of the lip have been divided into three categories: (1) traumatic lesions, (2) lesions that require excision, and (3) functional abnormalities.

Traumatic Injuries

A fresh, clean laceration of the lip is handled in a routine fashion. If the wound is linear, the edges are freshened, the mucocutaneous border is apposed first, and the remainder of the wound is sutured. If the wound is irregular in contour, if a triangular avascular flap is present, or if the normal architecture of the mucocutaneous border of the lip is distorted, conversion to a linear wound by excision of the wound edges is suggested. This conversion is best accomplished by making a "V" or wedge-shaped excision of the upper or lower lip (Fig. 33-41A). Whether the resection is carried through all three layers of the lip is determined by the depth of the laceration. Figure 33-41B illustrates a resection through cutaneous, muscular, and mucosal layers. After excision of the lesion, the muscular and submucosal layers are sutured as one layer with fine absorbable suture material (Fig. 33-41C). Care is taken not to penetrate the buccal mucosa. This precaution prevents suture material from being in direct contact with the oral cavity. Either 3-0 or 4-0 chromic catgut is usually adequate. As previously stated, the first suture in all layers should be the one nearest the mucocutaneous border. Because this area is constantly subjected to movement, a simple interrupted suture pattern is recommended for greater security. The cutaneous layer is then sutured with nonabsorbable suture of the veterinary surgeon's choice (Fig. 33-41D). An excisional debridement of the wound is recommended when wounds are more than 6 to 8 hours old or infected (Fig. 33-41). In my experience, rarely do wounds about the lip require delayed primary closure, partly because of the excellent vascularity of this area.

Wedge-type resections can also be performed in the area of the lip commissure with excellent results. The

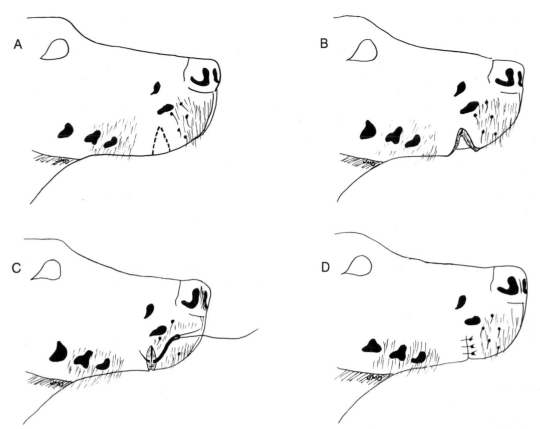

Fig. 33-41. *"V" or wedge-type cheiloplasty. A, Dotted line shows line of incision in upper lip. B, Wedge to be excised has been removed. C, Simple interrupted sutures being placed into muscularis and submucosa. The knots will be buried when the skin is closed. D, Skin sutures in place; wedge resection is completed.*

veterinary surgeon should be aware that an asymmetrical deformity of the mouth may result if the resection is extensive.

Lip Lesions Requiring Excision

Three types of lesions of and about the lips may require excisional cheiloplasty. These are lesions involved in certain infectious processes, neoplasms of this area, and granulomas.

Cheilitis is an inflammation of the lips and surrounding tissue folds that is usually accompanied by infection of the folds of the lips. This condition may be due to (1) tartar accumulations on the teeth causing friction to the lip, (2) an extension of a gingivitis or pyorrhea, or (3) microcheilia or a prominent lateral furrow of the lip, either of which may lead to excessive trauma and accumulation of food within the folds. In all instances, treatment must be directed at eliminating the causative factors predisposing the patient to this infection. This treatment may involve scaling of the teeth, frequent cleansing of accumulated foodstuffs in the furrows of the lips, the administration of topical as well as systemic antibiotics, and the use of astringents. Many of these conditions resolve with medical management.

In patients in which these forms of therapy are unsuccessful, excision of the prominent lateral lip fold is indicated (Fig. 33-42A). The entire lateral lip fold or furrow, as well as all infected tissue, must be resected by using an elliptical incision (Fig. 33-42B). This incision usually involves the mucocutaneous border only for a small segment cranially. The muscular and submucosal layers are sutured with fine 3-0 or 4-0 chromic catgut in an interrupted pattern. In most cases, the resection does not include the mucosa itself. For the cutaneous layer, 3-0 or 4-0 monofilament stainless-steel wire sutures are recommended (Fig. 33-42C).

Benign neoplasms of the lip are uncommon, but most are readily resectable by use of the "V" resection previously described (see Fig. 33-41).

The most common malignant neoplasms of the lip are squamous cell carcinoma, malignant melanoma, mast cell tumor, basal cell carcinoma, and fibrosarcoma that extends from the mouth. In many instances, the animals are first seen by the veterinarian when local invasion has already occurred. Often, these lesions are not resectable, but when the procedure is attempted, the animal is left with a gross deformity of the lip and mouth. More advanced techniques such as cryosurgery are now being used and may present a more effective way of managing these extensive tumors. Some squamous cell carcinomas have been responsive to radiation therapy. One hopes that these advanced techniques will become more readily available in the future.

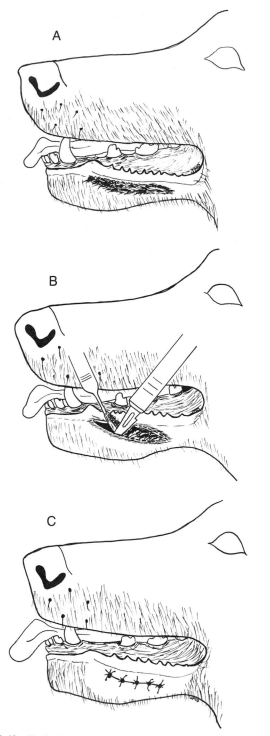

Fig. 33-42. *Cheiloplasty for lip-fold dermatitis. A, Prominent, infected lateral lip fold of the lower lip (heavily shaded area). B, A scalpel is used to remove all infected tissue. Elliptical incision. C, Skin sutures in completed cheiloplasty.*

When a potentially malignant neoplasm of the lip is seen by the veterinary surgeon in its early stages of development, prompt resection is indicated. Early resection often improves the prognosis and invariably leads to a more pleasing cosmetic result than later attempts at resection, when the lesion has been allowed to progress. The wedge resection described earlier (see

Fig. 33-41) is the preferred method of treatment. When more extensive tumors are presented at an early stage, elaborate plastic surgical techniques are available to facilitate closure of the large defect created in excision. In these cases, "Z" plasty, sliding graft, or other standard plastic surgical techniques may be required.

Eosinophilic granulomas (rodent ulcers) in the cat have traditionally been treated in one of three ways: (1) radiation therapy, which is often beneficial; (2) intralesional injection of repository corticosteroids, probably the most widely accepted form of therapy; and (3) surgical resection, which is used when the first two therapeutic measures have been unsuccessful. In my opinion, surgical resection is of little value and usually has a poor cosmetic result.

Megestrol acetate*, at a dose of 5 mg every other day for 10 to 14 doses, in combination with Depo-Medrol†, has been reported to be successful.[1]

Functional Abnormalities of the Lip

Though uncommon, cheiloschisis, or cleft lip, may occur, especially in the brachiocephalic breeds. The cleft may be located centrally at the philtrum of the upper lip, or it may be paramedian. The paramedian variety may be unilateral or bilateral. These clefts may be limited to the lip itself, or they may be associated with extension into the nares or combination with a cleft palate. The multiple variations of the "Z" plasty used to repair cleft lips in children are rarely necessary in the simple cleft lip that occurs in small animals. Elaborate techniques are primarily designed for optimal cosmetic effect and are not of primary concern here. A simple wedge resection (see Fig. 33-41) with meticulous layered closure is usually adequate. In extensive clefts, the veterinary surgeon should prepare by reviewing some of the literature related to clefts in man prior to attempting repair.

In certain breeds of dogs, an overabundance of everted lower lip may be seen just rostral to the commissure. This condition permits excessive drooling and interferes with the normal retention of saliva in the mouth. Functional problems such as moist dermatitis of the lower lip and adjacent structures may occur. In severe cases, the hair may mat along the neck and shoulders. In addition, owners may become exasperated by the distribution of saliva when the animal shakes its head. This problem is distasteful and may interfere with household cleanliness. The breeds most commonly affected are the St. Bernard, the boxer, and the cocker spaniel. Nerve palsies of the lower lip may also cause an acquired form of excessive drooling. A plastic procedure to correct this malady has been devised by Dr. Arthur North. The operation may be performed on one or both sides of the mouth, as the case requires. Its purpose is to affix the everted portion of the lower lip in a dorsally suspended position from the upper lip and thereby to eliminate the abnormal loss of saliva.

*Ovaban, Shering Corp., Kenilworth, NJ 07033
†Upjohn Co., Box 4000, Kalamazoo, MI 49001

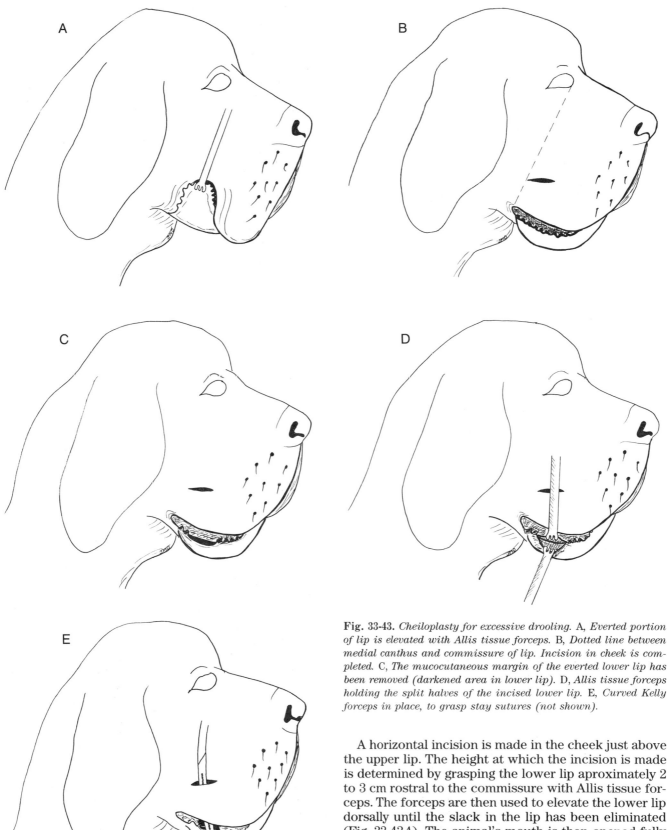

Fig. 33-43. *Cheiloplasty for excessive drooling. A, Everted portion of lip is elevated with Allis tissue forceps. B, Dotted line between medial canthus and commissure of lip. Incision in cheek is completed. C, The mucocutaneous margin of the everted lower lip has been removed (darkened area in lower lip). D, Allis tissue forceps holding the split halves of the incised lower lip. E, Curved Kelly forceps in place, to grasp stay sutures (not shown).*

A horizontal incision is made in the cheek just above the upper lip. The height at which the incision is made is determined by grasping the lower lip aproximately 2 to 3 cm rostral to the commissure with Allis tissue forceps. The forceps are then used to elevate the lower lip dorsally until the slack in the lip has been eliminated (Fig. 33-43A). The animal's mouth is then opened fully while the lower lip is held in this position, to ensure that when the lower lip is ultimately fixed in this position, no interference with the full range of motion of the jaws will exist. The height to which the lower lip

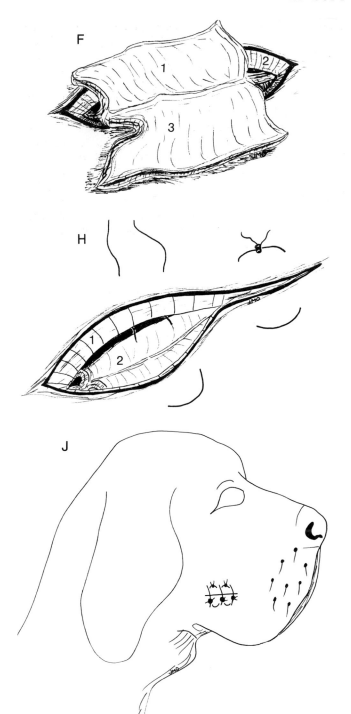

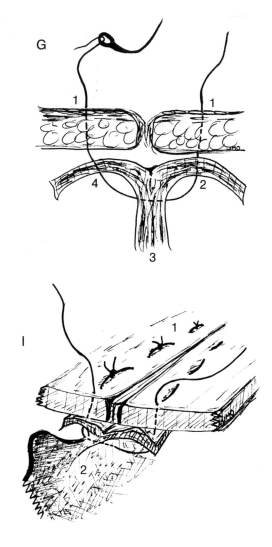

Fig. 33-43. *(cont.)* F, *Schematic of eversion of the two halves of the split lower lip through cheek incision (2). 1, Mucous membrane half of split lower lip; 3, cutaneous half of split lower lip. G, Cross-sectional diagram of suturing pattern after the split lower lip is replaced inside cheek. The first half of a horizontal mattress suture is in place. 1, Full thickness of cheek; 2, mucosal half of split lower lip; 3, full thickness of lower lip; 4, cutaneous half of split lower lip. H, The first horizontal mattress suture is in place. The second is ready to be tied. 1, Raw surface of cheek incision; 2, raw surface of everted lip incision. I, Cross-sectional view of mattress sutures in place. The first simple interrupted suture is just being placed. 1, Cheek; 2, lower lip. J, The completed cheiloplasty.*

has been elevated is marked with a scalpel blade on the upper cheek. The length of the incision is determined by visualizing a line between the medial canthus of the eye and the commissure of the lip. The point at which this line crosses the level predetermined to be the proper height marks the caudal end of the incision (Fig. 33-43B). This point usually corresponds to the level of the caudal root of the upper carnassial tooth. The incision is carried rostrally for approximately 2.5 cm in a horizontal plane and at the predetermined height. It is carried through all layers of the cheek, en-

tering the buccal vestibule. Care should be taken to avoid the cutaneous branch of the dorsal labial vein which lies just rostral and dorsal to this area.

Curved Metzenbaum scissors are used to remove a thickness of approximately 2 mm of the mucocutaneous border of the lower lip. This resection is started about 2 to 2.5 cm rostral to the commissure in large breed dogs (1 cm in smaller breeds) and is carried rostrally for 2 cm (1 cm in small breeds) (Fig. 33-43C). The raw edge of this mucocutaneous border is split to a depth of 0.5 cm with a scalpel (Fig. 33-43D). A stay suture is placed at the rostral and caudal angles of the incision in the lower lip. Kelly forceps are passed through the cheek incision into the vestibule of the mouth and then to the exterior (Fig. 33-43E). The two stay sutures are grasped with the Kelly forceps, the exposed portion of the lower lip is elevated along the mucosal face of the upper lip, and the previously prepared raw surfaces of the lower lip are exteriorized through the cheek incision.

The raw surfaces of the lower lip are everted (Fig. 33-43F) prior to placing the first suture. The initial layer of closure consists of horizontal mattress sutures placed in a through-and-through fashion (Fig. 33-43G). The needle first passes through all layers of the cheek; it then passes through the mucosal half of the lower lip, the combined thickness of all layers of the lower lip, and, finally, through the cutaneous half of the lower lip and back through all layers of the cheek. The entire procedure is repeated to complete the other half of the mattress suture (Fig. 33-43H). Medium (2-0) Vetafil sutures, as well as 1-0 and 2-0 stainless-steel wire, have been successfully used for this layer. Heavy suture material and a through-and-through suture pattern are employed to provide maximal holding power of the suture line, because it will be subjected to constant motion as soon as the animal awakens from anesthesia. When this layer is complete, some puckering may be noted at the incision site. A second layer of through-and-through simple interrupted sutures is used to oversew the original line (Fig. 33-43I). This suturing is done to approximate the skin edges closely, as well as to strengthen the site of the anastomosis.

The sutures are not removed for 3½ to 4 weeks, to allow the tissues to gain maximal strength. Some wrinkling of the cheek may be noted for several weeks postoperatively. The skin accommodates in time, and the end result is cosmetically pleasing as well as functionally corrective (Fig. 33-43J).

Reference and Suggested Reading

1. Dillon, R.: The oral cavity. *In* Current Veterinary Therapy. Edited by R. W. Kirk. Philadelphia, W. B. Saunders, 1980.

34 * Heart and Great Vessels

Patent Ductus Arteriosus

by Ralph A. Henderson

and William F. Jackson

Postnatal patency of the ductus arteriosus is the most common pathologic cardiac or vascular condition requiring surgical intervention in the dog. In the fetus, both right and left ventricles pump equal quantities of blood at a pressure of about 60/40 mm Hg. The unaerated pulmonary tissue provides high resistance to flow, and the blood leaving the right ventricle normally bypasses this nonfunctional tissue through the fetal ductus arteriosus.

At birth, the lungs inflate, pulmonary vascular resistance drops, and undefined mechanisms cause specialized smooth muscle fibers in the wall of the ductus to contract and to close the channel. Thus, decreased pulmonary resistance, closure of the ductus, and high pressure demands of the systemic circulation cause the well-known postnatal anatomic and biomechanical changes that distinguish the right and left ventricles.

If the ductus fails to close, the autonomy of the pulmonary and systemic circuits is not established, and a vicious cycle begins in that a portion of the systemic (left ventricular) cardiac output shunts into the pulmonary circulation with each cardiac cycle. The pulmonary system becomes hyperperfused (Fig. 34-1), and the increased pulmonary venous return increases the

volume load returning to the left ventricle (Fig. 34-2). The left ventricle accommodates for volume overloading initially by hypertrophy and, later, by a decompensating dilatation.

Concomitantly (the rapidity of progression depends on the flow across the patent ductus arteriosus) increased intrapulmonary vascular pressures and flows stimulate pulmonary arterial hypertrophy and inelasticity to counteract the acquired pulmonary overcirculation. Acquired pulmonary hypertension and pressure overloading of the right ventricle stimulate further myohypertrophic responses to complete the vicious cycle.

Advanced compensatory changes in the right heart caused by pumping against a fibrotically stenosed pul-

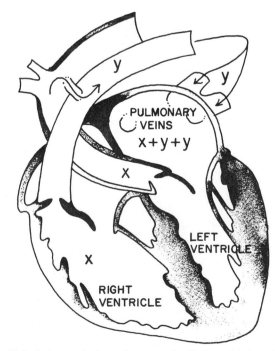

Fig. 34-2. *Left ventricular volume overloading results from the increased pulmonary venous return (x+y+y) (see Fig. 34-1). The left ventricle accommodates for the increased volume poorly, but this accommodation is defeated because of the chronic escape of systemic blood into the pulmonary circulation (y) through the patent ductus arteriosus during each pulse wave.*

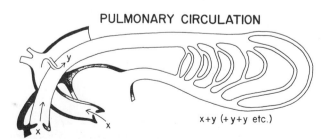

Fig. 34-1. *Mechanism of hyperperfusion of lungs with patent ductus arteriosus. Normally, the cardiac outputs (x) of the right and left ventricle are equal. In the presence of a patent ductus, however, the flow from the left to right (y) enters the pulmonary circulation during each repetitive pulse wave. The lungs become hyperperfused with this additional volume (x+y (+y+y etc.)).*

monary vasculature and the decompensating left heart may eventually cause the left-to-right shunt to reverse. When right-to-left shunting is present, the pulmonary circulation becomes minimally competent and the cyanotic patient is partially dependent on the shunt for systemic perfusion from the right ventral. Death is likely following surgical intervention in right to left shunts due to acute right heart pressure overload which precipitates ventricular failure. It has also been stated that right to left shunting can occur at birth rather than being acquired.

In summary, early changes in patent ductus arteriosus are associated with left ventricular enlargement, pulmonary hypertension, and usually a continuous murmur. Late changes associated with patent ductus arteriosus are biventricular enlargement, pulmonary fibrosis, and a variable murmur status depending on the degree of shunting and heart failure. Diagnostic interpretation and recommendations to the owners are given based upon these findings. Other congenital heart or physical anomalies may also be present.

Diagnostic Protocol and Preoperative Management

In the young dog with no other apparent abnormalities, the minimum data base includes the patient's medical history, a physical examination, an examination for parasites, a complete blood count and total protein and blood urea nitrogen determinations, a urinalysis, an electrocardiogram, and thoracic radiographs.

Young dogs with exercise intolerance, weight loss, cyanosis, and ascites should be suspected of having multiple anomalies or right-to-left shunting. These patients should receive a more thorough workup including determinations of liver enzymes, electrolytes, arterial and venous blood gases, and acid-base balance. Cardiac catheterization and angiography should be considered in these patients and in dogs older than 2 years of age. The contraindications to closure of a patent ductus arteriosus include right-to-left shunting and the presence of tetralogy of Fallot, or the association of the patent ductus arteriosus with an inoperable cardiovascular anomaly.

Acceptable surgical candidates should be subjected to operation between 3 and 6 months of age or as soon as practical after diagnosis. The patient's size is of little consequence, except fluid and anesthetic administration, ventilation, and control of body temperature are more critical in smaller patients.

Anesthesia

Our technique for anesthesia is to give intramuscular acetylpromazine (0.4 mg/kg) 30 minutes prior to anesthetic induction. This technique aids in a relaxed induction, promotes antiarrhymogenicity during anesthesia, and potentiates postoperative narcotic analgesics.

Atropine is not given because it blocks the reflex slowing of the heart following ligation of the ductus arteriosus and it precludes the emergency use of intravenous acetylcholine for temporary cardioplegia if hemorrhage or dissection complications are encountered.

Of the many anesthetic regimens available, we prefer to use thiopental, halothane, and controlled ventilation. If nitrous oxide is used, it is discontinued 5 minutes prior to the beginning of the thoracotomy closure.

A jugular catheter and a slow, continuous intravenous drip of lactated Ringer's solution should be maintained as an administration route for emergency therapy.

Surgical Techniques

Only operative closure of patent ductus arteriosus has proved effective in animals. Two general classes of closure exist: occlusion and division. Methods of occlusion include clips or ligatures, but we prefer double ligation because of its security and reduced potential for recanalization. The decision between occlusion or division is made at operation, when the ductus size is visualized. Occlusion requires less time and usually reduces operative risk. We feel, however, that aortico-pulmonary windows must be divided and sutured.

All operations for obliteration of ductus arteriosus patency require that the medial aspect of the ductus be exposed or otherwise dissected to allow passage of ligatures, clips, or vascular forceps. The dissection of this area is the most difficult and delicate portion of the procedure and deserves special consideration of pertinent anatomic features (Fig. 34-3).

The main pulmonary artery bifurcates at the opening of the ductus arteriosus. The origin and course of the right pulmonary artery is invisible to the veterinary surgeon, but the conjoining of the ductus and the right pulmonary artery forms an abrupt right angle that is thin and fragile when aneurysmic dilatation has occurred (Fig. 34-4).

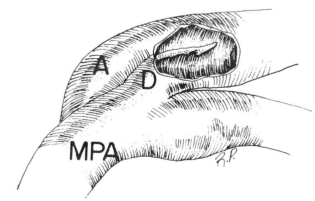

Fig. 34-3. *Anatomy of patent ductus arteriosus. The patent ductus (D) blends with the aorta (A), but its actual opening is caudal to its apparent union because of an intra-aortic shelf (seen with left lateral aortic wall removed). The fetal blood flow from main pulmonary artery (MPA) into the aorta is not obstructed by this shelf, but the flow is turbulent when the flow is from left (aorta) to right (pulmonary arteries). This turbulence is responsible for vascular dilatation of the aorta, patent ductus, and pulmonary arteries.*

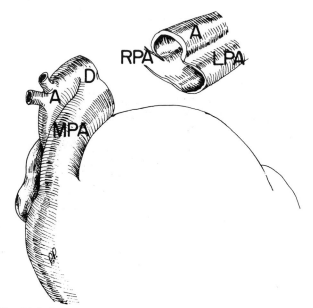

Fig. 34-4. *Anatomy of the patent ductus arteriosus with transverse section through main pulmonary artery (MPA), patent ductus (D), and aorta (A). The intra-aortic shelf of the ductus (Fig. 34-3) has been omitted. The right pulmonary artery (RPA) arborizes from the main pulmonary artery at the level and immediately ventromedial to the patent ductus. The angle of the right pulmonary artery-patent ductus junction is the most common location of tearing during dissection. LPA, left pulmonary artery.*

The conventional approach to dissection of the medial aspect of the patent ductus arteriosus requires the separation of the mediastinal pleura, the retraction of the phrenic and vagus nerves, and the careful avoidance of the left recurrent laryngeal nerve. When pleura has been removed from the lateral aspects of the aorta, the pulmonary artery, and the patent ductus arteriosus, right-angled forceps are used to dissect from caudal to cranial between the left pulmonary artery and the aorta. When dissecting medial to the patent ductus arteriosus, the medial aspect of the ductus may stretch and tear at the right pulmonary arterial junction. Additionally, the natural tendency is to try to dissect as superficially and conservatively as possible. In fact, deeper, more dorsal dissection placed toward the medial side of the aorta puts less stress on the patent ductus arteriosus. Additional hazards in conventional dissection include variations in toughness of the ductus and differences in pleural reflections. These dissection techniques are mentioned in the next section of this chapter.

MODIFIED TECHNIQUE FOR LIGATURE PLACEMENT AND OCCLUSION OF PDA

The patient's left shoulder, brachium, and hemithorax are routinely prepared for left lateral thoracotomy. Following thoracotomy, the mediastinal pleura dorsal to the aorta, but ventral to the thoracic duct, is incised with scissors from the left subclavian artery to the first aortic intercostal artery, which branches at the fifth rib. This wound is deepened by digital dissection to the medial (right) side of the aorta, and the aortic arch is freed (Fig. 34-5A). The ventral incised border of the mediastinal pleura is elevated with forceps, and dissection is continued to expose the lateral aspect of the descending aorta and the patent ductus arteriosus to the main and left pulmonary arteries. The mediastinal pleura is retracted ventrally; this maneuver retracts and protects the vagus and phrenic nerves. The left recurrent laryngeal nerve is not an obstacle, but may be tagged if the veterinary surgeon desires. The pericardium is avoided entirely.

When the ductus arteriosus is plainly visualized, a pair of ligatures is readily placed by passing a fine, blunt, curved hemostat from ventral to dorsal around the medial aspect of the aorta cranial to the ductus. Elevation of the aortic arch with an index finger while keeping the hemostat close to the aorta aids the initial passage. The instrument picks up the midpoint of a ligature on the dorsomedial aspect of the aortic arch (Fig. 34-5B). The ligature is drawn to the lateral aspect of the aortic arch. Care should be taken that the forceps are not opened too widely to receive the looped end or a tear could result. The jaws of the forceps should be sufficiently long that the instrument does not engage tissue in the vascular triangle as they are closed.

The forceps are introduced a second time, medial to the descending aorta and caudal to the ductus. The instrument grasps and withdraws the free ends of the ligature (Fig. 34-5C). The ductus arteriosus has now been loosely encircled, and preparation is made to slide the ligatures into position medial to the ductus. The ends of the suture should not be intertwined or the ligature will not be separated on the medial aspect of the ductus and will not allow proper double ligation.

The looped cranial and free caudal ends of the ligature are next placed under traction to advance the ligature from the dorsomedial aspect of the aorta to the aorta and right pulmonary artery. The ligature thus dissects the loose stroma between the vessels and incorporates a small amount of cushioning areolar tissue on the medial aspect of the ductus arteriosus (Fig. 34-5D).

The looped end is divided to form two complete ligatures. The occlusion procedure is completed by tying the ligatures slowly. The aortic side is closed first. One should observe the patient's heart rate for possible bradycardia and allow compensation for the change in vascular dynamics. Prior to replacing the left cranial lung lobes, the heart and major vessels are palpated to be certain that no fremitus due to an incompletely closed ductus remains.

DUCTUS DIVISION

If a ductus arteriosus is too short to ligate with a double or single ligature, or if iatrogenic trauma has caused hemorrhage, the ductus must be divided and sutured.

Technical skill in dissection and suturing and adequate instrumentation are important. Dissection may be conducted rapidly by passing a ligature as with the

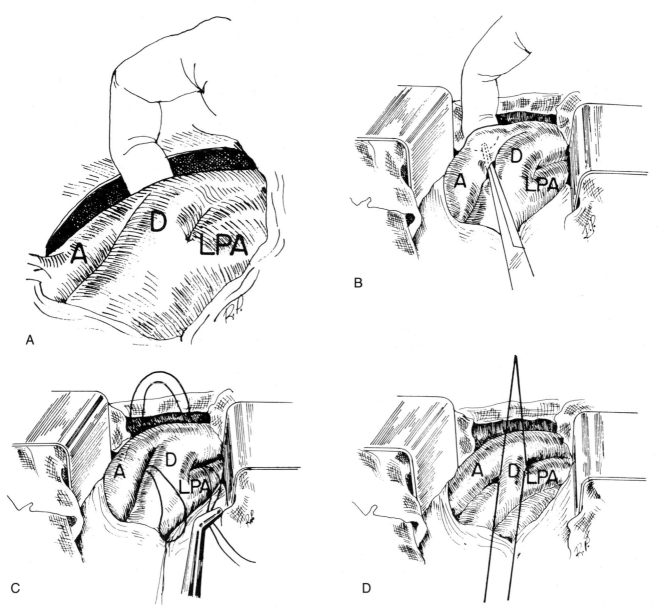

Fig. 34-5. A, *Dissection prior to ligature placement for patent ductus arteriosus. Following incision of the mediastinum dorsal to the aorta, the dissection to the medial aspect of the aorta (A) is performed digitally. Between the left subclavian and first intercostal vessels (at the fifth space) there are no vessels, nor are there fragile structures medial to the aorta in the mediastinum. The aorta is thoroughly mobilized on its medial aspect. D, patent ductus; LPA, left pulmonary artery. B, Ligature placement for patent ductus arteriosus. A pair of blunt, smooth hemostats are passed ventral to the aortic arch (A) aided by the index finger. The tips of the instrument should be kept close to the aorta. The instrument should be thin enough to insure that stretching of the patent ductus and pulmonary artery is minimal. Once passed, the instrument grasps the midpoint of a suture, which is drawn to the lateral aortic aspect. (D), patent ductus; LPA, left pulmonary artery. C, The maneuver used in B is repeated caudal to the ductus (D) around the descending aorta (A), and the two free ends of the looped ligature are pulled laterally. Care is taken to prevent the ligatures from becoming entwined. LPA, left pulmonary artery. D, The suture is placed under tension, and the medial aortic lengths are gently placed by traction medial to the ductus (D). The looped cranial suture is cut in two, forming two separate ligatures encircling the ductus that are carefully and slowly tied. A, aorta; LPA, left pulmonary artery.*

modified ligation technique, but one must remove the ligature after placing vascular clamps. If manual dissection is preferred, the dissection is carried more along the aorta than against the ductus arteriosus or pulmonary arteries. In ductus division, the main and left pulmonary arteries should be dissected more completely on their lateral aspect, and the aortic arch should be isolated early by digital dissection.

Patent ductus or coarctation forceps* specifically designed for this application are applied with the tips directed cranially. Alternately, a Pott's-Smith aortic clamp† may be used on the aortic side (Fig. 34-6). These instruments should be available even when liga-

* Pediatric cardiovascular forceps, American V. Mueller, 6600 West Touhy Avenue, Chicago, IL 60648
† American V. Mueller, 6600 West Touhy Avenue, Chicago, IL 60648

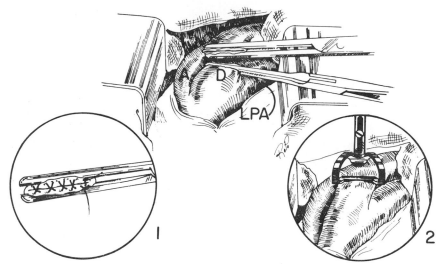

Fig. 34-6. *Ductus division and control of hemorrhage. Patent ductus or coarctation forceps are applied with the tips directed cranially. Modern instruments have fine teeth that are atraumatic and prevent slippage. A, aorta; D, ductus; LPA, left pulmonary artery. Inset 1, The ductus may be sutured with the simple continuous overlap (baseball or shoelace pattern), as shown, or with a fine simple continuous pattern. Small leaks are best managed with cruciate (X) mattress sutures. Inset 2, An alternate instrument, especially for short "windows," is the Pott's aortic clamp. This instrument includes a section of aortic wall, which is especially useful if the ductus has torn. Various sizes are made, and one size is not satisfactory for all dogs.*

tion is intended in the event the patent ductus arteriosus tears.

The occluding forceps are placed to allow at least 2 to 3 mm of vessel to lie between the forceps. The ductus arteriosus is divided, and the forceps are rolled laterally to expose the cut ductus edge for suturing. Size 5-0 silk suture swaged onto a cardiovascular needle and a fine simple continuous suture pattern or the over-and-over pattern are adequate (Fig. 34-6). The needle is passed carefully; one should follow its natural curve with an arced wrist motion to prevent vascular tearing. The clamps are removed slowly to check for bleeding. Slight seepage is anticipated and stops with pressure. Pulsatile hemorrhage is inhibited by cruciate or simple interrupted sutures. A small piece of oxidized cellulose sponge is interposed between the suture lines before closure to minimize suture abrasion.

Rarely is continuous thoracic drainage necessary; however, a thoracic catheter may be placed prior to rib closure, if desired. The ribs are approximated with heavy absorbable suture material, and the muscle, fascias, subcutis, and skin are closed in layers.

Complications

The complications associated with operations for patent ductus arteriosus include tearing of the major vessels, air embolization, central nervous or myocardial hypoxia, hypothermia, and hyper- or hypocapnea and the attendant respiratory acidosis or alkalosis, respectively. Anesthesia management is the same as any for any thoracic procedure, and vital changes must be monitored and corrected as they occur. Ductal or pulmonary arterial tearing may cause fatal intraoperative hemorrhage, and several procedures are commonly

used to avoid this complication. One method includes preparation of the patient with preplaced occluding tapes on the cranial and caudal venae cavae as for inflow occlusion. The aorta proximal and distal to the ductus arteriosus can be prepared in the same manner. In the event of severe hemorrhage, suction is essential, and digital pressure should be immediately applied to clear the operative field and to retard bleeding. The aorta cranial and cranial to the patent ductus and the main pulmonary artery may be occluded or temporarily cross-clamped. The inflow tapes are tightened. Pulmonary ventilation should cease. Ductus forceps should then be rapidly positioned to occlude only the torn ductus arteriosus. Major-vessel occlusion is then released.

Temporary cardioplegia with a bolus of intravenous acetylcholine (2 mg/kg) also allows better visualization. Retrograde flow from the systemic and pulmonary circulations causes blood to flow slowly from the tear, however.

Postoperative complications include recanalization, congestive heart failure, lung torsion, infection, thromboembolism, pneumothorax, cardiac tamponade, and adhesions. Careful technique and attention to detail limit these sequelae.

Postoperative Care

If severe pneumothorax is present following the thoracotomy closure, general atelectasis may cause hypoxia and hypercarbia, even in the presence of assisted ventilation. A temporary thoracic catheter is placed during closure, and thoracentesis is initiated as soon as closure sutures provide an airtight thoracic seal. Immediately following skin closure, thoracentesis is again

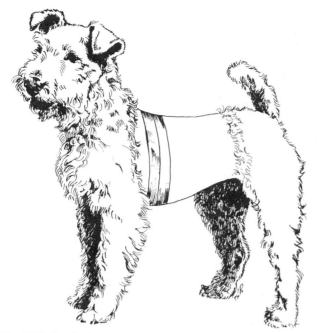

Fig. 34-7. *Bandaging the chest. Following a routine surgical procedure for patent ductus arteriosus, the functions of a bandage are to: (1) protect the wound, (2) apply pressure to prevent hematoma, and (3) mechanically stabilize to minimize pain and assist sutures. These functions can be performed by a snug bandage over only the surgical site. Tape is applied directly to the hair of the right side to prevent slippage. The narrow bandage improves respiration and allows aseptic preparation for thoracentesis without removing a full chest wrap.*

References and Suggested Readings

Breznock, E. M.: Patent ductus arteriosus. *In* Current Techniques in Small Animal Surgery. Edited by M. J. Bojrab. Philadelphia, Lea & Febiger, 1975.

Buchanan, J. W., and Lawson, D. D.: Cardiovascular system. *In* Canine Surgery. 2nd Ed. Edited by J. Archibald. Santa Barbara, CA, American Veterinary Publications, 1974.

Ettinger, S. J., and Suter, P. F.: Congenital heart disease. *In* Textbook of Veterinary Internal Medicine: Diseases of the Dog and Cat. Vol. 2. Edited by S. J. Ettinger. Philadelphia, W. B. Saunders, 1975.

Eyster, G. D.: Patent ductus arteriosus in the dog: characteristics of recurrence and results of 100 consecutive cases. J. Am. Vet. Med. Assoc., *168:*435, 1976.

Weirich, W. E., Blevins, W. E., and Rebar, A. H.: Late consequences of patent ductus arteriosus in the dog. A report of six cases. J. Am. Anim. Hosp. Assoc., *14:*40, 1978.

Surgical Correction of Patent Ductus Arteriosus: Conventional Method

by WALTER WEIRICH

Patent ductus arteriosus is the most common congenital cardiovascular defect in the dog. For the diagnostic features and presenting clinical signs of this disorder, the reader is invited to review the publications in the suggested reading list. Surgical correction should be performed as soon as the diagnosis is established.

Surgical Technique

A standard left fourth thoracotomy is performed. The veterinarian should review the anatomic features of the chest wall, to determine the least traumatic surgical approach (Figs. 34-8 and 34-9). When the chest is entered and the retractors are in place, the left lung is packed caudally with a moistened gauze sponge. This maneuver results in collapse of the lung, which causes no difficulty to the patient during the operation, yet facilitates visualization of thoracic organs.

The ductus arteriosus can be located beneath the vagus nerve where it interconnects the aorta to the pulmonary artery (Fig. 34-10). The phrenic nerve is seen running well below the area of the ductus. The mediastinum is opened, and the vagus nerve is retracted dorsally with 2-0 silk suture. The recurrent laryngeal nerve is identified where it branches from the vagus and passes around the caudal aspect of the ductus arteriosus. With minimal care, the recurrent laryngeal nerve can be avoided.

Several instruments should be available to make the dissection around the ductus arteriosus. Right-angle Meeker hemostatic forceps* (90° hemostatic full-horizontal serrated forceps) may be useful in making the dissection. A ligature carrier can be used to pass the suture material around the ductus. In the extremely

* Edward Weck & Co., Research Triangle Park, NC 27709

performed, bilaterally, and the volume is recorded. In the postoperative period, any deterioration in ventilation should cause clinical re-evaluation for pneumothorax. The routine evaluations of temperature, pulse rate and quality, and respiratory rate and quality are continued at 15-minute intervals until the dog's condition is stable.

Mechanical stabilization of the thoracic wound is important, and sterile dressings are applied over the wound. Full thoracic bandages are contraindicated in that they prevent full thoracic excursions and they make thoracentesis difficult. Instead, one or two strips of two-inch tape should compress the sterile dressing tightly over the wound and should circumferentially encompass the torso from the third through the fifth rib spaces (Fig. 34-7).

Postoperative thoracotomy pain may be significant and in some instances can induce dyspnea or apnea. In most patients, significant improvement in the quality of respiration and ventilation follows administration of analgesics. Meperidine may be given intravenously (1 mg/kg) and is repeated each 15 minutes until the desired effect is reached. Pallor is easily corrected by the administration of lactated Ringer's solution or other crystalloids, but total fluid administration in the routine correction of patent ductus arteriosus usually should not exceed 20 to 40 ml/kg.

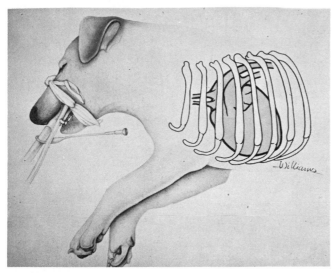

Fig. 34-8. *The relation of the great vessels and heart to the ribs indicates that the best site for the incision is in the left fourth intercostal space. (From Weirich, W. E., and Eyster, G.: Basic Cardiac Surgery.* In *Cardiology I. South Bend, IN, American Animal Hospital Association, 1976.)*

small patient, curved Halsted mosquito forceps may be sufficient for the dissection and the passage of the ligature. The instrument I prefer is the 45° Lahey gall duct forceps* both for dissection and as a ligature carrier.

The dissection must be done alternately from the cranial and caudal aspects in order to achieve a breakdown of medial tissue to isolate the ductus arteriosus. Gentle dissection is required when medial to the ductus. The point of the Meeker forceps should always be oriented toward the medial aorta and not the thin pulmonary artery.

The key to "gentle dissection" is that it must be carried out with small movements. If a tear should occur in one of the vessels, direct pressure nearly always stops the bleeding and allows the surgical procedure to be carried out at a subsequent time. Seven days later, the dissection can be safely attempted.

The final instrument passage on the medial aspect is generally made from the caudal aspect. When instrument tips can be seen cranial to the ductus arteriosus, the suture material can then be passed into the jaws of the clamp and pulled through. Larger (size 1-0) silk suture material is ideal for the ligature, but ⅛-inch cotton umbilical tape has also been used. The center of a doubled strand is passed into the jaws of the instrument. When this strand has been drawn medially around the

* American V. Mueller, 6600 West Touhy Avenue, Chicago, IL 60648

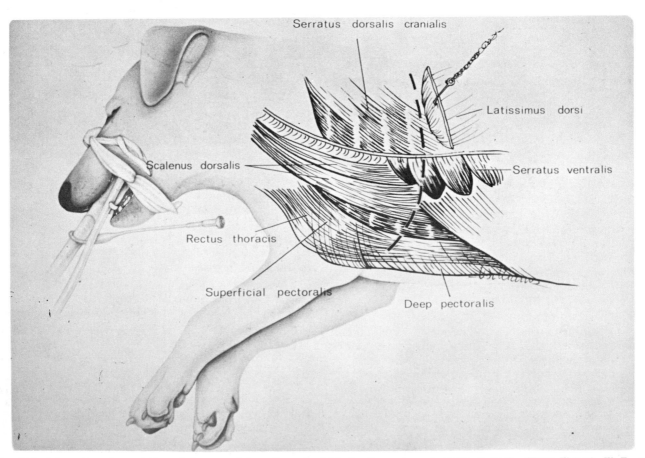

Fig. 34-9. *Schematic representation of the musculature through which the thoracotomy incision is made. (From Weirich, W. E., and Eyster, G.: Basic Cardiac Surgery.* In *Cardiology I. South Bend, IN, American Animal Hospital Association, 1976.)*

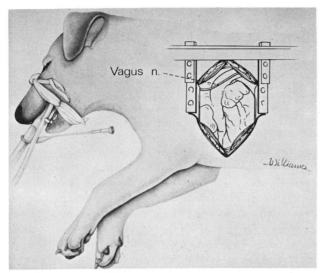

Fig. 34-10. *The vagus nerve is seen at the base of the heart in the area of the ductus arteriosus. (From Weirich, W. E., and Eyster, G.: Basic Cardiac Surgery. In Cardiology I. South Bend, IN, American Animal Hospital Association, 1976.)*

ductus arteriosus, it may be cut in the center, so that two strands are available to doubly ligate the ductus (Fig. 34-11).

Once the ligature material has been placed around the ductus arteriosus, a single throw on one ligature should be drawn down to occlude the ductus slowly. The usual response is a slowing of the patient's heart rate. On rare occasions, the patient's heart begins to beat erratically. Should this occur, the ligature should be released and drawn up slowly over a few minutes.

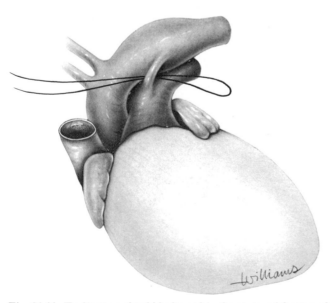

Fig. 34-11. *The ligature should be looped in the center of the strand and passed medial to the ductus arteriosus. It can then be cut at the loop and the ductus doubly ligated without a second passage of suture material. (From Weirich, W. E., and Eyster, G.: Basic Cardiac Surgery. In Cardiology I. South Bend, IN, American Animal Hospital Association, 1976.)*

The second ligature should be drawn up and tied with two separate square knots.

Following ligation of the ductus arteriosus, the fremitus in the pulmonary artery should disappear; however, this should be confirmed by palpation. The ligatures are cut close to the knot, and a chest drain is placed; one must ensure that multiple holes along the tube cross the mediastinal space so that both hemithoraces have adequate drainage. The thoracotomy is closed in a routine manner, and the air is evacuated gradually from the chest by the chest drain tube with an aspirating bulb syringe and a Heimlich valve. The chest drain tube may be removed as soon as the air stops draining and when the amounts of fluid are minimal, usually within 30 to 60 minutes after recovery from the surgical procedure.

The patient should be turned frequently to be sure that all the air has been removed from the thorax and to prevent hypostatic congestion. During the immediate postoperative period, the surgical incision should be covered with a sterile sponge, and the patient should recover from the operation with the incision side down. This technique allows the right lung, which is 50% larger than the left in the dog, to be uppermost and to provide the best ventilatory function during the early period of recovery. The animal should remain at cage rest until the lameness caused by incising the latissimus dorsi muscle is no longer evident. Postoperative care at home includes restricted activity (leash exercise) for 3 weeks, after which the animal can return to normal physical activity.

References and Suggested Readings

Weirich, W. E.: Patent ductus arteriosus. Pract. Vet., *47*:8, 1975.
Weirich, W. E., Blevins, W. E., and Rebar, A. H.: Late consequences of patent ductus arteriosus in the dog: a report of 6 cases. J. Am. Anim. Hosp. Assoc., *14*:40, 1978.

Surgical Correction of Persistent Right Aortic Arch

by JERRY A. GREENE

Persistent right fourth aortic arch is a common congenital vascular ring anomaly of the dog and cat. The normal fate of the embryologic brachial arch system is that the left fourth arch persists as the dorsal aorta, which is located to the left of both the esophagus and the trachea (Figs. 34-12 and 34-13). If the right fourth aortic arch becomes the functional adult aorta, and the left ductus arteriosus remains connected to the pulmonary artery, postnatally this band becomes the ligamentum arteriosum, which traps the esophagus between the heart base, the pulmonary artery, and the trachea (Figs. 34-14 and 34-15). This externally constricting band causes a functional esophageal obstruction (Fig. 34-16).

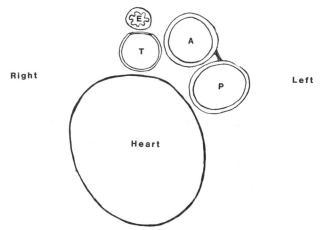

Fig. 34-12. *Schematic drawing of normal fate of embryologic brachial arch system. E, esophagus; T, trachea; A, dorsal aorta; P, pulmonary artery.*

Diagnosis

The German shepherd, Irish setter, and Weimaraner breeds of dogs and Siamese and Persian cats have a breed-specific predisposition for the persistent right fourth aortic arch anomaly. Other canine and feline breeds are affected less frequently.

Clinical signs usually commence with regurgitation upon weaning to a solid diet at 3 to 10 weeks of age. The regurgitated food is usually undigested, slime covered, and nonfetid. The patient's physical condition is dependent upon the degree and duration of the esophageal obstruction and the presence of aspiration foreign body pneumonia.

Barium paste esophagrams allow differentiation between congenital megaesophagus and the cranial thoracic esophageal dilatation due to a vascular ring obstruction. The latter causes a discrete, sudden termination of the esophageal lumen, usually at the fourth to fifth interspace. Early diagnosis and surgical correction render a more favorable prognosis. When surgical correction is delayed, secondary changes in the esophagus and lungs are greater, and therefore, the prognosis is poorer.

Preoperative Considerations

Ideally, the patient should be in the best physical condition possible prior to surgical correction. Broad-spectrum antibiotics are administered preoperatively because of susceptibility to infection. In patients with severe pneumonia, a tracheal wash culture and sensitivity test aid in the choice of antibiotics. An operation should not be delayed pending these test results, however, because delays in surgical procedures can cause continued dilatation of the esophagus. Prolonged dilation destroys nerve endings and renders the esophagus totally flaccid. In such patients, normal, rapid peristaltic-type movements do not develop, and the esophagus may remain dilated even after successful sectioning of the ligamentum arteriosum.

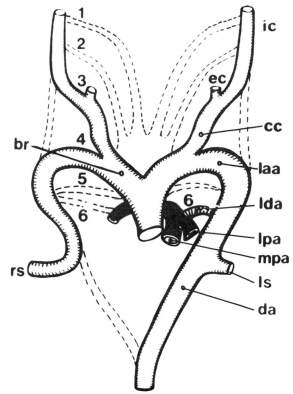

Fig. 34-13. *Schematic drawing of the normal embryologic development of the aortic arch system, ventrodorsal view. The uninterrupted lines represent the portions of the embryologic arch system that normally persist after birth, and the broken lines indicate the rudimentary or transient aortic arches. The first and second arches have involuted and do not contribute significantly to the permanent arterial system. The common carotid (cc), internal carotid (ic), and external carotid (ec) arteries originate from the third pair of arches and the aortic sac. The left aortic arch (laa) is derived from the left fourth arch and portions of the left dorsal aorta. The brachiocephalic artery (br) and the right subclavian artery (rs) originate from the right fourth aortic arch and portions of the right dorsal aorta. The fifth pair of aortic arches disappears in embryonic life, as does the dorsal right sixth aortic arch. The ventral right sixth aortic arch forms the pulmonary artery. The left ductus arteriosus (lda) originates from the left sixth or pulmonary arch and normally closes after birth to become the ligamentum arteriosum. It connects the left pulmonary artery (lpa) with the descending aorta (da). The main pulmonary artery (mpa) develops as the truncus arteriosus splits. The descending aorta (da) originates from the merged dorsal right and left aortas. The left subclavian artery (ls) normally arises from the descending aorta. (From Ettinger, S. J., and Suter, P. F.: Canine Cardiology. Philadelphia, W. B. Saunders, 1970.)*

Anesthesia

Because the vagus nerves are disturbed in the surgical correction of this condition, atropine sulfate and a preanesthetic agent are given to reduce excitability and to decrease the total amount of anesthetic to be given. Anesthesia is induced with either a short-acting intravenous barbiturate or a combination of halothane, nitrous oxide, and 50% oxygen administered by mask. A

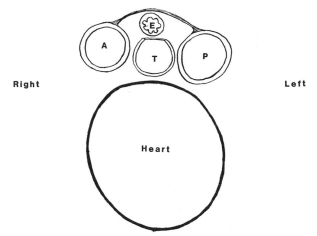

Fig. 34-14. *Schematic representation of the abnormal anatomic features found with a persistent right aortic arch. E, esophagus; T, trachea; A, dorsal aorta; P, pulmonary artery.*

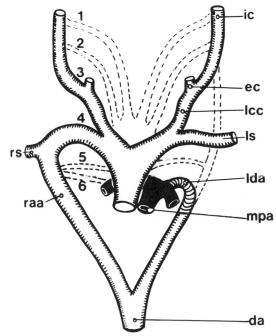

Fig. 34-15. *Schematic drawing of the embryologic arrangement of the vessels in persistent right aortic arch, ventrodorsal view (compare with normal development in Fig. 34-13). Uninterrupted lines illustrate the persistent portions of the embryologic arch system, and the broken lines indicate the transient or rudimentary portions. The transformations of arches 1, 2, 3, 5, and 6 and their respective branches, namely the internal carotid artery (ic), the external carotid artery (ec), and the common carotid artery (lcc), are the same as if development had been normal; however, the right fourth aortic arch (raa) persists instead of the left fourth arch, which in this case serves only as the origin of the left subclavian artery (ls). The left ductus arteriosus (lda) persists and remains connected to the right aortic arch and the descending aorta (da), thereby forming a closed vascular ring around the esophagus. The length of the left ductus arteriosus is schematically much longer than it is anatomically in order to show the proper relationship and development of the vessels. rs, Right subclavian artery; mpa, main pulmonary artery. (From Ettinger, S. J., and Suter, P. F.: Canine Cardiology. Philadelphia, W. B. Saunders, 1970.)*

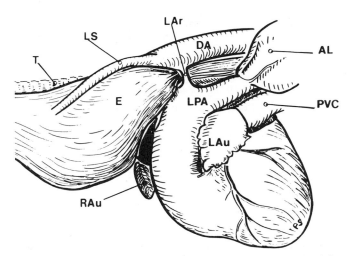

Fig. 34-16. *Schematic drawing from a dog with persistent right aortic arch and a vascular ring abnormality producing a stricture of the esophagus, viewed from the left side. T, trachea; LS, left subclavian artery; E, esophagus with precardiac saccular dilatation; LAr, ligamentum arteriosum; DA, descending aorta; LPA, left pulmonary artery; AL, left apical lobe of the lung; PVC, caudal vena cava; LAu, left auricle; RAu, right auricle. (From Ettinger, S. J., and Suter, P. F.: Canine Cardiology. Philadelphia, W. B. Saunders, 1970.)*

cuffed endotracheal tube is placed to prevent tracheal irritation from esophageal fluids. The esophagus is suctioned to remove fluids and food.

Controlled ventilation is started immediately following induction of anesthesia and is continued throughout the surgical procedure. Warmed fluids should be administered intravenously, and a heating blanket should be placed under the patient throughout the operation to prevent cooling.

Surgical Technique

The patient is positioned in right lateral recumbency with the left foreleg drawn slightly forward. The left thoracic wall, from the dorsal spinous processes to the sternebrae and from the shoulder to the last rib, is prepared for an aseptic surgical procedure.

The approach for a persistent right fourth aortic arch is through the fourth intercostal space. (See the section in Chapter 20 on thoracotomy.) The esophagus, the heart, the descending aorta, the main pulmonary artery, and the left vagus nerve are identified. The vagus nerve is retracted ventrally. Occasionally, a persistent left cranial vena cava is encountered and requires gentle retraction in a ventral direction.

The mediastinal pleura over the esophagus is incised until the aorta and the ligamentum arteriosum are located. The ligamentum arteriosum is encircled with two 2-0 silk ligatures. One ligature is tied close to the aorta and the other close to the main pulmonary artery. A transfixation suture is placed on the aortic side, and the ligamentum arteriosum is incised.

The stricture in the esophagus should be identified, and the surrounding mediastinal pleura and adventitia should be dissected, both cranial and caudal to the obstruction. A Foley catheter is then introduced through the mouth into the esophagus and is passed down to the constriction. The catheter is inflated and is then passed back and forth at the site of stricture, to identify any remaining constricting bands and to ensure that the lumen's size is sufficient.

Resection of the dilated cranial esophagus is not advisable because of its thin walls and its tendency to leak. Plication of the esophagus is only advocated when extreme dilatation is present. Care must be taken so that the sutures do not penetrate through the mucosa. Plication has no effect on the return of esophageal peristalsis.

A thoracic drain is placed prior to closure of the chest. The chest is thoroughly lavaged with warmed lactated Ringer's solution, and an opening is made in the cranial mediastinum to remove trapped air or fluid on the opposite side. The lung lobes are gently reinflated and repositioned. The chest is closed in a routine fashion. A light, nonconstrictive wrap is placed over the incision for support.

Postoperative Care

The chest drain is aspirated with a three-way stopcock and syringe. If no air or fluid are removed in the first hour postoperatively, the chest drain is removed. Should air or fluid be obtained, intermittent pressure or continuous suction is applied. Postoperative antibiotics are not usually administered unless an aspiration pneumonia is being treated concurrently.

The basic goals of postoperative management are to establish an adequate plane of nutrition and to prevent regurgitation. Small portions of solid food are given on the first postoperative day. The patient is fed in an upright position, and the position is maintained for several minutes once feeding is complete. The patient is gently rocked back and forth so that food and fluids do not pocket in the cranial esophagus. Multiple daily feedings are more easily handled by the patient than a single daily meal. Elevated feedings are recommended for the first 2 to 3 weeks. A follow-up esophagram is then performed to determine the status of the dilated esophagus. In some cases, elevated feedings may have to be continued indefinitely.

Prognosis for complete recovery is dependent on early diagnosis and surgical correction.

References and Suggested Readings

DeHoff, W. D.: Persistent right aortic arch. *In* Current Techniques in Small Animal Surgery. Edited by M. J. Bojrab. Philadelphia, Lea & Febiger, 1975.

Ellison, G. W.: Vascular ring anomalies in the dog and cat. Compend. Contin. Ed. *2*:693, 1980.

Helphrey, M. L.: Vascular ring anomalies in the dog. Vet. Clin. North Am., *9*:207, 1979.

Pulmonic Stenosis

by George Eyster

Pulmonic valve stenosis has long been recognized as a major congenital cardiac defect in the dog. The lesion is hereditary, although its exact genetics have not been fully elucidated. A breed predilection exists for English bulldogs, terriers, schnauzers (particularly giant schnauzers), beagles, Samoyeds, Chihuahuas, and keeshonds.

The majority of animals with pulmonic stenosis are not so severely affected as to produce signs of disease and, consequently, probably live a normal life. In the severely affected animal, however, early death is expected. As a result, a variety of surgical techniques have been used in veterinary medicine to correct or to alleviate pulmonic stenosis. Each technique has certain advantages, and most of the procedures can be easily accomplished in the veterinary practice.

Four basic types of pulmonic stenosis have been described (Fig. 34-17). Supervalvular pulmonic stenosis, the most rare, is generally seen as a membrane in the pulmonary artery distal to the pulmonary valve. This condition is probably not hereditary. Valvular pulmonic stenosis involves thickening or fusion of the valve cusps. Subvalvular pulmonic stenosis has a fibrous membrane just proximal to the pulmonic valve that obstructs the right ventricular outflow tract. Because valvular and subvalvular pulmonic stenosis are sometimes difficult to distinguish, the term pulmonic valve dysplasia has been recently used to describe a fibrous valvular and subvalvular lesion. The fourth type of pulmonic stenosis, infundibular, may be present as a single entity, but it is usually secondary to one of the previous three types. In this case, muscular hypertrophy encroaches on the right ventricular outflow tract. Muscular infundibular pulmonic stenosis is technically the most difficult type for the veterinary surgeon to correct.

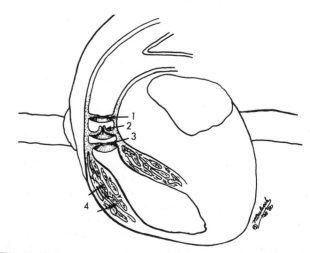

Fig. 34-17. *Types of pulmonic stenosis: (1) supravalvular, just caudal to the valve; (2) valvular, involving the valve structure; (3) subvalvular, fibrous ring just beneath the valve; and (4) muscular infundibular, involving the right ventricular outflow tract.*

Pathophysiology

With obstruction to blood outflow, pressure builds in the right ventricle and results in right ventricular hypertrophy. If the obstruction is minimal, the hypertrophy is adequate to produce a normal outflow from the right ventricle without compromising ventricular function, and the animal functions normally. If the obstruction is severe, right ventricular hypertrophy becomes marked, and ventricular filling is compromised. Cardiac output is reduced, and congestive heart failure of the right side may result. Clinical signs are particularly evident if the tricuspid valve fails with a secondary production of ascites. More frequently, arrhythmias brought about by hypertrophy cause a chief complaint of syncope. As with any disease of which low cardiac output is a feature, weakness, exercise intolerance, and perhaps failure to thrive may be found.

Diagnosis

The diagnosis of pulmonic stenosis is established by the patient's medical history, by physical findings, and by radiographic, electrocardiographic, and laboratory tests. The patient's history might indicate a perfectly normal animal without the signs of failure previously described. On physical examination, the animal may have ascites, but may generally be normal, except for the presence of a crescendo-decrescendo systolic murmur that is usually localized in the cranial left thorax and may radiate to the right. Electrocardiographic recording demonstrates right axis deviation and right ventricular hypertrophy. Thoracic radiographs indicate the presence of an enlarged right side of the heart and enlargement of the main pulmonary artery segment with normal peripheral lung fields.

The diagnostic test for pulmonic stenosis is angiography. Fortunately, in congenital stenoses, the venous angiogram is an ideal and simple diagnostic test. The radiopaque contrast medium is injected into the jugular vein as a bolus, and radiographs are taken 1 or 2 seconds later to reveal the right ventricular outflow tract, the pulmonic valve, and the pulmonary arterial tree. Poststenotic dilatation is diagnostic of pulmonic stenosis (Fig. 34-18). This technique is effective, simple, diagnostic, and available to the veterinary practice.

Indications for Surgical Treatment

These diagnostic tests are, at best, only indicative of the severity of the disease. A mean electrical axis on an electrocardiogram of greater than 180° is probably seen only in surgical cases. Additionally, animals demonstrating syncope or ascites need surgical treatment. Angiographic evidence of severe obstruction also indicates a lesion requiring a surgical procedure. The majority of pulmonic stenosis patients fall into a "gray zone," however, and pressure measurements should be performed. Unfortunately, direct pressure measurements require cardiac catheterization and recording techniques. Direct-needle cannulation of the right ven-

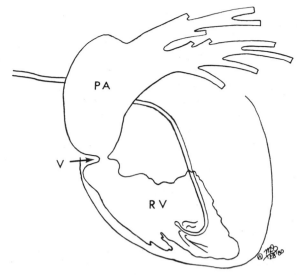

Fig. 34-18. *Angiogram of pulmonic stenosis. The outline of the right ventricular cavity is identified (RV). The area of the obstruction at the pulmonary valve is identified with the arrow at (V), and the poststenotic dilatation of the pulmonary artery is seen caudal to the obstruction (PA).*

tricle has been performed, but is not recommended. Instead, a catheter is introduced into the jugular vein and is passed into the right ventricle to measure pressure and preferably to pass through the obstruction into the pulmonary artery. The catheter is then withdrawn, and the position of the obstruction is documented as well as the gradient across the pulmonic obstruction (Fig. 34-19). At Michigan State University, the criteria for pulmonic stenosis corrective operations are as follows: (1) a symptomatic patient with ascites or syncope; (2) an electrocardiographic mean electrical axis greater than 180°; and (3) cardiac catheterization pressures, that is, right ventricular pressure greater than systemic (120 mm Hg) in any age dog, a pressure gradient between the pulmonary artery and the right ventricle of 100 mm Hg in any age dog, right ventricular pressure 90 mm Hg or greater in an immature dog, and a pressure gradient between the pulmonary artery and the right ventricle of 70 mm Hg in an immature dog.

Anesthesia

Atropine is administered preanesthetically to minimize bradycardia. Anesthesia is induced with a short-acting thiobarbiturate (thiamylal) to allow endotracheal intubation and is maintained with halothane delivered in oxygen. Anesthesia is maintained at minimal levels of halothane, and ventilation is manually controlled throughout the thoracotomy. Anesthesia is reduced during manual ventilation, with jaw tension and pulse pressure as the major criteria for determining the depth of anesthesia. All animals are monitored by electrocardiogram. Blood pressures are monitored by palpation of the aorta by the veterinary surgeon, and arterial blood gases are taken as needed from the lingual

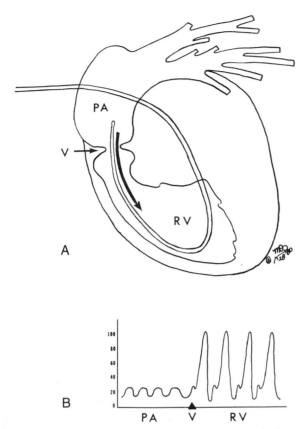

Fig. 34-19. *Catheterization pressure recording of valvular pulmonic stenosis. A, The catheter is shown being withdrawn from the pulmonary artery (PA) across the valve (V) into the right ventricle (RV). B, The simultaneous pressure recording is shown as recorded from the pulmonary artery across the valve into the right ventricle. The abrupt change from pulmonary artery pressure in the normal range to the elevated ventricular pressure contour identifies the lesion as discrete valvular pulmonic stenosis.*

artery. Anesthesia is reduced during the closure period. Most animals are ambulatory within 15 minutes of completion of the surgical procedure. No tranquilizers or analgesic agents are given in the postoperative period, and the animals are encouraged to ambulate, thereby minimizing postoperative respiratory complications.

Critically ill small patients may be anesthetized with halothane in an induction chamber. Anesthesia may be induced in extremely sick animals with intravenous diazepam and with halothane by face mask. Muscle relaxants are used occasionally to eliminate competition with manual ventilation.

Surgical Correction

The surgical procedure used for correction of pulmonic stenosis is dictated by two factors. First and most important is the type of pulmonic stenosis in the patient. For each of the four forms of pulmonic stenosis, an advantageous surgical technique exists, and some techniques are not effective for certain types of pulmonic stenosis. We describe five procedures: (1) the

Bistoury technique for valvular or discrete subvalvular lesions; (2) the modified Brock procedure for subvalvular lesions; (3) inflow occlusion pulmonary arteriotomy (Swan procedure) for valvular and some subvalvular lesions; (4) the outflow patch (Breznock modification) for wide area obstruction, especially useful in young dogs; and (5) an open-heart surgical technique for severe obstructive lesions. A less-common procedure is conduit construction for supervalvular stenosis.

With the exception of the open-heart procedures, all pulmonic stenosis operations are performed through a routine left lateral thoracotomy in the fourth intercostal space. Minimal bleeding is encountered if the scalenus medius muscle is separated at its insertion and the serratus ventralis thoracis is separated between muscle bellies. Care is taken not to cut the intercostal artery or vein. The incision should stop a centimeter from the sternum, so as not to incise the internal thoracic artery. The chest wound is retracted with a rib spreader to visualize the cardiac structures (Fig. 34-20). Direct pressure recordings made by a needle connected to a pressure transducer should be obtained if at all possible from the right ventricle and pulmonary trunk.

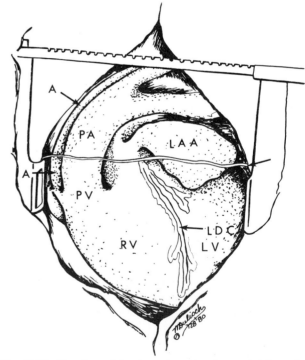

Fig. 34-20. *The view of the thoracic cavity from a left lateral approach in the fourth intercostal space. The lungs have been reflected caudally. The aorta (A) is visualized dorsally and cranially. The pulmonary artery (PA) is easily seen, and the area of the pulmonary valve marks a distinct change from arterial to heart tissue. The vagus nerve courses over the pulmonary artery in the pericardium. With the pericardium removed, the left descending coronary artery (LDC) marks the separation between the right and left ventricles (RV and LV). The left auricular appendage (LAA) can be visualized dorsally, and a pink color would indicate adequate ventilation and pulmonary function.*

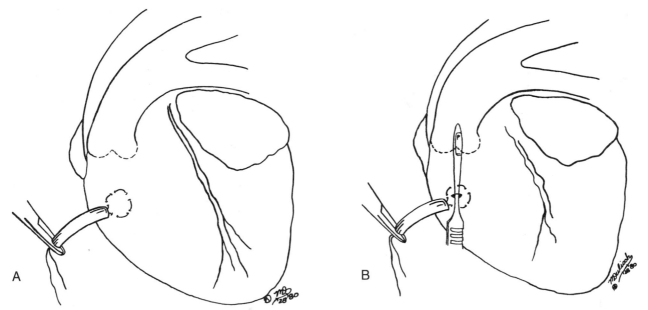

Fig. 34-21. *Bistoury technique. A, Pursestring suture and Rumel tourniquet on the right ventricular outflow tract. B, A Lichty's teat knife introduced through the pursestring suture into the right ventricle to cut and open an obstructed pulmonary valve.*

The Bistoury technique and modified Brock procedure are accomplished in an identical manner. These simple techniques provide access to the heart through a pursestring suture in an avascular portion of the right ventricular outflow tract. An 8-mm-diameter pursestring suture using 2-0 suture material is placed, and a Rumel tourniquet* is passed over the ends of the pursestring to control bleeding (Fig. 34-21 *A*). A small stab wound is carefully made through the epicardium and into the heart. A Lichty's teat knife† or similar instrument is introduced through the stab wound into the pulmonary artery. Appropriate sections are then made in the pulmonary valve or subvalvular obstruction (Fig. 34-21 *B*).

In the Brock modification, a rongeur is passed through the pursestring into the heart, and the offending tissues are rongeured and removed (Fig. 34-22). The instruments are withdrawn, and the pursestring is closed. Repeated direct pressure measurements of the right ventricle should reveal a 50% reduction in right ventricular pressure. The advantages of the Bistoury or modified Brock procedures are simplicity of technique and equipment and a generally effective outcome. The disadvantage of the technique is that the closed repair is accomplished by blind instrument passage, and if a pressure measurement cannot be obtained, evaluation of the effectiveness of the procedure is poor.

Pulmonary arteriotomy with venous inflow occlusion is a preferred method for repair of pulmonic stenosis in mature or nearly mature dogs with valvular or subvalvular lesions. The procedure allows direct visualization of the valve and immediate subvalvular struc-

tures. The disadvantages are that the technique is not effective in infundibular disease, is more time consuming than the Bistoury or modified Brock technique, and requires the completion of a major surgical manipulation in less than 3 minutes. A major additional disadvantage of the inflow occlusion technique is that, because of surgical scarring, the pulmonary annulus does

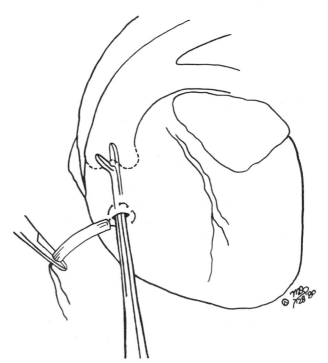

Fig. 34-22. *Modified Brock procedure. Infundibular rongeurs are introduced through the pursestring suture into the right ventricle to remove obstructed tissue from the right ventricle or pulmonary valve.*

*Available through American V. Mueller, 6600 West Touhy Avenue, Chicago, IL 60648

†Jensen-Salsbury Laboratories, 520 West 21st Street, Kansas City, MO 64141

not grow beyond the size of the opening left at the time of operation. Thus, in young animals of large breeds, progressive stenosis may develop as the animal matures.

First, the cranial and caudal vena cava are isolated from a left lateral thoracotomy. The cranial vena cava is found by blunt dissection in front of the heart and ventral to the brachiocephalic artery. Because the vena cava is far to the right of the midline, it may be difficult to locate. The structure is dark and, once visualized, is easily looped with an umbilical tape using right-angle forceps. A Rumel tourniquet is loosely applied. The caudal vena cava is identified by breaking the mediasti-

num caudal to the heart and by rotating the heart slightly cranially. Care is taken that a pulmonary vein is not inadvertently included within the loop of umbilical tape (Fig. 34-23 A).

The pericardium is then opened over the pulmonary artery, and 2 3-0 or 4-0 mattress sutures are placed in the pulmonary artery on either side of the intended opening (Fig. 34-23 B). The animal is ventilated with 100% oxygen for approximately 1 minute, and the tourniquets are tightened onto the venae cavae. The heart is allowed to empty, and the pulmonary artery is opened between the stay sutures. The blood is suctioned from the pulmonary artery to reveal the ob-

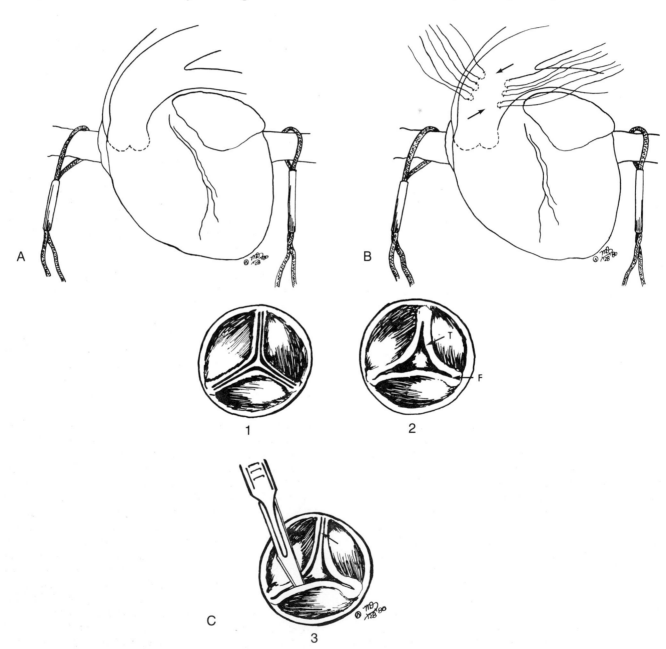

Fig. 34-23. A, *Umbilical tape and Rumel tourniquets placed on the cranial and caudal vena cava for inflow occlusion. B, Pulmonary artery stay sutures preplaced on either side of the intended incision line (identified between the two arrows). C, The pulmonic valve: 1, normal; 2, in pulmonic stenosis. The valve cuspids are fused at the edges (F) and are thickened along the commissures (T). 3, Direct visualization of surgical repair. The scalpel is opening the fused commissures. A previous cut has been made (arrow) separating two valve cusps.*

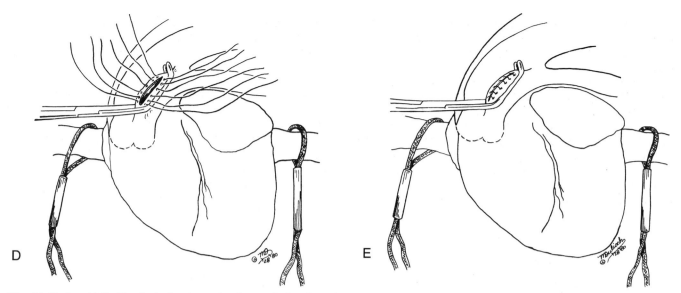

Fig. 34-23. (cont.) D, *The Satinsky clamp in place occludes the pulmonary artery opening. The tourniquets on the vena cava have been relaxed.* E, *The pulmonary artery is closed.*

structed pulmonary valve (Fig. 34-23 *C*). A No. 11 blade is used to incise, to excise, or to reconstruct the obstructed pulmonary valvular lesion (Fig. 34-23 *C*). Scissors may be used if preferred. If the lesion is subvalvular, the obstructing tissue is grasped by thumb forceps or hemostats and is excised with scissors or with the scalpel. Upon completion of the opening of the outflow tract, the stay sutures are lifted, and a Satinsky* clamp is placed to occlude the arteriotomy yet allow blood passage through the artery (Fig. 34-23 *D*). As the tourniquets are removed from the venae cavae, ventilation and blood flow are re-established. It is my opinion that the inflow time should be under 2 minutes and never over 3 minutes because complications are directly related to the length of occlusion time. After re-establishment of the circulation, the pulmonary artery is closed with 4-0 suture material (Fig. 34-23 *E*), and the clamp is removed. Chest closure is routine.

The closed patch-graft technique (Breznock modification) allows the veterinary surgeon to open the right ventricular outflow tract to any predetermined size. In this technique, the outflow tract can be opened without inflow occlusion or an open-heart procedure by using a cutting suture. This technique is preferred in extremely young animals of the large breeds where major growth is anticipated after surgical correction. It is also an effective technique in infundibular pulmonic stenosis. A long, slightly curved, atraumatic needle, with fine polyfilament stainless steel wire (2-0), is passed through a previously placed (3-0) catgut pursestring suture into the right ventricle, between the valve cusps inside the origin of the vessel, and is made to emerge through the lateral wall of the pulmonary artery. *Extreme care* must be taken to ensure that the wire has, in fact, penetrated into and passes from the lumen of the ventricle (Fig. 34-24 *A*). An elliptical Dacron patch† is then placed over the pulmonary artery across the area of the pulmonary stenosis down onto the right ventricle covering the cutting suture (Fig. 34-24 *B*). The size of the elliptical patch must be large enough to cover both entry and exit points of the cutting suture. The patch is sutured with 3-0 silk in a continuous pattern in such a way that both strands of the cutting suture emerge between the same continuous suture, so that when the cutting is complete, the cutting suture can be easily retrieved. The wire is withdrawn with a sawing motion, cleanly incising, in order, the pulmonary artery, the pulmonary valve, and the subpulmonic myocardium. The blood is diverted through the channel cut beneath the patch and from the right ventricle to the pulmonary artery (Fig. 34-24 *C*). Digital pressure over the patch to the ventricular wall controls bleeding if it occurs when the cutting wire is removed. Hemorrhage can be reduced by preclotting the Dacron patch with the patient's own blood.

In supravalvular pulmonic stenosis, the outflow patch may again be used, or a Dacron conduit‡ may be placed to bridge the obstruction. A great advantage of the conduit is maintenance of the normal pulmonary valve. The main pulmonary artery is dissected free of fat distal and proximal to the stenosis. Using a Satinsky clamp, the main pulmonary artery is partially occluded at the level of the poststenotic dilatation. A 12-mm pulmonary arteriotomy is made longitudinally. A 6-cm segment of Dacron arterial conduit 10 mm in diameter is preclotted with 5 ml of the dog's own blood. The conduit is anastomosed to the pulmonary artery, using 5-0 polyethylene§ cardiovascular suture (Fig. 34-25 *A*). The clamp partially occluding the pulmonary artery is released when the conduit has been completely occluded (Fig. 34-25 *B*). The proximal end of the conduit is appropriately shortened and is obliquely trimmed for

*American V. Mueller, 6600 West Touhy Avenue, Chicago, IL 60648
†Available U.S.C.I. Division, C. R. Bard, Inc., Billerica, MA 01821

‡Available U.S.C.I. Division, C. R. Bard, Inc., Billerica, MA 01821
§Dermalene, Davis & Geck, Inc., Manati, PR 00701

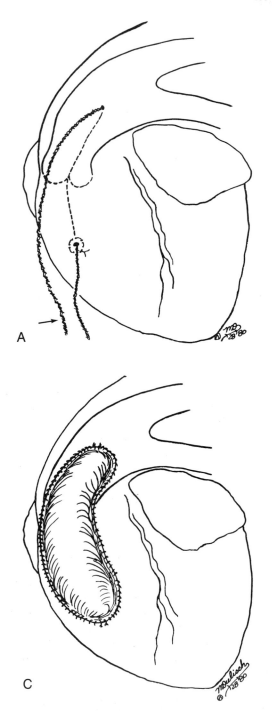

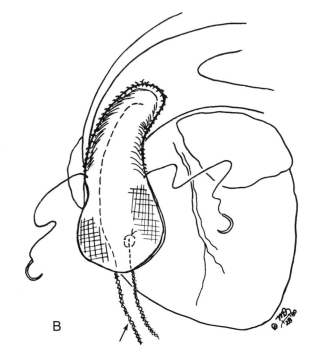

Fig. 34-24. A, *A wire cutting suture (arrow) is placed into the right ventricle through the pulmonary valve and exits through the pulmonary artery.* B, *An outflow graft patch is sutured from the pulmonary artery across the obstructed pulmonary valve to the right ventricle. The wire suture (arrow) is included under the patch graft.* C, *The outflow patch graft in place, when one has pulled the cutting wire suture out, opening the right ventricular outflow tract.*

anastomosis. A second Satinsky clamp is positioned for arteriotomy distal to the pulmonic valve and proximal to the stenosis. On completion of the proximal anastomosis (Fig. 34-25 *C*), blood flow is immediately detectable within the conduit.

Closure from the left lateral thoracotomy is accomplished in a routine manner. A chest drain tube should be introduced subcutaneously 1 or 2 rib spaces caudally to withdraw air and to monitor postoperative bleeding. In patients with Dacron implantation, the chest drain tube should be maintained for a minimum of 24 hours because the foreign material produces an effusion. The effusion can continue for several days until the Dacron has been endothelialized. For patients undergoing inflow occlusion, the Brock modification, or the Bistoury technique, the drain tube should be removed after completely withdrawing all thoracic air. Postoperative bleeding is not a problem with these techniques, yet problems associated with the maintenance of a drain tube may be difficult.

All types of pulmonary stenosis are amenable to open-heart surgical repair, which offers the advantage

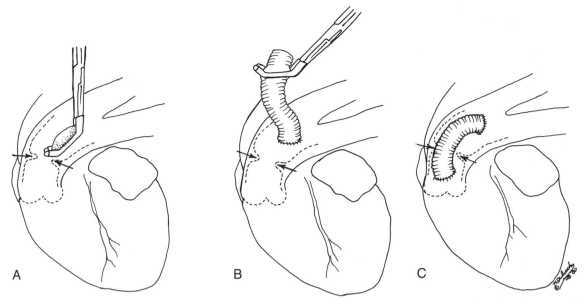

Fig. 34-25. A, *The Satinsky clamp grasping the pulmonary artery caudal to the obstruction (arrows).* B, *The Satinsky clamp is removed from the pulmonary artery when distal anastomosis of the conduit is accomplished.* C, *Completed Dacron graft between the pulmonary artery caudal to the obstruction (arrows) and that cranial to the obstruction.*

of direct visualization and reconstruction. Animals are placed on the heart-lung machine after either a right thoractomy or a median sternotomy. Blood from the venae cavae is diverted to the pump oxygenator, which returns oxygenated blood to the patient by a systemic artery. The right ventricle or pulmonary artery can be opened when total cardiopulmonary bypass is established and direct visualization and resection of the of-

fending tissue can be accomplished. If a patch is necessary to restore the outflow tract, it can be placed; the right ventricle is then closed with a continuous suture pattern (Fig. 34-26). Although open-heart techniques are performed in veterinary medicine, the procedures are long, arduous, and require extensive equipment, time, and postoperative care. These techniques are currently not practical in private practice, owing to financial considerations.

In summary, pulmonic stenosis, a sometimes fatal congenital heart defect in the dog, is amenable to surgical repair. Diagnosis must be established, and it is imperative that the type of pulmonic stenosis be identified. In patients with severe gradients of clinical signs, a variety of surgical techniques have been successfully used in veterinary medicine. With an effective repair for pulmonic stenosis, the patient should recover and should lead a normal life. Animals with this congenital cardiac defect, however, should not be used for breeding.

References and Suggested Readings

Breznock, E. M., and Wood, G. L.: A Patch-graft technique for correction of pulmonic stenosis. J. Am. Vet. Med. Assoc., *169:*1090, 1976.

Brock, R. C.: Pulmonary valvulotomy for the relief of congenital pulmonary stenosis. Br. Med. J., *1:*121, 1948.

Ford, R. B., Spaulding, G. L., and Eyster, G. E.: Use of an extracardiac conduit in the repair of supravalvular pulmonic stenosis in a dog. J. Am. Vet. Med. Assoc., *172:*922, 1978.

Himmelstein, A., Jomeson, A. G., Fishman, A. P., and Humphreys, G. H., II: Closed transventricular valvulotomy for pulmonic stenosis. Surgery, *42:*121, 1957.

Ott, B. S., Raymond, B. A., North, R. L., and Pickens, G. E.: Diagnosis and surgical repair of congenital pulmonic stenosis in the dog. J. Am. Vet. Med. Assoc., *144:*851, 1964.

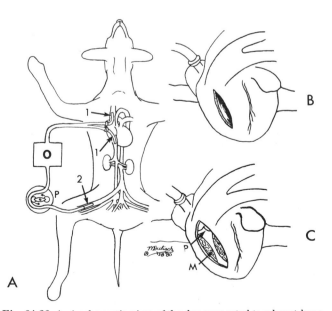

Fig. 34-26. A, *A schematic view of the dog connected to a heart-lung machine. The venous blood is diverted from the vena cava (1) to an oxygenator (0), is oxygenated, and is pumped (P) back to the dog by way of a convenient arterial cannulation (2).* B, *The right ventricle is opened, revealing the area of obstruction.* C, *Visualization of the muscular enlargement (M) or the obstructed pulmonary valve (P).*

Surgical Management of Pericardial and Intramyocardial Diseases Including Chemodectomas

by Stanley D. Wagner

and Eugene M. Breznock

Although probably applicable to the cat, we have clinically applied the surgical techniques described only to the dog.

Anatomic Features

The pericardium is a transparent, cone-shaped, fibroserous sac that is divided into an outer fibrous layer and an inner serosal layer.[11] The serosal layer is further divided into the parietal pericardium, which is firmly fused to the inner surface of the fibrous pericardium, and the visceral pericardium (epicardium), which is firmly attached to the surface of the heart. Histologically, the pericardium consists of an innermost mesothelial layer resting on a thin layer of loose connective tissue, and an outer, thick, resistant layer of collagen bundles and elastic fibers crossing each other at various angles.

The base of the fibrous pericardium joins the adventitia of the proximal portion of the great vessels. Dorsally, dense attachments to the aortic arch are seen. At the apex, the fibrous pericardium is attached to the ventral portion of the muscular periphery of the diaphragm by the thin sternopericardiac ligament.[11] Caudally, the fibrous pericardium is attached to the diaphragm by pleural reflections or ligaments.[4,8,11,24]

The parietal and visceral pericardium form a closed pocket, the pericardial cavity. No evidence exists of movement of isotopes or contrast materials between the pericardial and pleural cavities.[3] The pericardial cavity of the dog contains from 0.5 to 15 ml of a serous fluid that is probably an ultrafiltrate of blood serum.[14] In the absence of disease, the optimal quantity and composition of pericardial fluid is well maintained by osmosis, diffusion, and lymphatic drainage across the serosal surface.

The blood supply to the pericardium in the dog is from the pericardial branch of the internal thoracic artery, the pericardiacophrenic artery. Nerve fibers from the vagus nerve, the left recurrent laryngeal nerve, the phrenic nerve, and terminal branches of the esophageal plexus also penetrate the pericardium.[11] The lymphatic drainage of the pericardium is predominately into the retrosternal lymph node.[26]

Functions of the pericardium include lubrication of the heart and protection from extension of pleural infection and inflammatory changes. Maintenance of the heart in a semifixed position within the thorax, prevention of overdilation of the heart chambers, and limitation of right ventricular stroke volume (work) under conditions of increased left ventricular outflow resistance are other functions aiding homeometric autoregulation by maintaining balance in cardiac outflow between the cardiac chambers over several heart beats.[1,2,14]

Pathophysiology of Pericardial Disease

Reduction of the pericardial cavity by fluid, space occupying masses or fibrous tissue leads to compromise of cardiac function. Physical limitation of pericardial volume causes compression of the cardiac chambers and the venae cavae and restricts the ability of the heart to fill with blood during diastole. Venous pooling, increased central venous pressure, and a progressively decreasing cardiac output and stroke volume result.[17]

Inflammation of the pericardium may result in either a constrictive or a restrictive pericarditis. Constrictive pericarditis (epicarditis) results in an obliteration of the pericardial cavity by visceral contraction and an extension of the inflammatory process into the myocardium. The resulting myocardial fibrosis impedes both the filling and contraction of the cardiac chambers. In restrictive pericarditis, inflammatory changes associated with a thickened pericardium and increased pericardial fluid do not involve the heart muscle extensively, and only diastolic filling of the ventricles is hindered. Constrictive pericarditis is more difficult to treat surgically because visceral pericardium must be completely resected and myocardial tissue may need to be partially removed (Fig. 34-27). Restrictive pericarditis responds to the surgical removal of the fibrous and parietal pericardium alone; the visceral pericardium is left attached to the myocardium (Fig. 34-28).

Inflammatory changes in the pericardium have been attributed to mycotic, bacterial, and viral infections, to trauma, and to foreign bodies.[25] The origin of an idiopathic pericardiopathy that causes a serosanguineous to blood-tinged pericardial effusion is equivocal at this time, but the condition does respond to pericardiocentesis alone.

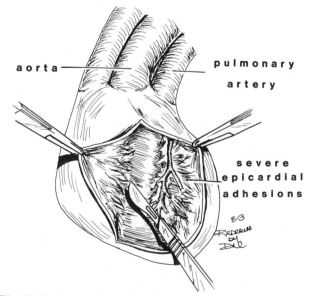

Fig. 34-27. *Constrictive pericardium being removed from the heart through a sternotomy incision.*

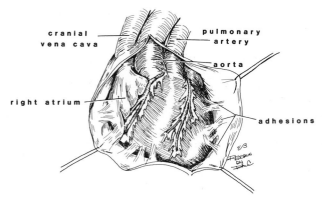

cranial
vena cava

pulmonary
artery

aorta

right atrium

adhesions

Fig. 34-28. *Restrictive pericardium being removed from the heart through a sternotomy incision.*

Granulomas variously affecting the atria, the ventricles, and the pericardium have been reported, as well as mesothelioma, hemangiosarcoma, and aortic body tumors.[15,19,28] Other reported causes of pericardial disease in the dog are congestive heart failure, hypoproteinemia, uremia, toxins, certain drugs, pericardial cysts, peritoneopericardial hernia with herniation, and incarceration of cardiac structures through a pericardial defect.

Clinical Signs of Pericardial Disease

The classic triad of increased venous pressure, decreased peripheral arterial pressure, and muffled heart sounds is usually present in pericardial disease.[5,10] Disease of the pericardium usually results in an outpouring of fluid into the pericardial cavity. Pericardial fibers have been shown to be poorly distensible when submitted to sudden stretching.[13,22] Chronic pericardial distension is accompanied by stretching of the elastic fibers, but excessive dilatation is hindered by the collagen fibers. Thus, if the pericardial fluid has accumulated rapidly in the pericardial cavity, as with a lacerated coronary artery, death may occur suddenly even with small amounts of pericardial fluid (cardiac tamponade). For example, 30 ml fluid impairs cardiac filling in a 10-kg animal when the fluid is rapidly infused into the pericardial cavity.[6,13] Gradual accumulation of fluid allows some adaptation by the pericardium until the clinical signs of congestive heart failure become evident from increased venous pressure (distended peripheral veins, pulsus paradoxus, abdominal ascites).

Diagnosis

A variety of diagnostic procedures can be used to differentiate pericardial disease from a dilated, failing heart. Radiography, electrocardiography, fluoroscopy, echocardiography, radionuclide imaging, cardiac pressure measurement by catheterization, and angiocardiography may confirm the presence of fluid or a space-occupying mass within the pericardial cavity.[4,5,6,10,12,29]

Some of these techniques are readily available in veterinary practice and are detailed in standard texts.

When the presence of pericardial fluid has been adequately demonstrated, a pericardiocentesis should be performed, and the pericardial fluid should be analyzed. Pericardiocentesis is a valuable diagnostic and prognostic procedure and may be therapeutic in selected cases. The minimum analysis of the pericardial fluid should include a measurement of specific gravity, bacterial and mycotic cultures, and cytologic study of the cells. If the fluid appears to be bloody, packed cell volume, plasma protein content, and clotting ability determinations should be obtained.[10,20,21,23]

Surgical Techniques

PERICARDIOCENTESIS

Although study of the thoracic radiographs may indicate a preferred location for pericardiocentesis, an area near the apex is generally selected in order to reduce the chance of lacerating a coronary artery.

Pericardiocentesis may be performed on the recumbent or standing patient. Although better physical control is obtained in recumbency, hemodynamic compromise may occur.[9] Monitoring the animal is best accomplished with an electrocardiogram during pericardiocentesis. The electrocardiogram may show premature ventricular contractions if the epicardium is irritated, and an increase in wave amplitude may be seen when the fluid is removed.

A 6 to 8 inch (16 to 18 gauge) intravenous catheter of polyethylene or Teflon over a needle should be used for pericardiocentesis. The catheter should have multiple fenestrations carefully made in the sidewall to facilitate fluid removal. Following routine surgical preparation and local anesthesia of the fourth, fifth, or sixth intercostal space, the catheter needle unit is attached to a 3-way stopcock and syringe and is introduced into the pericardium about one-fourth the distance between the costochondral junction and the sternum.

If the pericardium is thickened, some resistance may be met before entering the pericardial cavity. Once fluid is obtained, the needle should be drawn out, and the catheter should be advanced and secured in place. The majority of pericardial fluid can be removed, but loculated areas within the pericardial cavity may preclude aspiration of some fluid and debris. If the hematocrit of the pericardial fluid approaches the animal's peripheral venous hematocrit, discretion is used when withdrawing large volumes of the pericardial fluid. In any case, withdrawal of large volumes of pericardial fluid necessitates careful monitoring of the patient's vital signs.

Dark fluid that does not clot usually represents long-term third-space fluid losses that can be completely removed. While the catheter is still in place, a pneumopericardiogram can be done to evaluate the amount of fluid remaining and to verify the existence of a space-occupying mass within the pericardium.[9]

Careful insufflation with carbon dioxide is recommended for the pneumopericardiogram.

Following pericardiocentesis the patient should be observed for any signs indicative of the inadvertent laceration of a coronary artery (tamponade) or continued myocardial irritation (arrhythmias). Depending on the volume of pericardial fluid removed, the complication of a coronary arterial laceration may result in delayed tamponade or in clinical signs referable to blood loss.

PERICARDIECTOMY

Conservative treatment, consisting of two or three pericardial evacuations and specific antibiotic therapy following a positive bacterial culture, should be initially attempted for pericardial effusions. Pericardiectomy is indicated if fluid reaccumulates following repeated pericardiocentesis or if evidence suggests a space-occupying mass within the pericardium. The procedure is also performed for the treatment of restrictive and constrictive pericarditis.

Four surgical approaches are used for pericardiectomy. The left intercostal thoracotomy, right intercostal thoracotomy, and the median sternotomy are the most common. A transverse sternotomy is indicated in rare cases to increase surgical exposure.[7] If the diagnostic evaluation indicates the presence of a right side mass, a right intercostal thoracotomy or a median sternotomy should be performed. If pressure measurements in the caval atrium and right ventricle and angiocardiographic or endocardial-pericardial separation studies indicate a constrictive pericarditis (epicarditis), a complete pericardiectomy is indicated. Removal of fibrous, parietal, and visceral pericardium from all four heart chambers should be approached by median sternotomy. Either a right or a left intercostal thoracotomy is usually adequate for surgical excision of only the fibrous and parietal pericardium in cases of restrictive pericarditis or pericardial effusion. Because the edges of a pericardial window may later adhere to the cardiac muscle and may thereby form a new closed cavity, we prefer to perform a complete rather than a partial (window) pericardiectomy when treating pericardial effusion. Pericardial tissue samples should always be taken for histopathologic examination.

Chronic disease may obscure and may distort anatomic landmarks. If the phrenic nerve is enveloped by fibrosis and chronic inflammation, it can be traced cranially from the diaphragm to the point at which it crosses the pericardium. If the phrenic nerve cannot be bluntly elevated from the pericardium prior to pericardiectomy, parallel incisions dorsal and ventral to the nerve are initially made in the pericardium, and the nerve is retracted from the surgical site with Penrose drains. The vagus nerve can be traced as it courses the craniodorsal reflection of the fibrous pericardium within the mediastinal pleura. Because of its more dorsal anatomic location, the vagus nerve is not likely to be inadvertently severed during pericardiectomy.[11] The initial pericardial incision is continued, cranially and caudally, to the point at which the pericardium curves

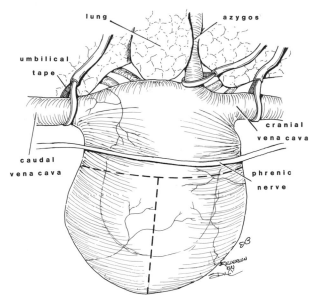

Fig. 34-29. *Umbilical tapes enclosed in rubber tubing have been placed around the great veins prior to incision of the pericardium (dashed lines). Pericardial effusion is evident.*

medially around the heart. A second pericardial incision, perpendicular to the midpoint of the first incision, extends past the apex of the heart and creates two wedge-shaped pericardial flaps (Fig. 34-29). Dissection in a cranioventral or caudoventral direction elevates each flap from the ventricular base to the apex and completes the removal of the pericardium from the right side of the heart. An assistant veterinary surgeon should then elevate the heart in a sling of moistened laparotomy sponges while the pericardium is removed from the left side of the heart. Visibility on the left side of the pericardium is impaired, so the pericardium should be excised only to the level of the phrenic nerve.

Because control of heavy hemorrhage may be difficult, electrocautery should be the principal method used in excising the pericardium. Electrocautery limits blood loss and expedites the operative procedure. Although inadvertent fibrillation of the heart has not been associated with the use of a properly grounded electrosurgical device, the veterinarian may wish to employ blunt and sharp surgical dissection in areas close to the visceral pericardium or myocardium.

Constrictive pericarditis (epicarditis) necessitates the removal of areas of the visceral pericardium and possibly the myocardium. Manometric readings of central venous pressure may be serially recorded during the surgical procedure to determine whether the visceral pericardium should be freed from around the atria and great vessels. Resection of the contracted pericardium by sharp and blunt dissection is performed with great difficulty (see Fig. 34-27). Coronary vascular trauma may result during decortication or "peeling" of visceral pericardial adhesions and plaques. Coronary vessel trauma or myocardial hemorrhage may be controlled by pressure or with small-caliber suture ligatures placed by fine swaged-on needles.

Once the pericardiectomy is completed, a chest tube is placed, and the thoracotomy incision is closed in a routine manner. Animals can function without a pericardium, but cardiac function is altered as compliance of the ventricles is altered. This altered compliance leads to dilation of the cardiac chambers during stress and an increase in heart weight and transverse diameter that radiographically appears as a rounding of the apex and a prominence of the atria.[14]

EXCISION OF PERICARDIAL CYSTS

Pericardial cysts, reported to be fibrous tissue or organized hematoma, should be dissected along with the thickened, adherent pericardium; the cysts are not usually attached to the surface of the heart.[16] Because pericardial cysts may recur, it is advisable to perform a subtotal pericardiectomy ventral to the phrenic nerves.

EXCISION OF CHEMODECTOMAS

Chemodectomas (aortic body tumors, chemoreceptor tumors) can arise from several sites within or outside the pericardium. Aortic bodies are normally present in the adventitial tissue between the aorta and the pulmonary artery, between the pulmonary artery and the left atrial appendage, and between the aorta and the right atrial appendage.[18]

Chemodectomas should be surgically approached from a fourth intercostal thoracotomy on the involved side or by a median sternotomy. If the pericardium is not involved, it may be used to form a pericardial cradle. Chemodectomas occur as single or multiple nodules; although not highly metastatic, they may be locally invasive and may displace the trachea and the vena cava as these tumors enter the right atrium.[15,19] The majority of the single chemodectomas experienced by one of us (Breznock and others[27]), however, have proved to be noninvasive and easy to resect by careful sharp and blunt dissection. The prognosis for palliation of pericardial effusion is favorable following excision of well-defined chemodectomas.

EXCISION OF MASSES INVOLVING
THE ATRIUM OR VENTRICLE

Unless diagnostic information such as radiographs and contrast angiocardiographic studies suggest otherwise, surgical exposure to the atria and ventricles should be through a fifth intercostal thoracotomy on the involved side. Although rare, the masses most commonly excised from the atria and ventricles are granulomas and neoplasms.

Umbilical tapes should be placed around the cranial and caudal vena cava, and around the azygos vein if operating on the right side, and should be passed through rubber tubing prior to incision of the pericardium (Fig. 34-29). The pericardium can be incised below and parallel to the phrenic nerve; a second incision, perpendicular to the first, creates a "T"-shaped pericardial incision. Other pericardial incisions, verti-

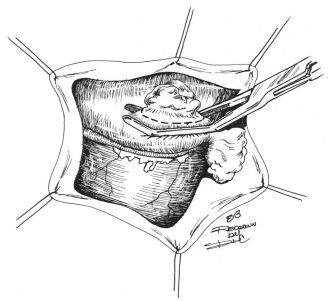

Fig. 34-30. *A partial occluding clamp encompasses the right atrial mass. Dashed line indicates the excision line.*

cal or horizontal, at different levels may increase the initial exposure as needed. If total exposure to one side of the heart is desired, one should completely reflect the phrenic nerve from the pericardium and extend a second pericardial incision from the apex to the level of the atrium. The creation of this pericardial "cradle" by multiple stay sutures elevates and stabilizes the heart in a satisfactory operating position. One must be careful not to obstruct the inflow and outflow of the heart.

Small perforations or tears in the atrial or ventricular wall may be identified and oversown with suture material. Small atrial masses may be encompassed by a partial occlusion clamp,* they may be widely excised, and the defect may be closed (Fig. 34-30). Blood flow through major vessels such as the coronary sinus or pulmonary veins should not be occluded when placing the partial occluding clamp. Suture material used in cardiac muscle should be of the nonabsorbable monofilament type. If the pericardium is not diseased, it can be sutured closed, removed, or left open. If the defect in the pericardium is left open, it should be left widely open to prevent incarceration of the heart or a lung lobe.

Large atrial masses and ventricular masses located in the free-wall or the apex of the heart that are too large to be encompassed under a partial occlusion clamp can be removed under normothermic venous occlusion. The disadvantage of venous occlusion is that the veterinary surgeon has only approximately 3 minutes to excise the mass and to suture the resulting defect.

After preparation for venous inflow occlusion and creation of the pericardial cradle, the area to be excised is delineated in the cardiac muscle (Fig. 34-31A).

*Satinsky cardiovascular clamps, available from American V. Mueller, 6600 West Touhy Avenue, Chicago, IL 60648

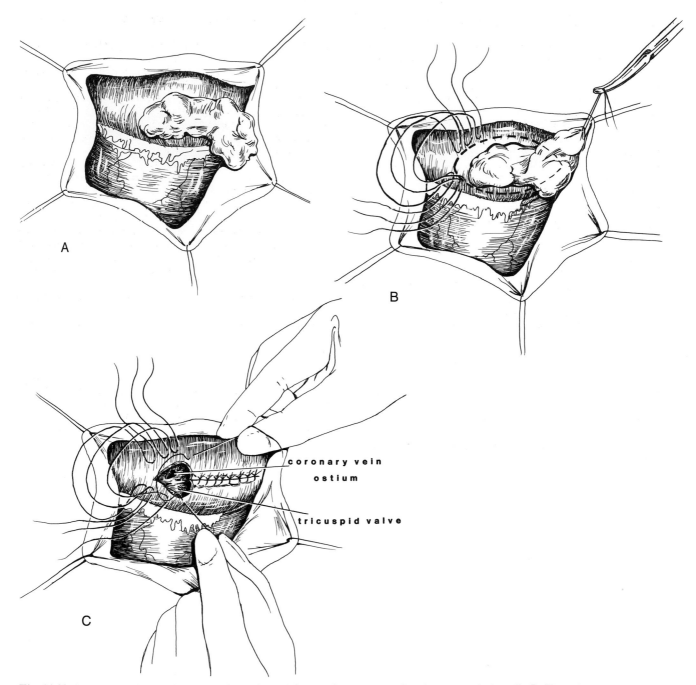

Fig. 34-31. A, *A large right atrial mass involving the atrial appendage is exposed with a pericardial cradle. B, The right atrial appendage is retracted dorsally. Lembert sutures are preplaced peripheral to the anticipated line of excision (dashed line) of the larger atrial mass. C, Under venous occlusion, the right atrial mass has been excised and many of the preplaced Lembert sutures have been tied.*

Masses extending across the coronary groove usually cannot be resected without major damage to the coronary arteries and the atrioventricular valve. Interrupted Lembert sutures are preplaced at the margins of the area to be sutured (Fig. 34-31B). The sutures usually need not enter the ventricular lumen and should not entrap underlying structures such as a cusp of the atrioventricular valve, papillary muscle, or chordae tendineae. Following placement of the Lembert sutures, venous return is inhibited by the preplaced umbilical tapes, the heart is allowed to empty, the mass is ex-

cised, and the defect is quickly closed (Fig. 34-31C). Intracardiac air is evacuated, and the umbilical tapes on the venae cavae are released following closure of the heart cavity. The suture line is examined for leakage following restoration of circulation.

If more time is needed for the completion of the surgical procedure, a more sophisticated method of blood diversion such as cardiopulmonary bypass or cardioplegia under hypothermic conditions must be employed. These techniques are beyond the scope of this discussion.

References and Suggested Readings

1. Bartle, S. H., et al.: Effect of the pericardium on left ventricular volume and function in acute hypervolaemia. Cardiovasc. Res., *3*:284, 1968.
2. Berglund, E., Sarnoff, S. J., and Isaacs, J. P.: Ventricular function, role of the pericardium in regulation of cardiovascular hemodynamics. Circ. Res., *3*:133, 1955.
3. Bhargava, A. K., Powers, T. E., and Rudy, R. L.: Pleural and pericardial fluid dynamics in dogs. Indian J. Vet., *49*:496, 1972.
4. Bhargava, A. K., Rudy, R. L., and Diesem, C. D.: Radiographic anatomy of the pleura in dogs as visualized by contrast pleurography. J. Am. Vet. Radiol. Soc., *10*:61, 1969.
5. Bolton, G. R.: Pericardial diseases. *In* Textbook of Veterinary Internal Medicine: Diseases of the Dog and Cat. Vol. 2. Edited by S. J. Ettinger. Philadelphia, W. B. Saunders, 1975.
6. Buchanan, J. W., and Kelly, A. M.: Endocardial splitting of the left atrium in the dog with hemorrhage and hemopericardium. J. Am. Vet. Radiol. Soc., *5*:28, 1964.
7. Buchanan, J. W., and Lawson, D. D.: Cardiovascular system. *In* Canine Surgery. 2nd Ed. Edited by J. Archibald. Santa Barbara, CA, American Veterinary Publications, 1974.
8. Burk, R. L.: Radiographic definition of the phrenicopericardiac ligament. J. Am. Vet. Radiol. Soc., *17*:216, 1976.
9. Ettinger, S. J.: Pericardiocentesis. Vet. Clin. North Am., *4*:403, 1974.
10. Ettinger, S. J., and Suter, P. F.: Canine Cardiology. Philadelphia, W. B. Saunders, 1970.
11. Evans, H. E., and Christensen, G. C.: Miller's Anatomy of the Dog. 2nd Ed. Philadelphia, W. B. Saunders, 1979.
12. Feigenbaum, H., Waldhausen, J. A., and Hyde, L. P.: Ultrasound diagnosis of pericardial effusion. JAMA, *191*:711, 1965.
13. Fineberg, M. H.: Functional capacity of the normal pericardium. Am. Heart J., *11*:748, 1936.
14. Holt, J. P.: The normal pericardium. Am. J. Cardiol., *26*:455, 1970.
15. Jubb, K. V. F., and Kennedy, P. C.: Pathology of Domestic Animals. Vol. 1. 2nd Ed. New York, Academic Press, 1970.
16. Marion, J., et al.: Pericardial effusion in a young dog. J. Am. Vet. Med. Assoc., *157*:1055, 1970.
17. Nerlich, W. E.: Determinants of impairment of cardiac filling during progressive pericardial effusion. Circulation, *3*:377, 1951.
18. Nonidez, J. F.: Distribution of aortic nerve fibers and the epithelioid bodies (supracardial paraganglia) in the dog. Anat. Rec., *69*:299, 1937.
19. Patnaik, A. K., Liu, S. K., Hurvitz, A. I., and McClelland, A. J.: Canine chemodectoma (extra-adrenal paragangliomas): a comparative study. J. Small Anim. Pract., *16*:785, 1975.
20. Perman, V., Alsaker, R. D., and Riis, R. C.: Cytology of the dog and cat. J. Am. Anim. Hosp. Assoc. [Suppl.], 17, 1979.
21. Perman, V., Osborne, C. A., and Stevens, J. B.: Laboratory evaluation of abnormal body fluids. Vet. Clin. North Am. *4*:255, 1974.
22. Rabkin, S., Berghause, D. G., and Bauer, H. F.: Mechanical properties of the isolated canine pericardium. J. Appl. Physiol., *36*:69, 1974.
23. Rebar, A. H.: Handbook of Veterinary Cytology. Saint Louis, Ralston Purina, 1978.
24. Schebitz, H., and Wilkens, H.: Atlas of Radiographic Anatomy of the Dog and Cat. 3rd Rev. Ed., Berlin, Verlag Paul Parey, 1977.
25. Schwartz, A., et al.: Constrictive pericarditis in two dogs. J. Am. Vet. Med. Assoc., *159*:763, 1971.
26. Thanikachalam, S., et al.: Lymphatic drainage of the heart muscle and pericardial sac in the dog. Indian Heart J., *30*:287, 1978.
27. Thomas, W. P.: Personal communications, 1980.
28. Thrall, D. E., and Goldschmidt, M. H.: Mesothelioma in the dog: six case reports. J. Am. Vet. Radiol. Soc., *19*:107, 1978.
29. Viamonte, M.: Carbon dioxide angiocardiography in the dog. J. Am. Vet. Radiol. Soc., *4*:18, 1963.

35 * Peripheral Vessels

Catheter Embolectomy for Arterial Occlusion

by DENNIS T. CROWE

An embolus is an intravascular obstruction brought by the blood from another vessel (arterioarterial embolus) or the heart (cardioarterial embolus) to obstruct the circulation. In contrast, a thrombus is an obstruction that is attached to that location. A thrombus may dislodge at its point of attachment and may embolize further distally, however, to become a thromboembolus.

Significant vascular occlusion with resulting ischemia is not unfamiliar to the majority of practicing veterinarians. The prevalence of acute vascular embolization or thrombosis in the dog and cat population is unknown, but the most commonly recognized location is the distal aorta and the iliac artery bifurcation in cats. Surgical and postmortem observations have also confirmed acute occlusions involving the celiac, splenic, hepatic, left gastric, cranial mesenteric, brachial, renal, segmental lumbar, and pulmonary arteries.

In recent years, the use of the Fogarty balloon-tipped catheter* has simplified the emergency removal of arterial emboli. The success of treatment depends on the early diagnosis and complete removal of the embolus or thrombus before the onset of irreversible myoneuronecrosis. Because the latter disorder may occur rapidly, primary treatment rather than referral is usually indicated. With only a few instruments and sutures commonly used for extraocular ophthalmic procedures, and with embolectomy catheters, the procedure can be done simply and safely without the need for general anesthesia.

Pathophysiology

The majority of feline arterial emboli originate from a cardiac thrombus. Thus, a patient presented to the veterinarian with acute embolic occlusion should be assumed to have significant underlying heart disease until proved otherwise. Idiopathic cardiomyopathy with accompanying myocardial hypertrophy and a

*Edwards Laboratories, Division of American Hospital Supply Corp., Santa Ana, CA

functional subaortic stenosis are common in the cat. Loosely attached thrombi develop in the poorly contracting, enlarged left atrium. Other predispositions are due to congestive heart failure and atrial fibrillation.

Endocardiosis with mitral insufficiency is common in the dog. Heartworm disease, indwelling intravenous or arterial catheters, and bacteremia may also be incriminated as causes of vascular thrombosis. Hypercoagulopathy and disseminated intravascular coagulopathy have been suggested as a cause of thrombosis in association with infection, trauma, or malignant disease.

Intra-Arterial Thromboembolic Disease

Emboli usually lodge at bifurcations of major arteries where the diameter abruptly narrows. Because of the large size of the thrombi found in the atrium, a common site is the bifurcation of the aorta and the iliac arteries. An embolus occurring at this site is commonly known as a saddle embolus. The severity of the ischemia produced depends on the acuity and the degree of occlusion, subtracting the amount of collateral circulation present. It is assumed that an unknown number of emboli occur in other "silent areas" of the circulation where collateral circulation is substantial.

Vasoactive substances released by the thromboembolic clotting process and hypoxic tissue changes distal to the obstruction are also damaging. Simply ligating the distal aorta in the cat does not produce the clinical signs of ischemia seen with a natural saddle embolization because the collateral circulatory channels are adequate. These channels include the lumbar arteries at the level of the fifth and sixth lumbar vertebrae and the caudal superficial epigastric arteries. Clinical signs of ischemia do result, however, from the introduction of a supernatant from lysed autologous red blood cells or a fresh autologous blood clot between two ligatures at the distal aorta's bifurcation. Clinical signs may also be produced by the addition of thrombin at the site of experimental ligation. It is likely that vasoactive substances liberated in the coagulation process and thrombus formation are responsible for an inadequate response by the collateral circulation to prevent hind-limb ischemia. For example, 5-hydroxytryptamine (serotonin) and prostaglandins $F_{2\alpha}$ cause intense constriction of the smooth muscle walls of the small arteries and arterioles and also enhance further thrombus formation. Factors affecting the rate of onset of necrosis include the size of the artery occluded, the collateral circulation, blood pressure, and temperature.

The major physiologic consequence of a large arterial embolus is the immediate onset of severe ischemia of the tissues normally supplied by the occluded artery. If untreated, an embolus causes neuronecrosis in about 50% of patients. Prominent early signs are pain, paralysis, and paresthesia, which result from the great sensitivity of peripheral nerves to oxygen deprivation. Striated muscle is also susceptible to hypoxemia, and necrosis may appear as early as 4 to 6 hours after the onset of ischemia.

Distal aortic embolectomy is generally successful if it can be performed before muscle necrosis develops. Occasionally, only moderate ischemia is present, and necrosis does not develop despite neurologic signs and vascular occlusion. This phenomenon is presumed to be due to the persistence of a sufficient amount of functional collateral circulation.

Unfortunately, sluggish arterial blood flow distal to the embolus predisposes a patient to secondary thrombus propagation further down the arterial tree. Secondary thrombi may join the original embolus or may develop in areas of severe stasis. Secondary thrombi further occlude major collateral channels and intensify the ischemia. As time progresses, effective therapy becomes more difficult because both the primary and secondary thrombi must be removed. Eventually, the progressive circulatory stasis becomes complicated by extensive capillary and venous thrombosis.

Following occlusion, an ascending deposit of platelets, fibrin, leukocytes, and erythrocytes may obstruct arterial branches proximal to the original site of occlusion.

Diagnosis

PHYSICAL EXAMINATION. Pain, paralysis, paresthesia, pulselessness and pallor (the 5 "P"s) are abrupt in onset. In 75 to 80% of patients, pain is severe and unremitting in the affected extremities. Palpation of the gastrocnemius muscle reveals hard, turgid muscle bellies. The nail beds and toe pads are pale or cyanotic, and perfusion is poor or nonexistent. The extremities are cold, and femoral arterial pulses are diminished or absent. Sensory disturbances vary from anesthesia to paresthesia.

A crucial prognostic sign for neuronecrosis is the loss of deep pain sensation. Few patients with this ominous sign recover. Conversely, if motor and sensory functions are intact, the patient's extremity may survive even though chronic ischemia may persist.

Another important prognostic sign is concerned with muscle turgor. Shortly after the onset of ischemia, the muscles are soft. With continuing ischemia, edema appears and gradually progresses to necrosis and finally to a functional rigor mortis. Early ischemic edema creates a "doughy" sensation on palpation. The importance of this physical finding is that as long as the muscles feel soft when palpated, the limbs and their function can possibly be saved with effective embolectomy and thrombectomy, regardless of how long the embolus has been present. Conversely, the presence of noncompliant muscles means that necrosis is taking place. Complete muscular rigor is an ominous sign, and treatment is not recommended.

An additional and important aspect of physical examination is the cardiac examination for underlying heart disease. In many patients, murmurs, arrhythmias, or pulmonary edema are apparent on auscultation. Dyspnea, cyanosis, and other signs of congestive heart failure are common.

OTHER DIAGNOSTIC TECHNIQUES. The diagnosis of acute arterial occlusion is readily made from the patient's medical history and the physical findings. An electrocardiogram and chest radiographs should be used to evaluate the presence of heart disease. An arteriogram should be performed if surgical therapy is not to be delayed beyond 4 to 6 hours from the onset of clinical signs. In most instances, a simple intravenous manual bolus injection, through a jugular vein catheter, of a tri-iodinated contrast medium* (2 ml/kg) confirms the diagnosis and defines the proximal extent of the obstruction. One or two lateral radiographs are taken in rapid sequence, beginning approximately 7 seconds from the completion of the injection.

Preoperative Considerations

Because patients with arterial emboli usually have serious heart disease and recurrence of vascular occlusion is common, discussion of prognosis and risks with the pet's owner is mandatory.

If treatment is elected, the prompt intravenous administration of heparin is recommended to inhibit the development of thrombi proximal and distal to the embolus. In the cat, 20 IU/kg intravenously along with 250 IU/kg subcutaneously have been recommended for the initial treatment. The subcutaneous doses should be repeated every 8 hours. Not only does heparin inhibit further formation of thromboemboli, but also it antagonizes some of the deleterious effects of sertonin on the collateral circulation. For heparin therapy in dogs, the drug should be started intravenously at 50 IU/kg. A subcutaneous injection of 250 IU/kg should also be given and repeated every 8 hours. Activated coagulation times are monitored to ensure a 1.5- to 2.5-fold increase from base line.

Relief of pain is also important. In addition to humane considerations, tachycardia decreases coronary blood flow and may further injure a hypertrophied myocardium. Low intravenous doses of ketamine hydrochloride (0.1 to 0.5 mg/kg) in cats or oxymorphone (0.05 to 0.2 mg/kg) in dogs are recommended to control pain. Intravenous diazepam (0.1 to 0.2 mg/kg), along with the ketamine or oxymorphone, may also be useful.

*Conray 400, Mallinckrodt Pharmaceuticals, St. Louis, MO

Surgical Technique

In most animals, local anesthesia is all that is necessary for catheter placement. Patients requiring celiotomy may be given epidural anesthesia or a balanced combination of ketamine and nitrous oxide and a muscular blocking agent.

Removal of aortic, iliac, and femoral arterial emboli is performed with the Fogarty balloon-tipped embolectomy catheter from incisions in either femoral artery or through an incision in the distal aorta. The approach(es) used depend on the location of the embolus and the size of the animal. The artery through which the catheter is introduced must be of sufficient size to permit catheter advancement proximal to the embolus and removal of the embolus with the catheter's withdrawal. Femoral arteriotomy alone is generally not large enough to accomplish this in animals weighing below 4 kg. Even in larger individuals, an approach through the aorta may be necessary.

The animal is placed in dorsal recumbency, and the femoral arteries are exposed. Each artery is dissected free from connective tissues and is encircled with moistened cotton tapes (Fig. 35-1A) or suture material (Fig. 35-1B). A 1% lidocaine-saline solution is used to keep the area moist and to help prevent arteriospasm. Adventitia is stripped away from the arteriotomy site with ophthalmic forceps, and a transverse incision is made through the vessel with fine ophthalmic scissors (Fig. 35-1C). The tip of a mosquito hemostat is gently introduced into the vascular lumen as a dilator, and the intima of the vessel is secured to the tunica adventitia of the vessel wall with 1 or 2 sutures of 6-0 or 7-0 suture material on each side of the incision (Fig. 35-2). The purpose of this fixation is to avoid intimal tears or dissections. In tiny vessels, this step is omitted because of size limitations.

The Fogarty arterial embolectomy catheter is a single-lumen, balloon-tipped catheter designed specifically to remove arterial emboli and thrombi. The catheters are available in 6 sizes, ranging from 2 to 7 French. The recommended maximum inflated balloon diameters are 4, 5, 9, 11, 13, and 14 mm, respectively. Each delicate, thin-walled, and compliant latex balloon holds a specific amount of fluid, and it is important that this volume not be exceeded. The most commonly used sizes are 2 or 3 French for cats and small dogs and 4 to 6 French for medium to large dogs. The balloon (of the 3- to 7-French catheters) is inflated with saline solution before it is introduced into the artery, to obtain an idea of the size of the filled balloon and to check the balloon's integrity. Air or carbon dioxide is used to inflate the balloon in the 2-French catheter.

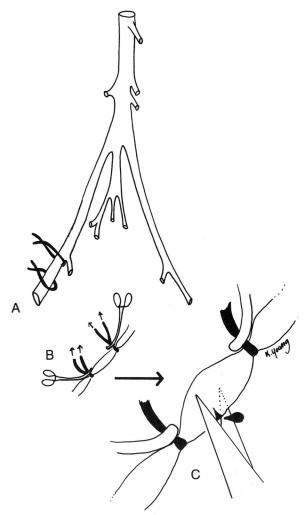

Fig. 35-1. A, *The femoral artery is exposed circumferentially 2 to 4 cm in length and is encircled with saline-moistened cotton tapes. One is placed approximately 1.5 cm proximal to the proposed arteriotomy site and the other is placed approximately 1.5 cm distal to the arteriotomy site. B, Suture material and curved mosquito hemostats are used to complete an atraumatic occlusive ring around the artery. C, When the adventitia of the artery has been stripped away from the arteriotomy site, a transverse incision through the vessel is made using fine ophthalmic scissors.*

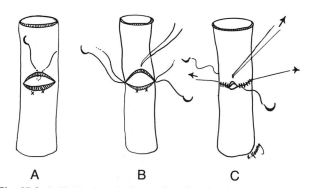

Fig. 35-2. A, *The intima is fastened to the other layers of the artery wall with one or two stitches on each side of the incision to prevent intimal tears and dissection when the catheter is passed into the arteriotomy site. B, Single 6-0 or 7-0 sutures are placed through the arterial wall at each end of the arteriotomy site to avoid further disruption of the artery during catheter passage and thromboembolus extraction. The ends of the sutures can also be left long and tagged with mosquito hemostats to facilitate later closure of the arteriotomy site. C, Following arterial embolectomy, the arterial incision is closed with simple continuous sutures. Notice that the closure is facilitated by traction placed on the two corner sutures and the middle "intimal securing suture."*

It is important to use a well-lubricated glass syringe to inflate the balloon rather than a plastic disposable syringe, because frictional forces between the plastic barrel and plunger reduce the critical control of balloon size. Additionally, the smallest syringe that holds the stated maximum fluid capacity should be used because less-subtle plunger displacements are required to make a given change in a balloon diameter. In the smaller sizes (2- to 4-French catheters), this is generally a 1-ml tuberculin or insulin syringe.

The deflated balloon catheter is passed distally into the arteriotomy site, if size permits, past thrombi, and is guided gently down the femoral artery until some resistance is met. The balloon is then carefully inflated and is gradually withdrawn to extract the emboli or thrombi (Fig. 35-3). The catheter is then directed proximally into the distal aorta proximal to the cranial extent of the blockage (Fig. 35-4). If this location is not known, the catheter should be advanced to the level of the thoracic aorta. The balloon is then inflated and is then carefully withdrawn. As the catheter is withdrawn, some of the fluid in the balloon must be removed to reduce its size as the balloon enters the iliac and femoral arteries. The embolus is forced ahead of the balloon and is extracted through the arteriotomy incision as the catheter is withdrawn. Successful embolectomy is indicated by a pulsatile flow from the proximal artery. Occasionally, several proximal and distal passes with the catheter are necessary to remove the emboli and the propagating thrombosis. If the procedure fails, aortotomy by means of celiotomy becomes necessary.

If successful, the procedure is then repeated in the opposite femoral artery to ensure that all fragments of clot have been removed. Following embolectomy, the artery is irrigated proximally and distally, with heparin-

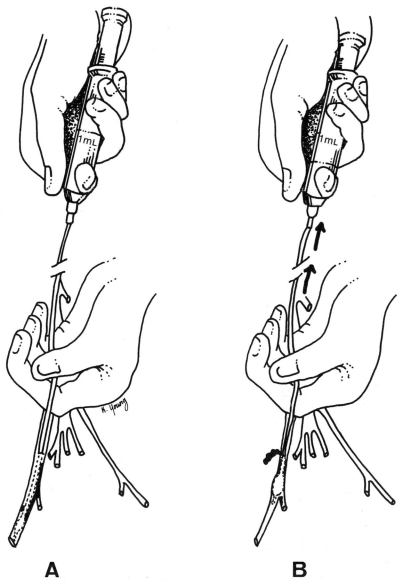

A **B**

Fig. 35-3. A, *The deflated balloon catheter is passed gently into the arteriotomy site and guided distally down the femoral artery until some resistance is met.* B, *The balloon is then inflated until resistance is felt and is gradually withdrawn.*

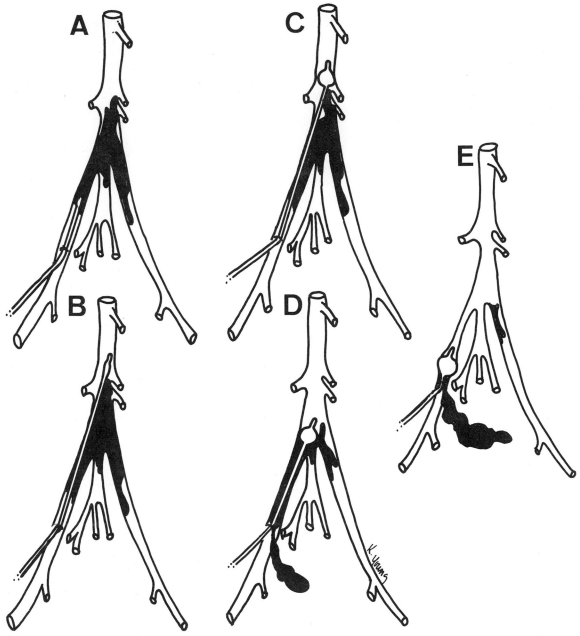

Fig. 35-4. A *and* B, *The deflated balloon catheter is passed proximally past the cranial extent of the blockage.* C *and* D, *The balloon is then inflated and is gently withdrawn.* E, *An extensive thromboembolus is being expelled from the arteriotomy site.*

ized saline solution (2 IU/ml). The arteriotomies are closed with continuous 6-0 or 7-0 sutures from the ends of the arteriotomy (see Fig. 35-2*C*). Polypropylene is the suture of choice, and magnification with surgical loupes is recommended.

Minor blood leakage between the sutures can usually be controlled by applying pressure for 5 minutes with the finger tip. If it is impossible to suture the arteriotomy site, simple ligation of the femoral artery just above and below the arteriotomy site is recommended; however, the ligatures should be placed below the branches of the deep femoral artery and approximately 3 to 4 other small tributaries that provide collateral circulation to the extremity. Complications in the use of

the Fogarty catheter are: (1) rupture of the artery by the inflated balloon; (2) perforation of the artery by the tip of the catheter; (3) tear of the intima and subsequent subintimal dissection; and (4) rupture of the balloon; (5) dislodgment of the embolus and pushing of it proximally as the tip of the catheter is being advanced. This complication can be avoided by using the appropriate-size catheter and not reusing it for this purpose. Resterilization increases the thickness of the balloon and roughens its surface. Other precautions to reduce the complications are as follows: (1) the catheter should *never* be forced against a resistance when passed into the artery; and (2) a small amount of air (preferably carbon dioxide, which can be aspirated from under a glass in which a match has been burning) can also be added to the fluid to improve balloon compliance, thus making arterial rupture or tearing of the intima less likely. When using the 2-French catheter, carbon dioxide and not saline solution is the medium recommended for inflation.

The operator must control the pressure in the balloon directly and carefully. When resistance increases, fluid is withdrawn to reduce pressure. A lag time exists between the manipulation of the syringe and the response at the balloon end of the catheter. One operator must control both the movement of the catheter and the diameter of the balloon.

Postoperative Care

Immediately following restoration of circulation, alterations in the patient's electrolytes and acid-base balance may occur. Systemic metabolic by-products are suddenly released. The administration of sodium bicarbonate and antiarrhythmic agents should be considered.

Heparinization of the patient is also recommended for the first postoperative week while the intimal defect is healing. Although debate exists on the safest and most economical and effective means of maintaining anticoagulation, the importance of continued anticoagulant therapy cannot be overemphasized. Because recurrence of embolization is common in the cardiomyopathy syndrome, 25 mg/kg aspirin, given every 3 to 4 days in the cat and daily in the dog for the duration of the patient's life, is advocated. Preliminary data also suggest that higher doses of aspirin given more frequently in cats may also be safe; for example, 25 mg/kg given once daily.

Cyproheptadine*, a 5-hydroxytryptamine antagonist, given intravenously (1 mg/kg) may also be beneficial in restoring collateral circulation to patients with acute arterial occlusion. Although its use has been documented, this agent has not been used extensively in clinical veterinary medicine.

Regardless of the drug regimen chosen, the single most important aspect of postoperative care is to be certain that the patient's circulation remains intact. Bi-

*Periactin, Merck, Sharp & Dohme, Division of Merck & Co., Inc., West Point, PA 19486

lateral, palpable femoral pulses are the best clinical sign of improvement. These pulses should be identified immediately after the operation, and their presence should be periodically confirmed by palpation. Disappearance of a previously palpable pulse may be an indication to repeat either the arteriogram or the surgical procedure.

References and Suggested Readings

Buchanan, J. W., Baker, G. J., and Hill, J. D.: Aortic embolism in cats: prevalence, surgical treatment and electrocardiography. Vet. Rec., 79:496, 1966.

Fogarty, T. J., et al: Experience with balloon catheter technique for arterial embolectomy. Am. J. Surg., 122:231, 1971.

Fogarty, T. J., et al: A method for extraction of arterial emboli and thrombi. Surg. Gynecol. Obstet., 116:241, 1963.

Frederick, W. C., and Olymbitis, J. T.: Fogarty embolectomy catheters in portal vein thrombosis. NY State J. Med., 69:2157, 1969.

Green, R. A.: Activated coagulation time in monitoring heparinized dogs. Am. J. Vet. Res., 41:1793, 1980.

Greene, C. E., and Meriwether, E.: Activated partial thromboplastin time and activated coagulation time in monitoring heparinized cats. Am. J. Vet. Res., 43:1473, 1982.

Greene, C. G.: Unpublished data. Preliminary investigations of platelet aggregation and clotting times in cats following aspirin and heparin therapy.

Holzworth, J., Simpson, R., and Wind, A.: Aortic thrombosis with posterior paralysis in the cat. Cornell Vet., 45:468, 1955.

Middleton, D. J., and Watson, A. D. J.: Activated coagulation times of whole blood in normal dogs and dogs with coagulopathies. J. Small Anim. Pract., 19:417, 1978.

Moncure, A. C., and McEnany, M. T.: Cardiovascular emergencies. In MGH Textbook of Emergency Medicine. Edited by E. W. Wilkins. Baltimore, Williams & Wilkins, 1978.

Olmstead, M. L., and Butler, H. C.: Five-hydroxytryptamine antagonists and feline aortic embolism. J. Small Anim. Pract., 18:247, 1977.

Sabiston, D. C.: Disorders of the arterial systems. In Textbook of Surgery. 11th Ed. Edited by D. C. Sabiston. Philadelphia, W. B. Saunders, 1977.

Schaub, R. G., Meyers, K. M., Sande, R. D., and Hamilton, G.: Inhibition of feline collateral vessel development following experimental thrombolic occlusion. Circ. Res., 39:736, 1976.

Weirich, W. E.: Vascular occlusion. In Current Techniques in Small Animal Surgery. Edited by M. J. Bojrab, Philadelphia, Lea & Febiger, 1975.

Yeary, R. A., and Swanson, W.: Aspirin dosages for the cat. J. Am. Vet. Med. Assoc., 176:1177, 1973.

36 * Lymph Nodes and Spleen

Tonsillectomy

by ROBERT L. PEIFFER, JR.

The success of surgical treatment of any disease process depends on an understanding of the anatomy, physiology, and pathology of the organ or tissue involved. Knowledge of the physiology of the tonsils is limited, as is the correlation of clinical and pathologic findings in tonsillar disease. The lymphoid tissues of the pharynx are generally acknowledged to play a protective role in the humoral and cellular immunologic response to disease involving not only the oral and pharyngeal region, but also the body as a whole. At this time, however, that role has not been clearly defined.

Surgical Anatomy

The anatomy of the palatine tonsils is similar in both the dog and the cat. The tonsils are paired, elongated structures of compact lymphoid tissue located in the lateral wall of the oral pharynx caudal to the palatoglossal arch. They lie in the tonsillar sinuses and are partially obscured from direct observation by the tonsillar fold, a thin extension of soft palate that overlies the medial aspect of the sinus.

The tonsils are attached to the dorsal wall of the sinus along their entire dorsal margin. In addition to the main fusiform portion, a minor layer of lymphoid tissue extends both medially and laterally in the dorsal mucosa of the sinus at the cranial pole of the tonsil. This minor portion of the tonsil can be visualized and removed only by adequate elevation of the tonsil from the sinus.

The blood supply to the tonsils comes from two or three branches of the tonsillar artery (a branch of the lingual artery) that enter the tonsil near its midpoint. Elevation of the tonsil from the sinus must be sufficient to remove all lymphoid tissue; however, excessive traction severs the main artery rather than its branches and results in unnecessary hemorrhage.

The palatine tonsils receive no afferent lymphatic vessels and drain variably into the deep cervical, medial retropharyngeal, and mandibular lymph nodes. Sensory innervation is provided by branches of the glossopharyngeal nerve. Additional tonsillar tissue can be found scattered throughout the mucosa of the nasopharynx and the base of the tongue, but is not identifiable as a surgical entity.

Indications

Tonsillectomy is indicated in animals with chronic recurrent tonsillitis or pharyngitis that is unresponsive to antibiotic therapy and in those with acute tonsillitis in which the physical presence of the enlarged tonsils contributes to difficulty in respiration or swallowing. The latter condition is most frequently observed in brachycephalic dogs. The rationale for removal is that (1) in chronic cases, the tonsillar tissue may be harboring a source of infectious organisms, and (2) the enlarged, inflamed tonsils themselves are primarily responsible for the prominent clinical signs and discomfort of the patient.

Removal of the tonsils may be indicated in neoplastic disease for therapeutic or diagnostic reasons. Squamous cell carcinoma and malignant lymphoma are the most common tonsillar neoplasms in the dog and cat.

Tonsillectomy may be employed as a diagnostic tool for chronic pharyngeal disease using cultures, impression smears, and histopathologic studies.

The operation should be preceded by complete physical examination, including an evaluation of the patient's clotting capabilities and fluid and electrolyte balance to determine surgical risk and to eliminate the possibility of the presence of systemic disease or other primary causes of secondary tonsillar involvement (such as a tonsillar sinus foreign body). Enlarged tonsils in healthy young dogs are not an indication for their removal because a variation in the size and in the position of the tonsil in relation to the sinus is normal, and the tonsils hypertrophy during the first year of life. Physiologic involution of tonsillar lymphoid tissue occurs after maturity.

Preoperative Considerations

Acute infections should be controlled by administering antibiotics preoperatively. The procedure is not sterile, but should be as aseptic as possible. Following induction of anesthesia and endotracheal intubation, the surgical area should be swabbed with povidone-iodine.* Operators should wear gloves. Elective operation should, of course, be preceded by a 12-hour fast.

Anesthesia

The choice of preanesthetic and anesthetic agents remains a matter of the veterinary surgeon's personal preference. Heavy sedation, in combination with local infiltration of anesthetic agent at the base of the tonsil, can be selected for tonsillectomy in high-risk patients and has the advantage that the swallowing reflexes remain intact. Because of the manipulative procedures, however, general anesthesia is preferable. A short-acting barbiturate or an inhalation anesthetic or a combination of both is acceptable. Endotracheal intubation with a cuffed tube is essential to prevent aspiration of blood, lymphoid tissue, and oral secretions; to ensure an open airway; and to assist in adequate ventilation and control of depth of anesthesia if a gas anesthetic is employed. Packing the laryngeal area around the tube with gauze further minimizes the possibility of aspiration. A rapid recovery from anesthesia and the return of swallowing reflexes are desirable.

If epinephrine is used for hemostasis in conjunction with halothane anesthesia, one must be aware of the sensitizing effect of this drug on the myocardium, one must use dilute solutions (1 : 10,000 to 1 : 100,000), and one must monitor cardiac function closely.

Positioning the Patient

The operating table may be tilted at 15°, with the patient's head down, to use gravity to help prevent aspiration. The patient can be placed in the lateral, dorsal, or sternal recumbent position; I prefer dorsal recumbency with the table tilted slightly. An assistant or a pair of tongue forceps are helpful to exert cranial and ventral traction on the tongue to maximize the surgical field and partially to elevate the tonsils from the sinuses. An oral speculum and adequate illumination are prerequisites for a successful operation, and a suction apparatus is handy for keeping the surgical field free of hemorrhage.

Surgical Technique

Several techniques for removal of the tonsils are acceptable. Principles common to all are complete removal of lymphoid tissue with minimal tissue trauma and maximal hemostasis (Fig. 36-1). The tonsils are grasped with forceps and are elevated from the sinus. Allis forceps are satisfactory; however, tonsillar forceps or small vulsellum forceps more effectively hold the friable tissue. Both the major and minor portions of the tonsil are identified. Epinephrine may be injected into the base of the tonsil at this time. The vasoconstrictive effect of epinephrine is transient, however, and secondary postoperative hemorrhage may occur if

*Betadine, Purdue Frederick Co., 50 Washington Street, Norwalk, CT 06856

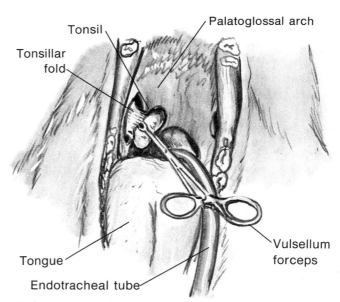

Fig. 36-1. *The adequately exposed tonsil is prepared for removal by one of several described techniques.*

epinephrine is relied upon as the sole method of hemostasis.

The tonsil may be sharply or bluntly dissected from the underlying mucosa with Metzenbaum scissors and an elevator or raspatory. Removal in a cranial to caudal direction facilitates complete removal of the minor tonsillar tissue. Hemorrhage is controlled as encountered with electrocautery, catgut ligature (4-0), direct pressure, topical application of epinephrine or astringents, by suturing the epithelial surfaces with 4-0 catgut, or by suturing the tonsillar fold over the sinus in a continuous or interrupted pattern with 4-0 catgut.

Alternately, the tonsil can be ligated dorsal to its base with a transfixion suture of 3-0 catgut, and the tonsillar tissue may be excised distal to the ligature with Metzenbaum scissors, a scalpel blade, or an electroscalpel.

A tonsil snare can be used; this instrument contributes to hemostasis by its crushing action. The loop of the snare is placed around the tonsil, the tonsil is grasped with forceps and is elevated, and the snare is positioned and is closed. Additional control of hemorrhage is usually required. The use of a tonsillotome based on similar principles has been described. In my experience, a diathermy snare or an electrotonsil snare is the ideal instrument for facilitating complete tonsil removal with minimal bleeding.

Tonsillectomy is incomplete without a blood agar culture, a stained impression smear biopsy, and a fixed histopathologic section interpretation of the involved tissue.

Postoperative Care

The patient should be kept in a head-down position, the endotracheal tube should be left in place until swallowing reflexes return, and the animal should be closely observed until it recovers completely from anesthesia. A liquid diet for the first 24 to 48 hours postoperatively facilitates ease of swallowing. In animals with infectious tonsillitis, the postoperative administration of antibiotics is indicated. Corticosteroids in combination with antibiotics may be beneficial if severe pharyngeal inflammation is present.

Complications

Operative and postoperative hemorrhage and aspiration of blood or lymphoid tissue with subsequent hypoxia or pneumonia are the two primary complications of tonsillectomy. Both are preventable when the described anesthesia and surgical techniques are employed. If incompletely removed, the tonsils may reappear by hyperplasia and hypertrophy; reoperation is performed in these animals if the disease process persists. Soft-tissue trauma due to poor surgical technique may be a complication of tonsillectomy. Subacute local pharyngitis may occur in the postoperative period and can be controlled medically. Occasionally, a chronic infectious pharyngitis persists in spite of tonsillectomy. In man, it has been suggested that removal of the tonsils predisposes the patient to future local infections and certain systemic neoplastic diseases, owing to immunologic deficiencies; these theories remain conjecture at this time.

Comments

Tonsillectomy is a tool that the veterinary surgeon has at his disposal; however, it is not an innocuous procedure and should not be approached as such. Cryodestruction of the tonsillar tissue, the use of electrotherapy and ultrasound to treat chronic pharyngeal disease, and greater understanding of tonsillar physiology and the body's immune response may alter the clinical approach to tonsillar disease in the years ahead.

References and Suggested Readings

Crouch, J. E.: Atlas of Cat Anatomy. Philadelphia, Lea & Febiger, 1969.

Evans, H. E., and Christensen, G. C.: Miller's Anatomy of the Dog. 2nd Ed. Philadelphia, W. B. Saunders, 1979.

Jones, T. C., and Hunt, R. D.: Veterinary Pathology, 5th Ed. Philadelphia, Lea & Febiger, 1982.

Jubb, K. V. F., and Kennedy, P. C.: Pathology of Domestic Animals. Vol. II. New York, Academic Press, 1970.

Kornblut, A. D.: Non-neoplastic diseases of the tonsils and adenoids. In Otolaryngology. Vol. III., Edited by M. M. Paparella and D. A. Shumrick. Philadelphia, W. B. Saunders, 1973.

Kornblut, A., and Kornblut, A. D.: Tonsillectomy and adenoidectomy. In Otolaryngology. Vol. III. Edited by M. M. Paparella and D. A. Shumrick. Philadelphia, W. B. Saunders, 1973.

Leonard, E. P.: Fundamentals of Small Animal Surgery. Philadelphia, W. B. Saunders, 1968.

Smith, C. R., and Hamlin, R. L.: Microcirculation and lymph. In Dukes Physiology of Domestic Animals. Edited by M. J. Swenson. Ithaca, NY, Cornell University Press, 1970.

Thordahl-Christensen, A.: Neck, pharynx, tonsils, and larynx. In Canine Surgery. Edited by J. Archibald. Santa Barbara, CA, American Veterinary Publications, 1965.

Techniques for Lymph Node Biopsy

by DENNIS J. MEYER

Indications

Lymph node biopsy is indicated for local or generalized lymphadenopathy of undetermined origin. It is often possible to distinguish between neoplastic and non-neoplastic disease by means of aspiration biopsy. Excisional lymph node biopsy is indicated for the histologic classification of lymphosarcoma and for the evaluation of metastatic disease.

Contraindications

Needle aspiration of a lymph node that contains a malignant neoplasm might be considered a contraindication, owing to the potential for dissemination. Fortunately, this is not an actual contraindication, and as outlined in this discussion, diagnostic needle aspiration of a malignant lymph node can be safely performed.[5]

Biopsy Site

A general knowledge of the areas drained by lymph nodes[2,4] is relevant to selecting a biopsy site (Table 36-1). The popliteal and the prescapular lymph nodes are the preferred biopsy tissues in generalized lymphadenopathy. Removal of a peripheral lymph node may result in localized, transient lymphedema. This complication may be accentuated when a lymph node, such as an inguinal node, is removed from a dependent area. The size of the lymph node is also a consideration in the selection of a biopsy site. A large lymph node may yield misleading information because it frequently contains necrotic or hemorrhagic tissue (Fig. 36-2). A slightly enlarged lymph node is preferred, and a sample from more than one location is desirable.

Surgical Techniques

Two techniques for sampling the lymph node are discussed: aspiration and excisional biopsy. These techniques fulfill the diagnostic needs of the clinician.

ASPIRATION BIOPSY

A 20-, 22-, or 25-gauge, 1- to 1.5-inch disposable needle is used for aspiration of the lymph node. The final choice of needle size is based on personal preference. The needle is firmly fixed to a 6- or 12-ml plastic syringe. Anesthesia is seldom required unless the patient is uncooperative. Discomfort to the patient is limited to skin penetration.

The skin over the lymph node is prepared as for a surgical procedure. The lymph node is firmly immobilized, usually between the veterinarian's thumb and forefinger. The needle is directed into the parenchyma

Table 36-1. *Selected Peripheral Lymph Nodes of the Dog and Their Drainage Sites*

Lymph Node	Location and Drainage
Buccal facial	Located rostroventral to the eye in a small percentage of dogs; drains buccal, dorsal nasal, narial, lateral nasal, and superior labial regions
Mandibular	Bilateral group of 2 or 3 nodes ventral to the angle of the jaw; drain eyelids and their glands, dorsal skin of the cranium, temporomandibular joint, and most other parts of the head
Superficial cervical	Bilateral group of 2 or 3 nodes located in front of the supraspinatus muscle; drain caudal part of head (pharyngeal and part of the pinna included), most of the thoracic limb, and the cranial part of the thoracic wall
Axillary	One or 2 nodes located caudal and medial to the shoulder joint; drains most of the thoracic wall, deep structures of the thoracic limb and neck, and the thoracic and cranial abdominal mammary glands
Popliteal	Oval node located at the divergence of the medial border of the biceps femoris muscle and the lateral border of the semitendinosus muscle; drains all parts distal to the node
Superficial inguinal	Two nodes located in the furrow between the abdominal wall and the medial surface of the thigh; drain caudal abdominal and inguinal mammary glands, ventral half of the abdominal wall, penis, prepucial and scrotal skin, ventral part of pelvis, tail, medial side of the thigh, stifle joint, and crus

(Data from Evans, H. E., and Christensen, G. C.: Miller's Anatomy of the Dog. 2nd Ed. Philadelphia, W. B. Saunders, 1979; and Shelton, M. E., and Forsythe, W. B.: Buccal lymph node in the dog. Am. J. Vet. Res., *40*:1638, 1979.)

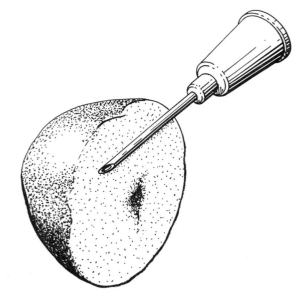

Fig. 36-2. *Diagram of a sectioned lymph node demonstrating the appropriate aspiration technique. The shaded area near the center of the lymph node represents a necrotic or hemorrhagic focus.*

held at right angles and sliding them in opposite directions. The smears should be thin and should appear slightly opaque to allow for proper staining and interpretation. Smears should be dried rapidly with a hair dryer.

EXCISIONAL BIOPSY

Superficial lymph nodes, especially the popliteal, can be removed using local anesthesia. General anesthesia is used when the patient's disposition is unstable and when removing deep lymph nodes, usually in association with a major operation. The skin over the superficial lymph node is prepared for an aseptic procedure, and local anesthesia is infiltrated into the skin.

The lymph node is firmly but gently immobilized with the thumb and forefinger. A skin incision is made over the lymph node, and the node is gently manipulated with the fingers. Efferent (hilar) vessels are ligated when readily apparent. Frequently, the superficial lymph node can simply be "shelled" out with digital manipulation and blunt dissection. One must take care not to place too much digital pressure on the node because the cells can be distorted and may thus appear pathologic on microscopic examination. Tissue dead space is obliterated during closure.

The lymph node is handled aseptically if it is to be cultured. The lymph node is sectioned, and one section is placed in a 10% buffered formalin solution and is submitted for histopathologic study. The remaining section is used to make impression smears: The cut surface of the lymph node is blotted on a paper towel and is gently touched to a glass microscope slide so that a slightly opaque imprint remains. Several slides are submitted for cytologic evaluation as an adjunct to histopathologic study.

of the lymph node. Negative pressure is then applied by pulling on the plunger (about 3 or 4 ml marks). With this negative pressure maintained, two or three back-and-forth movements of the needle in the lymph node should yield an adequate sample. Care should be taken always to keep the tip of the needle within lymph node tissue while suction is being applied to avoid blood and tissue contamination (especially perinodal fat). During the procedure, one feels a firm, cutting sensation, and the needle meets mild resistance. The plunger is gently returned to the starting position *before* the needle is removed from the lymph node.

The lymph node aspirate normally appears creamy white and watery to viscous. Smears are made by gently expelling the sample onto a glass slide. A watery sample can be spread by the technique used to make blood smears on glass microscope slides. If small chunks of aspirate are present, squash preps can be made by pressing the sample between two glass slides

Comment

Lymph node aspiration is a simple, often rewarding, antecedent diagnostic procedure to excisional biopsy. Information gained from smears of lymphoid tissue, however, may be compromised by one or more of the following:

1. A smear that is too thick. A technique that alternates areas of thin and thick is useful. A small amount of lymph node aspirate is placed on a glass slide and is drawn across the slide with the end of a second glass slide at a 45° angle using a side-to-side movement. The squash prep technique also yields consistently reliable results.

2. Slow drying of smears. The use of a hair dryer accelerates drying.

3. Rupture of the cellular elements due to unrefined smear-making technique. The problem is accentuated in lymphosarcoma; smears made from an aspirate of neoplastic tissue frequently contain ruptured lymphoid elements, presumably bcause of increased cell fragility.

4. Inadequate amount of lymphoid tissue. This problem may result when a plug of skin or other nonlymphoid tissue obstructs the needle lumen. Perinodal fat is often confused for lymph node tissue during aspiration and contaminates the sample. Smears appear greasy, and "glistening bubbles" are prominent. A rapid stain reveals the absence of lymphoid material. Contamination with blood also compromises cytologic interpretation.

5. Aspiration of a salivary gland instead of the lymph node. Glandular cell types obtained from a salivary gland aspirate mistaken for a lymph node might suggest metastatic disease. Because mandibular lymph nodes are frequently exposed to antigens in the naso-oropharyngeal area, mandibular lymphadenopathy is common. Interpretation of aspiration samples from this area must be done cautiously and is best performed by an experienced cytologist. When in doubt, one should repeat the aspiration or supplement it with an excisional biopsy.

A lymph node aspiration or impression smear should be evaluated with a rapid stain, such as new methylene blue, prior to submission to a commercial laboratory. This technique ensures that an adequate specimen has been obtained for diagnostic purposes and optimizes the cost benefit for the client.

The cytologic evaluation of lymph node tissue and the classification of lymph node disorders is excellently reviewed elsewhere.[1,3]

References and Suggested Readings

1. Duncan, J. R., and Prasse, K. W.: Veterinary Laboratory Medicine: Clinical Pathology. Ames, Iowa State University Press, 1977.
2. Evans, H. E., and Christensen, G. C.: Miller's Anatomy of the Dog. 2nd Ed. Philadelphia, W. B. Saunders, 1979.
3. Perman, V., Alsaker, R. D., and Riis, R. C.: Cytology of the dog and cat. J. Am. Anim. Hosp. Assoc. [Suppl.], 1, 1979.
4. Shelton, M. E., and Forsythe, W. B.: Buccal lymph node in the dog. Am. J. Vet. Res., 40:1638, 1979.
5. Soderstrom, N.: Fine-Needle Aspiration Biopsy. New York, Grune and Stratton, 1966.

Surgical Techniques of the Spleen

by SHARON STEVENSON

Anatomy and Physiology

The spleen is situated in the left hypogastric region, approximately parallel to the greater curvature of the stomach. The location of the organ is dependent on the size and position of other abdominal organs, particularly the stomach, to which it is loosely attached by the gastrosplenic ligament. The size and weight of the spleen are influenced by its blood content.

The splenic artery, which arises from the celiac axis, divides into dorsal and ventral branches several centimeters from the spleen. Prior to the bifurcation of the left gastroepiploic artery, the ventral branch supplies several small segmental arteries to the left limb of the pancreas. The dorsal branch terminates in the short gastric arteries after sending several end arteries to the dorsal extremity of the spleen (Fig. 36-3). Venous drainage is through the splenic vein to the gastrosplenic vein, which drains into the portal vein.

The spleen's functions are: (1) blood storage, (2) elimination of abnormal blood cells and particulate matter, (3) iron storage, and (4) immunologic functions including the elaboration of specific antibodies and opsonins. It has been shown that in the asplenic state, a normal immunologic response exists to bacteria injected subcutaneously, but not intravenously.[16] Activation and efficiency of the macrophage system are complicated and may be seriously affected in the asplenic patient. Thus, the veterinarian should try to maintain the patient's splenic function. In contrast to previous practices, the trend is away from total splenectomy whenever possible.

Indications for Surgical Treatment

The most common indication for splenectomy in small animals is neoplasia. Usually, splenectomy is performed to remove a primary splenic tumor. In the dog, hemangioma and hemangiosarcoma accounted for 50% of the splenectomies performed in 2 institutions in a recent retrospective study.[6] The study excluded splenectomies for splenic trauma, torsion of the splenic pedicle, or gastric volvulus. Other primary splenic tumors are fibrosarcoma, lymphosarcoma, plasma cell sarcoma, mast cell sarcoma, and reticular cell sarcoma. Metastasis of tumors from distant sites to the spleen is not common.[8]

Normal conditions that may be mistaken for neoplasia include splenosis, the presence of siderotic plaques (Gamna-Gandy bodies), and nodular hyperplasia. Splenosis may be either congenital or traumatic and is defined as the presence of multiple nodules of normal splenic tissue in the peritoneal cavity. These nodules are most commonly found on the greater omentum and the gastrosplenic ligament. Siderotic plaques, which are brownish encrustations on the splenic capsule composed of iron and calcium deposits, are common in older animals. Nodular hyperplasia is the occurrence of

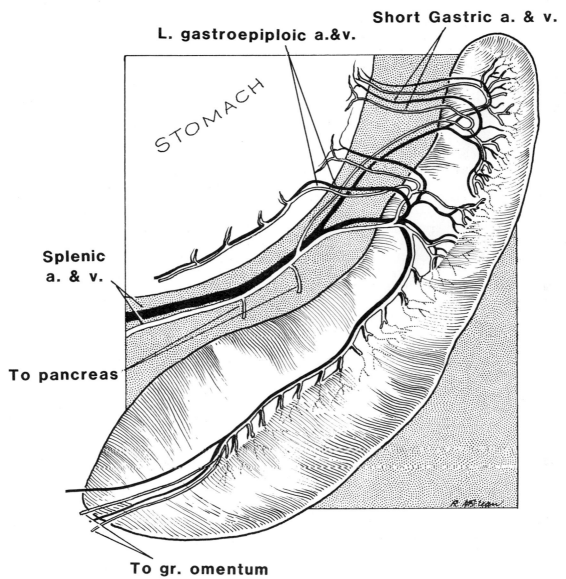

Fig. 36-3. *Blood supply to the spleen. Note the small branches to the left limb of the pancreas and the origin of the left gastroepiploic artery and vein, as well as the arrangement of small, segmental end arteries to the splenic pulp.*

discrete parenchymal foci of hyperplastic splenic tissue. The foci are symmetrical nodules, 2 cm or less in diameter, that are raised from the capsular surface. These nodules are not malignant changes.

Systemic mastocytosis is the most common indication for splenectomy in the cat, and remissions of over a year have been reported following splenectomy for this disorder.[10] Non-neoplastic conditions for which total splenectomy is indicated are torsion of the splenic pedicle, splenic rupture, and severe splenic trauma. Large subcapsular hematomas may also necessitate partial or total splenectomy. Refractory cases of autoimmune hemolytic anemia and idiopathic thrombocytopenia purpura are sometimes treated by splenectomy.

Splenomegaly in itself is not sufficient reason for splenectomy. The differential diagnoses of splenomegaly are sizable and are considered elsewhere.[1] Because

the veterinary surgeon must make a subjective intraoperative decision when confronted with a grossly enlarged spleen, it should be remembered that drugs are the most common cause of splenomegaly in the anesthetized animal. Tranquilizers derived from phenothiazine (acepromazine) and butyrophenone (droperidol), thiobarbiturates (thiamylal and thiopental), and oxybarbiturates (pentobarbital) produce passive congestion of the spleen.

Torsion of the splenic pedicle or congestion of the spleen may occur as a part of the gastric dilatation and volvulus syndrome. If large vessels are thrombosed, the spleen should be removed. It may be difficult, however, to decide whether damage to the spleen as a result of congestion is reversible or not. If the spleen begins to contract after repositioning, it should not be removed. If it remains large and blue to black in color, it is probably safer to remove it.

Partial splenectomy should be considered for abscesses, small hematomas, and localized trauma. Splenorrhaphy is preferred for lacerations that do not penetrate deeply into the hilus.

Preoperative Considerations

The chief concerns in the preoperative period are adequate hydration, acid-base balance, evaluation of the hemostatic mechanism, and total erythroid mass. A routine evaluation consisting of a hemogram, serum electrolyte and enzme determinations, a platelet count, and clotting time is recommended. A significant volume of blood may be lost during surgical removal of an enlarged spleen. Blood loss should be replaced with a balanced electrolyte solution or with blood. If the preoperative evaluation of total erythroid mass indicates anemia, then transfusions should be considered.

Intrasplenic injection of epinephrine has been recommended to stimulate splenic contraction and autotransfusion prior to removal of the spleen.[1] This practice is not recommended because it may release endotoxins or cardiac-depressant factors into the circulation from the congested spleen.[7,9] Thrombocytosis occurs following splenectomy and persists for approximately 16 weeks.[2] Thrombosis or disseminated intravascular coagulation occasionally occurs after splenectomy. Maintaining a normal acid-base balance and avoiding hypotension by the administration of preoperative fluids helps to prevent disseminated intravascular coagulation.

Surgical Techniques

SPLENORRHAPHY

Splenorrhaphy is defined as the suturing of the splenic capsule and is the technique of choice for lacerations. Deep hilar lacerations that cause uncontrollable hemorrhage necessitate partial or total splenectomy.

Celiotomy is performed through a ventral midline incision. Moderate hemorrhage can be controlled by ligation of individual end arteries within the splenic pulp. The application of a microfibrillar collagenous hemostatic agent* and the approximation of the splenic capsule with simple interrupted sutures of absorbable material on an atraumatic needle also control the majority of splenic bleeding (Fig. 36-4). Any combination of these methods can also be used. Deep lacerations or severe trauma may necessitate ligation of the local branch of the splenic artery.

Although the splenic artery branches are variable, bifurcation almost always occurs outside the spleen itself. This characteristic allows for easy control of the blood supply to a particular segment and for temporary control of the main artery. The end branches of the splenic artery are arranged along the longitudinal axis of the spleen and divide it into small transverse segments (see Fig. 36-3). Therefore, hemostasis may be achieved by reducing the arterial inflow to a given area and by suturing the capsular laceration. If the laceration is large, the main artery can be ligated with nonabsorbable suture, and the laceration may be sutured. A collateral arterial network quickly develops. Isotope scans 3 weeks following ligation of the splenic artery have demonstrated normal splenic perfusion.[10,11]

PARTIAL SPLENECTOMY

Partial splenectomy is the preferred technique for localized severe trauma to the spleen, for biopsy, or for a localized non-neoplastic lesion such as an abscess or a hematoma (Fig. 36-5A). The blood vessels to the portion of the spleen selected for resection are clamped, are cut, and are ligated as close to the spleen as possible (Fig. 36-5B). Arterial ligation results in ischemia of a discrete portion of the spleen. Pressure is applied

*Avitene, Avicon, Inc., Fort Worth, TX 76134

Editor's note: This product is extremely expensive, but has the advantage of leaving little debris. Other available products such as Surgicel (Johnson & Johnson) and Gelfoam (Upjohn) are not as completely or as quickly absorbed by the body.

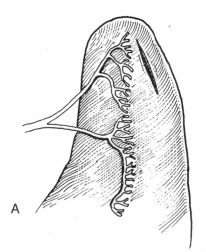 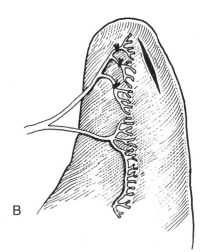 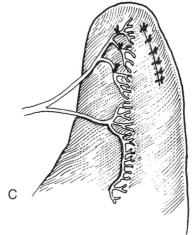

Fig. 36-4. *Splenorrhaphy is the technique of choice for splenic lacerations (A). B, Hemorrhage may be controlled by ligation of end arteries.*
C, *The lacerated splenic capsule is approximated with simple interrupted sutures of absorbable material on an atraumatic needle.*

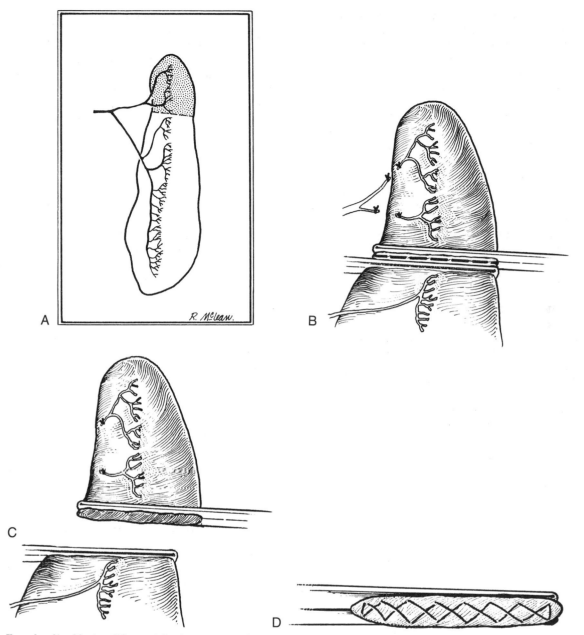

Fig. 36-5. *For a localized lesion (A), partial splenectomy is the preferred technique. B, The blood vessels to the portion of the spleen selected for resection are clamped, cut, and ligated. The margin of the newly created ischemic portion of the spleen is manually flattened, and forceps are then placed across the thinned spleen. C, The spleen is divided between the clamps. D, The cut edges of the splenic capsule are apposed using 3-0 absorbable suture material with a swaged-on tapered needle. A continuous cruciate pattern is illustrated.*

with the veterinarian's thumb and forefinger at the margin of the ischemic portion of the splenic pulp in order to create a flattened area devoid of pulp. The spleen is then divided between 2 clamps (Fig. 36-5C). The proximal clamp is removed, and the cut edges of the spleen are closed by suturing the edges of the splenic capsule together with 3-0 absorbable suture material with a swaged-on tapered needle (Fig. 36-5D). A continuous cruciate or continuous horizontal mattress suture pattern placed 2 to 3 mm from the edge can be used. The edges should then be oversewn with a simple continuous suture pattern. Digital pressure can be used for 5 minutes if further hemostasis is necessary. Omen-

tum can be incorporated in the sutures to cover the raw edges if desired. Hemorrhage must be controlled prior to closure.

SPLENECTOMY

Splenectomy is performed using a ventral midline approach large enough for easy visualization and handling of the organ. The enlarged or neoplastic spleen should be handled with great care because it is easily ruptured. The hilar vessels should be ligated as close to the spleen as possible, to avoid the small segmental arteries to the left lobe of the pancreas as well as to retain the left gastroepiploic artery. Because the collateral circulation of the stomach is adequate, the left gastroepiploic artery may be ligated if necessary, but it is preferable to save this vessel. Forceps or metal clips may be used on the splenic side of the vessels because they will be removed with the spleen, but individual nonabsorbable ligatures should be placed on the remaining vessels, the gastrosplenic ligament, and omentum. Care should be taken when clamping and ligating the short gastric vessels not to include stomach wall, because this maneuver predisposes the patient to avascular necrosis and fistulation. As much of the greater omentum as possible should be saved, and a thorough examination of abdominal viscera should be performed. This examination is easier when the spleen has been removed. When splenic neoplasia is present, the liver and splenic lymph nodes should be inspected for metastases, and a biopsy should be performed. Following removal of the organ, the splenic bed should be lavaged with warm saline solution and should be inspected for hemorrhage. Because of an increased incidence of infection, drains are not recommended unless the pancreas or its blood supply has been damaged.[3]

Splenectomy for torsion of the splenic pedicle requires special surgical techniques.[15] The spleen should be left twisted, and the vascular pedicle should be mass-ligated at the level of the torsion; the spleen is then removed intact, in order to reduce the possibility of sepsis and to prevent the release of endotoxins or cardiac-depressant factors into the circulation.[7,9] The pedicle is then untwisted, and individual components are religated separately to ensure control of hemorrhage. Nonabsorbable suture material should be used for ligations, and the left limb of the pancreas should be examined for avascular necrosis and for iatrogenic trauma.

Postoperative Care and Complications

The most frequent immediate postoperative problem is hemorrhage, which is generally a result of inadequate ligation of vessels and may be complicated by disseminated intravascular coagulation. Serial hematocrit and total protein determinations should be made postoperatively. If the hematocrit and total protein determinations steadily drop, if the patient's abdominal girth enlarges, or if abdominocentesis or lavage indicates hemorrhage, the abdomen should be surgically re-explored. The splenic bed should be lavaged with saline solution, and blood clots should be removed. If no splenic vessel is found to be bleeding, the splenic bed should be packed with gauze sponges for approximately 10 minutes. This maneuver is generally sufficient to control the bleeding. Other, less-frequent operative complications may be seen later, including abscessation, gastric fistulation, and traumatic pancreatitis. The onset of pancreatitis may occur 5 to 7 days postoperatively.

Overwhelming postoperative infection is a known complication of splenectomy in humans. Although such infection has not been reported in the veterinary literature, it should be considered in cases of acute postoperative collapse. An increased incidence of hemobartonellosis and babesiasis has been reported in dogs that have undergone splenectomy. Thrombocytosis after removal of the spleen is usually asymptomatic.

Other physiologic sequelae of splenectomy are mild anemia, slight reduction in blood volume, and increased reticulocyte count.[17] As a result of these changes (as well as the absence of the splenic reservoir), animals that have undergone splenectomy are unable to respond efficiently to increased demands for oxygen. Thus, such dogs fatigue more easily with exercise than intact dogs and are less able to respond to hypoxia under anesthesia.[5]

References and Suggested Readings

1. Brody, R. S.: The spleen. *In* Canine Surgery. 2nd Ed. Edited by J. Archibald. Santa Barbara, CA, American Veterinary Publications, 1974.
2. Butler, M. J., et al.: The coagulation and fibrinolytic response to splenectomy. Surg. Gynecol. Obstet., *142*:731, 1976.
3. Cerise, E. J., Pierce, W. A., and Diamond, D. L.: Abdominal drains: their role as a source of infection following splenectomy. Ann. Surg., *17*:764, 1970.
4. Cooney, D. R., et al.: Relative merits of partial splenectomy, splenic reimplantation, and immunization in preventing postsplenectomy infection. Surgery, *86*:561, 1979.
5. Ffoulkes-Crabbe, D. J. O., et al.: The effect of splenectomy on the circulatory adjustments to hypoxaemia in the anaesthetized dog. Br. J. Anaesth., *48*:639, 1976.
6. Frey, A. J., and Betts, C. W.: A retrospective study of splenectomy in the dog. J. Am. Anim. Hosp. Assoc., *13*:730, 1977.
7. Glode, L. M., Mergenhagen, S. E., and Rosenstreich, D. L.: Significant contribution of spleen cells in mediating the lethal effects of endotoxin in vivo. Infect. Immun., *14*:626, 1976.
8. Jubb, K. V. F., and Kennedy, P. C.: Pathology of Domestic Animals. New York, Academic Press, 1970.
9. Lefer, A. M.: Blood-borne humoral factors in the pathophysiology of circulatory shock. Circ. Res., *32*:129, 1973.
10. Liska, W. D., MacEwen, E. G., Zaki, F. A., and Garvey, M.: Feline systemic mastocytosis: a review and results of splenectomy in seven cases. J. Am. Anim. Hosp. Assoc., *15*:589, 1979.
11. Keramidas, D. C.: The ligation of the splenic artery in the treatment of traumatic rupture of the spleen. Surgery, *85*:530, 1979.
12. Mishalany, H., and Nassar, V.: Results of suturing of experimental blunt trauma to canine spleens. Leb. Med. J., *27*:329, 1974.
13. Osborne, C. A., Perman, V., and Stevens, J. B.: Needle biopsy of the spleen. Vet. Clin. North Am., *4*:311, 1974.
14. Sherman, N. J., and Asch, M. J.: Traumatic splenic injury: splenectomy vs. repair. Am. Surg., *45*:631, 1979.
15. Stevenson, S., Chew, D. J., and Kociba, G. J.: Torsion of the splenic pedicle in the dog: a review. J. Am. Anim. Hosp. Assoc., *17*:239, 1981.
16. Sullivan, J. L., et al.: Immune response after splenectomy. Lancet, *1*:178, 1978.
17. Waldman, T. A., Weissman, S. M., and Berlin, N.: The effect of splenectomy on erythropoiesis in the dog. Blood, *15*:873, 1960.

37 * Bone Marrow

Technique of Bone Marrow Biopsy

by DENNIS J. MEYER

Bone marrow biopsy is a simple procedure that is used as a diagnostic adjunct to the hemogram when a peripheral blood disorder is identified and in certain neoplastic conditions. Nonregenerative anemia, thrombocytopenia, leukocyte dyscrasia, hyperglobulinemias, radiographic bone lesions (as with plasma cell tumors), occult neoplasia, and fever of unknown origin are some of the clinical conditions in which a bone marrow biopsy may be indicated.

Contraindications to bone marrow biopsy are few. The most common are coagulation disorders and thrombocytopenia. Disseminated intravascular coagulopathy, as evidenced by thrombocytopenia, is frequently associated with disseminated neoplasia in human patients.[1] The frequency of coagulation disorders has not been completely evaluated in the dog and cat, but coagulopathies are probably associated with neoplasia in many patients.[6] Although skin bruising may be noted following the biopsy procedure, digital pressure controls incisional hemorrhage.

The three techniques discussed are aspiration, punch, and incisional bone marrow biopsy.

Bone marrow sampling is most commonly accomplished with the use of a Rosenthal* needle for aspiration biopsy (Fig. 37-1). The 2 sizes, which are 16 gauge by 1⁵⁄₁₆ inch and 18 gauge by 1 inch, suffice for dogs and cats. The shorter needle is easier to manipulate during the biopsy procedure; the longer needle can be used for large or obese patients.

Bone marrow core biopsy specimens can be obtained with the Jamshidi biopsy needle† (Fig. 37-2). An optional adapter for the handle is available and is recommended to facilitate the biopsy procedure. Two needles of each type should be available for use because they are easily bent or dulled in hard tissues. Careful technique results in prolonged use of the biopsy instruments.

Biopsy Sites

Common sites for bone marrow biopsy in dogs and cats are the wing of the ilium and the proximal femur. Ribs and sternebrae are also active bone marrow sites and are often used in horses and cows; however, these sites should be avoided in dogs and cats because of the potential for slipping past the bone and penetrating thoracic viscera. The wing of the ilium is the preferred

*Becton Dickinson and Co., Rutherford, NJ
†Kor Med Corp., 2950 Metro Drive, Minneapolis, MN 55420

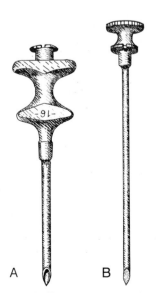

Fig. 37-1. *A drawing of a Rosenthal needle (A) and its stylet (B).*

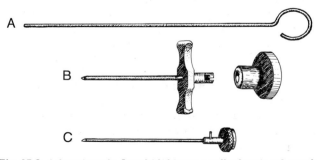

Fig. 37-2. *A drawing of a Jamshidi biopsy needle showing the probe (A), the needle and the round handle that fits the hub of the needle (B), and the stylet (C).*

491

site for bone marrow biopsy. In cats and in small dogs (under 7 kg), the femur may be technically easier.

Surgical Techniques

It is common to perform an aspiration biopsy in docile animals without local anesthesia. Infiltration with a local anesthetic agent causes discomfort and may upset the animal for the ensuing biopsy procedure. Generally, the most painful part of the bone marrow biopsy coincides with the aspiration of the bone marrow sample. Ketamine or other chemorestraint may be required in uncooperative cats.

The biopsy site is clipped and is surgically prepared; local anesthesia, if used, is infiltrated to the level of the periosteum. A small nick is made in the skin with a No. 11 scalpel blade. The animal is placed in lateral recumbency for both biopsy sites. Sternal recumbency can also be used for biopsy of the iliac crest in larger dogs.

ASPIRATION BIOPSY

ILIAC CREST. The biopsy needle is placed parallel to the long axis of the wing of the ilium (Fig. 37-3). The stylet should be locked in place. The needle is gripped firmly, so that the veterinarian's thumb and forefinger are on the hub of the needle and the flat head of the stylet is in contact with the medial aspect of the middle

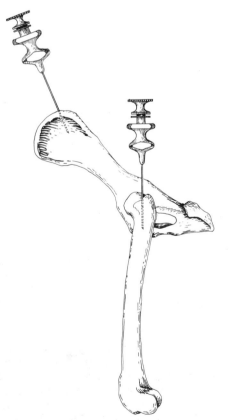

Fig. 37-3. *A diagram of the ilium and femur illustrating the sites for bone marrow biopsy. The angle of the needle is variable for the ilial site. The needle may approach a more vertical position in larger bones, in which case the needle is started more caudally on the wing of the ilium.*

finger. The needle is twisted through the cortex into the marrow cavity with short, clockwise-to-counterclockwise movements until firmly seated. In older animals, considerable effort may be required, owing to sclerosis of the bone. One should concentrate on the direction of the needle during the procedure. The vigorous effort necessary to seat the needle may move the hub of the needle right or left and may cause the marrow cavity to be missed. Once the needle is firmly seated, the stylet is removed, and a 12- to 20-ml syringe is securely attached to the needle.

Negative pressure is created by quickly moving the syringe plunger several times. When the first hint of red marrow appears in the tip of the syringe, the negative pressure is gently released, and the needle and syringe are quickly removed with movements similar to those used in seating the needle. Continued aspiration after the appearance of the bone marrow specimen results in an undesirable dilution by blood from the damaged sinusoids. As previously mentioned, pain, occasionally marked, is expressed by the patient at the time of aspiration. The response suggests that the needle is in the bone marrow.

When bone marrow does not appear in the syringe, two possibilities exist: (1) a problem exists with the technique; or (2) a primary bone marrow disturbance—hypoplasia or aplasia of the bone marrow cells or myelophthisis—is present. To evaluate the first possibility, the stylet is securely replaced, and the needle is advanced 1 or 2 mm. The stylet is then removed, and negative pressure is reapplied. If no marrow appears, the needle, with the syringe attached, is *slowly* removed by gradual clockwise-to-counterclockwise movements while continuous suction is maintained until marrow appears. If bone marrow still does not appear in the hub of the syringe, the syringe and needle are removed; one should release the plunger prior to removal from the patient. An attempt should be made to expel any bone marrow material gently from the lumen of the needle. Failure to obtain a sample is an indication to: (1) attempt at another biopsy site; or (2) perform a punch or incisional biopsy.

FEMUR. The dog or cat is placed in lateral recumbency. Local anesthesia is generally recommended for bone marrow aspiration biopsy of the femur except for the most docile animal. The tissue immediately medial to the greater trochanter, including periosteum of the trochanteric fossa, should be infiltrated with the local anesthetic agent, and a nick should be made in the skin.

For the right-handed person, the left stifle is firmly gripped with the left hand to immobilize the joint in a slightly flexed position. The thumb is placed along the lateral long axis of the femur. Control of the leg is attained, and the relative location of the shaft of the femur is identified with the left thumb. The greater trochanter is again identified with the right hand. The bone marrow needle (Fig. 37-3), held as previously described, is firmly directed along the medial aspect of the greater trochanter until contact is made with the trochanteric fossa. The procedure for obtaining a bone marrow specimen is similar to that previously described. The tip of the needle tends to "slip" out of the trochanteric fossa when the procedure is initiated. Counterpressure to the driving force of the needle is maintained with the palm of the veterinarian's left hand against the stifle. The long axis of the needle is maintained parallel to the long axis of the femur, as defined by the position of the left thumb. Once the needle is firmly seated in bone, an attempt is made to aspirate bone marrow. In larger dogs, the technique is modified by gripping the femur higher up and by placing the thumb along the femur's lateral long axis.

PUNCH BIOPSY

The punch biopsy is used to obtain a core of bone marrow for histopathologic examination: (1) when a sample is not obtained by aspiration biopsy; (2) to evaluate bone marrow cellularity as a supplement to aspiration biopsy; and (3) to evaluate for primary or secondary neoplasia, usually as an adjunct to aspiration biopsy. The femur and the crest of the ilium are the preferred sites for punch biopsy of the bone marrow.

The biopsy site is prepared as previously described. The Jamshidi needle, with its stylet securely in place, is firmly seated in cortical bone. The stylet is removed, and the needle is slowly but purposefully advanced 1 to 2 cm with the same clockwise-to-counterclockwise movements used to seat the needle. The needle is then *rotated* along its long axis, with the needle's tip as the pivot, and is removed from the body. The bone marrow core that is "broken" off by the rotational motion is held in the needle by its tapered construction, because the lumen of the needle narrows toward the tip. The needle is removed from the bone by using clockwise-counterclockwise twists. The sample is *gently* removed with the probe provided with the needle. The probe is inserted at the *distal* end (tip) of the needle, and the sample is expelled out the handle of the needle. An aspiration biopsy is then taken with a clean needle from another site to supplement the histopathologic evaluation.

INCISIONAL BIOPSY

On rare occasion, bone marrow for cytologic and histologic evaluation must be obtained by incisional biopsy using the wing of the ilium. A standard surgical approach to the crest of the ilium is used. An osteotome or a rongeur is used to expose the bone marrow. An 18-gauge needle attached to a syringe is used to aspirate bone marrow material from the exposed cavity, and smears are quickly made. A sample should also be submitted for histopathologic examination. The Jamshidi needle can be used for this purpose. It is imperative for the bone marrow sample to be free of crush artifact. Careful surgical manipulation is required.

Postoperative Care

Postoperative concerns are minimal following bone marrow biopsy. Potential complications are mainly related to iatrogenic damage of anatomic structures adjacent to the biopsy site. Such injury is usually due to inexperience of the veterinarian. Possible problems include damage to the sciatic nerve (femur), laceration of the intercostal artery (rib), and penetration of the thorax (rib and sternebrae).

Handling the Sample

The accuracy of information from a bone marrow biopsy is dependent on: (1) obtaining an adequate sample; (2) proper postoperative management of the sample; and (3) interpretation by an experienced clinical pathologist. Because the first two conditions depend on the individual who obtains the biopsy, the procedure should be performed by the clinical pathologist whenever possible. In private practice, in which this ideal is frequently impractical, the submission of an adequate biopsy sample is often the limiting step to a successful bone marrow biopsy.

It is paramount that the preparation for handling the bone marrow biopsy be completed *before* the actual biopsy is performed. The materials include glass microscope slides and a hair dryer. Clean glass microscope slides are laid out on a flat, clean surface. One or two drops of bone marrow are *quickly* placed on one slide, which is then angled so that the specimen slowly flows down the glass. Bone marrow appears granular or "sandy" because of the bone marrow "spicules." Several of these particles are transferred to another glass slide by pushing them off with a disposable needle. A squash prep (gently compressing the spicules between two glass slides at right angles and pulling them in opposite directions) results in an excellent smear.

A satisfactory smear generally has small dense spots (spicules) surrounded by thinner smeared material. The smears are quickly dried with a hair dryer. Because the bone marrow sample usually clots rapidly, in 15 to 30 seconds, a rapid, coordinated slide-making effort is necessary. If the sample clots prior to completing the smears, a portion of the clot can be smeared with the squash prep technique; however, sample quality is variable.

The remaining clotted bone marrow can be placed in a 10% buffered formalin solution and may be submitted along with the smears. Bouin's fixative maintains more accurate bone marrow cell morphologic features for histologic examination and is preferred to formalin fixation. A bone marrow punch biopsy sample is placed in a 10% buffered formalin solution or, preferably, in Bouin's fixative. Slides for cytologic evaluation can be made by *gently* rolling the core of bone marrow between two glass slides before placing it in the fixative, if an aspiration biopsy has been unsuccessful.

A representative smear should be rapidly stained to confirm the presence of bone marrow elements. New methylene blue stain is ideal, but other quick stains are also adequate. Wright's stain or Wright-Giemsa stain is recommended to stain the smears for cytologic detail and is best accomplished by the laboratory responsible for their interpretation. When samples are submitted to commercial laboratories, the laboratory should be consulted *prior* to the procedure, and an inquiry should be made into the specifics of sample management.

References and Suggested Readings

1. Bick, R. L.: Disseminated intravascular coagulation and related syndromes: etiology, pathophysiology, diagnosis, and management. Am. J. Hematol., 5:265, 1978.
2. Brynes, R. K., McKenna, R. W., and Sundberg, D.: Bone marrow aspiration and trephine biopsy. An approach to a thorough study. Am. J. Clin. Pathol., 70:753, 1979.
3. Collings, J. L.: Experience with Jamshidi needle biopsy of marrow in a community hospital. J. SC Med. Assoc., 74:284, 1978.
4. Fong, T. P., et al.: An evaluation of cellularity in various types of bone marrow specimens. Am. J. Clin. Pathol., 72:812, 1979.
5. Ieland, J., and MacPherson, B.: Hematologic findings in cases of mammary cancer metastatic to bone marrow. Am. J. Clin. Pathol., 71:31, 1979.
6. Madewell, B. R., Feldman, B. F., and O'Neill, S.: Coagulation abnormalities in dogs with neoplastic diseases. Thromb. Haemost., 44:35, 1980.
7. *Perman, V., Alsaker, R. D., and Riis, R. C.: Cytology of the dog and cat. J. Am. Anim. Hosp. Assoc. [Suppl.], 1, 1979.
8. Singh, G., Krause, J. R., and Breitfeld, V.: Bone marrow examination for metastatic tumor—aspirate and biopsy. Cancer, 40:2317, 1977.
9. Valli, V. E., McSherry, B. J., and Hulland, T. J.: A review of bone marrow handling techniques and description of a new method. Can. J. Comp. Med., 33:68, 1969.

*Recommended veterinary reference

38 * Muscles and Tendons

Surgery of Muscles and Tendons

by JAMES L. MILTON

and RALPH A. HENDERSON

Muscle and tendon injuries in the dog and cat are frequently caused by trauma, but are often masked by concurrent injuries, such as fractures and dislocations. Additionally, muscle injuries accompany all types of hernias and are created and repaired in almost every surgical procedure.

Muscle-tendon injuries of the limbs that cause significant disability and require surgical treatment are infrequently observed. Consequently, the anatomic, histologic, and physiologic features of the muscle-tendon unit and the clinical signs and methods of treatment for individual muscle injuries have not been emphasized in veterinary orthopedics.

For the purposes of discussion, muscle-tendon injuries are divided into four categories, based on anatomic location: (1) muscle belly, (2) musculotendinous junction, (3) tendon, and (4) tendinosseous junction (Fig. 38-1). The general techniques and principles of muscle and tendon surgery are presented, but emphasis is placed on the treatment of specific problems.

Muscle Belly

ANATOMY

Skeletal (striated) muscles are formed by bundles or fasciculi of individual muscle fibers (cells, sarcomeres) that are surrounded by connective tissue (Fig. 38-2). The connective tissue binds and integrates the action of the individual fibers and fasciculi, but simultaneously allows freedom of motion among individual muscle components and muscles. Blood vessels and nerves pass in these connective tissue septa to the fasciculi and fibers.[15] Muscle fibers have been divided into types based on their anatomic appearance, physiologic behavior, biochemical properties, and histochemical features.[7] The populations and ratio of these fiber types are altered by physical activity and various endocrine, neurologic, vascular, and muscle diseases. Each fiber contains many myofibrils that are responsible for contraction of the fiber and, ultimately, the muscle.

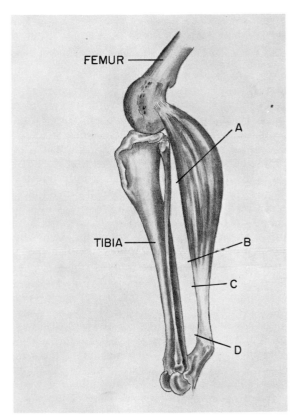

Fig. 38-1. *Classification of injuries based on anatomic location. Muscle belly (A), musculotendinous junction (B), tendon (C), and tendinosseous junction (D).*

REPAIR

Muscle tissue possesses an intrinsic capability of regeneration, but a limited ability for self-repair. Individual muscle fibers do not undergo cell division and do not contribute to the healing process. A small population of morphologically undifferentiated (satellite) cells that lie adjacent to the muscle fibers may form myoblasts and may contribute to muscle regeneration. The myofibrils of muscle fibers are capable of regeneration if the muscle is anatomically apposed so that scar tissue development is minimal and the muscle fiber is not strangulated by fibrous tissue. The ability of the muscle to regenerate is greater when its continuity is

495

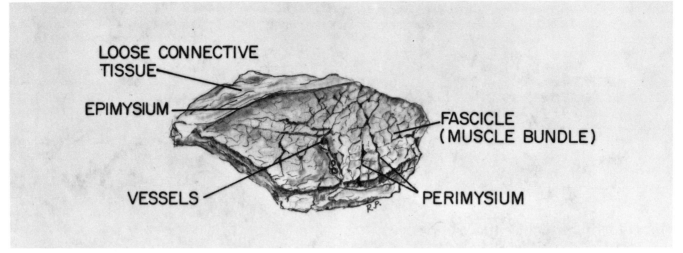

Fig. 38-2. *Muscle anatomy: cross section of a segment of the biceps femoris muscle.*

not completely disrupted, as in bruises or crushing injuries, than when the muscle is completely ruptured.[24]

Repair of transected muscle occurs predominately by invasion of the wound and hematoma with capillaries and fibroblasts from the muscle or surrounding tissue. Fibrous proteins are deposited and result in scar tissue and adhesion formation. Careful apposition of the muscle segments so that fibrous tissue replacement does not occur enhances healing by maximum muscle regeneration, minimum scar tissue, and minimum adhesions. Stress or movement during the early stages of repair may increase the amount of fibrous tissue deposition, scar tissue, and adhesions.[24]

CONTUSIONS

Contusions (bruises) accompany most traumatic injuries and rarely require special treatment. Massive contusions that result in inflammation, edema, and dysfunction should receive treatment. Such treatment includes (1) initial cold water packs for 24 hours followed by warm-water compresses or baths, (2) regional compressive wraps, (3) protective bandaging, and (4) immobilization.[13] Additionally, tension-relieving incisions, the local application of dimethyl sulfoxide (DMSO),[21] and the systemic administration of antibiotics and corticosteroids may be beneficial.

STRAINS

A strain is an overstretching or an overextension of any part of the muscle-tendon unit that results in structural alterations and signs of inflammation, especially discomfort, pain, and lameness.[13] The diagnosis is based on the history, the absence of disease in other structures of the limb, and local signs of inflammation upon palpation or movement of the muscle. Signs may be subtle, and the diagnosis may be difficult to substantiate. Treatment includes immobilization of the limb and enforced rest. The length and degree of treatment vary with the severity of the injury and the animal's

response. Warm-water soaks and the topical application of DMSO may be of value.

Difficulty may be encountered in distinguishing a strain from a rupture. Ruptures are characterized by greater dysfunction, greater disruption of the muscle, and more severe signs of inflammation. Exploration of the muscle is indicated when a rupture is suspected and when the function of the muscle is essential to normal use of the limb.

LACERATIONS

Lacerations of muscle should be surgically closed if a loss of function is evident or seems inevitable because of fibrous healing. The principles of treating open wounds should be followed, including liberal irrigation, adequate debridement, and administration of systemic antibiotics. Muscles with sufficient fibrous tissue sheaths should be closed with permanent suture material, such as nylon, polypropylene, or polyester fiber, placed through the muscle sheath in a horizontal mattress pattern (Fig. 38-3A). Muscles with inadequate fibrous tissue or deep lacerations may have to be reinforced with synthetic materials (button)[5] or fascial grafts to prevent suture pullout (Fig. 38-3B).

Transections of muscle tissue during a surgical procedure should be avoided. Muscle retraction for surgical exposure can be facilitated by adequate isolation and mobilization of the muscle, subperiosteal elevation of the muscle from the bone, and tenotomy or, preferably, osteotomy at its point of insertion. If muscle has to be incised, it should be incised in the direction of the fibers to minimize damage to the functional unit, the sarcomere.

RUPTURE

Rupture of a muscle belly with tearing and separation of its segments is rarely observed in the pet small animal. Ruptures of the gracilis (dropped thigh), triceps (dropped shoulder), and gastrocnemius (dropped

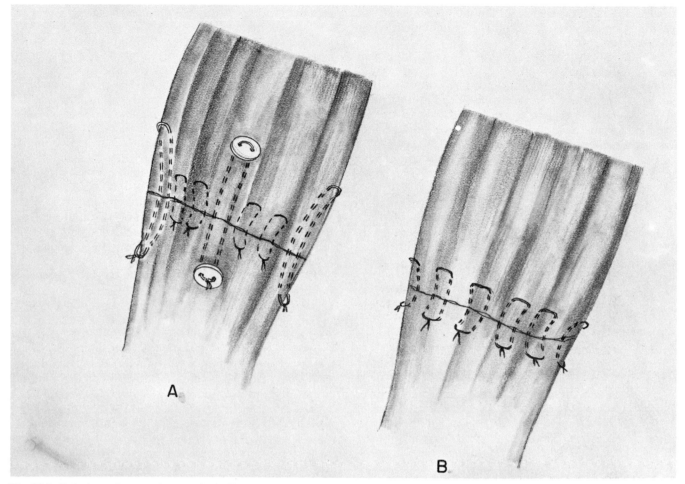

Fig. 38-3. *Techniques for suturing muscle. A, Closure with tension sutures and interrupted horizontal mattress sutures. Various bolsters, in this case a button, can be used for reinforcement. B, Closure with interrupted horizontal mattress sutures.*

hock) muscles have been reported in the racing greyhound.[16,31] Muscle ruptures occur secondary to dislocations, for example, a hip luxation with damage to the deep gluteal, gemelli, and internal obturator muscles, and displacement of fracture segments, for example, a distal femoral fracture with rupture of the quadriceps femoris muscle.

The signs exhibited by the animal vary with the severity of the rupture (strain, partial, complete) and the functional importance of the muscle. Accordingly, affected animals may have signs ranging from extreme dysfunction to a subtle lameness. The diagnosis is difficult to substantiate in the absence of an obvious disorder. The most common signs of muscle rupture are: (1) inflammation and hematoma in the region of the muscle, (2) discontinuity of the muscle belly (dropped muscle), (3) deformity of the limb, and (4) alteration of the gait from loss of muscle function. An obvious separation of the muscle is usually not evident on palpation because portions of the sheath may remain intact.

Partial ruptures, like strains, are best treated conservatively by immobilization and enforced rest, the length and degree of which are dictated by the severity of the injury and the functional importance of the muscle. Complete rupture of the muscle with substantial loss of function should be treated surgically for reasons presented previously. In the racing greyhound, complete ruptures or dropped muscles are treated predominately by conservative methods that often yield unsatisfactory results. Surgical repair of these muscles may improve and provide more predictable results.

A surgical procedure should be performed as soon as possible after diagnosing muscle rupture because delay results in contracture of the muscle segments and strangulation of the muscle fibers with fibrous tissue. Surgical treatment involves reapposition of the muscle segments. Muscle tissue offers limited strength in holding suture material, and suture pullout poses a problem when tension is applied to align the muscle segments. This problem has been combated by using tension sutures anchored to the muscle with bolsters (buttons) and by using a large-diameter (1-0 to 2) permanent suture material such as nylon, polypropylene, or polyester fiber (Fig. 38-3). Following apposition of the muscle segments, the sheath at the anastomotic site is closed circumferentially with horizontal mattress sutures of a nonabsorbable material and a small diameter (3-0 nylon). Postoperatively, immobilization and enforced rest are provided for at least 2 weeks, followed by limited activity for an additional 4 to 6 weeks. A guarded prognosis should be rendered for working dogs that must be returned to competition or performance.

Atrophy, fibrosis, and varying degrees of dysfunction are common sequelae to muscle injuries. In man, surgical resection of scar tissue followed by muscle-to-muscle anastomosis has been advocated to improve function. Freeing the muscle from surrounding adhesions has been used to restore function. Fibrotic and contracted muscles that interfere with the function of a joint or surrounding structures and are not essential to normal function of the limb can be resected or excised.

MUSCLE CONTRACTURE AND FIBROSIS

Injury to muscle fibers, nerves, or blood vessels may produce irreversible degenerative changes in the muscle: alterations of the number and type of fibers, fibrosis, adhesions, atrophy, and contracture. Trauma has been incriminated as the initiating factor in most cases, but the etiopathogenesis is poorly understood. Muscle contracture with significant dysfunction is observed most frequently in the infraspinatus and quadriceps femoris muscles in the dog.

INFRASPINATUS MUSCLE CONTRACTURE. This condition occurs almost exclusively in hunting breeds of dogs and causes a characteristic lameness manifested by limited movement of the shoulder, outward rotation of the brachium, adduction of the elbow, and lateral circumduction of the distal limb with a carpal flip (Fig. 38-4A).[18,31] Atrophy of the shoulder muscles may be observed or palpated. Manipulation of the shoulder reveals a reduction in range of motion during flexion and extension. The history often reveals a previous incidence of trauma with the development of an acute lameness that gradually subsides. Excision of the capsular portion of the infraspinatus tendon relieves the restriction of movement and successfully alleviates the lameness (Fig. 38-4B to D). This tenectomy provides an almost immediate return to normal function. Postoperative care consists of restricting the dog's activity for 10 to 14 days.

QUADRICEPS FEMORIS MUSCLE CONTRACTURE. Contracture of the quadriceps femoris muscle group with hyperextension of the knee (hyperextension syndrome, stiff-stifle syndrome) occurs primarily in the actively growing dog following fracture of the distal femur and prolonged immobilization, whether voluntary or enforced, of the limb in extension (Fig. 38-5A). The initial joint stiffness probably develops secondary to adhesions between the quadriceps femoris muscle and the distal femur. In chronic cases, the pathologic features become more complex as degenerative changes occur in the muscle tissue and articular structures of the knee. Treatment varies with the complexity of the problem, as does the prognosis. Surgical management is directed at restoring movement to the knee by: (1) freeing adhesions between the quadriceps femoris and the distal femur, (2) breaking adhesions between or around the femorotibial joint, (3) lengthening the quadriceps femoris mechanism, and (4) releasing the restrictive action of other extensor muscles (sartorius and tensor fasciae latae).

A lateral approach to the stifle and femur is used to isolate the quadriceps femoris muscle and free adhesions (tenolysis). Additional exposure of the quadriceps mechanisms may be achieved by a medial arthrotomy that is extended proximally along the caudal border of the vastus medialis muscle. A sheet of Silastic has been used between the femur and the quadriceps femoris muscle to prevent the recurrence of adhesions. Following isolation of the quadriceps femoris muscle, the patella is luxated medially, and the femorotibial joint is forcibly flexed. The patella is reduced, and flexion is repeated. In immature animals, care should be taken to avoid avulsion of the tibial tuberosity. If adequate flexion cannot be achieved with reasonable force, restrictive muscles must be incised or lengthened.

The cranial belly of the sartorius muscle is incised near its insertion on the patella. The quadriceps femoris muscle can be lengthened by various myoplasty procedures. We have used a sliding myoplasty technique to lengthen the mechanism of this muscle (Fig. 38-5 B and C). The rectus femoris muscle is isolated from the vastus group of the quadriceps femoris muscle and is transected near the patella. Branches of the femoral nerve and cranial femoral vessels are avoided. The vastus lateralis, intermedius, and medialis muscles are isolated as a unit and are elevated from their origin on the proximal femur. Flexion of the stifle produces a sliding effect between the rectus femoris and the vastus muscle group. The rectus femoris muscle slides proximally, and the vastus muscle group slides distally. The rectus femoris muscle and the cranial belly of the sartorius muscle are sutured to the vastus group of the quadriceps femoris muscle with the stifle positioned in flexion. Relief incisions may be required in the tensor fasciae latae. Alternate procedures for lengthening the quadriceps mechanism include partial quadriceps myotomy.[31] "Z" myoplasty, inverted "V-Y" myoplasty, and proximal transposition of the tibial crest.

Postoperatively, the leg is maintained in partial flexion, and passive movement of the limb is initiated in 3 to 5 days. Periodic sedation or anesthesia and forced flexion of the stifle may be required. Physical therapy and swimming should be encouraged. These corrective procedures have improved function and use of the limb, but, in the severely affected animal, restoration of the limb to near normal function has not been achieved. Alternate procedures include percutaneous pins with elastic bands, arthrodesis of the knee in a functional position and amputation of the limb.

A similar disorder may develop as a result of malunion of the distal femur with overriding of the proximal segment. The protruding end of the proximal segment acts as a mechanical barrier and, along with the adhesions, prevents movement of the patella. Resection of the protruding segment of bone and freeing of adhesions between the femur and the quadriceps femoris muscle has resulted in a significant improvement in function of the knee, especially in mature individuals.

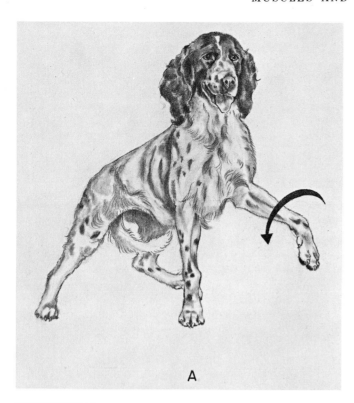

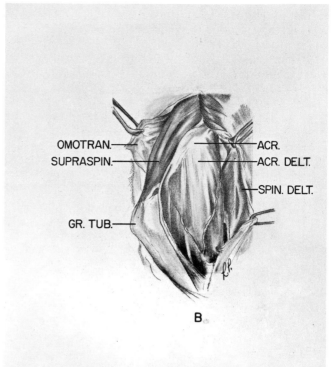

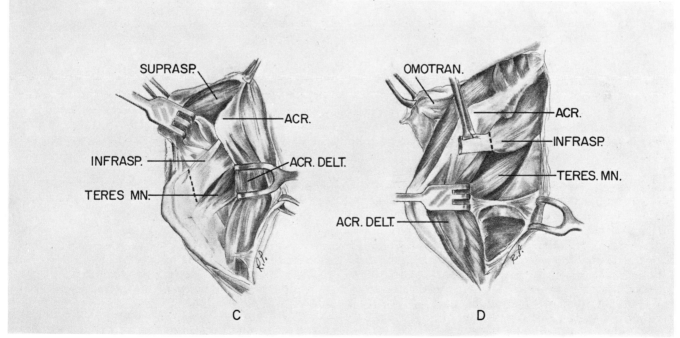

Fig. 38-4. *Infraspinatus muscle contracture. A, Characteristic lameness illustrated by adduction of the elbow and outward rotation of the antebrachium. B, C, and D, Technique for infraspinatus tenectomy: B, Superficial muscles of the shoulder; the omotransversarius muscle has been reflected from the acromion process to expose the supraspinatus muscle for illustration purposes and is not required during the operation; C, Exposure and transection of the tendon of the infraspinatus muscle near the greater tubercle is facilitated by caudal retraction of the acromial portion of the deltoideus muscle; D, Retraction of the acromial portion of the deltoideus muscle cranially and the spinous portion caudally exposes the infraspinatus muscle and tendon for tenectomy. OMOTRAN., omotransversarius m.; SUPRASPIN., supraspinatus m.; ACR., acromion; ACR. DELT., acromial portion of the deltoideus m.; SPIN. DELT., spinous portion of the deltoideus m.; INFRASPIN., infraspinatus m.; TERES. MN., teres minor m.; and GR. TUB., greater tubercle of humerus.*

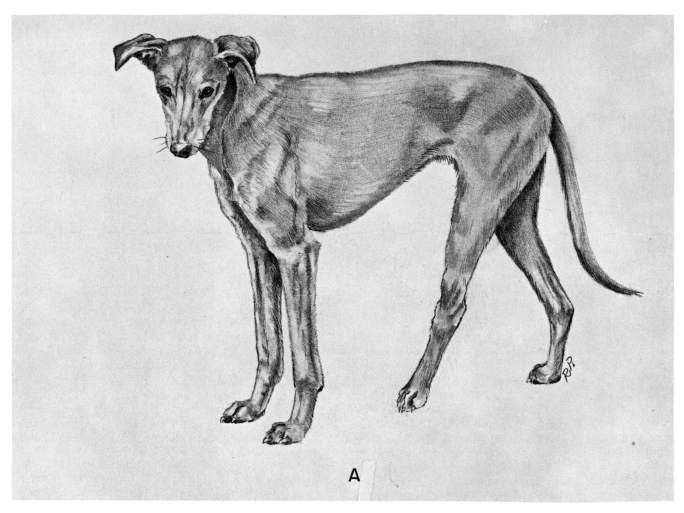

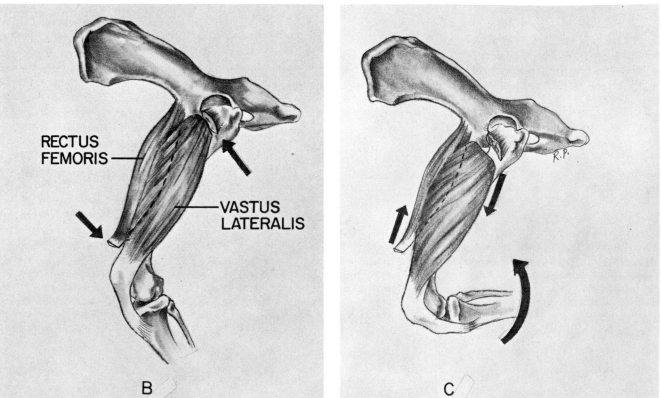

RECTUS FEMORIS

VASTUS LATERALIS

B

C

Fig. 38-5. *Quadriceps muscle contracture. A, Characteristic limb deformity depicted by hyperextension of the affected limb. B and C, Sliding quadriceps myoplasty technique for lengthening the quadriceps mechanism: B, Isolation of the rectus femoris muscle and transection distally near its insertion on the patella; elevation of the vastus muscle group from the femoral shaft and transection of their origin on the proximal metaphysis; C, Flexion of the stifle produces sliding of the rectus femoris muscle proximally and the vastus muscle group distally; the vastus lateralis and medialis muscles are sutured together distally and to the rectus femoris in its more proximal location.*

Congenital hindlimb hyperextension has been observed in littermates with myopathy secondary to Toxoplasma gondii polyradiculoneuritis. Both rear limbs are usually affected. The diagnosis is most often dependent on necropsy examination. Treatment is not recommended.

MUSCLE BIOPSIES

The histologic, histochemical, and electron-microscopic examination of muscle tissue provides information for establishing the pathologic process and for differentiating the myopathies according to their origin: inflammatory, degenerative, neoplastic, neurogenic, ischemic, or endocrine-related. The procedure for collection of the biopsy specimen varies with the examination to be conducted and with the individual techniques of the pathologist. For this reason, the pathologist should be consulted prior to collection of the tissue, so that proper procedure is followed. Muscle biopsy clamps are recommended to prevent contraction and alteration of the muscle fibers. For our laboratory, specimens for histologic and histochemical studies are wrapped in a moist surgical sponge for 30 minutes at room temperature prior to cryofixation. Special fixatives such as glutaraldehyde and paraformaldehyde are required for electron-microscopic studies.

Muscle-Tendon

ANATOMY

The transition from muscle to tendon occurs gradually over a broad area of the terminal portion of the muscle as muscle fibers decrease and connective tissue increases. The connective tissue elements of the muscle (endomysium, perimysium, and epimysium) are continuous with the connective tissue elements (collagen) of the tendon. Additionally, the collagen fibers of the tendon attach directly to the terminal portion of the cell membrane (sarcolemma) of the muscle fiber (sarcomere)[15] (Fig. 38-6).

REPAIR

Healing is primarily dependent upon capillary invasion and fibroblast proliferation in the wound. The amount of scar tissue and of adhesions depends upon a number of factors, including the amount of damage, the size of the wound, the method of treatment, and the amount of movement or stress on the damaged area. Following rupture, contraction causes separation of the muscle and tendon segments. Healing by fibroplasia re-establishes the continuity of the muscle and tendon, but may not re-establish the action of the muscle because of the increased muscle-tendon unit length.

STRAINS

See the discussion of strains in the foregoing section of this chapter, under "Muscle Belly."

LACERATIONS

Lacerations of the musculotendinous junction are treated in essentially the same manner as those of muscle. The suture pattern may vary because of tendon involvement. (See the following paragraphs.)

RUPTURES

Ruptures of the musculotendinous junction occur more frequently than ruptures of the muscle belly. The signs and treatment vary with the severity of the rupture and the function of the muscle. Separation or shearing of the musculotendinous segments causes loss of muscle function, and the inflammatory response causes pain and swelling. Separation of these segments

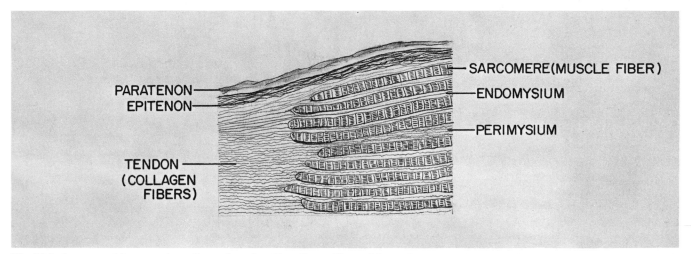

Fig. 38-6. *Anatomy of the musculotendinous junction. The collagen fibers of the tendon are continuous with the collagen fibers of the muscle and attach directly to the ends of the muscle fibers. (Modified from Ham, A. W.: Histology. 8th Ed. Philadelphia, J. B. Lippincott, 1980.)*

is usually not palpable because the rupture occurs over a broad area and portions of the muscle sheath and tendon remain intact. The diagnosis of a rupture is based on conformational changes and a lameness that reflects loss of muscle function. The rupture is localized to the musculotendinous area by the inflammatory changes—heat, swelling, and pain.

The objective of treatment is adequate apposition of the musculotendinous segments so that healing occurs with minimal loss of function. In most cases, this objective is best achieved surgically. The operation should be performed immediately because a significant delay allows contraction of the muscle and tendon segments and obliteration of the wound by fibroplasia.

With acute injuries, the tendon and muscle segments are isolated and are sutured. The suture material and pattern vary with the personal preference of the surgeon, but they must provide adequate anchorage in both the muscle and the tendon. A Bunnell or modified Bunnell suture pattern is most frequently used. A bed may be prepared in the muscle for the tendon, and a button may be used to anchor the suture to the muscle. Simple interrupted or mattress sutures are used to reinforce the line of anastomosis (Fig. 38-7).

Chronic injuries that have healed may require shortening of the musculotendinous unit to re-establish the action of the muscle. (See the section later in this chapter on tendon shortening). Most important in the treatment of an acute or chronic injury is postoperative care. The limb should be immobilized, with the joints positioned so that stresses are not transferred to the anastomotic site. The most common site of musculotendinous rupture in the dog is the gastrocnemius muscle.

GASTROCNEMIUS MUSCULOTENDINOUS RUPTURES. Rupture of the gastrocnemius musculotendinous junction occurs predominately in mature dogs of the working and hunting breeds. The history often includes trauma from lunging or jumping on the rear limbs. The condition frequently occurs bilaterally. The clinical signs include hyperflexion of and inability to extend the tarsus forcefully (dropped hock) (Fig. 38-8). Palpation of the common calcanean tendon and gastrocnemius muscle reveals inflammatory changes along the musculotendinous junction manifested by increased size and firmness. Manual extension of the tarsus produces excessive laxity of the common calcanean tendon.

In acute cases, treatment is directed at apposing the musculotendinous segments and preventing stress on the musculotendinous unit during healing. These objectives can best be achieved by surgical repair of the musculotendinous junction and immobilization of the tarsus and knee. Immobilization has been used successfully. External and internal fixation procedures have been used to stabilize the tarsus in partial extension, with the knee in partial flexion. Immobilization of the limb with a Schroeder-Thomas splint is perhaps the oldest and most traditional method of treatment. A more rigid stabilization of the tarsus can be achieved by fixation of the tuber calcanei to the distal tibia with a bone screw[3,6] or a full-pin splint (Fig. 38-9A).[12] Compression screw techniques are used with the bone screw (Fig. 38-9B). The size and type of screw are dictated by the size of the dog. These fixation procedures can be supplemented with casts, splints, and coaptation bandages.

Most patients treated by us have chronic cases of this disorder and have previously been treated by immobilization with a Schroeder-Thomas splint. In chronic cases, one must shorten the common calcanean tendon to re-establish function of the gastrocnemius and superficial digital flexor muscles. A doubling-over technique is preferred for shortening the tendon. (See the section of this chapter on tendon shortening). The tarsus is stabilized with the compression screw procedure, and the limb is immobilized for

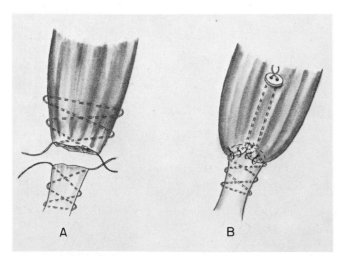

Fig. 38-7. *Suture techniques for musculotendinous ruptures. A, Bunnell-Mayer. B, Modified Bunnell with a bolster (button) for reinforcement. The tendon is pulled into a bed prepared in the muscle. The muscle-tendon junction is sutured with simple interrupted or mattress sutures.*

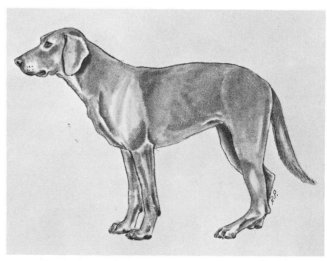

Fig. 38-8. *Injury to a portion of the gastrocnemius or superficial digital flexor muscle (Achilles complex). The characteristic deformity of the affected limb is illustrated by hyperflexion of the tarsus (dropped hock) with weight bearing.*

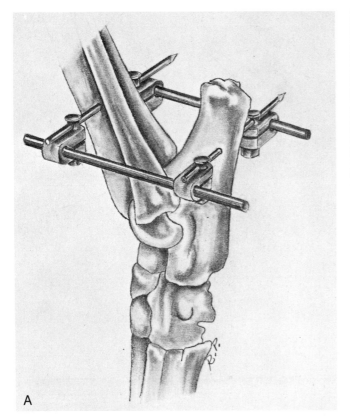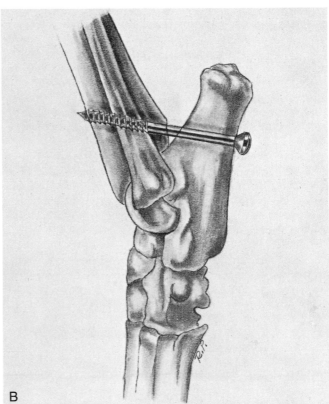

Fig. 38-9. *Techniques for stabilization of the tarsus: A, Full-pin splint; and B, Compression screw stabilization.*

2 weeks with a coaptation bandage or splint. The screw is removed 4 to 8 weeks postoperatively. This procedure has been the most consistently successful for returning normal function to the limb. We believe that rigid immobilization of the tarsus is an important aspect of the treatment of patients with acute or chronic cases of this disorder.

RUPTURE OF THE SUPERFICIAL DIGITAL FLEXOR. Rupture of the superficial digital flexor musculotendinous junction has been reported without simultaneous rupture of the gastrocnemius muscle.[4] The superficial digital flexor muscle lies deep to the gastrocnemius muscle. The superficial digital flexor tendon passes distomedial over the caudal aspect of the gastrocnemius tendon and the tuber calcanei and forms part of the common calcanean (Achilles) tendon. The clinical signs and treatment are essentially the same as those described for musculotendinous ruptures of the gastrocnemius.

Tendon

ANATOMY

Tendons are composed primarily of bundles and fascicles of dense connective tissue (collagen). Fibroblasts or tenocytes are the main cells in tendons and are interspersed in parallel rows between the collagen bundles. Tendons are covered and are separated from other tissues by loose areolar connective tissue (paratenon) or synovial sheaths. The paratenon and synovial sheaths facilitate the free gliding movement of the tendon (Fig. 38-10). Directional changes in the action of a tendon are achieved by transverse or annular ligaments, which are usually associated with synovial sheaths.

The major blood supply to tendons is derived from extrinsic vessels that pass longitudinally in the paratenon. Within the digital flexor synovial sheaths, the extrinsic (extratendon) vessels are supplied by a vinculum or a mesentery system of vessels that pass to the tendons through the mesotendon of the synovial sheath. The intrinsic (intratendon) vessels run longitudinally between the fascicles to supply the collagen bundles and cells and to anastomose freely with each other and with the extrinsic vessels.[10]

REPAIR

Tendons heal mainly by invasion of the wound with capillaries and cellular elements (fibroblasts) from the surrounding tissues (principally paratenon) and not usually by intrinsic cellular response. The adhesions that develop are part of the healing process. The wound of the tendon and the surrounding tissues heal as a unit; one wound, one scar. In the initial stages of healing, collagen fibers are deposited randomly in and about the tendon wound. As healing progresses and as remodeling occurs, collagen fibers become longitudinally oriented and continuous with the fibers of the tendon. Adhesions are remodeled and gradually weaken as movement and function return.[20,24]

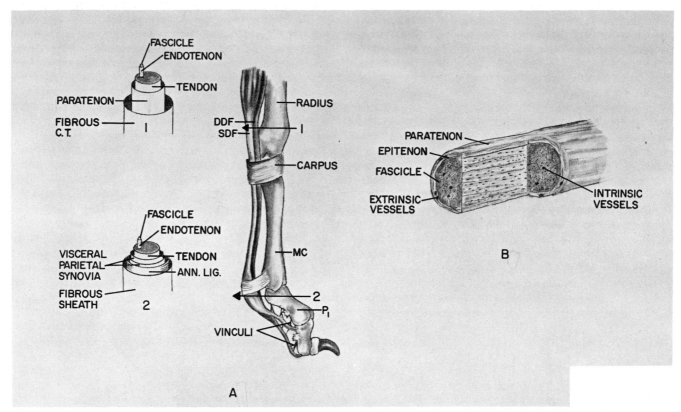

Fig. 38-10. *Anatomy of tendon.* A, *Diagram of the flexor tendons showing the various investing layers around the tendons: (1) Cross section of the tendon in the metacarpal or distal antebrachial regions reveals paratenon and fibrous sheath covering; and (2) Cross section of the tendons in the digital area at the level of the proximal annular ligament shows parietal and visceral synovial lining that facilitate gliding within the fibrous sheath. Blood supply to the tendons through the synovial sheaths is by mesentery-type vessels (vinculi) that arise from the periosteal surface of the adjacent bone. C. T., connective tissue; ANN. LIG., annular ligament; DDF, deep digital flexor; SDF, superficial digital flexor; MC, metacarpal; P₁, first phalanx. (Modified from Entin, M.: In Accident Surgery. Vol. 2. Edited by H. F. Moseley. New York, Appleton-Century-Crofts, 1964.)* B, *Section of tendon, with paratenon covering, illustrating tendon structure.*

The reduction of adhesions becomes an important consideration in tendons that must glide or move freely to provide normal function of a part. The prevention of permanent adhesions is critical to the success of tendon operations on the fingers in man. Manual dexterity is not required in the dog, however, and adhesions assume a less-important role in the surgical considerations. Various synthetic materials have been used as cuffs about the anastomotic site. These cuffs retard the healing process by preventing the invasion of the wound with fibroblast and capillaries from the surrounding soft tissues. Adhesions can be minimized by proper surgical technique, that is, atraumatic handling of the tissues and anatomic apposition and stabilization of the tendon segments, and proper postoperative care.

The rate and tensile strength of healing following the repair of tendons have been studied experimentally and are important in providing proper postoperative care.[20] During the early stage of healing, the strength of repair is primarily due to the holding power of the suture. The tendon ends soften for the first 4 to 5 days, when the tissue's integrity or holding power for the suture is at its lowest level. The strength of repair gradually increases as healing proceeds and, in 2 weeks, is dependent upon the strength of union and of the suture material. Early active use of the tendon increases separation of the segments and promotes excessive scar tissue formation. The results of experimental studies indicate that immobilization of the limb should be provided for at least 2 to 3 weeks so that stresses are not applied to the anastomotic site. Use of the leg after 3 weeks should be controlled in order to ensure a gradual return to normal activity by 6 weeks. Swimming is an ideal initial exercise because joints are used freely, but no weight is borne.

GENERAL PRINCIPLES OF TENDON SURGERY

Surgical procedures of the tendon should be performed with aseptic and atraumatic technique. Whenever possible, the skin incision should not be made directly over the tendon. Tendon segments should be atraumatically manipulated, preferably with the gloved fingers of the surgeon. Straight needles inserted through the tendon can be used to aid manipulation. The use of forceps to grasp tendons should be avoided. When the tendon must be held with forceps for suture placement, the traumatized end of the tendon should be grasped, and following placement of the suture, the damaged end of the tendon should be excised.[8,9] Hemostasis should be controlled by ligation, electrocoagulation, or a tourniquet. Tourniquets work best on the distal extremity of the limb. An Esmarch's nonadhesive elastic bandage (Vetrap) provides excellent hemostasis for surgical procedures involving the foot, carpus or tarsus.

The suture material and pattern for surgical procedures of the tendon vary with the size and shape of the tendon, the surgical technique employed, and the personal preference of the surgeon.[5,8,9,20,29,30] The suture materials for tendon operations should be strong, nonreactive, easy to handle, and nonabsorbable. A number of materials meet these basic requirements, including stainless steel wire, braided polyester fiber, monofilament nylon, and polypropylene. Stainless steel is strong and inert, but can be difficult to handle. Braided polyester is strong, inert, and easy to handle. Nylon is inert and easy to handle, but is comparatively weak. We prefer to use stainless steel and monofilament nylon suture material. The suture pattern should provide adequate anchorage of the suture material in the tendon with minimal damage to the tissue. Several techniques and patterns have been described. The Bunnell, Bunnell-Mayer, horizontal mattress, and Kessler or modified Kessler patterns are most frequently used in the dog (Figs. 38-11 and 38-12). The technique of anastomosis should provide a strong anastomosis, anatomic apposition, and proper tendon length and diameter. End-to-end, side-to-side, and interlacing or weaving techniques have been described (Figs. 38-12 and 38-13).[5,9,30]

REPAIR OF SEVERED TENDONS

Severed tendons are the most common indication for tenorrhaphy. Tendons rarely rupture. Tendon repair should be performed with minimal delay when the environment at the site of the injury is suitable: recent injury, minimal trauma, minimal contamination. The best time (golden period) for primary closure is 4 to 6

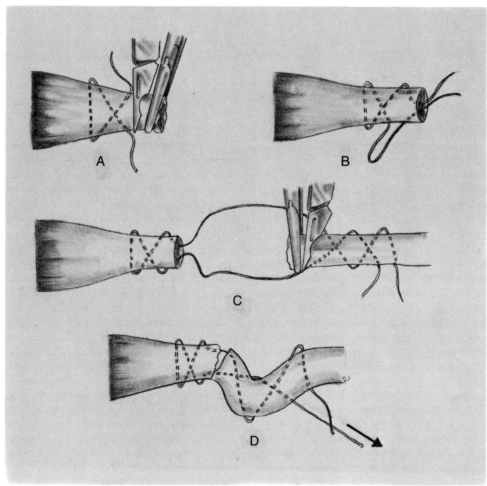

Fig. 38-11. *Bunnell's suture technique for tendon anastomosis. A, Placement of the cruciate suture. Forceps stabilize the tendon, and the damaged end of the tendon is excised. B, The cruciate suture is passed into the cut edge of the tendon. The tendon is held by digital pressure, and the suture is pulled tight. C, Forceps maintain the position of the opposing segment, and the cruciate pattern is started through the paratenon above the forceps. The tendon end is excised adjacent to the entrance point of the suture. D, The free ends of the suture are alternately pulled tight while the tendon segments are forced together by digital pressure. As the suture tightens, it is drawn into the anastomotic site. (Modified from Bunnell, S.: Surgery of the Hand. Philadelphia, J. B. Lippincott, 1944.)*

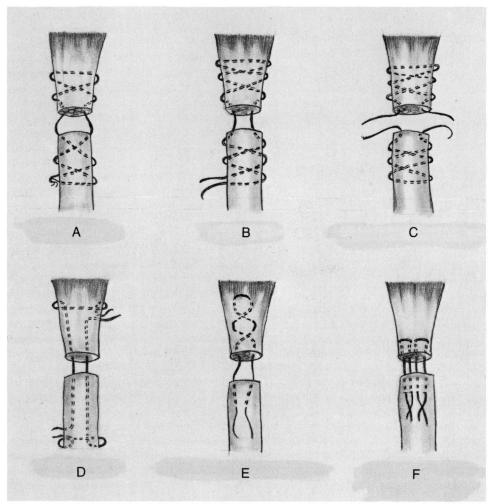

Fig. 38-12. *Suture techniques for end-to-end anastomosis:* A *and* B, *Bunnell;* C, *Bunnell-Mayer;* D, *Kessler;* E, *modified Bunnell; and* F, *interrupted mattress.*

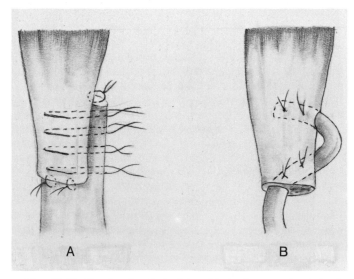

Fig. 38-13. *Overlapping techniques for tendon anastomosis:* A, *side-to-side;* B, *fish-mouth.*

hours after injury. This period can be extended if the wound is properly debrided and irrigated, if trauma and contamination are minimal, and if the tendon has adequate soft tissue surroundings and blood supply. Primary closure is subject to the discretion of the surgeon. The repair of severed tendons in infected and traumatized (degloving) wounds should be delayed until healing of the surrounding tissue occurs and a suitable environment is provided. In these patients, the leg is immobilized to reduce separation of the tendon segments.

The technique for anastomosis should provide anatomic apposition of the tendon segments, adequate strength of repair, and minimal tissue damage. The end-to-end anastomosis is most frequently used in the dog because it maintains the original length and diameter of the tendon and is comparatively simple to perform (see Fig. 38-12). Overlapping techniques, such as side-to-side, end-weave, or buttonhole overlapping procedures, provide a stronger anastomosis, but require greater tendon length and increase the diameter of the final anastamosis (see Fig. 38-13). In round or semiround tendons, such as the common calcanean tendon, a Bunnell or modified Bunnell suture pattern is most frequently used (see Fig. 38-12 *A*, *B*, and *C*). In small or flat tendons, other techniques may be more applicable (see Fig. 38-12 *D*, *E*, and *F*). Interrupted mattress sutures are commonly used in flat tendons. In an experimental study in dogs comparing different suture techniques for end-to-end anastomosis of the digital flexor tendons, the Kessler pattern provided the greatest strength of repair (Fig. 38-12 *D*).[30] A carbon fiber implant has been used to reinforce the line of anastomosis. (See the discussion later in this chapter on carbon fiber implants).[31] Following apposition of the tendon segments, the paratenon and epitenon are sutured at the anastomotic site in a simple continuous or interrupted pattern. Stresses on the tendon should be reduced by internal or external immobilization techniques.

SPECIAL INDICATION FOR TENORRHAPHY: SURGICAL TENOTOMIES. Tenotomies to facilitate surgical exposure usually involve muscles with short, flat tendons whose function is duplicated by surrounding muscles. Simple interrupted mattress sutures are used to reappose the tendon segments (see Fig. 38-12 *F*). An osteotomy is preferred when reflection of a major muscle or group of muscles is required.

SEVERED COMMON CALCANEAN (ACHILLES) TENDON. The common calcanean tendon is composed of the tendons of the gastrocnemius, superficial digital flexor, semitendinosis, gracilis, and biceps femoris muscles. The clinical signs and treatment for a severed calcanean tendon are essentially the same as those described for rupture of the gastrocnemius musculotendinous junction. A laceration is observed in the area of the tendon, and the tarsus drops into hyperflexion under the stress of weight bearing. With primary repair, the tendon segments are apposed with a Bunnell or Kessler-type suture pattern, and the paratenon is sutured over the anastomotic site. Tension on the musculotendinous unit is relieved by fixing the tuber calcanei to the distal tibia with a bone screw. A carbon fiber implant has been used to reinforce the anastomosis.[29] The implant is tied through a hole drilled in the tuber calcanei and is attached proximally to the gastrocnemius muscle belly. When chronic injuries heal in such a way that the common calcanean tendon is excessively long, the tendon will require shortening. An overlapping procedure is preferred. (See the discussion following on tendon shortening.)

SEVERED DIGITAL FLEXOR TENDONS. The superficial and deep digital flexor tendons insert on the proximal end of the second and third phalanges, respectively, and function in the foot by maintaining the toes in proper position so that the stresses of weight bearing are cushioned by the digital and metacarpal or metatarsal pads. The action of the tendons is facilitated in the digits by a synovial sheath and a system of annular ligaments (pulleys) Fig. 38-14.[12]

The tendon(s) are most commonly severed above and below the metacarpal and metatarsal pads, where they are least protected. Surgical exploration of a flexor tendon is indicated when clinical signs reflect a

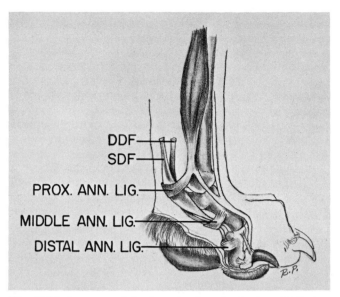

Fig. 38-14. *Anatomy of the flexor tendons in the foot. DDF, deep digital flexor; SDF, superficial digital flexor; PROX. ANN. LIG., proximal annular ligament.*

significant loss of function: flattening of one or more digits and elevation of the claw and digital pad with weight bearing. Injuries that require surgical treatment involve the superficial and deep digital flexor tendons in the metacarpal and metatarsal area and the deep digital flexor tendon in the digit. The deep digital flexor tendon is primarily responsible for the normal position of the toe.

The flexor tendons in the metacarpal and metatarsal area are covered and surrounded by adequate soft tissue and are more readily exposed and repaired than in the digital area. Isolation of the deep digital flexor tendon in the digits is complicated by the presence of synovial sheaths and annular ligaments, by the short length of the digit between the digital and metacarpal or metatarsal pad, and by the presence of thick foot pads. Tenorrhaphy is complicated when the proximal segment of the tendons retracts into the synovial sheath beneath the annular ligament and superficial digital flexor tendon. The annular ligament may be incised to expose the proximal segment if flexion and milking of the proximal tissue does not reveal it. In long-standing injuries, reapposition of the tendon segments may not be possible. A carbon fiber implant or a tendon graft can be used to bridge the gap between the tendon ends.[31] In small breeds of dogs, the size of the tendons further complicates the surgical repair.

The suture size and pattern vary with the size of the tendon. Bunnell, Kessler, or mattress suture patterns may be used. In the digit, transected annular ligaments or synovial sheaths should be sutured.

Postoperative care is aimed at preventing weight-bearing stresses on the tendons for at least 3 weeks. The leg is initially placed in a flexion bandage, with the tarsus or carpus and digits in a flexed position. Support is continued with a splint or cast. The prognosis is guarded because of the constant trauma and stresses of weight bearing that must be supported by the tendon. We have had limited success in restoring the integrity and function of the deep digital flexor tendon in chronic injuries.

TENDON LENGTHENING AND SHORTENING

Lengthening or shortening a tendon is indicated in chronic cases of lameness or in alteration of conformation due to contracture of or increase in musculotendinous unit length, respectively.

Contracture or laxity of the musculotendinous unit is most frequently observed in actively growing dogs, 3 to 4 months of age, that are subjected to various stresses including parasitism, malnutrition, and improper environment. The clinical signs include "buckling" or dropping of the carpus or tarsus. Correction of the husbandry practices and improvement in the physical condition of the animal usually restore normal function. Support bandages or splints aid in the management of patients with severe disorders. Rarely is surgical treatment required.

Several techniques for relieving contraction of a musculotendinous unit and for restoring normal function have been described (Fig. 38-15).[5,9] When the function of a muscle can be sacrificed, a simple tenotomy or tenectomy is indicated. (See the previous discussion of infraspinatus muscle contracture.) When the function of the muscle must be preserved, a lengthening procedure is required. (See the previous discussion of quadriceps femoris muscle contracture.) Tenoplasty techniques for lengthening include the "Z" tenotomy, the oblique or gliding technique, and the accordion technique. The "Z" tenotomy is most frequently employed. The elongated "Z" incision is made in the center of the tendon. It is most accurately performed by

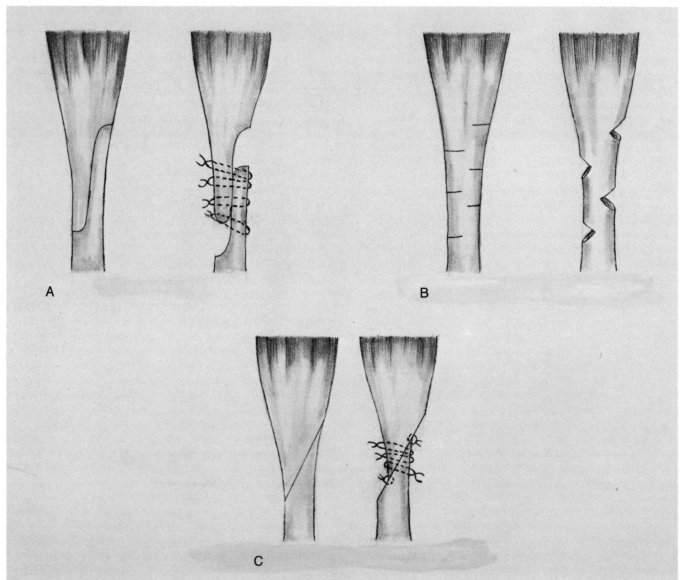

Fig. 38-15. *Tendon-lengthening techniques:* A, *"Z" tenotomy;* B, *accordion partial tenotomy;* C, *oblique or gliding tenotomy. (Modified from Butler, H. C.: Tendon, muscle and fascia. In Canine Surgery. 2nd Ed. Edited by J. Archibald. Santa Barbara, CA, American Veterinary Publications, 1965.)*

first splitting the tendon, then incising the "arms" of the "Z." The opposing segments can be sutured by an end-to-end or a side-to-side technique (Fig. 38-15 A).

Tendon-shortening techniques include the doubling-over method, the "Z" tenotomy, Hoffa's suture technique, and segmental excision (Fig. 38-16). The doubling-over method is preferred because it does not require a tenotomy, it provides a strong union, and it is comparatively simple to perform. The tendon or tendon segment must be sufficiently pliable, however, to allow folding, and the surrounding tissue must be able to accommodate the increased tendon size (Fig. 38-16A).

Improper healing of a rupture of the gastrocnemius musculotendinous junction or a laceration of the common calcanean tendon may result in a musculotendinous unit that is too long and in significant dysfunction.

(See the previous discussion of rupture of the musculotendinous junction.) Shortening of the common calcanean tendon by the doubling-over technique is preferred. Following any of these tenoplasty procedures, stresses on the tendon should be relieved by internal and external fixation procedures until sufficient healing has occurred.

TENDON GRAFTING

Tendon grafts are rarely indicated and performed in small animal surgery. Tendon autografts or allografts are indicated when tendon substance has been lost or when muscle contraction prevents the reapposition of tendon ends.[4,33] These techniques are more commonly used in man, and the reader is referred to our suggested reading list for further information on the sub-

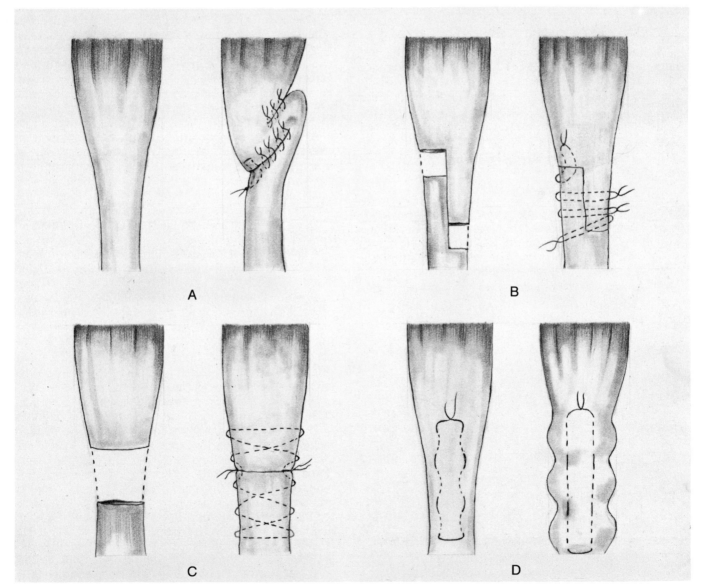

Fig. 38-16. *Techniques for tendon shortening: A, Doubling-over; B, "Z" tenectomy; C, segmental tenectomy; D, Hoffa's suture technique. (Modified from Butler, H. C.: Tendon, muscle and fascia. In Canine Surgery. 2nd Ed. Edited by J. Archibald. Santa Barbara, CA, American Veterinary Publications, 1965.)*

ject. Recently, filamentous carbon has been shown to be a suitable substitute for tendon grafts.[31]

CARBON FIBER IMPLANTS

Carbon fiber implants have been used experimentally as a substitute for tendon and clinically to reinforce conventional suturing of tendon and to fill gaps between tendon ends. The plaited strand of carbon fiber is sutured to the surface of the tendon with polyglycolic acid sutures. Specific clinical indications include ruptures of the deep digital flexor and common calcanean tendons. With injuries to the common calcanean tendon, the fiber is tied through a hole in the tuber calcanei and is sutured proximally to the gastrocnemius muscle.[31]

Tendinosseous Junction

ANATOMY

At the tendinosseous or cartilage junction, the connective tissue sheath and collagen fibers of the tendon blend with the periosteum and the collagen fibers of the bone or cartilage. The collagen fibers of the tendon that anchor into the bony substance are called Sharpey's fibers (Fig. 38-17).[15] The periosteal vessels are continuous with the extrinsic vessels of the tendon.

REPAIR

Most tendons insert or originate on the metaphyseal or epiphyseal areas of long bones. Injuries at the tendinosseous junction frequently involve bone in the form of avulsion fractures. Regardless of the type of injury, whether a fracture or a tendinosseous separation, the process of repair in tendon and bone is closely related and requires essentially the same environment to pro-

mote healing and a return to normal function. The local environment at the tendinosseous area is conducive to healing because it possesses a rich blood supply and a reliable source of fibroblasts and osteoblasts. Additionally, these injuries occur predominately in immature animals with an active metabolism and a rapid repair potential. Biomechanical forces that are normally transferred by the tendon and bone are most detrimental to the repair process, however. Tension from muscle contraction and movement of the bone (joint) causes separation of the injured tissues and must be combated if tendinosseous or fracture repair is to occur.

GENERAL SURGICAL CONSIDERATIONS

Three types of injuries are observed at the tendinosseous junction: (1) separation of tendon from bone, (2) separation of tendon from bone with a small avulsion segment(s) of bone, and (3) avulsion fracture. The objectives of repair are the same, regardless of the injury, and include anatomic alignment, stable fixation, and minimal tissue damage. Which technique is best varies with the location and the type of injury. Treatment should be initiated without delay because contracture of the muscle makes apposition of the segments more difficult.

Tendon separations with or without small bone segments are treated by suturing the tendon to the bone. A Bunnell, Kessler, or mattress-type suture with stainless steel wire is preferred in tendons of substantial size. Following placement of the suture in the tendon, the free ends of the wire are passed through small drill holes in the bone and are tightened to secure the tendon. Small bone chips can be excised or aligned and left with the tendon. Substantial segments of bone should be fixed with wire or pins to provide additional stabilization.

Avulsion fractures occur predominately in immature dogs of the large breeds. A traumatic origin is suspected, but is rarely confirmed, by the history. The fractures commonly involve traction epiphyses or processes: greater trochanter, tibial tuberosity, tuber calcanei, and supraglenoid tubercle. Tendon avulsions and fractures on the large pressure epiphyses (condyles) usually involve a superficial layer of bone and cartilage: long digital extensor and popliteus tendons.

The clinical signs, in most cases, are nonspecific and include a weight-bearing lameness and pain on manipulation of the associated joint. An obvious conformational deformity is observed with avulsions in major tendons such as the gastrocnemius tendon. Radiographic examination provides the diagnosis by revealing the segment of avulsed bone at the point of attachment of the tendon. A periosteal reaction is observed in chronic cases at this site. When clinical and radiographic signs are obscure, comparative radiographs and synovial fluid analysis (if a joint is involved) are helpful in establishing the diagnosis. The technique of fixation of these fractures depends on the size of the avulsed segment of bone. Small pins, wire, and screws

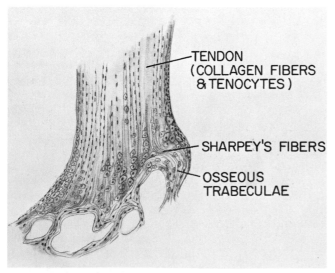

Fig. 38-17. *Tendinosseous junction anatomy. Collagen fibers of the tendon are continuous with the collagen fibers of the bone (Sharpey's fibers).*

TENDON
(COLLAGEN FIBERS
& TENOCYTES)

SHARPEY'S FIBERS

OSSEOUS
TRABECULAE

are commonly used for internal fixation. Spiked washers may be used with screws to prevent fracturing of small fragments.

TENDON-AVULSION FRACTURES

BICEPS BRACHII TENDON OF ORIGIN—SUPRAGLENOID TUBERCLE. The biceps brachii tendon arises from the supraglenoid tubercle of the scapula and passes distally across the cranial aspect of the shoulder, through the intertubercular groove, to its muscle belly on the cranial aspect of the humerus. Avulsion of the biceps brachii tendon with fracture of the supraglenoid tubercle occurs predominately in immature dogs, 4 to 8 months of age, of the large breeds. Clinical signs include a weight-bearing lameness and evidence of pain or discomfort on manipulation of the shoulder. Radiographic examination of the shoulder is essential to establishing a diagnosis and reveals the avulsed segment of bone.

Open reduction and internal fixation are the recommended treatment. The biceps brachii tendon and the supraglenoid tubercle are exposed through a craniomedial approach to the shoulder.[25] The craniomedial border of the supraspinatus muscle is isolated, and the muscle is retracted laterally. The suprascapular nerve should be avoided. The tubercle is aligned and is fixed to the scapula with a small Steinmann pin(s) and tension band wire or a small (2.7 or 3.5 mm) bone screw, using the compression principle (Fig. 38-18).

GREATER TROCHANTER—DEEP GLUTEAL, CAUDAL HIP MUSCLES. Avulsion fractures of the greater trochanter occur most frequently in combination with other traumatic injuries of the proximal femur and hip: femoral head and neck fractures and hip dislocations. The reader is referred to Part II of this book for further information.

LONG DIGITAL EXTENSOR TENDON OF ORIGIN—LATERAL FEMORAL CONDYLE SEGMENT. The long digital extensor tendon arises from the lateral condyle of the femur and passes distally across the craniolateral aspect of the stifle, through the extensor notch of the tibia, to its muscle belly, which lies deep to the cranial tibial muscle. Avulsion of the long digital extensor tendon occurs primarily in immature large-breed dogs, 4 to 6 months of age. Clinical signs include a weight-bearing lameness and pain or discomfort on manipulation of the stifle. The diagnosis is made by radiographic examination of the stifle. The lateral radiographic view best demonstrates the avulsed segment of the lateral condyle. This thin segment of bone and cartilage may not be visible in less-mature individuals, and exploration of the stifle is indicated to establish the diagnosis when lameness is persistent.

Reattachment of the avulsed tendon and fragment of bone is the recommended treatment.[1,22,25,29] A lateral approach is made to the stifle. The avulsed segment of the lateral condyle is aligned and is fixed with a cortical bone screw(s), using compression techniques.[26] A spiked washer prevents fracturing of the avulsed segment from the pressure of the screw head. Alternate techniques of treatment include wiring or stapling the fracture, excising the avulsed segment of bones and then suturing the tendon to the joint capsule and connective tissue near its point of origin,[21] and removal of the bone chip[23] (Fig. 38-19).

INSERTION OF POPLITEUS TENDON—FRAGMENT OF THE LATERAL FEMORAL CONDYLE. The popliteus tendon arises from the lateral condyle, slightly cranial and distal to the lateral epicondyle. The tendon passes caudally, beneath the lateral collateral ligament adjacent to the caudal horn of the lateral meniscus, to its muscle belly on the caudal aspect of the proximal tibia. A sesamoid bone is located in the caudal portion of most tendons.

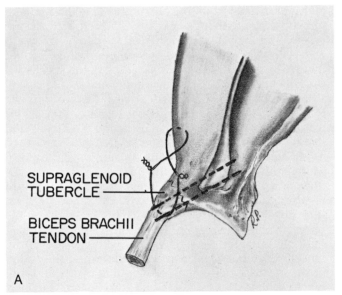

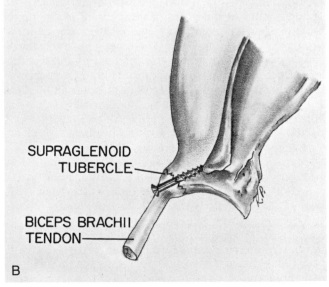

A

B

Fig. 38-18. *Technique for repair of avulsion fracture of the supraglenoid tubercle: A, Multiple small pins and tension-band wire; B, Compression screw fixation.*

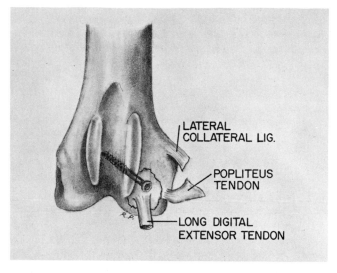

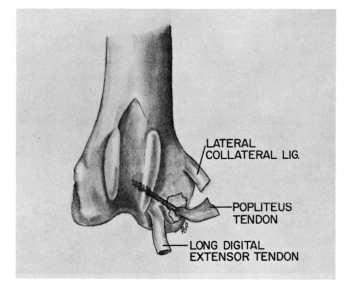

Fig. 38-19. *Avulsion of the long digital extensor tendon with a segment of the lateral femoral condyle. Reduction and stabilization of the avulsed segment of bone are maintained with a compression screw. A spiked washer (inset) can be used to prevent fragmentation of the avulsed segment of bone. See text for alternate methods of treatment.*

Fig. 38-20. *Avulsion of the popliteus tendon and fragment of the lateral condyle treated by compression screw fixation. A spiked washer (inset) is optional.*

Avulsion of the popliteus tendon with a fragment of the lateral condyle has been reported in a 3-year-old male husky.[27] We have treated this injury in a 5-month-old Irish setter. In both cases, the injury was chronic.

Clinical signs include weight-bearing lameness, muscle atrophy, and pain on manipulation of the joint. Radiographic examination reveals distal displacement of the popliteal sesamoid bone and a bone fragment positioned caudal to the point of attachment of the popliteus tendon. The lateral condyle is surgically exposed through a lateral approach. The biceps femoris muscle is reflected caudally to expose the lateral collateral ligament, the joint capsule, the popliteus tendon, and the lateral head of the gastrocnemius muscle. The tendon and the fracture segment are repositioned with a small cortical bone screw (2.7 or 3.5 mm) (Fig. 38-20). A spiked washer with the screw is optional.

ORIGIN OF THE GASTROCNEMIUS MUSCLE—LATERAL OR MEDIAL FABELLA. The lateral and medial fabellae articulate with and are bound by ligamentous tissue to the caudal aspect of the respective femoral condyles. Avulsion of the medial head of the gastrocnemius muscle and the medial fabella has been reported in a 7-year-old fox terrier.[11] Avulsion of the lateral fabella and head of the gastrocnemius muscle has been reported in a 5-year-old Alsatian.[31] We have treated avulsion of the lateral fabella in a 10-month-old Labrador retriever that jumped out of a moving truck. Both the Labrador retriever and the Alsatian exhibited hyperflexion of the

hock (dropped hock) with weight bearing. Radiographs of the stifle reveal distal displacement of the fabella on the affected side. Surgical reattachment of the fabella is essential to the return of normal function of the gastrocnemius muscle. The ligamentous tissue of the fabella and muscle are sutured, and an antitractional suture is placed around the fabella. A strand of carbon fiber was used to reinforce the repair in the Alsatian. We used a transarticular pin placed through the fabella and femur in addition to the sutures (Fig. 38-21). The pin subsequently broke and was replaced with a bone screw. The Labrador retriever gained almost immediate use of the limb following both operations. Proper immobilization of the limb is essential to the success of the procedure in large, active individuals.

INSERTION OF THE GASTROCNEMIUS TENDON—TUBER CALCANEI. The gastrocnemius muscle forms a major part of the common calcanean tendon (Achilles) and inserts on the proximal aspect of the tuber calcanei. Avulsion of the gastrocnemius tendon with a fracture of the tuber calcanei occurs primarily in immature dogs of the large breeds. In immature dogs, the entire epiphysis commonly fractures with the tendon. In mature dogs, only a small fragment of the epiphysis is observed with the tendon. The clinical signs are essentially the same as those observed with rupture of the musculotendinous junction or laceration of the tendon of the gastrocnemius muscle. The dog is unable forcibly to extend the tarsus, which drops into a hyperflexed position with weight bearing (dropped hock). Like the musculotendinous rupture, this condition may

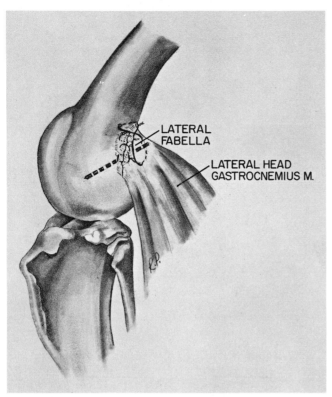

Fig. 38-21. *Avulsion of the lateral fabella treated by transarticular pinning, tension-band wiring, and suturing of the tendon of origin of the lateral head of the gastrocnemius muscle.*

occur bilaterally. Radiographs of the distal tibia and tarsus isolate the injury to the tendinosseous junction by revealing the avulsed fragment or epiphysis of the tuber calcanei. Lateral radiographs are most diagnostic.

Surgical reattachment of the avulsed tendon and bone is recommended. A caudolateral approach is made to the common calcanean tendon and the tuber calcanei. The lateral insertion of the superficial digital flexor tendon to the tuber calcanei is transected, and the superficial digital flexor tendon is retracted medially to expose the proximal end of the tuber calcanei and the tendon of the gastrocnemius muscle. When a substantial segment of bone has been avulsed, small pins and tension band wire are used to reattach the tendon and to fix the fracture. With a small fragment of bone, the tendon must be sutured to the tuber calcanei (Fig. 38-22). Stainless steel wire (4-0) is the preferred suture material. A Bunnell suture pattern is used to engage the tendon. With physeal fractures, the tuber calcanei frequently displaces or slips medially. The plantar ligament prevents proximal displacement. In these cases, simple suturing of the lateral supportive fascia is adequate to maintain reduction. The surgical procedure should be performed with minimal delay because contracture of the gastrocnemius muscle makes reapposition of the tendon more difficult and increases the incidence of failure. External and internal fixation procedures must be used to alleviate weight-bearing stresses on the gastrocnemius tendon.

OTHER TENDON AVULSIONS. We have treated others, but they are not discussed here because of the rarity of the problem and the similarity of the treatment to that already presented. These avulsions include: (1) Insertion of the triceps brachii tendon (medial head) with or without a fragment of the olecranon process; (2) Origin of the carpal and digital flexor tendons, avulsed with or without a fragment of the medial epicondyle of the humerus; (3) Insertion of the biceps brachii and brachialis tendons, with or without fragmentation of the

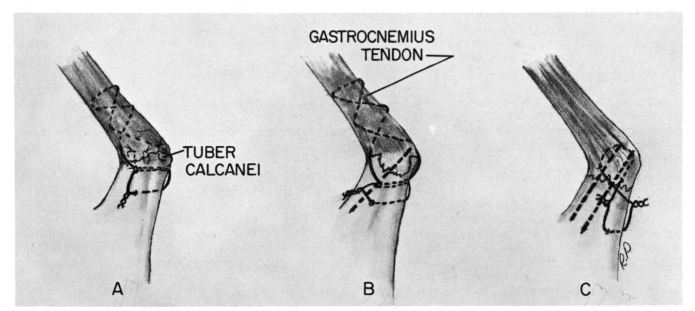

Fig. 38-22. *Avulsion-fracture of the gastrocnemius tendon and tuber calcanei. The superficial digital flexor tendon has been removed. A, The avulsed tendon is anchored to the tuber calcanei with a stainless steel wire using a modified Bunnell pattern. B, The avulsed tendon and small fragment of bone are treated with a Kirschner wire and modified Bunnell suture. C, The avulsion fracture of the tuber calcanei is stabilized with multiple Kirschner wires and tension-band wiring.*

proximal metaphysis of the ulna; and (4) Insertion of the extensor carpi radialis tendon, with or without a fragment from the proximal metaphysis of metacarpal bones II and III.

TENDON TRANSPOSITION

The action or function of a muscle can be transferred or altered by tendon transposition. The procedure is used in the treatment of joint dislocations and instabilities and in nerve paralysis, such as seen in hip dislocation, patella luxation, cranial cruciate rupture, and radial, sciatic, or peroneal nerve paralysis. The reader is referred to the chapters in this book on those specific conditions for further information.

TENDON DISPLACEMENT

Displacement of a tendon from its normal position can cause significant lameness and dysfunction. This condition has been reported with the tendons of the superficial digital flexor, biceps brachii, and long digital extensor muscles.

SUPERFICIAL DIGITAL FLEXOR TENDON. The superficial digital flexor forms part of the common calcanean tendon. It passes over the caudal aspect of the tuber calcanei, where it becomes broad and flat like a "cap." It is bound to the caudal aspect of the tuber calcanei by collateral insertions of dense connective tissue. An extensive synovial bursa, the bursa calcanea, lies between the superficial digital flexor tendon and the tuber calcanei and gastrocnemius tendon.

Displacement of the tendon of the superficial digital flexor muscle has been reported in mature dogs of the Shetland sheepdog, collie, greyhound, English setter, and terrier breeds.[2,32] Clinical signs include a weight-bearing lameness, palpable displacement of the tendon upon flexion of the tarsus, and tuber calcanei bursitis. The lateral collateral insertion usually ruptures, and the tendon displaces medially. Surgical repair of the collateral insertion restores normal use of the limb (Fig. 38-23).

TENDON OF ORIGIN OF THE BICEPS BRACHII. The tendon of origin of the biceps brachii muscle is held in the intertubercular groove by a transverse band of connective tissue that extends between the humeral tubercles. Medial displacement of the tendon has been reported in an 8-year-old border collie.[1] We have treated this condition in a 5-year-old miniature poodle. Clinical signs include a mild, intermittent lameness, palpable displacement of the tendon upon flexion of the shoulder, and cranial subluxation of the shoulder. Surgical treatment in the border collie consisted of passing a wire suture in a mattress pattern between the humeral tubercles to hold the tendon in place. We deepened the intertubercular groove and placed bone staples across this groove (Fig. 38-24).

TENDON OF ORIGIN OF THE LONG DIGITAL EXTENSOR. Caudal displacement of the long digital extensor from the muscular groove of the tibia has been reported in a year-old whippet with a malunion of the femoral shaft.[1]

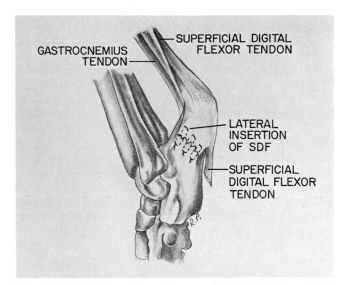

Fig. 38-23. *Medial luxation of the superficial digital flexor (SDF) tendon. The lateral retinacular tissue is sutured (plicated) in a horizontal mattress pattern.*

Clinical signs included a leg-carrying lameness and palpable displacement of the tendon upon flexion of the stifle. Surgical treatment involved placing a wire suture across the muscular groove of the tibia, to maintain the tendon in position.

Complex Muscle-Tendon Injuries

Complex muscle-tendon injuries involve more than one muscle and more than one area of the musculotendinous units. Upward or dorsal displacement of the scapula is the most common injury in this category.

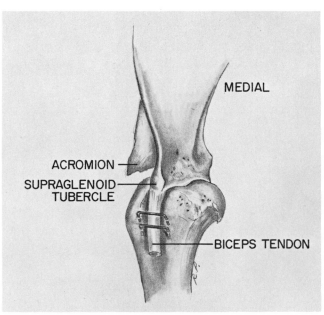

Fig. 38-24. *Dislocation of the biceps brachii tendon. The tendon is stabilized with two bone staples that bridge the intertubercular groove but do not bind the tendon.*

DORSAL DISPLACEMENT OF THE SCAPULA

The scapula is supported to the trunk primarily by the large, fan-shaped serratus ventralis muscle. Additional support and movement of the scapula are provided by the trapezius and rhomboideus muscles. Upward or dorsal displacement of the scapula occurs as a result of rupture or avulsion of the serratus ventralis muscle. Rupture of the trapezius and rhomboideus, teres major, and latissimus dorsi muscles and associated fractures of the scapula contribute to the instability. Mature dogs of medium and large breeds are most commonly affected. The history invariably reveals a traumatic origin, such as being hit by a car. The diagnosis is based on clinical signs of dorsal displacement of the scapula, which is evident upon weight bearing (Fig. 38-25). In some cases, the caudal border of the scapula is unstable and rotates laterally. The instability can be duplicated by manual manipulation of the limb and scapula. Radiographs may reveal fractures in association with the muscle avulsions. Stress radiographs demonstrate the displacement. Brachial plexus injury is not commonly associated with this injury, but a thorough neurologic examination should be conducted.

Surgical repair of the ruptured muscles provides the best results and is the recommended treatment. A caudolateral approach is made to the caudal and dorsal region of the scapula and the supportive muscles. Muscle segments are reapposed with mattress or cruciate sutures of 1-0 nylon. Avulsed muscles are sutured to the bone with stainless steel wire. Fracture segments are aligned and are stabilized by interfragmentary wiring. Postoperatively, the leg is placed in a flexion bandage for 2 to 3 weeks, and the dog's activity is controlled for 6 weeks. Chronic displacement of the scapula is treated in essentially the same manner. When the muscles cannot be reapposed by suturing, the scapula is wired to an underlying rib to maintain normal position.[17] Surgical treatment has resulted in a return to normal function in patients with both acute and chronic displacement.

Acknowledgment:

We wish to thank Mrs. Rhoda Pidgeon, A.M.I., for preparation of the illustrations.

References and Suggested Readings

1. Bennett, D., and Campbell, J. R.: Unusual soft tissue orthopaedic problems in the dog. J. Small Anim. Pract., 20:27, 1979.
2. Bernard, M. A.: Superficial digital flexor tendon injury in the dog. Can. Vet. J., 18:105, 1979.
3. Bloomberg, M. S., Hough, J. D., and Howard, D. R.: Repair of severed Achilles tendon in a dog: a case report. J. Am. Anim. Hosp. Assoc., 12:841, 1976.
4. Braden, T. D.: Fascia lata transplants for repair of chronic Achilles tendon defects. J. Am. Anim. Hosp. Assoc., 12:800, 1976.
5. Braden, T. D.: Tendons and muscles. In Current Techniques in Small Animal Surgery. Edited by M. J. Bojrab. Philadelphia: Lea & Febiger, 1975.
6. Braden, T. D.: Musculotendinous rupture of the Achilles apparatus and repair using internal fixation only. VM SAC, 69:729, 1974.
7. Braund, K. G.: Personal communication. Auburn University, Auburn, Alabama, 1980.

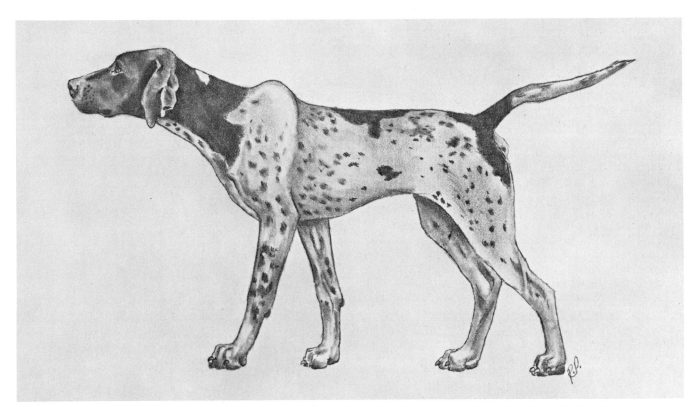

Fig. 38-25. *Upward luxation of the scapula. Characteristic deformity of the affected limb is observed with weight bearing.*

8. Bunnell, S.: Primary repair of severed tendons: the use of stainless steel wire. Am. J. Surg., *47*:502, 1940.

9. Butler, H. C.: Tendon, muscle and fascia. *In* Canine Surgery. 2nd Ed. Edited by J. Archibald. Santa Barbara, CA, American Veterinary Publications, 1974.

10. Caplan, H. S., Hunter, J. M., and Merklin, R. J.: Intrinsic vascularization of tendons. *In* American Academy of Orthopaedic Surgeons: Symposium on Tendon Surgery in the Hand. St. Louis, C. V. Mosby, 1975.

11. Chaffee, V. W., and Knecht, C. D.: Avulsion of the medial head of the gastrocnemius in the dog. VM SAC, *70*:929, 1975.

12. Evans, H. E., and Christensen, G. C.: Miller's Anatomy of the Dog. 2nd Ed. Philadelphia, W. B. Saunders, 1979.

13. Farrow, C. S.: Sprain, strain and contusion. Vet. Clin. North Am. *8*:169, 1979.

14. Gleeson, L. N.: Treatment of traumatic lesions of tendo-Achilles by joint fixation with a Stader splint. Vet. Med., *41*:442, 1946.

15. Ham, A. W.: Histology. 8th Ed. Philadelphia, J. B. Lippincott, 1980.

16. Hickman, J.: Greyhound injuries. J. Small Anim. Pract., *16*:455, 1975.

17. Hoerlein, B. F., Evans, L. E., and Davis, J. M.: Upward luxation of the canine scapula: a case report. J. Am. Vet. Med. Assoc., *136*:258, 1960.

18. Hufford, T., Olmstead, M. L., and Butler, H. C.: Contracture of the infraspinatus muscle and surgical correction in two dogs. J. Am. Anim. Hosp. Assoc., *11*:613, 1975.

19. Lammerding, J. J., Noser, G. A., Brinker, W. O., and Carrig, C. B.: Avulsion fracture of the origin of the extenser digitorum longis muscle in 3 dogs. J. Am. Anim. Hosp. Assoc., *12*:764, 1976.

20. Mason, M. L., and Allen, H. S.: The rate of healing of tendon. An experimental study of tensile strength. Ann. Surg., *113*:424, 1941.

21. O'Brien, T. J.: The use of DMSO in traumatic musculo-skeletal injuries in racing greyhounds. Anim. Hosp. *1*:272, 1965.

22. O'Donoghue, D. H.: Treatment of Injuries to Athletes. Philadelphia, W. B. Saunders, 1976.

23. Olmstead, M. L., and Butler, H. C.: Surgical correction of avulsion of the origin of the long digital extensor muscle in the dog: a case report. VM SAC, *71*:608, 1976.

24. Peacock, E. E., and Van Winkle, W. V.: Surgery and Biology of Wound Repair. Philadelphia, W. B. Saunders, 1970.

25. Piermattei, D. L., and Greely, R. G.: An Atlas of Surgical Approaches to the Bones of the Dog and Cat. 2nd Ed. Philadelphia, W. B. Saunders, 1979.

26. Pond, M. J.: Avulsion of the extensor digitorum longus muscle in the dog: a report of four cases. J. Small Anim. Pract., *14*:785, 1973.

27. Pond, M. J., and Losonsky, J. M.: Avulsion of the popliteus muscle in the dog: a case report. J. Am. Anim. Hosp. Assoc., *12*:60, 1976.

28. Smith, K. W.: Achilles tendon surgery for correction of hyperextension of the hock joint. J. Am. Anim. Hosp. Assoc., *12*:848, 1976.

29. Srugi, S., and Adamson, J. E.: A comparative study of tendon suture material in dogs. Plast. Reconstr. Surg., *50*:31, 1972.

30. Urbaniak, J. R., Cahill, J. D., and Mortenson, R. A.: Tendon suturing methods: analysis of tensile strength. *In* American Academy of Orthopaedic Surgeons: Symposium on Tendon Surgery in the Hand. St. Louis, C. V. Mosby, 1975.

31. Vaughan, L. C.: Muscle and tendon injuries in dogs. J. Small Anim. Pract., *20*:711, 1979.

32. Vaughn, L. C., and Faull, W. B.: Correction of a luxated superficial digital flexor tendon in a greyhound. Vet. Rec., *67*:335, 1955.

33. Vierheller, R. C.: Surgical repair of severed tendons and ligaments in the dog. Mod. Vet. Pract., *53*:35, 1972.

39 * Selected Procedures in Exotic Species

Onychectomy in the Exotic Feline

by JAMES PEDDIE

A current technique for onychectomy in exotic large cats is to remove the claw with its germinal tissue. One should retain the flexor process of the third phalanx to which the deep digital flexor tendon is attached. Amputating the claw in this manner preserves the normal anatomic and functional activities of the feline paw.

Surgical Technique

Anesthesia is induced with a combination of Ketamine hydrochloride, acepromazine maleate, and atropine sulfate. Endotrachael intubation and inhalant anesthesia are used to maintain an adequate depth of anesthesia. Surgical preparation consists of clipping the patient's hair on the nail sheath and liberally cleansing the extended claw with alcohol, to remove dirt and debris around the base of the nail.

An Esmarch tourniquet* is applied to the leg, starting at the paw and extending above the elbow on the foreleg and to above the hock on the rear leg. The proximal end of the Esmarch tourniquet is secured with a conventional tourniquet (Fig. 39-1A). After securing the proximal tourniquet, the Esmarch bandage is unwound to expose the paw up to the region of the carpus or the tarsus (Fig. 39-1B).

The claw is removed using a White's nail trimmer on the smaller exotic felids or a scalpel and a Gigli wire saw on the larger felids. Two cuts are made, both with the patient's nail extended (Fig. 39-1C). The first cut is on the dorsal surface of the digit at the articulation between the second and third phalanges. This articulation can be palpated as a depression proximal to the

nail bed on the dorsal surface of the digit. The second cut is made parallel to the bottom of the foot, to the depth of the first cut, forming a 90° angle at the point where the two cuts intersect (Fig. 39-1D). Care must be taken with the second cut to ensure that a margin of skin is excised with the claw. If this is not done, germinal nail tissue will remain and will lead to the development of scars and subsequent abscessation.

When the two cuts are made as described, the flexor process of the third phalanx, with its attaching deep digital flexor tendon, remains. Preservation of this structure results in a paw that is anatomically more correct and is better functioning. Several horizontal mattress sutures using an absorbable suture material are usually required to bring the edges of the skin flaps into apposition.

Bandages are applied to promote hemostasis and postoperative hygiene. Another objective of bandaging is to "milk" the skin of the digits distally down over the site of the amputation. A piece of two-inch tape, long enough to encircle the leg, is folded lengthwise so that the adhesive surface is exposed on both sides. The folded tape is placed loosely around the leg just proximal to the carpal or tarsal area. Tube gauze† is then applied by passing the foot and lower leg through the center of the applicator and by attaching the end of the gauze to the folded band of adhesive tape. With an assistant holding the gauze, anchoring it to the tape, firm, even pressure is applied to the gauze as it is pulled distally over the paw (Fig. 39-1D). The tube gauze is secured immediately distal to the paw by rotating the applicator. The applicator is returned with a loose application of gauze, and the previous steps are repeated three to six times. The direction of increasing tension is always distal. Elasticized tape‡ is then applied over the

---

*A tourniquet consisting of a piece of strong, flat rubber bandage that, when the blood has been forced from the limb, is wound about the proximal part of the limb to arrest circulation.

†Tubegauz, Scholl Mfg. Co., Inc., Chicago, IL 60610
‡Conform Tape, Kendall Co. Veterinary Products, One Federal Street, Boston, MA 02101

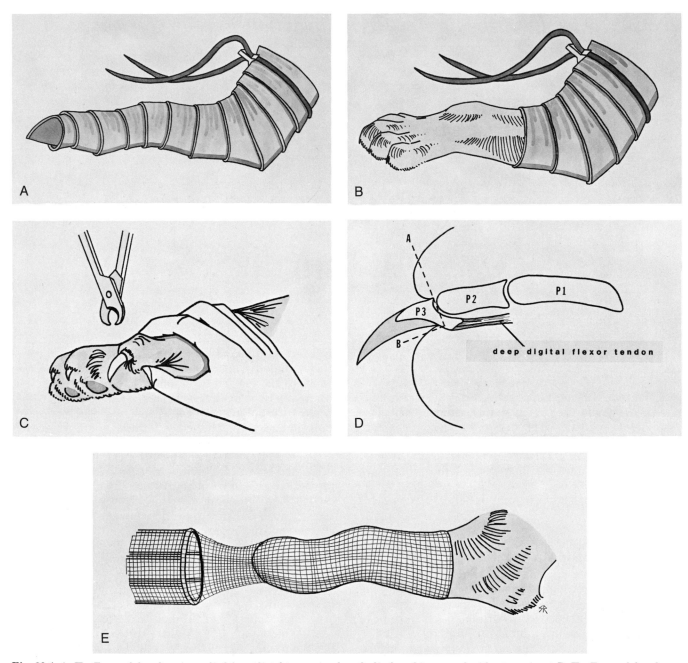

Fig. 39-1. A, *The Esmarch bandage is applied from distal to proximal on the limb and is secured with a tourniquet.* B, *The Esmarch bandage is unwound to expose the distal end of the limb.* C, *The claw is extended by applying pressure to the digital pad, and a White's nail trimmer is used to make the two cuts to remove the nail.* D, *The sequence, location, and angle of the two cuts used to remove the nail with its germinal tissue are illustrated by the lines A and B. Note that the flexor process of the third phalanx (P3), with its attachment of the deep digital flexor tendon, is left intact.* E, *Tube gauze of an approximate size is anchored proximally and is applied to the paw while continuous pressure is applied to milk the skin distally.*

gauze and is extended upward to attach to hair proximal to the gauze. Following this maneuver, the tourniquet should be removed; it is desirable to see a small amount of hemorrhage, which indicates adequate perfusion of the digits. If bleeding becomes profuse, one must reapply the tourniquet and retape the paw with slightly more pressure.

Postoperative care consists of an injection of benzathine penicillin G and the recommendations that: (1) the patient should be well bedded with dry sawdust or straw for the next 10 days; and (2) if the patient has not removed the bandages by the fifth postoperative day, the tape on the proximal end of the bandage should be cut, leaving the gauze intact; the patient usually removes the bandages prior to this time.

References and Suggested Readings

Fowler, M. E.: Zoo and Wild Animal Medicine. Philadelphia, W. B. Saunders, 1978.

Stunkard, J. A., and Miller, J. C.: An outline guide to general anesthesia in exotic species. VM, SAC, *69*:1181, 1974.

Avian Surgery

by ROBERT D. ZENOBLE

Restraint and Physical Examination of Pet Birds

An avian patient presented to a veterinarian should be brought to the office in its own cage if possible. The cage volume and bar spacing should be examined for proper proportion to the bird. The character and number of droppings should be noted because the number of stools per day is a reflection of food intake. The food cup should be observed for the type of food. Inexperienced owners do not realize that birds often drop the seed hulls into the food container, so that the seed cup appears full even though all the seed has been eaten. Cuttlebone should be positioned so the soft side is toward the bird. Grit is not necessary for the pet bird's health. Sandpaper-covered perches are not recommended because of irritation to the feet. The presence of too many toys and other objects in the cage can prevent the bird from moving freely around without damaging its feathers.

Before the patient is removed from the cage, it should be observed as it stands quietly. The bird's general appearance should be noted. A depressed bird stands quietly and allows its eyelids to close partially. The feathers may be ruffled. The rate and depth of ventilation should be assessed. A healthy bird breathes quietly, and any respiratory sounds should be considered abnormal. Any bird that stands on the floor of the cage instead of its perch is judged to be weak and in a critical state of poor health.

Before any bird is removed from its cage, the room door should be closed and window curtains should be drawn, to prevent an escaped bird from flying from the door or into window glass. Removal from its cage can be frightening and stressful to the bird. If the bird is tame, the owner should remove the bird. Many owners are inexperienced, however, and should not be allowed to catch the bird. All perches and toys should be taken out of the cage before attempting to remove the bird. Small birds such as parakeets, finches, cockatiels, and mynah birds should be caught with the bare hands. If the room lights are darkened, small birds can be quickly caught without excessive flight around the cage (Fig. 39-2).

Parrots should be caught using a lightweight glove or a light towel. The bird should be pinned against the side of the cage. The head should be grasped quickly from behind and should be held firmly by the lower beak. The head is held by the mandible between the thumb and forefinger (Fig. 39-3). One should not restrict the movement of the sternum. Because a bird does not have a diaphragm, restricting sternal movement can be dangerous (Figs. 39-2 and 39-3). The wings should be quickly grasped or wrapped in the towel to prevent damage by the excited bird. Cockatoos and macaws should be approached cautiously and gloves should be used because these larger birds can seriously injure the careless handler (Fig. 39-4).

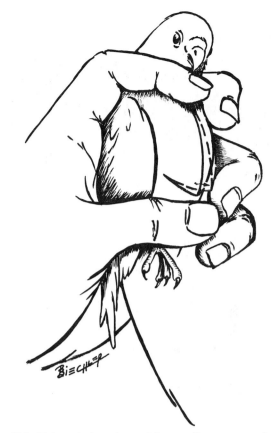

Fig. 39-2. *This technique is used for small, nonaggressive birds. Note that sternal movement is not restricted. (Courtesy of Iowa State University Veterinarian and Dr. D. Graham.)*

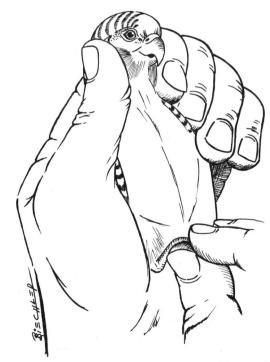

Fig. 39-3. *To hold a bird's head securely, one should grasp the lower mandible between the forefinger and thumb.*

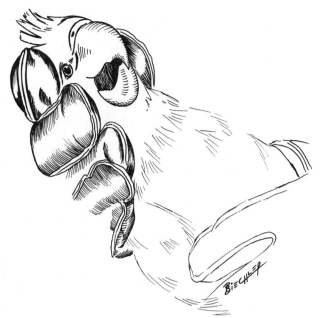

Fig. 39-4. *Large birds should be held with gloves. One should hold the head by the mandible in one hand and control the feet and wings with the other hand. A towel wrapped around the body is excellent for preventing wing feather damage and for protecting the handler from the claws.*

The physical examination should be gentle, quick, and thorough. The first assessment is the strength of the bird. A normal bird struggles when caught, whereas a sick bird is subdued. Weight loss should be judged from palpating the breast musculature. It can be quickly determined that a bird is in critical condition from marked breast-muscle wasting and a prominent keel. One should observe the eyes for conjunctivitis, corneal ulcers, pox lesions, and swelling of the periorbital tissue (sinusitis). The nares should be examined for discharges. The cere and commissure of the mouth are prime sites of Knemidokoptes mite infestation in the parakeet. (See the discussion later in this chapter.) The oral cavity should be examined for abscesses and plaque lesions of hypovitaminosis A. The commissure of the mouth should be examined for pox lesions and for proliferative, hyperkeratic lesions caused by mites. The abdomen should be palpated for the swelling of ascites and for firm distension suggesting a tumor. The vent should be examined for evidence of soiling of feathers indicating diarrhea.

The patient's legs and feet should be examined for Knemidokoptes mite lesions, evidence of articular gout, uneven wearing of scale tissue, bacterial infection, or calluses on toes.

The body should be rotated, and the dorsal and ventral aspects of the wing should be examined, along with the back of the body. Auscultating of the heart, lungs, and air sac may be attempted in larger birds. It is difficult to assess the pulmonary system and the air sacs accurately by auscultation alone. After a complete physical examination, the bird should be carefully released into its cage.

Preoperative Preparation

The avian patient should not be fasted prior to anesthesia. Feathers should be plucked and not cut. Empty feather follicles regrow feathers quickly, whereas cut feathers are replaced only at the normal molting time. Avian skin is thin and fragile. The skin should be gently washed and not scrubbed. Using large amounts of water should be avoided because it cools the bird's body temperature. A weak iodine solution should be used to disinfect the skin. A lightweight drape should be used to maintain sterility. It is, in fact, difficult to maintain optimum surgical sterility in a small patient, but aseptic surgical techniques should be attempted in all instances.

Blood collection can be safe and simple. The most practical and least stressful method of blood collection is cutting a toenail short and allowing the blood to drip into a capillary tube or collection vial treated with heparin. A styptic powder, such as ferric subsulfate or silver nitrate, can be packed into the end of the nail when it has been wiped free of blood (Fig. 39-5).

Surgical Equipment

Fingers are often too large for accurate manipulation in small birds. Ophthalmic instruments, including thumb forceps, strabismus scissors, an orbital speculum, and fixation clamps can be used. Sterile applicator sticks and cotton-tipped swabs are useful for applying disinfectants, for maintaining surgical hemostasis, and for sponging capillary blood. Gelfoam* absorbable gelatin sponge is also useful for hemostasis. Suture material should be absorbable and of small caliber (3-0 to 5-0). Electrocautery can be used for hemostasis, but excessive damage is difficult to prevent.

*Upjohn Co., Kalamazoo, MI

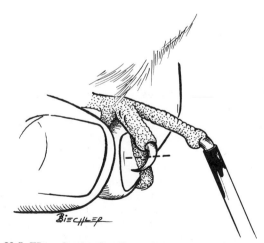

Fig. 39-5. *When elongated nails are trimmed, one should avoid cutting the blood vessel. When collecting blood, one should cut the vessel within the nail and collect the blood in a heparinized capillary tube. One should not hold the leg tightly enough to impede blood flow. The bird should be observed for bleeding when it has been returned to the cage.*

Anesthesia

Before a bird is anesthetized, it must be concluded that potential benefits outweigh possible risks. Birds apparently have a high tolerance to pain, and simple procedures should be conducted with manual restraint only.

Birds should not be fasted before anesthesia because hypoglycemia can occur rapidly in small avian species. Anesthesia should not be performed on a debilitated bird, if possible. Nutrition and energy should be provided by tube feeding preoperatively if the patient is anoretic. Fluids can be easily administered subcutaneously to combat dehydration. Loss of body heat is considerable during anesthesia. Heating pads during operation and heated recovery cages postoperatively are necessary.

Atropine may be administered at the dose of 0.04 to 0.1 mg/kg or 0.0012 to 0.003 mg/30 g to decrease respiratory secretions. Atropine is not necessary for short procedures.

In medium-sized and large birds, an endotracheal tube should be placed for all but short diagnostic procedures. The tracheal opening is easily identified in the bird's mouth, and intubation is simple. A small endotracheal tube or polyethylene tubing attached to an endotracheal tube adapter can be used on birds larger than cockatiels. If the bird is too small for intubation, its head can be kept elevated to prevent refluxed crop fluid from being aspirated. A cotton-tipped swab can be used to absorb accumulated fluid away from the tracheal opening.

Ketamine hydrochloride is widely used and is safe for anesthesia in caged birds. The advantages of this agent are that it is safe, one may administer more of it if a deeper plane of anesthesia is needed, and anesthetic induction is smooth. The disadvantages of ketamine are that its duration is variable, it is a poor muscle relaxant, and it stimulates fluttering and tremors. Suggested intramuscular dosages of ketamine are .03 to .05 mg/g and 10 to 25 mg/kg. Examples of doses for various species are: parakeet, 1 to 3 mg; cockatiel, 3 to 5 mg; parrot, 10 to 20 mg, and macaw, 15 to 45 mg. The drug is injected into the bird's pectoral muscle with a 25-gauge needle. Induction takes 3 to 5 minutes, and anesthesia lasts 10 to 30 minutes. Recovery time is variable and may take from 30 minutes to several hours. The patient's recovery from anesthesia is often associated with uncoordinated flapping of wings and righting attempts. Xylazine hydrochloride* (20 mg/ml) can be mixed with ketamine hydrochloride in a 1 : 1 ratio by volume, and this combined product can be used as general anesthesia. Xylazine reduces the vigorous, uncoordinated recovery resulting from ketamine alone. The dosage for the xylazine-ketamine combination is calculated from the ketamine in the product at a 50% reduction of the dosage previously given.

To decrease excitement during recovery, one should

wrap the patient in tissue paper and lightly tape it. One should allow the patient to recover in a quiet, darkened room. The bird lies quietly until it is awake and then wiggles out of the paper wrap. By that time, the bird is able to stand and perch.

Inhalation anesthesia is frequently used on avian patients. Halothane has the advantage of rapid induction and recovery time. Induction may be easily accomplished within 1 to 4 minutes using a face mask or an anesthesia box. An endotracheal tube is then placed, and anesthesia is maintained on a nonrebreathing system at 0.5 to 1.0-liter-per-minute flow of oxygen and a concentration of 0.5% to 1.5% of halothane. Recovery on 100% oxygen usually takes 3 to 8 minutes.

Methoxyflurane can also be used successfully to anesthetize birds. The induction and recovery times are longer than for halothane. Induction requires a 3 to 4% concentration with a 2 to 3-liter-per-minute oxygen flow. Maintenance requires a 1.5% to 2% concentration with a .5 to 1.0-liter-per-minute oxygen flow. Methoxyflurane is the agent I prefer for chemical restraint of birds for short diagnostic or surgical procedures. One should saturate a tiny piece of cotton with methoxyflurane, put it into a paper cup (or syringe barrel for smaller birds), and force the bird's head into the cup. This method of induction requires several minutes; when the bird's eyelids just begin to remain closed, one should remove the cup for 5 to 15 seconds at a time. Manual restraint must be maintained with this method because the bird seemingly can go from being anesthetized to being "wide awake" within seconds. This method may be used for examination, drawing blood, radiologic examination, and short surgical procedures.

Common Surgical Conditions and Treatment

INTEGUMENTARY DISORDERS AND PROCEDURES

BROKEN FEATHERS. Confinement in a cage that is too small results in damaged feathers. The feathers break as they strike the sides of the cage. Whereas damaged feathers mar the appearance of the bird, they are generally not harmful to its health and are replaced as the bird molts. If the bird continually picks at a broken flight feather, it should be removed by plucking it out. The feather should be pulled in the direction of growth. General anesthesia is seldom required.

HEMORRHAGING FROM FEATHERS. If a feather is in the process of growing and the quill is cracked or broken to the depth of the papilla, hemorrhage results. The affected feather shaft should be pulled from its follicle by gentle traction. The broken blood vessel retracts into the follicle and clots.

CLIPPING WING FEATHERS TO CONTROL FLIGHT. If a bird's flight is to be restricted for a short training period (6 to 8 weeks), the feathers should be plucked; new feathers soon regrow. If feathers are cut, then a new feather will not replace the cut feather until the bird molts (up to 6 months to a year).

*Rompun, Haver-Lockhart, Cutter Laboratories, Inc., Shawnee, KS 66201

Clipping feathers can be done so that the defect is least noticeable. On the upper and lower surfaces of the wing are overlapping feathers that cover the quills of the primary and secondary flight feathers. These are called contour feathers, and help to complete the flight surface. One should not cut these feathers, but rather one should lift them up or brush them aside to reveal the underlying quills of the flight feathers. All secondary flight feathers should be cut at the quill; the primary flight feathers are also cut, except for the last three feathers at the tip of the wing. Leaving the feathers at the tip gives the bird a normal appearance while standing. This clipping procedure should be performed on one wing only. The bird can still jump and fly short distances but its flight is uncoordinated and it can be easily caught. If a growing feather is cut and bleeds, one should pluck that quill (Fig. 39-6).

FEATHER CYSTS AND EPIDERMAL INCLUSION CYSTS. These manifest as focal, nonpainful swellings. The cyst should be incised, and the contents should be gently removed. The lining should be removed or cauterized.

CUTANEOUS AND SUBCUTANEOUS NEOPLASIA. Lipomas and lipogranulomas are common benign subcutaneous tumors. Benign tumors usually have a soft consistency, are well circumscribed, and shell out easily during a surgical procedure. Grossly, they are difficult to differentiate from cysts, granulomas, or abscesses. Malignant tumors such as fibrosarcomas and adenocarcinomas may be found and are usually firm, broad-based, and difficult to excise surgically. A swelling of the uropygeal gland (preen gland) could result from ductal obstruction, abscess, or neoplasia. The uropygeal gland is a common site of benign papillomas and malignant adenocarcinomas.

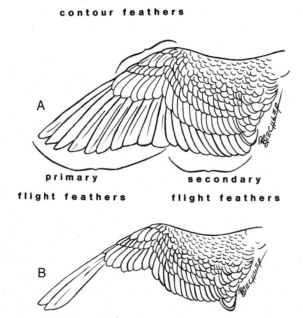

contour feathers

A

primary
flight feathers

secondary
flight feathers

B

Fig. 39-6. A, *When clipping wing feathers to restrict flight, one should cut only the primary and secondary feathers as illustrated. B, A more natural appearance is maintained if the last two to three feathers are not removed.*

SUBCUTANEOUS EMPHYSEMA. This condition may result from a ruptured air sac or a broken pneumatic bone. The air should be aspirated only if the amount is great and distressful to the bird. The ruptured air sac usually seals spontaneously.

TIGHT LEG BAND. Lameness and even ischemic necrosis of the foot may result from a tight leg band. These bands should be cut off carefully.

ELONGATED TOENAILS. Most birds do not require trimming of toenails. In parakeets, the blood vessel can usually be seen, and the nail may be clipped safely. The blood vessel extends far into the nail's length; therefore, pigmented nails should be shortened in small, gradual clips to avoid excessive bleeding. Styptic powder or a similar agent can be used to aid coagulation. The use of sandpaper-covered perches to keep nails trimmed should be discouraged because of excessive trauma to the surface of the bird's foot.

LAMENESS DUE TO FOOT TRAUMA. The undersurface of the foot is sensitive, and if erythema and inflammation is found, the perches should be padded and should be covered with soft tissue paper until the inflammation resolves.

DISEASES OF THE CERE. The scaly-face mite (Knemidokoptes pilae) is common in the parakeet and the canary. The mite attacks the nonfeathered parts of the bird: cere, skin surrounding the beak and eyelids, legs, and cloacal opening. The mite spends its entire life cycle on the host, burrowing into the skin and keratinized tissue. The lesion has a characteristic honeycomb appearance. Occasionally, the proliferation of keratin at these sites causes the owner to think there are fungal or neoplastic growths on the cere or legs. The diagnosis is confirmed by identifying the mite on skin scraping. In advanced cases, the mite injures the germinal part of the upper beak and causes distorted growth that may result in malocclusion.

Treatment for Knemidokoptes infestation involves the topical application of benzoate crotamiton* or mineral oil. Orthophenylphenol and rotenone† is occasionally toxic to individual birds. Mineral oil or Eurax is applied in small amounts to the lesions; it fills the burrows and thereby kills the mites. Crusts gradually soften and flake away. The owner should apply medication 2 to 3 times weekly for 4 to 5 weeks. The owner should observe the bird for months following treatment and should reinstitute treatment if new lesions are seen. If mites are found in one area, other nonfeathered areas should be continually examined for lesions. If excessive oily material is applied to the lesions, the bird will wipe the oil onto its wings and will coat the feathers. To avoid this potentially severe complication, one should use only small amounts of medication at each application.

Brown hypertrophy of the cere is a poorly understood problem of female parakeets in which the normally brown cere becomes thickened with accumu-

*Eurax, Westwood Pharmaceuticals, Inc., 468 Dewitt Street, Buffalo, NY 14213

†Goodwinol ointment, Goodwinol Products Corp., Huntington Station, NY 11746

lated keratin. This condition is benign, but removal of the excessive keratin can be attempted by first applying mineral oil to soften the keratinous material and then gently flaking away the layers of keratin.

TRIMMING BEAKS. Two types of beaks are found in pet birds. The soft-billed birds and the nonpsittacine seed-eating species have straight bills of varying length, with the upper mandible overlapping the lower. The second type is the hooked, heavy bill seen in seed-eating psittacines.

The most common deformity is simple overgrowth resulting from malocclusion. In the soft-billed and nonpsittacine seed-eaters, overgrowth occurs at the tip and along the nonoccluding edges of the upper mandible. This is easily trimmed with a pair of cuticle nippers. Problems of malocclusion occur more frequently in the psittacine species. In parrots and large psittacines, both the point of the bill and the lateral edges must be trimmed if they are overgrown. In birds with a light-colored beak, the line of demarcation between the vascular and avascular portions of the beak can be seen when the bird is held between the examiner's eye and a bright light source (transillumination). Trimming should be done as frequently as necessary. Should hemorrhage occur, it can be controlled with ferric subsulfate solution.

RESPIRATORY DISORDERS

Surgical treatment is not generally indicated for avian respiratory disorders. Sinusitis is common in cage birds, however, and occasionally results in abscess formation close to the eye or cere. Signs include periorbital swelling, closure of the lid(s), and nasal discharge. Because purulent material in birds is caseous and does not flow from an incised abscess, it must be curetted from the abscess. The base of the abscess should be carefully cauterized. Culture and sensitivity tests of the exudate and treatment with the appropriate antibiotic are indicated.

Birds may be presented to the veterinarian for dyspnea secondary to abdominal distension. Ascites, abdominal tumors, and retained eggs are conditions that cause dyspnea without primary involvement of the respiratory system. A general examination should be given to any bird with dyspnea in order to rule out abdominal disease.

DIGESTIVE TRACT DISORDERS

MOUTH LESIONS. Small, papilloma-like lesions at the commissures of the mouth may be true papillomas or pox lesions. Pox lesions usually regress spontaneously, but can serve as a source of pathogenic bacteria that may cause fatal septicemia. Knemidokoptes mites cause hyperkeratosis and small nodules of keratin at the commissure of the mouth. These lesions slough off as the mite infestation is treated. (See the previous discussion of diseases of the cere.)

Lingual and palatine abscesses are seen in large psittacine birds such as parrots. They are a sequela to upper respiratory infection and hypovitaminosis A. These lesions may interfere with prehension of food and mastication. Treatment requires surgical curettage and antibiotic therapy. Proper diet is essential to prevent symptoms of hypovitaminosis A. Candida albicans frequently colonizes abscesses. Drug therapy should be used to eliminate this opportunist if it is present.

CROP FISTULAS. Crop fistulas can result from lacerations or pressure necrosis and require surgical correction. The edges of the crop fistula must be debrided and sutured together. The skin should be sutured if it is a fresh, clean wound. If infection is well established, the skin laceration should be left open.

Although a surgical procedure may be required to relieve crop impaction, such an impaction is often relieved by lavage and gentle external massage.

ABDOMINAL SURGICAL CONSIDERATIONS

DIAGNOSTIC CELIOTOMY. Abdominal distension can result from ascites, retained egg, neoplasms, and egg-yolk peritonitis. Accurate diagnoses, prognoses, and therapy of intra-abdominal disease often require celiotomy.

The approach for celiotomy offering the greatest intra-abdominal exposure is a transverse incision halfway between the caudal end of the sternum and the cloacal opening. The incision can extend from one leg to the other. As the combined abdominal muscles and peritoneum are incised, care should be taken not to lacerate the underlying viscera. Although it is necessary to rupture the abdominal air sacs, one should attempt to maintain as much air sac integrity as possible. The extent of air sac disruption depends on the type of procedure performed. The abdomen is closed with two suture lines. The peritoneum and abdominal muscles are closed with a simple continuous suture using 3-0 to 5-0 polyglycolic acid or chromic gut. The skin is closed in the same manner.

EGG-BOUND BIRDS. An egg-bound bird should always be radiographed because more than one egg may be in the oviduct. If an egg is in the oviduct and is not presented into the cloaca and the patient is not stressed, medical therapy (cloacal lubrication, heated cage, force feeding) should be tried before considering surgical treatment. If the egg has not been presented in 24 to 48 hours, surgical intervention should be considered. If the oviduct and egg have prolapsed through the cloaca, the length of time the oviduct tissue has been exposed determines the correction. If the prolapsed oviduct is fresh, without drying of tissues, the exposed tissue should be cleansed with antibiotic ointment. A small incision is made in the least vascular area over the pole of the egg. The incision should be gently dilated with an instrument, and the oviduct should be separated from the surface of the egg. Gentle digital pressure behind the egg forces it through the opening. Once the egg has been removed, the incision is sutured, and the oviduct is placed back into the cloaca. One should attempt to replace the prolapsed oviduct back through the oviduct-cloacal opening.

If the oviduct has been prolapsed and shows severe drying and damaged tissue, the devitalized tissue must be excised. This devitalized tissue may be adhered to the egg and must be removed with it. The remaining oviduct should be sutured and replaced into the cloaca. If the defect is too large to suture, one should replace the oviduct without suturing. The bird should receive systemic antibiotics during the recovery period.

If the egg is in the cloaca or at the oviduct-cloacal opening, dilation of these structures occasionally permits passage of the egg. If dilation is inadequate and the shell membranes can be visualized through the orifice, the contents of the egg should be aspirated with an 18-gauge needle and syringe. The eggshell can be gently compacted by digital pressure through the abdominal wall. The egg compresses, with particles of shell clinging to the shell membrane, and it can be withdrawn through the cloaca with small forceps. Lubrication should be used to prevent damage to the oviduct mucosa. The oviduct should be irrigated with warm saline solution to remove all pieces of eggshell and to avoid egg-yolk peritonitis. All these techniques can be performed without anesthesia. These patients are severely stressed, and anesthesia adds a significant risk.

If the egg cannot be removed as described, celiotomy is performed. An incision over the egg through the oviduct easily produces the egg, and the incision is sutured. If necrosis of the oviduct is present, the oviduct and ovary are removed.

PROLAPSED OVIDUCT OR INTESTINE. Prolapse of the oviduct or the intestine may result from tenesmus. The underlying cause may be the patient is egg-bound, or it may be parasitic, enteritic, or idiopathic. The prolapsed tissue should be cleansed, lubricated, and covered with a topical anesthetic cream to reduce sensation. One should place a pursestring suture in the cloacal ring. This suture should be tight enough to prevent prolapse but loose enough to permit the passage of droppings. The suture can be left in place for several days. Systemic antibiotics should be administered for 5 to 7 days.

EMERGENCY CONDITIONS

CONCUSSION. Birds fly directly into window glass, and severe neurologic damage may result. The prognosis is grave if the bird does not recover within several hours. The bird should be kept warm and cushioned during recovery. Steroid therapy is suggested, but its value is uncertain.

DYSPNEA. A bird showing dyspnea is in critical condition. The bird should be kept quiet and undisturbed. Oxygen therapy may be of value. Extreme dyspnea (acute) is often caused by nonrespiratory disease such as abdominal distension from ascites or abdominal masses.

HEMORRHAGING FEATHERS. Acute hemorrhaging is often due to broken feathers. Birds should be treated immediately by plucking the affected feathers.

SEVERE DEBILITATION. A bird showing weakness and emaciation is in critical condition and must be handled carefully. Heat and other supportive care is needed before the diagnostic workup is instituted.

Postoperative Care

After a surgical procedure, the avian patient should be wrapped in tissue paper, kept in a dark, warm (27 to 30° C), quiet area, and allowed to recover slowly. Larger parrots anesthetized with inhalation agents can be held in a nurse's arms until recovered. As soon as the patient can stand on a perch, food should be replaced in the cage.

Birds healthy before the anesthetic episode usually begin to eat soon after recovering from anesthesia. If the bird was ill prior to anesthesia and does not eat after recovering from anesthesia, tube feeding should be begun in 2 to 4 hours. A "wait and see" approach to feeding an anoretic bird is dangerous.

General principles of mammalian antibiotic therapy should be followed in birds. Antibiotic therapy is suggested for established infections, in certain orthopedic procedures, for abscesses, and for surgical procedures of the gastrointestinal tract. Antibiotic therapy is not needed for routine procedures. Although most antibiotics are safe in birds, active therapeutic blood and tissue levels have not been adequately documented. The doses used are empirical. Oral administration is more practical than injectable therapy, unless the veterinarian is familiar with microdose equipment and techniques. Antibiotics can be administered in drinking water, but consumption is hard to assess. Some avian species originate from arid areas and normally drink only small amounts of water. Examples of antibiotics and selected dosages are provided in Table 39-1.

Hospital Techniques

Hospitalized birds must be provided with additional heat, either by heat lamps or by using human infant

Table 39-1. *Antibiotics in Avian Practice*

Oral	
Chloramphenicol palmitate (150 mg/5 ml)	100 mg/kg tid
Ampicillin	150-200 mg/kg tid
Cephalexin (Keflex) (250 mg/5 ml)	35-50 mg/kg qid
Injectable	
Gentamicin	.5 mg/30 g bid
Chloramphenicol succinate	100 mg/kg tid
Cephalothin	100 mg/kg qid
Dissolved in Drinking Water	
Tylosin plus vitamins (400 mg/tsp)	1 tsp/5 oz water
Erythromycin (450 mg/tsp)	1 tsp/pt water
Chloramphenicol succinate (100 mg/ml)	6 drops/oz water

incubators as cages. The temperature should be kept at 27 to 30° C. Fresh food should be supplied daily, in the form of seed, peanuts, fruits, and vegetables. The cage is cleaned daily so that consumed seed can be estimated by discarded seed hulls. The number of stools produced daily is roughly related to food intake. If a bird is not eating well, it should be weighed daily.

Force-feeding is important supportive care in avian medicine. Even if a bird appears to be eating adequate amounts, if its weight is decreasing, tube feeding is necessary. Patients that are underweight but are eating and are maintaining weight may not require force-feeding. Approximate weights of common cage birds are as follows: parakeet, 30 g; cockatiel, 100 g; Amazon parrot, 325 to 500 g; and macaw, 600 to 1000 g. Feeding tubes 5 French in diameter are recommended for parakeets and canaries; 10-French tubes are recommended for cockatiels and medium-sized parrots; and 15-French tubes are suggested for large parrots and macaws. A speculum may be necessary to pass a tube in large species. The bird should be gently restrained while the tube is passed, and the material is gently deposited into the crop. Accidental passage into the trachea is possible but unlikely. One should not overfill or palpate the crop after feeding.

A thick solution of protein nutritional supplement* and a milk-free soy formula† provide practical diets for tube feeding. Alternate foods are blended baby cereals or domestic chicken starter ration. Birds should be fed 2 to 3 times daily, depending on weight loss. Parakeets can be fed 1 to 2 ml, cockatiels 3 to 4 ml, average parrots 10 ml, large parrots 15 to 30 ml, and macaws up to 35 to 50 ml at each feeding.

Oral antibiotics can be easily administered by cutting and smoothing the tip of an 18-gauge needle. The bird can be allowed to bite the needle while the antibiotic is slowly given orally. This technique can be effective for home care.

References and Suggested Readings

Altman, R. B.: General principles of avian surgery. Compend. Contin. Ed. Practicing Vet., *3*:177, 1981.

Altman, R. B.: Avian anesthesia. Compend. Contin. Ed. Practicing Vet., *2*:38, 1980.

Ensley, P.: Caged bird medicine and husbandry. Vet. Clin. North Am., *9*:499, 1979.

Fowler, M. E. (ed.): Diseases of caged birds and exotic pets. *In* Current Veterinary Therapy VII. Edited by R. W. Kirk. Philadelphia, W. B. Saunders, 1980.

Fowler, M. E. (ed.): Zoo and Wild Animal Medicine. Philadelphia, W. B. Saunders, 1978.

Petrak, M. L. (ed.): Diseases of Cage and Aviary Birds. 2nd Ed. Philadelphia, Lea & Febiger, 1982.

Steiner, C. V., Jr., and Davis, R. B. (eds.): Caged Bird Medicine. Ames, Iowa State University Press, 1981.

*Gerval, Lederle Laboratories, Division of American Cyanamid Co., Berdan Avenue, Wayne, NJ 07470

†Neo-Mull-Soy, Syntex Laboratories, Inc., 3401 Hillview Avenue, Palo Alto, CA 94304

Adjunct Surgical Techniques for Avian Surgery

by Nancy A. Leiting

Avian surgery differs from mammalian surgery in several aspects, including the need to maintain the high avian body temperature during operation, the importance of hemostasis, and the absolute need to minimize stress in any other form. The technique of clamping and then incising tissue can be employed to remove superficial tumors and abscesses and to facilitate dissection in major abdominal surgical procedures.

In preoperative preparation, a vitamin K supplement is administered to facilitate clotting, because many companion birds are deficient in this vitamin, owing to improper nutrition. If feasible, the bird is given therapeutic doses of an oral vitamin supplement in its drinking water for a week before an elective procedure.‡ Intramuscular injections of vitamin K are also useful.

The sterile surgical pack consists of cotton-tipped swabs, 2- by 2-inch gauze sponges, curved and straight mosquito forceps, and fine-pointed scissors. The surgical site is prepared by plucking the feathers one at a time, by applying traction in the same direction as their growth. This is done with care so as not to tear the bird's paper-thin skin. A surgical scrubbing agent is not used because most are too irritating to avian skin. Instead, a gauze sponge soaked in warm water is used to remove superficial debris from the skin. The use of alcohol is contraindicated because it serves to increase heat loss from the skin. A dilute aqueous iodine solution may be used to promote local antisepsis. Heat loss is of utmost concern, owing to the normally high avian body temperature (40 to 43°C), and a heating pad should be placed under the patient during prolonged procedures.

Before an incision is made, such as around a mass on the wing (Fig. 39-7A), the skin is clamped with a straight mosquito hemostat (Fig. 39-7B). The hemostat is left in place for approximately 10 seconds to crush skin capillaries. The hemostat is then removed, and a scissor incision follows in the line of the crushed tissue (Fig. 39-7C and D). If a larger incision is required, the original incision can be lengthened by placing one jaw of the hemostat above the skin and the other jaw between the skin and the underlying tissue. The crush and incision processes are then repeated.

The nature of the mass, its vascularity, and the configuration of the attachment determine how it must be removed. Many subcutaneous lipomas are quickly peeled out with blunt dissections. If a pedicle attachment is present, a hemostat is placed on the stalk of tissue, which is then ligated with 3-0 or 4-0 chromic gut suture material. Wide-based tumors are crushed then excised, if possible, according to the technique outlined in the previous paragraph. Because hemostasis is

‡Avitron, Lambert-Kay Laboratories, Division Carter-Wallace, Cranbury, NJ 08512. Apply 16 to 18 drops per tablespoon of drinking water.

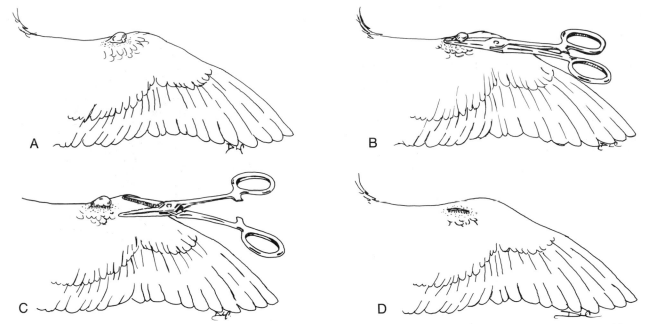

Fig. 39-7. A, *An abcess or tumor on the lateral aspect of a wing. The site is prepared for operation by gently removing the feathers adjacent to and surrounding the growth. B, The thin skin is clamped with a mosquito hemostat. C, The hemostat is removed; the clamped area is easily discernible from the mass and the unclamped skin. D, The skin is incised along the creases left by the hemostat. Suturing of the incised skin is easily performed and does not retard healing.*

of the utmost importance, clamping and ligation of all vessels are mandatory. Even slight capillary oozing should not be left to clot on its own. A cotton-tipped swab soaked in epinephrine (1 : 1000 without lidocaine) and direct pressure should be applied to the area until the seepage ceases. Subcutaneous sutures are not required. A simple continuous pattern using a fine, taper-point needle with swaged-on 4-0 chromic gut suture is used to close the skin.

Oral antibiotics may be given for 5 to 7 days postoperatively when the procedure involves a contaminated wound or abscess. Ointment or cream should not be applied to any avian wound, whether sutured or not, because this type of medication causes the feathers to be "glued together" and thereby prevents the feathers from performing a major function of retaining body heat. Antibiotic powders designed for application to mammalian wounds are also contraindicated. Such topical medications are rarely necessary because the naturally high body temperature of birds deters postoperative infection. Sutures are absorbed within 10 to 14 days of the surgical procedure.

Complications of avian surgical procedures consist of: excessive heat loss resulting in a prolonged recovery time; excessive blood loss causing the demise of the patient; and tearing of the skin during the passage of suture needles. These factors are controlled by the veterinarian's consideration of operative detail and careful surgical technique.

References and Suggested Readings

Brownell, J. R.: Diagnosis and Treatment of Caged Bird Diseases in the Veterinary Practice. Ames, Iowa State University Press, 1968.

Fowler, M. E.: Restraint and Handling of Wild and Domestic Animals. Ames, Iowa State University Press, 1978.

Lint, K. C., and Lint, A. M.: Diets for Birds in Captivity. Bandford Books, 1981.

Petrak, M. L.: Diseases of Cage and Aviary Birds. 2nd Ed. Philadelphia, Lea & Febiger, 1982.

Steiner, C. V., and Davis, R. B.: Caged Bird Medicine. Ames, Iowa State University Press, 1981.

Sturkie, P. D. (ed.): Avian Physiology. New York, Springer-Verlag, 1976.

Anal Sac Resection in the Ferret

by JAMES E. CREED

The ferret is becoming a popular housepet, but odor emitted from the anal sacs of both sexes is often objectionable. Like nearly all carnivores[2] and all mustelids,[4] the ferret has an anal sac on each side of the anus. The ducts open at 4- and 8-o'clock positions on the inner cutaneous zone of the anus, adjacent to the mucocutaneous junction. The sacs are interposed between the internal and external anal sphincter muscles. Material stored within the sac is secreted by a glandular complex surrounding the neck of the sac and 3 to 4 mm of the duct. This complex is evident without magnification, but a binocular loupe enhances visualization. The sebaceous gland component surrounding the distal part of the duct is covered asymmetrically by an apocrine gland component.[1] Surgical removal of the anal sacs and their ducts eliminates the odor of anal sac secretions, but some odor from sebaceous and apocrine tubular glands in the perianal region may remain.

Indications

Request by the client is the principal indication for performing this procedure. Veterinarians should recommend this operation for all ferrets at 6 to 8 months of age, however, to make them more acceptable pets. Neutering should be recommended at this age in both sexes to reduce odor further. Neutering also prevents the development of aplastic anemia in nonbreeding females, which can develop from hyperestrinism associated with prolonged estrus.[1,3] The client must be made aware that anal sac resection and neutering do not eliminate all "musky" odor, because of sebaceous and apocrine glands in the ferret's perianal skin.

Preoperative Considerations

In addition to a complete physical examination, it is wise to determine the patient's packed cell volume of blood and total serum protein level. One study of 11 healthy male ferrets reported an average packed cell volume of 52.4% and an average total serum protein of 6.0 g/dl.[1] Food should be withheld for 12 hours. Prior to anesthesia, atropine (.04 mg/kg) is administered subcutaneously. Anesthesia is induced with oxygen and methoxyflurane in an anesthesia chamber and is maintained with a mask or an endotracheal tube 2.5 mm in inner diameter.* An alternate method is intramuscular injection of ketamine hydrochloride (26 mg/kg) and acepromazine (1.1 mg/kg).

The ferret may be positioned for anal gland resection in dorsal or ventral recumbency. Because neutering is frequently performed and is best accomplished in dorsal recumbency, it is advisable to position all ferrets this way, to provide consistent orientation of anatomic structures. The ferret is placed at the end of a table on a sandbag or a similar pad to prevent loss of body heat, with its pelvic limbs pulled cranially and its tail dropped. The scrotal or ventral abdomen and perianal regions are prepared and are draped for the surgical procedure. Aseptic neutering is accomplished, and then the surgical drape is shifted to expose the ferret's anal region.

Surgical Technique

A binocular loupe should be used to locate the minute end of each anal sac duct and to aid visualization throughout the procedure. The end of each duct and 2 mm of skin and mucous membrane are grasped with mosquito forceps. A circumferential incision is made with a No. 15 Bard Parker scalpel blade immediately distal to the forceps tip; one must be careful not to incise too deeply. Using a gentle scraping action with the blade, skin and mucosa are reflected from the duct (Fig. 39-8). The glandular complex surrounding the terminal 3 to 4 mm of the duct makes dissection difficult (Fig. 39-8, C). This complex has a nodular surface with skeletal muscle fibers inserting into the glandular tis-

*12-French outer diameter Cole, Intermountain Veterinary Supply, Inc., 3950 Holly Street, Denver, CO 80207

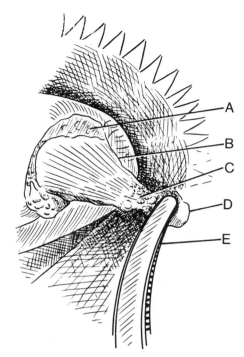

Fig. 39-8. *Resection of anal sac.* A, *External anal sphincter muscle;* B, *wall of anal sac;* C, *nodular glandular complex surrounding duct;* D, *end of anal sac duct;* E, *tip of mosquito forceps grasping skin, mucous membrane, and terminal duct.*

sue. One should not attempt to find a fascial plane at this time, and dissection should be superficial with respect to overlying tissue. Shifting the mosquito forceps to clamp them across skin, mucous membrane, and terminal duct should prevent tearing the duct as caudal traction is applied with the forceps (Fig. 39-8, E). Applying parallel, second forceps provides even more support.

A fascial plane is encountered as dissection is carried beyond the glandular complex (Fig. 39-8, B). The anal sac can be removed readily by reflecting sphincter muscles off the sac wall with a scraping action of the scalpel blade. Staying on the proper fascial plane not only enhances sac removal, but it also minimizes hemorrhage and damage to the internal and external anal sphincters. If the fascial plane is followed, little muscle will be left on the sac wall. The wall appears yellowish white; it is thin, and glandular secretions are yellow. It is easy to rupture the duct and the sac, particularly if the veterinary surgeon is inexperienced. Trying to establish a fascial plane before dissecting beyond the nodular glandular complex is particularly hazardous, because it is easy to cut into the duct lumen. If the duct or sac is incised, surgical extirpation can still be accomplished, but absence of a distended sac makes the operation more tedious; the odor is obnoxious, but not overwhelming.

Intraoperative hemorrhage is negligible, although sterile cotton-tipped applicator sticks work well to clear the surgical field of oozing blood. Sutures are not required, and it is not necessary to administer local or systemic antibiotics.

Postoperative Care

The patient is normally discharged when recovery from anesthesia is complete. Although no serious postoperative sequelae have been observed, complications can occur. Persistent minor hemorrhage may develop postoperatively, but this ceases spontaneously. Potential complications include prolapsed rectum and fecal incontinence due to excessive trauma to the anal sphincter muscles. Staying on the proper fascial plane minimizes both trauma and the possibility of these serious sequelae.

References and Suggested Readings

1. Creed, J. E., and Kainer, R. A.: Surgical extirpation and related anatomy of anal sacs of the ferret. J. Am. Vet. Med. Assoc., *179*:575, 1981.
2. Ewer, R. F.: The Carnivores. Ithaca, NY, Cornell University Press, 1973.
3. Kociba, G. J., and Caputo, C. A.: Aplastic anemia associated with estrus in pet ferrets. J. Am. Vet. Med. Assoc., *178*:1293, 1981.
4. Ryland, L. M., and Gorham, J. R.: The ferret and its diseases. J. Am. Vet. Med. Assoc., *173*:1154, 1978.

40 * Traumatic Wounds

Initial Management of Traumatic Wounds

by PAUL B. JENNINGS, JR.

Small animal veterinary practitioners see many traumatic injuries; thus, they should have an aggressive and systematic approach to wound treatment. This chapter presents methods of evaluating the treatment of traumatic wounds and their complications in small animals. Swaim has published an excellent text for in-depth reading on this subject.[17]

Instructions over the telephone should attempt to reassure the animal's owner, as well as to prevent the well-meaning owner from doing unintentional harm to the animal while enroute to the hospital. The owner may notice severe lacerations or extensive burns, but may not be aware of the main systemic physiologic problems that are more life-threatening than the external injury. Instructions should include the following:

1. Do not give the animal anything by mouth.
2. Refrain from using a tourniquet, but do place a gauze pad or a clean towel over the bleeding sites and apply direct pressure.
3. If the description of the injury suggests spinal cord trauma, have the owner place the animal on a board or other firm surface to transport.
4. Cover sucking chest wounds with a vaseline gauze pad while enroute to the clinic.
5. Do not put greasy ointments on chemical or flame burns. Flush the area with cold water and transport the patient immediately.

The veterinarian should evaluate the entire animal and should administer emergency care before treating the specific wound(s). The patient must have a patent airway, bleeding must be controlled, and the cardiovascular system must be stabilized.[9,14]

Inspection of the Wound

The animal must be restrained and must be free of pain for inspection and definitive treatment. General anesthesia or sedation with or without local anesthesia is required if the animal's condition permits use of such agents.

The area around the wound must be closely clipped to allow proper inspection and cleaning, especially in feline bite injuries, in which multiple puncture wounds are readily obscured. To prevent hair from spilling into the wound, sponges moistened with saline solution may be placed over the open wound. Hair matted with blood or tissue debris may need to be softened with water or combed before clippers will work. Depilatories or safety razors should not be used close to the wound edges because the irritation they cause may increase the wound's susceptibility to infection.

Following clipping, the skin around the wound should be prepared in the same manner as for an aseptic surgical procedure. If dirt and grease are present, a surgical scrub brush is used in conjunction with surgical soap. Imbedded particles of dirt, asphalt, or glass may have to be picked out with sterile forceps.

Cleansing the Wound

Hydraulic flushing with sterile saline solution effectively removes remaining particulate matter and bacteria. Saline solution may be delivered under pressure by use of an intravenous infusion bottle elevated above the patient, a bulb syringe, a large hypodermic syringe, or a pulsating water-jet lavage device designed for the purpose* (Fig. 40-1). This water-jet device is a surgical modification of the dental Water Pik†. The pulsating action of the device loosens debris, and the copious flow of fluids floats this material from the wound. Pressures of up to 60 pounds per square inch at the tip of the nozzle provide excellent penetrating ability. As recesses of the wound are lavaged, a gloved index finger may be used to probe for hidden pockets in the wound, to ensure complete exposure of the open tissue (Fig. 40-2).

Additions to lavage solutions have included hydrogen peroxide, nitrofurazone, povidone-iodine, and various antibiotics.[4] These combinations may enhance the effectiveness of the lavage solutions. More important than any additive, however, is the principle that a lavage solution must provide the needed physical cleansing and flushing of the wound without creating additional trauma.

*SurgiLav, Stryker Corp., Kalamazoo, MI
†Teledyne Aquatec, Fort Collins, CO 80521

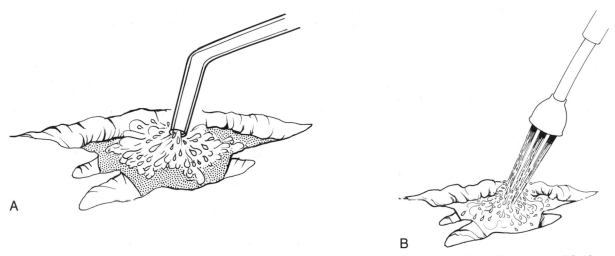

Fig. 40-1. *Pulsating water lavage may be delivered by a tip delivering either single (A) or multiple (B) streams of fluid.*

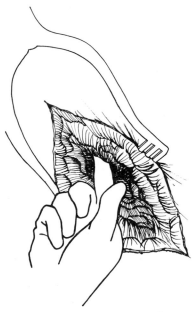

Fig. 40-2. *The gloved index finger is an excellent probe to explore hidden recesses of the wound.*

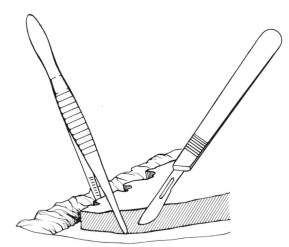

Fig. 40-3. *Sharp scalpel incisions are used to remove devitalized tissue.*

Technique of Wound Debridement

Dead tissue must be removed to prevent decomposition and enhancement of bacterial growth. Dark, friable muscle and shredded fascia are excised by clean, sharp scalpel incisions back to bleeding muscle and viable fascia (Fig. 40-3). The tissue should be grasped gently with thumb forceps and should be debrided using even strokes of the scalpel blade. Sawing movements should be avoided because such movements produce ragged edges. The veterinarian should be meticulous in providing hemostasis as the wound is debrided.

A conservative approach is adopted for debridement of vascular and nerve tissues. One should leave as much viable tissue as possible while removing frayed edges, so as to facilitate reanastomosis. Wet saline dressings can be used for gradual physiologic debride-

ment. These dressings must be changed daily until a granulation bed is achieved. Then the wound is protected by Telfa Wet-Pruf pads*, which can be changed less frequently.

An important decision is whether or not a bone fragment can be left for incorporation into a fracture repair. Large bone fragments that have not been severely displaced and have a viable blood supply through periosteal attachment should be left in place. Small, displaced bone fragments or splinters should be removed, using copious lavage and curettage if necessary.

Closure of Traumatic Wounds

Minor wounds under 6 to 8 hours old are closed primarily following cleaning and debridement. Wounds with extensive tissue destruction, pockets of dead space, incomplete hemostasis, or excess tissue fluids are left open under sterile dressing coverage. In some cases, portions of the wound may be closed to provide

*Kendall Co. Veterinary Products, One Federal Street, Boston, MA 02101

coverage while dependent portions of the wound are left open to drain. If the wound granulates to the satisfaction of the veterinarian within 4 to 7 days, a delayed primary closure of skin and subcutaneous tissue is performed. In wounds with massive tissue avulsions, the clinician may provide as much debridement, drainage, and closure as possible in one sitting and may repeat this treatment as the wound progressively drains, granulates, and shrinks in size.[2]

Suture selection should include fine monofilament material for vessel ligation, anastomosis of vessels and nerves, and for layered closure of debrided wounds. Chromic catgut and polyglycolic acid absorbable sutures also work well for layered fascial closures.[3] Where tension may be a factor, or where the animal may molest the wound postoperatively, fine stainless steel wire sutures are excellent.[9]

Bite wounds (including cat-fight cellulitis and abscesses), gunshot wounds, open fractures, penetrations of the intestinal tract, and any contaminated wound that can be only incompletely cleaned should *not* be closed primarily.

WOUND DRAINAGE

Drains may be needed to assist in the liberation of tissue fluids. The use of drains may be dangerous if they are retained too long or if they allow contamination of the wound cavity.

In veterinary patients, soft rubber drains are readily adaptable to varying needs. Penrose-type drains can be cut to size, inserted into wound crevices, and sutured to the skin at a remote point of exit to prevent removal by the animal. If possible, drains should be dressed with Telfa Wet-Pruf pads and bandaged to prevent retrograde contamination, exudate skin maceration, and removal by the patient. In large, contaminated traumatic wounds with ample surrounding skin, the skin over the upper portion of the wound may be closed over a drain while the dependent portions are left unsutured for the gravity flow of discharges. Occasionally, wounds must be drained through "windows" in casts or splints to protect fractured skeletal elements and to prevent automutilation, while allowing proper daily wound care. Although gauze or other bandage material is sometimes used for drain material, the potential of cotton fibers to remain as foreign bodies when the drain has been removed and the action of these materials as a potent wick into the cavity make these drains less desirable than those composed of latex rubber.[3]

The placement of a drain does not preclude daily wound irrigation. If an intractable animal prohibits the use of a drain, frequent lavage of the wound with isotonic fluid may have to be substituted for drains.

BANDAGES AND DRESSINGS

The primary purposes of bandages and dressings are to protect the wound from additional external trauma, to provide a means of retaining adequate wound moisture, and to absorb wound exudate. Additional purposes are to provide adequate immobilization without impairing circulation and temporary coverage to wounds awaiting later closure. Clean, bulky, nonocclusive dressings of the Robert Jones variety are ideal for many extremity injuries. Encompassing pressure dressings are useful in sizable trunk wounds, whereas "patch bandages" attached to the animal's hair with adhesive tape and ether are useful in small body wounds.

In extremity wounds accompanying fractures, immobilization is required to ensure proper skeletal alignment while soft tissues heal. Open fractures of the radius, ulna, tibia, or fibula may be treated with Thomas splints or Kirschner external fixation devices to allow access to the wound site. Metacarpal, metatarsal, carpal, tarsal, or phalangeal open fractures are amenable to aluminum or plastic splints. Modified Thomas splints or plaster casts do not provide stability for many humeral and femoral fractures. The Kirschner external fixation apparatus is especially well suited to stabilizing long bone fractures because the transfixation pins can be situated away from the open fracture site. The device provides rigid immobilization while allowing local treatment.[6] Detailed information regarding the treatment of open fractures is available in Part II of this book.

Special Wounds

GUNSHOT WOUNDS. The amount of damage produced in a gunshot wound is directly proportional to the mass of the missile times the square of the velocity of the projectile.[8] Most gunshot wounds in veterinary medicine are made by low-velocity missiles, that is, velocities of under 1200 feet per second. The wound tract produced by missile penetration is surrounded by varying amounts of injured tissue, but the hole of entrance does *not* give the clinician any clue as to the amount of damage along the tract.

Gunshot wounds are considered contaminated, with a high potential for aerobic and anaerobic infection. Thus, all gunshot wounds should be explored, and the basic principles of debridement, lavage, and drainage are important. Abdominal gunshot wounds require exploratory celiotomy through an incision long enough to provide access to the entire cavity.

In the thorax, correction of the pneumothorax or hemothorax produced by the penetrating missile is the first concern. Thoracentesis or tube drainage of the chest are important corrective measures (see Chap. 21). Continuing hemorrhage requires immediate exploratory thoracotomy. Because of the relative sterility of the organs of the thoracic cavity, as compared with the abdominal viscera, more time is available following emergency measures to stabilize the patient's condition before deciding whether or not surgical exploration is necessary.

Shotgun pellets frequently can be seen in radiographs of hunting dogs. When fired at close range, shotguns produce massive damage with large tissue defects. Standard principles of emergency treatment and management should prevail, and methods of covering the defects should include immediate (dressings, partial skin closure) and long-term (muscle transposition, sliding grafts) treatment. Shotgun pellets fired from a distance may do no more than penetrate the skin. Although the most accessible pellets may be removed, they are usually difficult to locate and are thus left alone unless they cause problems.

DOG BITE WOUNDS. Because of the skin penetration and the immense amount of force generated from a bite, the skin wound may not reflect the severe amount of tissue damage below the skin.[9] Bite wounds are contaminated with the biting animal's oral bacterial flora, the victim's skin bacteria, and probably soil and other environmental organisms. Gram-positive cocci and anaerobic bacteria are the most common organisms found in these wounds. Thus, penicillin is recommended as a first choice to administer in patients with bite wounds, as an adjunct to debridement, drainage, and wound coverage.

TRAP WOUNDS. Animals whose legs have been caught in steel traps frequently have metacarpal or metatarsal fractures.[6] If the animal has been held in the trap for a prolonged period, necrosis and gangrene are usually present, and the animal may show signs of systemic toxicity. Following cleaning and debridement of the limb, tetanus antitoxin should be considered to complement high doses of antibiotics. Soaking the leg is beneficial to reduce swelling and remove devitalized tissue. Amputation should be considered only as a last resort for total devitalization of the distal extremity.

Wound Infections

Bacterial contamination of a wound implies that microorganisms have "soiled" the disturbed tissues.[15] When bacterial infection of a wound occurs, the body has reacted to the presence of microorganisms and their toxins. Factors influencing the infection of a contaminated wound include: (1) time elapsed since contamination; (2) the numbers of organisms introduced, their invasive capacity, velocity of penetration, and virulence; (3) factors influencing the host defenses, including state of dehydration, pre-existing infection, shock, diabetes mellitus, or an altered immune status; and (4) the presence of foreign bodies, clotted blood, necrotic tissue, fluids, and excessive dead space within the wound.

Most wound infections can be prevented if the veterinarian treats wounds promptly, using the principles of debridement and lavage previously outlined. Antimicrobial therapy alone is not enough to prevent wound contamination from progressing to infection if necrotic tissue, blood, or debris are allowed to exist in the wound.

Bacterial quantitation is a means to differentiate contaminated from infected wounds. Where fewer than 10^5 bacteria/g tissue are present, the wound may be considered contaminated; more than 10^5 bacteria/g tissue suggests infection.[12] An exception is β-hemolytic streptococci; wounds containing fewer than 10^5 organisms/g tissue are clinically significant, that is, are

associated with infection.[13] Thus, wounds known to contain β-hemolytic streptococci should not be closed. When a wound infection is established, proper surgical techniques must be supplemented with clinical microbiologic methods, to identify the offending organism(s) and to provide specific treatment.

A primary method of evaluating an infected wound includes identifying the offending organism(s) by a simple Gram-stained impression smear of a piece of tissue excised from the wound or wound exudate.[7] Microscopic examination of the Gram-stained slide gives information on its general bacterial category and on whether the infection involves one or more species of bacteria. For quantitation and identification of the specific wound pathogen, the rapid slide test of Robson and Heggers[11] allows the clinician to categorize and to estimate the quantity of bacteria present in the wound. The test takes 15 minutes to perform, uses the Gram stain to categorize the organism, and is calibrated to measure either greater or fewer than 10^5 organisms/g tissue[5] (Table 40-1).

Two specimens of wound debris should also be taken for culture. One is streaked onto blood agar, and the other is placed into thioglycollate broth and is incubated for 24 hours at 37° C. Wound biopsy material may also be inoculated into thioglycollate. Because the surface of the wound should be cleaned before the biopsy, an alternate method is to excise a tissue specimen, dip it into alcohol, and flame the surface to destroy surface contaminants. Using a sterile scalpel blade and forceps, one may cut the specimen in half and drop it into

Table 40-1. *Rapid Slide Test for Quantitative Wound Cultures*

1. Perform a biopsy of the open wound, using a 4-mm dermal punch, or cut a tissue specimen with a scalpel. The specimen should weigh at least 250 mg.
2. Dip the specimen in alcohol and flame the surface. Weigh the specimen and dilute it in supplemented thioglycollate broth (or supplemented brain-heart infusion broth) at the ratio of 1 g tissue to 9 ml diluent.
3. Mince the tissue and homogenize with tissue homogenizer.*
4. Draw a 15-mm-diameter circle on a microscope slide with a wax pencil. Deliver 0.02 ml of the suspension to the glass slide, using a 20-lambda Sahli pipette.
5. Air-dry the slide in an oven at 75° C for 15 minutes.
6. Stain with the Gram stain.
7. Examine the slide under a microscope, using a 1.8-mm objective (97×). If even a single organism is present, the bacterial count is greater than 10^5 organisms/g tissue. An absence of organisms on the slide indicates a count of fewer than 10^5/g tissue.
8. Prepare serial dilutions of the homogenate (1 : 100, 1 : 1000, and so on) to prepare pour plates using standard methods of tube dilution and serial plating. These plates should be incubated at 37° C for 18 to 24 hours. The exact number of bacteria present can now be determined by counting the numbers of bacterial colonies.

*Pestle No. S-64, Tube No. S-74: Tr1-R Instruments, Inc., Rockville Center, NY 11570
(Adapted from Heggers, J. P., Robson, W. C., and Ristroph, J. D.: A rapid method for performing quantitative wound cultures. Milit. Med., *134*:666, 1969; and Heggers, J. P.: University of Chicago, Personal communication, 1980.)

Table 40-2. *Microorganisms Frequently Found in Infected Wounds and the Antibiotics of Choice for Treatment*

I. Gram-Positive Bacteria

Organism	Primary Antibiotic and Dose*	Secondary Antibiotic and Dose
Staphylococcus aureus	Penicillin (20,000–40,000 U/kg q6h)	Cephalothin (10 mg/kg q6h)
Staphylococcus aureus, penicillinase-producing	Methicillin (20 mg/kg q6h) or oxacillin (10 mg/kg q6h)	Cephalothin
Streptococcus pyogenes	Penicillin	Erythromycin (10 mg/kg q6h)
Streptococcus, viridans group	Penicillin	Cephalothin
Streptococcus, enterococcus group	Ampicillin (10–20 mg/kg q8h) plus streptomycin (10–20 mg/kg q6h) or kanamycin (6 mg/kg q12h)	Kanamycin
Streptococcus, anaerobic	Penicillin	Clindamycin (4 mg/kg q6h)
Pasteurella multocida	Penicillin	Tetracycline (20 mg/kg q8h)
Corynebacterium	Erythromycin	Penicillin
Clostridium	Penicillin	Chloramphenicol (20–50 mg/kg q8h)

II. Gram-Negative Bacteria

Organism	Primary Antibiotic and Dose	Secondary Antibiotic and Dose
Escherichia coli	Gentamicin (4 mg/kg q12h)	Ampicillin or Cephalothin
Enterobacter	Gentamicin	Carbenicillin (150 mg/kg q8h)
Proteus mirabilis	Ampicillin	Gentamicin
Proteus, other species	Gentamicin	Carbenicillin
Pseudomonas aeruginosa	Gentamicin	Carbenicillin
Pseudomonas fluorescens	Gentamicin	Polymyxin B (2 mg/kg q12h)
Bacteroides, enteric strains	Clindamycin or Tetracycline	Chloramphenicol
Bacteroides, oral strains	Penicillin	Clindamycin
Leptotrichia buccalis (Fusobacterium fusiforme)	Penicillin	Tetracycline

*The antibiotic dose is presented only the first time it appears in this table.
(Adapted from Haller, J. A., and Soto, D. S. Y.: Trauma. *In* Antimicrobial Therapy. Philadelphia, W. B. Saunders, 1974; Watson, A. D. J.: Antimicrobial therapy. *In* Current Veterinary Therapy VI. Philadelphia, W. B. Saunders, 1977; Heggers, J. P.: Personal communication, 1980; Jang, S. S., Biberstein, E. L., Hirsh, D. C.: A Diagnostic Manual of Veterinary Clinical Bacteriology and Mycology. Davis, University of California, 1978.)

thioglycollate broth. After incubation in thioglycollate, the organisms are inoculated onto blood agar plates. Anaerobically, incubation may be performed by the GasPak*. Incubation time varies from 12 to 48 hours, depending upon the organism. Following incubation of the specimen, the veterinarian should select isolated bacterial colonies from the blood agar plates, prepare Gram stains, and compare the predominating organism(s) with those seen on the initial Gram stain and rapid slide test.

Antimicrobial susceptibility testing is an important component of therapeutic decision-making. The disk-diffusion (Kirby-Bauer) method† is the most practical for clinical application in veterinary medicine. In clinical veterinary practice, it is convenient to use small, prepared plate systems for application of antibiotic sensitivity discs.

Mixed bacterial cultures should not be used for antimicrobial susceptibility testing. Rather, each potential pathogen grown on blood agar should be isolated, and its antibiotic sensitivity should be tested separately if the zones of inhibition are to be interpreted accurately.

*BBL Microbiology Systems, Cockeysville, MD 21030
†Bactassay, Pitman Moore, Inc., Washington Crossing, NJ 08560

To initiate treatment pending results of testing, the veterinarian should select an antibiotic that covers the category of organisms identified in the initial Gram stain. For gram-positive organisms, penicillin remains the drug of choice for all but the penicillinase-producing bacteria. Some organisms are susceptible to high doses of penicillin, but not to low doses. Gentamicin is effective against a wide range of gram-negative bacteria, but is largely ineffective against anaerobic bacterial genera. Table 40-2 lists infecting organisms and the antibiotics recommended for treatment.

The veterinarian may need to modify the antibiotic therapy when the results of the cultures and sensitivities become available. One should use as specific an agent as possible and should reserve the broad-spectrum agents for animals with overwhelming infections of unknown type.

References and Suggested Readings

1. Bhaskar, S. N., Cutright, D. E., and Hunsuck, E. E.: Pulsating water jet devices in debridement of combat wounds. Milit. Med., *136*:264, 1971.

2. Eger, C. E.: Management of wounds with severe tissue loss: a case report. J. Am. Anim. Hosp. Assoc., *12*:834, 1976.

3. Furneaux, R. W.: Management of contaminated wounds. Canine Pract., *2*:22, 1980.

4. Gross, A., Cutright, D. E., and Larson, W. J.: The effect of antiseptic agents and pulsating jet lavage on contaminated wounds. Milit. Med., *137*:145, 1972.

5. Heggers, J. P., Robson, W. C., and Ristroph, J. D.: A rapid method for performing quantitative wound cultures. Milit. Med., *134*:13, 1969.

6. Herron, M. R.: Care of trap wounds. Canine Pract., *4*:4, 1977.

7. Jennings, P. B.: Surgical techniques utilized in the presence of infection. Arch. Am. College Vet. Surg., *4*:43, 1975.

8. Lipowitz, A. J.: Management of gunshot wounds in the soft tissues and extremities. J. Am. Anim. Hosp. Assoc., *12*:813, 1976.

9. Neal, T. M., and Kay, J. C.: Principles of treatment of dog bite wounds. J. Am. Anim. Hosp. Assoc., *12*:657, 1976.

10. Neuman, N. B.: Management of contaminated wounds of the extremities. VM SAC, *69*:1275, 1974.

11. Robson, M. C., and Heggers, J. P.: Surgical infections. I. Single bacterial species or polymicrobic in origin. Surgery, *65*:608, 1969.

12. Robson, M. C., Krizek, T. J., and Heggers, J. P.: Biology of surgical infections. Current Probl. Surg., *10*:1, 1973.

13. Robson, M. C., Duke, W. F., and Krizek, T. J.: Rapid bacterial screening in the treatment of civilian wounds. J. Surg. Res., *14*:426, 1973.

14. Roush, J. C.: Trauma of the extremities. Canine Pract., *2*:38, 1975.

15. Sherman, J. J., and Bradley, R. L.: Emergency care of skin trauma: case report and discussion. VM SAC, *74*:1141, 1979.

16. Stone, J. L.: Evaluation and immediate management of the trauma patient. Canine Pract., *2*:19, 1975.

17. Swaim, S. F.: Surgery of Traumatized Skin: Management and Reconstruction in the Dog and Cat. Philadelphia, W. B. Saunders, 1980.

41 * Burns

Current Techniques for the Initial Management of Burns

by CHARLES G. MCLEOD, JR.

Fortunately, serious burn injuries are rare in animals. Veterinarians are qualified, however, by virtue of their experience with other forms of trauma, to handle treatable cases of burn injury. Initial management should be directed at stabilizing the animal, accurately estimating the extent of injury, and protecting the wound from infection. The outcome of a serious burn injury often depends on the attention given to these aspects of treatment.

Causes of Burns

Burns in companion animals are usually accidental. Flame, scald, chemical, electrical, and friction burns cause similar but variable degrees of necrosis of the epidermis and underlying structures. House fires, ignition of fuels, spilling of hot food, and hot bath water may all cause burn injuries in pets. Chemical burns may occur following the use of various home remedies in treating skin conditions in pets. Serious burns of the feet may be seen when an unleashed pet strays onto hot tar or uncured cement. Young dogs frequently suffer burns of the mouth and tongue when they chew through electrical cords. Additionally, a cruel segment of our society maliciously inflicts burns upon defenseless animals. The odor of kerosene or gasoline should alert the clinician to this possibility.

Burn Management Techniques

PREVENTION OF BURN SHOCK

It is rarely practical to salvage an animal with burns over more than 30% of its total body surface (TBS). Smaller burns (20 to 30% TBS) require careful fluid therapy, generally 8 to 10 ml/kg/hour, as initial treatment, of fluid replacement. Burns of under 10% TBS usually require no fluid replacement therapy in initial treatment.

Lactated Ringer's solution is the fluid of choice, and the dose should be closely adjusted according to burn size, urine output, hematocrit, changes in body weight, and oral fluid intake.[3] Animals instinctively drink fluids after being burned, and care must be taken to regulate replacement therapy to avoid fluid overload. The grave "postburn complications" related to shock and fluid loss, including renal dysfunction and pulmonary edema, are virtually eliminated when replacement therapy is adequate, but not excessive.

It may be necessary to control pain (especially in partial-thickness burns) with narcotics or narcotic derivatives. Full-thickness burns are usually insensitive, except at their margins where a mixed zone of partial- and full-thickness injury is found.

COOLING OF THE WOUND

Complete agreement does not exist as to the value of skin cooling on the development of burn injury.[2,4,6] It is likely that cooling is useful in reducing pain and the depth of injury if it is applied immediately or within a few minutes following exposure. Burns of the feet and extremities may be immersed in cold-water soaks, and ice bags may be applied to larger areas of injury. The length of time for cooling is partly a matter of the clinician's patience, but at least 20 minutes are required to provide subsequent reduction in pain and swelling. The patient's body temperature should be monitored carefully to avoid excessive cooling.

WOUND CLEANSING

It is especially important in the initial management of chemical burns to cleanse the wound. Chemicals that remain on the wound, especially if they are trapped under heavy ointments or bandages, may continue to cause epithelial loss. Strong acids should be removed with dilute basic soap solutions, followed by thorough rinsing with water. Caustic basic materials may be removed with soapy water to which a small quantity of vinegar has been added. In reality, however, the identity of the chemical causing the burn is usually unknown, and "elbow grease," soap, and water are the obvious remedies.

Hair should be gently clipped from the area of burn injury to allow for close examination of the skin and to facilitate the application of topical ointments.

DETERMINATION OF THE EXTENT AND DEPTH OF THE BURN

Burn injuries present several immediate clinical challenges. The clinician must decide whether treatment is feasible. Although each patient is considered individually, an important step in making this determination is to estimate the extent of burn injury (Table 41-1). Diagrammatic estimations of the burn injury are useful, but require arbitrary adjustment for the shape (breed), age, and size of the animal.

The depth of the burn wound must also be determined. *Full-thickness* or third-degree burns have a dry, "waxy" appearance, a firm texture, and are insensitive to all but deep finger pressure. Wounds of this type have no potential for healing except through contraction and often require extensive grafting. *Partial-thickness* or second-degree burns are painful, wet, hyperemic, and usually have extensive swelling. Blistering is not a consistent finding in partial-thickness burns of animals. Such burns have a good prognosis and generally heal within 2 weeks if adequately protected from infection with topical antibiotics. Minor burns, such as sunburn of a clipped poodle, usually require no topical treatment.

Regardless of the original estimates of the extent and depth of burn injury, the injury should be reassessed after 24 hours when the demarcation between necrotic and viable tissue becomes more evident. The clinician must consider, in addition to burn size and depth, the animal's age and general health in making decisions regarding treatment or euthanasia.

PROTECTION OF THE WOUND

The principal local management problem in serious burns is infection, because necrotic tissue and exudates serve as a rich medium for bacterial growth.[7] Thus, burn therapy is aimed at reducing the bacterial population on and within the burn wound. Serious invasive burn wound infections result from overwhelming gram-negative bacterial growth. Infection impairs or stops healing, increases scar formation, and causes graft failure. Systemic antibiotics are of little value in controlling this bacterial growth because they have no significant concentration within the necrotic tissue of the burn wound.[1] Topical antibiotics should be applied as soon as other supportive therapy is completed. Acceptable antibiotics include silver sulfadiazine, nitrofurazone, and mafenide although the last-named drug causes significant pain when applied to second-degree burns. Small burns of the feet and extremities may be covered with light bandages. Bandages should be loosely applied and changed daily. Proper nursing practices, including bathing and air exposure of the wound prior to rebandaging, reduce incidences of infection and decrease the amount of convalescence time.

Larger areas of injury heal well when treated as open wounds if they are protected to prevent removal of the topical agents. Animals have a remarkable capacity to close their wounds through granulation, epithelialization, and contraction. In long-haired breeds, scarring is of little concern. The healthy wound, when cleaned, should have a reddish pink color and a granular surface. With maturation, the surface is pale pink, owing to the reduction in capillaries and the increase in fibrous connective tissue. The burn wound should be examined a week after injury for evidence of invasive infection. Discrete zones of secondary hemorrhage and necrosis within or at the margin of the burn wound suggest this complication. Pseudomonas aeruginosa is the most common invasive organism. Although Staphylococcus and Candida species are frequently cultured from burns, they are usually not the cause of true tissue invasion and subsequent bacteremia.

Inhalation Injury

Victims trapped in fires are exposed to numerous noxious products of combustion, including several oxides of nitrogen and sulfur, hydrochloric acid, formaldehyde, hydrocyanide, carbon monoxide, soot, and hydrocarbons. These substances can cause immediate or delayed necrosis of respiratory tissues[8] and seriously complicate an otherwise manageable burn case. The diagnosis of inhalation injury in animals is usually made from clinical signs and is confirmed by thoracic radiographs. Immediate respiratory distress is usually

Table 41-1. *Body-Weight-to-Surface-Area Conversion**

Body Weight in Kilograms	Surface Area in Centimeters
2	1,600
4	2,500
6	3,800
8	4,000
10	4,600
12	5,200
14	5,800
16	6,400
18	6,900
20	7,400
22	7,900
24	8,300
26	8,800
28	9,200
30	9,700
32	10,100
34	10,500
36	10,900
38	11,300
40	11,700
42	12,100
44	12,500
46	12,800
48	13,200
50	13,500

* Percentage of total body surface burned is calculated by dividing area burned (in centimeters squared) by the surface area and multiplying by 100.
(Data from King, T. C., and Zimmerman, J. M.: First aid cooling of the fresh burn. Surg. Gynecol. Obstet., *120*:1271, 1965.)

related to hypoxia or to carbon monoxide poisoning. Prompt administration of high concentrations of oxygen usually relieves this immediate distress. Later, alveolar and interstitial pulmonary infiltrates are seen in thoracic radiographs. Larger airway obstruction may also develop and is usually related to obstructive casts at the bronchiolar and bronchial level. Humidified oxygen, intermittent positive-pressure ventilation, and frequent mechanical clearing of the airways through suction are additional supportive measures that may be used in the presence of an endotracheal or tracheostomy tube. Systemic antibiotic therapy is indicated if bronchopneumonia develops.

Electrical Burns

Electrical injuries are characterized by small areas of cutaneous or oral mucosal necrosis and deep necrosis of soft tissues. Patients that receive severe electric shock may immediately require artificial ventilation. Initial care is also directed at treating the deep and often disfiguring wounds of the tongue or mouth in animals that chew through electric cords. Deep necrosis of muscle and occasionally partial or complete paralysis of the tongue may occur. Thus, management involves surgical debridement of tissues coagulated by the thermal energy generated when the electric current courses through tissues of varying resistance. Rarely, one finds an exit wound on an extremity that represents the site of current grounding. These wounds and the proximal muscle compartments of the affected extremity should be periodically observed for evidence of deep muscle and bone necrosis caused by the current coursing through these tissues.

Nutritional Requirements

Significant burn injury and the ensuing repair mechanism induce a poorly understood state of hypermetabolism.[9] Nutritional requirements are increased and are monitored by following the changes in body weight. Adequate caloric and protein intake is necessary to avoid pronounced catabolism.

In summary, small burns respond well to simple therapy. Animals, especially young, healthy dogs, have a tremendous capacity for healing large, open, cutaneous wounds, including burns.

In large burns, the clinician faces the same problems seen in critically burned human patients. These areas have been addressed in detail by experienced authors in the list of references and suggested readings. With proper initial management and stabilization of the burned animal, veterinary clinicians and surgeons who elect to treat larger burns may be more successful using principles known to be effective in human burn therapy.

References and Suggested Readings

1. Bruck, N. M.: The management of small burns. In Burns: A Team Approach. Edited by C. P. Artz, J. A. Moncrief, and B. A. Pruitt, Jr. Philadelphia, W. B. Saunders, 1979.
2. King, T. C., and Zimmerman, J. M.: First aid cooling of the fresh burn. Surg. Gynecol. Obstet., 120: 1271, 1965.
3. Moncrief, J. A.: Replacement therapy. In Burns: A Team Approach. Edited by C. P. Artz, J. A. Moncrief, and B. A. Pruitt, Jr. Philadelphia, W. B. Saunders, 1979.
4. Piller, N. B.: The resolution of thermal edema at various temperatures under coumarin treatment. Br. J. Exp. Pathol., 56:83, 1975.
5. Pruitt, B. A., Jr., and Moylan, J. A.: Current management of thermal injury. Surgery, 6:237, 1972.
6. Shulman, A. G.: Ice water as primary treatment of burns. JAMA, 173:1916, 1960.
7. Teplitz, C.: The pathology of burns and the fundamentals of burn wound sepsis. In Burns: A Team Approach. Edited by C. P. Artz, J. A. Moncrief, and B. A. Pruitt, Jr. Philadelphia, W. B. Saunders, 1979.
8. Welch, G. W., et al.: The use of steroids in inhalation injury. Surg. Gynecol. Obstet., 145:539, 1977.
9. Wilmore, D. W.: Nutrition. In Burns: A Team Approach. Edited by C. P. Artz, J. A. Moncrief, and B. A. Pruitt, Jr. Philadelphia, W. B. Saunders, 1979.

Part II

Bones and Joints

42 * Cervical Spine

Caudal Cervical Spondylopathy and Myelopathy in Large Breed Dogs

by STEPHEN J. WITHROW

and HOWARD B. SEIM, III

Cervical spondylopathy and resultant myelopathy are being recognized and diagnosed at an increasing rate. Cervical spondylopathy has been chosen as the name for this entity because it implies no specific cause. Other names that have become more or less synonymous include wobbler syndrome, cervical vertebral instability, spondylolisthesis, spondylosis, and cervical vertebral malformation. Although many variations exist in this syndrome, the emphasis of this discussion is on caudal cervical lesions that result in ventral cord compression.

The etiology of this syndrome is still obscure, even though heritable, congenital, traumatic, nutritional, and degenerative causes have been suggested. Undoubtedly, as our knowledge of this disease improves, we shall be able to define its cause more precisely. We feel that most cases of this disorder result from chronic instability or degenerative disk disease with secondary ligamentous impingement of the spinal cord.

Myelography is absolutely essential in determining the site of the lesion. Apparent "tipping" of vertebrae or coning of the vertebral canal has been notoriously misleading in demonstrating the involved interspace(s). Typical myelographic findings are schematically depicted in Figure 42-1. If the spinal cord compression does not disappear with strong linear traction, actual disk herniation, although rare, can be suspected.

Pathophysiologic Features

An understanding of the pathophysiology is required in order to understand the rationale for surgical treatment. The instability of the lower cervical vertebrae (as a cause *or* an effect of disk disease) may result in enlargement or redundancy of the dorsal anulus fibrosus (disk protrusion) and dorsal longitudinal ligaments (Fig. 42-1). Rarely, overt disk herniation occurs. Because most dogs have a slowly progressive myelopathy, they can compensate well. It is at this point, where the spinal cord is compressed, that minor trauma can induce significant spinal cord injury. Decompression and, probably more important, stabilization allow the spinal cord to recover in most cases. Most dogs have a slowly progressive (weeks to months) history of tetraparesis. Motor signs are generally more pronounced in the rear limbs. Pain is rarely a presenting sign.

Surgical Technique

The surgical procedure that we advocate is a ventral slot (described in the following section of this chapter), a corticocancellous bone graft, and ventral plating of the involved interspace.

The dog is premedicated with dexamethasone (2 mg/kg) several hours prior to the surgical procedure. The entire ventral neck, including sternum and both proximal humeri, is clipped. The dog is then positioned in dorsal recumbency and is secured to the table. A standard ventral approach to the affected interspace is made, and a ventral transdiskal slot procedure is performed. The slot is carried about 75% of the distance to, but not into, the spinal canal. Bleeding cancellous bone must be reached at each end of the slot. The slot is made just wide enough to accept the bone graft, roughly two-thirds of the width of the vertebral body. The length of the slot needs to be about half as long as the proposed bony implant. Before traction, most slots are 1 cm^2 for the average Doberman pinscher.

The ventral slot is not carried into the spinal canal for several reasons. It is our experience that removal of the ligament and anulus is not necessary as long as they can be stretched flat. If they are placed in traction, they will lie flat on the floor of the spinal canal and the spinal cord will be decompressed. Moreover, entrance into the canal and attempted ligament removal may endanger the cord, may prolong the operation, and may result in significant sinus hemorrhage and, in our experience, incomplete decompression. Once the slot has been drilled, the patient's head is grasped firmly behind the base of the skull, and rigid longitudinal traction is applied. With this traction, the slot should approximately double in length.

The veterinary surgeon can then measure the exact length of the bone graft to be inserted. The ideal im-

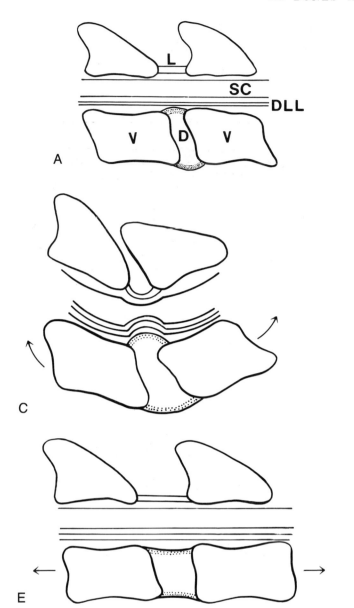

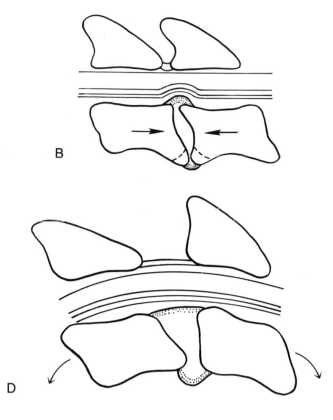

Fig. 42-1. A, *Normal anatomy of involved structures. L, Ligamentum flavum; SC, spinal cord; DLL, dorsal longitudinal ligament; V, vertebrae; and D, intervertebral disk. B, A collapsed interspace and spondylitic changes on the ventral end plates of the vertebrae (as depicted in this drawing) occur in fewer than half the cases seen. C, Hyperextension of the neck accentuates the compression both dorsally and ventrally and must be done with caution. D, Ventral flexion of the neck usually alleviates the compression. E, Linear traction also alleviates compression and is the key to therapy.*

plant should be strong yet should allow ingrowth of host bone. We have used pelvic autografts, tibial allografts from a frozen bone bank, and currently, bovine heterografts* with equal success. Heterografts have a tendency to compress and fragment, however. If hollow grafts from the tibia are used, cancellous bone is packed tightly into the medullary cavity before the graft is inserted.

The ideal choice of a grafting material is still under investigation. If one chooses an autogenous ilial graft, as much cortex as possible should be salvaged. Even then, these grafts often partially crush and collapse, resulting in loss of the decompression. The main advantage of an autogenous pelvic graft is speed of fusion. If cortical tibial grafts are used, the fusion is often delayed, up to a year or more in some cases, and the

* Kiel Surgibones, Unilab, Inc., Hillside, NJ 07205

graft may push into the vertebral bodies and cause partial loss of decompression. If tibial grafts are used, they should be packed into the medullary cavity with fresh autogenous cancellous bone in an attempt to enhance early fusion. Attempts are being made to find a graft with the same viscoelasticity as the cervical vertebrae.

Because slight collapse of the graft or vertebrae is evident on many 3-month rechecks, and the dogs are doing well, it may be that stability is more important than decompression in the long term. It is our opinion that the enlarged, hypertrophied ligament and anulus may actually atrophy once stability is attained. Graft choice then becomes less critical.

When the graft has been measured and cut to size, it is tapped into place while longitudinal traction is applied to the neck (Fig. 42-2). If any space remains in the slotting hole, it may be packed with freshly harvested cancellous bone taken from the proximal humerus. A

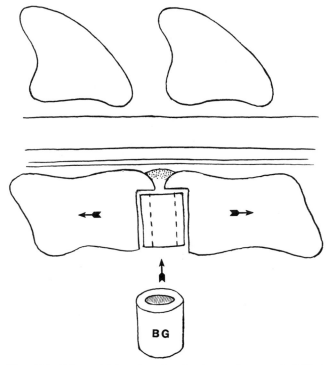

Fig. 42-2. *Schematic drawing showing how a bone graft (BG) is fitted into a ventral cervical slot with the interspace distracted.*

medium-sized plastic plate* is then applied across the interspace. Two cortical, 3.5-mm screws are placed in each vertebral body. The screw holes are drilled at angles away from the canal and are inserted without tapping the holes. Screw length is estimated by measuring the radiographs. Care must be exercised not to enter the spinal canal with the screws (Fig. 42-3).

Attempts at placing the graft snugly in place without a plate, as is done in man and the horse, have regularly caused the graft to be dislodged ventrally. We therefore routinely place a plate ventrally to keep the graft in place as well as to aid in maintaining distraction. With rigid steel plates, screws frequently pull out of the vertebral bodies. For this reason, we have used the more flexible Lubra plates, which can be cut to the needed length on the operating table. The plates are only faintly visible on radiographs, and no screw pullout or plate breakage has been noted to date. Any remaining cancellous bone is then packed lateral to the plate and over the intervertebral space. Closure of soft tissues is routine.

Postoperative Considerations

The dogs are allowed to recover from anesthesia and are then put in a neck brace. This brace may take several forms (Fig. 42-4), but should attempt to immobilize the neck *and* the thoracic cage as a unit. Braces that incorporate the cervical region alone do not stop movement of the caudal cervical vertebrae.

* Lubra plate, Lubra Co., 1905 Mohawk, Fort Collins, CO 80525

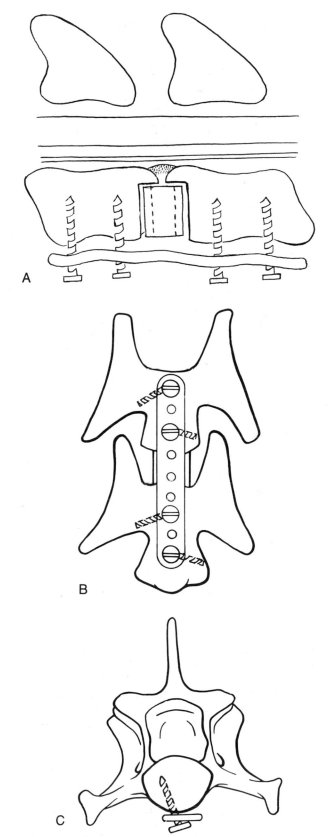

Fig. 42-3. A, *Postoperative view with plastic plate, screws, and bone graft in place.* B, *Plate and screws as seen from ventral aspect. Note that screws diverge away from the canal.* C, *Cross-sectional view showing appropriate angulation of screws to avoid injury to the spinal cord.*

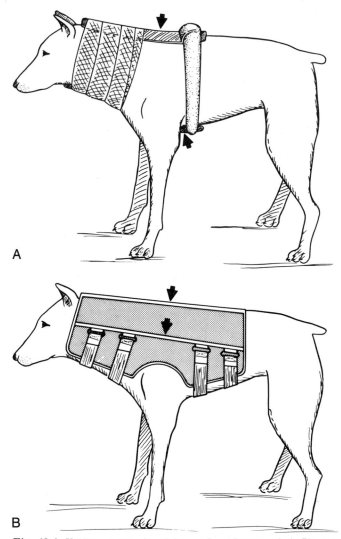

Fig. 42-4. *Various types of neck braces have been used. A, Plaster splints (arrows) supplemented with bandage material may be used. B, A human orthopedic knee brace with steel rods (arrows) may also be adapted for use.**

The administration of corticosteroids is discontinued unless the dog is worsened postoperatively, in which case the dose is halved daily for a week.

Activity is restricted for 3 months; then the collar is removed and radiographs are taken. Depending on the dog's temperament, the owner's degree of responsibility, and radiographic evidence of fusion, the collar may be permanently removed or replaced for another few months.

Several months may be required to note the final degree of neurologic improvement.

References and Suggested Readings

Chambers, J. M., and Betts, C. W.: Caudal cervical spondylopathy in the dog: a review of 20 clinical cases and the literature. J. Am. Anim. Hosp. Assoc., *13*:571, 1977.

*Canine Orthopedics Custom Designs, 107 7th Street, Broadmoor, Colorado Springs, CO 80906

Denny, H. R., Gibbs, C., and Gaskell, C. J.: Cervical spondylopathy in the dog—a review of thirty-five cases. J. Small Anim. Pract., *18*:117, 1977.

Gage, E. D., and Hoerlein, B. F.: Surgical repair of cervical subluxation and spondylolisthesis in the dog. J. Am. Anim. Hosp. Assoc., *9*:385, 1973.

Hurov, L. I.: Treatment of cervical vertebral instability in the dog. J. Am. Vet. Med. Assoc., *175*:278, 1979.

Maston, T. A.: Cervical vertebral instability (wobbler syndrome) in the dog. Vet. Rec., *104*:142, 1979.

Seim, H. B., and Withrow, S. J.: Pathophysiology and diagnosis of caudal cervical spondylo-myelopathy with emphasis on the Doberman pinscher. J. Am. Anim. Hosp. Assoc., *18*:241, 1982.

Selcer, R. R.: Cervical spondylopathy: wobbler syndrome in dogs. J. Am. Anim. Hosp. Assoc., *11*:175, 1975.

Trotter, E. J., deLahunta, A., Geary, J. C., and Brasmer, T. H.: Caudal cervical vertebral malformation-malarticulation in Great Danes and Doberman pinschers. J. Am. Vet. Med. Assoc., *168*:917, 1976.

Wright, F., Rest, J. R., and Palmer, A. C.: Ataxia of the Great Dane caused by stenosis of the cervical vertebral canal: comparison with similar conditions in the basset hound, Doberman pinscher, ridgeback and the thoroughbred horse. Vet. Rec., *92*:1, 1973.

Parker, A. J., et al.: Cervical vertebral instability in the dog. J. Am. Vet. Med. Assoc., *103*:71, 1973.

Ventral Decompression for Treatment of Herniated Cervical Intervertebral Disk in the Dog

by HOWARD B. SEIM, III

and STEPHEN J. WITHROW

Herniated cervical intervertebral disks in dogs are manifested by neck pain, tetraparesis, or both. Critical neurologic examination, coupled with radiographic examination, frequently reveals the affected interspace. Occasionally, myelography is necessary when apparently more than one lesion could be causing the problem, when a lesion is seen that is not compatible with the neurologic examination, or when no sign of a lesion is seen on plain radiographic survey films.

The neurosurgical procedures described for treatment of cervical disk disease in the dog include fenestration, dorsal laminectomy, hemilaminectomy, and ventral decompressive techniques.[2,3,4,7,8] The selection of one of these neurosurgical procedures has been dictated by the neurologic signs exhibited by the patient. Fenestration had been advocated for patients with pain alone, especially dogs with recurrent attacks. Dorsal laminectomy and hemilaminectomy have been used in those patients exhibiting chronic recurrent exacerbations of neck pain, and especially in patients with moderate to severe tetraparesis. Recently, it has been shown that ventral decompression without concurrent fenestration results in both rapid (48 hours for pain and 1 week for pain and tetraparesis) and sustained relief of signs.[6]

Fenestration has been shown to be effective for eventual pain relief in some patients, but remains an inadequate procedure for removal of disk material from impingement on the spinal cord and nerve roots.

With fenestration, one hopes to prevent further disk extrusion, and the veterinary surgeon hopes the dog will recover from its current attack and will not experience a recurrence. Patients that undergo fenestration for cervical disk disease exhibit a longer morbidity than those treated with ventral decompression.

Dorsal decompressive laminectomy and hemilaminectomy for the treatment of cervical disk disease are rarely indicated and have several inherent disadvantages. The severe disruption of hard and soft tissues, prolonged operating time, poor visualization of ventrally and ventrolaterally dislocated disks, and the excessive manipulation of the spinal cord necessary to remove the disk material result in prolonged morbidity. Laminectomy without mass removal may not always achieve maximal effect and has been compared to removing the roof of a house to let the water out of the basement. Dorsal laminectomy has been shown to be effective in the removal of massive lateral disk protrusions, which occur rarely with spontaneous cervical disk disease in the dog. Recently, the dorsal laminectomy and hemilaminectomy approach to patients with cervical disk protrusions exhibiting signs of severe recurrent pain or pain and tetraparesis has been increasingly abandoned in favor of the ventral decompressive procedure.[1,6,7,8]

The ventral approach better fulfills the criteria for an effective surgical procedure: minimal dissection through normal tissue planes, little disruption of normal anatomic structures, adequate visualization of ventral and ventrolateral disks, certain removal of the disk, minimal manipulation of the spinal cord, quick recovery, few complications, relatively rapid operating time, and sustained relief of signs.

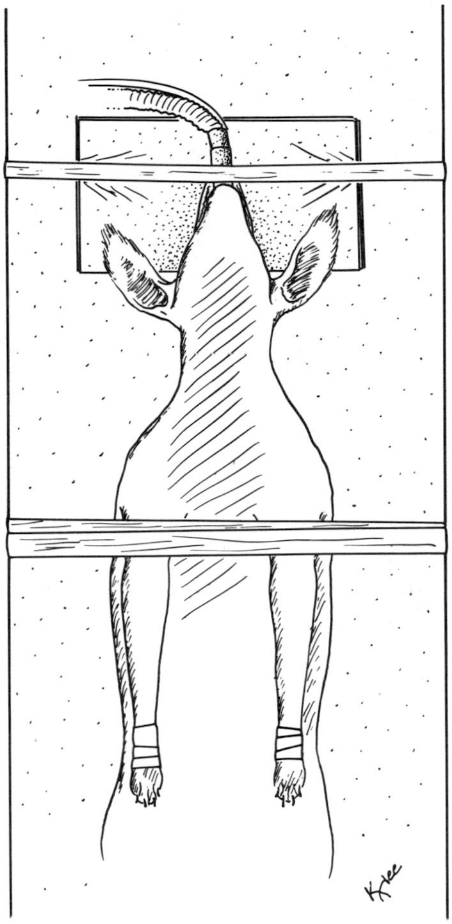

Surgical Technique

The dog is premedicated with dexamethazone phosphate (2 mg/kg body weight). Broad-spectrum antibiotics are given 24 hours preoperatively, at the time of the procedure, and 2 days postoperatively. Anesthesia is induced with an ultrashort-acting barbiturate, and endotracheal intubation is performed. An inhalation anesthetic agent is used for maintenance of anesthesia. Lactated Ringer's solution is administered intravenously throughout the procedure. Patients with any degree of tetraparesis either should be placed on a Bird respirator* or should have intermittent positive-pressure respiration during anesthesia.

The ventral neck is clipped and is prepared for an aseptic surgical procedure. The dog is positioned in dorsal recumbency with the chest in a "V"-trough. The front legs are taped caudally, and the head is taped cranially. Mild linear traction is placed on the neck to hold the intervertebral spaces apart (Fig. 42-5).

A midline ventral exposure is used, as described for cervical disk fenestration[5] (see the next section of this chapter). The location of the affected intervertebral space is determined by palpating the prominent trans-

*Bird Corp., Mark 7 Lane, Palm Springs, CA

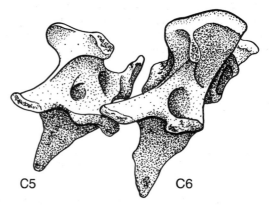

Fig. 42-5. *Positioning the patient for the surgical procedure.*

verse process (wings) of C6. On the midline and just off the most cranial aspect of the process is the C5–C6 intervertebral space (Fig. 42-6). An alternate technique is to palpate the prominent ventral spinous process of the first cervical vertebra and then to count caudally (Fig. 42-7). It is often wise to count in both directions to be sure of operating the correct interspace.

Once the involved space has been located, the longus colli muscles are incised along their median

C5   C6

Fig. 42-6. *Palpation of the sixth cervical vertebra to determine the affected intervertebral space.*

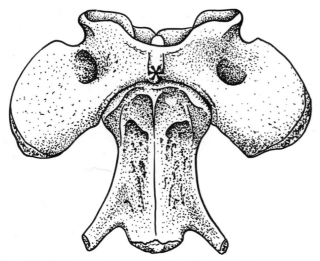

Fig. 42-7. *Palpation of the atlas (asterisk), followed by counting, to determine the affected intervertebral space.*

raphe, and the tendinous insertions on the ventral spinous processes are cut with scissors. The muscle is then subperiosteally elevated off the ventral surface of the two vertebral bodies directly adjacent to the involved intervertebral space. Self-retaining retractors are inserted to hold the longus colli muscles apart (Fig. 42-8A). Care should be taken at this point to protect the structures of the carotid sheath and the esophagus from inadvertent damage by the retractors. Meticulous control of hemorrhage is extremely important to prevent pooling of blood in the "slot" to be created. The ventral spinous process is removed with a rongeur. The ventral anulus fibrosus is then excised with a No. 11 scalpel blade. It must be appreciated that the intervertebral space has a slight caudal-to-cranial angle that must be compensated for when making the cut (Fig.

42-8B). The anulus fibrosus and any disk material present are removed with a disk rongeur or a dental scraper.

A high-speed pneumatic drill with a bone bur* is used to create a rectangular defect in the bodies of the two involved vertebrae. Frequent irrigation with physiologic saline solution is used to dissipate heat and to prevent burning of bone and drying of tissue.

The defect should extend no farther than three-quarters the width of the interspace (Fig. 42-9). Because of the caudal-to-cranial angle of the cervical intervertebral spaces, the defect should be centered slightly towards the cranial vertebral body, so that when the spinal canal is reached, the slot will be directly centered over the intervertebral space (Figs. 42-10 and 42-11). The defect should not extend more than one-quarter the length of the vertebra cranially or caudally.

The depth of the defect can be gauged by visualizing three distinct layers of bone as one drills (Fig. 42-12A). First, the hard outer cortical layer of the vertebral body is penetrated. Second, the softer, more hemorrhagic marrow layer is visualized. This layer is more easily drilled than the cortical layer. Finally, the inner cortical layer of the vertebral body is seen. Once this layer is reached, drilling must be done carefully so as not to break into the spinal canal abruptly. It is imperative to remain on the midline throughout the procedure, to ensure that the laterally located vertebral artery and vein (in the vertebral body) and the vertebral venous sinuses (on the floor of the spinal canal) are not lacerated.

Once the drill has penetrated in the inner cortical layer, a 3-0 bone curette can be used to enlarge the defect. Dorsal anulus fibrosus should be curetted away

---

* Hall International Inc., 3M Co., P.O. Box 4307, Santa Barbara, CA 93103

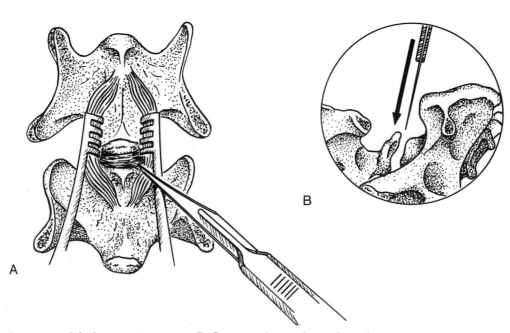

Fig. 42-8. A, *Retraction of the longus colli muscles.* B, *Compensating angle cut (arrow).*

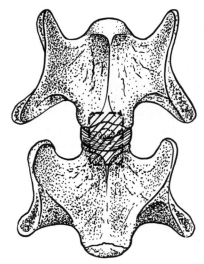

Fig. 42-9. *Creation of a rectangular defect between the two affected vertebrae.*

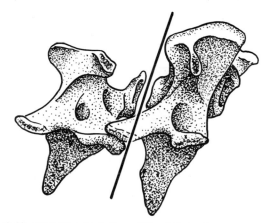

Fig. 42-10. *Cranial orientation of the defect cut.*

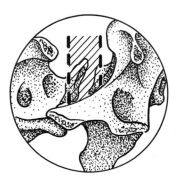

Fig. 42-11. *Centering of the defect over the intervertebral space.*

to expose the dorsal longitudinal ligament. The inner cortical layer of bone should then be curetted to a diameter in which the veterinary surgeon can work. Care must be taken to avoid excessive lateral curettage and subsequent laceration of the venous sinus. Once the exposure is adequate, careful removal of the dorsal longitudinal ligament is performed with fine forceps and a No. 11 scalpel blade, allowing access to and re-

moval of disk material (Fig. 42-12*B*). It is best to remove disk material located on the ventral midline first. Removal of laterally located disk material results in a greater chance of injuring the venous sinus. A dull, flat dental spatula is best suited for removal of the disk material (Fig. 42-12*C*). This instrument enables the veterinary neurosurgeon to remove laterally extruded disk material with less fear of lacerating the venous sinus. Special care should be taken when old, calcified disks are encountered. They may be adherent to venous sinus or dura. Disk material should be removed until the veterinary surgeon can visualize the dural tube (Fig. 42-12*D*).

During the entire procedure, meticulous hemostasis, using bipolar cautery, bone wax, Gelfoam,* Cottonoid† or sponges, and suction, is mandatory to allow adequate visualization. An understanding of the proper method of using each specific device helps in controlling hemorrhage, the major complication of this procedure.

Bipolar cautery is used to control hemorrhage in the soft tissue surrounding the bony defect. Prior to drilling, the bone should be easily visualized to ensure accuracy. Hemorrhage in bone may be encountered as the cancellous layer of the vertebral body is reached. If the bleeding is excessive, bone wax pressed into the bleeding surface provides adequate hemostasis. Once the canal has been reached, the biggest problem is to avoid the vertebral venous sinus while retaining the appropriate exposure. If the venous sinus is lacerated or is inadvertently cut, suction, Gelfoam, and a Cottonoid or sponge can be used effectively to stop the hemorrhage. A piece of Gelfoam is cut to approximately half the size of the slot. A piece of Cottonoid or sponge is soaked in physiologic saline solution and is made ready for use.

The following sequence of events must occur if venous sinus hemorrhage is encountered. Suction is initially used to control and to locate more accurately the point of hemorrhage. Once the hemorrhage has been located, the suction device is removed, and the previously cut piece of Gelfoam is quickly placed at the site of hemorrhage. The sponge or Cottonoid is then placed over the Gelfoam, and the suction tip is replaced on top of the Cottonoid or sponge to evacuate the excess blood from the surgical site. Suction on the Cottonoid or sponge is continued until the hemorrhage subsides. In 2 minutes, the sponge or Cottonoid is gently removed, and further disk removal can continue. It is important not to apply suction directly on the Gelfoam because the material will disappear into the suction device and hemorrhage will resume.

If the laceration of the venous sinus is so severe that hemorrhage continues in spite of the previously mentioned techniques, the veterinary surgeon can use the suction device to remove blood continuously from the surgical site and at the same time to remove the remaining disk gently. This procedure should be at-

* Upjohn Co., Kalamazoo, MI
† Johnson & Johnson Products, Inc., New Brunswick, NJ, 08903

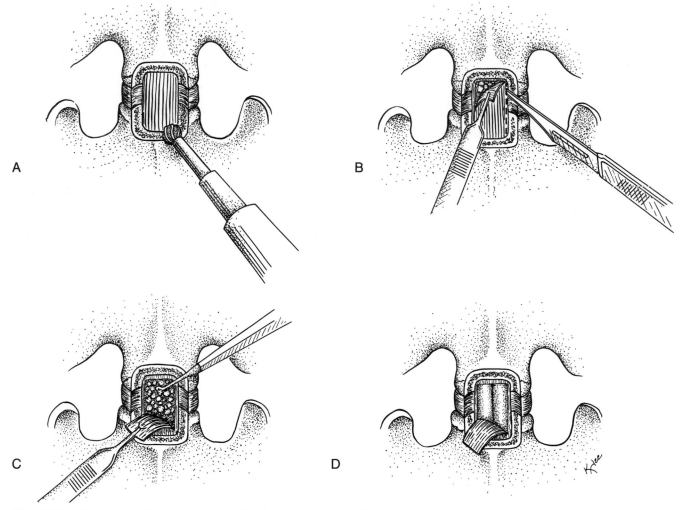

Fig. 42-12. A, *Depth of the defect.* B, *Removal of the dorsal longitudinal ligament.* C, *Removal of disk material.* D, *Termination of the disk removal when the dural tube is visualized.*

tempted only if the suction device can keep pace with the hemorrhage, and if visualization of structures is adequate.

Prior to closure, all hemorrhage should be controlled. Multiple flushing with physiologic saline solution is done to dislodge any remaining bone dust from the soft tissues. Closure of the soft tissue is routine.

Postoperative Considerations

Corticosteroid administration should be discontinued gradually over a 3- to 7-day period. Early and sustained recovery from neurologic signs is the rule rather than the exception.

The only disadvantages to this technique are the creation of too wide a defect, which results in instability and collapse of the innerspace, and potential rupture of the vertebral venous sinus during manipulation of the intervertebral foramen and along the floor of the spinal canal with the dental tool. Good surgical technique and proper neurosurgical instrumentation can help to avoid such problems.

References and Suggested Readings

1. Coppola, A. R.: Anterior cervical discectomy without fusion. Va. Med., *106*:297, 1979.
2. Denny, H. R.: The surgical treatment of cervical disc protrusions in the dog: a review of 40 cases. J. Small Anim. Pract., *19*:251, 1978.
3. Funquist, B., and Svalastoga, E.: A simplified surgical approach to the last two cervical vertebrae in the dog. J. Small Anim. Pract., *20*:593, 1979.
4. Gilpin, G. N.: Evaluation of three techniques of ventral decompression of the cervical spinal cord in the dog. J. Am. Vet. Med. Assoc., *168*:325, 1976.
5. Piermattei, D. L., and Greely, R. G.: An Atlas of Surgical Approaches to the Bones of the Dog and Cat. 2nd Ed. Philadelphia, W. B. Saunders, 1979.
6. Seim, H. B., and Prata, R. G.: Ventral decompression for the treatment of cervical disk disease in the dog: a review of 54 cases. J. Am. Anim. Hosp. Assoc., *18*:233, 1982.
7. Swaim, S. F.: Ventral decompression of the cervical spinal cord in the dog. J. Am. Vet. Med. Assoc., *164*:491, 1979.
8. Swaim, S. F.: Ventral decompression of the cervical spinal cord in the dog. J. Am. Vet. Med. Assoc., *162*:276, 1973.

Atlantoaxial Instability

by PETER SHIRES

Atlantoaxial instability is one cause of high cervical spinal cord compression in the dog. Young, small breed dogs are most commonly affected. Clinical signs include high cervical pain and variable proprioceptive and motor dysfunction in one or more limbs.

Surgical Anatomy

The atlas (C1) articulates with the occipital condyles by means of two laterally placed, cupped diarthrodial joints. The articular conformation restricts movement between the occipital condyle and the atlas to the dorsoventral plane. Conversely, the atlas and axis (C2) have a multifaceted articulation that allows rotational and some lateral movement. Rotation is centered around the odontoid process, which projects cranially from the axis into the bony ring formed by the atlas around the spinal cord. The odontoid process is secured to the ventral arch of the atlas and is separated from the cord by a tough, fibrous sheet, the transverse ligament. The cranial end of the odontoid process is attached to the occipital condyles by the alar ligaments and to the ventral aspect of the foramen magnum by the apical ligament (Fig. 42-13). All these ventral ligaments tether the odontoid process and hence the axis to the ventral arch of the atlas. The dorsal arch of the atlas and dorsal spine of the axis are joined by the tough dorsal atlantoaxial ligament, which helps to stabilize the atlantoaxial joint.

The head, through the occipital condyles, rests on the atlas, which, in turn, articulates with the axis. The axis is primarily supported by the "bow string" of the nuchal ligament and "bow" of the cervical spine. The nuchal ligament attaches to the axis, thus allowing free movement of the head by pivoting at the occipitoatlantoaxial articulation. With head flexion, the occipitoatlantal joint is moved through its full range of motion. With continued forced flexion, the atlantoaxial joint becomes stressed. The odontoid process, ventral ligaments, and dorsal atlantoaxial ligament are the center of stress in forced head flexion (Fig. 42-14).

Pathophysiologic and Etiologic Features

The clinical signs of cervical pain and limb motor dysfunction are due to pressure on the spinal cord. With atlantoaxial instability, spinal cord pressure is a result of narrowing of the neural canal by downward displacement of the atlas relative to the axis (Fig. 42-15) or by forward tilting of the atlas relative to the axis (Fig. 42-16). A number of etiologic factors may bring about these two conditions:

1. Congenital (Fig. 42-17)

   Absence of the odontoid process and hence a lack of ventral ligamentous support

   Separation of the apical ossification center from the remainder of the odontoid process leading to impaired ventral ligamentous support; this condition is probably due to traumatic separation after delayed closure of the physis

   Malformation (angulation) of the odontoid process, endangering the cord by its proximity alone

   Lack of ventral or dorsal ligamentous support between the atlas and axis leading to axial instability

2. Traumatic (Fig. 42-18)

   Rupture of the atlantoaxial or occipitoaxial ligamentous support

   Fracture of the odontoid process and rupture of the dorsal atlantoaxial ligament

   Fractures of the atlas or axis

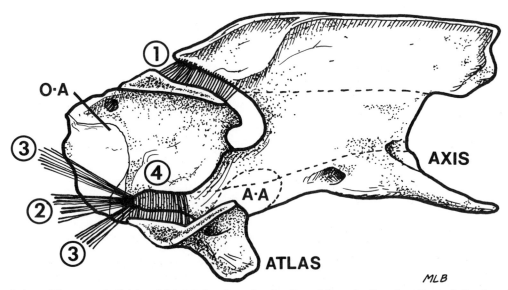

Fig. 42-13. *Lateral view of the normal atlantoaxial joint showing a hemisection of the axis, the atlas, the occipitoatlantal joint (O-A), the atlantoaxial joint (A-A), the dorsal atlantoaxial ligament (1), the apical ligament (2), the paired alar ligaments (3), and the transverse ligament (4).*

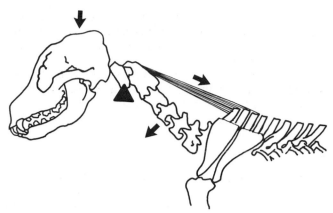

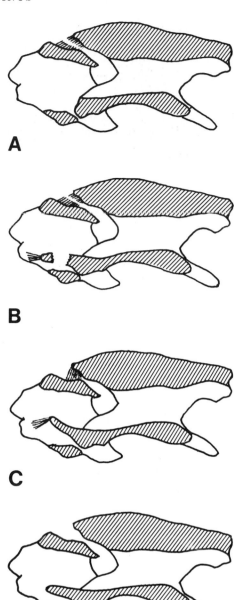

Fig. 42-14. *Diagrammatic representation of the forces around the atlantoaxial joint when downward pressure is applied to the head. The "bow" of the cervical spine and the "string" of the nuchal ligament absorb most normal flexion forces (arrows). Excessive force concentrates stresses at the atlantoaxial fulcrum (solid triangle).*

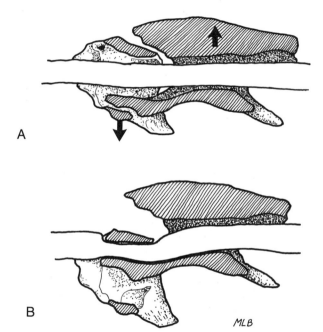

Fig. 42-15. *A, and B, Cross-sectional diagrammatic representation of cord compression in the atlantoaxial area after downward displacement of the atlas relative to the axis.*

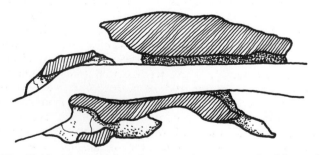

Fig. 42-16. *Atlantoaxial cord compression as a result of forward tilting of the atlas relative to the axis.*

Fig. 42-17. *Cross-sectional diagrammatic representation of some congenital causes of atlantoaxial cord compression. A, Absence of the odontoid process and secondary weakening of the dorsal atlantoaxial ligaments. B, Ununited odontoid apex and secondary dorsal atlantoaxial ligament rupture. C, Dorsal angulation of the odontoid process. D, Lack of ventral or dorsal ligamentous atlantoaxial support.*

Whatever the origin, the result is instability of the atlantoaxial joint and pressure on the spinal cord in that area. The degree of pressure depends on the distortion stress placed on the head and the presence and angulation of the odontoid process. An intact odontoid process severely traumatizes the spinal cord if the

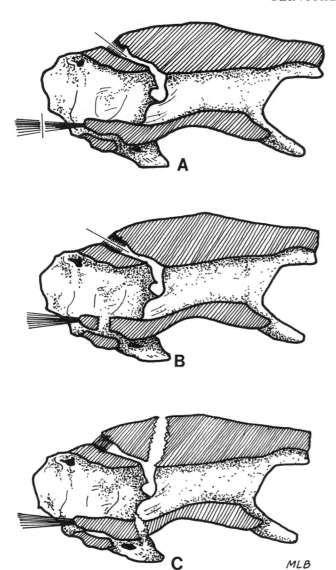

Fig. 42-18. *Some traumatic situations leading to atlantoaxial cord compression. A, Ligamentous rupture. B, Odontoid process fracture and dorsal ligamentous rupture. C, Axis fractures.*

process deviates dorsally during neck flexion (see Fig. 42-16). Congenital dorsal angulation of the odontoid process reduces the distance between the spinal cord and the bony canal and thereby increases the risk factor in cases of instability (see Fig. 42-17C).

Clinical cases of atlantoaxial subluxation are usually the result of a combination of congenital and traumatic factors. An animal with congenital lack of support to the odontoid process has progressive stretching and weakening of the dorsal atlantoaxial ligament. Eventually, little trauma is needed to rupture the ligament and to precipitate a subluxation. A dog with normal atlantoaxial anatomic features requires considerable flexion force to the head to rupture the supporting ligaments or fracture the odontoid process.

Two clinical syndromes are seen. The congenital form is usually seen in young, small breed dogs of both sexes, in which the head size and weight are disproportionate to the strength of ligamentous support. A his-

tory of trauma is not always evident, although careful questioning often traces the onset to a minor incident that would be uneventful in an animal with normal anatomic configurations.

The traumatic form may be seen in any breed, age, or sex of dog with a history of sudden, powerful downward flexion of the head, such as a head-first fall or running into a wall.

Diagnosis

Presenting signs vary from localized upper cervical pain to terminal respiratory and tetraparalysis. Most frequently the characteristic signs include cervical pain, especially with flexion of the head and neck, and mild-to-moderate upper motor neuron signs to the fore- and hind legs.

Signalment and clinical signs are identical to signs seen when the upper cervical cord is compressed for any reason. It is essential to differentiate between atlantoaxial subluxation and other cervical cord disorders, such as intervertebral disk herniation and fractures, for therapeutic and prognostic reasons. A positive diagnosis of atlantoaxial subluxation can be made if the space between the dorsal spine of the axis and the dorsal arch of the atlas is wider than normal. A good-quality radiograph taken with the animal in lateral recumbency and the neck in a "normal" position may be sufficient to demonstrate an increased dorsal atlantoaxial space. If not, a flexed lateral view has been advocated, bearing in mind that hyperflexion of an unstable atlantoaxial joint can severely traumatize the spinal cord, especially if the odontoid process is intact. Ventrodorsal and open-mouth views allow visualization of the odontoid process and permit evaluation of lateral displacement of the process. (Note: Open-mouth views also necessitate some flexion of the neck and could induce spinal cord trauma.) Absence of positive radiographic evidence does not exclude the possibility of an atlantoaxial instability. It is not uncommon to make a diagnosis, based on clinical signs alone, after ruling out all other possibilities.

Medical Treatment

Conservative therapy has been advocated when neurologic involvement is minimal and displacement is not severe. The head should be supported in an extended neck position for at least 6 weeks with a neck brace made of suitable material such as x-ray film or Orthoplast* (Fig. 42-19). Concurrent therapy with intravenous mannitol or dexamethasone is recommended initially to reduce and control spinal cord edema. Cage rest is essential for 1 to 3 weeks. Analgesics are used if necessary. Clients should be informed of possible recurrence because stability is dependent on atlantoaxial scar tissue. Newly formed fibrous tissue is weaker than the original ligaments. Protective management should be advocated for the remainder of the dog's life.

* Johnson & Johnson Products, Inc., New Brunswick, NJ 08903

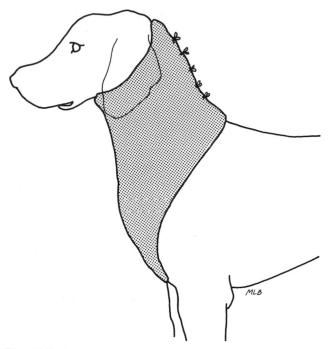

Fig. 42-19. *A lateral view of a padded neck brace made of exposed x-ray film.*

Surgical Treatment

Surgical therapy is recommended for all patients showing neurologic involvement. Two surgical techniques are currently used; both aim to stabilize the atlantoaxial joint in the normal position, and both allow decompression when indicated.

DORSAL APPROACH

After routine surgical preparation and general anesthesia, the dog is placed in sternal recumbency with the head and neck supported in a partially flexed position (Fig. 42-20A). A dorsal midline approach is made through the skin and paraspinal muscles from the nuchal crest to the dorsal spine of the third cervical vertebra. All musculature is gently reflected from the dorsal arch of the atlas and the dorsal spine of the axis. Self-retaining retractors aid in maintaining exposure. The dorsal membranes joining the atlas and axis and the occiput and atlas are incised with a No. 12 Bard-Parker blade (Fig. 42-20B). The atlantoaxial ligament must be incised bilaterally to allow symmetric suture placement between the atlas and the axis.

When spinal cord compression is severe, the area may be decompressed by removing part of the cranial dorsolateral lamina of one side of the axis with small rongeurs. The caudal aspect of the dorsal arch of the atlas can also be removed to add to the decompression (Fig. 42-20C). Removal of more than one-third of the dorsal atlantal arch weakens the structure and compromises fixation.

Two widely separated, small holes are drilled in the dorsal spine of the axis. The dorsal arch of the atlas is secured to the dorsal spine of the axis with heavy suture material or orthopedic wire. Heavy suture is preferred by some veterinary surgeons because of difficulties encountered in passing 20- to 22-gauge wire under the arch of the atlas without traumatizing the spinal cord and because of wire breakage from cyclic stresses.

To place the suture extradurally, a loop of fine wire is passed from the atlantoaxial space under the dorsal arch of the atlas. A loop of heavy, nonabsorbable suture is threaded through the wire (Fig. 42-20D), and the suture is carefully drawn under the atlantal arch. The suture is cut, creating a double strand. The atlantoaxial joint is gently aligned, and the cranial suture is passed through the cranial hole in the axis and is tied. The caudal suture is passed through the caudal hole and is tied (Fig. 42-20E).*

The paraspinous musculature, subcutaneous tissue, and skin are closed by standard methods. Postoperative care should include steroid and antibiotic therapy, cage rest for 5 to 7 days, and a neck brace for 2 to 3 weeks.

Complications of this technique are (1) wire or suture breakage with resultant reluxation, (2) fracture or incomplete fusion of the dorsal arch of the atlas that renders fixation to the axis impossible, (3) fracture of, or insufficient bone in, the dorsal spine of the axis that makes caudal fixation impossible, and (4) rotation of the axis on the atlas by tying the sutures too tightly.

VENTRAL APPROACH

A permanent resolution to atlantoaxial instability can be achieved by fusing the two vertebrae in anatomic alignment. Decompression, when required, can

* Editor's Note. An alternate single-wire dorsal technique is successfully used by the editor. Two holes are drilled in the dorsal arch of the atlas and one is drilled in the cranial half of the dorsal spinous process of the axis. The large canal at this point allows the 20-gauge wire to be threaded through the holes in the atlas without compressing or compromising the spinal cord. The wire is then passed through the hole in the dorsal spinous process of the axis and is tightly twisted (Ed. Note Fig. 1). This technique provides stability and eliminates the impaction and resulting angulation that may occur with other dorsal approaches using the cranial pull stabilization. The major complication involves a fracture of the dorsal arch of the atlas in small or miniature dogs. If this should happen, a ventral approach can be attempted.

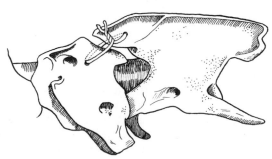

Ed. Note Fig. 1. *An alternate single-wire technique. Two holes are drilled in the dorsal arch of the atlas and one in the cranial half of the spinous process of the axis.*

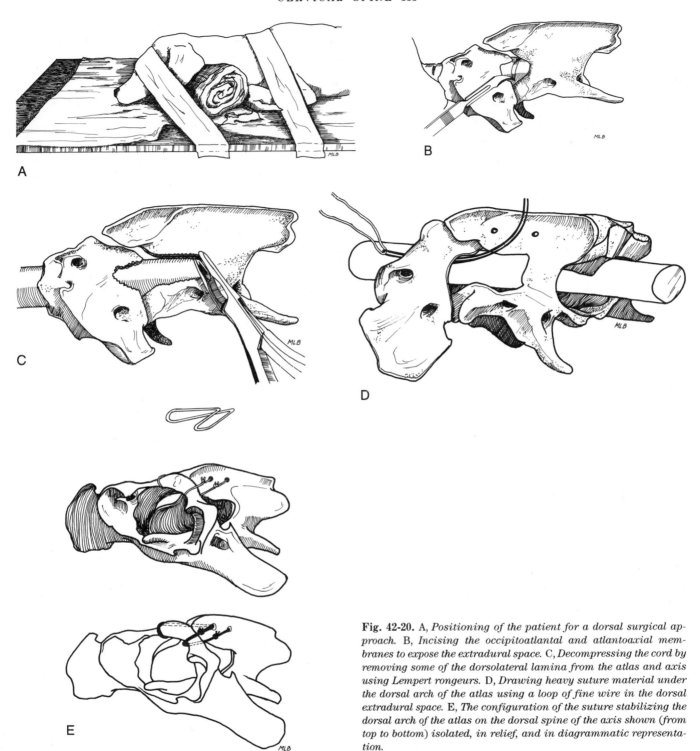

Fig. 42-20. A, *Positioning of the patient for a dorsal surgical approach.* B, *Incising the occipitoatlantal and atlantoaxial membranes to expose the extradural space.* C, *Decompressing the cord by removing some of the dorsolateral lamina from the atlas and axis using Lempert rongeurs.* D, *Drawing heavy suture material under the dorsal arch of the atlas using a loop of fine wire in the dorsal extradural space.* E, *The configuration of the suture stabilizing the dorsal arch of the atlas on the dorsal spine of the axis shown (from top to bottom) isolated, in relief, and in diagrammatic representation.*

be performed by removing the fractured or malaligned odontoid process during the ventral fixation procedure.

The surgical approach is made through a ventral midline incision with the dog in dorsal recumbency. The head and neck are extended and supported by a pad under the upper cervical area (Fig. 42-21*A*). The paired sternothyrohyoid muscles are separated, and blunt dissection is used to mobilize and reflect the tra-

chea, carotid artery, vagus nerve, and esophagus. These structures are gently retracted to expose the ventral cervical musculature. The wings and ventral prominence of the atlas are palpated, and muscular attachments to the atlas and axis are reflected away from the midline. The ventral pouches of the joint capsules are removed from the paired atlantoaxial joints (Fig. 42-21*B*). Self-retaining retractors aid in visualization of the area.

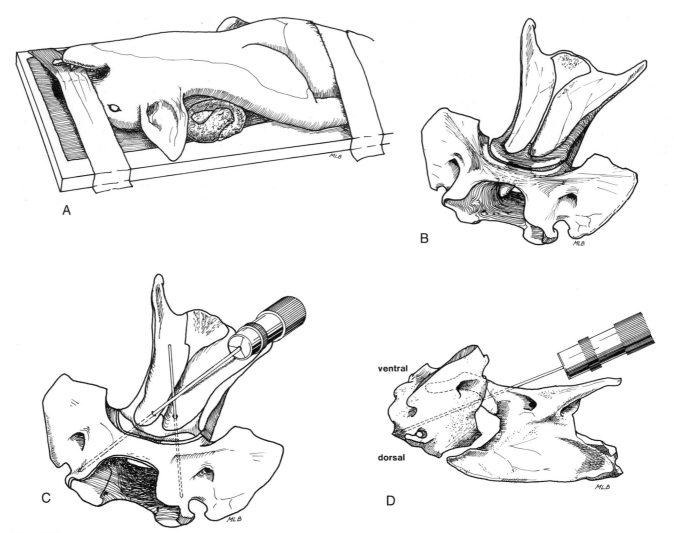

Fig. 42-21. A, *Positioning of the patient for a ventral approach to the atlantoaxial joint.* B, *The ventral aspect of the atlantoaxial joint seen from a craniolateral view.* C, *Pin placement through the atlantoaxial joints from the ventral body of the axis. Accurate seating of the pins into the medial side of the alar notch is essential.* D, *A lateral view of the stabilization pin placement from the ventral body of the axis, through the atlantoaxial joint, and into the heavy bone surrounding the neural canal.*

Using small rongeurs or a power drill, the odontoid process is separated from the cranial end of the axis if it is pressing on the spinal cord. Ligaments attached to the apex of the odontoid process are exposed through a ventral opening in the fascia covering the foramen magnum. The odontoid process is removed after incising the ligaments. Removal decompresses the spinal cord in that area and alleviates a potentially dangerous situation should instability recur. This step is unnecessary if spinal cord compression is not severe.

The atlantoaxial joints are separated to allow removal of the articular cartilage with a No. 15 Bard-Parker blade. A cancellous bone graft taken from the proximal humerus is packed into the joint spaces. The atlantoaxial segment is carefully aligned and is stabilized with small-fragment forceps placed over the atlantoaxial joint. Two small Steinmann pins or large Kirschner wires are premeasured, and the desired length is marked. The pins are driven from the center

of the axis across the scarified atlantoaxial joint and are seated in the atlas just medial to the alar notch (Fig. 42-21*C*). The point of each pin must be kept as ventral as possible to avoid penetrating the dorsal surface of the thin wings of the atlas (Fig. 42-21*D*). The length of the pins is premeasured from the point of entry into the axis to the palpable medial aspect of the alar notches on the atlas. When both pins are seated, they are cut off close to the body of the axis. If the protruding ends can be bent without compromising the fixation, this maneuver will prevent cranial migration of the pins into the occipital condyles. A power drill facilitates pin placement and is recommended. The small-fragment forceps are removed, and the ventral spinal musculature, sternothyrohyoideus muscles, subcutaneous tissues, and skin are closed routinely.

Postoperative therapy with antibiotics, 3 to 5 days of cage rest, and application of a neck brace for 2 to 3 weeks are advisable. Dexamethasone may be used if preoperative neurologic signs are severe. Early bone bridging of the joint space should be radiographically visible in 6 to 8 weeks. Complications include inappropriate pin placement leading to instability, pin migration, vertebral artery puncture, or neural canal penetration.

In conclusion, atlantoaxial instability is an infrequent problem seen usually in small breeds of dogs. Accurate diagnosis allows rehabilitation by conservative or surgical methods. Surgical fixation allows early and more reliable return to normal function. A ventral surgical approach may only be used when the necessary instrumentation is available, but it does afford a reliable, permanent solution to atlantoaxial instability.

References and Suggested Readings

Chambers, J. N., Betts, C. W., and Oliver, J. E.: The use of nonmetallic suture material for stabilization of atlantoaxial subluxations. J. Am. Anim. Hosp. Assoc., *13*:602, 1977.

Gage, E. D., and Smallwood, J. E.: Surgical repair of atlantoaxial subluxation in a dog. Small Anim. Clin., *65*:583, 1970.

Geary, J. C., Oliver, J. E., and Horlein, B. F.: Atlantoaxial subluxation in the canine. J. Small Anim. Pract., *8*:577, 1967.

Parker, A. J., and Park, R. D.: Atlantoaxial subluxation in small breeds of dogs: diagnosis and pathogenesis. Small Anim. Clin., *68*:1133, 1973.

Sorjonen, D. C., and Shires, P. K.: Atlantoaxial instability: A ventral surgical technique for decompression, fixation and fusion. Vet. Surg., *10*:22, 1981.

43 * Thoracolumbar Spine

Intervertebral Disk Fenestration

by JAMES E. CREED

and DANIEL J. YTURRASPE

The herniated intervertebral disk syndrome remains an enigma for a significant number of dogs and causes clinical signs ranging from pain to death from diffuse myelomalacia. Degeneration of intervertebral disks is a systemic disease of the musculoskeletal system occurring primarily in, but not limited to, chondrodystrophoid breeds of dogs. In itself, this disease is of little significance. It is the secondary manifestation of spinal cord injury associated with protrusion or extrusion of the degenerate disk into the spinal canal that becomes clinically significant.

Various methods have been advocated for treating intervertebral disk disease in dogs. Although many dogs respond favorably to nonsurgical methods of treatment, a significant number have recurrent attacks. In chondrodystrophoid breeds, such attacks of varying severity are often a characteristic feature of intervertebral disk disease. The interval between attacks varies, and one or more disks may be responsible for producing clinical signs. When one attack closely follows another, the second is frequently due to the extrusion of additional material from the disk responsible for the previous attack. When clinical signs referable to disk disease are separated by a long interval, it is more likely that multiple disks are responsible. Although rare, almost simultaneous prolapse of three disks has been observed. Little or no correlation exists between the severity of one attack with that of succeeding attacks of disk disease. Mild clinical signs of pain may be followed by disk herniation producing irreversible damage to the spinal cord.

The role of surgery in treating intervertebral disk disease in dogs is well established, and every method can generally be classified into one of two groups, based on its primary objective: (1) the nucleus pulposus can be removed from the intervertebral disk to prevent its subsequent prolapse (that is, disk fenestration); or (2) the spinal cord or nerve roots can be surgically decompressed. Both procedures are frequently indicated as a part of treatment.

Removal of the nucleus pulposus from the intervertebral disk by fenestration must be considered primarily prophylactic; it does not alter existing conditions within the spinal canal resulting from prior extrusion of disk material. Intervertebral disk fenestration may have potential therapeutic value when the inflammatory reaction within the spinal canal has been perpetuated by slow extrusion of nuclear material.[4]

It is reported that 93.8% of cervical disk herniations occur between C2 and C6,* and 98% of the thoracolumbar disk herniations occur between T10 and L5.[2] Proper fenestration of multiple disks accomplishes two purposes: (1) it prevents subsequent herniation of additional nucleus pulposus from the partially herniated disk and precludes further exacerbations of the disease; and (2) it reduces, to a negligible level, chances of the subsequent herniation of another disk. To achieve these objectives, selected multiple disks, including ones that are radiographically normal and abnormal, are fenestrated in addition to the offending disk.

Diagnosis of intervertebral disk disease is based on the patient's medical history, clinical signs, breed, and neurologic, radiographic, and laboratory examinations. Because clinical signs of disk herniation are related either to pain or to loss of neurologic function, they are nonspecific and serve only as a guide in selecting appropriate diagnostic methods. Diagnostic objectives include not only confirming that clinical signs are due to disk herniation, but also precisely locating the lesion. Location of the herniation, an essential prerequisite for surgical treatment, requires high-quality radiographs.

Intervertebral disk fenestration should be used as the sole surgical treatment of disk disease only when one is reasonably sure, based on clinical and neurologic signs, that the existing neurologic deficit is reversible without decompressing the spinal cord. Recovery in such cases can be expected with medical treatment alone, provided disk herniation is not progressive. If the reversibility of a neurologic deficit without surgical intervention is doubtful or questionable,

---

* Vertebrae and intervertebral disks are referred to by letter and number (e.g., first and second lumbar vertebrae are L1 and L2 and the disk between them is L1–L2; cervical is C and thoracic is T.

disk fenestration should be combined with spinal cord decompression. Regardless of the severity of clinical signs, if radiographic evidence suggests that an intervertebral disk has completely herniated (that is, the nucleus pulposus is no longer present in the disk space), fenestration of that disk will not alter the course of the disease.

Cervical Disk Fenestration

INDICATIONS

Dogs having one or more recurrent episodes of cervical pain or impairment of motor function within a few weeks and that are otherwise in good health are candidates for this procedure. If radiographs indicate that most or all of the nucleus pulposus has herniated into the spinal canal or the patient is tetraparetic, fenestration will not be beneficial. Such patients should be considered for ventral spinal cord decompression at the affected site, with fenestration of other unherniated disks between C2 and C7.

Advanced age, in itself, is not a contraindication for disk fenestration, but the low incidence of cervical disk herniation in dogs 10 or more years of age limits the prophylactic value of this procedure. Fenestration is performed in this group of patients only when clinical signs persist for several weeks in spite of medical treatment or when multiple attacks within a short time can be attributed to an unstable disk.

PREOPERATIVE CONSIDERATIONS

Corticosteroids and antibiotics are administered presurgically. When preanesthetic drugs have been administered, anesthesia is induced with a short-acting barbiturate and is maintained by endotracheal administration of an acceptable volatile agent. Intravenous fluids are administered during the surgical procedure. The ventral cervical region is surgically prepared in a manner consistent with antiseptic technique. The dog is positioned in perfect dorsal recumbency, with the neck arched over a rolled pad or a bottle to open the intervertebral spaces ventrally, making them more accessible. The patient's muzzle is secured to the table, and the forelimbs are pulled caudally and are tied loosely to the table in a "slump" position.

INTRAOPERATIVE CONSIDERATIONS

A ventral cervical midline skin incision extends from the caudal border of the larynx to the manubrium sterni. The operation is performed from the side of the patient corresponding with the veterinary surgeon's "handed" ability. Access to the ventral aspect of the spinal column is gained by dividing the paired sternohyoideus muscles[3,5] or by digitally dissecting between the sternothyroideus and sternocephalicus muscles.[1] The trachea and the esophagus are retracted to the left, and the adventitia is digitally divided to expose the paired longus colli muscles lying on the ventral aspect

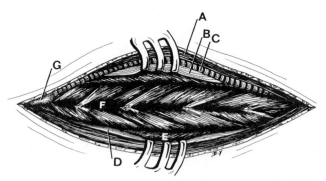

Fig. 43-1. *Anatomic features relevant to intervertebral disk fenestration. A, Sternohyoideus m.; B, esophagus; C, trachea; D, carotid sheath; E, longus capitis m.; F, longus colli m.; G, thyroid gland.*

of the spinal column. Retraction of muscles, trachea, and carotid sheath with a self-retaining retractor aids visualization (Fig. 43-1).

Knowledge of the regional anatomy permits the surgeon to locate and identify each intervertebral space and thus avoid considerable frustration. The paired longus colli muscles converge on the midline in a "V"-shaped configuration, the apex of which points toward the head of the dog (Fig. 43-1). These muscles insert by small, distinct tendons on the ventral protuberances of the vertebral bodies. The ventral midline protuberances are formed principally by the caudoventral aspect of the end plate of the vertebral bodies and are easily palpable. The white, glistening anulus fibrosus of each disk can be exposed just caudal to the ventral protuberances by bluntly separating the longus colli muscles at this level. Although unnecessary for disk fenestration, the ventral aspects of the disks can be more completely exposed by transecting the small tendons of the longus colli muscles where they insert on the ventral protuberance.

Two landmarks, the wings of the atlas and the large distinct transverse processes of C6, are used to identify each cervical disk; both are easily palpable from the surgical field. The first cervical disk (C2–C3) is located by palpating the caudal aspect of the wings of the atlas with the thumb and second finger. With the hand in this position, the index finger is moved to the midline and slightly caudally to the ventral protuberance of C2 immediately cranial to the first cervical disk. The disk between C5 and C6 (fourth cervical disk) is located using the transverse processes of C6. The thumb and second finger are used to palpate the rostroventral aspect of these processes, and the index finger is moved to the ventral midline and slightly rostrally to locate the ventral protuberance of C5. The disk lies immediately caudal to this process. Correlation of these two methods and counting of ventral protuberances are used to identify precisely each cervical disk. Access to a skeleton is also useful for anatomic orientation.

Normally, five cervical disks (C2 to C7) are fenestrated. The disk between C6 and C7 can be fenestrated with slightly more difficulty, and fenestration of the disk between C7 and T1 is difficult from this approach.

Because of the difficulty in fenestrating the latter disk and its low incidence of prolapse, fenestration is not recommended unless clinical signs referable to the disk are demonstrated.

The sequence of disks fenestrated is unimportant. When the ventral anulus fibrosus has been exposed, it is incised transversely with a No. 11 Bard-Parker scalpel blade, or an elliptical section of the anulus is excised. Disk contents are removed with a modified dental-claw tartar scraper, commercial disk fenestration excavator*, or the eye portion of a large suture needle held in a needle holder. The nucleus pulposus is removed using a circular motion. The dorsal anulus should not be penetrated to avoid injuring the overlying spinal cord. Referring to the diameter of the intervertebral space on radiographs helps one to estimate the distance the instrument can be safely inserted into the disk space.

The consistency of the nucleus pulposus varies from gelatinous in normal disks to white, cheesy, and granular in calcified degenerate disks. Correlation of calcified disk material removed with calcified disks visible on radiographs confirms the location of any such disk being fenestrated. It is not imperative all disk material be removed, except that of the offending disk; here removal of nucleus pulposus should be accomplished carefully and completely. Reckless fenestration of a partially herniated, unstable disk can force additional nucleus into the spinal canal and can exaggerate clinical signs.

With proper surgical technique, it is unnecessary to debride tissue or to suture the longus colli muscles. If the sternohyoideus muscles are divided for exposure, they should be approximated with absorbable suture material. Subcutaneous tissues are opposed in a like manner, and skin is closed with any dermal suture.

POSTOPERATIVE CONSIDERATIONS

Although little morbidity results from the surgical procedure, fenestration is not likely to bring about a sudden clinical improvement because disk material previously herniated remains in the spinal canal. Failure to explain this situation to the client before the procedure can lead to strained veterinarian-client relations and to considerable frustration for the veterinary surgeon.

Depending on clinical signs, the patient receives corticosteroid, antibiotic, and, if indicated, analgesic medication for at least 3 to 4 days postoperatively. When the patient goes home, close confinement is unnecessary because impending or progressive disk herniation is prevented by fenestration.

Thoracolumbar Disk Fenestration

INDICATIONS

This procedure is appropriate for patients of any breed predisposed to disk herniation (such as dachs-

*Richards Manufacturing Co., Inc., 1450 Brooks Road, Memphis, TN 38116

hund and Pekingese), with clinical signs ranging from lumbar pain to partial caudal motor paralysis, otherwise in good health, and less than 8 years of age. One study indicated only 5% of dogs with thoracolumbar disk herniations are over this age.[2] It is not known whether older dogs are less likely to have recurrent problems, but in such dogs a conservative approach seems advisable initially. Fenestration should be considered when signs of disk herniation are first evident, and the operation is definitely recommended if signs progress in severity or on the first recurrence. Dogs presented to the veterinary surgeon with sudden caudal motor paralysis should undergo spinal cord decompression. If pain can still be perceived in the rear toes, fenestration should also be accomplished. Fenestration can be performed within a variable period following disk herniation; however, we prefer to operate within the first 2 to 3 days. The patient can then recuperate from the surgical procedure while hospitalized to treat signs produced by that herniation.

PREOPERATIVE CONSIDERATIONS

Corticosteroids and antibiotics are administered prior to the procedure. The anesthetic regimen is the same as that outlined for cervical disk fenestration. An area of the back extending from the vertebral border of each scapula to the crest of each ilium is clipped and is prepared for the surgical procedure. The dog is positioned in ventral recumbency on an insulating pad to conserve body heat. The veterinary surgeon should operate from the side of the patient opposite that of his "handed" ability. Radiographs and a skeleton should be available for reference.

INTRAOPERATIVE CONSIDERATIONS

A dorsolateral approach[6] is used to gain access to the eight intervertebral disks between T10 and L5. Disks between T9 and T10 and L5 and L6 can also be fenestrated if they are calcified or partially herniated. These disks are not routinely fenestrated because of their low incidence of herniation and remote location, making fenestration more difficult. Not only is the L5–L6 disk more difficult to fenestrate, but considerable risk exists of creating a femoral nerve deficit if the adjacent ventral nerve branch is damaged.

The skin incision extends from a point 1 to 2 spinous processes rostral to the anticlinal vertebra (T11) to a point 1 vertebra rostral to the ilium. This incision may be made directly on the dorsal midline or 1 to 2 cm lateral to the midline on the side from which the disks are to be fenestrated. The cutaneus trunci muscle, subcutaneous fat, and superficial fascia are incised in the same plane and are reflected sufficiently to expose the lumbodorsal fascia 1 to 2 cm lateral to the dorsal midline (Fig. 43-2A). The lumbodorsal fascia and the aponeurosis of the longissimus thoracis et lumborum muscle are incised along an imaginary line drawn from a point 5 mm lateral to the spinous process of T9 to a point 1 to 2 cm lateral to the comparable process of L6 (Fig. 43-2B). In the rostral portion of the surgical field,

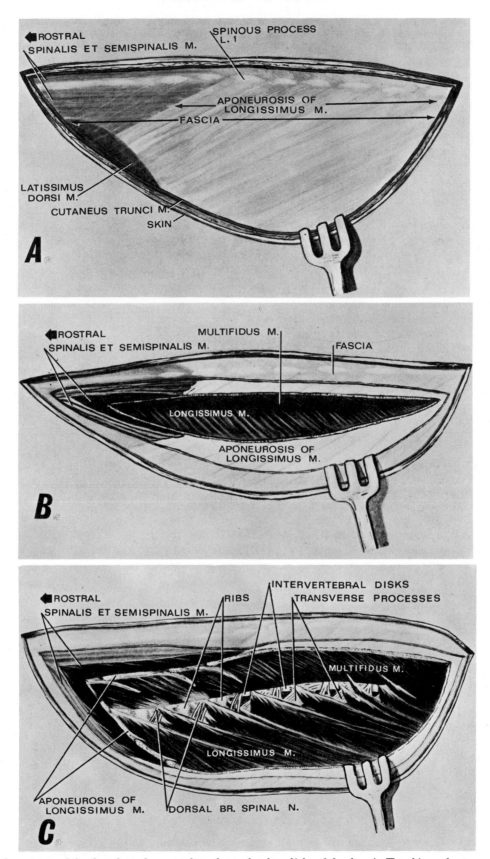

Fig. 43-2. *Surgical anatomy of the dorsolateral approach to thoracolumbar disks of the dog. A, The skin, subcutaneous fascia, fat, and cutaneus trunci muscle have been incised and reflected laterally on the left side of the dog. B, The deep external fascia of the trunk, the aponeurosis of the longissimus thoracis muscle, and the caudal edge of the spinalis et semispinalis muscles have been incised to expose the underlying multifidus and longissimus muscles. C, The multifidus muscle is separated from the longissimus thoracis muscle by blunt dissection to expose the thoracolumbar spine for intervertebral disk fenestration.*

the caudal border of the spinalis and semispinalis thoracis muscles, interposed between the lumbodorsal fascia and the aponeurosis of the longissimus thoracis muscle, is also incised (Figs. 43-2*B* and 43-3).

Access to the intervertebral disks is gained by opening the intermuscular septum between the multifidus lumborum and thoracis muscles medially and the longissimus dorsi and sacrococcygeus dorsalis lateralis muscles laterally (Figs. 43-2*C*, 43-3, and 43-4). This septum is the first one lateral to the dorsal spinous processes; it is easiest to locate in the midlumbar region where fat is interposed superficially between the muscles. Division of the muscles is easily accomplished by blunt dissection in the lumbar region; however, the septum is less distinct over the ribs. All blunt dissection is accomplished with an Adson semisharp, or comparable, periosteal elevator in each hand. Tubercles of the last four ribs are exposed; one must take care not to disturb the small nerves and vessels coursing craniolaterally immediately dorsolateral to each tubercle. Separation of the musculature is carried to the base of the lumbar transverse processes.

The novice should completely separate muscles to this level and should be careful to avoid dorsal branches of the spinal nerves (Fig. 43-2*C*). This maneuver provides good visualization of the intervertebral disks and adjacent structures. The experienced veterinary surgeon can "tunnel" down to each transverse lumbar process and can thereby avoid considerable tedious dissection and trauma. The short transverse process of L1 lies adjacent to the last rib, assuming the thirteenth rib is present, and is used as an anatomic reference point. All other lumbar transverse processes can be "tunneled" down to by referring to the lateral radiograph and by estimating the distance between each process. If judgment is correct, the veterinary surgeon will never see the dorsal branch of each rostral

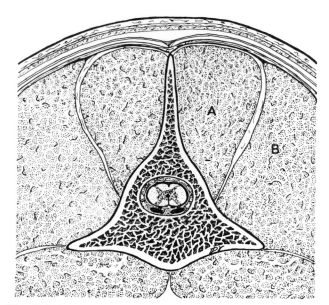

Fig. 43-4. *Cross section through L4. A, Multifidus lumborum m.; B, longissimus lumborum m.*

spinal nerve or its allied vessels. As the operation proceeds caudally from T13 to L1, succeeding transverse processes are situated progressively deeper.

After exposing each lumbar transverse process (L1 to L5), the lumbar disks are exposed. In the lumbar region, the lateral anulus of the intervertebral disk lies immediately rostral to the base of each transverse process (Fig. 43-5). In the caudal thoracic area, the disk lies rostromedial to the head of each rib; the T10–T11 disk is difficult to expose because it is situated 1 to 2 cm ventromedial and is partially covered by the rib tubercle. Each disk can be visualized by elevating tissue off the lateral anulus with a periosteal elevator. The

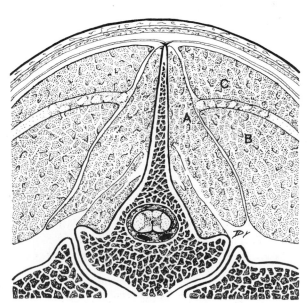

Fig. 43-3. *Cross section through T12. A, Multifidus thoracis m.; B, longissimus thoracis m.; C, spinalis et semispinalis mm.*

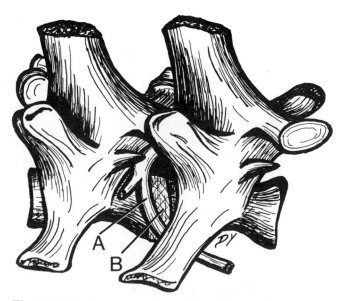

Fig. 43-5. *L3–L4, showing the relation of the spinal nerve to the intervertebral disk. A, Ventral branch of L3 spinal nerve; B, intervertebral disk.*

use of a small self-retaining retractor (Gelpi or Weitlaner) or hand-held retractors enhances visualization. Caution should be exercised so as not to invade the intervertebral foramen, which lies immediately dorsal to each disk and contains a spinal nerve and allied vessels. The inexperienced veterinary surgeon may overcompensate in avoiding the intervertebral foramen and may work too far ventrally where considerable risk of injuring the ventral branch of the spinal nerve exists. Ventral branches of spinal nerves pass adjacent to the ventrolateral aspect of each disk (Fig. 43-5).

In the lumbar area, ventral branches of spinal nerves are located under the intertransverse fascia and are not visible in the surgical field unless an attempt is made to expose them. To ensure that a ventral branch is not traumatized, it is helpful to introduce the tip of a curved mosquito hemostat into the intertransverse fascia adjacent to the ventrolateral border of the anulus and to spread the jaws gently. This maneuver exposes the ventral nerve branch occasionally, and the tissue defect also creates a landmark for the veterinary surgeon to avoid. If the L5–L6 disk is fenestrated, the ventral branch of the fifth lumbar nerve should be identified and avoided to ensure that it is not damaged.

The disk's lateral anulus is visualized best for fenestration if adjacent muscle is retracted rostrodorsally with a curved periosteal elevator. This retractor also protects the dorsal branch of the spinal nerve and associated vessels. A pointed scalpel blade is used either to incise or to remove an elliptical section of the anulus fibrosus. The anulus should not be cut where it cannot be visualized. Fenestration is accomplished, in a manner similar to that described for the cervical region, using the same instruments. The tip of the hook is directed upward, with care taken not to break through the dorsal anulus. The partially herniated disk must be fenestrated cautiously to avoid forcing additional nucleus pulposus into the spinal canal (Fig. 43-6).

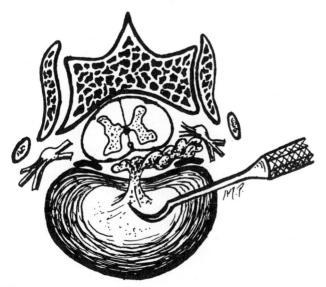

Fig. 43-6. *The correct position of a modified dental claw tartar scraper to fenestrate a disk, in this case a partially herniated disk.*

Fenestrating the T10–T11 disk requires special care to avoid creating pneumothorax; the pleura, directly ventral to this disk, rises and falls with respiratory movement. If the existence of pneumothorax is in question, irrigation of the area with saline solution and expansion of the lungs by compressing the ventilation bag should provide an answer; air bubbles will appear in the surgical field if significant pneumothorax exists.

Minimal hemorrhage associated with exposure and fenestration of thoracolumbar disks can be controlled usually by topical pressure on bleeding tissue with a periosteal elevator. Rarely, hemostatic forceps or electrocautery will be required to control bleeding.

Every disk fenestrated should be identified anatomically to ensure that no disks are missed between T10 and L5. If clinical signs merit decompression of the spinal cord, it is best to perform spinal cord decompression and then to follow with disk fenestration. Fenestration is less compatible with dorsal decompression. Hemilaminectomy and fenestration can be performed from the same side; although the multifidus muscle is badly traumatized, no adverse clinical signs have been observed. Lateralization of signs often dictates that a decompressive surgical procedure and fenestration be performed on opposite sides of the spinal column.

Debridement of tissue is not necessary when the "tunnel" technique is used to expose the lumbar disks. Performing a hemilaminectomy on the same side, or division of the multifidus and longissimus dorsi muscles down to the transverse processes for improved exposure, likely necessitates some debridement. The aponeurosis of the longissimus muscle and the overlying thoracolumbar fascia are approximated with one suture line of absorbable suture material. Subcutaneous tissues are apposed with similar material, catching the underlying fascia occasionally to obliterate dead space. The skin incision is closed with any dermal suture, and a light-pressure bandage may be applied around the trunk of the dog and may be left in place for 4 to 7 days.

POSTOPERATIVE CONSIDERATIONS

Corticosteroid and/or analgesic agents should be administered for 1 to 3 days postoperatively because most dogs experience some discomfort. Thereafter, treatment depends on clinical signs. Because corticosteroids are used in association with this operation, skin sutures should not be removed for at least 3 weeks to avoid incisional dehiscence. Dogs routinely go home 48 to 72 hours postoperatively or as soon as voluntary urination is evident. In addition to preventing subsequent attacks of disk prolapse, fenestration eliminates the need for prolonged confinement of dogs with functional ambulatory ability, and physical therapy can be initiated within a day or so of the surgical procedure in the patient with caudal paralysis.

The degree of paresis, if present, remains unchanged in most animals in the immediate postoperative period following disk fenestration. Occasionally, clinical signs are more severe immediately following the procedure, and because of this possibility, the client must be forewarned. Deterioration in neurologic status may be, but is not necessarily, associated with the operation. If pathologic changes in the spinal cord, which may or may not be known, are progressive at the time of the surgical procedure, disk fenestration need not be faulted for a worsened neurologic state. Such a condition could result from spontaneous herniation of additional nucleus pulposus while the dog is anesthetized for radiographs or for the operation, or overzealous fenestration of a partially herniated disk could force additional material into the spinal canal. Trauma to the spinal cord from the fenestration hook is an unlikely cause for an increased neurologic deficit. The client should be advised that some dogs suddenly deteriorate neurologically without radiographs or operation.

The most likely potential surgical complications include: (1) failing to fenestrate a disk; (2) creating pneumothorax; (3) injuring spinal nerves; (4) damaging the spinal cord; and (5) cutting spinal arteries.

In most dogs, evidence of some degree of spinal nerve injury exists for at least a few days postoperatively. Dogs may have slight scoliosis, with deviation to the operated side, and sag (paralysis) of abdominal muscles ipsilateral to the operated side may be noticeable. If the ventral branch of the fifth lumbar nerve (L5–L6) has been damaged, the dog will have at least a temporary femoral nerve deficit. The severity of these signs has been directly correlated with the expertise of the veterinary surgeon.

We are aggressive in promoting thoracolumbar disk fenestration because it is impossible to predict the severity of a recurrent disk attack. Herniation of disks in the cervical region has not been observed to cause permanent caudal paralysis or death from diffuse myelomalacia; in the thoracolumbar region, however, such a sequela is not unusual. Fenestration, properly performed, should minimize the chance of a subsequent disk attack, and the dog's locomotion should not be compromised.

The dorsolateral approach is preferred for the fenestration of thoracolumbar disks because: (1) it permits decompression by hemilaminectomy when this procedure is also indicated; (2) minimal trauma is inflicted; and (3) relatively easy access to nine disks is provided. Thoracolumbar intervertebral disk fenestration is considerably more difficult than cervical disk fenestration, and the potential for severe and possibly permanent neurologic injury cannot be overemphasized. It requires a thorough understanding of anatomy and basic surgical principles. Consequently, the novice should perform this surgical procedure successfully on an experimental animal before attempting it on a clinical patient.

References and Suggested Readings

1. Cechner, P. E.: Ventral cervical disc fenestration in the dog: a modified technique. J. Am. Anim. Hosp. Assoc., *16:*647, 1980.
2. Gage, E. D.: Incidence of clinical disc disease in the dog. J. Am. Anim. Hosp. Assoc., *11:*135, 1975.
3. Hoerlein, B. F.: Canine Neurology, Diagnosis, and Treatment. 3rd Ed. Philadelphia, W.B. Saunders, 1978.
4. Pettit, G. D.: Intervertebral Disc Protrusion in the Dog. New York, Appleton-Century-Crofts, 1966.
5. Piermattei, D. P., and Greeley, R. G.: An Atlas of Surgical Approaches to the Bones of the Dog and Cat. 2nd Ed. Philadelphia, W.B. Saunders, 1979.
6. Yturraspe, J. D., and Lumb, W. V.: A dorsolateral muscle separating approach for thoracolumbar intervertebral disk fenestration in the dog. J. Am. Vet. Med. Assoc., *162:*1037, 1973.

Thoracolumbar Disk Disease

by ERIC J. TROTTER

In recent years, the practicing veterinarian has been deluged with data supporting various authors' opinions on the most suitable treatments for paraparesis or paraplegia due to thoracolumbar disk disease in the dog.[5, 7-9, 11, 12, 14, 16-19, 23, 26, 27, 33] The veterinary medical literature contains many conflicting claims regarding the relative safety and efficacy of a wide variety of therapeutic regimens, both surgical and nonsurgical. Most of these regimens have merit when applied rationally to individual patients on a selected basis. In most instances, the specific technique varies with the severity, and frequently, the chronicity of the neurologic deficit, because most are based on early decompression of the spinal cord and the removal of the compressive mass of disk material. Many of the variations in operative technique, instrumentation, and ancillary therapy are due more to personal preferences than to fundamental differences of opinion regarding the rationale of therapy.

The very nature of the intervertebral disk "syndrome" has been responsible for much of the controversy. Numerous ingenious methods have been devised to induce both acute and chronic spinal cord compression artificially, with varying degrees of impact injuries, and to study the efficacy of various medical and surgical procedures. Experimental reproduction of the entire "vicious cycle" often responsible for the spinal cord lesion in spontaneous intervertebral disk protrusion or extrusion has, however, eluded investigators and has therefore precluded a controlled evaluation of therapeutic techniques.

Objective analysis is further clouded by many other factors, such as the extreme variability of spinal cord lesions, both in type and severity, the high incidence of spontaneous and often unpredictable recoveries, particularly in mildly affected animals, the impressive compensatory abilities of the canine spinal cord, the simultaneous use of medical and surgical therapy, the frequently inadequate documentation of history of acuteness of onset, progression of signs, and duration of the neurologic deficit, and the absence of a standard neurologic classification. Most veterinary surgeons agree, however, on the superiority of surgical to nonsurgical therapy when disk protrusion or extrusion has resulted in severe paresis or paraplegia.

Pathologic Features of Thoracolumbar Disk Disease

Except for the fortunately small percentage of patients with thoracolumbar disk extrusions that result in ascending-descending myelomalacia, the basic lesion in the thoracolumbar intervertebral disk syndrome is a compressive myelopathy of varying degree that usually involves from one to four segments of the spinal cord. The spinal cord lesion has been attributed to a number of factors. These include mechanical distortion or derangement of the nervous elements, microvascular and vasoactive chemical changes that result in decreased perfusion, venous stasis, hemorrhage, edema, ischemia and anoxia and the resultant demyelination, axonal loss, gliosis, focal malacia, and cavitation. The severity, extent, and, in fact, type of spinal cord lesion are influenced by many factors. The magnitude, consistency, and rate of extrusion of the intervertebral disk are critical. A small, rapidly occurring protrusion or extrusion usually causes a much more severe spinal cord lesion and, thus, neurologic deficit than does a large, slowly progressive protrusion.

The rate of development of the spinal cord compromise also appears to be critical in the reversibility or irreversibility of the lesion. It has been stated that slowly progressive mass lesions produce neurologic dysfunction due to progressive demyelination of intact axons by direct pressure or by vascular deprivation with edema and hypoxia that are often reversible.[27] Peracute impact injuries to the spinal cord caused by acute disk extrusion, however, frequently result in a "vicious cycle" of traumatic spinal cord autodestruction, with far less reversibility. The "dynamic force" with which the disk extrudes, or the resultant impact on the spinal cord, the inflammatory reaction in the epidural space, the specific location of the extrusion with respect to the diameter of the vertebral canal in relation to the diameter of the spinal cord, and the persistence of mechanical compression also govern the type, extent, and reversibility of the spinal cord lesion. Thus, the spinal cord lesion in intervertebral disk extrusions in the thoracolumbar region may vary from persistent mechanical compression with minimal demyelination and axonal loss to complete focal spinal cord malacia.

In contrast to this focal compressive myelopathy, thoracolumbar disk extrusion may result in a diffuse, necrotic myelopathy. This disorder has previously been referred to as hematomyelia, ascending syndrome, hemorrhagic myelomalacia, and ascending cord necrosis. Because of the progressive nature of the lesion and the predominance of hemorrhage and necrosis, it may be better designated ascending-descending myelomalacia.

The pathogenesis of myelomalacia is largely unknown, although numerous mechanisms have been proposed, including release of catecholamines, vasospasm, thrombosis, venous occlusion, and rupture of medullary vessels with resultant ischemia and anoxia.

The onset is typical of that of a focal compressive myelopathy subsequent to thoracolumbar disk extrusion. Usually within 24 hours of the almost invariably peracute onset of clinical signs, however, the spinal cord lesion begins to progress.

The spread of the lesion may consist of both ascension and descension, or either component may predominate. Analgesia and areflexia become more extensive as the multisegmental hemorrhagic necrosis continues. The neck is often held in extension, contributing to the general impression of extreme apprehension and exquisite pain. Affected dogs frequently are pyrexic and aggressive. Extensor rigidity of the forelimbs (Schiff-Sherrington phenomenon), owing to the destruction of ascending inhibitory neurons, precedes thoracic limb motor deficits. As the myelomalacia continues, Horner's syndrome may be observed. Respirations are diaphragmatic due to loss of innervation of the intercostal muscles and are easily observed as such because of atony of the abdominal muscles. The level of analgesia may be seen to ascend from the original level. The necrotic phenomenon may spontaneously arrest, but in most cases, death from respiratory failure ensues within 4 days of onset. At necropsy, extradural and intradural hemorrhage are often extensive. Examination of transverse sections of involved segments of spinal cord reveals varying degrees of hemorrhage, necrosis, and cavitation. The ascending or descending lesion may "skip over" some segments, or it may involve all segments of the spinal cord from conus medullaris to medulla.

It is not known whether immediate decompression can prevent the occurrence of myelomalacia or whether it can be modified or arrested by the administration of anticatecholamine drugs, but the disorder has occurred postoperatively in dogs in spite of early decompression and medical therapy. When these signs become apparent, euthanasia is recommended because of the extensive, irreparable nature of the spinal cord lesion, the animal's acute suffering, and the hopeless prognosis. Only careful neurologic examination can aid in the differentiation between descending myelomalacia with an irreversible lesion and a focal compressive myelopathy of the lumbosacral intumescence with a reversible lesion.

Neurologic Examination

Protrusions or extrusions of the thoracolumbar disks most often result in an upper motor neuron and general proprioceptive lesion, with varying degrees of pain and bilaterally symmetric pelvic limb paresis and ataxia. Pain may be diskogenic or radicular. Hind-limb and perineal segmental reflexes are usually normal or hyperreflexic. Muscle tone in the pelvic limbs and abdomen may be normal, hypotonic, or hypertonic. The crossed-extensor reflex may be present. The Schiff-Sherrington phenomenon is not commonly associated with thoracolumbar disk protrusion, even with paraplegia, unless myelomalacia ensues. Conscious perception of pain caudal to the lesion, not to be confused with the flexor or withdrawal reflex, may be normal, decreased, or absent; such perception classifies the patient as eugesic (normogesic), hypalgesic, or analgesic. Postural reactions of the pelvic limbs may be absent or poorly performed. Bladder function may be normal or "spinal" (retention or retention-reflex). Defecation is rarely affected. The approximate site of the lesion may often be localized by the level of analgesia, the panniculus reflex, or the animal's hyperesthetic response to digital pressure applied to the dorsal spines (hyperpathia). In severe cases, a line of analgesia to noxious stimuli may be traced on the abdominal wall.

Further classification of the degree of paresis or paralysis has proved useful. The grading system is as follows:

Grade 5—Normal strength
Grade 4—Supports,* minimal paresis and ataxia
Grade 3—Supports, frequently stumbles, moderate paresis and ataxia
Grade 2—Supports with assistance, stumbles, and falls
Grade 1—No support, slight movement when supported by tail
Grade 0—Absence of purposeful movements

In some cases of lumbar disk protrusion or extrusion, the lesion may be a mixed upper and lower motor neuron type. These lesions result from a compressive myelopathy involving the spinal cord segments containing the cell bodies of the lower motor neurons to the perineum, tail, or pelvic limbs. The previously described neurologic signs of the upper motor neuron lesion are complicated by lower motor neuron signs such as hyporeflexia or areflexia. Disk protrusions or extrusions at L2–L3, L3–L4, L4–L5, and L5–L6 may result in varying degrees of dysfunction of the spinal cord segments or roots of the femoral, sciatic, perineal, and caudal neurons evidenced by altered muscle tone and segmental spinal reflexes. The prognosis in these patients is not as favorable as in those with pure upper motor neuron lesions due to the involvement of the cell bodies themselves rather than of the axons alone. Differentiation of these lower motor neuron lesions from myelomalacia is essential because of the radical differences in prognosis and treatment. The tone of the abdominal musculature, the cranial extent of the line of analgesia, the patient's ability to support the trunk, and the character of the respirations may be considered in the differential diagnosis.

Continual recording of the neurologic status of the patient from the time of admission through the preoperative and postoperative periods is essential for optimum care and objective evaluation of therapeutic techniques.

Radiographic Evaluation

Myelography is only rarely necessary because most lesions due to thoracolumbar disk protrusion or extru-

*Support in this context means voluntary motor activity to reach a standing position.

sion can be adequately localized through a combination of accurate neurologic examination and plain roentgenographic films of the thoracolumbar spine. High-quality diagnostic films require precise positioning of the patient under general anesthesia and multiple, well-collimated exposures to eliminate artificial disk space narrowing due to parallax. The offending disk frequently demonstrates a combination, or any of the following changes: uniform narrowing, wedging, opacification with protrusion or extrusion into the vertebral canal, and subsequent narrowing of the intervertebral foramen or synovial joints from collapse of the intervertebral space. The diagnosis is usually made on the basis of the lateral views (centered over T11–T12 and L1–L2), and is confirmed by the ventrodorsal view. Because of the presence of the transverse intercapital ligament on all but the last two pairs of ribs, disk extrusions cranial to this point are uncommon. Accurate localization of an upper motor neuron and a general proprioceptive lesion between T3 and L3, localized hyperpathia, and critical evaluation of plain roentgenographic films usually suffice to localize the lesion.

Medical Therapy

Partial resorption of compressive extruded disk material, the formation of a stable fibrosis in the offending disk, the impressive compensatory ability of the canine spinal cord, the resolution of edema, the restoration of microvasculature, and remyelination may account for the high incidence of spontaneous improvements in cases with mild-to-moderate neurologic dysfunction. Medical therapy is used in *mild* cases mainly as supportive treatment for these reparative mechanisms. Analgesics, muscle relaxants, antiarthritic preparations, and corticosteroids should, however, be used with caution during the healing stages of the disk. Overzealous administration of these medications, even with strict exercise restriction, may lead to complete relief of the beneficial self-limiting pain. Overactivity at this stage may result in the extrusion of further disk material and a worsening of the patient's neurologic dysfunction. Excessive pain should be lessened with medication, but should not be completely relieved. Enforced cage rest, preferably under the supervision of a veterinarian, is advisable during the administration of these preparations.

Surgical Techniques

Various authors have alluded to the greater incidence of recurrence of both cervical and thoracolumbar disk protrusions following medical rather than surgical therapy.[17,18, 28] Experience here confirms this observation. At present, initial attacks of pain, or pain and *minimal* paresis, are treated with cage rest and corticosteroid administration. Most *recurrent* or medically nonresponsive cases with these mild signs have responded well to fenestration of the offending and adjacent disks (see the previous section of this chapter). If signs persist following fenestration, decompression and mass removal are employed. The mechanism of action of fenestration, according to Olsson, is the production of an acute inflammatory reaction that stimulates phagocytosis, resorption of necrosis, and the formation of a stable fibrosis in the disk.[26] Little, if any, *immediate* decompressive effect exists, but further protrusion of degenerate disk material is probably prevented. The technique may thus be both therapeutic and prophylactic in cases of mild paresis or pain and paresis. With minimal operative trauma, all the "high-incidence" disks may be fenestrated by the ventral, dorsal, or dorsolateral approach (Figs. 43-7 and 43-8).[7,12,17, 26, 37] As with cervical disk fenestrations, however, neurologic recovery in thoracolumbar disk fenestrations is frequently not immediate.

Because of the proposed mechanism of action, the technique of disk fenestration should probably be employed more as a prophylactic than a therapeutic procedure in those dogs with a history of repeated episodes of pain and minimal paresis with spontaneous recovery. In cases of significant paresis and ataxia, a more direct approach is indicated: direct spinal cord decompression and removal of the compressive mass. Basically, two techniques are commonly employed for the direct relief of spinal cord compression due to in-

tervertebral disk protrusion in the thoracolumbar region. These are hemilaminectomy and dorsal laminectomy.

Hemilaminectomy and hemilaminectomy with concurrent fenestration of adjacent disks have been well described and practiced with excellent results (Fig. 43-9).[12,13,16,17,19] Hemilaminectomy provides direct decompression of the spinal cord with easy removal of extruded disk material from the vertebral canal on the side of the hemilaminectomy. Significant difficulty may be encountered with removal of extruded disk material if the side (right versus left) of extrusion is not delineated by myelography. Marked hemorrhage is frequently encountered from the internal vertebral venous plexus and the vertebral arteries. Cranial or caudal extension of the decompression over the full length of traumatized spinal cord is often more difficult than with dorsal laminectomy.

DORSAL LAMINECTOMY

A significant difficulty in dorsal laminectomy techniques in dogs has been that of providing the necessary exposure and decompression of the spinal cord without predisposing the patient to postoperative constrictive fibrosis.

In the dog, the laminectomy defect appears to heal similarly to a fracture of a long bone, with organization of the hematoma that fills the defect and formation of a fibrous callus or scar, which, to a varying degree, often changes to cartilage and then to bone. This progression appears similar to endochondral bone formation, variably arrested as fibrous nonunion. Asymptomatic dural adhesions and perineural fibrosis often result. Spinal cord compression and subsequent neurologic dysfunction may also occur. Depending on the occurrence and extent of secondary spinal cord compression as a result of this scar, the phenomenon has been termed constrictive fibrosis, laminectomy membrane, epidural scar formation, or postlaminectomy stenosis. With some laminectomy techniques in dogs, the laminectomy membrane causes no significant problems. In others, the rapid filling of the laminectomy defect with dense scar tissue results in disastrous secondary compression of the spinal cord against the ventral aspect of

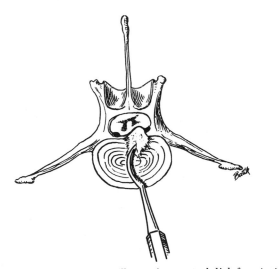

Fig. 43-7. *Transverse section illustrating ventral disk fenestration with a tartar scraper.*

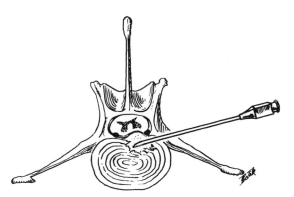

Fig. 43-8. *Transverse section illustrating dorsal disk fenestration with a blunt, 14-gauge needle.*

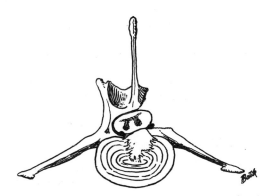

Fig. 43-9. *Transverse section through area of hemilaminectomy prior to ablation of the offending disk.*

the vertebral canal during maturation of the laminectomy membrane. In man, re-exploration or reoperation for recurrence of intervertebral disk protrusion is complicated by this phenomenon.

Many studies have been performed to elucidate the mechanism of formation of the laminectomy membrane and to investigate various methods for its prevention following laminectomy in both man and the dog.[3,15,21,22,24] In the dog, in which occurrence of this phenomenon has been a major limitation to decompressive techniques of the thoracolumbar spine, the problem has been investigated in the extensive works of Funkquist and Schantz and others.[3,10,20,29,35]

In the Funkquist type A laminectomy (Fig. 43-10A), the vertebral arches, including the articular processes, are excised to a level corresponding approximately to that of a dorsal plane through the middle of the spinal cord. Secondary spinal cord compression occurs because of the proliferation and maturation of connective tissue across the laminectomy defects. Retention of the cranial articular processes, portions of the caudal articular processes, and the outer compact bone of the dorsolateral portions of the vertebral arches in the Funkquist type B laminectomy (Fig. 43-10B) result in less spinal cord exposure, but prevent the complication of spinal cord compression during the healing stages of the laminectomy defect.

Removal of the protruded disk material is not recommended with the Funkquist type B laminectomy unless the extrusion is dorsal or dorsolateral to the spinal cord. Owing to the narrow width of this laminectomy, removal of protruded disk material from the ventral or ventrolateral aspect of the vertebral canal can be accomplished only with traumatic spinal cord manipulation.

The decompressive efficacy of the hemilaminectomy and the dorsal laminectomy (performed in a manner similar to the Funkquist type B procedure) have been determined to be approximately equal in dogs subjected to spinal cord compression with inflatable balloons.[13] Thus, the distinct, major advantage of the hemilaminectomy, if performed on the side of disk extrusion, is the ready access to the ventral aspect of the vertebral canal to allow for the direct removal of the compressive mass.

A modification of the Funkquist type B laminectomy (Fig. 43-10C) has several advantages. It provides more spacious decompression of the spinal cord than either of the previously described techniques, with sufficient exposure of the entire vertebral canal for the removal of extruded disk material even from the ventral midline. It thus satisfies the basic criteria of decompression and mass removal.

MODIFIED DORSAL LAMINECTOMY

As with any extensive surgical procedure, adequate preoperative physical and neurologic examination, aseptic technique, assisted ventilation with inhalation anesthesia, intravenous fluid support, and accurate monitoring of the patient are essential.

The dog is positioned in sternal recumbency with sandbags or vacuum positioners. No padding is placed under the abdomen, because partial occlusion of the caudal vena cava results in shunting of venous return through the internal vertebral venous plexuses. The dorsum of the patient's back is prepared for an aseptic surgical procedure. Self-adhesive, incise plastic draping material* is used to supplement the usual four-quadrant draping technique to ensure a waterproof barrier against contamination.

The skin incision, centered over the area of involvement, is made slightly lateral to the dorsal midline in order to avoid delayed skin healing due to pressure from the underlying dorsal spines. For adequate exposure with minimal operative trauma, the incision should be extended at least two vertebrae cranial and caudal to the offending disk. Following incision of the superficial fascia of the trunk and the fat layer of the dorsal lumbar region, the thoracolumbar fascia is incised either sharply or by electrocautery immediately lateral to the spinous processes. Periosteal elevators are used for blunt and sharp dissection of the epaxial musculature ventrally to a level just ventral to that of the accessory processes (Fig. 43-11). Elevation of the epaxial musculature, under tension from self-retaining retractors, is performed caudally to cranially. Small branches of either the paired lumbar or intercostal arteries are cauterized by means of bipolar cautery to prevent the return of electrical impulses through the

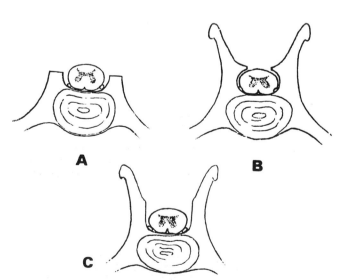

Fig. 43-10. *Transverse sections through areas of dorsal laminectomies to illustrate relative spinal cord exposure. A, Laminectomy similar to Funkquist type A with excision of the vertebral arches, including the articular processes to a level corresponding to that of a dorsal plane through the middle of the spinal cord. B, Laminectomy similar to Funkquist type B, with retention of the cranial articular processes, and portions of the caudal articular processes. C, Modified dorsal laminectomy with complete excision of the caudal articular processes and excavation of the pedicles.*

*Steri-Drape, Animal Care Products, 3M Co., 3M Center, St. Paul, MN 55101

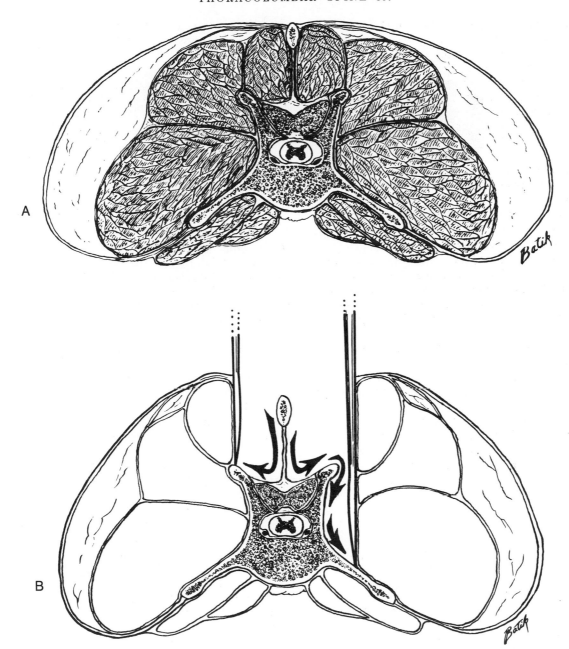

Fig. 43-11. A, *Transverse section caudal to the disk at L1–L2 to illustrate the relationships of the superficial fascia of the trunk, the thick lumbar fat layer, the superficial and deep portions of the thoracolumbar fascia, and the epaxial and hypaxial musculature. B, Periosteal elevation of the epaxial musculature prior to dorsal laminectomy or dorsal fenestration. Arrows indicate the direction of force applied to the elevator for atraumatic periosteal elevation.*

spinal cord. Careful periosteal resection is absolutely essential for minimal hemorrhage and muscle trauma. Moist laparotomy tapes or neurologic sponge strips are used to cushion the self-retaining retractors and to maintain a clear surgical field (Fig. 43-12).

A readily identifiable landmark for determining the proper site of the laminectomy is the dorsocaudally directed thirteenth rib, which is also located more superficially than the cranioventrally directed first lumbar transverse process. The spinous processes of the vertebrae cranial and caudal to the involved disk space

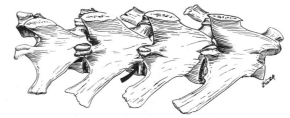

Fig. 43-12. *Careful periosteal elevation of epaxial musculature results in excellent exposure of the vertebral column to the level of the accessory processes (arrow).*

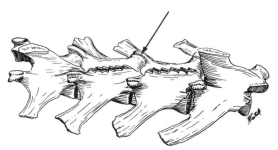

Fig. 43-13. *The dorsal spines cranial and caudal to the offending disk have been excised. The arrow indicates the joint space between the cranial and caudal articular processes, which is used as a guideline for the lateral extent of the laminectomy.*

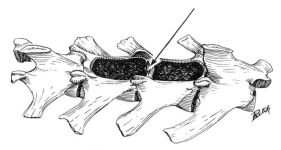

Fig. 43-15. *The outer cortical bone and most of the middle layer of cancellous bone, including that of the caudal articular processes, has been removed. The arrow indicates the dense cortical bone at the intervertebral space and the interarcuate ligament.*

are gently resected by means of bone rongeurs (Fig. 43-13). En bloc excision of these processes with bone cutters can be extremely hazardous. Minimal torsional forces may result in vertebral subluxation in small dogs.

The outer cortical bone of the dorsal laminas is removed with a high-speed air drill with a 4-mm, egg-shaped bur with notched flutes. The bone structure and color are a reliable index of the depth of drilling: (1) outer cortical bone is dense and white, (2) middle cancellous bone is spongy and red, (3) inner cortical bone is dense, white, and *thin*. The key to the increased exposure with this type of laminectomy is the width. The drilling is continued laterally to the joint spaces between the lateral aspects of the caudal articular processes of the cranial vertebra and the medial concave surfaces of the cranial articular processes of the caudal vertebra (Fig. 43-13, arrow). The cranial articular processes are left intact, except for their most craniomedial portions. The caudal articular processes are removed entirely, however, to increase spinal cord exposure and to allow for undercutting of the laminectomy edges.

The middle layer of cancellous bone is removed by drilling (Fig. 43-14). At the area of the intervertebral space, only dense cortical bone and the interarcuate ligament are present (Fig. 43-15, arrow). Caution must be exercised when drilling in this area to prevent slipping of the drill into the vertebral canal. When the thin layer of inner cortical bone begins to sag under the pressure of the drill, a 2.3- or 1.6-mm, round carbide-tip bur is substituted.

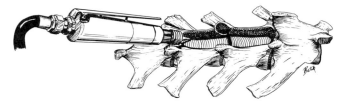

Fig. 43-16. *Angled drilling into the cancellous bone around the periphery of the thin plate of inner cortical bone avoids drilling directly over the spinal cord and results in smooth, deeply undercut edges. This procedure increases both exposure and decompression and facilitates the removal of disk material.*

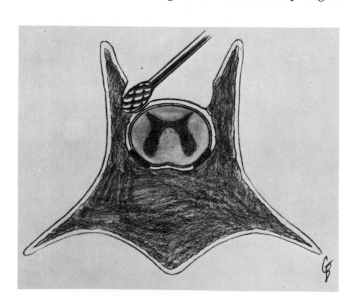

Fig. 43-14. *Following excision of the middle layer of cancellous bone over the spinal cord, excavation of the pedicles is begun with the 4-mm-diameter bur. The spinal cord is protected by the inner layer of cortical bone during the undercutting procedure.*

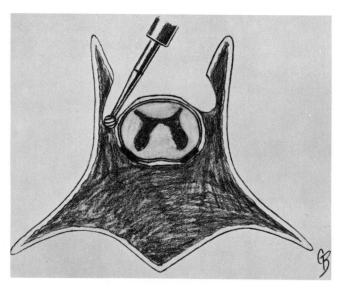

Fig. 43-17. *Additional excavation of the middle layer of cancellous bone of the lateral lamina is performed with the small round burs. This maneuver further isolates the thin layer of inner cortical bone over the spinal cord.*

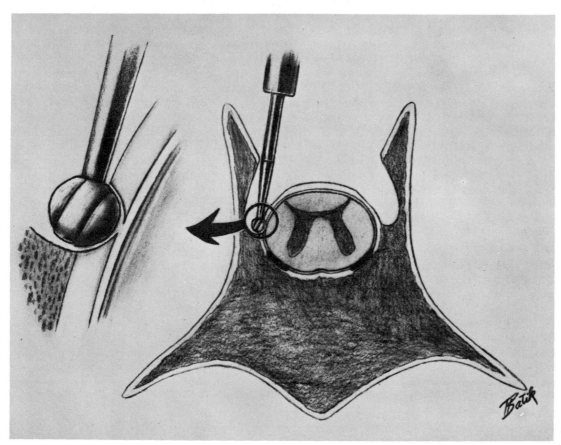

Fig. 43-18. *With the smallest round bur, the inner cortical shelf is cut free, resulting in smooth, deeply undercut edges of the laminectomy.*

Up until this point, the spinal cord has been protected from the drill by the inner cortical bone in all areas of the laminectomy. This thin plate of bone is now isolated by drilling around the periphery of the laminectomy with the small drill at approximately a 45° angle away from the spinal cord (Figs. 43-16 to 43-18). The inner cortical shelf is elevated and is removed by grasping the interarcuate ligament with a fine hemostat (Fig. 43-19). The angled drilling with the smaller bur avoids drilling directly over the spinal cord and results

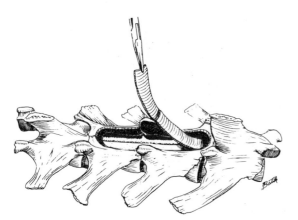

Fig. 43-19. *The thin, isolated shelf of inner cortical bone is elevated with a fine hemostat and is removed.*

in smooth, deeply undercut edges of the laminectomy with excellent exposure of the full width of the vertebral canal (Fig. 43-20). With the smallest bur, the pedicles may be further excavated laterally while still preserving the *outer* layer of cortical bone of the pedicle to prevent constrictive fibrosis. In ventrolateral disk extrusions, the compressive mass of disk material acts as a self-retaining retractor of the spinal cord during this additional excavation of the pedicles (Fig. 43-21).

Intermittent flushing of lactated Ringer's solution through a plastic slide washing bottle and fluid removal with suction effectively remove the bone dust and dissipate the minimal heat produced by the high-speed air drill. A clear surgical field with adequate visualization of bone structure and color is essential to accurate drilling. To prevent thermal and vibratory necrosis of both the spinal cord and remaining pedicles, a new, ultrasharp air-drill bur should be used for each patient. On an experimental basis, the sharpness of the bur appears to be more important than the speed of the air drill.

The amount of fat in the epidural space is an index of decompression. The laminectomy is continued cranially and caudally until a normal amount of epidural fat, which is squeezed from the vertebral canal by the edematous spinal cord, is visualized around the spinal cord; this fat indicates decompression of the entire length of traumatized spinal cord. The laminectomy

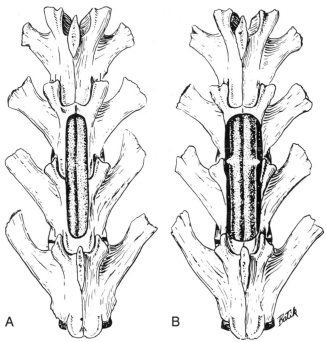

Fig. 43-20. *Dorsal view of laminectomies, to illustrate relative exposure of the spinal cord and epidural space. A, Narrow dorsal laminectomy similar to the Funkquist type B in which portions of the caudal (inner) articular processes are spared. B, Modified dorsal laminectomy in which the caudal articular processes are completely excised to increase spinal cord exposure and to allow for atraumatic removal of extruded disk material.*

extends from interarcuate ligament to interarcuate ligament; this technique facilitates atraumatic elevation of the thin layer of inner cortical bone. In most instances, laminectomy over two to three vertebrae is sufficient. Although some instability occurs with complete excision of the caudal articular processes, this factor has presented no problems to date.

Complete excision of the caudal articular processes and excavation of the lateral laminas and pedicles facilitate removal of extruded disk material with minimal, if any, direct spinal cord manipulation. Disk removal is possible even with the minimal epidural space of the frequently affected chondrodystrophic dogs with relative vertebral canal stenosis. Radiculotomy or rhizotomy often expedites removal of extruded disk material from the ventral or ventrolateral aspects of the vertebral canal. "Sling sutures" of 5-0 cardiovascular silk may be placed in the dura mater to allow for atraumatic retraction or rolling of the spinal cord should this prove necessary during disk removal. Tartar scrapers, such as those used for disk fenestration, fine tip suction, and various other ophthalmic and dental instruments (lens spoon, lens loop, iris spatula, microrongeurs, and dental explorer No. 3) have proved useful for the removal of the compressive mass of disk material from the vertebral canal.

In peracute cases in which intramedullary spinal cord edema or hemorrhage is likely, if inadvertent surgical spinal cord trauma has occurred or if the prognosis is in doubt, even in chronic cases, a full-length durotomy is performed. By means of Potts-Smith 60° angled cardiovascular scissors or a bent, disposable 20-gauge needle, the dura mater is incised on the dorsal midline for the full length of the laminectomy. Early incision of the inelastic dural sheath is thought to result in greater intramedullary decompression of the spinal cord. Such an incision also permits the formulation of a more accurate prognosis because either superficial or deep *focal* malacia, as opposed to ascending-descending myelomalacia, and thrombosis, disappearance, or rupture of the superficial spinal cord vasculature, as well as the absence of normal spinal cord pulsations, are readily observable.

In chronic cases, loss of spinal cord substance and glial scarring may be seen in irreversible lesions. Myelotomy, either superficial or deep, is only performed in patients with severe paraplegia without intact pain perception when the prognosis is in question. Although not totally innocuous, full-length durotomy in

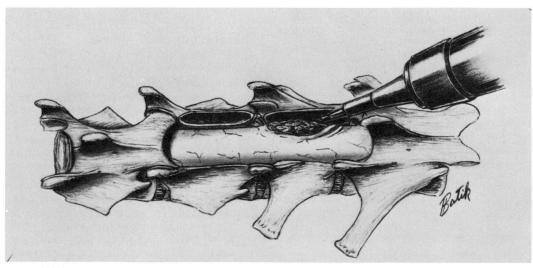

Fig. 43-21. *The pedicle adjacent to the compressive mass may be further excavated to facilitate removal of the extruded disk material.*

the dog is not associated with the disastrous complications of spinal cord herniation through the dural defect and continued leakage of cerebrospinal fluid that have been reported in man. A mild, transient neurologic deficit may be associated with durotomy in dogs.

Following durotomy in those patients in which edema or hemorrhage has been considered a significant component of the spinal cord lesion, or in which intentional or accidental spinal cord manipulation has occurred, selective regional spinal cord hypothermia is used. The entire laminectomy defect is gently filled with lactated Ringer's slush to effect the hypothermic episode. The slush is melted with room-temperature lactated Ringer's solution after 20 minutes of direct spinal cord contact and is removed with suction prior to a secure closure of the dorsal lumbar fascia. The slush is produced in wide-mouth, autoclaveable centrifuge bottles of 250 ml nylon that are partially filled with lactated Ringer's solution and are placed in a deep freeze (−80° C) for 40 minutes. Vigorous shaking of the chilled bottles produces a fine ice-crystal slush similar to that of commercial "Sno-Cones."

Both experimental and clinical data have indicated the efficacy of the foregoing simple and practical technique for the production of spinal cord hypothermia. During this brief hypothermic episode, internal spinal cord temperatures of 6° C have been realized. The exact mechanism of action of local spinal cord hypothermia can only be postulated, but it appears to ". . . allow doing extensive dissection, manipulating, and unavoidably causing surgical trauma—heretofore prohibitively dangerous."[4]

Although used here mainly for its beneficial effects in reducing *intrasurgical* spinal cord trauma, spinal cord hypothermia has been previously proved in both experimental and clinical investigations to be of great benefit in the *early* treatment of impact injuries of the spinal cord.[1, 2] In one particularly applicable investigation in dogs, weights were dropped a known distance through a virtually frictionless Teflon tube onto an impounder that rested on the exposed spinal cord (Fig. 43-22).[1] With this technique, a predictable, reproducible force, measured in g/cm, could be applied to the spinal cord. With known degrees of impact injury, the protective effects of selective regional spinal cord hypothermic perfusion were evaluated. The results indicated encouraging and significant differences between the neurologic recoveries of control and of perfused animals.

Immediate and delayed cooling techniques of the injured spinal cord have been extensively investigated by numerous authors. The postulated mechanism of action of selective regional spinal cord hypothermia, as with brain hypothermia, is based on a reduction in the metabolic requirements and reactions of cooled nervous tissue. By reducing the inflammatory response to injury, ischemia due to edema and vasospasm should be minimized, and the cooled spinal cord should be more resistant to the ischemia. The adverse effects of vasoactive substances accumulating in the area of spinal cord wounding may also be decreased by hypother-

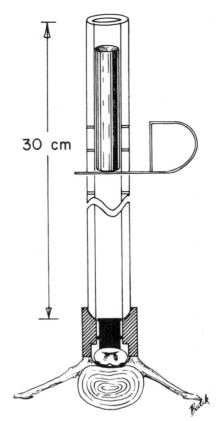

Fig. 43-22. *Line drawing to illustrate mechanism of Albin[2] and colleagues for producing known amounts of impact injury to the exposed canine spinal cord.*

mia. By these mechanisms, local spinal cord hypothermia, if used immediately after extrinsic or intrasurgical trauma to the spinal cord, will, one hopes, arrest or aid in the prevention of hemorrhagic necrosis of the spinal cord.

In other studies, normothermic perfusion appeared to be superior to hypothermic perfusion.[30,31] The mechanism proposed was that of perfusion dialysis, in which the toxic vasoactive catecholamines released after impact injury to the spinal cord were physically diluted or were removed during the irrigation process. These vasoactive amines have been previously reported to be at least partially responsible for the autodestructive sequence of events resulting in hemorrhagic necrosis.

No adverse effects have been seen with this brief hypothermic episode, but such effects have been reported following prolonged spinal cord hypothermia.[30] Perhaps, during this brief hypothermic episode for protection during surgical manipulation, both cooling and dialysis are important.

Supportive Therapy

"Improvement in neurosurgical results has been achieved not only with perfection of operative techniques, however, but also because of increased ability to protect the central nervous system during and after surgical procedures."[25] Through extensive investigations of the pathophysiologic response of the spinal cord to impact injury, more rational ancillary protective measures for the spinal cord have become a reality.[6] Although numerous experimental drugs, such as dimethyl sulfoxide, epsilon-aminocaproic acid, alpha-methyl-p-tyrosine, phenoxybenzamine, naloxone, ethacrynic acid, gamma-hydroxybutyrate, and crocetin, have been suggested for the therapy of impact injuries, their clinical use awaits further documentation. Previously proved techniques are, however, routinely used to protect the already-traumatized spinal cord during invasive neurosurgical procedures.

In *peracute* cases in which edema is believed to be a prominent factor in the spinal cord compression, a 20% solution of mannitol in water is administered through a filtered fluid administration apparatus at a dosage of 2 g/kg body weight. The calculated amount is given over a 10- to 20-minute period to achieve maximum osmotic effect. This infusion may be repeated once in 3 to 4 hours. The administration of mannitol is usually begun once all soft tissue dissection has been completed, because of its tendency to increase hemorrhage. The hypertonic solution of inert, nontoxic mannitol effectively lowers cerebrospinal fluid pressure, brain mass, and probably spinal cord mass with little rebound effect.

Large doses of corticosteroids are administered intravenously at the time of the surgical procedure, or in the early preoperative period if an immediate decompressive operation is not possible. Dexamethasone is frequently administered at a dosage of 2 mg/kg body weight. The calculated dose of dexamethasone is mixed into a balanced electrolyte solution, which is administered during the operative procedure. The beneficial effects, reported by various authors, of corticosteroids in neurosurgical patients result primarily from the reduction of inflammation and edema of the nervous tissues; these agents may even stabilize lysosomal membranes and re-establish vascular integrity. Broad-spectrum antibiotics are administered preoperatively and are mixed into the balanced electrolyte solution administered during the surgical procedure. Balanced electrolyte solutions are administered in the intraoperative period to maintain normovolemia and to offset the dehydrating effect of the potent osmotic diuretic, mannitol.

Hyperventilation is achieved by means of mechanically assisted respiration, in order to produce a mild respiratory alkalosis. This technique has proved to be an effective means of preventing central nervous system (CNS) edema due to acidosis; it is also a safeguard in the prevention of inadvertent laceration of the internal vertebral venous plexus. The undercutting procedure of the laminectomy is continued only during the expiration phases of the ventilator when the sinuses are collapsed from decreased intrathoracic pressure and subsequent increased venous return to the right heart.

Proper positioning of the patient is essential for the prevention of venous engorgement and possible CNS

edema due to stasis. It has been shown that occlusion of the external jugular veins or caudal vena cava increases the flow through the internal vertebral venous plexuses.

Some veterinary surgeons recommend fenestration of the offending and adjacent disks at the time of the decompressive surgical procedure. Owing to the extremely low incidence of disk extrusion at another interspace in dogs subjected to laminectomy at this and other institutions, concomitant prophylactic disk fenestration is not performed. (See the next section of this chapter, by Bojrab.)

Immediately prior to closure, a piece of absorbable gelatin sponge (Gelfoam*) creased on the midline and carefully cut to conform to the laminectomy is placed in the laminectomy defect. This sponge is "tented" dorsally by the crease to simulate the normal roof of the vertebral canal. The cut edges are placed in direct apposition with the remaining pedicles. Following a final check for hemostasis, the exposure is closed by layers.

In recent years, other materials have been recommended for placement in the laminectomy defect for the prevention of dural scarring, constrictive fibrosis, perineural fibrosis, and the elimination of cosmetic defects. An absorbable gelatin sponge has been praised and later blamed for an exaggerated and deleterious fibrous tissue response.[3,15,21,22,24] The effects of a particular type of implant appear to be related to the specific surgical technique, if not to the specific surgeon, because results appear to vary with various implants in the different laminectomy defects. With the modified dorsal laminectomy technique, the implantation of this sponge has given excellent results, both on an experimental and a 10-year clinical basis. Research in progress has shown that scarring (laminectomy membrane formation) is not prevented to a significant degree by the implantation of gelatin sponge in this particular surgical technique. The sponge implantation results in a predictable and seemingly innocuous healing pattern without any clinical or experimental evidence of significant secondary spinal cord compression (constrictive fibrosis), however. The underlying dural incision seals rapidly by "neomembrane formation." The cut edges of the dura mater that retract toward the remaining pedicles heal in association with the overlying, *noncompressive* laminectomy scar. Implantation of Gelfoam, muscle, and free fat transplants, as well as the absence of an implant, have met with variable and often unsatisfactory results with this technique. Pedicle fat grafts, rather than free fat grafts, to prevent the laminectomy scar and its subsequent metaplasia to cartilage and then bone appear promising, as described by Kiviluoto and colleagues in lumbar laminectomies in young rabbits.[15,22] Evaluation of my current experimental work with implantation of pedicle fat grafts in laminectomies performed by the technique described herein in the thoracolumbar region of mature dogs may indicate the advisability of a change from Gelfoam to pedicle fat grafts. The healing process of the laminectomy defect

* Upjohn Co., Kalamazoo, MI 49001

appears to be influenced not only by the implant or lack of implant, but also by the specific surgical technique employed, the instrumentation used, the patient's age and species, the ancillary support measures, the durotomy, the anatomic region of the operation, and the length of the decompression.

With or without Gelfoam implantation or the use of wires between adjacent dorsal spines, cosmetically unacceptable scars or structural defects have not been a problem with this technique.

Postoperative Care

Corticosteroid therapy is continued in the postoperative period. Catastrophic gastrointestinal complications have been seen infrequently in both human and veterinary medicine during corticosteroid therapy following neurosurgical procedures.[32,36] Because of the low incidence of these complications and the overwhelming experimental and clinical evidence supporting the beneficial effects of corticosteroids, however, their administration is still recommended. Clinical studies in man have shown that the decrease in mucous viscosity and the increase in gastric acidity and pepsin do not develop before the seventh day of ACTH administration; therefore, corticosteroids should not be administered for more than 6 days.[36] In the postoperative care of laminectomy patients, the doses of corticosteroids are gradually decreased over the first 4 to 5 postoperative days to prevent suppression of adrenal function due to the exogenous steroid administration. Parenteral administration of dexamethasone appears to result in fewer gastrointestinal complications than does oral administration. With minor variations, according to the cause and severity of the preoperative neurologic dysfunction and the patient's postoperative response, the following regimen of postoperative corticosteroid administration is used:

Postoperative day	Dose of dexamethasone (mg/kg/day) (administered in divided dose, tid.)
1–2	0.5–1.0
3–4	0.25–0.5
5–6	0.125–0.25

Broad-spectrum antibiotic therapy is continued for at least 3 days after the discontinuance of steroid therapy, and longer in dogs with persistent urinary incontinence.

The use of foam-rubber cage pads, air mattresses, small water beds, or cedar shavings reduces the incidence of decubitus in paralyzed patients. Whirlpool baths reduce muscle spasticity, improve circulation, promote paddling movements of the pelvic limbs, help to prevent muscle atrophy, and add to the general sense of well-being of the patient. The addition of a whirlpool concentrate of povidone-iodine solution is beneficial for the prevention of urine scald, superficial pyodermas, and infection of decubital sores.

Well-lubricated, aseptically maintained indwelling urinary catheters decrease the bladder trauma associated with repeated manual expressions and aid in the prevention of retention cystitis and urine scald. Vitamin C is often administered to maintain a low urine pH.

Maintenance of a high plane of nutrition to overcome negative nitrogen balance, enthusiastic nursing care, and generous amounts of affection cannot be overemphasized.

Exercise carts, easily constructed from inexpensive aluminum rod and lawn mower wheels, aid in the prevention of pressure sores and in the stimulation of early postoperative pelvic limb activity. Tailing exercises are substituted in the occasional animal that begins to develop a dependence on the exercise cart.

Paralyzed patients are discharged from the hospital as soon as conscious control of micturition is regained. Most owners are delighted to participate in the rehabilitation program. Early return to familiar surroundings promotes enthusiasm on the part of the patient and an early return to normal function.

Discussion

Because of the extreme variability of spinal cord lesions subsequent to thoracolumbar disk extrusion in the dog, postoperative recovery varies in both extent and duration. It has been said that the duration of the recovery period seems to be *directly proportional* to the duration of spinal cord compression and *inversely proportional* to the rapidity of onset of neurologic dysfunction. Probably as a result of fiber size and myelination, the larger, more myelinated fibers usually recover more slowly. Thus, during recovery, the first-affected pathways responsible for proprioception are the last to recover, and the last-affected pathways responsible for pain perception are frequently the first to recover. Voluntary motor function is usually regained shortly after recovery of pain perception and urinary continence.

Reversibility or irreversibility of the spinal cord lesion can be predicted with a fair degree of accuracy by evaluation of the patient's medical history and neurologic examination. It can be confirmed only by surgical exploration or postmortem examination. As has been so aptly stated recently, ". . . the age-old question of when to operate and with what prognosis will always be controversial."[27] Based on the clinical experience of myself and many others, however, certain generalizations regarding prognosis and anticipated recovery times may be made.

In most instances of mild to moderate paresis and ataxia, regardless of the acuteness of onset, full recovery can be anticipated if a decompressive procedure and mass removal are performed within a reasonable period of time. In cases of chronic paraparesis, with persistent, long-standing spinal cord compression, however, permanent or irreversible spinal cord damage may be present. This damage may be observed at the time of operation. Removal of the frequently indurated disk extrusion that causes the chronic pressure on the spinal cord only rarely improves the neurologic dysfunction. Following durotomy, such dysfunction is often evidenced by an easily observable loss of spinal cord substance, syrinx formation, or glial scarring.

Even in cases of acute complete motor paralysis, most patients recover to a functional status following prompt surgical intervention, as long as pain perception is intact. The prognosis is not as favorable in those dogs with complete sensorimotor paralysis (grade 0 with dense analgesia). The rapidity of onset of neurologic dysfunction is highly significant in these cases. Those patients in which the disorder has a gradual onset and progressive deterioration have a far more favorable prognosis than those with a peracute onset of complete sensorimotor paralysis. The recovery period also, as previously mentioned, is inversely proportional to the rapidity of onset of neurologic dysfunction and is directly proportional to the duration of paralysis. In these most severely affected dogs, euthanasia is performed at the time of operation if durotomy reveals irreversible spinal cord damage incompatible with functional recovery. Myelotomy may be necessary to differentiate superficial from deep spinal cord malacia because superficial malacia does not preclude functional recovery. Complete sensorimotor paralysis is not, however, a contraindication for surgical treatment. In my experience, at least half the completely paralyzed, densely analgesic dogs have recovered completely following therapy by the methods described.

References and Suggested Readings

1. Albin, M. S., White, R. J., Yashon, D., and Harris, L. S.: Effects of localized cooling on spinal cord trauma. J. Trauma, *9*:1000, 1969.
2. Albin, M. S., et al.: Localized spinal cord hypothermia—anesthetic effects and applications to spinal cord injury. Anesth. Analg., *46*:8, 1967.
3. Barbera, J., et al.: Prophylaxis of the laminectomy membrane—an experimental study in dogs. J. Neurosurg., *49*:419, 1978.
4. Brasmer, T. H., and Lumb, W. V.: Lumbar vertebral prosthesis in the dog. Am. J. Vet. Res., *33*:499, 1972.
5. Brown, N. O., Helphrey, M. L., and Prata, R. G.: Thoracolumbar disk disease in the dog: a retrospective analysis of 187 cases. J. Am. Anim. Hosp. Assoc., *13*:665, 1977.
6. De La Torre, J. C., Johnson, C. M., Goode, D. J., and Mullan, S.: Pharmacologic treatment and evaluation of permanent experimental spinal cord trauma. Neurology, *25*:508, 1975.
7. Flo, G. L., and Brinker, W. O.: Lateral fenestration of thoracolumbar discs. J. Am. Anim. Hosp. Assoc., *11*:619, 1975.
8. Funkquist, B.: Decompressive laminectomy in thoracolumbar disc protrusion with paraplegia in the dog. J. Small Anim. Pract., *11*:445, 1970.
9. Funkquist, B.: Thoracolumbar disc protrusion with severe cord compression in the dog I, II, III. Acta Vet. Scand., *3*, 1962.
10. Funkquist, B., and Schantz, B.: Influence of extensive laminectomy on the shape of the spinal canal. Acta Orthop. Scand. [Suppl.], *56*, 1962.
11. Gage, E. D.: Incidence of clinical disc disease in the dog. J. Am. Anim. Hosp. Assoc., *11*:135, 1975.
12. Gage, E. D.: Modifications in dorsolateral hemilaminectomy and disc fenestration in the dog. J. Am. Anim. Hosp. Assoc., *11*:407, 1975.
13. Gage, E. D., and Hoerlein, B. F.: Hemilaminectomy and dorsal laminectomy for relieving compressions of the spinal cord in the dog. J. Am. Vet. Med. Assoc., *152*:351, 1968.
14. Gambardella, P. C.: Dorsal decompressive laminectomy for treatment of thoracolumbar disc disease in dogs: a retrospective study of 98 cases. Vet. Surg., *9*:24, 1980.
15. Gill, G. G., Sakovich, L., and Thompson, E.: Pedicle fat grafts for the prevention of scar formation after laminectomy. Spine, *4*:176, 1979.
16. Hoerlein, B. F.: Comparative disk disease: man and dog. J. Am. Anim. Hosp. Assoc., *15*:535, 1979.
17. Hoerlein, B. F.: Canine Neurology: Diagnosis and Treatment. 3rd Ed. Philadelphia, W. B. Saunders, 1978.
18. Hoerlein, B. F.: The status of the various intervertebral disc surgeries for the dog in 1978. J. Am. Anim. Hosp. Assoc., *14*:563, 1978.
19. Hoerlein, B. F.: Further evaluation of the treatment of disc protrusion paraplegia in the dog. J. Am. Vet. Med. Assoc., *129*:495, 1956.
20. Horne, T. R., Powers, R. D., and Swaim, S. F.: Dorsal laminectomy techniques in the dog. J. Am. Vet. Med. Assoc., *171*:742, 1977.
21. Keller, J. T., et al.: The fate of autogenous grafts to the spinal dura—an experimental study. J. Neurosurg., *49*:412, 1978.
22. Kiviluoto, O.: Use of free fat transplants to prevent epidural scar formation. Acta Orthop. Scand. [Suppl.], *164*:1, 1976.
23. Knecht, C. D.: Results of surgical treatment for thoracolumbar disc protrusion. J. Small Anim. Pract., *13*:449, 1972.
24. LaRocca, H., and MacNab, I.: The laminectomy membrane. J. Bone Joint Surg. [Am.], *56B*:545, 1974.
25. Matson, D. V.: Treatment of cerebral swelling. N. Engl. J. Med., *272*, 1965.
26. Olsson, S. E.: On disc protrusion in the dog. Acta Orthop. Scand. [Suppl. 8] 1951.
27. Prata, R. G.: Neurosurgical treatment of thoracolumbar disks: the rationale and value of laminectomy with concomitant disk removal. J. Am. Anim. Hosp. Assoc., *17*:17, 1981.
28. Russell, S. W., and Griffiths, R. C.: Recurrence of cervical disc syndrome in surgically and conservatively treated dogs. J. Am. Vet. Med. Assoc., *153*:1412, 1968.
29. Swaim, S. F., and Vandevelde, M.: Clinical and histologic evaluation of bilateral hemilaminectomy and deep dorsal laminectomy for extensive spinal cord compression in the dog. J. Am. Vet. Med. Assoc., *170*:407, 1977.
30. Swaim, S. F., et al.: Comparison of hypothermic and normothermic spinal cord perfusion in the dog. Vet. Surg., *8*:119, 1979.
31. Tator, C. H., and Deecke, L.: Value of normothermic perfusion, hypothermic perfusion, and durotomy in the treatment of experimental acute spinal cord trauma. J. Neurosurg., *39*:52, 1973.
32. Toombs, J. P., Caywood, D. D., Lipowitz, A. J., and Stevens, J. B.: Colonic perforation following neurosurgical procedures and corticosteroid therapy in four dogs. J. Am. Vet. Med. Assoc., *177*:68, 1980.
33. Trotter, E. J.: Canine intervertebral disk disease. *In* Current Veterinary Therapy VI. Edited by R. W. Kirk. Philadelphia, W. B. Saunders, 1977.
34. Trotter, E. J.: Modified dorsal laminectomy and selective spinal cord hypothermia in the treatment of thoracolumbar disk disease. *In* Current Techniques in Small Animal Surgery. Edited by M. J. Bojrab. Philadelphia, Lea & Febiger, 1975.
35. Trotter, E. J., Brasmer, T. H., and deLahunta, A.: Modified deep dorsal laminectomy in the dog. Cornell Vet., *65*:402, 1975.
36. Valergakis, F. E., Critides, S., and Winakur, G. L.: Gastrointestinal complications in neurosurgical patients treated with steroids. Am. J. Gastroenterol., *58*: 441, 1972.
37. Yturraspe, D. J., and Lumb, W. V.: A dorsolateral muscle-separating approach for thoracolumbar intervertebral disk fenestration in the dog. J. Am. Vet. Med. Assoc., *162*:1037, 1973.

Prophylactic Thoracolumbar Disk Fenestration

by M. Joseph Bojrab

Surgical fenestration of the intervertebral space provides a means of prophylaxis in disk disease. If protrusion exists, surgical removal of the nucleus remaining in the intervertebral area will eliminate the pressure causing the protrusion. At the same time, if all other disks that are potential problems (T9–T10 to L5–L6) are fenestrated, complete prophylaxis against future disk protrusions is achieved. The material already extruded into the canal cannot be removed by disk fenestration alone; however, fenestration is encouraged for the removal of other degenerated disks that are potential problems in order that vigorous physical therapy, such as hydrotherapy and cart walking, can be prescribed without fear of causing another protrusion or even extrusion. Ventral fenestration facilitates access to all the potentially offending disks with a minimum amount of surgical trauma. Ten disks are fenestrated (T9–T10 to L5–L6). The thoracic disks are exposed through a tenth intercostal thoracic approach and the lumbar disks through a paracostal abdominal incision.

Surgical Procedure

The patient is placed in right lateral recumbency, and the left lateral side is clipped and prepared aseptically. The skin incision is made over the thirteenth rib from the dorsal to the ventral midline. The subcutaneous tissue is then dissected, the incision is slid caudally, and a paracostal incision is made into the abdomen. The left kidney is located and is reflected ventrally with the peritoneum. Frazier laminectomy retractors are then positioned (Fig. 43-23A), and the abdominal viscera are packed off with a laparotomy pad. This retroperitoneal abdominal exposure affords access to the L1–L2 through L5–L6 intervertebral spaces. The iliopsoas muscle is then hooked with a muscle retractor and is retracted away from the ventral midline (Fig. 43-23B). The ventral intervertebral prominences can be palpated. The lateral transverse processes are then identified and are numbered for orientation. Medial to the first transverse process is the T13–L1 intervertebral space. This space is not easily exposed from the abdominal approach and thus is fenestrated from the thorax. The remaining intervertebral spaces (L1–L2 to L5–L6) are fenestrated. The ventral longitudinal ligament and ventral annular fibers are cut with a scalpel. The nucleus pulposus is then removed with a modified claw-type tartar scaler. An inward, upward, and outward motion is used to clear the intervertebral space of as much nucleus as possible. Once this maneuver has been completed, the retractors are removed, and the muscle layers are individually sutured with 2-0 synthetic absorbable suture material. The skin incision is then slid in the cranial direction, and an incision is made into the thorax between the tenth and eleventh ribs. The Frazier laminectomy retractors are placed, and resuscitation is instituted (Fig. 43-23C). The T9–T10 through T13–L1 intervertebral spaces are located and are dissected free of pleura; the sympathetic trunk and intercostal vessels are carefully avoided (Fig. 43-23D). When the dissection is complete, the disks are fenestrated in the same manner as already described. The thorax, latissimus dorsi muscle, and skin are closed in the routine manner.

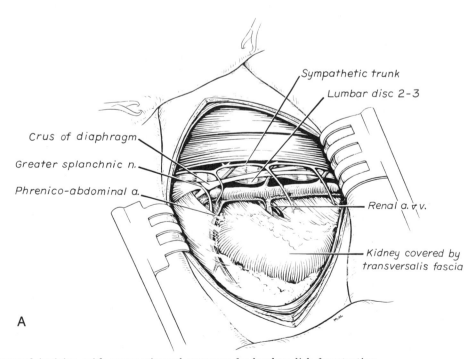

Fig. 43-23. A, *Paracostal incision with retroperitoneal exposure for lumbar disk fenestration.*

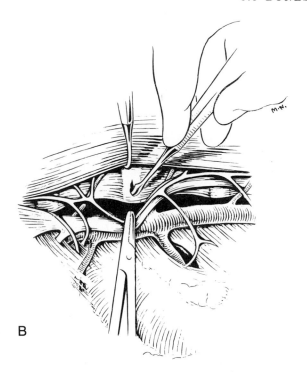

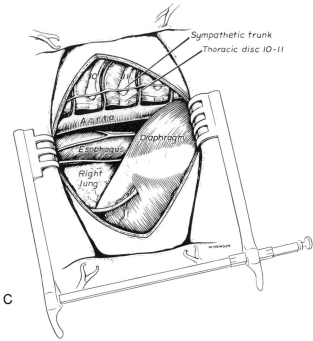

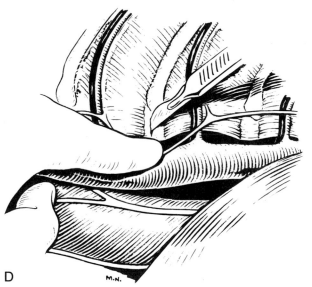

Fig. 43-23. *(cont.)* B, *Fenestration of a lumbar disk. The sublumbar muscles have been elevated and the crus of the diaphragm, aorta, and sympathetic trunk have been depressed. C, Exposure for thoracic disk fenestration. D, The aorta is depressed with the index finger, and the ventral longitudinal ligament is penetrated with a scalpel. (From Leonard, E. P.: Orthopedic Surgery of the Dog and Cat. 2nd Ed. Philadelphia, W. B. Saunders, 1971.)*

Postoperative Care

The animal is monitored closely during the anesthetic recovery period. Antibiotics are given, the bladder is kept evacuated, and intensive physical therapy is instituted. Physical therapy includes hydrotherapy and cart walking.

44 * Spinal Trauma

Spinal Trauma

by MELVIN HELPHREY

Fractures, luxations, and subluxations of the spine are forms of spinal injury that often need surgical repair. Although most of these injuries occur as a result of being struck by an automobile, gunshot wounds or high-rise accidents in metropolitan areas may also cause spinal trauma. The need for surgical treatment is based upon the neurologic status of the patient and the degree of instability of the spine. Numerous methods of surgical repair and stabilization of the spine are used today, and no one method may be used successfully in all cases.

The preoperative assessment, surgical technique, and postoperative management of spinal fractures, luxations, and subluxations are discussed.

Pathophysiologic Features

A brief discussion of the forces exerted on the spine helps in understanding the difficulty of maintaining adequate stabilization of the spinal column. The spine, like any other supporting structure of the body, is exposed to bending, shearing, and rotational forces (Fig. 44-1). The supporting structures of the spine include the paraspinal muscles (Fig. 44-2), the dorsal and ventral longitudinal ligaments, the supraspinous ligament, the anulus fibrosus of the intervertebral disk, the interspinous ligament, the intertransverse ligament, and the interarcuate ligament (ligamentum flavum or yellow ligament) (Fig. 44-3). Most important, the cranial and caudal articular processes of the vertebrae interdigitate with each other and prevent dorsal or ventral displacement (Fig. 44-4). The angle of articulation allows

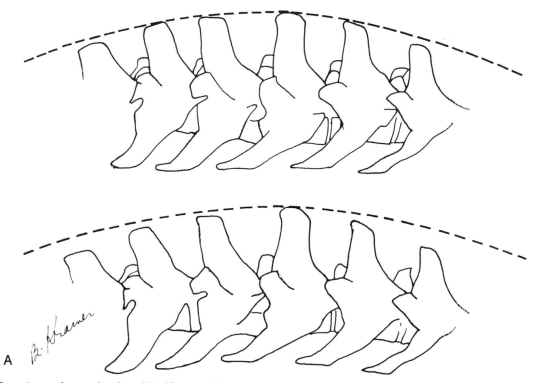

Fig. 44-1. *The spine undergoes bending* (A). *(Continued on next page.)*

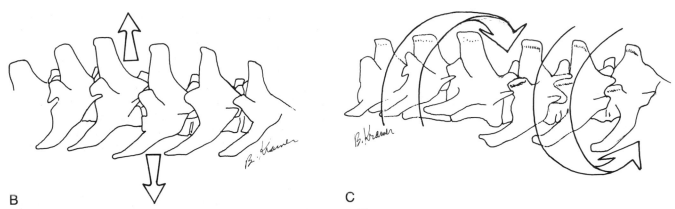

B   C

Fig. 44-1. *(cont.) The spine also undergoes shearing* (B) *and rotation* (C).

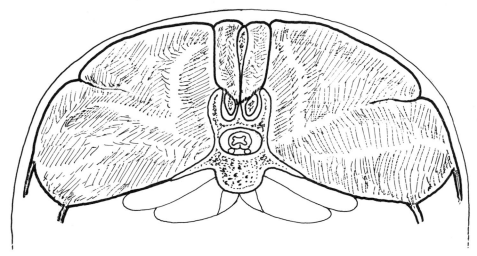

Fig. 44-2. *The paraspinal muscles provide stability to the spine by virtue of their mass effect.*

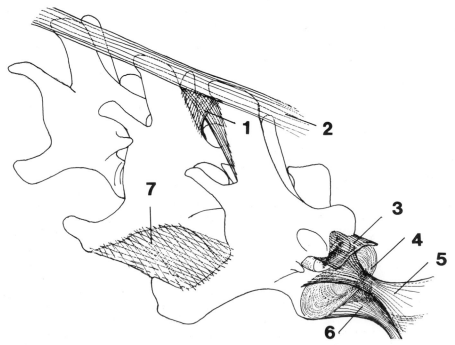

Fig. 44-3. *Ligamentous structures of the spine include: interspinous ligament (1), supraspinous ligament (2), interarcuate ligament (3), anulus fibrosus of the intervertebral disk (4), dorsal longitudinal ligament (5), ventral longitudinal ligament (6), and intertransverse ligament (7).*

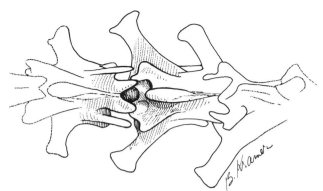

Fig. 44-4. *Normal articulation of the facets (cranial and caudal articular processes) is important in preventing injury from shearing forces.*

for normal ventral flexion of the spine with gliding movement of the articular facets, however.

The normal anatomic features may be interrupted with excessive bending, shearing, or rotational forces. Obviously, adequate stabilization of the spine requires neutralization of these forces. The center of movement of the spine is located in the intervertebral disk space, and therefore, any method of fixation applied dorsal to the vertebral body (that is, pedicle, lamina, or dorsal spinous process) may neutralize bending forces, and any fixation device placed through the intervertebral space (cross pins) may counter shearing forces. Rotational forces may be minimized by either method. When a repair fails, it is usually because of improper technique or failure of the implant to neutralize adequately those forces acting upon the spine.

Owing to the inherent stability of the thoracic spine, most traumatic lesions occur at the thoracolumbar area, where the lumbar vertebrae absorb considerable force. The second common area of involvement is the lumbosacral area. Immature dogs commonly suffer epiphyseal injuries to the vertebral bodies because their ligamentous supporting structures are stronger than bone. Fractures may be classified as either transverse or compression fractures with mild to severe displacement. The degree of radiographic displacement cannot always be correlated with the neurologic signs or prognosis. The neurologic injury may be due to spinal cord compression or contusion or to a ruptured intervertebral disk, especially in injuries causing flexion of the spine. A thorough medical and neurologic examination should be performed, and concurrent orthopedic and soft tissue injuries should be evaluated.

Indications for Surgical Treatment

A neurologic examination should be performed to determine: (1) whether the radiographic and clinical locations of the lesion are the same; (2) whether disease of the spinal cord (hematomyelia or myelomalacia) is widespread; and (3) the severity of the lesion.

Lateral and ventrodorsal radiographs should be taken to evaluate the spine accurately. Care must be taken in handling such patients because they may have considerable instability of the spine, and improper manipulation of the spine may produce further spinal cord trauma. Initial radiographs of the unanesthetized patient are easily taken in most instances. Hypotensive tranquilizers should be avoided until a thorough medical and neurologic evaluation is performed. If surgical treatment is anticipated, better-quality radiographs taken with the patient under anesthesia may provide a more accurate radiographic evaluation of the spinal trauma.

If the neurologic examination reveals no deep pain and displacement of the spinal canal is greater than one-third, the prognosis must be guarded, and surgical intervention may offer no advantage. On the other hand, some large breed dogs may benefit from surgical stabilization even though they are ambulatory. What then, are the criteria for surgical intervention of spinal injuries? Those dogs that are ambulatory but weakened may be treated medically by cage rest and administration of dexamethasone and analgesics, with daily neurologic examinations to determine whether their course is improving, static, or deteriorating. Patients that do not improve significantly with conservative therapy within 2 days should be operated. Those that are static but show evidence of instability of the spine, as determined by manual palpation of the injured area of the spine during ambulation and feeling or hearing a "click" of the unstable vertebrae, should be stabilized surgically. Patients whose conditions are deteriorating need rapid decompression and stabilization of the spinal column. Nonambulatory dogs with voluntary movement of the limbs are most likely to benefit from surgical decompression and stabilization of the spinal column.

Animals without voluntary movement or evidence of deep pain may not recover from the spinal shock and are presented to the veterinarian with a physiologically or anatomically severed spinal cord. The latter may be identified by examination of the spinal cord once a decompressive surgical procedure has been performed. A surgical procedure should not be performed from either the neurologic or radiographic evaluation alone.

Surgical Techniques

A multitude of surgical techniques are in use today to provide stability to the lumbar spine, including cross pins, cross pins and methyl methacrylate, intramedullary pins and wires, dorsal body plating, and dorsal spinal plating. The size of the animal, the location of the fracture, the equipment available, and the veterinary surgeon's experience dictate which method of fixation will be used. Generally, large dogs (greater than 20 kg) require rigid fixation because of the tremendous forces exerted on the unstable spine. Cross pins, body plates, and spinal plates alone or in combination are most commonly used in these patients. Such injuries in small dogs (less than 10 kg) may be repaired by using intramedually pins and wires and cross pins. Body casts may be used in conjunction with any method of repair, but are useful only in trauma of the thoracolumbar area. When possible, decompressive procedures should be performed to ensure relief of spinal cord compression. A fat graft should be placed over the spinal cord to prevent scar formation from causing further spinal cord compression. All surgical approaches are through a dorsal laminectomy incision.[5] All animals undergoing surgical repair should be treated with parenteral corticosteroids prior to and during the operation.

CROSS PINNING

Steinmann pins inserted in cross-pin fashion through the intervertebral space can provide adequate fixation for transverse fractures, luxations, and subluxations[1] (Fig. 44-5). After a decompressive dorsal laminectomy, and with visualization of the spinal cord, two Steinmann pins are inserted obliquely in a dorsal plane across the fractured site. The first pin is started at the base of the transverse process of the vertebral body and is directed cranially, 30° from the long axis of the spine. Care should be taken to avoid the spinal nerve root exiting the foramina. The pin is advanced across the fracture site and is embedded into the vertebral body cranial to the fracture. The cranial Steinmann pin is started just cranial to the base of the transverse process of the vertebra and is advanced in a medial and caudal direction, crossing the fracture site.

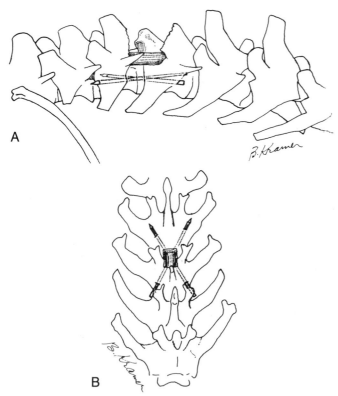

Fig. 44-5. *A and B, Intramedullary pins are placed through the vertebral bodies and cross the intervertebral space on the median plane.*

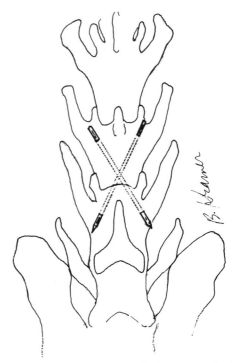

Fig. 44-6. *In the caudal lumbar spine, both pins may be placed in a caudal direction.*

If the pins are to be inserted through a dorsal laminectomy incision, their passage must be in a more ventral direction because insertion through the dorsal plane is not generally possible, owing to interference of the paraspinal muscles. The pins may be placed in a true dorsal plane by inserting the pins laterally through the paraspinal muscles and into the vertebral body. This method requires more care and experience for accurate placement of the pins. In the caudal lumbar spine, the wings of the ilia provide difficulty in placement of the caudal pin. Therefore, both pins may be placed from a cranial to a caudal direction (Fig. 44-6). The placement of pins in the thoracic spinal column is difficult because of the articulation of the head of the rib. If pins are to be used in this area, placement from a caudal to cranial direction on the left and right side of the spine is most convenient.

This technique is easy to perform; however, pin migration may be a problem if the dog is too active postoperatively. Application of a Kirschner apparatus helps to prevent pin migration, but also prohibits cutting the pins close to the vertebral bodies.

METHYL METHACRYLATE

Intramedullary pins and methyl methacrylate cement may be used in combination to stabilize fractures or luxations.[6] A dorsal laminectomy is performed to provide adequate decompression on the spinal cord, and four Steinmann pins are inserted into the vertebral bodies (Fig. 44-7). Two pins, one on each side, are inserted into the vertebral body cranial to the luxation. They are started from a dorsolateral point on the vertebral body and are directed caudoventrally and medi-

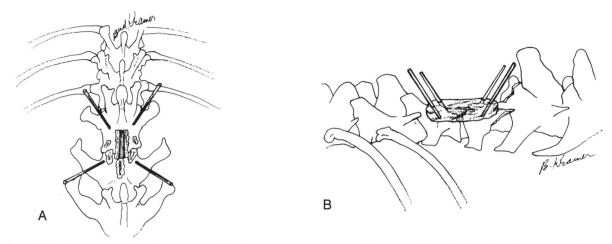

Fig. 44-7. *Dorsal (A) view of pins placed into vertebral bodies prior to encasement of the pins with methyl methacrylate cement. B, Lateral view after encasement of the pins.*

ally. The caudal two pins are again started in the dorso-lateral vertebral body and are inserted cranioventrally and medially. The pins are then cut at the level of the dorsal spinous processes.

A fat graft is placed over the dry surgical field in preparation for application of the methyl methacrylate cement. After mixing the cement, it is placed around the laminectomy site, incorporating the pins. Owing to the heat of polymerization, the cement should not be allowed to contact the spinal cord. Flushing with a cold saline slush helps to absorb the heat of polymerization. Because the methyl methacrylate cannot conveniently be removed, strict adherence to asepsis is essential if postoperative infection is to be avoided.

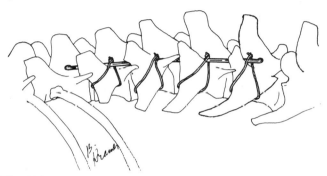

Fig. 44-8. *An intramedullary pin is placed through the dorsal spinous process, and orthopedic wire is passed around the transverse process bilaterally.*

INTRAMEDULLARY PINS AND WIRES

Injuries in dogs weighing less than 10 kg may also be stabilized by inserting an intramedullary pin through the dorsal spinous process and supporting the vertebral bodies to the pin with orthopedic wire placed around the transverse processes (Fig. 44-8), through the dorsal spinous process[2] (Fig. 44-9), or around the ribs (Fig. 44-10). Because this method of repair is less rigid than spinal plating or cross pinning, at least two interspaces on each side of the fracture should be included in the repair. A dorsal laminectomy or a hemilaminectomy should provide adequate decompression.

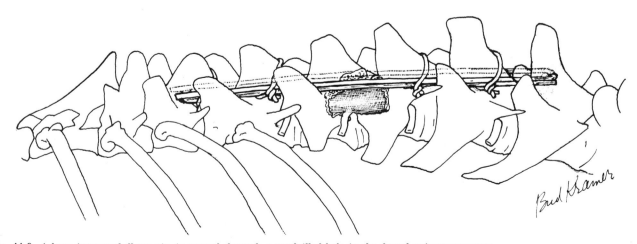

Fig. 44-9. *A bent intramedullary pin is passed through a predrilled hole in the dorsal spinous process.*

exists, however, a longer plate may be used to span three vertebrae.

Application of a plate in the thoracic spine is more difficult because temporary separation of the head of the rib must be performed. This maneuver may also result in iatrogenic pneumothorax. Application of a plate on the thoracic vertebrae requires contouring of the transverse process, so that the plate lies flat against the vertebral body. Rhizotomy of the spinal nerve roots above L4 may be performed to prevent nerve root pain subsequent to healing of the fracture. Plates have been applied to the lumbar spine without rhizotomies, however, and subsequent nerve root irritation has not been a problem.

DORSAL SPINAL PLATING

Two dorsal spinal plates are commonly used: a stainless steel plate*,[4] and a flexible vinylidene plate†.[3] These plates are applied to the dorsal spinous processes. Fractures of the dorsal spinous process or dorsal lamina severely jeopardize this method of repair. The vinylidene plate has multiple holes designed to fit between the dorsal spinous processes (Fig. 44-13). The inside surface of the plate should incorporate at least three intervertebral spaces on either side of the instability. Because the dorsal spinous process is tapered dorsally, the bolts are tightened securely to prevent the plate from migrating.

Stainless steel plates may be applied to the dorsal spinous processes, but the bolts are placed through the processes themselves (Fig. 44-14). Each hole in the plate is not directly in the middle of each process; therefore, maximum strength from the process may not be gained, and fracture of the spinous process may be a complicating factor. This plate should also be set as low on the spine as possible, it should span at least five interspaces, and it requires that the dorsal spinous processes be intact.

*Aurburn Spinal Plate, Richard Mfg. Co., Memphis, TN
†Lubra Plate, Lubra Co., Fort Collins, CO

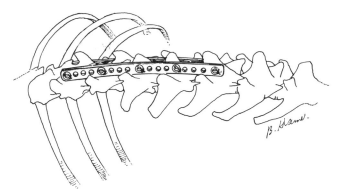

Fig. 44-14. *A stainless steel spinal plate is applied to the dorsal spinous processes.*

REPAIR OF SEVENTH LUMBAR FRACTURES

Fracture with luxation of the seventh lumbar vertebra is common in dogs. The neurologic signs may not be confined strictly to the sacral nerves. Trauma to the cauda equina may also injure the sciatic and femoral nerves. The sciatic nerve arises from L6, L7, and S1. The caudal rectal nerve arises from S2 and S3 and provides innervation to the bowel and bladder.

Reduction of the fracture or luxation is accomplished by traction on the head and tail, thus moving the sacrum caudally. The body of L7 is levered down onto the sacrum so that the articular processes of L7 are aligned with the cranial articular surface of the sacrum. Reduction is maintained by a transilial pin placed through the wings of the ilium, caudal to the base of the dorsal spinous process of L7 (Fig. 44-15). Once reduction has taken place, an exploration of the spinal canal may be performed with rongeurs to decompress the spinal cord adequately. Reduction of this type requires that the articular processes of L7 are intact. Migration of the Steinmann pin may be a complication.

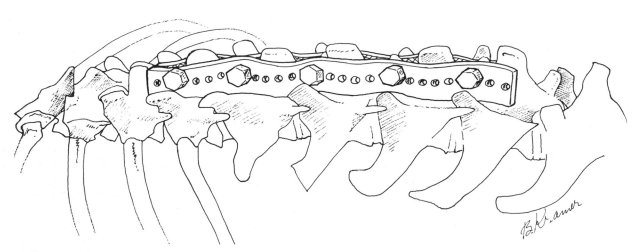

Fig. 44-13. *A vinylidene spinal plate is applied to the dorsal spinous processes.*

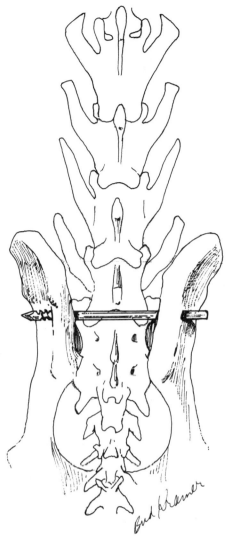

Fig. 44-15. *For a lumbosacral luxation an intramedullary pin is placed through the wings of the ilium caudal to the dorsal spinous process of L1.*

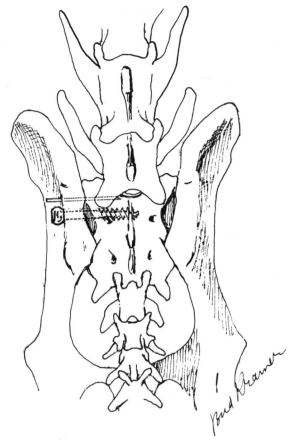

Fig. 44-16. *An intramedullary pin is placed through the ilium into the sacrum to provide stabilization. A lag screw is then placed through the ilium into the sacrum.*

REPAIR OF SACROILIAC LUXATIONS

Many sacroiliac luxations do not require stabilization. Stabilization should be recommended when early ambulation is desired or when concomitant fractures of the rear limbs or pelvis are present. Lag screw fixation provides the most secure repair (Fig. 44-16). A linear skin incision is made over the wing of the ilium, and the middle gluteal muscle is reflected laterally and ventrally. The caudal aspects of the iliocostalis and longissimus lumborum muscles may be reflected medially to visualize the sacrum. A small Kirschner wire is passed medially through the ilium and is imbedded into the sacrum to maintain reduction while a screw is inserted into the sacrum. A cortical or cancellous screw may be used. If a cortical screw is used, the drill hole through the ilium should be overdrilled to provide compression of the luxation.

REPAIR OF SACROCOCCYGEAL FRACTURES

Owing to the sacral innervation of the bowel and bladder (S2 and S3), repair of sacrococcygeal fractures and luxations should be recommended whenever moderate displacement or neurologic dysfunction is present. Displaced coccygeal vertebrae may cause traction on the nerve roots of the cauda equina.

Amputation of the tail may be indicated if deep pain is absent. Even with a tail amputation, repair of moderately displaced coccygeal vertebrae with stabilization by internal fixation is indicated because of potential or evident trauma to the sacral nerves. It must be remembered that the coccygeal vertebrae may not all be removed without involvement of the structures of the perineum, especially the external anal sphincter muscles.

Mild displacement of sacral or coccygeal vertebrae in a small dog may require only orthopedic wire through the facets (Fig. 44-17). Sacral fractures may be more adequately stabilized by using an intramedullary pin and orthopedic wire, similar to repair of thoacolumbar instabilities (Fig. 44-18); however, the "U"-shaped pin is inserted through the dorsal spinous process of L6 or L7 and is directed caudally on the dorsal

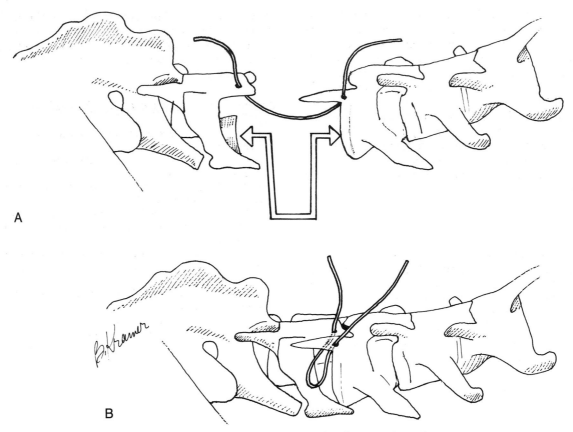

Fig. 44-17. A *and* B, *Orthopedic wire is used to wire the facets of the displaced coccygeal vertebrae.*

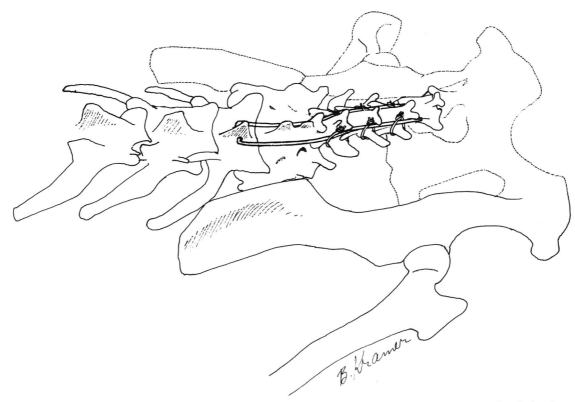

Fig. 44-18. *A "U"-shaped intramedullary pin is placed through the dorsal spinous process of L7 and is contoured to the lamina of the sacral and coccygeal vertebrae. Orthopedic wire is then used to secure the transverse processes to the pin bilaterally.*

vertebral lamina, medial to the articular facets. Because most sacral and coccygeal displacements are ventral, the vertebrae are supported with orthopedic wire from the transverse processes to the intermedullary pin. The facets should also be wired to prevent distraction. If the tail is completely anesthetic, amputation will not only relieve some of the traction on the fracture, but will also prevent soilage of the tail with fecal material. Even with amputation of the tail, a surgical procedure is recommended to repair greatly displaced sacral fractures because neurologic complications may accompany a large callous formation at the healed fracture site.

Postoperative Care

External bandages or support may be required for further stability of thoracolumbar trauma. If the surgical procedure has provided adequate stabilization, however, strict cage rest may be sufficient for the immediate postoperative management period (3 to 5 days). Corticosteroid administration should be continued postoperatively in tapering doses for 5 to 7 days. Antibiotics should be administered to prevent wound infection and cystitis from urine retention. Bladder expression in those animals that fail to retain bladder function is necessary. Neurologic evaluations should be performed daily for accurate assessment of the patient's condition.

References and Suggested Readings

1. Gage, E. D.: A new method of spinal fixation in the dog. VM SAC, 64:295, 1969.
2. Gage, E. D.: Surgical repair of spinal fractures in toy breed dogs. VM SAC, 66:1095, 1971.
3. Hoerlein, B. F.: Canine Neurology: Diagnosis and Treatment. Philadelphia, W. B. Saunders, 1978.
4. Lumb, W. V., and Brasmer, T. H.: Improved spinal plates and hypothermia as adjuncts to spinal surgery. J. Am. Vet. Med. Assoc., 157:338, 1970.
5. Piermattei, D. L., and Greeley, R. G.: An Atlas of Surgical Approaches to the Bones of the Dog and Cat. 2nd Ed. Philadelphia, W. B. Saunders, 1979.
6. Rouse, G. P., and Milton, J. I.: The use of methylmethacrylate for spinal stabilization. J. Am. Anim. Hosp. Assoc., 11:418, 1975.
7. Slocum, B., and Rudy, R. L.: Fractures of the seventh lumbar vertebra in the dog. J. Am. Anim. Hosp. Assoc., 11:167, 1975.
8. Swaim, S. F.: Vertebral body plating for spinal immobilization. J. Am. Vet. Med. Assoc., 158:1683, 1971.

45 * Pelvis

Management of Pelvic Fractures

by GUY B. TARVIN

Although the bones of the pelvic girdle (ilium, ischium, pubis, and sacrum) are well protected by muscles,[4] fractures of this area are common. In some studies, this injury accounts for 20 to 25% of the fractures seen in small animals.[1,3,10] The pelvis of the dog and cat has many functions, including support of the body on the rear limbs, attachment of several muscles, and as a canal through which pass numerous nerves, blood vessels, and other soft tissue structures (urogenital tract and colon). Fractures of the pelvis compromise these functions to varying degrees; therefore, proper management is a necessity in order to minimize undesirable sequelae. With this information as background, this discussion offers a rational approach to management of pelvic fractures, primarily sacroiliac dislocations and ilial fractures. Fractures of the sacrum and acetabulum are mentioned at several points in the text; however, the reader is referred to Chapter 44, on spinal surgery, and the section of this chapter on acetabular fracture repair, respectively, for more detail on these subjects.

Diagnosis

In order for a well-protected structure such as the pelvis to be injured, severe trauma must be inflicted. Such is almost always the case because most of these fractures are related to automobile accidents or falls from a great height. Trauma of this magnitude not only damages bones, but may also injure soft tissue. One recent study[6] showed a greater than 50% incidence of serious injuries, such as pulmonary contusions, ruptured bladder and urethra, nerve injury, or spinal and other fractures, associated with pelvic fractures. It is a good rule of thumb to assess the *entire* animal carefully before dealing with the pelvic fractures; otherwise, life-threatening problems may be overlooked. Once life-threatening problems are ruled out, a thorough examination of the rear limb can be performed. Pelvic fractures or dislocations should be considered in any traumatic episode from which the animal demonstrates rear limb dysfunction. Careful and subtle palpation of the limb should allow one to localize the source of the problem to the pelvis.

Palpation of the pelvis involves both external and internal (rectal) examinations. By placing one's hands over the pelvis and assessing bony landmarks such as the wings of the ilium, the greater trochanter, the ischial tuberosity, and the dorsal spinal processes of the sacrum, inconsistencies in location from one side to another can be appreciated. Such inconsistencies may indicate displacement of a portion of the pelvis. Manipulation of these landmarks can then be performed to assess for crepitation, instability, and pain.

Prior to conservative or surgical management, a thorough neurologic examination of the limb, anus, and perineal area is indicated. Anatomically, the pelvis is closely related to several nerves. The sciatic nerve is prone to injury in pelvic trauma because it courses along the medial aspect of the ilium and over the caudal portion of the acetabulum before continuing distally down the limb[4] (Fig. 45-1*). This position exposes the nerve to trauma at several locations. This nerve can quickly be assessed by applying a painful stimulus to the lateral digits of the rear leg. A positive response is for the dog to turn and to acknowledge the pain, for

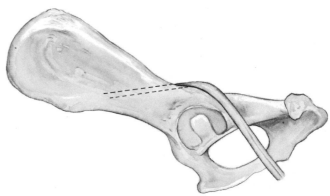

Fig. 45-1. *Diagram demonstrating the intimate relation of the sciatic nerve to the pelvis.*

*The illustrations in this section of Chapter 45 were drawn by Carol G. Prusa, Biomedical Communications Center, College of Veterinary Medicine, University of Illinois.

example, by trying to bite. Femoral nerve reflexes, sensation in the perineal area, and anal tone should also be assessed. Serial evaluations of the neurologic status should be made because examinations done early in the course of the injury or shock may give erroneous findings.

The time taken to assess neurologic function is often well spent. Unless neurologic function is intact, limb dysfunction and fecal and urinary incontinence may persist even though the pelvic fracture heals. This situation results in poor relations between client and veterinarian and wasted time and effort spent in the repair.

An internal or rectal examination is also important. Not only does it allow one to diagnose fractures by palpation, but also it provides useful information regarding the degree of compromise of the pelvic canal, the stability of the fracture fragments, the assessment of rectal wall perforations, and the degree of anal sphincter tone. The last observation may be especially important with pelvic fractures involving the sacrum, because injury to the pudendal nerve may thus be suspected. Ultimately, radiographic evaluation, with two or more plain roentgenograms, is necessary to confirm and to complete the diagnosis of pelvic fractures.

Medical Treatment

Treatment of pelvic fractures can be divided into two categories: nonsurgical and surgical. Nonsurgical management is based on the rationale that the soft tissue structures surrounding the pelvis, such as the muscle mass and the sacrotuberous ligament, act as an internal splint and support. This treatment may involve reduction of the fragments by rectal or external manipulation while the animal is under anesthesia. Whether such manipulation is done or not, the remainder of the treatment regimen includes cage rest, the appropriate supportive care (bladder expression and cleaning the animal, for example), and possibly the use of non-weight-bearing slings.[11] Treatment of this type is indicated in minimally displaced fractures that do not severely compromise the pelvic canal. Other indications for this type of therapy are when economics is a strong consideration and in those fractures so badly smashed that surgical repair may not be feasible. Even though most fractures involving a joint are best repaired and stabilized by internal fixation, some minimally displaced acetabular fractures can be treated by the nonsurgical method. As with all fractures treated nonsurgically, however, good communications with the client are necessary to success.

Dogs treated by the nonsurgical method should be evaluated frequently by physical examination. Although some exercise, in the form of short walks to defecate and urinate, may be allowed once the fractures are palpably stable on rectal and external examination, a complete return to activity should be discouraged until radiographic union is demonstrated, perhaps in 6 weeks or more.

Indications for Surgical Treatment

Surgical management is indicated when the following criteria are met:

1. Gross displacement, especially in fractures involving the acetabulum.
2. Compromise of the pelvic canal, especially in intact bitches.
3. Unstable, weight-bearing segment (see Fig. 45-3). The instability of this fracture type must be assessed by physical examination of the animal. Instability is often related to pain. If the animal is weight-bearing on the limb on the side of the fracture, the fragment is probably stable. Ultimately, a thorough physical examination is necessary to assess stability.
4. Other considerations for surgical intervention include an earlier return to function than with nonsurgical therapy, especially in large breed dogs, a better cosmetic appearance, especially for short-haired show dogs, and a need for an exploration to assess nerve or other soft tissue injury in the area.

Surgical Techniques

As previously mentioned, many patients require intensive care for other problems related to their trauma. Surgical treatment should not be attempted in these cases until the patient is considered a good surgical risk. On the other hand, delay or procrastination makes surgical reduction more and more difficult; therefore, the operation should be well timed.

In almost all pelvic fractures, a surgeon is dealing with multiple fractures within the pelvic girdle because of the architecture of the pelvis. The pelvis, when viewed from its dorsal aspect, has the appearance of a rectangular box. This structure is unique in that it prevents fewer than two fractures from occurring at one time in the pelvis (Fig. 45-2).

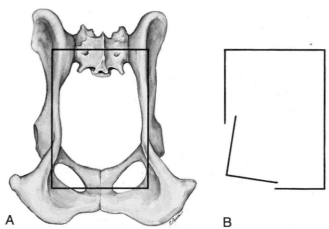

Fig. 45-2. A *and* B, *Illustration of the "box-like" structure of the pelvis demonstrating that fewer than two fractures seldom occur.*

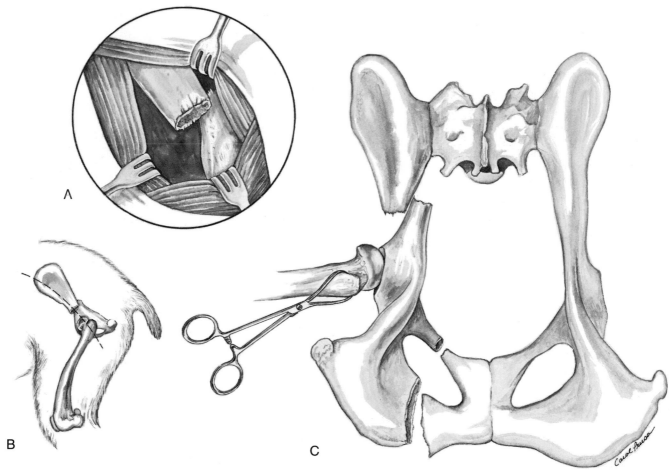

Fig. 45-3. A, *Lateral approach and exposure of ilial shaft with fracture.* B, *This pelvic fracture has an unstable weight-bearing segment.* C, *A Lewin clamp is attached to the greater trochanter to facilitate reduction.*

The purposes of performing a surgical procedure are to reduce the fragments and thus relieve compromise of the pelvic canal and to stabilize the weight-bearing segments. To accomplish this end, it is not necessary to reduce and fix all the fractures. Sufficient stability can often be achieved by proper repair of only one fracture. For example, in Figure 45-3, fractures have occurred through the pubis, ilium, and ischium, leaving a weight-bearing segment containing the acetabulum displaced into the pelvic canal. Such a set of fractures can often be adequately treated by fixation of the ilial fracture without fixation of the ischial or pubic fractures. With these thoughts in mind, surgical treatment of certain pelvic fractures is now discussed.

UNSTABLE SACROILIAC DISLOCATIONS

I prefer the dorsolateral approach[9] to the sacroiliac joint with the dog in lateral recumbency (Fig. 45-4A). Lateral recumbency allows easy manipulation of the limb to reduce the (usually) cranial dorsal luxation of the wing of the ilium and also allows easy application of the fixation devices. In bilateral cases, a dorsal approach is preferred because both sides can be exposed simultaneously.

Once the sacroiliac joint has been exposed, the limb is grasped, and caudal traction is applied. In acute cases this maneuver, as well as manipulation of the dorsal wing of the ilium with Kern bone-holding forceps, is usually sufficient to reduce the dislocation. In large dogs or in more chronic cases (greater than 4 days), more vigorous manipulation may be required. One technique employs inserting two small Steinmann pins or Kirschner wires.[1] One pin (wire) is inserted into the dorsal part of the ilium and the other into the wing of the sacrum (Fig. 45-4B). These pins can be used as "handles" to manipulate the ilium into position and also as landmarks to aid in reduction. These pins are removed when fixation is complete. Once the fracture has been reduced, fixation is accomplished by use of two screws or Kirschner wires. The screws are best applied in lag fashion.[7] One should overdrill the proximal cortex and tap the distal cortex or use a cancellous bone screw (Fig. 45-5). The screws or pins are applied through the ilium and into the wing of the sacrum (Fig. 45-5).

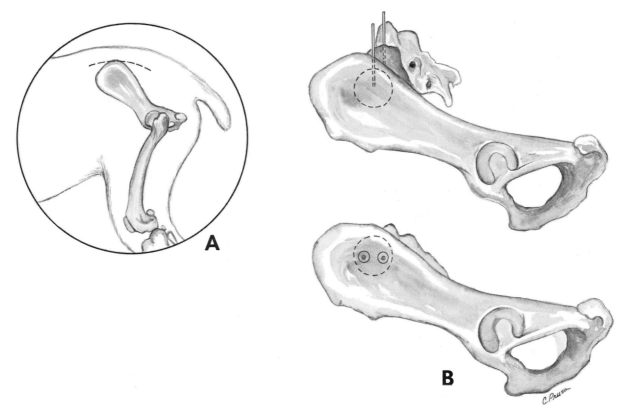

Fig. 45-4. A, *Lateral position and skin incision for repair of a unilateral sacroiliac dislocation.* B, *Placement of two pins directly dorsal to the articular surface of the sacral wing and ilium aids reduction and alignment; lateral view of screw fixation.*

FRACTURES INVOLVING THE ILIUM

I prefer a lateral approach to the ilium.[b]

Fractures of the ilium lend themselves to several modes of fixation. When the fragments are of sufficient length to allow at least two bone screws proximally and distally, I prefer bone plating. The ilium is a wide,

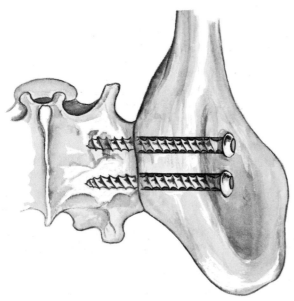

Fig. 45-5. *Lag screw fixation of the sacroiliac luxation.*

flat bone and lends itself readily to this technique. Reduction can sometimes be accomplished by grasping the fragment ends with Verbrugge forceps and bringing the ends into proper alignment; however, further manipulation is often needed. One technique that can be used when the hip joint is intact is to grasp the greater trochanter with Lewin forceps and to manipulate the distal fragment into reduction (see Fig. 45-3). Once the fracture has been reduced, a bone-holding forceps is applied, or the assistant maintains reduction while the plate is contoured and applied (Fig. 45-6A). In some cases, the aforementioned techniques of reduction are insufficient, owing to the muscle contracture. In these patients, the following procedure may be used. The plate is contoured, using the radiograph of the opposite side, when intact, as a guide, and is applied only to the distal fragment. The fragment ends are brought as close to reduction as possible. A Verbrugge clamp is applied as in Figure 45-6B and C to complete reduction.[2] The plate is then secured to the proximal segment. When drilling, gauging, and taping the screw holes, care must be taken not to injure the structures, such as the rectum and sciatic nerve, medial to the ilium. Screws in the proximal segment often engage the wing of the sacrum. Although this maneuver results in greater holding power, care should be taken, just as in repair of the sacroiliac dislocation, to avoid the spinal canal in this area.

Some fractures of the ilium can also be pinned. This technique seems to be most successful in fractures

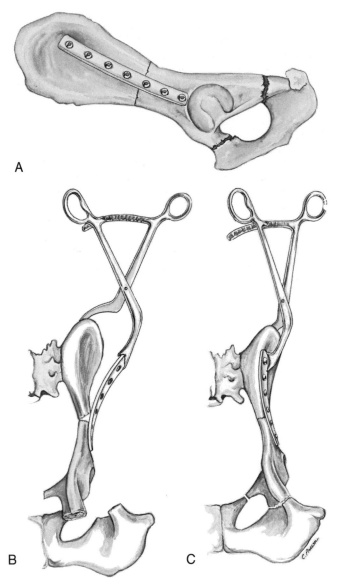

occurring proximal to or in the midbody area of the ilium. Fractures distal to the midbody area of the ilium do not often permit sufficient length of insertion of the pin(s) to provide adequate stability. The technique can be performed when the fracture has been exposed.

The pin(s) is started in the proximal fragment near the cranial dorsomedial aspect of the wing of the ilium. The pin(s) is driven down the shaft of the ilium and into the proximal segment (Fig. 45-7). A pin of identical length is used to check the distance coursed by the driven pin. The hip joint should also be palpated to discern whether the implant has entered the joint. If so, the pin is retracted until no palpable evidence of joint invasion is noted. Several pins should be driven in a similar manner to improve stability. This technique is technically difficult because the medullary cavity of the ilium is narrow, and in driving the pins the cortex is often penetrated. Although stability achieved by this technique is rarely as satisfactory as with plate fixation, it is mentioned here as an alternative when bone plating equipment is not available.

Fractures of the ilium near the acetabulum can also be treated with bone plates. If further exposure is needed, a trochanteric osteotomy may be used to reflect the gluteal mass dorsally[8] (Fig. 45-8).

Fractures of the ilium with concurrent sacroiliac luxations are best treated with plate fixation. The approach is a modification of the lateral approach to the ilium.[12] Once the ilium is exposed, the attachment of the iliacus muscle to the ventral border of the ilium is incised. Blunt dissection, preferably with the finger, is directed along the medial face of the ilium until the articular surface of the sacral wing and ilium are pal-

Fig. 45-6. A, *Reduced fracture and bone plate in place. B and C, Reduction by precontouring a plate and levering the distal fragment in place with a Verbrugge clamp.*

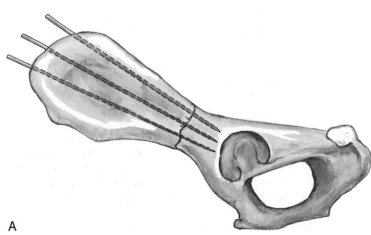

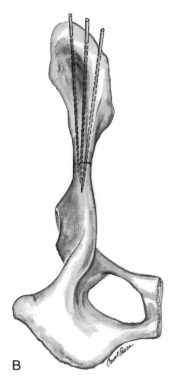

Fig. 45-7. A *and* B, *Pin placement for ilial fractures.*

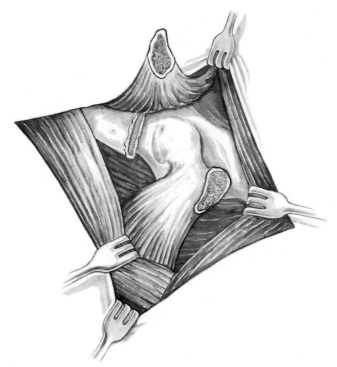

Fig. 45-8. *Trochanteric osteotomy is sometimes necessary to expose fractures near the acetabulum for repair.*

pated (Fig. 45-9). Once the fracture has been reduced, a small Kirschner wire is inserted through the ilium and into the sacral wing to maintain reduction. The plate is applied as previously described for ilial fractures. The screws over the sacroiliac joint are purposely applied in lag fashion to engage the wing of the sacrum.

Postoperative Care

Postoperative radiographs are indicated to evaluate the implant(s) and reduction. Appropriate steps should be taken if errors in reduction have occurred. If adequate fixation is accomplished, no special aftercare is required. Appropriate bedding and nursing care, along with confinement for 2 to 3 weeks is advised. In 2 to 3 weeks, physical and radiographic assessments are necessary to determine whether further confinement is needed.

Fractures involving both sides of the pelvis are dealt with individually. Surgical procedures can be staged approximately 2 days apart or as the animal's condition allows.

In summary, fractures of the pelvis are a common orthopedic problem. A "hands-on" approach is required throughout the care of these animals because a severe traumatic episode has occurred. Indications

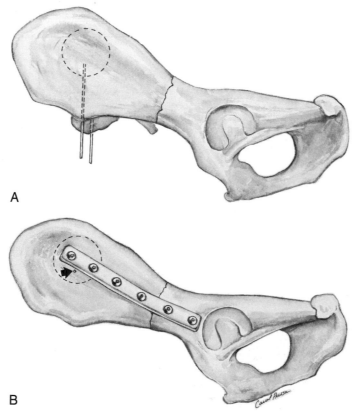

A

B

Fig. 45-9. *Exposure of concurrent fractured ilium and sacroiliac luxation by a lateral approach. The center of the articular surface of both joint components (sacrum and ilium) can be palpated. A, Pins may be inserted as shown to aid reduction. B, Reduction is initially held by a small pin (arrow) until a plate is applied.*

exist for both surgical and nonsurgical therapy. Although injuries in this area involve multiple fractures or dislocations within the pelvic girdle, surgical repair of the ilial fracture or the sacroiliac luxation is usually sufficient to achieve adequate stability of the weight-bearing segment and to correct the compromise of the pelvic canal. Acetabular fractures and sacral fractures are covered in later sections of this chapter.

References and Suggested Readings

1. Brinker, W. O.: Fractures of the pelvis. In Current Techniques in Small Animal Surgery. Edited by M. J. Bojrab. Philadelphia, Lea & Febiger, 1975.
2. Brown, S. G., and Biggart, J. F.: Plate fixation of ilial shaft fractures in the dog. J. Am. Vet. Med. Assoc., 167:472, 1975.
3. Denny, H. R.: Pelvic fractures in the dog: a review of 123 cases. J. Small Anim. Pract., 19:151, 1978.
4. Evans, H. E., and Christensen, G. C.: Miller's Anatomy of the Dog. 2nd Ed. Philadelphia, W. B. Saunders, 1979.
5. Hohn, R. B., and Janes, J. M.: Lateral approach to the canine ilium. Anim. Hosp., 2:111, 1966.
6. Jackson, D. A., and Brasmer, T. H.: Thoracic and non-thoracic injuries associated with pelvic fractures in dogs. In press.
7. Muller, M. E., Allgower, M., and Willenegger, H.: Manual of Internal Fixation. New York, Springer Verlag, 1970.
8. Piermattei, D. L., and Greeley, R. G.: Approach to the hip joint and body of the ilium biostiotomy of the greater trochanter. In Surgical Approaches to the Bones of the Dog and Cat. 2nd Ed. Philadelphia, W. B. Saunders, 1979.
9. Piermattei, D. L., and Greeley, R. G.: Approach to the wing of the ilium and sacroiliac joint. In Surgical Approaches to the Bones of the Dog and Cat. 2nd Ed. Philadelphia, W. B. Saunders, 1979.
10. Robins, G. M., Dingwall, J. S., and Sumner-Smith, G.: A plating of pelvic fractures in the dog. Vet. Rec., 93:550, 1975.
11. Robinson, G. W., and McCoy, L.: A pelvic limb sling for dogs. In Current Techniques in Small Animal Surgery. Edited by M. J. Bojrab. Philadelphia, Lea & Febiger, 1975.
12. Sinibaldi, K.: Personal communication.

Cauda Equina Compression Syndrome

by GUY B. TARVIN

and RAYMOND PRATA

The cauda equina is less frequently the site of neurologic dysfunction than the cervical or thoracolumbar spine in small animals. Disease of the low lumbar spine has a pronounced effect in that several nerves controlling locomotion, fecal and urinary continence, and sensation to the hind quarters can be involved simultaneously or individually. Therefore, the syndrome of cauda equina compression can result in diverse symptoms and is often difficult to diagnose. In order to understand diagnosis and treatment of the problem better, this discussion reviews the anatomic features, pathomechanics, diagnostic aids, and treatment of this syndrome.

Anatomic Features

The cauda equina is a leash of nerve roots of the low lumbar spine. These nerve roots descend from their spinal cord segment origins to their site of emergence from the spinal canal. Early in the development of the embryo, the spinal nerves leave the spinal cord at right angles to exit at the respective foramina. As the embryo continues to develop, the spinal cord ceases to grow before the vertebral column. It is because of this differential growth of the two structures that the spinal cord of the dog extends only to the level of the fifth or sixth lumbar vertebra. Thus, the spinal nerves of the mature dog have to course obliquely and caudally to exit at the respective foramina[4] (Fig. 45-10A).

Nerves included in the cauda equina are L7, S1 to 3, and coccygeal nerves 1 to 5. The L6, L7, and S1 nerve roots contribute fibers to the sciatic nerve. The pudendal nerve, which innervates the perineum, is composed

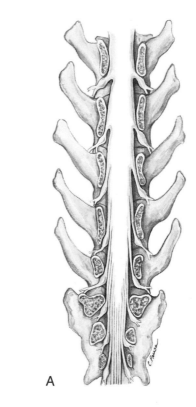

A

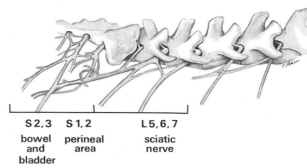

S 2, 3	S 1, 2	L 5, 6, 7
bowel and bladder	perineal area	sciatic nerve

B

Fig. 45-10. A, *Dorsoventral view of the cauda equina.* B, *Nerve distribution of the cauda equina.*

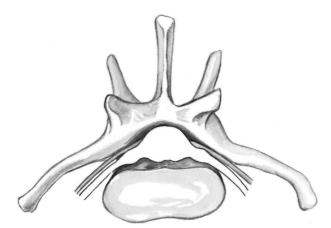

Fig. 45-11. *Normal cross section of the spine.*

of the S1 and S2 nerve roots. The pelvic nerve, which carries parasympathetic fibers to the bowel and bladder, is composed of fibers from S2 and S3. The tail is innervated by the nerve roots originating from the coccygeal segments[4] (Fig. 45-10*B*). The cauda equina is enclosed within the spinal canal whose boundaries are (1) dorsally, the lamina of the vertebrae, ligamentum flavum, and articular facets; (2) laterally, the pedicles of the vertebrae and ligamentum flavum; and (3) ventrally, the body of the vertebrae, dorsal longitudinal ligament, and the anulus fibrosus. The cross section of the spinal canal is triangular in shape, and the facets form lateral recesses in which nerves lie just prior to their exit through the foramina (Fig. 45-11).

The intervertebral foramina form short restricting canals for exit of spinal nerves and blood vessels to and from the spinal canal. Articular facets, ligamentum flavum, pedicles, vertebral bodies, and intervertebral disks make up the boundaries of the foramina. In the sacrum, the nerves exit through the foramina in the bone.[4] Deformities and injuries, whether congenital or acquired, of any of these structures comprising the canal or foramina may result in attenuation of the cauda equina and structures in the interverterbral foramina.

Causes of Compression

Attenuation of the cauda equina may have several causes.[10] Neoplasia, infection (intradiskal osteomyelitis), acute disk extrusion, spondylosis, trauma, or congenital spinal stenosis are among the lesions that may attenuate the cauda equina and may cause neurologic dysfunction. Infectious processes such as intradiskal osteomyelitis may be of bacterial or, less frequently, of fungal origin.[3] The source of these infections may be systemic or may be spread from local wounds in the area, such as from tail docking and bite wounds over and around the dorsum of the pelvis.[9] The subsequent inflammatory, destructive, and proliferative processes may cause instability as well as nerve root compression.

Although neoplasia is not commonly the cause of cauda equina compression, chondrosarcomas,[3] osteosarcomas,[9] and metastatic choroid plexus carcinoma[8] of the lumbosacral spine have been reported. Trauma from various causes can result in fracture dislocations of the lumbosacral spine.

Other than the aforementioned etiologic factors, spinal stenosis can be either acquired or congenital. Acquired forms of lumbar spinal stenosis can be caused by primary degenerative spondylosis (multifocal), focal spondylosis secondary to or associated with degenerative disk disease, spondylolytic spondylolisthesis, or pseudospondylolisthesis. These changes basically result from instability of one or more segments of the lumbar spine. In an effort to afford stability, the body responds to the proliferative changes in several structures (that is, thickened lamina, pedicles, facets, and ligaments). In veterinary medicine, some of the causes of acquired stenosis have been documented.[7]

Congenital stenosis can be subdivided into those episodes that occur in dogs with achrondroplasia[1] and those considered to be idiopathic.[2] Whatever the cause, congenital stenosis is characterized by a shortening of the pedicles, thickened and sclerotic apposition of the lamina and articular processes, infolding and hypertrophy of the ligamentum flavum adjoining the lamina, and sclerotic and bulbous articular facets that bulge into the dorsal half of the canal (Fig. 45-12). The most common sites of involvement in dogs are the L6–L7 and L7–S1 spinal cord segments.[10] Idiopathic lumbar spinal stenosis does not usually manifest itself until middle or late age. In these patients, the bony changes are present at birth with further attenuation, as evidenced by a thickened ligamentum flavum, occurring later in life and resulting in clinical signs.[10]

Spinal stenosis not only causes mechanical compression of the dural tube and nerve roots, but also produces intermittent ischemia of the nerve roots.[11] Dilation of the vessels of the nerve roots and spinal cord occurs subsequent to the increased demand imposed on neural function during exercise[11] (Fig. 45-13). The

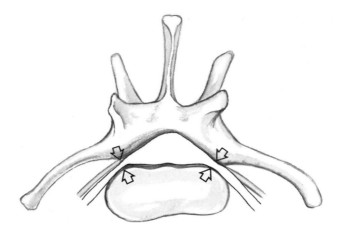

Fig. 45-12. *Stenosis of spinal canal. Not only is the dural tube pinched, but also the exiting nerves as they course through the narrowed foramina (arrows).*

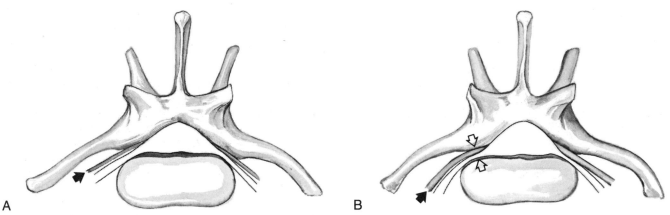

Fig. 45-13. *Stenosed spinal canal. Vessels (solid arrow) before (A) and after (B) exercise. B, Exercise causes vessels to dilate and increases pressure on nerve roots within the foramina (clear arrows).*

nerve roots and associated vessels, being abnormally confined by the stenosed canal or intervertebral foramen, are further attenuated when exercise is induced. The subsequent overall increased diameter of the nerve roots, confined by the stenotic canal, reduces the effective blood flow to roots and causes an ischemic phenomenon.[11]

Ischemia produces root pain and subsequent reflex pain (paresthesias, dysesthesias) to the part innervated by that nerve(s). Various states of paresis may also be associated with the ischemic and pressure phenomena. In each instance, early in the course of the disease, the referred pain or paresis is intermittent and is associated with exercise. The severity of pain or paresis progresses with increased stenosis, which is associated with degenerative disease of the ligamentous and bony structure of the stenotic canal. In the latter instance, the pain or paresis may be persistent. Therefore, adequate historical information is mandatory to establish the initial intermittency of the deficits. Signs referable to the extremities, tail, bowel or bladder function, and genitals have been reported.[10]

Diagnosis of Compression

Animals presented to the veterinarian with stenosis of the cauda equina usually exhibit intermittent lameness, fecal or urinary incontinence, or paresthesias and dysesthesias, such as evidenced by tail biting, leg biting, genital licking, conscious proprioception deficits, and motor weakness. These animals all have lumbosacral pain. The lameness is usually related to dysfunction of the nerve roots comprising the sciatic nerve, whereas fecal and urinary incontinence are the result of attenuation of the S2 and S3 nerve roots.

Paresthesias are unpleasant sensory disturbances that often manifest as referred pain (lameness) or in various forms of self-mutilation of the tail, leg, or extremity. More often than not, dogs are treated for various obscure dermatologic problems. Dysesthesias are even less pleasant sensory disturbances enhanced by manipulation of the affected part by the clinician. Each

condition has been demonstrated in previous literature.[10]

The cauda equina is unique because a large number of nerve roots are contained in a small area (L6 through S3). A single lesion can involve several nerves and may result in one or all of the aforementioned signs. Thus, the presenting symptoms are often bizarre and mimic other problems, such as orthopedic disorders, anal sacculitis, and tail-head dermatitis. In order to arrive at a correct diagnosis, a general examination of the entire animal and an orthopedic examination of the hind limbs should be performed first.

Once the more common causes are ruled out, a critical neurologic examination is indicated, including an evaluation of conscious proprioception, motor function, reflexes, sensory status, anal tone, and state of continence (from the patient's medical history). Most important, the clinician must manipulate the lumbosacral spine to establish the presence or absence of pain. This finding was the most consistent on all reported cases.[10]

Electromyographic studies have also been used to localize the lesions to specific nerves and segments in animals with this syndrome.[10] Whenever facilities are available, this tool can provide useful information to support a diagnosis. In our experience, however, confirmation with such studies is not the rule.

Having established historical and clinical neurologic signs referable to the cauda equina, plain radiographs, taken when the patient is under general anesthesia, are indicated to evaluate potential existing disease of the lumbosacral spine. Neoplasia, fractures, congenital lesions, herniated disks, spondylosis, intradiskal osteomyelitis, and lumbosacral stenosis can often be confirmed by radiographic means alone. In numerous cases of congenital stenosis, however, little if any bony pathologic tissue may be demonstrated. Myelographic studies in this area are of little value because it is often difficult to obtain an adequate dye column this far caudally. Intraosseous venography may be of value in some patients; however, it does not permit adequate study of the dorsal aspect of the canal.[6,10] Consideration should be given to epidural dye studies.

Surgical Treatment of Compression

In patients demonstrating neurologic dysfunction of the cauda equina, several factors should be considered in deciding the optimal mode of therapy:

1. Duration and severity of the dysfunction. An animal with mild proprioceptive deficits of short duration (1 to 2 days) has a better prognosis than an animal with no sensation to the hind quarters.

2. Etiologic factors. Neoplastic processes, such as osteogenic sarcoma, may offer a poor prognosis. Congenital stenosis[10] and some other disorders[7] offer a good prognosis if a surgical procedure is performed early in the course of the disease. Intradiskal osteomyelitis responds, in our experience, most favorably to analgesics, muscle relaxants, and antibiotics. Patients that respond poorly are candidates for surgical treatment, culture, and biopsy.

3. Economics and aftercare. Especially in the case of traumatic luxations or fractures of the area, surgical decompression, stabilization, and aftercare are costly and time-consuming. If the patient's owners are unwilling or unable to make financial commitments or fail to understand their role in postoperative care, surgical treatment is not warranted.

It should be remembered that each case is to be evaluated on an individual basis; not all are clear cut with regard to prognosis, and individual decisions must be made.

Surgical exposure of the cauda equina is best accomplished by laminectomy, facetectomy, and foraminotomy. The epiaxial musculature is subperiosteally elevated and is retracted laterally (Fig. 45-14). The dorsal spinous processes are removed with a ronguer. The dorsal lamina is removed with a ronguer or a high-speed bur. In cases of congenital stenosis, a thickened ligamentum flavum may be encountered. The ligament can be resected using a No. 11 Bard-Parker scalpel blade, as in Figure 45-15A. The extent of the laminectomy should continue cranially and caudally until the dural contents are free of compression. Laterally, the facets must be removed, effecting a foraminotomy and subsequently decompressing the nerve roots (Fig. 45-15B). Biopsy specimens can be taken in cases of suspected neoplasia or infection. Curettage and culture of the interspace in cases of intradiskal osteomyelitis can be accomplished by working lateral to the sheath of nerves (Fig. 45-16). Prior to closure, the spine is evaluated for stability. Rarely is instability a feature in patients with stenosis of the spinal canal. If the spine is unstable, the technique used in the repair of spinal fractures can be employed (see Chap. 44). The wound is copiously lavaged with normothermic saline solution. A free graft of fat is taken from the subcutaneous tissue near the incision and is placed over the laminectomy site to effectively decrease scar formation.[5] The lumbosacral fascia is closed on the midline with 2-0 or 3-0 monofilament nylon suture material. The remainder of the closure is routine.

Postoperative Care

As with all surgical cases, proper postoperative care is essential to obtain satisfactory results. Strict rest and confinement should be enforced especially in active dogs for 4 to 8 weeks. In dogs that are unable to ambulate, straw bedding helps to prevent decubitus ulcers and urine burns, and bladder expressions or intermittent catheterization and assisted fecal evacuation may be indicated to prevent adverse sequelae.

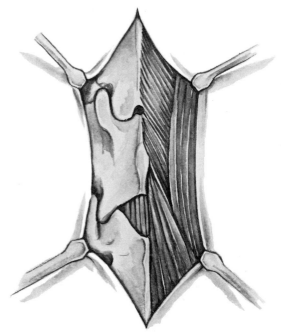

A

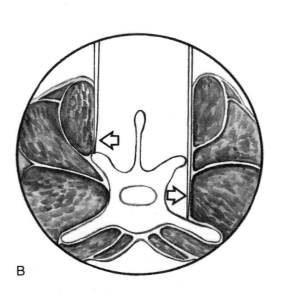

B

Fig. 45-14. A and B, *Muscle elevation for dorsal laminectomy.*

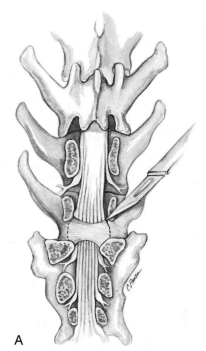

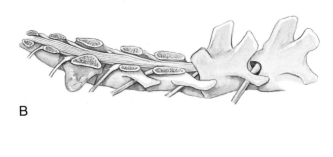

Fig. 45-15. A, *When the lamina has been removed, a thickened ligamentum flavum may be encountered. This structure can be resected as shown with a scalpel blade. B, A lateral view shows the extent of laminectomy, facetectomy, and foraminotomy.*

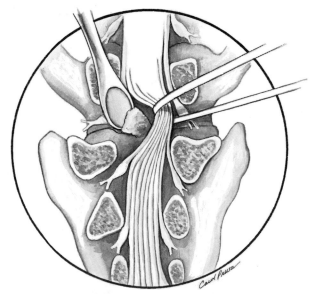

Fig. 45-16. *Intervertebral curettage can be performed with gentle retraction of the cauda equina.*

References and Suggested Readings

1. Alexander, E.: Significance of the small lumbar spinal canal. J. Neurosurg., *31*:513, 1969.
2. Armoldi, C. C., and Brodsky, J.: Lumbar spinal stenosis and nerve root entrapment syndromes. Clin. Orthop., *115*:4, 1976.
3. Berzon, J. L., and Dueland, R.: Cauda equina syndrome: pathophysiology and report of seven cases. J. Am. Hosp. Assoc., *15*:635, 1979.
4. Evans, H. E., and Christensen, G. C.: Miller's Anatomy of the Dog. 2nd Ed. Philadelphia, W. B. Saunders, 1979.
5. Gill, G. G., Sakovich, L., and Thomson, E.: Pedicle fat grafts for the prevention of scar formation after laminectomy: an experimental study in dogs. Spine, *4*:176, 1979.
6. McNeel, S. V., and Morgan, J. P.: Interosseous vertebral anography: a technique for examination of the canine lumbosacral junction. J. Vet. Radiol. Soc., *19*:168, 1978.
7. Oliver, J. E., Selcer, R. R., and Simpson, S.: Cauda equina compression from lumbosacral malarticulation and malformation in the dog. J. Am. Vet. Med. Assoc., *173*:207, 1978.
8. Patnaik, A. K., et al.: Choroid plexus carcinoma with meningeal carcinomatosis in a dog. Vet. Pathol., *17*:381, 1980.
9. Tarvin, G.: Cauda equina syndrome. Presented as a resident paper. New York, Animal Medical Center, March, 1976.
10. Tarvin, G., and Prata, R. G.: Lumbosacral stenosis in dogs. J. Am. Vet. Med. Assoc., *177*:154, 1980.
11. Wilson, C. D., Enhi, G., and Grollmus, J.: Neurogenic intermittent claudication. Clin. Neurosurg., *18*:62, 1971.

Acetabular Fractures

by DONALD A. HULSE

Incidence

Fractures involving the pelvic girdle are common in small animal practice. Pelvic fractures represent approximately 25% of all fractures and generally affect multiple sites of the pelvis. One area frequently involved either alone or in combination with other pelvic fractures is the acetabulum. The most common cause of pelvic fractures is automobile accidents, but isolated acetabular fractures may occur from a lesser degree of trauma, particularly in young patients with an open acetabular physis, which represents a weak link in the bony structure of the pelvis.

Clinical Signs and Diagnosis

The patient who has an acetabular fracture is likely to have concurrent soft tissue or other skeletal injuries and therefore requires a thorough physical examination. It is particularly important to evaluate the neurologic status of the patient prior to treating the obvious skeletal fractures. Evaluation of the coxofemoral joint generally elicits pain and crepitation with flexion, extension, and internal rotation of the hip joint. Such is not always the case with isolated acetabular fractures, however. If the patient is ambulatory, it will generally exhibit a non-weight-bearing lameness with the involved limb. Again, this statement is not always true in that some patients are presented to the veterinarian with a weight-bearing lameness if moderate trauma has resulted in an isolated acetabular fracture. The amount of soft tissue swelling varies according to the degree of trauma.

The swelling, pain, and crepitation noted with evaluation of the coxofemoral joint lead the veterinary surgeon to consider acetabular fracture as a differential diagnosis in a high percentage of cases. The veterinary surgeon must not delete acetabular fracture from his differential diagnosis, however, solely because pain and crepitation are not readily elicited with examination. Any suspicion of acetabular involvement must be included in the differential diagnosis and confirmed with radiographs. Radiographic evaluation must include ventrodorsal and lateral projections, and the patient must be properly prepared with an enema to empty the rectum. Oblique views of the acetabulum may be helpful to determine the degree of articular surface involvement in some cases.

Anatomy and Fracture Classification

The acetabulum is a deep, cotyloid (cup-shaped) cavity that forms a socket to receive the femoral head in creation of the hip joint. The acetabulum is composed of the ilium, the ischium, and the pubis, which all fuse during the twelfth postnatal week. The smooth articular surface of the acetabulum is widest cranially and extends from the acetabular lip three-fourths the distance to the depth of the acetabulum. The nonarticular area of the acetabulum is thin and quadrangular in appearance. This part of the acetabulum is the acetabular fossa, which is the site of attachment of the ligament of the head of the femur.

I prefer to classify fractures of the acetabulum according to the course of the fracture line as it crosses the articular surface of the acetabulum. Fractures of the acetabular fossa are always present, but anatomic reduction and stabilization are not necessary to restore function to the hip joint in most cases. Transacetabular fractures are classified into four groups (Fig. 45-17): cranial, central, caudal, and comminuted. Central transacetabular fractures are the most common, and comminuted transacetabular fractures are second in frequency. Preoperative radiographs must be interpreted carefully, in that a comminution of the acetabular fossa may be mistaken for a severely comminuted articular surface; such a mistake may lead one to believe that reconstruction of the articular surface is hopeless. The veterinary surgeon may choose a less satisfactory method of management in this case, when in reality, a single fracture line through the articular surface may be present.

Management

The veterinarian can manage acetabular fractures in three ways: (1) internal reduction and fixation; (2) conservative cage rest; and (3) excision arthroplasty.

An internal reduction and fixation procedure is the treatment of choice for acetabular fractures because malunion of an articular fracture can result in a painful degenerative joint. Short-term and long-term evalua-

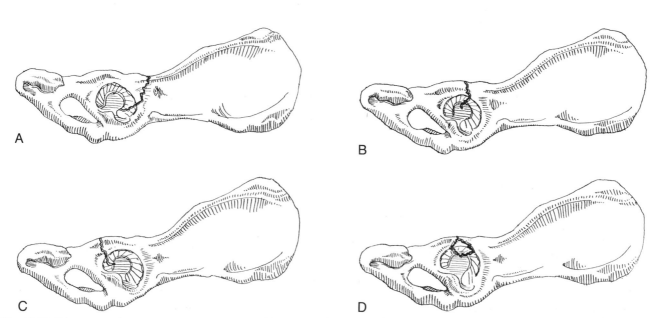

Fig. 45-17. *Diagrammatic representations of cranial* (A), *central* (B), *caudal* (C), *and comminuted* (D) *transacetabular fractures.*

tions of acetabular fractures in the dog treated with internal reduction and fixation revealed adequate function with little or no osteoarthrosis. Caudal acetabular fractures are treated conservatively unless marked displacement or instability of the fracture fragments is present. The surgical approaches to the acetabulum are well illustrated in the veterinary literature. The approach is left to the preference of the veterinary surgeon, but a trochanteric osteotomy is preferred at our hospital (Fig. 45-18).

The skin incision is centered over the cranial border of the greater trochanter and extends proximally toward the dorsal midline and ventrally along the cranial border of the femur. The subcutaneous tissues are incised along the same line, and the skin edges are toweled in. An incision is made through the biceps femoris fascia along its cranial border to facilitate caudal reflection of the biceps muscle. The sciatic nerve should be visualized at this point and followed proximally to the gluteal musculature. An incision is now made along

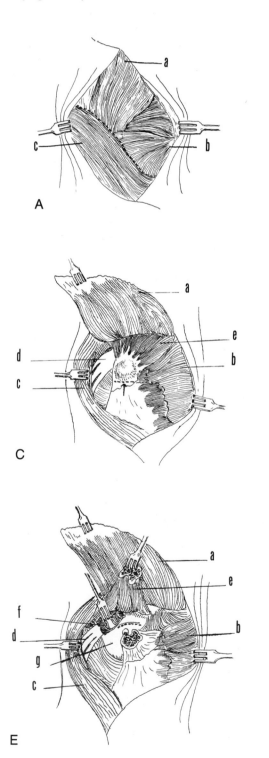

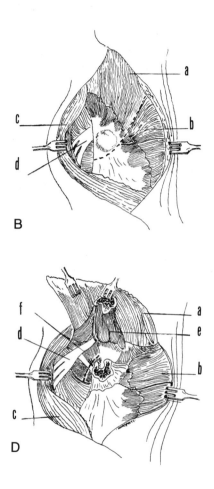

Fig. 45-18. A *to* E, *Diagrammatic representations of exposure of the hip joint through an osteotomy of the greater trochanter. a, Superficial gluteal muscle; b, tensor fasciae latae muscle; c, biceps femoris muscle; d, sciatic nerve; e, middle and deep gluteal muscles; f, internal obturator and gemelli muscles; g, joint capsule.*

the caudal border of the tensor fasciae latae muscle and is extended proximally along the cranial border of the superficial gluteal muscle. The insertion of the superficial gluteal muscle is isolated and is incised at the level of the third trochanter to allow proximal reflection of the muscle belly. The middle and deep gluteal muscles are visualized, and a straight hemostat is passed beneath the deep gluteal muscle from cranial to caudal, to act as a guide for osteotomy of the greater trochanter. Care is taken at this time to visualize the sciatic nerve. One then places the osteotome at the level of the third trochanter, positions the osteotome at 45° to the long axis of the femur, and guides the osteotome toward the prepositioned hemostat. The middle and deep gluteal muscles are reflected dorsally with the greater trochanter. A periosteal elevator is used to reflect the deep gluteal muscle from the joint capsule and the cranial half of the acetabulum.

Caudally, the gemelli muscles and tendon of the internal obturator muscle are incised as they insert into the trochanteric fossa. Once again, care must be taken to visualize the sciatic nerve. The gemelli muscles and internal obturator tendon are reflected with a periosteal elevator to expose the caudal aspect of the acetabulum. Bone-holding forceps are positioned on the caudal body of the ilium cranial to the acetabulum and on the ischiatic spine caudal to the acetabulum to facilitate reduction. Care must be taken not to damage the sciatic nerve when attempting reduction. With difficult reduction, a pin may be driven into the ischial tuberosity to provide a lever for caudal retraction. The joint capsule is now opened to remove debri such as small fragments and blood clots.

With the fracture satisfactorily reduced, as judged by direct visualization of the articular surface, two Kirschner wires are driven across the fracture line. If the articular surface is comminuted, the fragment is stabilized to the parent bone with Kirschner wires or a lag

screw. Additional stabilization is obtained with a small "L"- or "T"-shaped bone plate and screws (Fig. 45-19). The joint capsule and insertions of the gemelli muscles and the internal obturator tendon are repositioned and are sutured. The greater trochanter is reduced and is stabilized with three Kirschner wires. The insertions of the superficial gluteal and tensor fasciae latae muscles are repositioned and are sutured with an interrupted pattern. The fascia of the biceps muscle, the subcutaneous tissues, and the skin are sutured using standard methods.

Conservative treatment for acetabular fractures involves enforced cage rest and nursing care. Post-treatment evaluation of patients managed conservatively indicates that approximately 50% of these patients regain adequate function if fracture displacement is minimal.

Strict confinement with minimal exercise is important early in the course of treatment to prevent the further distraction of fracture fragments that may occur with premature weight bearing. Passive flexion and extension of the hip joint, together with muscle massage, are used to help the patient to retain the hip joint's range of motion and muscle integrity. A progressive exercise program is begun 3 to 4 weeks after trauma, but only when fracture stability has been assured by clinical and radiographic assessment. Swimming therapy is recommended to restore muscle strength. Nursing care is primarily concerned with the patient's comfort during the confinement period. A soft bedding that absorbs urine is used to prevent decubitus ulcers and urine scalding. The patient needs bathing frequently, and a mild laxative may be necessary to prevent constipation. In summary, the client must monitor the patient closely and must change management practices in accordance with the patient's need.

Excision arthroplasty is a common technique used for hip joint disorders including acetabular fractures,

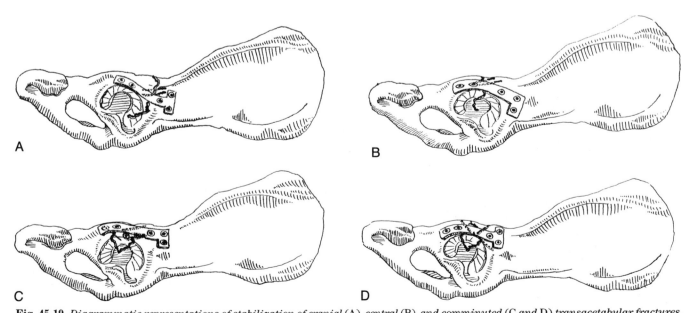

Fig. 45-19. *Diagrammatic representations of stabilization of cranial* (A), *central* (B), *and comminuted* (C and D) *transacetabular fractures.*

but the long-term results of excision arthroplasty do not support this procedure as a treatment of choice for acetabular fractures. Excision arthroplasty should be used only when surgical or conservative treatment has failed.

Postoperative Care

Whether the patient has been treated surgically or conservatively, proper nursing care is essential. Soft bedding and frequent bathing are necessary for the patient's comfort. If the patient is ambulatory, strict limitation of exercise is necessary until radiographic healing of the fracture is confirmed. Swimming is an excellent form of therapy that promotes muscle strength and hip joint mobility without an exertion of excessive weight-bearing forces on the fracture site. The prognosis for limb usage is good in patients with acetabular fractures.

References and Suggested Readings

1. Archibald, J. (ed.): Canine Surgery, 2nd Ed. Santa Barbara, CA, American Veterinary Publications, 1974.
2. Brinker, W. O.: Fractures of the pelvis. In Current Techniques in Small Animal Surgery. Edited by M. J. Bojrab. Philadelphia, Lea & Febiger, 1975.
3. Brown, S. G., et al.: Plate fixation of iliac shaft fractures in the dog. J. Am. Vet. Med. Assoc., *167:*472, 1975.
4. Denny, H. R.: Pelvic fractures in the dog: a review of 123 cases. J. Small Anim. Pract., *19:*151, 1978.
5. Duff, R., et al.: Long-term results of excision arthroplasty of the canine hip. Vet. Rec., *101:*181, 1977.
6. Gendreau, C., et al.: Excision of the femoral head and neck: the long-term results of thirty-five operations. J. Am. Anim. Hosp. Assoc., *13:*605, 1977.
7. Hulse, D. A., and Root, C. R.: Management of acetabular fractures: long-term evaluation. Compend. Contin. Ed., *2:*189, 1980.
8. Leighton, R. L.: Surgical treatment of some pelvic fractures. J. Am. Vet. Med. Assoc., *153:*1739, 1968.
9. Piermattei, D. L., and Greeley, R. G.: An Atlas of Surgical Approaches to the Bones of the Dog and Cat. Philadelphia, W. B. Saunders, 1979.
10. Robins G. M., et al.: The plating of pelvic fractures in the dog. Vet. Rec., *93:*550, 1973.
11. Singleton, W. B.: Limb fractures in the dog and cat—V fractures of the hind limb. J. Small Anim. Pract., *7:*163, 1966.
12. Steven, G. E., et al.: The use of a plastic bone plate in the repair of pelvic fractures in the dog. J. Am. Anim. Hosp. Assoc., *14:*597, 1978.
13. Wadsworth, P. L., et al.: Dorsal surgical approach to acetabular fractures in the dog. J. Am. Vet. Med. Assoc., *165:*908, 1974.
14. Wheaton, L. G., et al.: Surgical treatment of acetabular fractures in the dog. J. Am. Vet. Med. Assoc., *162:*385, 1973.

Sacroiliac Luxation

by William W. Ryan

Unilateral sacroiliac luxation is most common and is always associated with single or multiple fractures of the pelvic bones. These pelvic fractures generally spare the opposite sacroiliac joint from luxating. For example, fractures of the wing of the ilium on one side spare that joint from luxating, whereas the same trauma forces the other side of the pelvis cranially to disarticulate the sacroiliac joint.

Bilateral luxations can also occur, and these are usually unaccompanied by fractures of the pelvic bones.[3,4]

Diagnosis

A tentative diagnosis of sacroiliac luxation can sometimes be made by palpating the iliac crests to detect cranial displacement. This palpation should accompany complete pelvic palpation, including rectal evaluation, to detect other pelvic fractures. Because of the severity of soft tissue damage usually accompanying pelvic fractures and luxations, it is difficult to arrive at an accurate diagnosis by physical examination alone. Radiographic examination is imperative. Ventrodorsal and lateral radiographs must be taken to verify the diagnosis of sacroiliac luxation. The direction of these luxations is either craniodorsal or craniolateral.[3,4]

Conservative Treatment

Strict cage rest suffices in most cases of sacroiliac luxation and allows the animal to return to satisfactory function. This strict cage rest should be maintained for at least 4 to 6 weeks. The degrees of pain and reluctance to ambulate accompanying sacroiliac luxations, especially if bilateral, are usually so severe that surgical intervention for reduction and stabilization is recommended. Surgical treatment allows for a rapid return to normal function, minimizes undesirable fracture disease, and avoids prolonged hospitalization.

Surgical Treatment

APPROACH

The ilium and sacroiliac joint are best approached craniodorsally over the iliac crest. The skin incision is made over the crest of the ilium and extends caudally along the body of the ilium and terminates above and slightly medial to the greater trochanter. The cutaneus trunci muscle, subcutaneous fat, and deep gluteal fascia are then incised in line with the skin incision to expose the middle gluteal muscle and the crest of the ilium. The middle gluteal muscle is freed from the ilium by incising its origin along the crest and dorsal edge of the body of the ilium. This incision is then continued caudally in the same line to sever fibers of the middle gluteal muscle that originate dorsal and medial to the ilium. The cranial gluteal artery and vein enter the middle gluteal muscle in the deep caudal portion of this incision on the surface of the deep gluteal muscle. After subperiosteal elevation, the middle gluteal muscle is retracted laterally to expose the ilium.

Because the ilium is usually displaced cranially in sacroiliac luxations, the tissue between the iliac crest and the sacrum is already separated, and little additional blunt dissection is necessary to expose the area.

REDUCTION AND STABILIZATION

Following the surgical approach just described, the separated surfaces of both the sacrum and the wing of the ilium should easily be visualized. Reduction can be accomplished by manipulation and leverage applied with bone-holding forceps. A more accurate means of anatomic reduction has been described by Brinker.[1] It involves inserting 2 Kirschner wires or small Steinmann pins in the 12 o'clock position, one in the wing of the ilium and the other in the sacrum (Fig. 45-20). The separation is then aligned and is reduced by bringing the pins together.[1]

Surgical stabilization is accomplished by the use of two cancelleous screws (Fig. 45-21) or one cancellous screw and one Kirschner wire in small dogs or cats (Fig. 45-22).

It is difficult to maintain the two bones in anatomic reduction during the insertion of these screws; this problem can be eliminated by first inserting one or two Kirschner wires through the ilium and into the sacrum immediately after reduction is attained. These Kirschner wires are then removed following screw placement.

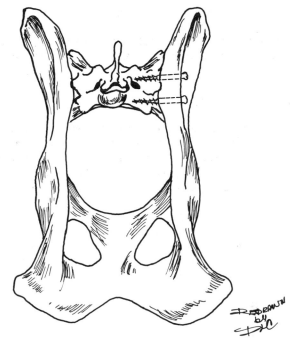

Fig. 45-21. *Surgical stabilization using two cancellous screws.*

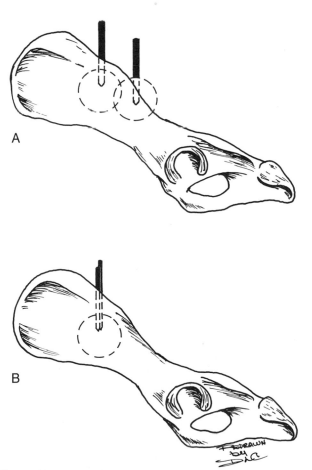

Fig. 45-20. A *and* B, *Insertion of 2 Kirschner wires or small Steinmann pins in the 12 o'clock position, one in the wing of the ilium and the other in the sacrum.* (*From Brinker, W. O.: The pelvis. Current Techniques in Small Animal Surgery. Edited by M. J. Bojrab. Philadelphia, Lea & Febiger, 1975.*)

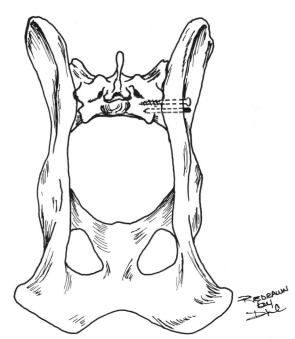

Fig. 45-22. *Surgical stabilization using one cancellous screw and one Kirschner wire.*

The length of the screws chosen must be slightly less than the distance to the spinal canal, to avoid serious neurologic complications. This length can be measured accurately by means of the preoperative radiographs.

Cortical screws can be used in place of cancellous screws if the ilium is overdrilled to the outside diameter of the screw thread and the sacrum is drilled to the diameter of the shank of the screw (lag-screw effect).[1,4]

After surgical repair, closure is accomplished by suturing the muscle sheath and gluteal fascia with simple interrupted or horizontal mattress sutures to pull the muscle back up against the ilium. The subcutaneous tissue and skin are then sutured in separate layers.[1,2,4]

Postoperative Care

Postoperative care should include strict excercise restriction for 2 weeks and the administration of broad-spectrum oral antibiotics for 1 week and analgesics if necessary.

References and Suggested Readings

1. Brinker, W. O.: The pelvis. *In* Current Techniques in Small Animal Surgery. Edited by M. J. Bojrab. Philadelphia, Lea & Febiger, 1975.
2. Piermattei, D. L., and Greeley, R. G.: An Atlas of Surgical Approaches to the Bones of the Dog and Cat. 2nd Ed. Philadelphia, W. B. Saunders, 1979.
3. Pettit, G. D.: Other joints of the pelvic limb. *In* Canine Surgery. 2nd Ed. Edited by J. Archibald. Santa Barbara, CA, American Veterinary Publications, 1974.
4. Pond, M. J.: Sacroiliac luxation. *In* Current Techniques in Small Animal Surgery. Edited by M. J. Bojrab. Philadelphia, Lea & Febiger, 1975.

46 * Pelvic Limb

Corrective Osteotomies for Treatment of Selected Hip Joint Disorders

by GUY B. TARVIN

Pelvic and femoral osteotomies are commonly employed by the orthopedist as one mode of therapy for degenerative joint disease of the hip.[8,15] Pelvic osteotomies are useful in the treatment of congenital luxation of the hip in older children (over 18 months of age.)[15] Because of the similarities between this human disease and canine hip dysplasia, the pelvic osteotomies used in human medicine[15,18,19] have been modified for use in the dog.[1,5,7,16,20] Although less commonly encountered, severe proximal femoral deformities can be corrected by derotational osteotomies. For the most part, pelvic and femoral osteotomies are used in large breed dogs; less heroic procedures such as excision arthroplasty may give adequate results in smaller breeds. With these thoughts in mind, this discussion deals with pelvic and femoral osteotomies used in the dog with special reference to rationale, indications, technique, and postoperative care.

Pelvic Osteotomies

INDICATIONS AND RATIONALE FOR TREATMENT

All dogs, whether they develop canine hip dysplasia or not, have radiographically normal hips at birth.[14] In order for normal development of the hip to continue, full congruity between the femoral head and the acetabulum is required.[4,14] In dogs that become affected with hip dysplasia, changes occur in the joint capsule and surrounding structures between the time of birth and 60 days of age.[14] These changes initially manifest themselves as joint laxity or instability. This initial joint instability upsets the normal weight-bearing forces across the articulation. As the disease progresses, these abnormal forces result in changes of the femoral neck angles,[21] acetabular inclination angles, and degenerative joint disease (Fig. 46-1). Each animal is affected to varying degrees, and some show few changes until mature (approximately 2 years of age). Various studies indicate that if the abnormal weight-bearing forces across the joint can be corrected early in the course of the disease, a "normal" articulation will develop.[17] Joint laxity in these cases usually does not recur because of improved contact of the joint components and the more mature muscular support that develops around the joint.[5] Although changes occur on either side of the joint, it is my opinion that, as with the human counterpart of this disease,[15] the acetabular changes are often the most severe. Moreover, it has been demonstrated that if the acetabular component is shifted so that normal congruity of the joint is maintained, the femoral changes will revert to normal limits with time.[17] With these thoughts in mind, certain select patients with hip dysplasia may be helped by a pelvic osteotomy. Criteria in selecting these patients are the following:

1. A young animal demonstrates clinical signs referable to canine hip dysplasia. One of the purposes of performing an osteotomy is to correct the abnormal weight-bearing forces.[12,13] If done early enough, many of the changes, such as femoral anteversion and acetabular inclination, can be reversed and corrected.[17] Although no definite data are available, the consensus of many workers supports 10 to 11 months as a cutoff time in dogs.[5,6,16,20] When the procedure is performed prior to this age, the bones of the acetabulum and proximal femur are still capable of responding.

2. Sufficient shape remains to the acetabulum and femoral head. If severe degenerative joint disease, characterized by periarticular osteophytes, a flat acetabulum, and a flat femoral head, is present, remodeling of the joint components into a useful articulation is unlikely. In these patients, excision arthroplasty or joint replacement may be indicated.

3. The joint is stable when the limb is placed in a position of 30 to 45° of abduction and 10 to 15° of internal rotation (Fig. 46-2). This position mimics the new relationship that can be accomplished by shifting the acetabulum by the osteotomy. One must be cautious when applying this technique clinically because further tightening and stability of the joint can be expected from ancillary techniques, such as joint capsule imbrication and greater trochanter transplantation. If severe instability persists after placing the limb in this position, however, one should question whether pelvic osteotomy will be sufficient therapy.

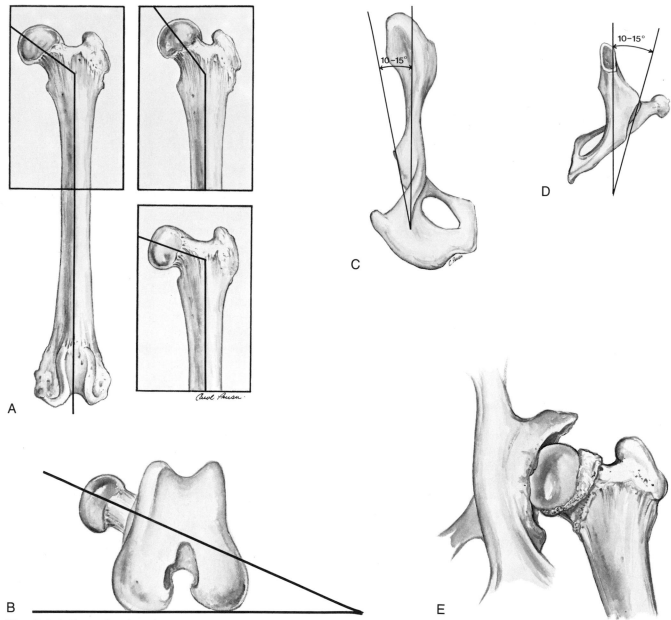

Fig. 46-1. A, *Femoral neck angles: top insert demonstrates coxa valga; bottom insert demonstrates coxa vara.* B, *View of femur for anteversion angle calculation; normal should be approximately 10 to 35°.* C *and* D, *Acetabular angles.* E, *Degenerative joint disease.*

If these criteria are met, a pelvic osteotomy can be considered.

SURGICAL TECHNIQUE

The dog is positioned and draped in a manner to allow exposure of both the ilium and the pubic symphysis (Fig. 46-3A). The pubic symphysis is first exposed by a midventral approach.[10] Using either a guarded osteotome or an oscillating saw, the symphysis is split (Fig. 46-3B). Care should be taken to protect deeper structures during the osteotomy. The incision is then packed with moist sponges, and the ilium is exposed by a lateral approach.[7] The hip joint at this time is also exposed using a trochanteric osteotomy.[3] Careful blunt dissection (with a finger) is performed medial

to the body of the ilium, and a malleable retractor is inserted immediately medial to the bone (Fig. 46-4A). A "stairstep" osteotomy is performed in the body of the ilium. The cuts running dorsally to ventrally are made perpendicular to the long axis of the bone while the horizontal cut is "beveled" dorsally (Figs. 46-4B and 46-5). Once complete, these osteotomies (in the pubis and ilium) create a free-floating, weight-bearing segment that can be easily manipulated. The entire acetabulum is translocated laterally and distally, and the dorsal rim is rotated "over" the femoral head (Fig. 46-4C). The ilium is fixed in the appropriate position with two lag screws, and the overlapped pubis is secured with cerclage wires (Fig. 46-4D). This procedure provides adequate stability. The joint capsule is opened, the joint is inspected, and the capsule is imbricated with

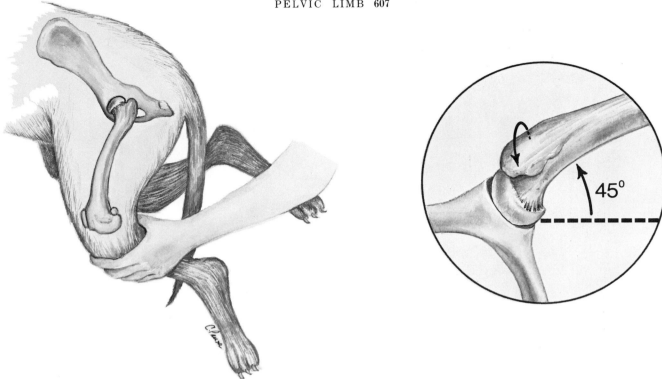

Fig. 46-2. *Position for preoperative evaluation to determine whether osteotomy will benefit the animal.*

heavy (size 1-0 to 1 chromic catgut) mattress sutures. The greater trochanter is then transplanted caudally and distally to add further stability to the hip[3] (Fig. 46-6). Closure of both incisions is routine.

POSTOPERATIVE CARE

The animal should be placed in an Ehmer sling until soft tissues have regained an adequate amount of strength to allow weight-bearing (2 to 3 weeks). After this period, restricted exercise or cage rest should be enforced until evidence of radiographic union is present.

SPECIAL CONSIDERATIONS

In patients with bilateral disease, a second operation can be performed in 4 to 6 weeks after the first. The procedure on the second site is similar; however, because of the callus at the previous pubic symphysotomy, it is easier to split the pubic and ischial rami on the cranial and caudal rings of the obturator foramen (Fig. 46-7). The remainder of the procedure and postoperative care are the same as for the first side.

Because hip dysplasia has been shown to have a genetic component in its etiology, neutering should be a prerequisite to the procedure.

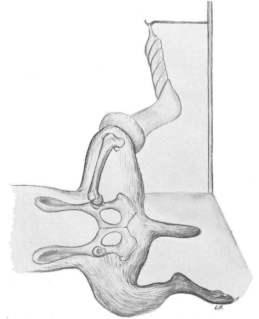

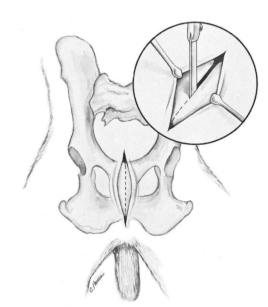

Fig. 46-3. A, *Positioning for the procedure.* B, *Approach and splitting (insert) of the pubic symphysis.*

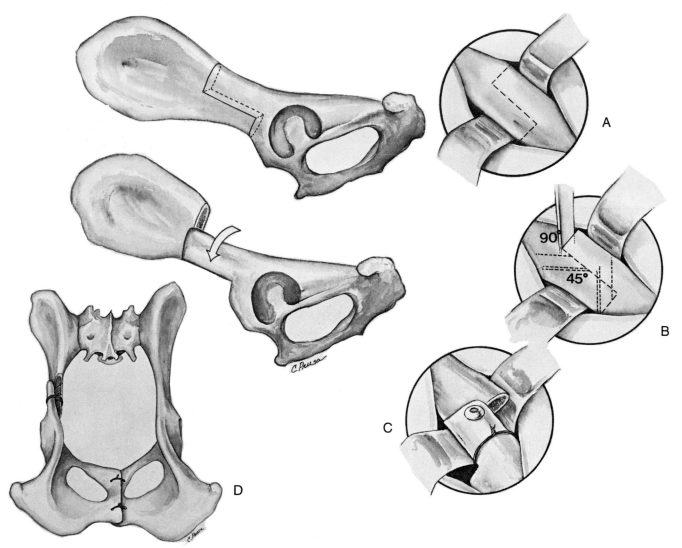

Fig. 46-4. *"Stairstep" osteotomy in ilium. A, A malleable retractor is placed medial to the ilium to protect the deeper structures. B, The horizontal portion of the osteotomy is beveled approximately 45° dorsally; a free-floating acetabular segment is created. C and D, After shifting the acetabulum, the ilium and the pubis are fixed in position.*

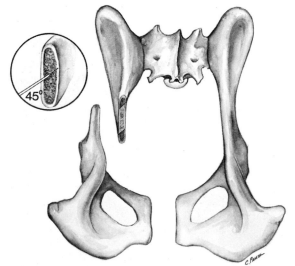

Fig. 46-5. *A free-floating acetabular component is formed; The inset demonstrates the level of the horizontal cut for the stairstep osteotomy.*

Proximal Femoral Osteotomies

Deformities of the proximal femur such as coxa valga, coxa vara, and large anteversion angles (see Fig. 46-1) may require osteotomies to improve limb function.[8] Although coxa vara is seen in many small breed dogs affected with medial patellar luxation,[11] it is rarely severe enough to cause clinical signs and to require surgical correction. Coxa valga and large anteversion angles are often seen in hip dysplasia. From the previous discussion on pelvic osteotomies, correction of these deformities in the young dog (under 10 months) is probably not indicated unless the disorder is severe. (In these cases, if the acetabular component is corrected, many of the proximal femoral deformities will revert to normal.)[14] Guidelines have not yet been established regarding the point at which canine femoral deformities become severe enough that reversion to normal after a pelvic osteotomy becomes unlikely. Recommendations for human patients, however, suggest that, if femoral anteversion angles are greater than 70°

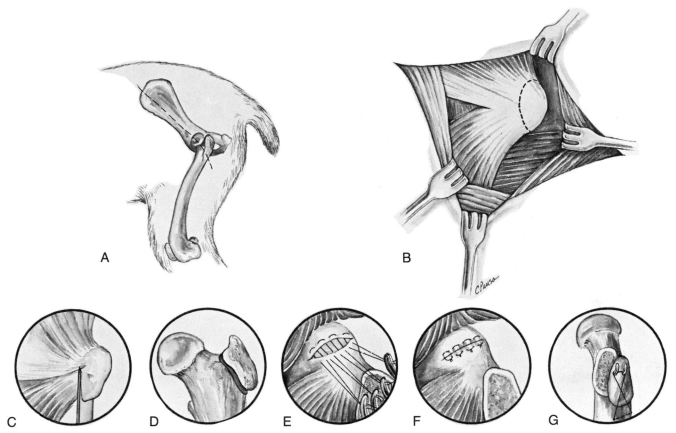

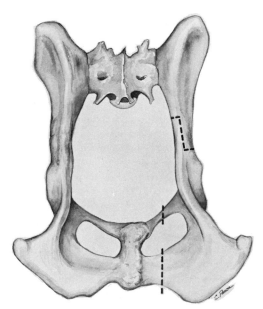

Fig. 46-6. A *to* G, *Transplantation of greater trochanter and capsular imbrication are performed.*

and coxa valga greater than 160°, concurrent femoral osteotomies be done along with pelvic osteotomies.[17] My experience is in accord with these recommendations.

Large anteversion angles or coxa valga in the more mature animal do not respond as well to pelvic osteot-

omies, and in these patients, proximal femoral osteotomies may be necessary to improve joint function. As with pelvic osteotomies, a prerequisite for this procedure is a femoral head and acetabulum of sufficient shape.

SURGICAL TECHNIQUE

The surgical approach to the proximal femur is a modified Watson-Jones (craniolateral) approach.[2] Once exposed, parallel small Steinmann pins are driven into the proximal femur and shaft (Fig. 46-8). The femur undergoes osteotomy just distal to the level of the lesser trochanter and is derotated as indicated (Fig. 46-9). The osteotomy is fixed with a compression plate. It is recommended that the osteotomy site be packed with a fresh autogenous cancellous bone graft.[9]

POSTOPERATIVE CARE AND SPECIAL CONSIDERATIONS

If rigid fixation is achieved, passive range-of-motion exercises can be begun after the initial pain of the operation has subsided (3 to 4 days). A minimal amount of weight-bearing can be allowed; however, exercise should be restricted until evidence of bony union is demonstrated radiographically.

In patients with bilateral disease, the second side may be staged as soon as the animal's condition permits. One should realize, however, that operating on the patient's second side before the first is capable of

Fig. 46-7. *Dotted lines indicate osteotomy done on the second side.*

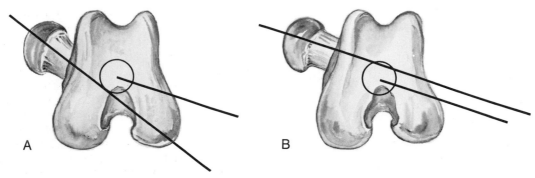

Fig. 46-8. *Placement of pins for derotation for excessive anteversion.* A, *Abnormal result;* B, *desired result.*

supporting the animal's weight may result either in failure of the plates or osteotomies to heal or in a permanently nonambulatory dog that requires extensive nursing care.

In conclusion, in addition to the techniques of canine pelvic and femoral osteotomy described in this section, several other pelvic osteotomy procedures are available.[1,5,6,16] These other operations use the stairstep osteotomy in the ilium, but differ from the technique described here in their method of freeing the rest of the bony attachments of the acetabular segment. I prefer the technique described here because it allows a more freely movable acetabular segment than the other procedures and allows fixation at both the ilium and the pubis. Whichever technique is chosen, one must remember to evaluate the animal carefully prior to the procedure to determine whether it meets the aforementioned criteria. When these criteria are met, good results have been obtained.[5,6,16,20] It is my opinion that femoral osteotomies for proximal femoral deformities are less frequently indicated. Certain criteria must also be met to justify this procedure. Further research on pelvic and femoral osteotomies needs to be done to evaluate the biomechanical and biologic changes induced on the hip joint. Then new indications, such as use of these procedures in older dogs with degenerative joint disease, and a clearer understanding of hip disease and treatment may evolve.

References and Suggested Readings

1. Brinker, W. O.: Corrective osteotomy procedure for treatment of canine hip dysplasia. Vet. Clin. North Am. *1:*467, 1971.
2. Brown, S. G., and Rosen, H.: Craniolateral approach to the canine hip: a modified Watson-Jones approach. J. Am. Vet. Assoc., *159:*1117, 1971.
3. DeAngelis, M., and Prata, R.: Surgical repair of coxofemoral luxation in the dog. J. Am. Anim. Hosp. Assoc., *9:*175, 1973.
4. Harrison, T. J.: The influence of the femoral head on pelvic growth in acetabular form in the rat. J. Anat., *95:*12, 1961.
5. Henry, W. B., and Wadsworth, P. L.: Pelvic osteotomy in treatment of subluxation associated with hip dysplasia. J. Am. Anim. Hosp. Assoc. *11:*636, 1975.
6. Hohn, R. B., and Janes, J. M.: Pelvic osteotomy in the treatment of canine hip dysplasia. Clin. Orthop., *62:*70, 1969.
7. Hohn, R. B., and Janes, J. M.: Lateral approach to the canine ilium. Anim. Hosp., *2:*111, 1966.
8. Nunamaker, D. M., and Newton, C. D.: Canine hip disorders. *In* Current Techniques in Small Animal Surgery. Edited by M. J. Bojrab. Philadelphia, Lea & Febiger, 1975.
9. Olds, R. B., et al.: Autogenous cancellous bone grafting in small animals. J. Am. Anim. Hosp. Assoc., *9:*454, 1973.
10. Piermattei, D. L., and Greely, R. G.: An Atlas of Surgical Approaches to the Bones of the Dog and Cat. Philadelphia, W. B. Saunders, 1979.
11. Putnam, R. W.: Patellar luxation in the dog. Master's Thesis, University of Guelph, Ontario, Canada, January, 1968.
12. Rab, G. T.: Biomechanical aspects of Salter osteotomy. Clin. Orthop., *132:*82, 1978.
13. Radin, E. L., and Paul, I. L.: The biomechanics of the congenital dislocated hips and their treatments. Clin. Orthop., *98:*32, 1974.
14. Riser, W. H.: Growth and development of the normal canine pelvis, hip joints, and femur from birth to maturity. Vet. Pathol., *12:*264, 1964.

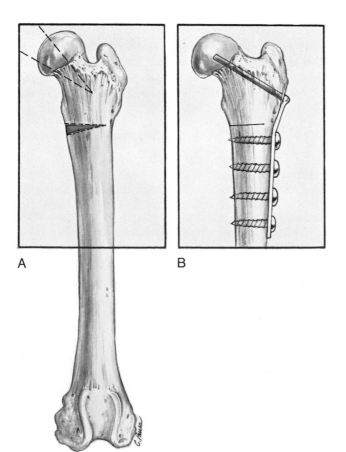

Fig. 46-9. A and B, *Osteotomy and plate fixation for excessive coxa valga.*

15. Salter, R. B.: Osteotomy of the pelvis—editorial comment. Clin. Orthop., *98*:2, 1974.

16. Schraeder, S.: Triple osteotomy for treatment of hip dysplasia: a preliminary report. J. Am. Vet. Med. Assoc., *178*:39, 1981.

17. Serafimov, L.: Biomechanical influence of the innominate osteotomy on the growth of the upper part of the femur. Clin. Orthop., *98*:39, 1974.

18. Steel, H. H.: Triple osteotomy of the innominate bone. Clin. Orthop., *122*:116, 1977.

19. Sutherland, D. H., and Greenfield, R.: Double innominate osteotomy. J. Bone Joint Surg., *59A*:1082, 1977.

20. Tarvin, G. B.: A veterinary orthopedist's view of canine hip dysplasia. *In* Proceedings of a Symposium on Canine Hip Dysplasia. Orthopedic Foundation for Animals. St. Louis, October 23 to 24, 1979.

21. Wilkinson, J. A.: Femoral anteversion in the rabbit. J. Bone Joint Surg., *44B*:386, 1962.

Pinning Techniques for Repairing Coxofemoral Luxations

by LARRY J. WALLACE

Traumatic luxations of the coxofemoral joint are more common in dogs over 11 to 12 months of age. Younger dogs with an open proximal femoral physis usually sustain a Salter-Harris fracture through that physis from the same type of trauma that causes a luxation in older dogs. Coxofemoral luxations are generally classified as craniodorsal, dorsal, caudodorsal, and ventral.[5,6] Craniodorsal luxations occur more frequently.[3,5,6]

It is essential to understand the causes, clinical signs, physical findings, diagnostic methods, and anatomic and pathologic features associated with coxofemoral luxations. This information is well described and is readily available in the literature.[3-6]

Although coxofemoral luxations are not regarded as emergencies, they should be treated as soon as possible. At least two radiographic views (lateral and ventrodorsal) are essential, not only to confirm or deny the clinical diagnosis, but also to identify potential complications, such as avulsion fractures to the femoral head, fractures of the dorsal acetabular rim, or associated pelvic fractures. Thoracic radiographic views should also be taken if the trauma responsible for the luxation either originates from the dog's being hit by a motor vehicle or is unknown. These radiographic views are to rule out such disorders as pneumothorax, traumatic lung syndrome, diaphragmatic hernia, or fractured ribs.

Coxofemoral luxations that have been present for no longer than 48 hours can generally be treated by closed reduction unless an indication for open reduction is known. Obvious indications for an open reduction include, but are not limited to, avulsion fractures of the fovea capitis, dorsal brim acetabular fractures, chronic luxations, and cases wherein closed reduction cannot be achieved. The success of closed reduction for luxations of more than 48 hours' duration decreases, owing to the presence of soft tissue in the acetabulum. Dogs with degenerative osteoarthrosis associated with hip dysplasia that sustain a traumatic coxofemoral luxation are generally candidates for an excision of the femoral head and neck or a total hip prosthesis.

Several different acceptable methods are available to treat coxofemoral luxations satisfactorily.[3-6] The method of repair is generally determined by the duration and extent of injury related to the luxation and by the preference of the veterinary surgeon. The veterinary surgeon must be familiar with more than one method because, on occasion, the preferred method cannot be used, and an alternate one must be employed. It is also important to be familiar with the various surgical approaches to the hip for obtaining the best exposure of different classes of luxations.[7]

The purpose of this discussion is not to cover all the different methods of repairing coxofemoral luxations, but rather to describe two pinning procedures that have been highly successful when done correctly. The pinning techniques described herein are the DeVita pin technique[1] and the use of a transacetabular pin.[2] Both techniques are applicable for treating any of the different classifications of traumatic coxofemoral luxations. The surgical approach may vary, depending on the type of luxation. The DeVita pin technique is unique in that it can be used in conjunction with either closed or open reduction. Because of their frequency, the treatments and surgical approach described here pertain to craniodorsal luxations.

DeVita Pinning Technique

This technique was first documented by DeVita in 1952.[1] It is easy to perform and, when done correctly, is effective in providing a barrier against lateral and dorsal movement of the femoral head out of the acetabulum following either closed or open reduction of the luxation. If the hip reluxates after applying some force to it following closed reduction of a recent luxation, additional fixation will be required to maintain the femoral head in the acetabulum. If the femoral head does not reduce well or easily reluxates from the acetabulum with little to no stress applied to it following closed reduction, an open reduction will be necessary.

SURGICAL PROCEDURE

Following closed reduction of the hip, the anesthetized patient is placed in lateral recumbency with the affected hip facing up. A sandbag or towels are placed between the stifles to prevent adduction of the affected limb. An area approximately 2 inches in diameter centered at the ventral edge of the ischial tuberosity on the affected side is clipped, and the skin is properly prepared for the surgical procedure. When the area has been draped, a 1-cm skin incision is made immediately ventral to the ischial tuberosity. Selection of the proper Steinmann pin size is important to provide adequate stability of the hip joint. In general, the following pin diameters are recommended, based on the dog's weight: A ⅛-inch pin is used for dogs under 10 kg, a ³⁄₁₆-inch pin for dogs 10 to 20 kg, and a ¼-inch pin for dogs weighing over 20 kg. A pin that is too small does not provide the stability necessary to maintain the femoral head in the acetabulum. A threaded intramedullary pin is used to decrease the possibility of pin migration. The tip of a sterile, trocar-pointed, threaded intramedullary Steinmann pin is inserted through the incision and is passed ventral to the ischial tuberosity (Fig. 46-10, (1)). As the pin is advanced, the veterinary surgeon should feel the pin contact the ischial tuberosity as it passes ventral to it.

It is important, when passing the pin under the ischial tuberosity, that the pin be directed at the femoral neck and not in too craniomedial a direction or it may hit the ischiadic (sciatic) nerve (Fig. 46-11). When passing the pin forward from the ischial tuberosity to the femoral neck, it should be advanced slowly and carefully. If the ischiadic (sciatic) nerve is touched by the point of the pin it will cause the leg to jerk slightly. If that should happen, one should withdraw the pin and

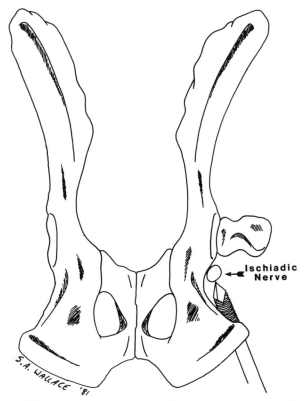

Fig. 46-11. *A pin placed ventral to the ischial tuberosity and improperly directed in a craniomedial direction toward the caudal aspect of the acetabulum increases the risk of hitting the ischiadic (sciatic) nerve.*

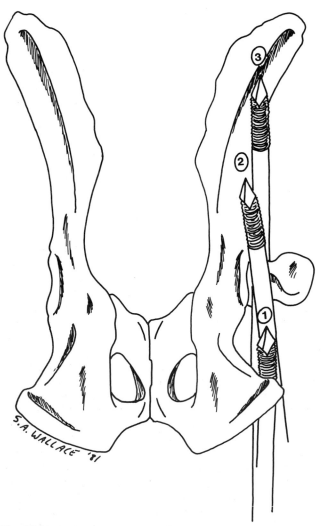

Fig. 46-10. *The pin is properly inserted ventral to and is advanced cranially from the ischial tuberosity (1) to cross over the femoral neck and contact the outer cortex of the ilium (2). Inward pressure, applied by the thumb of the opposite hand over the skin and muscles covering the lateral surface of the ilium, facilitates proper entry of the pin into the wing of the ilium (3).*

redirect it to miss the nerve. Then one should proceed with the placement of the pin. If the pin is started and is directed properly, the nerve will not be touched. Because a threaded pin is used, it should be pushed and not turned as it is being advanced until the pin's point has made contact with the ilium. This maneuver eliminates the possibility that the soft tissue near the ischiadic (sciatic) nerve will become entangled in the threads of the pin and will thus damage the nerve.

With the thumb and index finger of the opposite hand simultaneously grasping the greater trochanter as a guide, the veterinary surgeon carefully pushes the pin forward at an angle that allows it to pass medial to the greater trochanter and just dorsal to the femoral neck. For proper proximity to the femoral neck, the point of the pin should make contact with the femoral neck as it is advanced forward. When the pin makes contact with the femoral neck, it is slightly retracted. By placing downward pressure on the pin chuck, the point of the pin is slightly elevated. It is then pushed forward over the femoral neck. One should be able to feel the pin make contact with the femoral neck as the pin passes over its dorsal surface. When the point of the pin has been advanced approximately an inch cranial to the femoral neck, the thumb of one's opposite hand should be advanced from the greater trochanter to press inward on the skin and muscles over the lateral surface of the ilium. This maneuver aids in forcing the

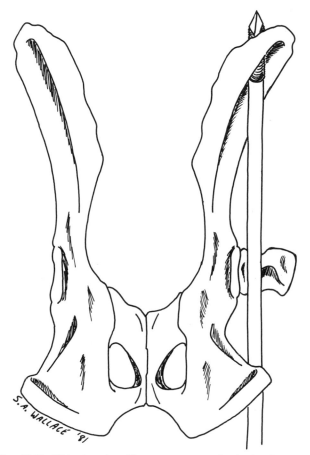

Fig. 46-12. *This drawing illustrates proper final pin placement under the ischial tuberosity, over the femoral neck, and into the wing of the ilium as seen in a ventrodorsal view of the pelvis.*

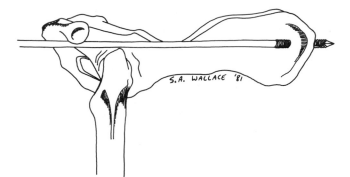

Fig. 46-13. *This drawing illustrates proper final pin placement under the ischial tuberosity, over the femoral neck, and into the wing of the ilium as seen in a lateral view of the pelvis.*

tip of the pin to make contact with the outer cortex of the ilium (see Fig. 46-10(2)). Contact of the pin with the outer cortex of the ilium can be felt as the pin is advanced forward.

At this time, the pin should be turned in a clockwise manner as it is being advanced to facilitate the point of the pin's cutting into the bone. It is important to continue pressing inward with the thumb of the opposite hand over this area to keep the pin as close as possible to the ilium. If pressure from the thumb is not applied, the pin may not seat in the bone and will thus slide past the wing of the ilium. When the point of the pin is advanced to the site where the wing of the ilium flares outward, it cuts into the wing and allows the threads to obtain a purchase in the cortex (see Fig. 46-10(3)). Once penetration is initially detected, the pin should be advanced about half an inch (Figs. 46-12 and 46-13). This maneuver provides an adequate purchase of the threaded part of the pin in the wing of the ilium. The pin is then cut off below the skin caudal to the ischial tuberosity. The skin incision is appropriately closed. The leg is then placed in an Ehmer sling, and postoperative ventrodorsal and lateral radiographic views of the pelvis are taken to ascertain reduction and proper pin placement.

POSTOPERATIVE CARE

The Ehmer sling is left on for 2 weeks, during which time the dogs activity must be restricted. At the end of the first postoperative week, the dog is examined to make sure that the hip has not reluxated and that the Ehmer sling fits properly. When the Ehmer sling is removed at the end of the second week, the stability of the hip is re-evaluated, and the sutures are removed. During each examination, one should check to make sure that the pin has not migrated. This check is done by palpating the end of the pin located under the skin ventral to the ischial tuberosity. The pin is left in place 4 to 6 weeks postoperatively. Fibrous connective tissue forms around the pin and provides additional stability to the hip joint once the pin has been removed. While the pin is in place, the dog's activity should be restricted. When outside, the dog should be kept on a short leash and should not be allowed to run free.

When it is time for pin removal, ventrodorsal and lateral radiographic views of the pelvis are taken to evaluate the coxofemoral joint and to ensure that the pin is still in its original position. For pin removal, the dog can be given either a narcotic analgesic or a general anesthetic agent. The dog is placed in lateral recumbency with the affected side up. An area ventral to the ischial tuberosity is clipped and is prepared as in the original pin placement. If the dog is given a narcotic analgesic, the skin over the pin should be infiltrated with a local anesthetic agent. A small incision is made over the pin, which is readily palpable ventral to the ischial tuberosity. The skin is pushed down to allow the cut end of the pin to protrude through the incision. A pin chuck is applied to the pin, which is then removed using counterclockwise rotations until its threaded end exits the wing of the ilium. Counterclockwise rotations of the pin are then stopped, and the pin is withdrawn through the incision. One or two sutures are used to close the incision. Following pin removal, the stability and range of motion of the coxofemoral joint are evaluated. At this time, the hip joint should be stable.

The dog can be sent home following recovery from the narcotic or anesthetic. For 2 weeks following pin removal, the dog should not be allowed any strenuous activity; then, its normal activity can gradually be resumed.

GENERAL COMMENTS

The two most common errors made when using this technique are starting the pin too far medial to the ischial tuberosity and using a pin that is too small. A pin that is too small does not provide proper contact with the dorsal aspect of the femoral neck when the pin is anchored in the wing of the ilium. Should this error occur, the barrier against lateral and dorsal displacement of the femoral head out of the acetabulum will be insufficient. If the pin is started medial to the ischial tuberosity, the pin will generally pass over the dorsal brim of the acetabulum; in such a case, nothing is there to prevent reluxation from occurring. Contact of the pin with the ischiadic (sciatic) nerve can be avoided by following the guidelines discussed under surgical procedures.

The DeVita technique can also be used to provide additional stability to the hip joint when an open reduction is necessary. When the femoral head and acetabulum have been carefully debrided of adhering soft tissue or avulsed bone fragments, the hip is reduced. If any joint capsule is present, it should be sutured for additional support. If no joint capsule is present, as in many chronic luxations, surrounding fascia should be sutured over the joint for additional stability. The veterinary surgeon may then proceed with placement of the pin as described for a closed reduction. Depending on the surgical approach used for open reduction, the pin can be observed or palpated as it is properly passed over the neck of the femur. The postoperative care is the same as described for a closed reduction.

Although this procedure is more frequently used in dogs, it can also be used in the domestic cat. The operation is more difficult in cats because of their straight pelvis that makes it difficult to seat the pin in the wing of the ilium. In the average, adult domestic cat, a pin size of $\frac{7}{64}$-inch or $\frac{1}{8}$-inch in diameter is most effective.

Transacetabular Pinning Technique

This procedure has been described for the treatment of coxofemoral luxation.[2] Although the technique can be employed in most dogs requiring an open reduction for repair of a coxofemoral luxation, its greatest indication is for use in dogs with recurrent or long-standing luxations. The caudal or craniolateral surgical approaches to the hip joint are used most commonly when using this technique. Because most hip luxations are craniodorsal, I prefer the caudal approach to the hip joint.[7]

SURGICAL PROCEDURE

The patient is positioned in lateral recumbency and is properly prepared for a caudal approach to the hip.

Once the ischiadic (sciatic) nerve has been isolated and the hip joint has been identified, one must isolate the femoral head and inspect it for viable articular cartilage and any defects that may not have been recognized on the preoperative radiographs. If any serious defects that would interfere with proper joint function are present, the veterinary surgeon can proceed with an excision arthroplasty or perhaps a total hip prosthesis. If the femoral head is in good condition, the fibrous tissue around it is carefully removed, and any part of the round ligament attached to the fovea capitis is excised.

Next, the fibrous tissue is carefully removed from the acetabulum, and its articular surface is examined for any defects. If the acetabulum is in good condition, one can proceed with the repair of the luxation. Special care must be taken to preserve any joint capsule that may be attached to the acetabulum or femoral neck. The femoral head must be exposed so the veterinary surgeon can clearly see the fovea capitis for proper pin placement. When using the caudal approach, this exposure is accomplished by adducting the limb and rotating it inward. A nonthreaded, double-trocar-pointed Steinmann pin is used for this procedure. The proper pin size is one with a diameter 50 to 75% of the diameter of the fovea capitis. For ease in passing the pin, about 2 inches of the pin should protrude from the end of a hand chuck or power drill.

The tip of the pin is placed in the center of the fovea capitis (Fig. 46-14A). It should pass from the fovea capitis down the center of the femoral neck and should emerge laterally at or slightly below the level of the third trochanter (Fig. 46-14B). The chuck is then repositioned on the pin emerging from the lateral side of the proximal femur and is carefully withdrawn until the proximal point of the pin is level with the fovea capitis (Fig. 46-14C). The pin chuck is advanced on the pin to a predetermined distance from the third trochanter, so that when the pin is driven through the acetabular fossa, its point is no more than 0.7 to 1.0 cm into the pelvic canal medial to the acetabulum. This distance can be predetermined from the preoperative ventrodorsal radiographic views. The femoral head is properly reduced into the acetabulum. With the limb held in a slightly abducted position, the pin is advanced to penetrate through the medial wall of the acetabulum to emerge 0.7 to 1.0 cm into the pelvic canal (Fig. 46-14D). The limb is maintained in an abducted position by a sterile towel. The pin chuck is then backed off on the pin about an inch and is used to bend the pin in an upward direction while the veterinarian holds the patient's leg steady. The pin is cut near the bend and is turned down against the bone (Fig. 46-14E) for easy removal at a later time. If any joint capsule is present from the acetabulum and femoral neck, it is closed with sutures. If the joint capsule is absent or is too severely damaged to hold sutures, the surrounding fascia should be sutured over the joint for additional stability. The various tissues are closed in a routine manner.

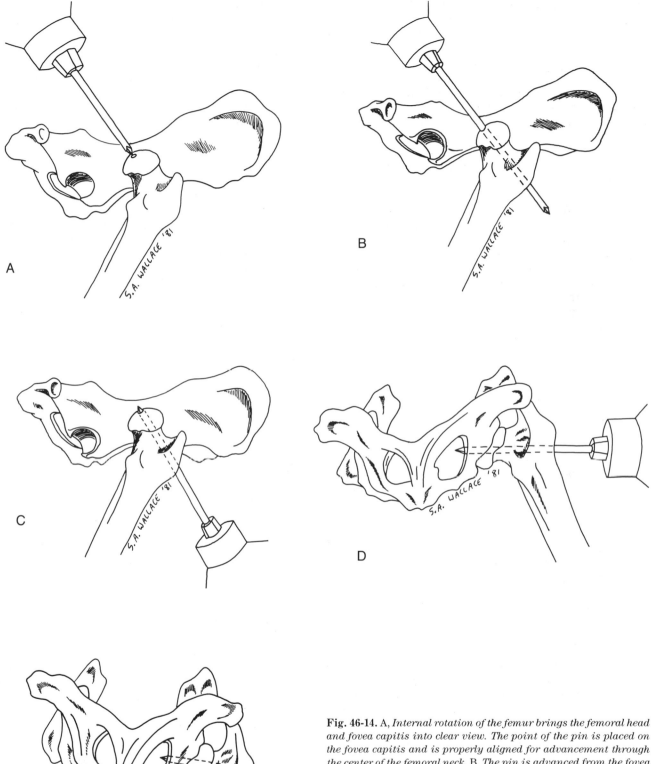

Fig. 46-14. A, *Internal rotation of the femur brings the femoral head and fovea capitis into clear view. The point of the pin is placed on the fovea capitis and is properly aligned for advancement through the center of the femoral neck. B, The pin is advanced from the fovea capitis through the center of the femoral neck to emerge on the lateral surface of the femur. C, The pin is to be withdrawn so the point will be level with the fovea capitis before reducing the femoral head into the acetabulum. D, The femoral head is reduced into the acetabulum and the pin is advanced across the acetabular fossa and through the medial wall of the acetabulum to emerge into the pelvic canal. E, The pin is bent, cut off, and turned down so the cut end rests against the lateral surface of the femur.*

POSTOPERATIVE CARE

The limb is placed in an Ehmer sling before removing the patient from the operating table. Postoperative ventrodorsal and lateral radiographs are taken to make sure that reduction and pin placement are correct. If the pin has been advanced too far or not far enough, the patient must be taken back to the operating room for proper positioning of the pin. The patient is generally released from the hospital on the second or third postoperative day.

The transacetabular pin should be left in place for 3 weeks. During this time, the patient's activity must be restricted and the Ehmer sling must be left in place. Weight-bearing is not allowed on the affected leg while the pin is in place. Therefore, if the sling comes off before the 3 weeks are up, the dog must be returned to the hospital for placement of a new sling. If everything goes well following the dog's release from the hospital, it should be returned on the tenth postoperative day to remove the skin sutures and to evaluate the Ehmer sling. At the end of the third postoperative week, the dog is returned to the veterinarian for removal of the pin. Pin removal is easily accomplished because the pin can be readily palpated lateral and distal to the greater trochanter. Before the procedure, ventrodorsal and lateral radiographic views of the pelvis should be taken.

Anesthesia for this pin removal procedure can be induced by using a narcotic intravenously, in addition to a local anesthetic in the skin and subcutaneous tissue around the pin, or one may use a general anesthetic. The patient is placed in lateral recumbency. The area over the pin is prepared for the surgical procedure and is draped. A small, skin incision, 2 to 3 cm long, is made over the pin, which is easily exposed. The pin is grasped with a pair of orthopedic pliers and is pulled straight out, with some rotational movement, in the same angle in which it was put in place. While the veterinary surgeon begins pulling on the pin, the thumb of the opposite hand must be used to push in on the greater trochanter, to avoid the possibility of pulling the femoral head out of the acetabulum. The skin incision is appropriately closed.

The patient can go home following recovery from anesthesia. The skin sutures are removed in 10 days. The patient's activity must be restricted for 2 weeks following removal of the pin. After this time, no restrictions to the patient's activity are needed.

GENERAL COMMENTS

When done correctly, this procedure has proved to be successful in the treatment of chronic coxofemoral luxations. The most common complication of this technique is breakage of the pin at the area of greatest stress in the acetabulum. This complication can be avoided by using a nonthreaded pin of the proper size and by keeping the limb in an Ehmer sling while the pin is in place. I have had no problems with breakage when using a nonthreaded pin that occupies 50 to 75% of the diameter of the fovea capitis. Another, less-frequent complication is postoperative hip subluxation or luxation. The incidence of this complication is greatly reduced when the pin protrudes no further than 0.7 to 1.0 cm from the medial wall of the acetabulum into the pelvic canal. It is important not to have the pin protrude any further into the pelvic canal or it may injure the rectum. On the other hand, the pin must protrude far enough into the pelvic canal so that the bevel of the trocar point is beyond the pin hole in the medial wall of the acetabular fossa. It must also be emphasized that, because this pin passes from the fovea capitis of the femoral head through the fossa of the acetabulum, it does not penetrate or injure the articular cartilage. Although this procedure is most frequently used in dogs, its use in the domestic cat has been documented.[2]

Acknowledgment

I wish to acknowledge and express my sincere thanks to my son, Mr. Steven A. Wallace, for preparing the drawings used to illustrate this discussion.

References and Suggested Readings

1. DeVita, J.: A method of pinning for chronic dislocation of the hip joint. In Proceedings of the 89th Annual Meeting of the American Veterinary Medical Association, 1952, p. 191.
2. Gendreau, C. L., and Rouse, G. P.: Surgical management of the hip. In Scientific Proceedings of the American Animal Hospital Association, 1975, p. 393.
3. Leonard, E. P.: Luxations in the pelvic limb. In Orthopedic Surgery of the Dog and Cat. 2nd Ed. Philadelphia, W. B. Saunders, 1971.
4. Olds, R. B.: Coxofemoral luxation. In Current Techniques in Small Animal Surgery. Edited by M. J. Bojrab. Philadelphia, Lea & Febiger, 1975.
5. Pettit, G. D.: Joints of the hind limb. In Canine Surgery. 2nd Ed. Edited by J. Archibald. Santa Barbara, CA, American Veterinary Publications, 1974.
6. Pettit, G. D.: Coxofemoral luxation. Vet. Clin. North Am., 1:503, 1971.
7. Piermattei, D. L., and Greeley, R. G.: An Atlas of Surgical Approaches to the Bones of the Dog and Cat. 2nd Ed. Philadelphia, W. B. Saunders, 1979.

Excision of the Femoral Head and Neck

by PHILIP B. VASSEUR

The veterinarian is often confronted with canine lameness arising from the coxofemoral joint. Degenerative arthrosis is frequently present, and conservative management is often indicated. Persistent pain and disuse may warrant surgical intervention, however, and numerous surgical options are available. Excision of the femoral head and neck is commonly performed, and if patients are carefully selected, satisfactory results can be expected in the majority of cases.

Preoperative Considerations

The establishment of a fibrous articulation (pseudo-arthrosis) in the coxofemoral joint can be achieved by removing the femoral head and neck. The results of this operation depend upon a number of factors. These considerations should be carefully evaluated for each individual patient, and the prognosis should be made clear to the patient's owner prior to the surgical procedure.

1. Body Size. Cats and small dogs generally do well, often with clinically normal function. These animals tend to be active, and their small size puts minimal stress on the fibrous articulation that forms. Any animal that is overweight should be dieted prior to operation, if possible. In large dogs (>25 kg) with hip fractures or luxations, every effort should be made to restore a normal articulation. Total joint replacement should be considered for selected patients if correction is not possible. In giant breeds, femoral head and neck excision is strictly a salvage procedure that should be performed only when other avenues of therapy have been exhausted.

2. Temperament. The aggressive, active dog uses the leg sooner and generally has a better result than a lethargic, less-active animal. The muscular 35-kg Labrador retriever has an entirely different prognosis from the 35-kg obese collie.

3. Surgical Technique. A minimally traumatic approach and smooth osteotomy afford early recovery and weight-bearing. Small bony irregularities are not critical, but larger projections resulting in significant crepitation should be avoided.

INDICATIONS FOR SURGICAL TREATMENT

1. Legg-Calvé-Perthes disease
2. Recurrent coxofemoral luxations
3. Severe fractures involving the coxofemoral joint
   a. Comminuted acetabular fractures
   b. Selected femoral head or neck fractures
4. Degenerative joint disease
5. Canine hip dysplasia

Surgical Techniques

MODIFIED CRANIOLATERAL APPROACH

Most patients can be operated on through a modification of the craniolateral approach that reflects the origins of the vastus musculature and thus gains increased exposure of the femoral neck.[2,8] With the animal under inhalant anesthesia, the entire limb is

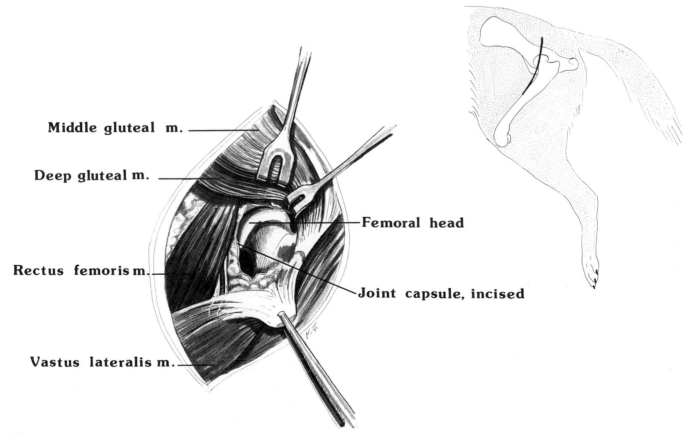

Fig. 46-15. *Modified craniolateral approach to the hip joint. Note the periosteal reflection of the vastus lateralis, medialis, and intermedius muscles to gain exposure of the femoral neck.*

Middle gluteal m.

Deep gluteal m.

Rectus femoris m.

Vastus lateralis m.

Femoral head

Joint capsule, incised

clipped from a point above the hock to the dorsal midline and is routinely prepared for an aseptic surgical procedure. The patient is placed on the operating table in lateral recumbency with the limb suspended. The leg is routinely draped, and a sterile stockinette is used to allow manipulation of the limb during the operation.

A slightly curved incision is started just cranial and 3 to 4 cm dorsal to the greater trochanter, to extend distally along the proximal fourth of the femoral shaft (Fig. 46-15). The incision is carried through the subcutaneous tissues to the level of the fascia lata, and the fascia is incised at the cranial border of the biceps femoris muscle. Cranial retraction of the tensor fasciae latae muscle and caudal retraction of the biceps femoris muscle expose the greater trochanter. Self-retaining retractors (Weitlaner or Gelpi) are helpful when one is working alone. Care should be taken not to damage the sciatic nerve with the retractor. The loose connective tissue around the trochanter is cleared away, and the insertions of the deep and middle gluteal muscles are retracted dorsally and caudally. The deep gluteal muscle is attached to the joint capsule, and some dissection is necessary to mobilize the muscle. The origins of the vastus medialis, intermedius, and lateralis muscles are reflected using a periosteal elevator, and the joint capsule, if intact, is incised to expose the femoral head and neck (Fig. 46-15). If necessary, the tendon of the deep gluteal muscle can be partially severed to gain additional exposure. The lesser trochanter can be palpated medially and should be preserved; it serves as the insertion of the iliopsoas muscle, an important flexor and external rotator of the hip.

If the hip is luxated, it is helpful to obtain reduction prior to or during the procedure. This reduction restores normal anatomic relationships and stabilizes the femoral head in the acetabulum during the osteotomy. If the luxation cannot be reduced, a retractor should be placed under the femoral head and neck to provide stabilization and to protect the surrounding soft tissues. The osteotome chosen should be of sufficient width to allow clean severance of the femoral neck without repeated cuts. Positioning of the osteotome is important. Figure 46-16 demonstrates the correct angle for the osteotomy. The osteotome is placed on the lateral surface of the femoral neck, and the handle is held cranially, directing the cut caudally and medially. A common error is to direct the osteotome directly medially, that is, perpendicular to the table. This error results in the incomplete excision of the medial femoral neck (Fig. 46-17). Several sharp blows are generally sufficient to complete the osteotomy.

The femoral head is then grasped with a towel clamp, and the round ligament, if intact, is severed with Mayo scissors. Any remaining capsular attachments are cut to allow removal of the femoral head and neck. Any bony projections or irregularities that remain on the cut surface should be removed with a rongeur or a bone rasp. If hemorrhage from the medullary surface is persistent, bone wax is used to achieve hemostasis. The wound is flushed, and the vastus muscles are sutured to the periosteum, if possible, using fine sutures of monofilament nylon. Alternatively, these muscles can be sutured to the deep gluteal muscle. The remaining tissue planes are closed routinely.

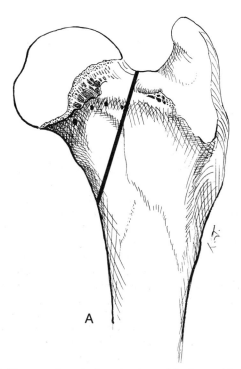 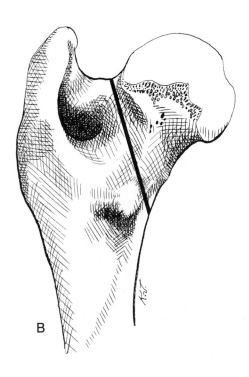

Fig. 46-16. *The correct angle for ostectomy of the femoral head and neck.* A, *Lateral view;* B, *medial view. Note the complete removal of the femoral neck with preservation of the lesser trochanter.*

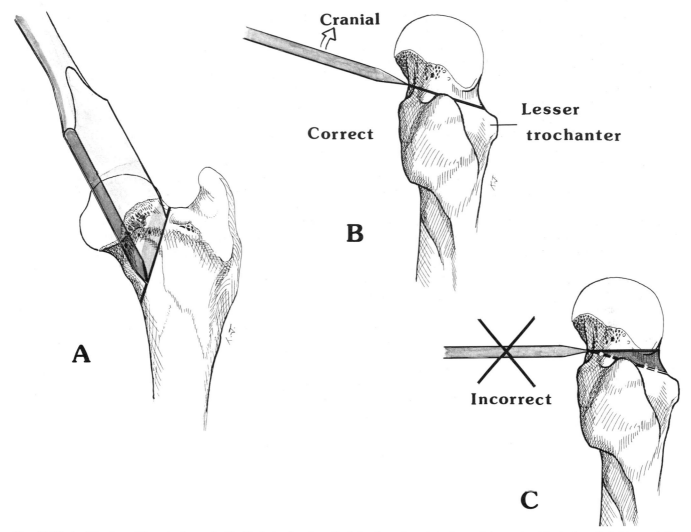

Fig. 46-17. *Positioning of the osteotome. A, The blade is placed on the lateral surface at the base of the neck with the handle held cranially. B, A dorsal view shows the correct angle for the osteotomy, providing complete excision of the femoral neck. C, A common error is to direct the osteotome perpendicular to the table; this maneuver results in incomplete excision of the femoral neck.*

DORSAL APPROACH

In heavily muscled dogs or in those with severe degenerative joint disease, additional exposure may be needed and can be obtained through severance of the middle and deep gluteal tendons.[1,8] The approach is made in the manner described previously. In addition, the tendons of the middle and deep gluteal muscles are severed, leaving adequate tissue on the greater trochanter to allow secure reattachment (Fig. 46-18). The osteotomy is completed in the manner described previously, and the tendons are sutured in a modified Bunnell pattern using 1-0 or 2-0 monofilament nylon. No attempt is made to close the joint capsule; the remaining tissue planes are closed routinely.

VENTRAL APPROACH

The ventral approach to the coxofemoral joint is rapid and is minimally invasive.[6,8] The exposure, however, is limited, and this approach finds use only in the cat and small dog.

Accurate positioning of the patient on the table is important. The animal is placed in dorsal recumbency with the hind legs abducted and firmly taped so that the legs form a right angle relative to the long axis of the body. This position tenses the pectineus muscle for easy identification and gives the operator a consistent anatomic framework, both of which are especially important for this approach.

The skin incision is made directly over the pectineus muscle, starting at the muscle's origin on the pubis and extends distally approximately one-fourth the length of the femur (Fig. 46-19A). The subcutaneous tissue and fascia are opened in line with the incision and are retracted cranially and caudally. The pectineus muscle is isolated and is severed near its origin on the pubis, with care taken not to damage the femoral artery, vein, and saphenous nerve, which run along the cranial border of the muscle. Under the pectineus muscle are the deep

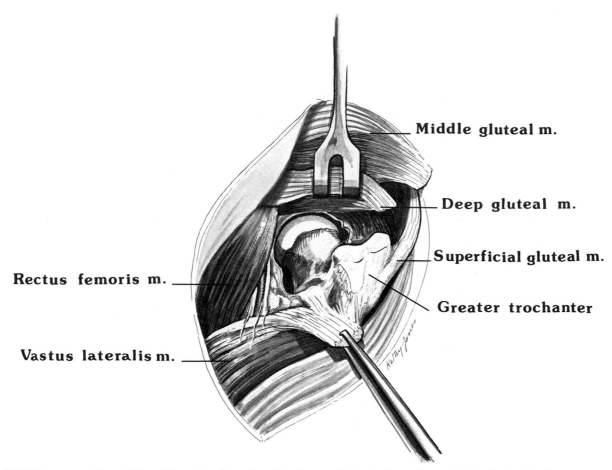

Fig. 46-18. *Tenotomy of the middle and deep gluteal muscles. Note the remaining tendon on the greater trochanter, to allow secure reattachment of the tendons during closure.*

femoral vessels, which run across the surface of the iliopsoas muscle. These vessels are preserved, and the iliopsoas muscle is bluntly separated from the adductor, which lies caudally (Fig. 46-19A). The iliopsoas muscle is retracted cranially and the adductor caudally, to expose the ventral aspect of the joint. Manipulation of the femur aids in locating the capsule, which is incised to expose the femoral head (Fig. 46-19B). Further retraction and elevation of the capsule gain exposure of the femoral head and neck. If the femoral neck has been fractured, the round ligament is severed, and the femoral head is removed. The fracture surface is palpated, and any irregularities are smoothed with a small bone rasp. If the femoral neck is intact, as in Legg-Calvé-Perthes disease, an osteotome is placed on the ventral surface of the neck and is directed toward the intertrochanteric fossa; one must take care to preserve the lesser trochanter (Fig. 46-19C).

Following the osteotomy, the round ligament is cut, and the fragment is removed. The medullary surface is checked for rough areas and is smoothed if necessary, the wound is lavaged, and the muscles are apposed with a minimum number of absorbable sutures. The pectineus muscle is reattached with several mattress sutures of monofilament nylon. The skin is closed routinely.

Postoperative Complications and Management

Complications that can occur following these procedures include shortening of the operated limb with prominence of the greater trochanter, decreased range of motion in the pseudoarthrosis as compared to the normal hip, and muscle atrophy.[5] Occasional lameness is a common finding, and larger dogs often have difficulty in jumping or in climbing stairs.

Postoperative physical therapy in the form of running, swimming, and whirlpool baths and weight reduction are all helpful in restoring early function, especially in the less-active dog.

Although many medium-sized and large dogs can achieve adequate function, one should not expect the excised hip to perform as well as the normal articulation. Many hunting dogs may return to the field, but they rarely return to top form, especially if operated bilaterally.

Analgesics can be of value postoperatively to encourage the patient's use of the limb. Aspirin is recommended in the dog at a dosage of 10 mg/kg bid.[3] Analgesics are seldom required in the cat.

Chronic lameness and disuse occasionally occur and are usually the result of bony crepitation, inadequate

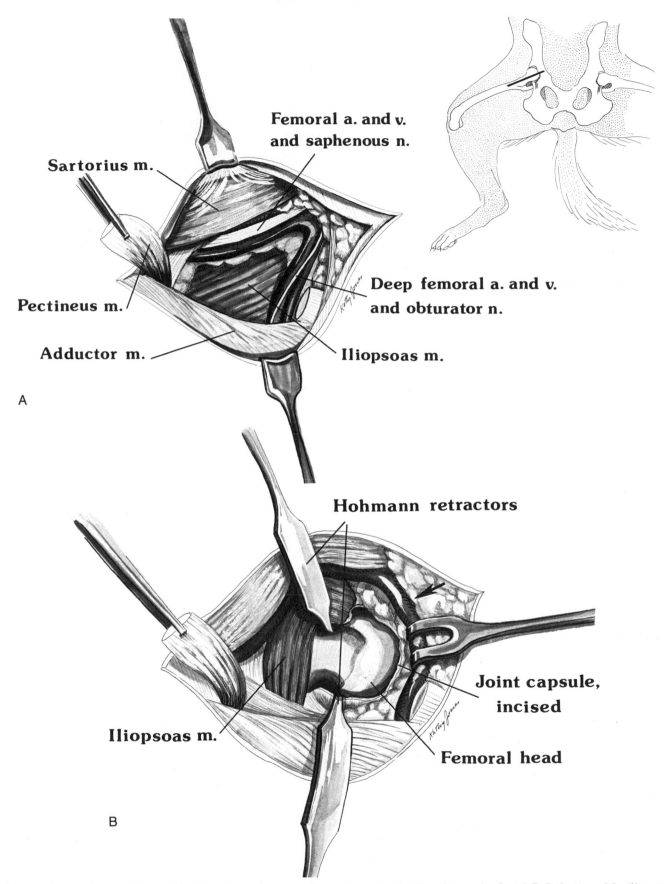

Femoral a. and v. and saphenous n.

Sartorius m.

Deep femoral a. and v. and obturator n.

Pectineus m.

Adductor m.

Iliopsoas m.

A

Hohmann retractors

Joint capsule, incised

Iliopsoas m.

Femoral head

B

Fig. 46-19. *Ventral approach to the hip joint; the pectineus muscle has been severed at its origin and reflected. B, Reflection of the iliopsoas muscle to gain exposure of the joint; the deep femoral vessels must be identified and gently retracted (arrow). (Continued on next page.)*

Osteotome

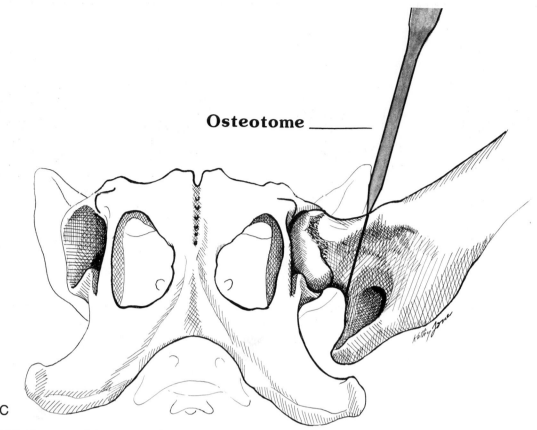

Fig. 46-19. *(cont.)* C, *Placement of the osteotome from the ventral approach; the blade is directed towards the intertrochanteric fossa with care taken to preserve the lesser trochanter.*

postoperative rehabilitation, or incorrect initial diagnosis. If no other cause for the lameness can be found, and if physical therapy and analgesics are ineffective, surgical exploration is indicated. Radiographs may be helpful in locating bony spurs, but the radiographic appearance is variable and does not correlate well with the clinical condition.[4] At operation, any bony irregularities should be removed, and the surface should be smoothed with a bone rasp or file. If infection is suspected, a culture should be taken. Severe muscle atrophy can result in significant bony contact that is difficult to avoid. In selected cases, the interposition of local soft tissues, such as fat or fascia, can be of benefit in preventing bony contact.[7] The prognosis in these patients is guarded, and aggressive postoperative physical therapy is critical to success.

References and Suggested Readings

1. Brown, R.E.: A surgical approach to the coxofemoral joint of dogs. North Am. Vet., *34:*420, 1953.
2. Brown, S. G., and Rosen, H.: Craniolateral approach to the canine hip: a modified Watson-Jones approach. J. Am. Vet. Med. Assoc., *159:*1117, 1971.
3. Davis, L. E.: Clinical pharmacology of salicylates. J. Am. Vet. Med. Assoc., *176:*65, 1980.
4. Duff, R., and Campbell, J. R.: Radiographic appearance and clinical progress after excision arthroplasty of the canine hip. J. Small Anim. Pract., *19:*439, 1978.
5. Duff, R., and Campbell, J. R.: Long term results of excision arthroplasty of the canine hip. Vet. Rec., *101:*181, 1977.
6. Evans, H. E., and Christensen, G. C.: Miller's Anatomy of the Dog. 2nd Ed. Philadelphia, W. B. Saunders, 1979.
7. Olds, R. B.: Personal communication, 1980.
8. Piermattei, D. L., and Greeley, R. G.: An Atlas of Surgical Approaches to the Bones of the Dog and Cat. 2nd Ed. Philadelphia, W. B. Saunders, 1979.

Meniscectomy

by Gretchen L. Flo

Meniscal injury in the dog usually occurs secondary to some form of cruciate ligament disorder, that is, a partial or full tear of the cranial or caudal cruciate ligament. A 53% incidence of meniscal injury concurrent with cruciate ligament damage has been reported.[4] Ninety-eight percent of the meniscal injuries involve the medial meniscus only. The lateral meniscus is rarely involved, unless excessive joint instability is present from significant trauma, such as from an automobile accident. In these patients, both menisci may be injured.

When the meniscus becomes extensively damaged, the caudal axial (inner) portion of the meniscus luxates under the weight-bearing surface of the femur and causes erosive damage to the articular surface as well

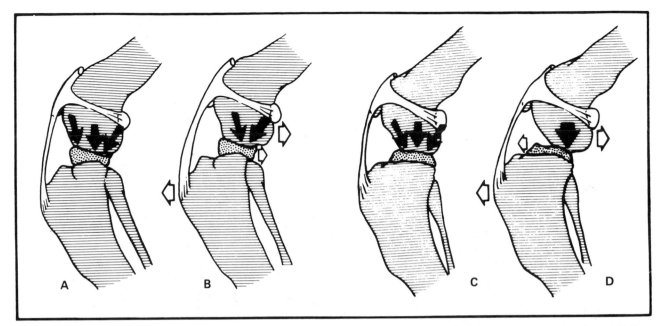

Fig. 46-20. *Mechanical explanation of medial meniscal tears. A, Lateral aspect of a normal stifle joint; the meniscus is stippled. B, Lateral stifle in cranial drawer position; the weight-bearing area on the lateral meniscus is still diffuse. C, Medial aspect of a normal stifle joint. D, Medial stifle in cranial drawer position; the weight-bearing area rests on the caudal horn of the medial meniscus and crushes it. Note: Dark arrows represent weight-bearing pressure on menisci; clear arrows represent tissue movement. (From Flo, G. L., and DeYoung, D.: Meniscal injuries and medial menisectomy in the canine stifle. J. Am. Anim. Hosp. Assoc., 14:683, 1978.)*

as increased discomfort to the animal. Meniscectomy, therefore, is indicated.

The reason for meniscal injury secondary to cruciate disease can be explained by abnormal sliding of the tibia on the femur (Fig. 46-20). The higher incidence of medial meniscal injury can be explained by anatomic differences between the medial and the lateral meniscus. Both menisci are attached to the tibia at each of their ends by ligaments. Their convex peripheries are attached by synovium and loose connective tissue. The lateral meniscus has fewer synovial attachments where the popliteal tendon crosses its caudal abaxial side. In

addition, a ligamentous attachment to the femur is present. The medial meniscus, however, is attached to the medial collateral ligament. Therefore, the medial meniscus is more rigidly attached. With abnormal craniocaudal movement of the tibia, the femoral condyle crushes the caudal rim of the more firmly attached medial meniscus while the lateral meniscus is pulled caudally with the femoral condyle by the femoral ligament.

The meniscus may be torn at the time of the original injury or subsequently from walking on an unstable stifle. Repeated trauma to the caudal horn of the menis-

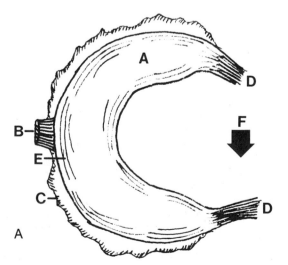
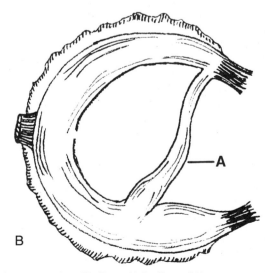

Fig. 46-21. *A, Area of meniscal stress during cranial drawer movement. (A, Stress area (crush); B, medial collateral ligament attachment; C, loose synovial membrane attachment; D, ligaments attaching the meniscus to the tibia; E, longitudinal fibers in meniscal parenchyma; F, direction of drawer movement.) B, Cranial luxation of torn axial portion. (A, Torn fragment.)*

cus results in a separation between fibers (Fig. 46-21A). Following cleavage, the axial portion may luxate cranially and caudally between the femoral and tibial condyles (Fig. 46-21B); this luxation gives rise to an audible or palpable snap. This longitudinal separation of the caudal horn is the so-called "bucket-handle" tear in human patients.

Diagnosis of Meniscal Injuries

Meniscal injuries are most frequently diagnosed by direct evaluation following arthrotomy; however, care-ful evaluation of the patient's medical history and physical findings may suggest meniscal involvement. A meniscal tear is suspected when a dog is still non-weight-bearing 2 weeks or more following cranial cruciate ligament rupture. Subsequent meniscal injury is suspected when weight-bearing returns following cruciate rupture, and the patient suddenly becomes non-weight-bearing at a later time. In addition, large breeds of dogs have a higher incidence of secondary meniscal involvement and should be closely evaluated.

The patient's owner also may hear a click or a snap when the dog ambulates. During flexion and extension

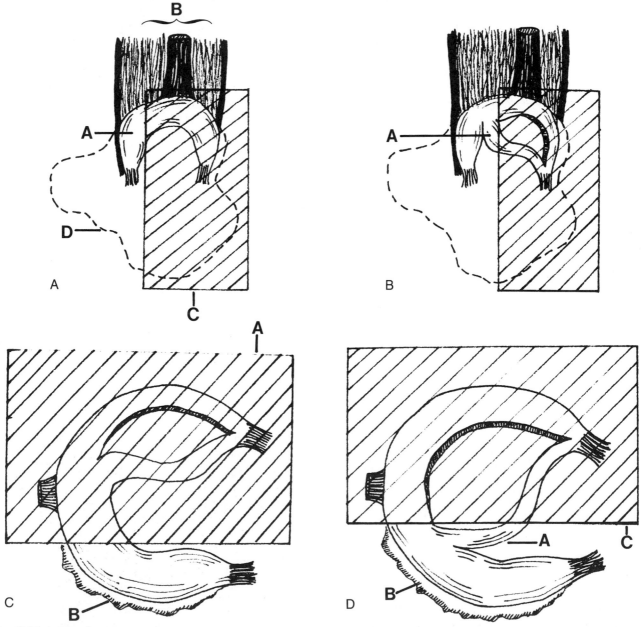

Fig. 46-22. A, *Dorsolateral view of medial meniscus in situ on the tibia. (A, Cranial horn of medial meniscus; B, synovial and collateral ligament attachments to the meniscus; C, shaded area represents vision obscured by the femur; D, tibia.) B, Dorsolateral view of a displaced torn meniscus in situ. (A, Axial fragment displaced cranially with no synovial attachment on its cranial surface.) C, Dorsocranial view of an undisplaced torn meniscus. (A, Shaded area represents vision obscured by femoral condyles; B, synovial attachments.) D, Dorsocranial view of a displaced torn meniscus in cranial drawer position. (A, Displaced fragment devoid of synovial attachments on its cranial surface; B, synovial attachment; C, shaded area represents vision obscured by femur.)*

of a stifle joint that has a torn meniscus, a click may sometimes be felt and heard. This meniscal click often disappears with the relaxation that accompanies anesthesia or sedation. The degree of drawer movement may also be lessened by wedging of the displaced meniscal tissue between the femoral and tibial condyles. A prominent, firm swelling may also be seen on the medial aspect of the joint over the area of the medial collateral ligament.

The definitive diagnosis of a torn meniscus is made upon surgical exploration. Recognizing a damaged meniscus may be difficult for those veterinary surgeons who are not familiar with meniscal disorders; therefore, I shall try to describe its appearance. With the patella luxated laterally, one cannot see the front edge of the cranial horn of the medial meniscus because it is covered by its synovial attachments. The cranial horn has to be visualized from a top or a side view, and only a small portion of it can be seen (Fig. 46-22A). If meniscal tissue is seen immediately adjacent to the cranial surface of the femoral condyle with no synovium attached to its cranial surface, it is the axial (inner) part of the torn caudal horn of the meniscus that is luxated forward (Fig. 46-22B). If the torn meniscus is not displaced into the cranial joint compartment (Fig. 46-22C), the tibia is then gently pulled into the cranial drawer position to facilitate its visualization. The cranial drawer movement is accomplished by manipulation of the extremity or by placing a curved hemostat under the cranial attachment of the medial meniscus and gently levering it against the distal femoral trochlea. This maneuver allows visualization of the cranial half of the meniscus. The meniscus is torn if a piece of tissue flips (Fig. 46-22D) cranially in front of the femoral condyle or if tiny cleavage lines, delineated by blood, are present within the white fibrocartilage.

A decision must be made at that time either to remove the luxated axial piece of the meniscus (partial meniscectomy) or to remove the meniscus in its entirety (total meniscectomy). This choice is discussed at the end of this chapter section.

Three complications associated with meniscectomy technique must be avoided. One is inadvertent laceration of the articular cartilage. The second is excision of the cranial half of the meniscus while leaving the damaged caudal half in the stifle joint. The third problem is overzealous excision of the meniscus that may lacerate the adjacent medial collateral ligament and fibrous joint capsule and may lead to medial joint instability. Detailed knowledge of the anatomic features and practice on a cadaver should eliminate these potential problems.

Surgical Technique

The affected limb is prepared for an aseptic surgical procedure and is draped in a routine manner. A medial parapatellar arthrotomy is performed, and the patella is luxated laterally (Fig. 46-23).[5] The use of a medial parapatellar arthrotomy results in better visualization of the medial meniscus and facilitates meniscectomy. If a medial meniscal tear is diagnosed through a lateral

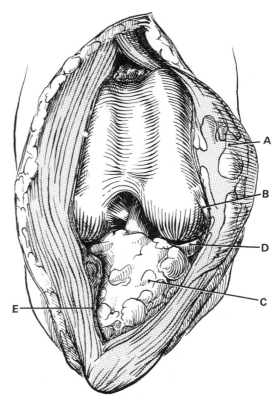

Fig. 46-23. *Medial parapatellar arthrotomy. (A, Patella; B, long digital extensor tendon; C, fat pad; D, lateral meniscus; E, cut edge of fibrous joint capsule.) (From Flo, G. L., and DeYoung, D.: Meniscal injuries and medial meniscectomy in the canine stifle. J. Am. Anim. Hosp. Assoc., 14:683, 1978.)*

arthrotomy, it is advisable to perform another arthrotomy on the medial side of the joint. Following the arthrotomy, the remains of the cruciate tags are debrided to improve inspection of the meniscus as well as to remove any irritation caused by degenerating tissue. If the meniscus still cannot be visualized well, a small

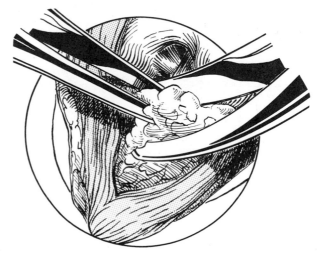

Fig. 46-24. *Partial excision of fat pad for exposure if necessary. (From Flo, G. L., and DeYoung, D.: Meniscal injuries and medial meniscectomy in the canine stifle. J. Am. Anim. Hosp. Assoc., 14:683, 1978.)*

amount of fat pad may be removed over the cranial insertion of the medial meniscus and the intermeniscal ligament (Fig. 46-24). The stifle joint is placed in cranial drawer position, and the lateral meniscus is inspected first, followed by inspection of the medial meniscus. If it is ascertained that the meniscus is extensively damaged, a total meniscectomy should be performed (Fig. 46-25, and see also Figs. 46-21*B* and 46-22*B* and *D*).

The meniscectomy is initiated by incising the intermeniscal and cranial tibial ligaments using a No. 15 Bard-Parker scalpel blade (Fig. 46-26*A*). To protect the underlying cartilage, a curved hemostat may be placed underneath these ligaments prior to incision. The meniscus is then held with thumb forceps while its synovial attachments are severed. During the excision, the width of the meniscus, as viewed ventrally, can be used as a guide to avoid removing too little or too much tissue. Kocher's forceps are then attached to the fibrous joint capsule adjacent to the medial meniscus, and Kocher's forceps (these work best on larger dogs) or a meniscal clamp* is attached to the free portion of the meniscus. Traction is then applied in opposite directions (Fig. 46-26*B*). This traction allows the meniscus and tibia to be drawn forward and allows dissection in front of the articular surface of the femur. A No. 15

* Carb meniscus clamp, Richards Manufacturing Co., Memphis, TN 38116

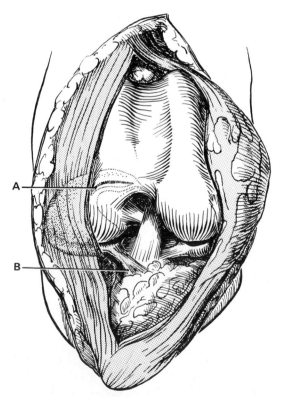

Fig. 46-25. *Position of undisplaced torn meniscus in relation to the femoral condyles. (A, Longitudinal tear of the medial meniscus in a reduced position; B, cranial ligamentous attachment of the medial meniscus.) (From Flo, G. L., and DeYoung, D.: Meniscal injuries and medial meniscectomy in the canine stifle. J. Am. Anim. Hosp. Assoc., 14:683, 1978.)*

Bard-Parker blade or a smaller No. 64 Beaver miniblade† can be used to separate the meniscus from the synovial attachments longitudinally. As the dissection proceeds around the medial side of the joint, Kocher's forceps on the joint capsule should be reattached closer to the remaining intact meniscus on the synovial side (Fig. 46-26*C*). This maneuver helps to bring the field of dissection into better view and prevents laceration to the articular cartilage. The synovial attachment to the femur should be carefully cut horizontally without cutting into the fibrous joint capsule or medial collateral ligament (Fig. 46-26*C*). Following completion of the medial dissection, the caudal horn must be freed. The caudal synovial attachments are generally stretched or torn and usually can be ripped free by applying lateral traction on the meniscal clamp. Once these synovial attachments are free, the entire meniscus lies in the interior of the joint with just the caudal tibial ligament intact (Fig. 46-26*D*).

The tibia is gently "drawered" forward by an assistant to allow exposure and visualization. A small scalpel blade is then placed under the meniscal attachment, and the meniscus is drawn over the blade. This maneuver severs the ligament without lacerating the surface of the articular cartilage and caudal cruciate ligament. Following meniscectomy, any remaining cruciate tags are debrided, and the arthrotomy is closed with simple interrupted nonabsorbable sutures. The joint is then stabilized with the stabilization technique of choice. I prefer the modified retinacular imbrication technique.[2]

Postoperatively, the limb should be supported for 1 to 2 weeks by a soft bandage or a splint, to reduce joint motion and to facilitate healing of the arthrotomy.

Discussion

Meniscal regeneration in conjunction with cruciate repair has been reported.[1] The regenerated tissue appeared anatomically similar to a normal meniscus and was composed of fibrocartilage.[1] Minimal articular cartilage degeneration was present. In another study,[3] the meniscus was removed without creating joint instability from cruciate ligament debridement. Both studies resulted in identical degrees of meniscal regeneration, and the latter study showed that total meniscectomy alone can result in some articular cartilage degeneration. Therefore, it is important not to remove normal menisci.

In a clinical situation, many patients with chronic stifle injuries (6 to 12 months' duration) remain lame until the degenerate meniscus is removed. A marked clinical improvement is often seen within 4 to 8 weeks, even in patients that require no stabilization procedure. This finding indicates to us that meniscectomy offers significant relief of pain and improves limb function.

Veterinarians who perform cruciate surgical procedure and who have never diagnosed or removed torn menisci have said they have not had poor results, so why should they start diagnosing and removing menisci now? The answer is that if they have had 100%

† Rudolph Beaver, Inc., Belmont, MA 02178

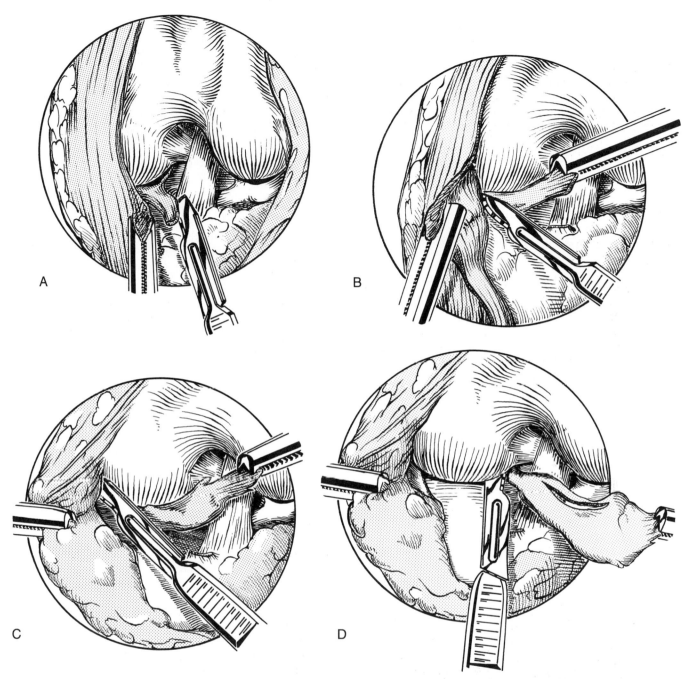

Fig. 46-26. A, *Severance of the cranial ligamentous attachment of the medial meniscus. (Note: In these drawings, the cranial cruciate ligament is left intact for orientation purposes.)* B, *Dissection of the medial meniscus sagittally from the peripheral synovium by retraction of the capsule medially and the freed meniscus laterally.* C, *Repositioning of Kocher's forceps closer to the intact medial meniscus; a small synovial attachment to the femur may have to be transected.* D, *Careful severance of the caudal ligamentous attachment of the medial meniscus. (From Flo, G. L., and DeYoung, D.: Meniscal injuries and medial meniscectomy in the canine stifle. J. Am. Anim. Hosp. Assoc., 14:683, 1978.)*

perfect results with their cruciate operations, then they are not doing many, or else they belong in a referral practice. Theoretically speaking, those joints stabilized early, within a few days of injury, do not have the degree of meniscal damage seen in our referral practice, where a 53% incidence is seen. Possibly, those patients stabilized with just a crushing of the caudal horn may clinically perform well. Those cases with "bucket-han-

dle" tears, however, probably do not do well, and such a possibility should be considered when re-evaluating those dogs. "He's just got too much arthritis" is not always the reason for poor limb function after the stabilization technique, and an exploration should be performed if the client is willing.

Much discussion exists in the human field as to whether a partial meniscectomy (removing the axial strip that is flipped in front of the femoral condyle) is better than a total meniscectomy, as described in this chapter. The advantage is that the thicker peripheral aspect of the meniscus is left intact, whereas in total meniscectomies some microinstability can arise from its absence, until regeneration stabilizes it. The disadvantages of partial meniscectomy include: (1) leaving in unseen secondary or tertiary tears (I have seen several menisci with multiple longitudinal lacerations); (2) greater chance of iatrogenic laceration to the articular cartilage; and (3) noninvasion of the vascular synovium where regeneration may be more complete. More research is needed to see which technique yields the best results.

References and Suggested Readings

1. DeYoung, D., and Flo, G. L.: Experimental medial meniscectomy in dogs undergoing cranial cruciate ligament repair. J. Am. Anim. Hosp. Assoc., 16:639, 1980.
2. Flo, G. L.: Modification of the lateral retinacular imbrication technique for stabilizing cruciate ligament injuries. J. Am. Anim. Hosp. Assoc., 11:570, 1975.
3. Flo, G. L., and DeYoung, D.: Meniscal regeneration and joint changes seen after total meniscectomy. Unpublished data. Presented at the annual meeting of the Veterinary Orthopedic Society, February, 1980.
4. Flo, G.L., and DeYoung, D.: Meniscal injuries and medial meniscectomy in the canine stifle. J. Am. Anim. Hosp. Assoc., 14:683, 1978.
5. Piermattei, D. L., and Greeley, R. G.: An Atlas of Surgical Approaches to the Bones of the Dog and Cat. 2nd Ed. Philadelphia, W. B. Saunders, 1979.

Collateral Ligament Injuries

by ERICK L. EGGER

The collateral ligaments are important stabilizing factors in the stifle joint. Injury to these ligaments is usually traumatically induced and is often associated with disruption of either the cranial or the caudal cruciate ligament.

Anatomic Features

The medial collateral ligament originates on the medial epicondyle of the femur and passes distally in the joint capsule. It passes over the medial lip of the tibial plateau, where an underlying bursa allows the ligament to slip back and forth as the joint moves. The ligament attaches to the medial shaft of tibia with a long, narrow insertion.[2] The medial collateral ligament is positioned over the central axis of the stifle so as to remain tight throughout flexion and extension of the joint.[1]

The lateral collateral ligament originates on the lateral epicondyle of the femur and passes distally in the joint capsule to insert on the fibular head.[2] The lateral collateral ligament is caudal to the central axis of the joint.[1] This position results in a tight ligament in extension that limits internal rotation and contributes to craniocaudal stability. The ligament then loosens as the joint flexes and allows the tibia to rotate internally.

Diagnosis

The clinical diagnosis of isolated collateral ligament injuries can be difficult. With the joint held in full extension, varus and valgus forces occasionally result in angulation away from the side with the ruptured ligament. If both cruciate ligaments are intact, however, they will greatly reduce or prevent this instability. Some increase in rotational movement may be seen. Evidence of a widened joint space on one side on radiographs taken while the joint is stressed may aid the diagnosis. Collateral ligament rupture in the presence of a cruciate ligament disruption is readily revealed by the presence of varus or valgus angulation of the joint when stress is applied and a dramatic increase in rotational instability with the stifle extended.

Treatment

Management of collateral ligament injuries varies with the severity of injury and the resultant instability. A stretched or isolated torn collateral ligament without gross instability can often be managed with external coaptation. A lateral splint fashioned of plaster or Hexcelite* in a padded bandage that is contoured is used to stress the joint toward the side of the injured collateral. This coaptation must be maintained for at least 3 to 4 weeks.

SURGICAL TECHNIQUES

Because the collateral ligaments are extrasynovial, the blood supply is sufficient to allow simple ruptures to heal if the ends are adequately apposed. A continuous, 3-loop pattern of monofilament nonabsorbable material such as nylon or polypropylene can be used to suture collateral ligaments (Fig. 46-27). Each pass of the suture is at a different distance from the torn ends and axially at a 120° rotation from the previous passage. This pattern tightens well, and these sutures rarely pull out of the torn ligament ends.

Suturing of severely traumatized ligaments may not provide adequate support. For these cases, a large figure-8 suture of nylon or polypropylene can be placed between bone screws seated at the collateral ligament's attachments, to provide additional support while the tissues heal (Fig. 46-28). Care must be taken to tighten a lateral collateral ligament repair only in extension because overtightening of this area prevents normal range of motion.

Patients in which the ligament has been torn away from the bone are best managed by fixation of the ligament with a bone screw. A spiked washer† can be used to trap the ligament without compromising its vascularity (Fig. 46-29). Any concurrent injury, such as a torn

* Hexcel Medical Products, 11711 Dublin Boulevard, Dublin, CA 94566
† Synthes, Ltd., 983 Old Eagle School Road, Wayne, PA 19087

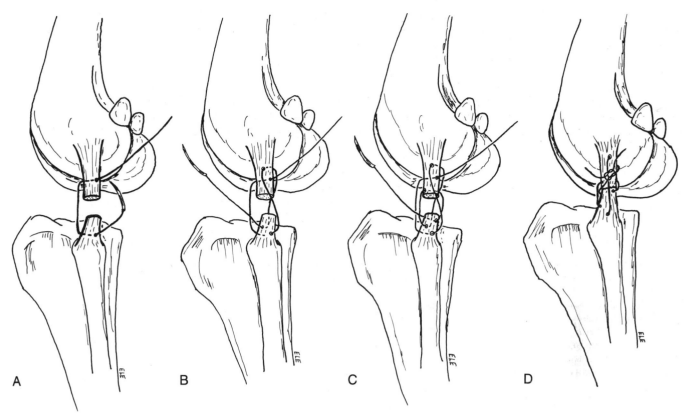

Fig. 46-27. *Primary suturing of a collateral ligament rupture. A, First loop of suture pattern. B, Second loop of suture placed at 120° rotation to first. C, Third loop of suture again rotated. D, Suture pulled tight and tied.*

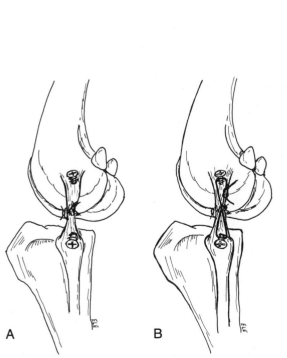

Fig. 46-28. *Figure-8 support of weak collateral ligament repair. A, Collateral ligament repaired as well as possible and bone screws placed at both attachments of the ligament. B, Figure-8 suture placed around screw head.*

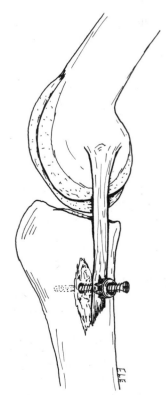

Fig. 46-29. *Reattachment of an avulsed ligament with a spiked washer and a bone screw.*

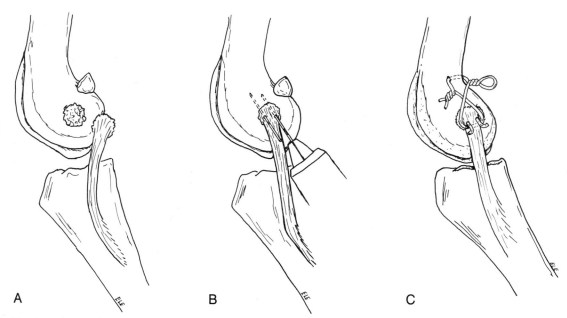

Fig. 46-30. *Fixation of an avulsion fracture of the attachment of a collateral ligament. A, Avulsion of the proximal attachment of the medial collateral ligament. B, Fixation of the fragment with two parallel Kirschner wires. C, Placement of a figure-8 wire to counteract the ligament pull.*

meniscus or cruciate ligament rupture, should be dealt with, and the joint should be externally supported with a lateral splint for 3 to 4 weeks while the collateral ligament heals.

Avulsion fractures of the ligament's bony attachments are best handled by surgical reduction and fixation (Fig. 46-30). One or two Kirschner wires are driven through the fragment to hold reduction. Then, a figure-8 tension-band wire is passed behind the Kirschner wires and through a transverse hole in the bone. This wire is tightened to counteract the pull of the ligament. The Kirschner wires should be cut off and bent back to reduce soft tissue irritation. Alternately, a bone screw can be used if the avulsion fragment is large enough.[1] Because internal fixation of a fracture should result in a stable repair, extended external coaptation is usually not indicated. A soft, padded bandage may be used for several days postoperatively to control soft tissue swelling, however.

References and Suggested Readings

1. Arnoczky, S. P., Tarvin, G. B., and Vasseur, P.: Surgery of the Stifle—The Menisci and Collateral Ligaments. The Compendium on Continuing Education II:395–399, 1980.
2. Evans, H. E., and Christensen, G. C.: Miller's Anatomy of the Dog. 2nd Ed. Philadelphia, W. B. Saunders, 1979.

Fractures of the Tibia

by Kenneth R. Sinibaldi

Fractures of the tibia occur most commonly in the bone's shaft. The normal anatomic twist and curves of the tibia are responsible for the usual spiral or oblique nature of these fractures, especially in the middle third of the bone. Proximal and distal epiphyseal fractures are more common in the young animal. The fibula is usually fractured when the tibia is fractured. In the young animal, however, the fibula is often spared and aids as an internal splint after reduction. In this discussion of tibial fractures, mention of fibular involvement is made only when pertinent.

As with any fracture, the primary concern should be with life-threatening injuries such as chest trauma and shock, because the patient will not die from a fractured bone. It is, however, important to assess the nature of the fracture injury as to soft tissue involvement, blood supply, neurologic involvement, and the presence of an open injury. Fractures of the tibia have a high tendency to be open, owing to decreased muscle mass covering the bone. The distal third is more prone to this type of injury. The sharp oblique nature of tibial fractures may lead to an open fracture if it is not administered properly. For this reason, all tibial fractures should be placed in a Robert Jones type of dressing or they should be splinted until the patient's condition is stable or until a decision has been made as to the definitive repair of the fracture.

Selection of a method of repair depends on the biomechanical forces that have acted upon the limb to cause a specific type of fracture and bone fragment displacement. This displacement is due to soft tissue forces acting on the bone and must be considered in manipulation to reduce the fracture. Basically, four forces act to create fractures: bending, rotational, shearing, and compressive forces (Fig. 46-31). Compressive forces are only detrimental in the young patient with epiphyseal injury. In most cases of simple fracture, only one force is involved, but combinations may occur and may thus lead to more involved frac-

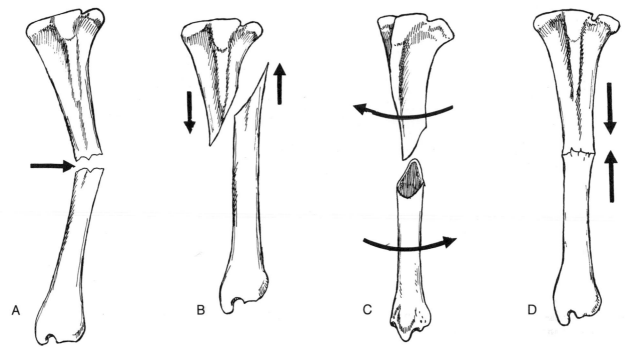

Fig. 46-31. *Biomechanical forces acting to create fractures.* A, *Bending;* B, *shearing;* C, *rotation;* D, *compression.*

tures. Knowing how a fracture occurs greatly helps in selection of repair methods and implants used.

Intramedullary pins work well against bending forces, but are poor against rotational and shearing forces because they are round and serve only to align the fracture axially. If the pin can be placed in the medullary cavity in a "dynamic" position, however, it may be adequate in some tibial fractures in combating these forces. Fractures that do not have the potential for rotational or shearing components can be successfully managed with intramedullary pinning. If an intramedullary pin is used in a fracture on which rotational and shearing forces are acting, some additional means of repair is necessary to stabilize the fracture. The use of full cerclage, hemicerclage, figure-8 wires, cross-pins, and Kirschner-Ehmer half-pin splints in combination with intramedullary pins works well (see Fig. 46-34).

The Kirschner-Ehmer apparatus and plating technique work well against all the forces mentioned, and for this reason are an excellent choice in repairing tibial fractures.

External coaptation is an alternative to open reduction and has worked well in some tibial fractures. It is also important to remember that certain types of coaptation are better suited in controlling biomechanical forces than others in fracture repair. As an example, a midshaft transverse tibial fracture with some jagged edges may be reduced adequately by closed reduction and held in position with a lateral splint. The lateral splint does not control rotational forces adequately, however. A cast crossing the joint above and below the fracture is more effective because it does negate rotational as well as bending forces and thus is superior to the lateral splint.

In the decision to use external coaptation as the sole method of repair, it is important to evaluate not only the mechanism of fracture, but also the nature of the patient. An aggressive, hyperactive, or uncontrollable chewer may destroy a cast or a splint shortly after its application. For this reason, some fractures that would heal well in a cast in one dog may not in another.

Diaphysis

Simple fractures of the tibial diaphysis can be handled with a cast. Pinning affords excellent axial alignment, but limited control over rotation. Bone plates and Kirschner-Ehmer splints are a better choice biomechanically because they control all bending, shearing, and rotational forces. The approach to the tibia is usually made from the medial side of the bone. Few vital structures (cranial branch of medial saphenous artery and vein and superficial peroneal nerve) are exposed. These structures can easily be identified and retracted. In essence, the approach to the tibia is a skin incision.

The tibia should be pinned in a normograde direction, that is, from the medial side of the proximal tibia distally. The site of pin introduction is a small depression on the medial side of the proximal tibia equidistant from both the medial collateral ligament and the straight patellar tendon (Fig. 46-32). The pin is introduced approximately at right angles to the tibial shaft until the point of the pin is embedded in the bone. At that point, the pin is angled dorsally and parallel to the axis of the tibia and is driven into its final position (Fig. 46-32). The pin meets some resistance initially as it enters the medullary cavity, little resistance through the

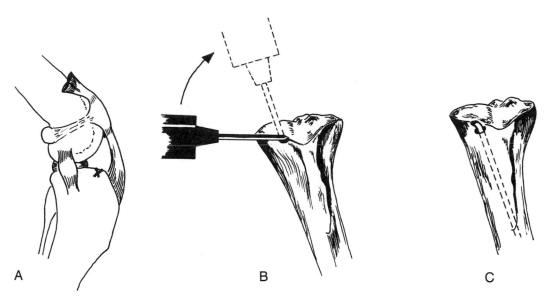

A   B   C

Fig. 46-32. *Normograde pinning of the tibia.* A, *Site of pin introduction* (*X*). B, *Pin started and moved parallel to axis of bone.* C, *Pin placement completed.*

medullary cavity, then resistance again as the pin is embedded in the cancellous bone of the distal tibia.

When the pin is placed properly, it is dynamic and has three points of contact: proximally at its entry point, against the lateral cortex of the diaphysis, and seated in the cancellous bone distally (Fig. 46-33). Once

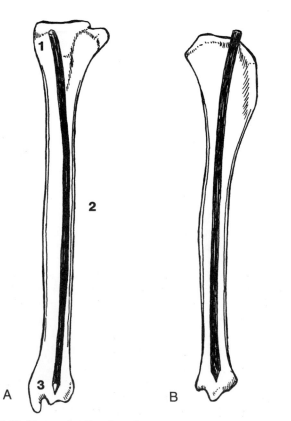

Fig. 46-33. *Three-point fixation of pin in a tibia.* A, *Craniocaudal view: entry point* (*1*), *lateral cortex* (*2*), *distal cancellous bone* (*3*). B, *Lateral view.*

the pin is in position, the proximal end can be bent to facilitate removal in the future and to ensure that no contact is made with the femur (see Fig. 46-32). If this technique is used, the pin will be outside the joint and will allow for normal free motion of the stifle. A flexible pin should be used because heavier pins do not give or allow for easy application. This technique can be used in combination with cerclage wires, cross-pins, and external Kirschner-Ehmer splints (Fig. 46-34).

No reason exists to pass the pin in a retrograde fashion in a tibial fracture repair because the risk of putting the pin into or close to the center of the joint as it exits the proximal tibia is great. This error occurs because of the anatomic shape of the tibia and the offset of the axial alignment of the medullary cavity in relation to the tibial plateau, particularly if heavy, nonflexible pins are used.

Intramedullary pins can be used in highly comminuted fractures as long as the tubular nature of the fractured bone is restored (Fig. 46-35).

Kirschner-Ehmer splints can be used on almost any type of tibial fracture provided enough room exists proximally and distally for application of the pins. This technique has proved to be of value in highly comminuted open fractures caused by gunshot wounds. The lateral side of the bone is the preferred side of application, but the medial side can also be used (Fig. 46-36). Pins should be placed at divergent angles approximately 40 to 60° to each other on both sides of the fracture. An angle of approximately 20 to 30° from a perpendicular to the axis of a line drawn parallel to the opposite cortex is ideal for the placement of the first pins (Fig. 46-36). In some cases, however, the angles may have to be changed to allow for placement of the pins, or another technique should be selected if adequate placement cannot be achieved. Pins should be driven by hand and not by power, to lessen the chance for loosening due to necrosis of bone from the heat

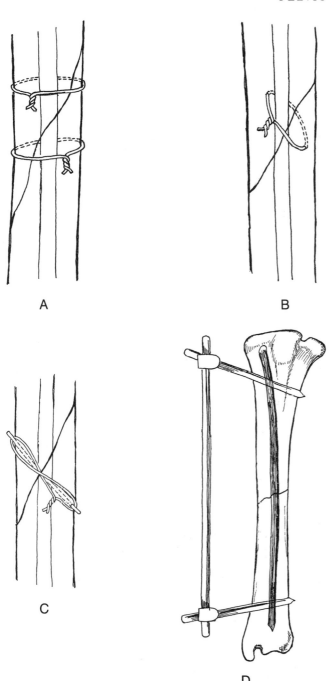

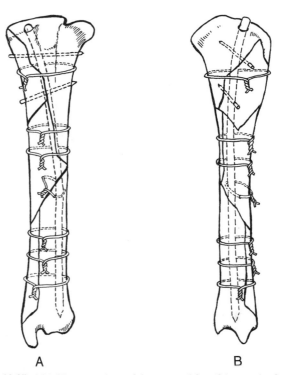

A   B

Fig. 46-35. *A highly comminuted fracture of the tibia repaired with an intramedullary pin, cerclage, hemicerclage, and small Steinmann pins. A, Craniocaudal view. B, Medial view.*

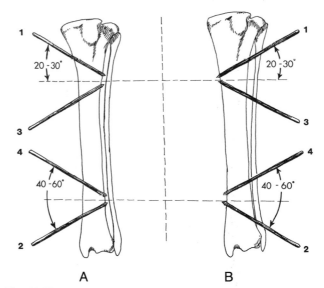

A   B

Fig. 46-36. *A and B, Kirschner-Ehmer pin placement. Note that the pin position can be modified to achieve stable reduction. The numbers 1 to 4 indicate the order of pin placement when a single attachment bar is used.*

Fig. 46-34. A, *Intramedullary pin and full-cerclage repair of an oblique fracture of the tibial diaphysis. B, The same fracture repaired with an intramedullary pin and hemicerclage wire. C, Oblique fracture of the tibial diaphysis repaired with an intramedullary pin, a cross pin, and figure-8 wire. D, The same fracture repaired by intramedullary pinning and external Kirschner-Ehmer half-pin splinting.*

produced by drilling. Both cortices should be penetrated by the pins. The pins should not cross as they exit. Threaded pins may have a better purchase than trocar-tip pins.

The order of placement, shown in Figure 46-36, allows freedom in cranial, caudal, dorsal, and ventral placement of pins 3 and 4 as they are positioned

through their respective clamps. Pins should always be placed with little pressure on the skin and underlying soft tissue. Increased pressure at the pin entrance causes necrosis of tissue and leads to infection and loosening. The pins should not enter the bone through the incision. When properly used, these pins can remain in place for more than 4 months.

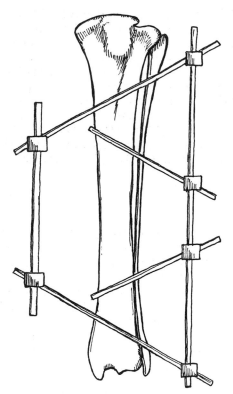

Fig. 46-37. *Modified use of a Kirschner-Ehmer splint with a full bar medially and laterally.*

advantage of rigid fixation and eliminates the use of coaptation, reduces the risk of fracture disease such as atrophy and stiffness, and allows for a more rapid return to function by the patient. It is beyond the scope of this paper to discuss the many principles of plating. Veterinary surgeons who elect to use such a method should become familiar with the principles, equipment, and techniques prior to its application to a patient.

Proximal Tibia

Most of these fractures occur in young animals and are of the Salter I and II classification of epiphyseal fractures. It is important to realize the age of the patient that sustains this type of fracture because of the possible growth potential at the epiphyseal plate. For this reason, techniques that compress the growth plate lead to premature epiphyseal closure with leg shortening and varus or valgus deformity.

These fractures can be handled by closed reduction in a cast if seen early after injury. Radiographs taken 2 to 3 weeks after casting in a young, growing dog allow for assessment of possible deformity because such a disorder usually occurs rapidly after closure of the growth plate. Correction or plan for correction can be undertaken at that time, depending on the age of the patient. It should be mentioned that perfect reduction is required in the closed management of epiphyseal fractures or malunions and deformity are possible.

Open reduction of these fractures requires application of Kirschner wires or small Steinmann pins. Usually, two pins are sufficient to hold the fracture in reduction. The pins should be placed as follows: one medial to lateral and one lateral to medial starting at the medial and lateral edges of the proximal tibia. When the tibial tubercle is avulsed with the epiphysis, a third pin can be used (Fig. 46-38).

The use of screws in lag fashion should be discouraged unless the growth potential is minimal at the time of repair. The limb is placed in a padded bandage post-

Added stability can be achieved by allowing the most proximal and distal pins to penetrate both cortices and by attaching these pins with a rod on the opposite side (Fig. 46-37). Postoperative care involves the use of a heavy padded bandage (modified Robert Jones), for several weeks and then a lighter protective bandage until the fracture has healed.

Bone plating techniques can be used on almost any diaphyseal fracture of the tibia, and in some instances a bone plate is the implant of choice. It does have the

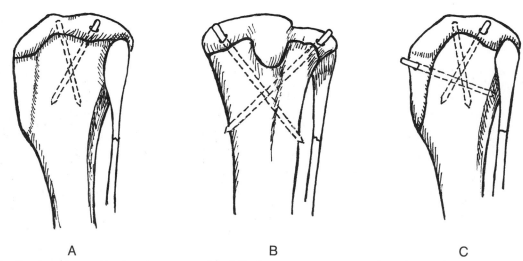

A   B   C

Fig. 46-38. *Pin fixation of a proximal tibial fracture. A and B, Cross-pin technique. C, Tibial tuberosity also fractured with proximal epiphysis; addition of another pin for stabilization.*

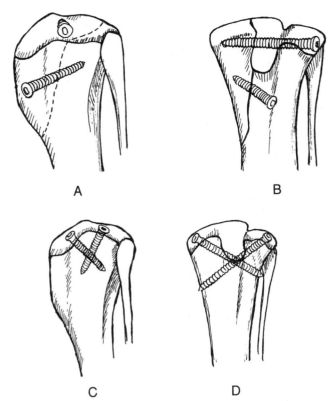

A   **B**

C   **D**

Fig. 46-39. *A and B, Intra-articular fracture of the proximal tibia repaired with screws used in a lag fashion. Craniocaudal (A) and lateral (B) views. C and D, Proximal tibial fracture repaired with two screws, one medial and one lateral, used in a lag fashion. This technique is used in older patients. Craniocaudal (C) and lateral (D) views.*

operatively for 10 to 14 days. Pins can be removed in 4 to 6 weeks, when radiographic evidence of healing or preservation of growth potential is obvious. Fractures of the proximal tibia in the older patient can be handled as previously described. In addition, screws can be used in a lag fashion, especially in cases of intra-articular fractures (Fig. 46-39). Avulsion fractures of the tibial tuberosity can be repaired with a single or a double pin, a tension band, or a lag screw. The single pin works well in toy breeds of dogs. The pin should be placed at an angle to counter the normal tensile (distracting) force of the patellar tendon (quadriceps pull) (Fig. 46-40). In medium-sized dogs, two pins or a tension band can be used to achieve the same results. A screw placed in a lag fashion can be used in larger breeds (Fig. 46-40). No matter what the nature of the proximal tibial fracture, it should be stressed that the stifle joint be examined for ligament and meniscal injuries.

Distal Tibia

These fractures not involving the articular surface can be handled in a cast if closed reduction can be achieved or with a Steinmann pin if adequate bone is present in the distal segment (Fig. 46-41). External co-aptation is usually needed with this technique. Cross-pinning techniques can be used (Fig. 46-42). It is important to start the pins medially and craniolaterally or just cranial to the fibula. Pins passing through the fibula may cause pain due to bone irritation from the pin several weeks later, even though the fracture looks healed radiographically.

In fractures that are extremely distal, several techniques can be used. Closed reduction is not impossible, and in some young animals with Salter I and II fractures, it is the treatment of choice. External compression clamps can also be used. A pin of adequate size is passed through the distal fragment; one should avoid the fibula if possible. A second pin is passed parallel to this first pin in the proximal segment. A third pin may also be used and passed parallel to the previous pins. Clamps are applied to the ends of the pins, and pressure is applied on the pins toward the fracture as the clamps are tightened (Fig. 46-43). The leg is placed in a heavy padded bandage for 10 to 14 days. After this time, the bandage is reduced to protect the pins and to allow flexion and extension of the tibiotalar joint. The

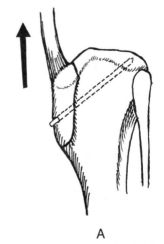   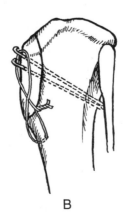   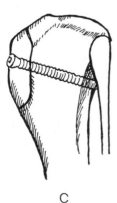

A   **B**   **C**

Fig. 46-40. *Avulsion fracture of the tibial tuberosity. A, Repaired by single pin fixation; note the direction of the pin and distraction force (arrow). B, Tension-band repair. C, Lag screw fixation.*

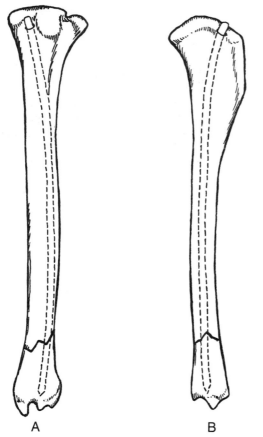

Fig. 46-41. A and B, *Intramedullary pin repair of a distal fracture of the tibia.*

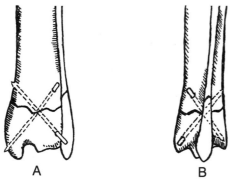

Fig. 46-42. A and B, *Distal tibial fracture repaired with cross pins, one medial to lateral and one lateral to medial, avoiding the fibula.*

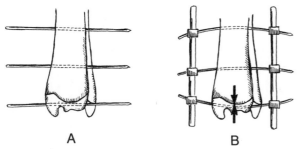

Fig. 46-43. *Distal tibial fracture repaired by the use of external compression clamps. A, Position of pins. B, Tension placed on pins to cause compression at the fracture site.*

pins can be removed when radiographic evidence of healing is present.

The retrograde passing of an intramedullary pin through the tarsus into the distal tibia and then up the shaft is an alternate method. Care must be taken to align the tarsal joint at a normal angle (115 to 125° in the cat; 125 to 145° in the dog). The pin is introduced medial to the fibular tarsal bone through the tibial tarsal bone. One should use the smallest pin possible to achieve an adequate and stable reduction. This technique also ensures minimal damage to the articular surfaces. It is imperative that the limb be casted to protect the pin from breaking. The pin should be removed 2 to 3 weeks postoperatively, and a cast or splint should be reapplied. At this time, the progression of healing or "stickiness" to the fracture should be adequate to allow removal without displacement. The limb is left in a splint for 1 to 2 weeks longer and then is placed in a padded bandage for an additional week or so. At the time of cast and or splint change, the patient's joints should be carefully taken through a range of motion to loosen them and to eliminate joint stiffness.

Fractures that involve half to three quarters of the bone may require combinations of the techniques described. Cancellous and cortical bone grafts may be beneficial in more complicated fractures and should be used.

The methods of repair described here are basic and, if used, lead to successful management of most tibial fractures. It should be noted that fractures more complicated than those presented can be repaired by combinations of the stated techniques. Veterinary surgeons should not limit themselves to one technique or method. The only impeding factor in repairing the most complicated fracture is a lack of imagination.

References and Suggested Reading

Archibald, J. (ed.): Canine Surgery. 2nd Ed. Santa Barbara, CA, American Publications, 1974.

Bojrab, M. J. (ed.): Current Techniques in Small Animal Surgery. Philadelphia, Lea & Febiger, 1975.

Evans, H. E., and Christensen, G. C.: Miller's Anatomy of the Dog. 2nd Ed. Philadelphia, W. B. Saunders, 1979.

Muller, M. E., et al.: Manual of Internal Fixation. New York, Springer-Verlag, 1970.

Piermattei, D. L., and Greeley, R. G.: Atlas of Surgical Approaches to the Bones of the Dog and Cat. 2nd Ed. Philadelphia, W. B. Saunders, 1979.

Whittick, D. G.: Canine Orthopedics. Philadelphia, Lea & Febiger, 1974.

Femoral Head and Neck Fractures

by DONALD A. HULSE

Fracture Classification

Fractures of the femoral head or femoral neck are common in dogs and cats. The fracture is commonly secondary to automobile accidents, but it may also be caused by other traumatic episodes such as gunshots or falls. In that the majority of patients will have undergone a severe traumatic episode, a thorough physical examination and stabilization of the patient is necessary before initiating diagnostic or surgical procedures.

Femoral head and neck fractures may be broadly classified into two categories, intracapsular and extracapsular (Fig. 46-44). Intracapsular fractures are further divided into: (1) capital physeal fractures, (2) foveal avulsion fractures, and (3) subcapital fractures. Extracapsular fractures are further divided into: (1) lateral fractures, (2) peritrochanteric fractures, and (3) subtrochanteric fractures.

The femoral capital physeal fracture is the most common type of femoral head fracture seen in small animal practice. This high incidence is due to the open physis, which is a weak link in the musculoskeletal system until closure of the growth plate occurs. Trauma that causes ligamentous injury in the adult is likely to result in a fracture line extending through the zone of cell hypertrophy of the growth plate in the young patient. Foveal avulsion fractures are seen with coxofemoral luxations in which stresses bring about a bone-ligament failure, rather than a failure of the ligament itself. Treatment of this type of injury is discussed in the second section of this chapter, on coxofemoral luxations. Subcapital fractures are not common, and therefore, discussion of these injuries is limited. Peritrochanteric and subtrochanteric fractures are also discussed elsewhere in the final section of this chapter. Lateral trochanteric fractures are common extracapsular fractures and are addressed in this section.

Anatomic Features

The hip joint is a ball-and-socket joint with a wide range of movement. The stability of the hip joint is maintained by the muscles, the joint capsule, and the

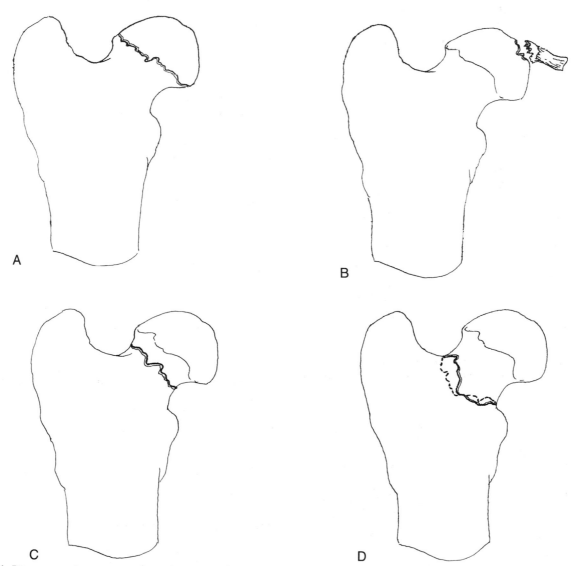

Fig. 46-44. *Diagrammatic representations of a capital physeal fracture* (A), *an avulsion fracture of the femoral head at the insertion of the round ligament* (B), *a subcapital fracture* (C), *and a lateral femoral neck fracture* (D).

ligament of the head of the femur. The joint capsule attaches medially a few millimeters from the edge of the acetabular lip and laterally on the neck of the femur 1 to 2 cm from the cartilage-capped femoral head. The ligament of the head of the femur is a heavy, flattened chord extending from the fovea in the head of the femur to the acetabular fossa and is the primary stabilizer of the hip joint. In the young dog, the proximal femoral growth plate is a continuous structure extending from the femoral head to the greater trochanter. With development, the single growth plate divides into the capital femoral growth plate and the trochanteric growth plate. The proximal femoral growth plate is thought to contribute approximately 25% of the total femoral length and to close normally between 9 and 12 months of age. The physis of the greater trochanter contributes to the normal architecture of the proximal femur, but adds little to the longitudinal growth of the femur.

The blood supply to the hip joint and associated musculature in the dog is provided by vessels that originate from the lateral circumflex femoral, medial circumflex femoral, and caudal gluteal arteries (Fig. 46-45). These vessels give origin to the ascending epiphyseal (cervical) arteries, which are divided into four groups: (1) cranial cervical ascending vessels, (2) dorsal cervical ascending vessels, (3) ventral cervical ascending vessels, and (4) caudal cervical ascending vessels. The ventral and dorsal cervical ascending vessels traverse the femoral neck in retinacular folds, in contrast to the cranial and caudal vessels, which do not ascend the femoral neck in retinacular folds. The dorsal, cranial, and ventral cervical ascending vessels

branch and anastomose with each other to form an intracapsular arterial ring at the edge of the articular cartilage. The dorsal and ventral cervical ascending arteries then penetrate the femoral head at the edge of the articular cartilage and course toward the center of the head of the femur just above the growth plate. These dorsal and ventral epiphyseal arteries branch and anastomose with each other to form an intraosseous arterial arch.

The metaphyseal vessels originate from the cervical ascending vessels and enter the bone close to the margin of the articular cartilage. The metaphyseal arteries may be divided into three groups: (1) dorsal, (2) ventral, and (3) cranial. The cranial group, the most numerous, is composed of three to five arteries. Apparently, no communication exists between the epiphyseal and the metaphyseal circulation in the immature dog. The ligament of the femoral head contains several small vessels throughout its length that terminate at the foveal attachment of the ligament without penetrating the bone.

Clinical Signs and Diagnosis

Patients with an intracapsular fracture of the proximal femur are usually presented to the veterinarian with a non-weight-bearing lameness. Examination of the coxofemoral joint elicits pain upon flexion, extension, and rotation. Bony crepitation may also be noted with manipulation of the coxofemoral joint. Patients with intracapsular fractures who sustain a mild degree of trauma may have a weight-bearing lameness and may exhibit only mild discomfort on examination of the coxofemoral joint. The definitive diagnosis of an intracapsular fracture of the proximal femur is confirmed by lateral and ventrodorsal radiographs.

Surgical Approach (Fig. 46-46)

A craniolateral approach or a trochanteric osteotomy may be used for exposure of the coxofemoral joint in the dog. Knowledge of the normal blood supply to the hip joint and preservation of the remaining arterial supply to the femoral head after trauma are important considerations for fracture healing. With a femoral capital physeal fracture, it is likely that severe trauma to the blood supply occurs at the time of fracture because the cervical ascending arteries cross the growth plate prior to entering the femoral head. Nevertheless, the veterinary surgeon must exercise care not to compromise the vasculature further with surgical trauma.

Our studies of the normal blood supply to the canine hip joint indicate that either a craniolateral approach or a trochanteric osteotomy may be used for surgical exposure of the canine hip joint without producing severe trauma to the existing blood supply. The arterial supply to the femoral head after trauma may not be the only factor influencing the prognosis for healing. Experimental studies in animals and clinical studies in man indicate that anatomic reduction and rigid fixation are as important, if not more important, than the re-

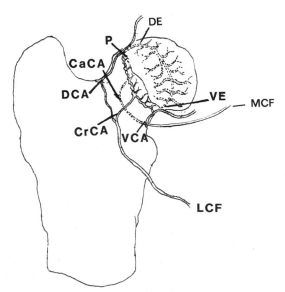

Fig. 46-45. *Diagrammatic representation of the normal blood supply to the femoral head in the immature dog. LCF, Lateral circumflex femoral artery; MCF, medial circumflex femoral artery; CrCA, cranial cervical ascending artery; DCA, dorsal cervical ascending artery; CaCA, caudal cervical ascending artery; VCA, ventral cervical ascending artery; DE, dorsal epiphyseal artery; VE, ventral epiphyseal artery; P, physis.*

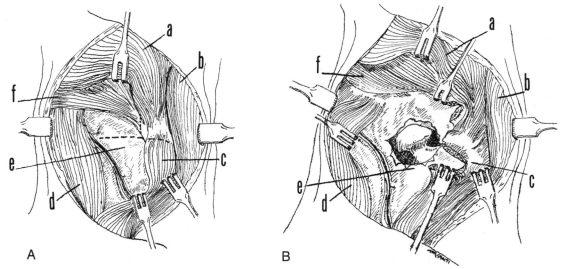

Fig. 46-46. A *and* B, *Diagrammatic representation of exposure to the hip joint through a craniolateral approach. a, Middle gluteal muscle; b, biceps femoris muscle; c, vastus lateralis muscle; d, rectus femoris muscle; e, joint capsule; f, deep gluteal muscle.*

maining blood supply to the femoral head at the time of the surgical procedure. Therefore, the surgeon should initially approach the coxofemoral joint through a craniolateral exposure and should stabilize the fracture if anatomic reduction and rigid fixation can be accomplished. If anatomic reduction or fixation is difficult through the craniolateral exposure, a trochanteric osteotomy should be performed to allow greater visualization of the fracture site. The important concepts in the management of intracapsular fractures of the proximal femur are gentle atraumatic technique and adequate exposure of the fracture site to achieve anatomic reduction and rigid fixation of the fracture.

Surgical Techniques

The veterinary surgeon is referred to the section of Chapter 45 on acetabular fractures for a description of the technique for osteotomy of the greater trochanter. The craniolateral approach to the hip joint is begun with a skin incision centered at the level of the greater trochanter passing over the cranial border of the greater trochanter and shaft of the femur. Proximally, the incision begins 3 to 4 cm from the dorsal midline and extends distally one-third the length of the femur. The subcutaneous tissue is incised along the same line, and the skin edges are toweled in to reduce bacterial contamination. The incision is carried through the superficial and deep layers of the fascia lata along the cranial edge of the biceps femoris muscle and superficial gluteal muscle. This allows caudal retraction of the biceps femoris and superficial gluteal muscles. The tensor fasciae latae muscle is separated from the border of the middle gluteal muscle; this maneuver allows proximal retraction of the middle gluteal muscle and visualization of the deep gluteal muscle. The deep gluteal muscle may be undermined and retracted dorsally, or a partial tendonotomy of its insertion may be performed to facilitate dorsal retraction of the muscle.

At this point, the joint capsule may be noted to be torn, and the femoral neck may be displaced craniodorsally through the torn capsule. If the joint capsule is not torn, an incision is made through it, following the longitudinal axis of the femoral neck. Fibrin and blood clots are then gently removed to expose the fracture surfaces. Reduction and stabilization of the fracture are now accomplished. If the veterinary surgeon encounters difficulty with reduction, an osteotomy of the greater trochanter is performed to allow increased visualization and ease of reduction. The technique for stabilization should provide rigid fixation, which can be achieved with multiple Kirschner wires or by the lag screw principle.

REPAIR OF CAPITAL PHYSEAL FRACTURES (FIG. 46-47)

With capital physeal fractures, multiple Kirschner wires or a lag screw may be used for stabilization. Kirschner wires are preplaced in the femoral neck by driving the pins from the fracture line laterally or from the greater trochanter toward the fracture line. The pins should be placed at different angles in a triangular pattern for increased rigidity. Reduction of the fracture is accomplished by exerting ventral and caudal traction on the femoral shaft and by stabilizing the femoral head with a Lewin clamp. With the fracture in exact anatomic reduction, the Kirschner wires are driven into the femoral head. Care must be taken not to penetrate the articular surface of the femoral head. This maneuver can be accomplished by measuring the depth of the femoral head on the preoperative radiograph and by using this measurement as a guide for the depth of pin penetration into the femoral head.

If a lag screw is used for stabilization of a capital physeal fracture, the principles outlined to achieve compression with screw fixation must be followed. To

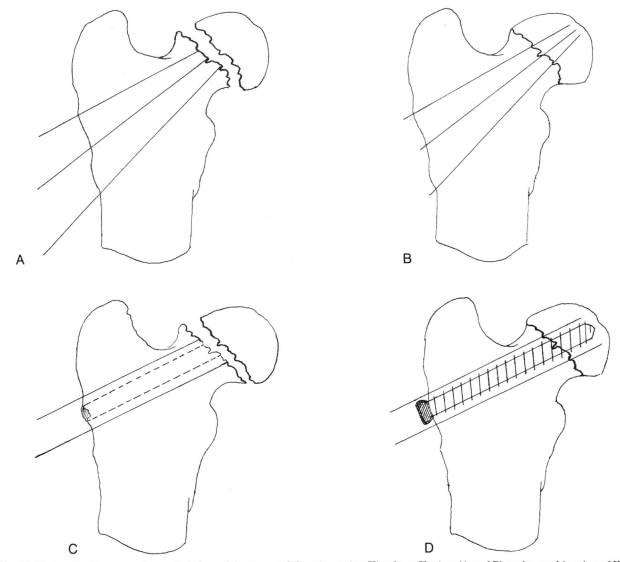

Fig. 46-47. *A to D, Diagrams of a capital physeal fracture stabilization using Kirschner K wires (A and B) and a combination of Kirschner wires and a compression screw (C and D). See text for details.*

achieve compression with a cortical screw, the veterinary surgeon must overdrill the femoral neck so that the threads of the screw do not purchase within the femoral neck. The veterinary surgeon may use a special drill guide or may drill from the fracture surface of the femoral neck toward the trochanter to ensure proper placement of the glide drill hole in the center of the femoral neck. At this point, a Kirschner wire is preplaced above and below the glide drill hole in the femoral neck. Care is taken to make sure that the Kirschner wires will not interfere with the screw placement through the femoral head and neck. The fracture is now anatomically reduced using the techniques described, and the preplaced Kirschner wires are driven into the femoral head.

Reduction of the fracture is checked, and if satisfactory, the femoral head is drilled with the proper-sized drill bit. A drill sleeve is inserted into the glide hole through the femoral neck to ensure proper positioning of the drill hole in the femoral head. A depth gauge is inserted to measure the proper screw length to be used, and the drill hole is tapped to receive the screw. The screw length should be 2 mm shorter than that measured by the depth gauge, to prevent penetration of the articular surface by the screw point. As the screw is tightened, the veterinary surgeon will note compression of the fracture line.

REPAIR OF AVULSION FRACTURES OF

THE FEMORAL HEAD

Trauma causing a coxofemoral luxation results in failure of the ligament of the head of the femur. In the majority of patients, the failure is within the ligament itself, but occasionally, a bone-ligament failure occurs. In such a case, a piece of bone from the ligament insertion on the femoral head is avulsed. The size of the bone chip is variable, but must be removed surgically along with the remnants of the ligament. The avulsed piece of bone originates from a non-weight-bearing surface, and its removal does not result in degenerative joint disease. The surgical exposure is accomplished with one of the techniques described. Methods for stabilizing the coxofemoral articulation may be found in the second section of this chapter, on coxofemoral luxations.

REPAIR OF SUBCAPITAL FRACTURES

This type of injury is not common, but does occur in mature dogs and cats. Surgical intervention with reduction and stabilization of the fracture is the treatment of choice. Excision arthroplasty may be used to treat small dogs and cats, but it should not be used in large or giant breeds of dogs. The surgical exposure is accomplished with a craniolateral approach, as previously described. If reduction is difficult through the exposure, an osteotomy of the greater trochanter can be used to facilitate visualization and reduction. Stabilization is best accomplished with a combination of Kirschner wires and a compression screw.

SURGICAL CLOSURE FOR THE CRANIOLATERAL APPROACH

With the fracture stabilized, the veterinary surgeon should flush the site with sterile saline solution to remove blood clots and debris from within the joint. The joint capsule is sutured using a simple interrupted pattern. If a partial tendonotomy of the deep gluteal muscle is performed, the tendon should be sutured with nonabsorbable material, using a cruciate suture pattern. The tensor fasciae latae and biceps femoris muscles are sutured with a continuous suture pattern; the subcutaneous tissue and skin are sutured by standard methods.

REPAIR OF EXTRACAPSULAR FRACTURES OF THE PROXIMAL FEMUR (FIG. 46-48)

Peritrochanteric and subtrochanteric fractures are discussed within the final section of this chapter, on fractures of the femur. Lateral fractures of the femoral neck occur in both mature and immature dogs and cats. The vascular supply to the hip joint is not compromised with extracapsular fractures to the degree seen with intracapsular fractures. Knowledge of the vascular anatomy and gentle, atraumatic surgical techniques are necessary to prevent iatrogenic vascular compromise and osteonecrosis of the femoral neck. The fracture is exposed through the craniolateral approach described previously. Exposure may be further increased by ventral reflection of vastus lateralis muscle. Stabilization is best achieved with a compression screw and Kirschner wires.

Postoperative Care

Strict confinement is recommended for the first 3 weeks postoperatively. After this time, exercise can be increased gradually. Even at this stage, the patient should be exercised with a leash and should not be allowed free activity. Normal activity cannot be instituted until radiographic healing of the fracture is confirmed. The majority of these fractures heal in a 4- to 7-week period. The screw or Kirschner wires should be removed 4 to 6 months after radiographic healing is confirmed.

References and Suggested Readings

Archibald, J. (ed.): Canine Surgery. Santa Barbara, CA, American Veterinary Publications, 1974.

Arnoldi, C. C.: Intraosseous pressures in patients with different types of fracture of the femoral neck. Angiology, *21*:403, 1970.

Arnoldi, C. C., and Lemperg, R. K.: Fracture of the femoral neck. Clin. Orthop., *129*:217, 1977.

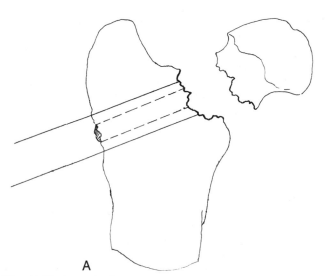

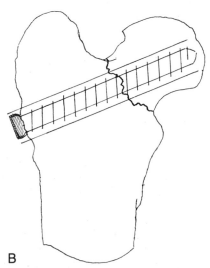

Fig. 46-48. A *and* B, *Diagram of a lateral femoral neck fracture using Kirschner wires and a compression screw. See text for details.*

Arnoldi, C. C., and Linderholm, H.: Fracture of the femoral neck. Clin. Orthop., *84*:116, 1972.

Aron, D. N., et al.: A review of reduction and internal fixation of proximal femoral fractures in the dog and man. J. Am. Anim. Hosp. Assoc., *15*:455, 1979.

Aune, S.: The early assessment of femoral head viability in cases of fracture of the neck of the femur. Anan method. Acta Chir. Scand., *135*:205, 1969.

Bojrab, M. J. (ed.): Current Techniques in Small Animal Surgery. Philadelphia, Lea & Febiger, 1975.

Clanton, T. O., et al.: Knee ligament injuries in children. J. Bone Joint Surg., *61*, 1979.

Daly, W. R.: Femoral head and neck fractures in the dog and cat: a review of 115 cases. Vet. Surg., *1*:29, 1978.

D'ambrosia, R. D., et al.: Vascularity of the femoral head. Clin. Orthop., *121*:143, 1976.

Glincher, M. J., and Kenzora, J. E.: The biology of osteonecrosis of the human femoral head and its clinical implications. Clin. Orthop., *140*:273, 1979.

Gorden, L. S.: Malreduction and avascular necrosis in subcapital fractures of the femur. J. Bone Joint Surg., *53*:183, 1971.

Hulse, D. A., et al.: Use of the lag screw principle for stabilization of femoral neck and femoral capital epiphyseal fractures. J. Am. Anim. Hosp. Assoc., *10*:29, 1974.

Hulth, A., and Johannson, S. G.: Femoral-head venography in the prognosis of fractures of the femoral neck. Acta Chir. Scand., *123*:287, 1962.

Johnson, J. H., and Crothers, O.: Revascularization of the femoral head. Clin. Orthop., *114*:364, 1976.

Mussbuchler, H.: Arteriographic studies in fractures of the femoral neck and trochanteric region. Type and incidence of findings in pre and post operative examinations, relation to fracture dislocation and prognostic value. Angiology, *21*:385, 1970.

Nunamaker, D. M.: Repair of femoral head and neck fractures by interfragmentary compression. J. Am. Vet. Med. Assoc., *162*:569, 1973.

Rhinelander, F. W., et al.: Bone vascular supply. *In* Skeletal Research: An Experimental Approach. Edited by D. J. Simmons and A. S. Kukin. New York, Academic Press, 1979.

Rivera, L. A.: Master's Thesis, Department of Veterinary Anatomy, School of Veterinary Medicine, Louisiana State University, 1979.

Ross, P. M., et al.: Slipped capital femoral epiphysis long-term results after 10–38 years. Clin. Orthop., *141*:176, 1979.

Salter, R. B.: Textbook of Disorders and Injuries of the Musculoskeletal System. Baltimore, Williams & Wilkins, 1970.

Schlonsky, J.: Radioisotope scanning of bone. A review of the literature. Ohio State Med. J., *68*:128, 1972.

Shoji, H., et al.: Scintimetry of intracapsular fracture of the hip: a preliminary report. Clin. Orthop., *86*:85, 1972.

Simon, W. H., and Wyman, E. T.: Femoral neck fractures. Clin. Orthop., *70*:152, 1970.

Caudal Cruciate Ligament Injuries

by ERICK L. EGGER

The caudal cruciate ligament provides much of the stability necessary for normal stifle function. Because of the relatively large size and position of this ligament within the joint, injury is usually caused only by severe trauma. Concurrent injury of associated supporting structures and even fractures are common; these complications make diagnosis and treatment of caudal cruciate ligament disorders challenging.

Anatomic and Physiologic Features

The caudal cruciate ligament originates in a fossa on the lateral aspect of the medial femoral condyle at the cranial limit of the intercondylar groove. It passes medial to the cranial cruciate ligament caudodistally to insert on the lateral edge of the popliteal notch of the tibia.[4] As the ligament passes through the joint, it is ensheathed in a fold of synovium. Like the cranial cruciate ligament, the caudal cruciate ligament is actually composed of two distinct fiber bundles, the cranial bulk and the caudal band. These bundles slide and twist around each other to provide support in both flexion and extension.[1,5]

The stabilizing influence of the caudal cruciate ligament has been determined by selectively cutting it or the associated supporting structures and stressing the joint. This ligament acts mainly to limit caudal subluxation of the tibia relative to the femur. This caudal movement becomes more apparent as the joint is flexed and is absent in complete extension. Rotational stability is also provided by the caudal cruciate ligament, particularly in flexion, as evidenced by the increase of up to 45° of internal rotation when this ligament is cut. With the ligament cut, the fully extended stifle has normal rotational and caudal stability. Cutting either the medial or the lateral collateral ligament causes a loss of this stability; this finding indicates that, at full extension, the collateral ligaments stabilize the joint. The influence of the collateral ligaments decreases as the joint is flexed because the lateral collateral ligament becomes loose.

Mechanism and Diagnosis of Injury

The caudal cruciate ligament can be injured in one of two manners. A caudally directed blow to the tibial crest with the stifle in flexion causes an isolated injury. If the stifle is in extension, one of the collateral ligaments must also yield if the caudal cruciate ligament is to give way. A severe rotational force can also injure the caudal cruciate ligament, particularly in stifle flexion.

Diagnosis of disruption of the caudal cruciate ligament can be challenging. When the ligament is disrupted and the joint is held at normal walking angles, the caudal thigh muscles pull the tibia into a caudal subluxated position (Fig. 46-49). Stressing the joint by palpation forces the tibia forward to its normal position. This movement resembles the "cranial drawer motion" that characterizes rupture of the cranial cruciate ligament. Injuries of the caudal cruciate ligament are frequently misdiagnosed as those of the cranial cruciate ligament for that reason. The two injuries can be differentiated by palpating for drawer motion in both flexion and extension. The disrupted cranial cruciate ligament reveals a positive drawer motion in both flexion and extension. The disrupted caudal cruciate ligament, on the other hand, shows drawer motion in flexion, but not in extension. A lateral radiograph of the flexed stifle confirms an injury to the caudal cruciate

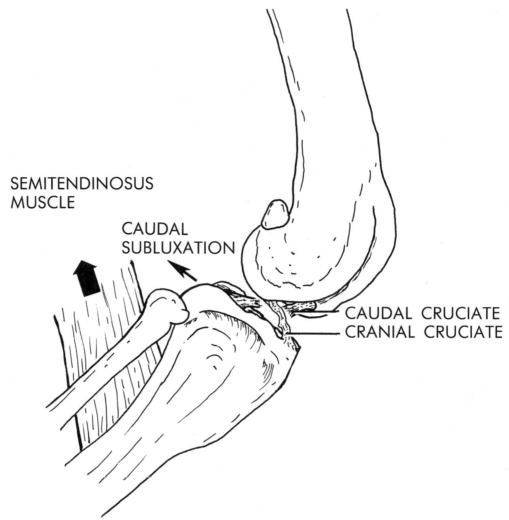

SEMITENDINOSUS
MUSCLE

CAUDAL
SUBLUXATION

CAUDAL CRUCIATE
CRANIAL CRUCIATE

Fig. 46-49. *Depiction of caudal cruciate ligament disruption with semitendinosus muscle pull resulting in caudal subluxation and loosening of the cranial cruciate ligament. (Modified from an illustration by Dean W. Biechler.)*

ligament by revealing caudal displacement of the tibia when compared to a radiograph of the normal joint.

The diagnosis of an injury of the caudal cruciate ligament is often complicated by the presence of other traumatic injuries. Concurrent disruption of one of the collateral ligaments, as evidenced by medial or lateral angular instability, is common. This disruption makes the differentiation of cranial from caudal cruciate ligament rupture difficult because drawer motion is apparent in both extension and flexion. An injury of the caudal cruciate ligament in the presence of a femur or tibia fracture often goes unnoticed on physical examination. This finding emphasizes the importance of palpating the integrity of the stifle joint after fixation of nearby fractures.

The injury to the caudal cruciate ligament can take one of three forms. If the animal is young, so that the ligament is stronger than the bone, an avulsion fracture of the ligament's bony attachment can be seen. In humans, this avulsion is usually of the tibial attachment; however, the veterinary literature and personal experience have revealed only the occurrence of femoral

avulsions. A total rupture of the caudal cruciate ligament can occur with an obvious disruption of the ligament and fraying of the ends that are apparent when surgically examined. A partial rupture, usually of the cranial bulk, with stretching of the remaining ligament can occur. Because the synovial sheath usually does not rupture, it may appear, surgically, to be intact. If, however, the cranial cruciate ligament is observed while the joint is manipulated, the synovial sheath can be seen to go taut and lax as the tibia subluxates back and forth.

Surgical Treatment

The ideal treatment for injuries of the caudal cruciate ligament would provide normal stability without limiting the normal angular and rotational range of motion. Except for avulsion fractures, a totally satisfactory treatment has not been developed. This discussion mentions the methods that have been explored and describes the surgical techniques that have shown clinical usefulness.

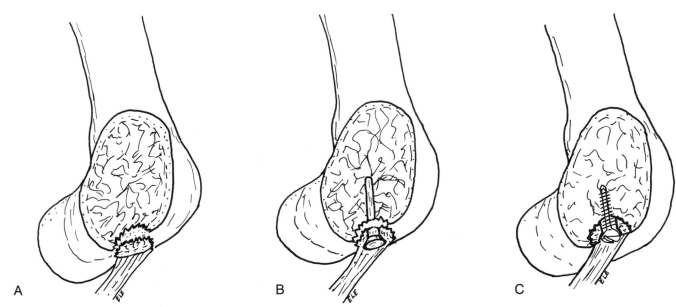

Fig. 46-50. *Fixation of caudal cruciate ligament avulsion with an interfragmentary screw. A, Avulsion fracture of the caudal cruciate ligament's femoral attachment (lateral condyle removed for illustration). B, The screw hole is drilled; the hole in the fragment is overdrilled and countersunk. C, The screw is applied, resulting in lag-type compression of the fracture.*

Avulsion fractures of the bony attachment of the caudal cruciate ligament are best treated by reattachment of the fractured fragment. If the patient and the fragment are large enough, this fixation can be achieved with an interfragmentary bone screw.[7] This screw should be applied in a lag fashion by overdrilling the fragment hole to the outside diameter of the screw threads or by using a partially threaded screw (Fig. 46-50). The fragment hole should be countersunk to allow adequate seating of the screw head and to reduce the chance of the fragment splitting.

If the patient or the fragment is too small to use screw fixation, the fragment can be fixed in reduction with Kirschner wires. Three small Kirschner wires are driven through the fragment at divergent angles to achieve triangulation. The wires should be cut off and driven in to lie flush with the bony surface (Fig. 46-51).

Rupture of the caudal cruciate ligament presents a different problem. Primary repair of the ligament has not proved to be a practical approach in dogs and cats. The complete synovial ensheathement leads to poor healing as a result of the limited blood supply. Furthermore, the frayed ligament ends are difficult to suture securely.

Some authors have elected not to treat this rupture surgically, but rather rely on development of fibrosis to stabilize the stifle joint.[6] One problem with this approach is frequent damage to associated structures, such as collateral ligaments or menisci, which requires surgical attention. Another concern is that the biomechanics of the joint dictate that the stifle caudally subluxates and then reduces each time the joint is put through its range of motion. Experimental transection of the caudal cruciate ligament without surgical stabilization in a group of 4 dogs resulted in slowly progressive osteoarthritic changes and restriction in range of

motion, with clinical drawer motion still apparent over a 4-month study.[3]

Extracapsular tightening procedures, using either imbrication sutures or fascial grafts, have been described.[2] Such an approach has been used in cats by placing 2 large horizontal mattress sutures of 1-0 monofilament polypropylene from the proximal patella to the fibular head laterally and to the fascia of the caudomedial tibial prominence on the medial aspect of the

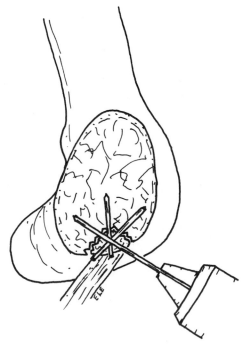

Fig. 46-51. *Fixation of caudal cruciate ligament avulsion by triangulating with Kirschner wires.*

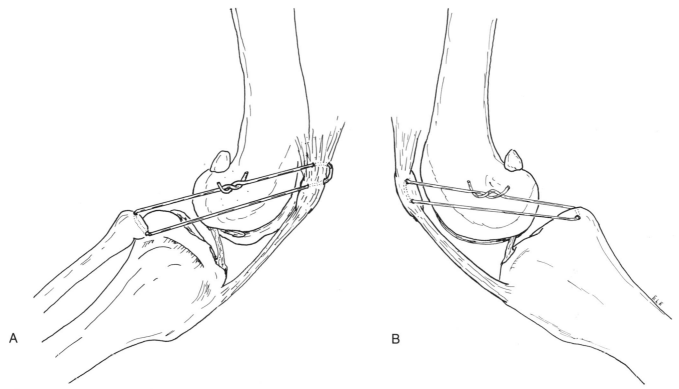

Fig. 46-52. *Extracapsular imbrication for stabilizing a ruptured caudal cruciate ligament. A, A lateral mattress suture runs from the proximal patella to the fibular head. (Modified from an illustration by Dean W. Biechler.) B, A similar medial suture runs from the patella to the caudomedial edge of the tibia.*

joint (Fig. 46-52). Postoperative stability and clinical leg use were satisfactory; however, 3-month rechecks found recurrence of the drawer motion and the presence of mild crepitus.[3] This technique was attempted on several large dogs using No. 2 polypropylene suture, but stifle stabilization could not be obtained without severe alteration of the femoral-patellar articulation.[3]

A "reverse Paatsama" procedure to replace the caudal cruciate ligament was experimentally evaluated (Fig. 46-53). A graft of fascia lata, patellar tendon, or long digital extensor tendon was used. Although stabilization could be obtained at the time of operation, clinical drawer motion was present within a few days, and secondary osteoarthritis soon became apparent.[3] This complication probably resulted from stretching of the graft due both to chronic muscle pull and to the difficulty in placing the graft in the correct functional position.

The current methods of stifle stabilization following rupture of the caudal cruciate ligament provide craniocaudal stability at the expense of some reduction in normal rotation.[3] By trapping its distal third behind a bone screw placed in the caudomedial corner of the tibial plateau, the medial collateral ligament is redirected to parallel the caudal cruciate ligament (Fig. 46-54).

The long digital extensor tendon is used in a similar manner in the lateral aspect of the fibular head, and a screw is placed just cranial to the femoral attachment

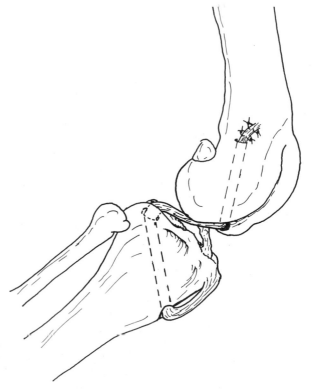

Fig. 46-53. *A "reverse Paatsama" technique for replacing a ruptured caudal cruciate ligament. Experimental trials were unsuccessful. (Modified from an illustration by Dean W. Biechler.)*

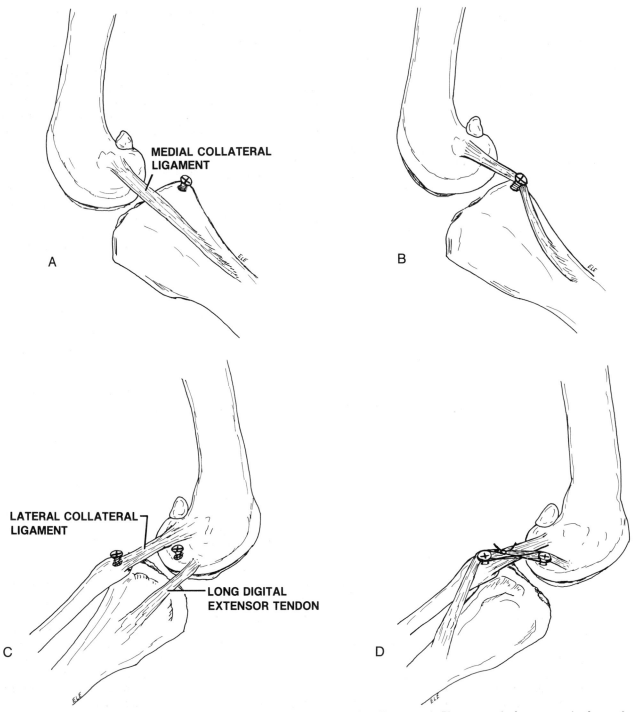

Fig. 46-54. *The current technique for treating a rupture of the caudal cruciate ligament. A, Placement of a bone screw in the caudomedial corner of the proximal tibia. B, Trapping the medial collateral ligament "behind" the bone screw. C, Placement of bone screws in the fibular head and midway between the long digital extensor origin and the proximal attachment of the lateral collateral ligament. D, Trapping the long digital extensor tendon "behind" the bone screws and stabilizing it with a figure-8 suture over the screw heads.*

of the lateral collateral ligament. A figure-8 suture of No. 2 polypropylene is placed between the 2 screws to provide additional immediate support. This method has the advantage of being simple, yet it can easily be modified to include the repair of other injuries that are commonly present. Following the operation, the patient's leg is placed in a heavy, padded bandaged (Robert Jones dressing) for 3 or 4 days to control swelling. A caudal splint, fashioned of plaster or Hexcelite* in a padded bandage, is applied and is maintained for approximately 6 weeks while the fibrous tissues heal.

* Hexcel Medical Products, 11711 Dublin Boulevard, Dublin, CA 94566

References and Suggested Readings

1. Arnoczky, S. P., and Marshall, J. L.: The cruciate ligaments of the canine stifle: an anatomical and functional analysis. Am. J. Vet. Res., *38:*1807, 1977.
2. DeAngelis, M. P., and Betts, C. W.: Posterior cruciate ligament rupture. J. Am. Anim. Hosp. Assoc., *9:*447, 1973.
3. Egger, E. L., Rigg, D. L., and Hoefle, W.: Experimental and clinical evaluation of posterior cruciate ligament repairs. Unpublished work, 1978 to 1980.
4. Evans, H. E., and Christensen, G. C.: Miller's Anatomy of the Dog. 2nd Ed. Philadelphia, W. B. Saunders, 1979.
5. Girgis, E. G., Marshall, J. L., and Monajem, A. L.: The cruciate ligaments of the knee joint: anatomical, functional, and experimental analysis. Clin. Orthop., *106:*216, 1975.
6. Hohn, B. R., and Newton, C. D.: Surgical repair of ligamentous structures of the stifle joint. *In* Current Techniques in Small Animal Surgery. Edited by M. J. Bojrab. Philadelphia, Lea & Febiger, 1975.
7. Knecht, C. D., Crise, R., and Cechner, P. E.: Repair of avulsion of the caudal cruciate ligament in a dog using a bone screw. J. Am. Anim. Hosp. Assoc., *12:*784, 1976.

Cranial Cruciate Ligament Repair

by STEVEN P. ARNOCZKY

Surgical repair of the cranial cruciate ligament has undergone considerable development in the past 25 years,[7] and a comprehensive review[7-10] of the techniques and materials used for the repair and reconstruction of the ligament can leave one bewildered and confused. Although the surgical procedures may vary, the basic principle of repair remains the same, the reestablishment of joint stability.

Pathophysiology

The cranial cruciate ligament functions to constrain joint motion.[3] It prevents cranial subluxation of the tibia on the femur (cranial drawer sign), hyperextension of the stifle joint, and along with the caudal cruciate ligament, excessive internal rotation of the tibia on the femur.[3] Excessive forces during extremes of any of these movements damage this ligament.[1,2] Although excessive trauma causes acute rupture of the cranial cruciate ligament, it is thought that the majority of cruciate ligament lesions are a result of chronic degenerative changes within the ligaments themselves.[1,2] Variations in conformation, valgus (knock-knee) and varus (bowleg) deformities of the stifle, and repeated minor stresses can result in progressive degenerative joint disease. As these joint changes develop, the cruciate ligaments undergo alterations in their microstructure and may be more susceptible to damage from minor trauma.

Surgical Techniques

It is well established that rupture of the cranial cruciate ligament results in progressive degenerative changes within the joint.[2] For this reason, most such injuries should be repaired. In some chronic conditions of cranial cruciate ligament rupture, however, severe degenerative joint changes may dictate a less-favorable prognosis following surgical repair. In these patients, conservative management with anti-inflammatory drugs and somatic pain relievers may provide adequate palliative care. Moreover, concurrent joint disease, such as rheumatoid arthritis and systemic lupus erythematosus, may obviate the repair of the ligament insufficiency.

As noted previously, many techniques are described for the repair of cranial cruciate ligament rupture. It has been my experience, however, that no one technique produces consistently good results in all sizes and breeds of dogs. The following procedures have shown to be consistently effective in the repair of cranial cruciate ligament insufficiency in the specified cases.

LATERAL RETINACULAR IMBRICATION

This *extra-articular* repair "stabilizes" the joint by altering (tightening) extra-articular tissues.[6] Although such a repair does alter normal joint motion,[5] it is well tolerated in dogs weighing up to 15 kg and provides excellent joint stability.

The animal is placed in lateral recumbency, and the affected limb is routinely prepared for an aseptic surgical procedure. The joint is approached through a routine lateral arthrotomy and is inspected thoroughly for additional pathologic features, such as meniscal tear. The remnants of the ruptured ligament should then be removed, and the joint should be thoroughly irrigated with lactated Ringer's or saline solution.

A single mattress suture of heavy (No. 1 or 2) Teflon-impregnated Dacron* is placed on the lateral aspect of the joint, to prevent the excessive internal rotation of the tibia on the femur as well as the cranial subluxation of the tibia on the femur associated with cranial cruciate ligament insufficiency. The skin and subcutaneous tissues are retracted caudolaterally, and the lateral fabella is located by palpation.

The suture material is passed behind the lateral fabella and into the dense connective tissue surrounding it (Fig. 46-55A). The suture is then directed craniodistally, where it is passed into the lateral third of the patellar ligament just proximal to its insertion on the tibial tuberosity. The suture material is then reinserted into the ligament about 3 mm from its point of emergence and is directed so as to exit near the original point of entry (Fig. 46-55B). The limb is then placed in a functional position, and the suture is tightened (Fig. 46-55C). This suture should eliminate the drawer movement completely. If a slight cranial drawer movement is still present, an additional mattress suture, placed parallel and as close as possible to the first suture, can be used to eliminate the remaining drawer movement. If appreciable drawer movement exists after placement of the first suture, the suture should be

* Polydek, Deknatel Inc., 110 Jericho Turnpike, Floral Park, NY 11001

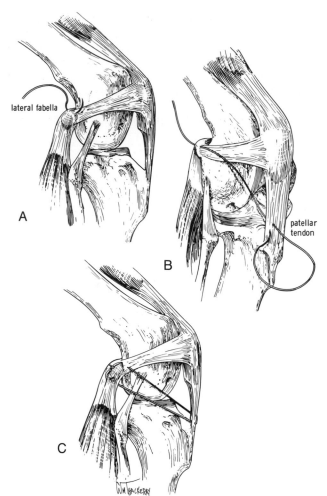

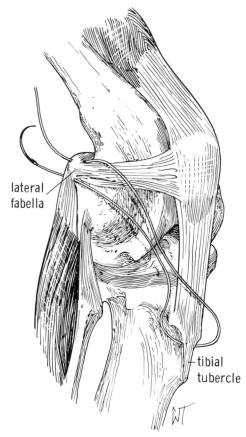

Fig. 46-56. *The lateral imbrication suture can also be placed through a drill hole in the tibial crest. (From Arnoczky, S. P.: Surgery of the stifle: the cruciate ligaments. Compend. Contin. Ed. Practicing Vet., 2:106, 1980.)*

Fig. 46-55. *Lateral retinacular imbrication. A, Placement of imbrication suture in the connective tissue surrounding the lateral fabella. B, The suture is directed craniodistally and into the lateral third of the patella just proximal to the tibial tuberosity. See text for details. C, The suture is passed into the connective tissue caudoventral to the lateral fabella and is tied with the limb in a functional position. (From Arnoczky, S. P.: Surgery of the stifle: the cruciate ligaments. Compend. Contin. Ed. Practicing Vet., 2:106, 1980.)*

removed and replaced. It should be noted that the fibular nerve passes caudally to the lateral fabella, and appropriate caution should be used when placing the suture in this area.

If the patellar ligament is damaged or for some reason does not support the imbrication suture, a drill hole can be placed in the proximal aspect of the tibial crest, and the suture can be passed through it (Fig. 46-56). The arthrotomy, subcutaneous tissues, and skin are closed in a routine manner.

Postoperatively, the limb is placed in a soft, padded bandage for 2 weeks, and the animal's activity is restricted for a total of 4 weeks. Although the confined activity during this period allows the operated tissues to heal, it also serves to limit the stresses on the weight-bearing unoperated leg. In the case of degenerative cruciate lesions, it is not uncommon for the cranial cruciate ligament of the opposite limb to rupture,

owing to the additional forces placed on the "normal" stifle by an altered gait and weight-bearing.

"OVER-THE-TOP" REPAIR

This *intra-articular* repair anatomically replaces the cranial cruciate ligament with a patellar tendon graft.[4] This procedure was designed for use in dogs weighing more than 15 kg. In my experience, most extra-articular repairs do not produce long-term joint stability in the larger dogs. The over-the-top technique provides a functional replacement for the cranial cruciate ligament and thereby limits any abnormal joint motion.

The animal is placed in lateral recumbency, and the affected limb is routinely prepared for an aseptic surgical procedure. A lateral parapatellar incision extends from the midshaft of the femur to the proximal tibia. The subcutaneous and fascial tissues are dissected free, and the patellar ligament is clearly defined. The patellar ligament is incised longitudinally between the junction of the middle and medial thirds of its width. The incision is extended over the patella and into the patellar tendon, where it is directed in a proximal lateral direction to incorporate the fascia lata (Fig. 46-57A). The incision proximal to the patella should be made 1 to 1.5 times the distance from the patella to the tibial tuberosity (Fig. 46-57A); this incision ensures an adequate length of graft in dogs of all sizes.

An osteotome is then placed in the groove of the patella created by the scalpel blade, and a craniomedial wedge of bone is removed, with the medial third of the patellar tendon and ligament attached (Fig. 46-57B). Extreme care should be taken during the osteotomy to preserve the entire articular surface of the patella. The medial third of the patellar ligament is then dissected free to the level of the tibial tuberosity. An incision through the infrapatellar fat pad is necessary to mobilize the graft, but the fat pad should not be stripped from its ligamentous attachments because it provides much of the blood supply to the patellar ligament. An incision extending proximally and parallel to the initial

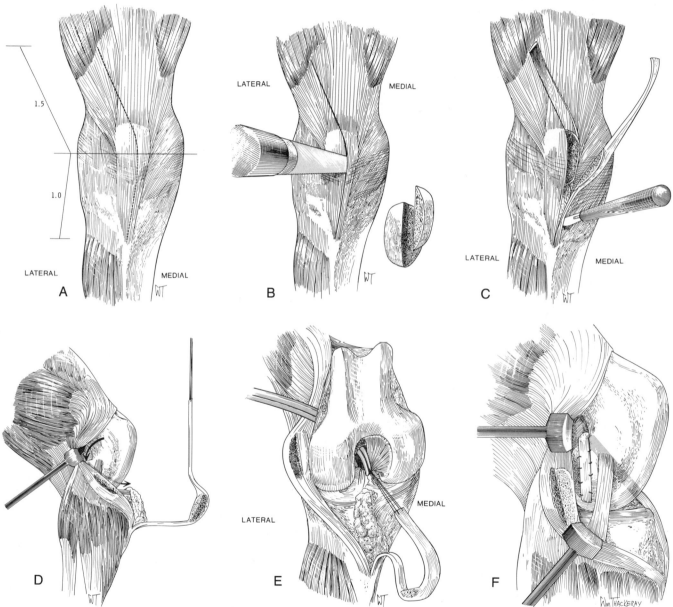

Fig. 46-57. *Over-the-top repair technique. A, Cranial view of the stifle showing the location of the initial incision for the proposed graft. Note that the proximal portion of the incision is directed laterally to incorporate the fascia lata. B, Placement of the osteotome to remove the craniomedial wedge of patella with accompanying soft tissue. (Inset), cranial view of the patella showing the extent of the osteotomy. Note that the osteotomy does not extend to the caudal articular surface of the patella. C, The graft is completed by incising the joint capsule, patellar tendon, and fascia lata parallel to the initial incision and by freeing the graft at its proximal end. D, Lateral view of the stifle showing retraction of the patella and soft tissues of the joint laterally to expose the lateral femoral condyle and fabella. Arrows indicate the path of the hemostatic forceps over the top of the lateral femoral condyle and into the joint. E, Cranial view of flexed stifle showing tips of the hemostatic forceps emerging lateral to the caudal cruciate ligament and grasping the sutures in the free end of the graft. F, Lateral view of the stifle showing the graft passing through the joint and over the top of the lateral femoral condyle. The graft is then sutured to the soft tissues of the lateral femoral condyle. (A to F, From Arnoczky, S. P., Tarvin, G. B., Marshall, J. L., and Saltzman, B.: The over-the-top procedure: a technique for anterior cruciate ligament substitution in the dog. J. Am. Anim. Hosp. Assoc., 15:283, 1979.)*

incision is then made in the joint capsule at the medial border of the patellar ligament, to free the proximal fascial portion of the graft. An autogenous graft consisting of fascia, patellar tendon, patellar bone wedge, and patellar ligament with a distal attachment to the tibial tuberosity is thus created (Fig. 46-57C).

The remnants of the ruptured cranial cruciate ligament are then removed through the medial arthrotomy, and the joint is inspected for further disease. The patella, joint capsule, and soft tissues are then retracted laterally to expose the lateral femoral condyle and fabella (Fig. 46-57D). The lateral fabella is located by palpation, and a small vertical incision is made in the femoral-fabellar ligament. With the joint in extreme flexion, curved hemostatic forceps are inserted into the incision and are passed over the top of the lateral femoral condyle and into the intercondylar notch; one must take care to preserve the caudal joint structures by staying close to the bone. The tips of the hemostatic forceps are gently manipulated until they can be seen within the joint (Fig. 46-57E). A Bunnel suture pattern of 3-0 stainless steel is placed in the free end of the graft, and the suture is grasped by the hemostat. The graft is gently pulled through the joint and over the top of the lateral condyle by gentle traction on the hemostat. Flexing and extending the joint during this maneuver facilitate the passage of the graft.

Once the graft has been pulled through the joint, it is held under gentle traction, and the joint is tested for craniocaudal stability. Once cranial drawer motion has been eliminated, the graft is attached to the lateral femoral condyle. With traction maintained and the leg held in a functional position (approximately 35 to 40° of flexion), the graft is sutured to the tissues of the lateral femoral condyle with simple interrupted sutures of 3-0 stainless steel (Fig. 46-57F). The incision in the femoral-fabellar ligament is also closed with simple interrupted sutures.

The arthrotomy is then closed in a routine manner. When closing the medial arthrotomy, the veterinary surgeon should take care to avoid excessive tension on the patella and patellar ligament, which may predispose the joint to a medial luxation of the patella. If tension is a problem, loose approximation sutures should be placed in the joint capsule, and the subcutaneous soft tissues should be used to cover the arthrotomy defect.

Postoperatively, the limb is placed in a modified Robert Jones dressing for 2 weeks and the animal's activity is restricted for a total of 4 weeks. In larger dogs (over 30 kg), a lateral plaster of Paris splint is added for the first 2 postoperative weeks, and activity is restricted for a total of 4 to 6 weeks.

In summary, successful repair of insufficiency of the cranial cruciate ligament is dependent upon the reestablishment of joint stability. Although this end can be accomplished by the aforementioned techniques, it must be stressed that other components of the stifle (patella, menisci, collateral ligaments) must not be overlooked when evaluating the joint. These structures work in concert to allow normal joint motion, and fail-ure to recognize concurrent patellar malalignment or meniscal injury in cranial cruciate ligament insufficiency may result in less than optimal postoperative function. The reader is therefore encouraged to refer to the other sections in this chapter relating to stifle surgery, in order to establish a comprehensive understanding of this complex joint.

References and Suggested Readings

1. Arnoczky, S. P.: Surgery of the stifle: the cruciate ligaments. Compend. Contin. Ed. Practicing Vet., 2:106, 1980.
2. Arnoczky, S. P., and Marshall, J. L.: Pathomechanics of cruciate and meniscal injuries. In Pathophysiology of Small Animal Surgery. Edited by M. J. Bojrab. Philadelphia, Lea & Febiger, 1981.
3. Arnoczky, S. P., and Marshall, J. L.: The cruciate ligaments of the canine stifle. An anatomical and functional analysis. Am. J. Vet. Res., 38:1807, 1977.
4. Arnoczky, S. P., Tarvin, G. B., Marshall, J. L., and Saltzman, B.: The over-the-top procedure: a technique for anterior cruciate ligament substitution in the dog. J. Am. Anim. Hosp. Assoc., 15:283, 1979.
5. Arnoczky, S. P., Torzilli, P. A., and Marshall, J. L.: Evaluation of anterior cruciate ligament repair in the dog. An analysis of the instant center of motion. J. Am. Anim. Hosp. Assoc., 13:553, 1977.
6. DeAngelis, M. P., and Lau, R. E.: A lateral retinacular imbrication technique for the surgical correction of anterior cruciate ligament rupture in the dog. J. Am. Vet. Med. Assoc., 157:79, 1970.
7. Knecht, C. D.: Evaluation of surgical techniques for cruciate ligament rupture in animals. J. Am. Anim. Hosp. Assoc., 12:717, 1976.
8. Rudy, R. L.: Stifle joint. In Canine Surgery. 2nd Ed. Edited by J. Archibald. Santa Barbara, CA, American Veterinary Publications, 1974.
9. Strande, A.: Repair of the Ruptured Cranial Cruciate Ligament in the Dog. Baltimore, Williams & Wilkins, 1967.
10. Whittick, W. G.: Canine Orthopedics. Philadelphia, Lea & Febiger, 1974.

Patellar Surgery

by Steven P. Arnoczky

and Guy B. Tarvin

Injuries and dysfunctions of the patella are frequent causes of rear limb lameness in small animals. Although medial patellar luxation and, to a lesser extent, lateral patellar luxation comprise the majority of patellar-associated lesions, fractures of the patella must also be considered in any discussion of patellar surgery.

Functional Anatomy

The patella can be described as the ossified portion of the quadriceps tendon. The patella itself is a passive structure in the body; however, it plays an important role in a dynamic system referred to as the extensor mechanism of the stifle. Movement of the patella is under direct influence of this mechanism, and knowledge of the mechanics of this system is essential in the treatment of dysfunctions of the patella.

The primary extensor group of muscles of the stifle is the quadriceps femoris.[5] Three of these four muscles, the vastus lateralis, the vastus medialis, and the vastus intermedius, originate from the proximal femur (the rectus femoris muscle originates from the ilium), and all four converge to form the quadriceps tendon.[5] This tendon primarily attaches to the proximal portion of the patella; however, a thin portion crosses over the cranial surface of the patella to blend with the patellar ligament.

The patellar ligament is a strong band of fibrous connective tissue that courses from the patella to the tibial tuberosity. When the quadriceps muscle group contracts, the resulting force pulls on the patella, the patellar ligament, and the tibial tuberosity and results in extension of the stifle. During this motion, the patella rides in the trochlear groove. A cross-section of the patella reveals a convex articular surface. The corresponding trochlear groove is concave and therefore allows for an intimate articulation between the femur and the patella. On either side of the patella and attached to the joint capsule are the parapatellar fibrocartilages. These structures articulate with the trochlear ridges and act to increase the surface area and thus to disperse the force of the quadriceps muscles.

Normal alignment of the extensor mechanism is necessary for stability of the stifle joint. Dysfunction of this mechanism results in abnormal joint mechanics and in joint instability.[1] Such instability not only causes degenerative joint disease, but also places increased stress on other supporting structures, such as the cranial cruciate ligament, the collateral ligaments, and the menisci.[13]

Repair of Patellar Luxation

MEDIAL PATELLAR LUXATION

Medial patellar luxation is one of the most common patellar problems presented to the veterinary practitioner.[7,13,15] This disorder can be either congenital or traumatic, with the congenital form more common. It is usually observed in small breed dogs[11] and may cause minimal to severe gait abnormalities. The clinical picture is often one of an obese animal with a varus (bow-legged) deformity of the rear limbs. The animal often crouches, owing to the inability to extend the stifles fully, with its toes pointed inward. Often, the owner describes a "skipping" or a "hopping" type of gait in which the animal skips one or more steps on the involved limb. This gait is usually transient and is caused by the patella's riding up and over the medial trochlear ridge and being "trapped" on the medial aspect of the joint. Medial patellar luxations, unless traumatic, rarely cause acute lameness. Although medial patellar luxations may be present in acute lameness, these luxations are usually chronic, and other causes of the lameness should be pursued. Those dogs with a history of patellar luxation and a sudden onset of pain in the siftle should be examined carefully to rule out cruciate ligament injury.

Various causes for congenital medial patellar luxation have been proposed.[8,9,12,13] The pathogenesis, however, is probably a combination of underlying bony abnormalities, any of which may be a cause or an effect of the disease. Any of the following abnormalities can result in congenital medial patellar luxation, but some degree of each deformity is probably present[12,13]: (1) coxa vara, (2) medial displacement of the quadriceps tendon, (3) external femoral torsion, (4) medial deviation of the distal femur, (5) shallow trochlear groove, and (6) internal rotation and medial deviation of the proximal tibia.

The presenting symptoms and signs of medial patellar luxation vary in severity, and therefore, each patient should be handled individually. Numerous methods exist for the repair of medial patellar luxation,[2,4,6,7,13-16] and a single technique does not work or is not indicated for all degrees of medial patellar luxation. The following discussion presents the treatment rationale that we advocate and that is based upon the grading system of Putnam.[12]

GRADE I. The stifle joint is almost normal, and the patella luxates only when the joint is extended and digital pressure is applied.

Animals with Grade I medial patellar luxation often have no clinical signs when presented. Indications for surgical treatment should be weighed carefully, because it is difficult to suggest operating on a clinically normal animal. That these asymptomatic animals may be prone to future ligamentous or bony abnormalities,[10] owing to the abnormal pull across the joint, may justify them as surgical candidates. It is our opinion, however, that these animals not be operated on until they become clinically symptomatic for the disease.

From the classification, the bony structures of the joint are nearly normal. This guideline suggests that the tibial tuberosity and the femoral trochlea are properly formed and have proper anatomic relationships within the joint. When surgical treatment is considered necessary, these two structures should be checked at the time of operation. A lateral parapatellar incision is made, and the extensor mechanism is visualized. Before opening the joint capsule, one should examine the alignment of the tibial tuberosity and the patella. These structures should be in a straight line parallel to the long axis of the limb when viewed from a craniocaudal direction. In Grade I medial patellar luxation, these structures usually line up well. The joint capsule is then opened, and the patella is retracted medially to permit visualization of the trochlear groove. The groove is examined for depth and any degenerative changes. If the groove is normal in appearance, no reconstructive procedures are needed.

In most cases of Grade I medial patellar luxation, the only requirement is the creation of a lateral restraint to prevent medial displacement of the patella. This restraint is accomplished by imbricating the lateral joint capsule with an interrupted Lembert suture pattern. In smaller animals (15 kg or less), 2-0 chromic gut is used, and in large animals, 1-0 chromic usually suffices. Another technique that has worked well is the use of a single suture of 1-0 or 2-0 nylon passed around the lateral fabella and through the quadriceps tendon just proximal to the patella. The suture is then directed distally along the medial border of the patella and is passed through the patellar ligament immediately distal to the patella. The suture is then tied on the lateral aspect of the joint and serves to restrict medial displacement of the patella. This technique works especially well in large dogs.[1]

The patella is now examined by placing a varus stress on the stifle and by internally rotating the tibia. If the patella does not luxate through a range of motion with the limb in this position and digital pressure applied to the patella, the repair is sufficient. If the patella still has a tendency to luxate, a medial releasing incision is performed by making a longitudinal parapatellar incision through the fibrous portion of the joint capsule. This incision is not closed. These procedures work well if the tibial tuberosity and femoral trochlea are normal. If these structures are abnormal, soft tissue procedures alone are not capable of overcoming the problem.

GRADE II. The patella usually lies in its normal position; however, it luxates upon flexion of the joint and remains luxated until relocated by manual pressure or extension of the joint.

These animals usually have some form of gait disturbance. Degenerative changes are more likely to develop, owing to the greater degree of malarticulation.

The tibial tuberosity and trochlear groove are evaluated as previously described. If the trochlear groove is shallow, it is corrected first. A trochleoplasty is performed by first making two parallel incisions into the trochlear cartilage with a scalpel blade. These incisions delineate the medial and lateral boundaries of the new trochlear groove. The groove should be wide enough to permit proper seating of the patella while maintaining an adequate lateral and, especially, medial trochlear ridge. The cartilage between the incisions is removed with a bone rongeur or a high-speed drill.[15] In younger dogs, the cartilage can easily be removed with a No. 15 scalpel blade. It is imperative that the groove be uniformly deepened to the level of bleeding subchondral bone to ensure the regeneration of fibrocartilage.[16] The new groove should be of sufficient width to accommodate the patella, it should have a well-developed medial ridge, and it should be of sufficient depth to discourage luxation (Fig. 46-58A).

If the tibial tuberosity is deviated medially, this deviation is corrected by transplanting the attachment of the patellar ligament to a more lateral position. This transplantation is done by osteotomy of the tibial tuberosity and lateral placement of the tuberosity under the cranial tibialis muscle.[2,6,7,13,14] The tibial tuberosity is then fixed in place by one or two small Kirschner wires (Fig. 46-58B and C). The patella is then tested in the previously described manner. Little, if any, tendency for luxation should be noted. If some tendency for medial luxation still exists, the tibial tuberosity can be moved farther laterally, or the joint capsule can be imbricated laterally. A medial releasing incision can be added if necessary (Fig. 46-58D and E).

GRADE III. The patella is luxated most of the time.

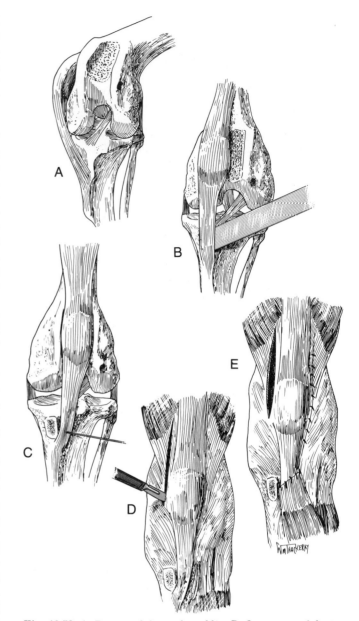

Fig. 46-58. A, *Regrooved femoral trochlea.* B, *Osteotomy of the tuberosity. Note that the fascial extension onto the tibial crest is left intact.* C, *Lateral transplantation and fixation of the tibial tuberosity with a Kirschner wire.* D, *Medial releasing incision.* E, *Lateral imbrication of the joint capsule.* (From Arnoczky, S. P., and Tarvin, G. B.: Surgery of the Stifle: the patella. Compend. Contin. Ed. Practicing Vet., 2:200, 1980.)

The patella may be reduced with the limb in the extended position.

All the techniques used in treating Grade II medial patellar luxations are probably needed to correct Grade III medial patellar luxation (Fig. 46-58). The same format for examining the structures should be followed to dictate the necessity of each procedure, however. If the tendency for luxation remains following correction with these techniques, it may be due to (1) an inadequate medial releasing incision or (2) a medial rotatory instability of the tibia. The medial re-

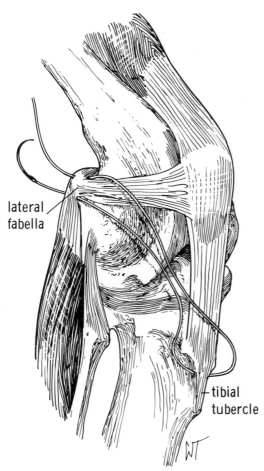

lateral
fabella

tibial
tubercle

Fig. 46-59. *Placement of the lateral derotational suture.* (*From Arnoczky, S. P., and Tarvin, G. B.: Surgery of the Stifle: the patella. Compend. Contin. Ed. Practicing Vet., 2:200, 1980.*)

leasing incision can be extended proximally to incise a portion of the sartorius and vastus medialis muscles. The rotational instability can be corrected with a lateral suture of heavy nonabsorbable material placed around the lateral fabella and through a drill hole in the tibial crest (Fig. 46-59). Usually, a combination of the aforementioned techniques corrects a Grade III medial patellar luxation.

GRADE IV. The patella is dislocated and cannot be reduced without surgical intervention.

This form of medial patellar luxation is the least common and should be corrected at an early age to prevent the resulting bony deformities of the femur and tibia. In most cases, the previously discussed techniques are inadequate to correct the disorder because of the severe bony deformities. These patients usually require osteotomies (derotational, cuneiform) of the tibia or femur to correct the anatomic structures and thereby the mechanics of the patella.[7,13]

LATERAL PATELLAR LUXATION

This problem is not as common as medial patellar luxation and is seen most often in the large breed dog.[7,13] The disorder may be congenital or traumatic in origin. In the congenital form, this condition is often associated with hip dysplasia or an isolated deformity such as genu valgum. The deformities causing lateral malalignment of the extensor mechanism are, for the most part, the opposite of those causing medial luxations: (1) coxa valga, (2) lateral displacement of the quadriceps tendon, (3) internal femoral torsion, (4) laxity of medial fascia and contraction of lateral fascia, and (5) external rotation and lateral deviation of the proximal tibia.

As in medial patellar luxation, the severity of the lesion varies widely. The animals usually have a valgus (knock-knee) deformity of the rear limbs and are first seen in a crouched stance with the toes pointing outward. Correction of this disorder is again based on the aforementioned grading system. In each case, the structures of the stifle are assessed and are corrected in the same stepwise manner as for medial patellar luxation. The obvious modifications to the procedures are: (1) *medial* imbrication, (2) *lateral* releasing incision, (3) *medial* transposition of the tibial tuberosity, and (4) *medial* derotational suture.

POSTOPERATIVE CARE

Postoperative considerations in both medial and lateral patellar luxations include a soft, padded bandage for 2 weeks and confined exercise for a minimum of 3 weeks. In the case of bilateral patellar luxations, the most severely affected limb is usually operated on first, and at least a 4-week healing period is observed before the second limb is treated.

Repair of Patellar Fractures

Patellar fractures are uncommon in veterinary practice and are associated with severe trauma to the stifle.[1] It is therefore imperative that all structures of the stifle be carefully evaluated when patellar fractures are encountered.

As noted previously, the patella plays an intricate role in the extensor mechanism of the stifle.[1] Removal of the patella consistently results in degenerative lesions within the stifle.[1] A general rule to follow in treating patellar fractures is that the patella should be preserved whenever possible. Patellectomy should be performed only as a salvage procedure and only when the patella is so completely destroyed that no fragment is large enough to contribute effectively to the extensor mechanism.

The patella is under great tensile force from the pull of the quadriceps muscles, and fracture fragments often distract. Internal fixation is the treatment of choice to restore normal anatomic structure and function. Fracture repair consists of reduction of the fragments, re-establishment of a smooth articular surface, preservation of the extensor mechanism, and fixation. The greatest chance for successful surgical treatment is with a simple transverse fracture through the patella that leaves two fragments of equal size. Fixation can be accomplished with a tension-band wire to neutralize the distractive forces of the quadriceps muscles. The patella is approached through a lateral arthrotomy, and the articular surface is examined as the fracture is reduced. Orthopedic wire (18- or 20-gauge wire) is passed laterally to medially through the quadriceps tendon just proximal to the patella (Fig. 46-60A). The wire is then brought across the cranial surface of the patella and is reinserted into the patellar ligament just distal to the patella in a lateral-to-medial direction (Fig. 46-60B). With the stifle in extension, the free ends of the wire are twisted on each other until the fracture is reduced (Fig. 46-60C and D). The wire is then cut, and the twisted portion is folded on itself. Another technique is to loop two wires around the patella, tightening one from the medial aspect and one from the lateral aspect of the patella. Following the surgical procedure, the animal is placed in a soft, padded bandage and is allowed only limited weight-bearing for 2 to 3 weeks.

In some patellar fractures, only the proximal portion of the patella can be salvaged. In such instances, the fracture fragments of the distal portion are resected.

Following this resection, the proximal portion of the patellar ligament is weakened or may actually be ruptured. Horizontal mattress sutures of 4-0 stainless steel are used to reinforce this attachment. If the tendon is torn, simple interrupted sutures can be used to approximate the torn ends (Fig. 46-61). The tension forces across this compromised portion of the patellar ligament must be neutralized to allow for adequate healing. This end is accomplished by passing 18- or 20-gauge orthopedic wire through the quadriceps tendon proximal to the patella and continuing it distally where it is passed through a drill hole in the tibial crest (Fig. 46-61). With the limb in extension, the wire is tightened until the stress on the patellar ligament is relieved. Thus, the wire transmits the force of the quadriceps tendon to the tibia and puts the patellar ligament at rest. The animal is placed in a soft, padded bandage and is allowed only limited exercise for 2 to 3 weeks. The orthopedic wire can be removed in 4 to 6 weeks.[3] It has been our experience[1] that these wires often break by the fourth postoperative week.

In cases of patellar ligament rupture, a similar technique can be employed. Following repair with mattress or Bunnell sutures of 4-0 stainless steel, a tension band of orthopedic wire is similarly placed around the patella and through a drill hole in the tibial crest. Postoperative considerations are as previously described.

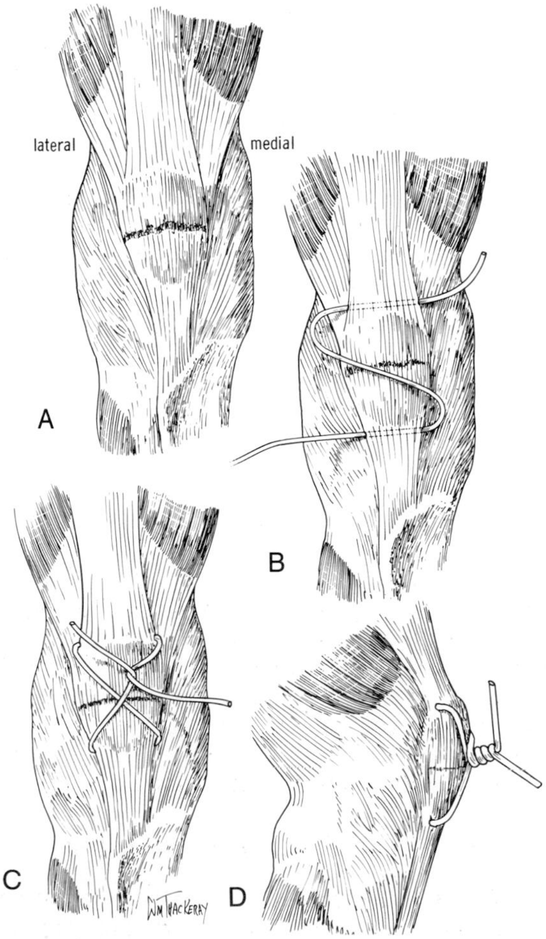

Fig. 46-60. A, *Placement of the wire proximal to the patella. B, Wire is brought across the cranial surface of the patella and is reinserted into the patellar tendon distal to the patella. C, The wires are tightened. D, Lateral view of a properly placed tension band. (From Arnoczky, S. P., and Tarvin, G. B.: Surgery of the Stifle: the patella. Compend. Contin. Ed. Practicing Vet., 2:200, 1980.)*

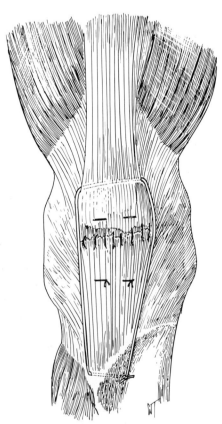

Fig. 46-61. *Placement of the mattress sutures and tension-band wire in partial patellectomy. (From Arnoczky, S. P., and Tarvin, G. B.: Surgery of the Stifle: the patella. Compend. Contin. Ed. Practicing Vet., 2:200, 1980.)*

Patellectomy

As previously noted, the patellar-femoral articulation plays an important role in the biomechanics of stifle motion. Removal of the patella alters this function, and severe degenerative changes result. Patellectomy is therefore indicated only when patellar damage is so severe that repair is impossible.

Patellectomy is most easily performed through a standard lateral arthrotomy. The fractured patella is retracted medially and is everted to expose its fragmented articular surface. The fracture fragments are then removed with a rongeur or a periosteal elevator and scalpel (Fig. 46-62A). Removal of the patella alters the biomechanics of the quadriceps pull[1] and also weakens that portion of the patellar ligament. For these reasons, mattress sutures of 4-0 stainless steel are used to "snug-up" the patellar ligament (Fig. 46-62B). This maneuver accommodates for the laxity in the extensor mechanism caused by the absence of the patella, as well as reinforces the weakened patellar tendon. The sutures are placed with the limb in extension, and the animal placed in a soft, padded bandage with restricted exercise for 2 to 3 weeks.

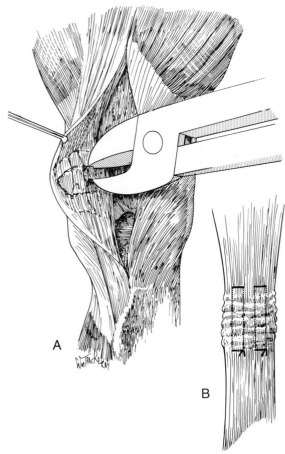

Fig. 46-62. A, *Removal of fractured patellar fragments from the articular surface of the patella with a rongeur. B, "Snugged-up" patellar ligament after patellectomy. (From Arnoczky, S. P., and Tarvin, G. B.: Surgery of the stifle: the patella. Compend. Contin. Ed. Practicing Vet., 2:200, 1980.)*

References and Suggested Readings

1. Arnoczky, S. P., and Tarvin, G. B.: Surgery of the stifle: the patella. Compend. Contin. Ed. Practicing Vet., *2*:200, 1980.
2. Brinker, W. O., and Keller, W. E.: Rotation of the tibial tuberosity for correction of luxation of the patella. Mich. State Univ. Vet., *22*:92, 1962.
3. Carb, A.: A partial patellectomy procedure for transverse patellar fractures in the dog and cat. J. Am. Anim. Hosp. Assoc., *11*:649, 1975.
4. DeAngelis, M. P.: Patellar luxations in dogs. Vet. Clin. North Am., *1*:403, 1971.
5. Evans, H. E., and Christensen, G. C.: Miller's Anatomy of the Dog. 2nd Ed. Philadelphia, W. B. Saunders, 1979.
6. Flo, G., and Brinker, W. O.: Fascia lata overlap procedure for surgical correction of recurrent medial luxation of the patella in the dog. J. Am. Vet. Med. Assoc., 156:595, 1970.
7. Harrison, J. W.: Patellar dislocation *In* Current Techniques in Small Animal Surgery. Edited by M. J. Bojrab. Philadelphia, Lea & Febiger, 1975.
8. Hobday, F.: Congenital malformation and displacement of the patella. Vet. J., *60*:216, 1905.
9. Lacroix, J. V.: Recurrent luxation and the patella in dogs. North Am. Vet., *2*:47, 1930.
10. O'Brien, T. R.: Developmental deformities due to arrested epiphyseal growth. Vet. Clin. North Am., *1*:441, 1971.
11. Priester, W. A.: Sex, size, and breed as risk factors in canine patellar dislocation. J. Am. Vet. Med. Assoc., *160:*740, 1972.
12. Putnam, R. W.: Patellar luxation in the dog. Master's thesis, University of Guelph, Ontario, Canada, 1968.
13. Rudy, R. L.: Stifle joint. *In* Canine Surgery. 2nd Ed. Edited by J. Archibald. Santa Barbara, CA, American Veterinary Publications, 1974.
14. Singleton, W. B.: Transplantation of the tibial crest for treatment of congenital patellar luxation. In Proceedings of the 27th Annual Meeting of the American Animal Hospital Association, 1960.
15. Trotter, E.: Medial patellar luxation in the dog. Compend. Contin. Ed. Practicing Vet., *2*:58, 1980.
16. Vierheller, R. C.: Grooving the femoral trochlea. *In* Proceedings of the 34th Annual Meeting of the American Animal Hospital Association, 1967.

Fractures of the Femur

by David Stoloff

The most frequently fractured bone in the dog is the femur. Fractures may result from external trauma caused by rotational, angular, distractional, or shearing forces or a combination of these forces. Because the strength of the femur is derived from its cortical structure, anatomic reduction and rigid internal fixation are imperative for proper healing.

Fractures of the Greater Trochanter

The physis of the greater trochanter closes between 6 and 12 months of age.[23] It is a traction physis and does not contribute to longitudinal bone growth. Injuries to this physis (Fig. 46-63A) may result in an early closure of this growth plate. Although in man and rabbits, injuries to this physis have been reported to cause valgus deformities, such may not be the case in the

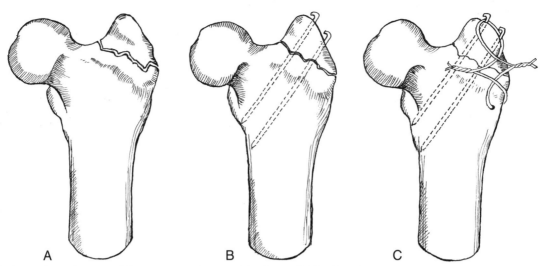

Fig. 46-63. A, *An avulsion fracture of the greater trochanter of the femur.* B, *Two Kirschner wires are inserted from the greater trochanter into the medial cortex of the femur.* C, *A hole is drilled distal to the fracture line, and a figure-8 tension-band wire is applied.*

dog.[14] Greater trochanter fractures are often seen along with proximal epiphyseal separations, femoral neck fractures,[10] and femoral head dislocations.[14]

APPROACH

A curved skin incision is made through the skin and subcutis along the craniolateral aspect of the proximal quarter of the femur cranial to the greater trochanter toward the midline of the back. The fascia lata is incised along the cranial border of the biceps femoris muscle. The origin of the vastus lateralis muscle, attached to the greater trochanter, is incised so to allow resuturing following fracture repair.

FIXATION TECHNIQUE

The method of fixation must overcome distractional and rotational forces present at the fracture site. Multi-ple Stille nails, Kirschner wires, or in cases where the epiphysis has closed, a cancellous screw may be used. Tension-band fixation, however, provides an ideal technique for fracture repair. Rotational stability is achieved, and distractional forces are neutralized and are converted to compressive forces with weight-bearing.

Two Kirschner wires are inserted through the greater trochanter and into the medial cortex of the femur, parallel to one another and at right angles to the fracture line (Fig. 46-63B). A hole is then drilled through the femoral shaft approximately 3 cm distal to the fracture line in a craniocaudal direction. Orthopedic monofilament stainless steel wire, 22-gauge wire for small dogs and cats and 18- to 20-gauge wire for larger dogs, is passed through the predrilled hole, around the proximal pins in a figure-8 fashion, and is tightened (Fig. 46-63C). An Ehmer sling may be applied and left in place for a week following this type of fixation.[3]

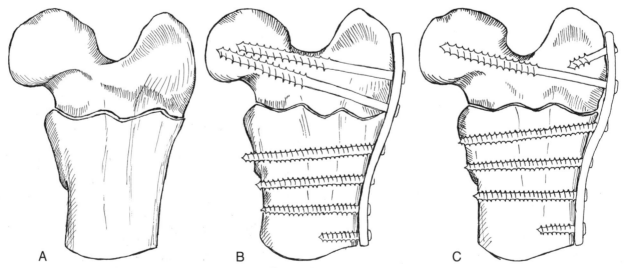

Fig. 46-64. A, *An intertrochanteric fracture of the femur.* B, *and* C, *An intertrochanteric fracture can be repaired with a bone plate.*

Intertrochanteric Fractures

These fractures occur between the greater and lesser trochanters (Fig. 46-64A). Fracture fixation may be successfully accomplished by using two Steinmann pins (a technique similar to that described for fixation of subtrochanteric femoral fractures) or a bone plate (Figs. 46-64B and C).

Subtrochanteric Femoral Fractures

This fracture occurs just distal to the lesser trochanter (Fig. 46-65A). Bending and rotary forces at the fracture site must be neutralized by the fixation technique selected.[19] A single pin and a half-Kirschner apparatus (Figs. 46-65B and C) or a double-Steinmann pinning technique can be used (Figs. 46-65D and E). Double

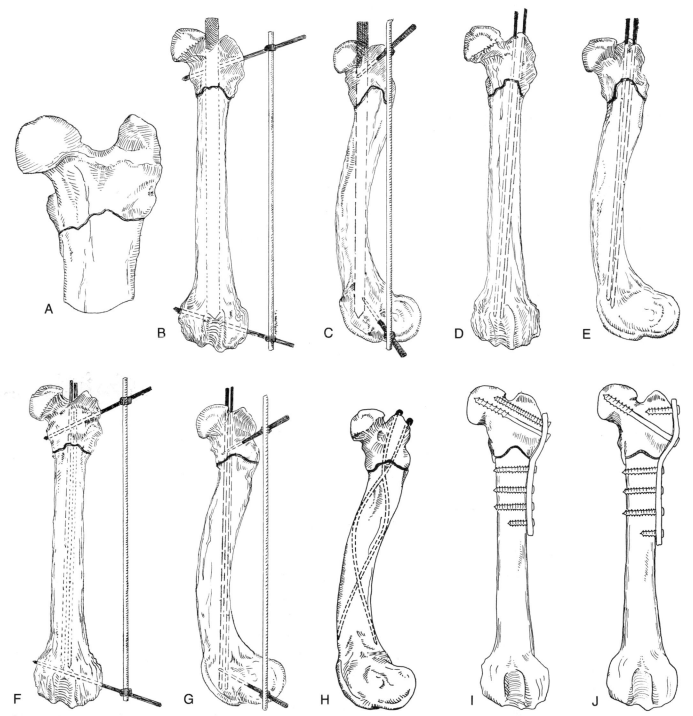

Fig. 46-65. *Subtrochanteric fracture* (A) *repaired with an intermedullary pin and a half-Kirschner apparatus (craniocaudal, B; lateral, C) double intramedullary pins (craniocaudal, D; lateral, E) double intramedullary pins and a half-Kirschner apparatus (craniocaudal, F; lateral, G) Rush pins (H), or a bone plate (I and J).*

pins in addition to a half-Kirschner apparatus (Figs. 46-65*F* and *G*), Rush pins (Fig. 46-65*H*), or a bone plate (Figs. 46-65*I* and *J*) also serve as adequate means of fixation. Pins should be inserted from the most proximal portion of the greater trochanter to achieve maximum stability.

Fractures of the Lesser Trochanter (Calcar)

Structurally, this area provides an important medial buttress for the femur. Varus deformity results from inadequate fixation of this bony segment. One or more lag screws (Fig. 46-66) or several small Kirschner wires and cerclage wires can be used for initial stabilization of this bony segment. Double or multiple pins or a bone plate (Fig. 46-66*C*) then can be used to complete the femoral repair.

Comminuted or Multiple Fractures Involving the Proximal Epiphysis, Neck, Greater Trochanter, or Shaft of the Femur

A dynamic compression plate makes an ideal implant for fractures of this type. Alternatively, angle plates may be employed in larger dogs. Dynamic compression plates provide an opportunity to obtain optimum anatomic fracture alignment by allowing screw insertion from a variety of angles. The plates may be prebent to conform to radiographs of the lateral aspect of the contralateral femur prior to application.

PLATE FIXATION

Butterfly fragments are lagged to major segments, and the femoral head and neck are initially stabilized using a small Kirschner wire. The plate is positioned so that the second screw hole is located just distal to the greater trochanter. A hole is then drilled through the second plate hole through the femoral neck into the most central portion of the femoral head. Exact anatomic fixation following screw insertion is imperative. A second screw is placed through the most proximal screw hole to fix the greater trochanter into position. Screws are then placed through the plate into the distal fragment. Lag screws are used where the screws cross fracture lines. A minimum of three screws should be placed through the plate into the distal fragment penetrating six cortices. The most distal screw should penetrate only one cortex, to decrease the stress concentration effect (Fig. 46-67).

Fractures Involving the Middle Third of the Femur

Increases in limb length have been reported in man following fractures that involve the femoral diaphysis, especially the middle third of the shaft where the physes have been open. A callus or metal implant (intramedullary pin or nail) within the intramedullary cavity stimulates the formation of a collateral blood supply from the epiphyseal vasculature. This development results in a hyperemia in the epiphyseal plate and increased longitudinal growth "proportional to the intensity and duration of the hyperemia in and around the fracture."[40] This phenomenon occurs in animals in which the physis is still open. Compensatory growth in other epiphyses, such as of the tibia of the same limb, may similarly result.

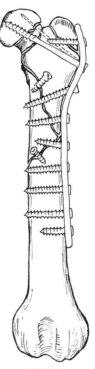

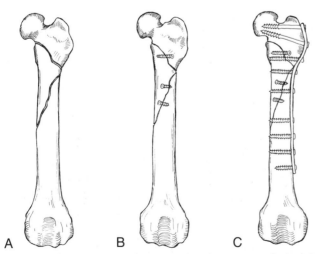

Fig. 46-66. A, *Fracture of the calcar.* B, *A lag screw technique is used for initial fixation.* C, *A bone plate is then applied.*

Fig. 46-67. *Multiple fracture of the femur repaired using lag screws and a dynamic compression plate.*

GREENSTICK FRACTURES

The periosteum and cortex on one side of the femur are fractured. The opposite cortex may be bent or compressed, but it has an intact periosteum.

The closed technique of intramedullary pin fixation described in the following paragraph is a suitable method of fracture repair.

Short Oblique or Transverse Fractures (Fig. 46-68)

CLOSED TECHNIQUE FOR INTRAMEDULLARY PINNING

With intramedullary pinning, one or more pins are driven into the medullary cavity. The pin or pins should be seated firmly in cancellous bone proximally and distally and should approximate the diameter of the medullary cavity at the fracture site. In the cat, the medullary canal can easily be filled by the pin at the fracture site. In the dog, however, because of the cranial bowing of the femoral shaft, this end cannot be achieved as easily.

Although angular forces at the fracture site are neutralized with a single intramedullary pin, rotational stability[2] must be achieved by using multiple, stacked pins or a half-Kirschner apparatus. Additional fixation is also used to neutralize shearing forces in oblique fractures, but this step is not always needed. Sciatic nerve injury from pin irritation may be a complication of this technique.

This technique[24] is especially useful in small dogs (12 kg or less) and in cats for fixation of greenstick fractures or stable transverse or oblique fractures. Fractures less than 5 days old that are easily palpated are most amenable to this technique. The possibility of introducing infection and of causing further vascular compromise to the bone at the time of operation is decreased. Failure to identify linear cracks and other bony defects, however, as well as the interposition of soft tissue structures during a closed procedure, may result in significant postoperative complications.

A small skin incision is made medial to the proximal portion of the greater trochanter (Fig. 46-69A). With the portion of the thigh containing the proximal fragment stabilized with one hand, a pin is inserted through the skin incision into the trochanteric fossa along the caudal border of the medullary canal until it protrudes .5 to 1 cm from the fracture site (Fig. 46-69B). The proximal fragment is then rotated in a craniolateral direction, and the distal fragment is levered into position by angulation or distraction (Fig. 46-69C). The pin is advanced in the distal fragment until it is seated securely in the cancellous bone of the distal epiphysis (Fig. 46-69D). The distal segment is overreduced, when indi-

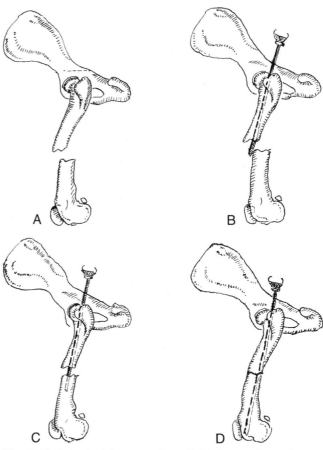

Fig. 46-69. A, *An incision is made medial to the greater trochanter.* B, *An intramedullary pin is inserted through the trochanteric fossa into the intramedullary canal until it protrudes .5 to 1 cm from the fracture site.* C, *The proximal fragment is levered craniolaterally, and the distal fragment is angled until the pin can be advanced into it.* D, *The pin is seated securely in the distal fragment.*

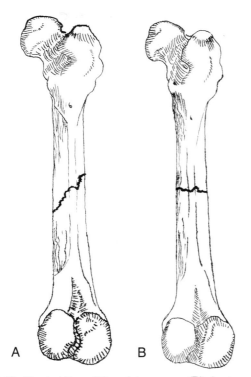

Fig. 46-68. *Short oblique (A) and transverse (B) fractures of the femur.*

cated, to gain a more secure purchase. The limb should be radiographed before the veterinary surgeon cuts the pin to an appropriate length.

CLOSED TECHNIQUE FOR PLACEMENT OF KÜNTSCHNER INTRAMEDULLARY NAILS

These nails, primarily used in larger dogs,[18] are available in clover-leaf, "V," "U," or "C" designs. An open slot in the nail provides an avenue for vascular invasion. These nails resist angular forces, and rotational stability is maintained by impingement of the ridges of the nail on the inner cortex. Although these nails are seated in man following cortical reaming, they are usually placed with little or no prior reaming in the dog because the curved diaphysis and thin cortex of the femur are not well suited for this procedure.

A stab incision is made through the skin on the medial aspect of the greater trochanter.[21,26,33] With a Steinmann pin, a hole is drilled through the trochanteric fossa, which is then enlarged if needed with an awl (Fig. 46-70A). The fracture is reduced and is temporarily held in position by using a guide pin (Fig. 46-70B). The Küntschner nail is then tapped along the guide pin the full length of the medullary canal (Fig. 46-70C). The guide pin is removed, and the nail is seated in the distal fragment (Fig. 46-70D). The pin is driven under compression to give spring-loaded ten-

sion on the endosteal surface of the bone. The nail should be as long as the shaft of the bone, and its proximal end should be approximately level with the greater trochanter, so that it may be removed following healing.

INDICATIONS AND APPROACH FOR OPEN REPAIR TECHNIQUES

In general, open repair techniques should be employed when debridement is needed, when closed reduction is not possible, or when callus revision or grafting is required.

A skin incision is made over the craniolateral aspect of the femoral shaft.[29] The fascia lata is incised along its attachment to the biceps femoris muscle. The vastus lateralis muscle is reflected cranially and the biceps femoris muscle caudally to expose the femoral shaft. If required, the adductor muscle may be reflected caudally by subperiosteal reflection.

SINGLE PIN FIXATION

Following a lateral approach to the femur, the proximal femoral segment is held in neutral[42] or slight internal rotation, it is adducted, and the hip joint is extended to avoid damage to the sciatic nerve while the pin is passed in a retrograde direction. With a hand

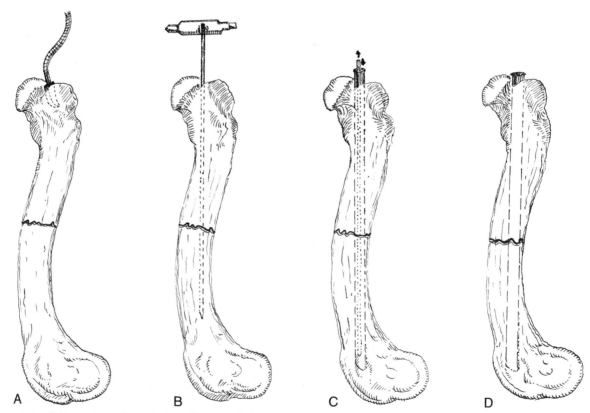

Fig. 46-70. *Küntschner nailing. A, The hole made with a Steinmann pin in the trochanteric fossa is enlarged with an awl. B, The fracture is reduced and is temporarily held in position with a guide pin. C, The nail is tapped along the guide pin into the medullary canal. D, The nail is seated in the distal fragment.*

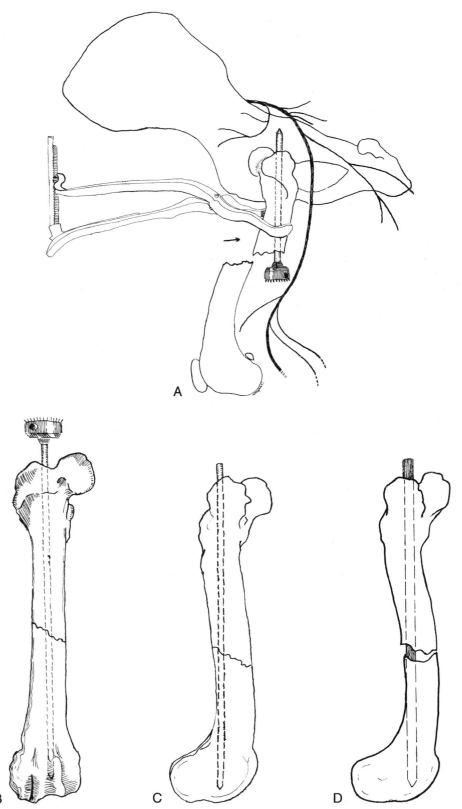

Fig. 46-71. *Open reduction and fixation of a transverse femoral fracture using an intramedullary pin. A, The proximal femoral segment is adducted and the hip joint is extended. The pin is passed in a retrograde direction up through the trochanteric fossa. The distal portion of the proximal segment of the femur (arrow) must be held in a caudal position so the proximal portion will be placed in a cranial position. The intramedullary pin will be thereby directed away from the sciatic nerve. B (craniocaudal view) and C (lateral view), A hand chuck is placed on the proximal portion of the pin. The pin is pulled proximal until parallel with the fracture site. The fracture is reduced, and the pin is driven distally along the caudal cortex and into the cancellous bone of the distal fragment. D, Sometimes, the distal fragment must be excessively reduced to seat the pin firmly in the distal fragment.*

chuck or a drill, the pin is directed in a retrograde fashion from the distal end of the proximal segment along the medullary canal and out through the craniolateral aspect of the trochanteric fossa and skin (Fig. 46-71A). The hand chuck or power drill is then placed on the proximal portion of the pin, and the pin is pulled proximally until the distal end of the pin is parallel with the fracture site. Alternatively, a pin may be passed in a normograde direction from the trochanteric fossa. The fracture is reduced with bone-holding forceps. In order to gain maximum stability, the pin is directed along the caudal cortex of the distal femur and is seated securely in the cancellous bone of the distal fragment with the aid of a bone chuck or a mallet (Figs. 46-71B and C). The subchondral bone is not penetrated. In some cases, the caudal portion of the distal fragment must be angled cranially, to create a gap on the caudal cortex, in order to seat the pin securely and to avoid penetrating the trochlear groove of the distal fragment (Fig. 46-71D). The depth of pin penetration should be checked radiographically before the pin is cut.

CROSSED INTRAMEDULLARY PINS[28]

The two pins pass from the trochanteric fossa and greater trochanter, across the fracture site, to the distal diaphysis. The pins selected do not fill the medullary cavity and cross after passing the fracture site (Fig. 46-72). The pins may be passed in a normograde or a retrograde direction from the fracture site. Additional fixation may be employed as indicated.

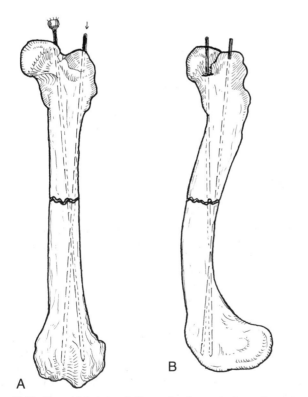

Fig. 46-72. *Crossed intramedullary pinning technique. Two pins are used. The pins do not fill the medullary cavity.* A, *Craniocaudal veiw.* B, *Lateral view.*

MULTIPLE OR STACKED PINS

In this technique, the pins completely fill the intramedullary canal to increase bone-to-pin contact and to improve rotational and angular stability (Fig. 46-73). For fractures of the middle or proximal third of the femoral shaft, the first pin maybe passed in a retrograde fashion through the medullary cavity of the proximal fragment until the pin's end is flush with the fracture line. The fracture is reduced, and the pin is driven distally to stabilize the reduction. Additional pins are passed in a normograde direction down the shaft starting at the trochanteric fossa or greater trochanter to increase stability.[9] If longitudinal fissures are present, the segments must first be held with cerclage wire prior to placement.

KÜNTSCHNER INTRAMEDULLARY NAILS

Following exposure of the fracture site, an intramedullary pin is directed in a retrograde fashion proximally through the trochanteric fossa. The procedure then follows the technique described under the closed method for placement of these nails.

HALF- OR FULL-KIRSCHNER
(HALF-PIN SPLINTING) APPARATUS

This external fixation apparatus can be applied following a closed or open fracture reduction and fixation. This device can be skillfully used to aid in neutralizing rotational and shear forces to maintain femoral length. The pins penetrate both near and far cortices and are positioned at a 35 to 45° angle to each other. For maximum stabilization, the pins should be placed close to the distal ends of the bone. During pin insertion, the skin and musculature should be in their normal anatomic positions (Fig. 46-74). When a full Kirschner apparatus is applied, all pins should be placed in linear alignment.

HEMICERCLAGE WIRE

Hemicerclage wire passes through and partially around the circumference of the bone. It can be used to prevent rotational instability in transverse and short oblique fractures.

FIGURE-8 ORTHOPEDIC WIRE

This type of wire fixation[7] is particularly useful in conjunction with intramedullary pin fixation for transverse fractures of the femur. The intramedullary pin is initially placed in the proximal fragment. Before the pin is seated in the distal fragment, 2 transverse holes are drilled with a Kirschner wire a distance equal to the width of the bone above and below the fracture site. These holes are drilled at 90° to the longitudinal axis of the femur and are positioned so that the wire, when tightened, encompasses and contacts the intramedullary pin. Orthopedic wire is twisted, and either end is

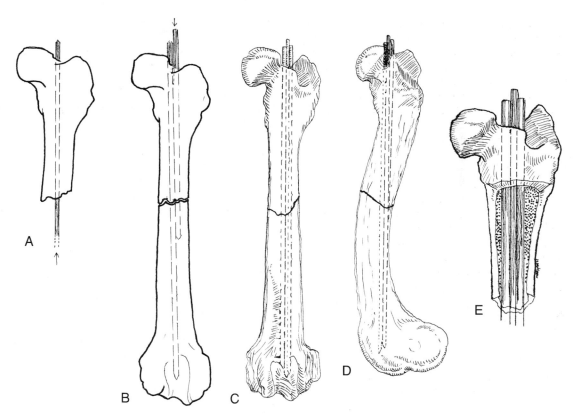

Fig. 46-73. *Stacked pinning technique. Pins fill the medullary canal.* A, *The first pin may be passed in a retrograde direction up the medullary cavity of the proximal fragment.* B, *Additional pins are directed in a normograde fashion.* C, *Craniocaudal view.* D, *Lateral view.* E, *Partial longitudinal section.*

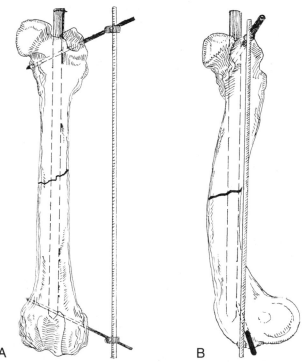

Fig. 46-74. *Half-Kirschner apparatus.* A, *Craniocaudal view.* B, *Lateral view.*

passed through the preplaced holes to form a figure-8 (Fig. 46-75A). The intramedullary pin is then firmly seated in the distal segment, and the wire is tightened (Fig. 46-75B). Increased stability can be achieved if the wire encloses a pin that can be pulled to the endosteal surface of the bone and can thereby increase pin-to-bone contact.[7,42]

KIRSCHNER WIRES AND FIGURE-8

TENSION-BAND WIRES

For short oblique fractures, these techniques may be employed. A detailed description of this technique is given in the discussion of repair of long oblique femoral fractures.

DOUBLE FIGURE-8 WIRING

This technique is useful for repair of transverse fractures. One Kirschner wire (.035 to .062 in. in diameter) is placed 90° to the longitudinal axis of the femoral shaft the width of the femur above and below the fracture line. Figure-8 wires are placed around the Kirschner wires and are alternately tightened, forming a cruciate pattern (Fig. 46-76).

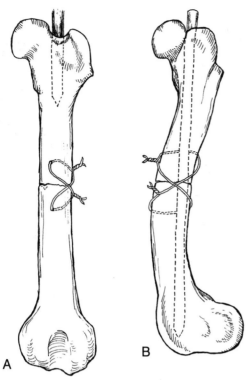

Fig. 46-75. A, *A Kirschner wire is used to drill transverse holes a distance equal to the width of the bone above and below the fracture site. Orthopedic wire is threaded through the holes to form a figure-8 pattern. B, The intramedullary pin is seated distally, and the wire is tightened. The wire encompasses the pin. Increased rotational stability is achieved.*

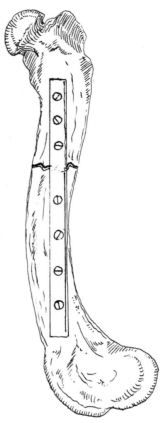

Fig. 46-77. *A bone plate used for fixation of a transverse midshaft femoral fracture.*

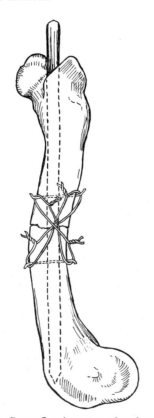

Fig. 46-76. *Two figure-8 wires are placed around transverse Kirschner wires and are tightened to form a cruciate pattern.*

BONE PLATES (FIG. 46-77)

A bone plate can be used for fixation of a transverse midshaft femoral fracture. A minimum of four cortices above and below the fracture line must be secured. Six cortices would be preferred.

Long Oblique Fractures or Fractures with Large Butterfly Fragments

KIRSCHNER WIRES AND LAG SCREWS

For long oblique fractures, figure-8 wires can be placed around the ends of Kirschner wires to aid intramedullary pin fixation (Fig. 46-78). A half-Kirschner apparatus maybe applied to increase stability further. Multiple pins can be used in place of a single intramedullary pin. Lag screws can be used in conjunction with bone plating initially to secure large butterfly fragments to a major segment.

CERCLAGE WIRING

Following intramedullary pin fixation, cerclage and hemicerclage wires can be employed to prevent rotation and overriding of bone fragments. A cerclage wire completely encircles the circumference of the bone

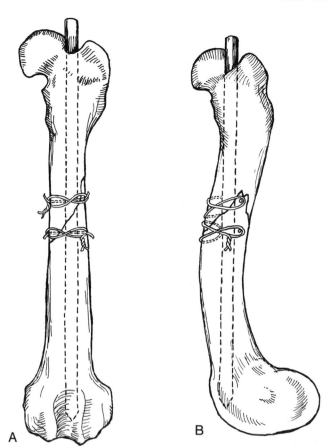

Fig. 46-78. *A long oblique fracture is repaired with an intramedullary pin and transversely placed Kirschner wires. A, Craniocaudal view. B, Lateral view.*

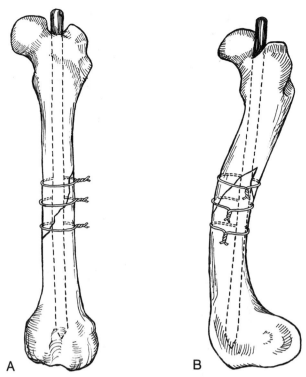

Fig. 46-79. *Full-cerclage wires and an intramedullary pin are used to fix a long, oblique, midshaft fracture of the femur. A, Craniocaudal view. B, Lateral view.*

(Fig. 46-79), whereas a hemicerclage wire incompletely encompasses this outer structure.

Full-cerclage wires are indicated in repair of longitudinal cortical or fissure fractures and spiral fractures and for stabilization of large butterfly fragments. Full-cerclage wires are used in long oblique fractures when the obliquity of the fracture is "equal to or greater than twice the cross-sectional diameter of the diaphysis."[44] Because the majority of the blood supply to cortical bone enters at right angles, and longitudinal blood flow through cortical bone runs for a distance of only 2 to 3 mm, cerclage wire does not pose a threat to the vascular supply of bone if properly applied.

Wires are placed around the periostium at 90° to the longitudinal axis of the femur. In general, 18-gauge wire is used for animals over 10 kg and 20- to 22-gauge wire for smaller animals.[43] A groove or a notch is placed in any area of changing diameter of bone to decrease the chance of wire slippage. The wire must not be kinked and must be twisted uniformly when it is applied. All wires should be secured with equal tension. A single wire should not be used, except possibly in cases of fissure fractures.[31] Two or more wires should always be used to eliminate a point of stress concentration caused by a single wire. A single wire can serve as a fulcrum "encouraging angular motion."[31] Multiple wires are placed 1 cm apart. One wire should be positioned approximately 0.5 cm from the "end of each oblique fracture."[16,43] The use of cortical bone tacks with a pull-out tension device has been demonstrated with cerclage wiring.[38]

Multiple or Comminuted Fractures or Fractures with Longitudinal Fissures

Repair of these fractures involves the reconstruction of smaller fragments into two larger segments that can then be joined (Fig. 46-80). During reconstruction, it may be necessary to decrease femoral length in order to decrease torsional stress and to achieve stability. Dogs over 20 kg can lose up to 1 cm in length without impairment of function. When it is not possible to reconstruct a severely comminuted fracture, a cancellous or corticocancellous graft[39] can be used. Cortical or corticocancellous grafts can be secured in position with cerclage wire, intramedullary pins, lag screws, or a bone plate.[15]

Many different types of fixation devices may be used: lag screws in addition to a full Kirschner apparatus, stacked pins, or an intramedullary pin in addition to cerclage or hemicerclage wires and a half-Kirschner apparatus. Half-pin splinting provides rotary stability and guards against collapse. With severely comminuted fractures with excessive soft tissue injury, a full Kirschner apparatus may be used as the sole means of fixation (Fig. 46-81). Küntschner nails are contraindicated

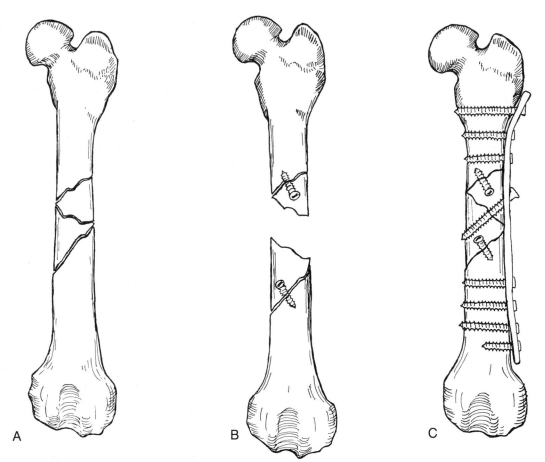

Fig. 46-80. A, *Multiple fracture of the femur.* B, *Lag screws are used to fix the smaller fragments to the larger segments.* C, *The two larger segments are then reduced and are fixed using a neutralization plate.*

in longitudinal and comminuted fractures and in fractures with butterfly fragments. Additionally, methyl methacrylate has been used as an intramedullary splint to aid fixation of these complex fractures.[38]

Plates are indicated for comminuted and other unstable types of fractures. Small fragments (butterfly, for example) are temporarily held to a major bone segment with a 0.045-cm Kirschner wire, with cerclage wires, or with bone-holding forceps and then are secured with lag screws. The bone is placed in normal anatomic alignment using the stifle, greater trochanter, and facies aspera (rough surface for the adductor magnus muscle) as reference points.[17] The two larger segments are then joined with a neutralization plate (bone plate). The plate should be contoured to provide proper internal fixation and to decrease implant fatigue and the possibility of failure. The plate can be contoured by using radiographs taken from the lateral aspect of the contralateral femur. Because bone is strongest in compression and weakest in tension, the plate is placed on the craniolateral aspect (tension-band side) of the femur. A dynamic compression plate is used so that screws can be angled to provide additional axial and intrafragmentary compression. Screws that cross a fracture line should be placed with a lag effect. The screws should penetrate at least 6 cortices above and below the fracture site.

Fractures Involving the Distal Third of the Femur

Fractures may occur in the distal diaphysis, metaphysis, or epiphysis or in several of these areas.

A curved incision is made through the skin and subcutaneous tissue to extend from the distal third of the femur, lateral to the patella and patellar ligament, to the tibial tuberosity. The fascia lata is incised along the cranial border of the biceps femoris muscle, as is the lateral fascia of the stifle joint. The biceps femoris muscle and the lateral fascia of the stifle joint are retracted laterally, and the joint capsule is incised lateral to the patellar ligament. The patella and the vastus lateralis muscle are reflected medially, and the stifle is flexed.

Supracondylar and Intracondylar Fractures

Because the hypertrophic chondrocyte layer of the growth plate is structurally weaker than adjacent bone, tendon, and ligaments,[25] and because the distal epiphysis of the femur closes between 7 and 13 months of age,[12] dogs between 4 and 11 months[4] of age most commonly experience intracapsular fractures through the

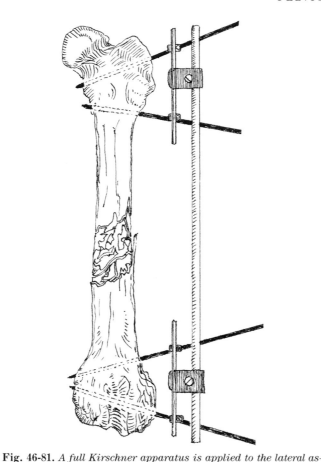

Fig. 46-81. *A full Kirschner apparatus is applied to the lateral aspect of the femur for repair of a severely comminuted midshaft fracture with extensive soft tissue injury.*

Fig. 46-83. ⟨
the origin o⟨

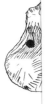

Fig. 46-84. ⟨
through the
normograde

epiphyseal plate. After 2 years of age, diaphyseal fractures are more common.[1]

The distal femoral physis is responsible for 75% of the longitudinal growth of the femur. An injury to the epiphyseal plate causes hyperemia and may lead to acceleration in longitudinal growth; however, slowing of growth is more characteristic[40] and results in premature closure of the growth plate. An eccentric closure of the growth plate can cause angular deformities of the femur. In man, it has been found that exact anatomic reduction and fixation can lead to revascularization of the germinative layer and healing without the formation of a callous bridge between the metaphysis and epiphysis;[40] thus is abnormal distal femoral growth avoided.

A simple epiphyseal separation through the hypertrophic zone occurs in Salter type I fractures. A fracture in a similar location in the growth plate, but extending into the metaphysis, is seen in Salter type II fractures. These fractures are caused by shearing or avulsion forces. Because the germinative layer is not disturbed in these fracture types and normal growth can be expected, a good-to-excellent prognosis has usually been given. Some authors, however, have observed a less favorable outcome following repair of these two fracture types and feel that a less-favorable prognosis is warranted.[18]

Salter type III fractures extend from the joint surface through the epiphysis and a portion of the physis. Salter type III fractures result from intra-articular shearing forces and can be given a good-to-fair prognosis[27] following anatomic reduction and fixation if the epiphyseal vasculature has not been seriously compromised[34] and if the germinative layer is undisturbed. Fractures extending from the joint surface through the epiphysis, across the growth plate, and through a portion of the metaphysis (Salter type IV) are given a guarded[25] or a poor[27] prognosis. Recently, it has been stated that these last two fracture types always involve the germinative layers,[40] and a poorer prognosis should be given.

In general, with distal femoral fractures, the distal fragment is displaced caudally and laterally while the proximal fragment rides cranial and slightly medial to the distal fragment. Because of the irregularity of the growth plate, shearing and rotational forces do not present major problems in repair, whereas angular forces must be neutralized.

CLOSED REDUCTION AND FIXATION

This type of reduction and fixation can be used soon after trauma in patients with nonarticular fractures (Salter types I and II). The technique involves flexing the stifle, applying traction over the proximal portion of the caudal aspect of the tibia, and forcing the distal end of the proximal fragment cranially. Following reduction, the limb is placed in a flexion[13] bandage for 10 to 14 days. Postoperative complications include intra- and extra-articular adhesions and stiff-stifle syndrome.

DOUBLE RUSH PINNING

When inserted in the medullary cavity, the Rush pin exerts three-point contact, provides spring-loaded tension against the endosteal cortex, and allows the surrounding musculature to cause "contact compression" at the fracture site.[22] Two pins are generally used to provide maximum compression, as well as to neutralize angular, rotational, and some torsional forces[35] at the fracture site.

The initial lateral guide hole is started in the distal end of the lateral condyle of the femur lateral to the trochlear ridge and cranial to the origin of the lateral digital extensor tendon or lateral collateral ligament. The exact point for starting the drill hole varies because of the curvature of the bone. Generally, the point of insertion is more proximal the more curved the bone. This guide hole is made with a pin or a reamer awl. The hole is started perpendicular to the longitudinal axis of the distal femur. When the pin or reamer awl is seated, the angle is changed to an angle of 30 to 40°[33,45] to a line bisecting the distal third of the femur (Fig. 46-82A and B). A second guide hole is similarly made beginning in the medial condyle proximal to the origin of the medial collateral ligament of the stifle. The pins should be of a 5/32-in. diameter or less[5] and can be prebent if indicated prior to insertion. The Rush pin is

of the proximal segment through the trochanteric fossa (Figs. 46-84A, B, C). The fracture is reduced and, with the stifle extended, the pin is passed in a normograde direction into the lateral epiphysis (Fig. 46-84D). Because of the cranial bow of the dog's femoral shaft, pins should be rotated through an arc of only 90 to 180° during insertion. The following pin sizes are suggested for this technique: animals less than 5 kg, 1/16 in.; 5 to 9 kg, 5/64 in.; 9 to 27 kg, 7/64 in.; 27 kg and over, 1/8 in.[32]

A half-Kirschner apparatus (half-pin splinting) is used in conjunction with intramedullary pinning, especially in patients with Salter types III and IV fractures, to overcome rotational instability. One pin is placed through the greater trochanter, and a second is placed through both femoral condyles (Fig. 46-85). The trochanteric pin may be fixed to the intramedullary pin.[18]

DOUBLE INTRAMEDULLARY PINNING

This technique (Fig. 46-86) can be used for repair of unstable fractures, especially in medium and large dogs, to achieve rotational, shearing, and some torsional stability.[35] For flexibility, pins of smaller diameter are used. Following reduction, pins can be driven from the lateral and medial condyles into the proximal segment,[41] or the pins can be passed in a retrograde direction from the caudal lateral and caudomedial cortex of the distal portion of the proximal fragment. Then, following reduction, these pins are directed in a

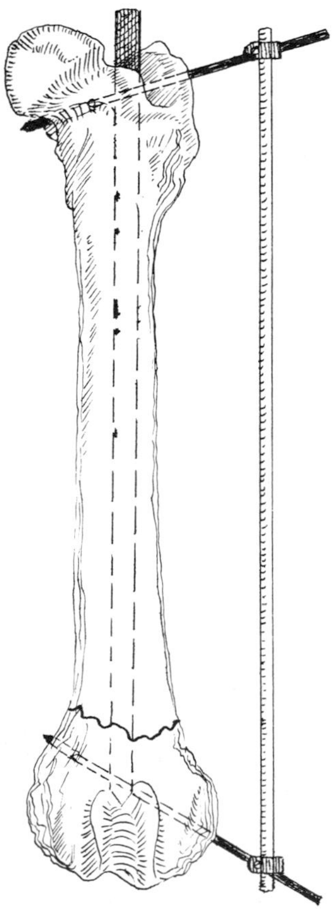

Fig. 46-85. *Supracondylar fracture repaired with an intramedullary pin and a half-Kirschner apparatus.*

normograde fashion into the subchondral bone[3] of the distal fragment. It is always important to overreduce the distal segment in order to anchor the pins securely.

CROSS-PINNING (FIG. 46-87)[11,37]

This type of fixation is used in cats and in small dogs to provide rotational, torsional, shearing, and distractional stability.[35] Stability is achieved by providing two-point fixation at different angles.[18]

Pins may be inserted by any of three basic techniques: (1) one pin is driven proximally from the craniolateral and another from the craniomedial aspect of the distal portion of the femoral shaft; the pins cross and pierce the opposite femoral cortex at the level of the origin of the articularis genus muscle (Fig. 46-87); the fracture is reduced, and the pins are seated into the condyles (Fig. 46-87B); (2) the femur can be reduced and the pins inserted lateral to the trochlear groove in a manner similar to that described in (1) (Fig. 46-87C); the pins are then seated under the condylar surface; (3) alternatively, one pin can be passed in a retrograde direction from the femoral condyle into the proximal shaft while a second pin can be directed in a normograde fashion from the shaft into the opposite condyle[35] (Fig. 46-87D). The pins, in any case, cross proximal to the fracture line. The proximal portion of the pins may be cut short or left long for purposes of removal following healing.

PLATE FIXATION (FIG. 46-88)

Plate fixation may be used if four cortices can secure screw purchase. This fixation is especially applicable to larger, mature dogs.

LAG SCREW FIXATION

Lag screw fixation is an ideal method for repair of intra-articular condylar fractures (Salter types III and IV fractures) when anatomic reconstruction is imperative.

The fracture is reduced and is held in position with reduction forceps. A Kirschner wire is inserted from the lateral or medial condyle through the cortex of the opposite condyle. One or two screws (cancellous or cortical) are inserted with a lag effect. With this technique, the screw threads either do not cross (cancellous screw) or do not secure the near fragment (cortical screw). The Kirschner wire may be left in place for its antirotational property (Fig. 46-89). Double pinning, plating, or cross-pinning must be used in conjunction with this technique.

Small medial condylar fractures having attached caudal cruciate and medial collateral ligaments that cannot be repaired with a transcondylar screw can be repaired using a proximal-to-distal, obliquely placed lag screw[14] (cancellous) (Fig. 46-90). The fractured condyle can be levered into position with a bone hook, and a drill guide can be used to aid drill positioning.

With fractures of the distal third of the femur, limited activity is recommended for 2 to 3 weeks.

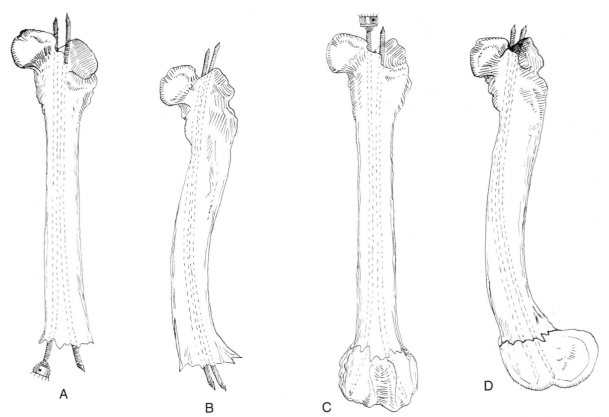

Fig. 46-86. *Double intramedullary pinning. One pin is passed in a retrograde direction from the caudolateral and another from the caudomedial cortex of the distal portion of the proximal fragment (A, craniocaudal, B, lateral views). The fracture is reduced, and the pins are driven distally (C, craniocaudal, D, lateral views).*

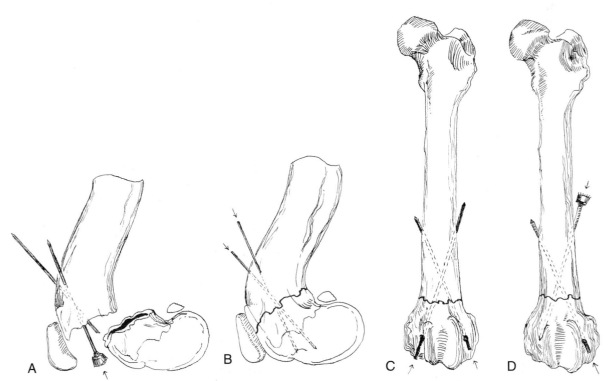

Fig. 46-87. *Crossed-pin technique for small dogs and cats. A, One pin is driven from the craniolateral and another from the craniomedial aspect of the distal portion of the proximal femur. B, Following fracture reduction, the pins are seated into the condyles. C, Alternatively, pins may be inserted from the distal condyles. D, One pin is directed in a retrograde fashion from the femoral condyle into the proximal shaft. A second pin is passed in a normograde direction from the shaft into the opposite condyle.*

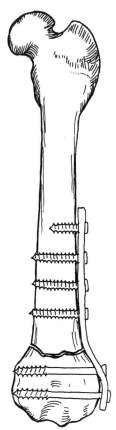

Fig. 46-88. *Plate fixation for supracondylar fracture repair.*

Acknowledgments

I wish to thank Drs. Y. Z. Abdelbaki and D. Hulse for reviewing this paper, Tom Morganti and Michael Broussard and Dr. Kay Schwink for the art work, Harry Cowgill for the photography, and Lynne Stoloff for the preparation of this manuscript.

References and Suggested Readings

1. Alcantara, P. J., and Stead, A. C.: Fractures of the distal femur in the dog and cat. J. Small Anim. Pract., *16*:649, 1975.
2. Braden, T. D., and Brinker, W. O.: Radiologic and gross anatomic evaluation of bone healing in the dog. J. Am. Vet. Med. Assoc., *169*:1318, 1976.
3. Brinker, W. O.: Small Animal Fractures. East Lansing, Michigan State University Continuing Education Service, 1978.
4. Brinker, W. O.: Fractures. *In* Canine Surgery. 2nd Ed. Edited by J. Archibald. Santa Barbara, CA, American Veterinary Publications, 1974.
5. Campbell, C. J., Grisola, A., and Zanconato, G.: The effects produced in the cartilagenous epiphyseal plate of immature dogs by experimental surgical traumata. J. Bone Joint Surg. [Am.], *41*:1221, 1959.
6. Chaffee, V. W.: Multiple (stacked) intramedullary pin fixation of humeral and femoral fractures. J. Am. Anim. Hosp. Assoc., *13*:599, 1971.
7. Creed, J. E.: Stabilization of unstable long bone fractures with pins and wire. Washington Crossing, NJ, Pitman-Moore Audiotutorial Program No. 13, 1977.
8. Culvenor, J. A., Hulse, D. A., and Patton, C. S.: Closure after injury of the distal femoral growth plate in the dog. J. Small Anim. Pract., *19*:549, 1978.
9. DeAngelis, M. P.: The femur. *In* Current Techniques in Small Animal Surgery. Edited by M. J. Bojrab. Philadelphia, Lea & Febiger, 1975.
10. Denny, H. R.: Simultaneous epiphyseal separations and fractures of the neck and greater trochanter of the femur in the dog. J. Small Anim. Pract., *12*:613, 1971.

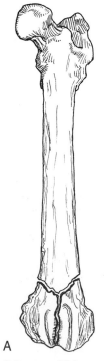

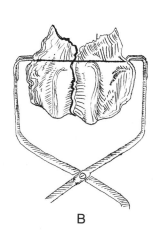

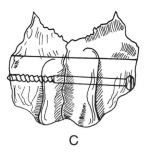

Fig. 46-89. A, *Salter type IV fracture of the distal femur.* B, *The intracondylar fracture is reduced and is temporarily held in reduction with vulsellum forceps and a transcondylar Kirschner wire.* C, *A lag screw is then inserted to secure the intracondylar fracture reduction. The remaining reconstruction is performed as previously described.*

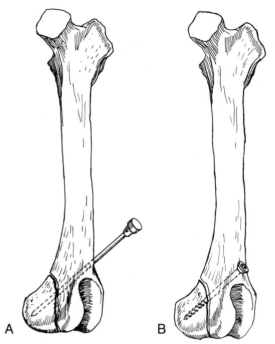

Fig. 46-90. *Medial condylar fracture. A, Using a drill guide, an oblique drill hole is made. B, A cancellous screw is used for fragment fixation.*

11. Endres, W. A.: Repair of bilateral supracondylar femoral fractures in a cat. VM SAC, *66*:990, 1971.

12. Gillette, E. L., Thrall, D. E., and Lebel, J. L.: Carlson's Veterinary Radiology. Philadelphia, Lea & Febiger, 1977.

13. Grahan, J. E. B., Ketchell, R. J., and Bodendistel, J. K.: Simple fixation for distal epiphyseal fractures of the femur in the cat and dog. Can. Vet. J., *1*:492, 1960.

14. Hauptman, J., and Butler, H. C.: Effect of osteology of the greater trochanter with tension band fixation on femoral conformation in beagle dogs. Vet. Surg., *8*:13, 1979.

15. Henrickson, P.: Clinical report: entire segment bone transplant in a cat. J. Am. Vet. Med. Assoc., *174*:826, 1979.

16. Hinko, P. J., and Rhinelander, F. W.: Effective use of cerclage in the treatment of long-bone fractures in dogs. J. Am. Vet. Med. Assoc., *166*:520, 1975.

17. Hohn, R. B.: Plate fixation of comminuted femoral shaft fractures in the dog. J. Am. Vet. Med. Assoc., *162*:646, 1973.

18. Horne, R., Milton, J. L., and Henderson, R.: Advanced small animal orthopedic surgery course notes. Auburn, AL, Auburn University, 1976.

19. Hulse, D. A.: Orthopedic surgery course notes. Baton Rouge, Louisiana State University, 1980.

20. Hurov, L., and Seer, G.: External Kirschner clamp fixation with intramedullary pinning for distal femoral epiphyseal fracture repair. Can. Vet. J., *9*:31, 1968.

21. Jenny, J.: Kneutscher's medullary nailing in femur fractures of the dog. J. Am. Vet. Med. Assoc., *117*:381, 1950.

22. Lawson, D. D.: The use of Rush pins in the management of fractures in the dog and cat. Vet. Rec., *70*:760, 1958.

23. Lee, G. T.: Rush pin techniques. Kirschner Orthopedic Appliances Instruments and Techniques for Veterinary Surgery. Catalog 80-1. Aberdeen, Kirschner Scientific, 1980.

24. Lesser, A. S.: Method of internal fixation of femoral fractures using intramedullary pins and a closed technique. J. Am. Anim. Hosp. Assoc., *12*:754, 1976.

25. Llewellyn, H. R.: Growth plate injuries—diagnosis, prognosis and treatment. J. Am. Anim. Hosp. Assoc., *12*:77, 1976.

26. Muller, M. E., Allgower, M., Schneider, R., and Willeneger, H.: Manual of Internal Fixation. New York, Springer-Verlag, 1979.

27. O'Brien, T. R.: Development deformities due to arrested epiphyseal growth. Vet. Clin. North Am., *1*:441, 1971.

28. Piermattei, D. L.: Canine orthopedics and treatment of fractures. *In* Proceedings of an Orthopedic Symposium. Toronto Academy of Veterinary Medicine. Toronto, 1971.

29. Piermattei, D. L., and Greeley, R. G.: An Atlas of Surgical Approaches to the Bones of the Dog and Cat. Philadelphia, W. B. Saunders, 1979.

30. Presnell, K. R.: Case report. Surgical repair of a comminuted distal femoral fracture in a dog. Can. Vet. J., *20*:196, 1979.

31. Rhinelander, F. W.: Minimal Internal Fixation of Tibial Fractures. Clin. Orthop., *107*:188, 1975.

32. Rouse, G. P.: Distal femoral epiphyseal fracture repair in the dog and cat. Washington Crossing, NJ, Pitman-Moore Auditorial Program No. 19, 1979.

33. Rudy, R. L.: Principles of intramedullary pinning. Vet. Clin. North Am., *5*:209, 1975.

34. Salter, R. B., and Harris, W. R.: Injuries involving the epiphyseal plate. J. Bone Joint Surg. [Am.], *45*:587, 1963.

35. Shires, P. K. and Hulse, D. A.: Internal fixation of metaphyseal growth plate fractures using the distal femur as an example. Compend. Contin. Ed. Practicing Vet., *2*:854, 1980.

36. Sumner-Smith, G.: Observations on epiphyseal fusion of the canine appendicular skeleton. J. Small Anim. Pract., *7*:303, 1966.

37. Sumner-Smith, G., and Dingwall, J. S.: A technique for repair of fractures of the distal epiphysis in the dog and cat. J. Am. Anim. Hosp. Assoc., *9*:171, 1973.

38. Sumner-Smith, G., and Waters, E. H.: The adjunctive use of methyl methacrylate bone cement in the stabilization of multiple fractures. J. Am. Anim. Hosp. Assoc., *12*:778, 1976.

39. Wadsworth, P. L., and Henry, W. B.: Entire segment cortical bone transplant. J. Am. Anim. Hosp. Assoc., *12*:741, 1972.

40. Weber, B. G., Brunner, C. H., and Freuler, F.: Treatment of Fractures in Children and Adolescents. New York, Springer-Verlag, 1980.

41. Whittick, W. G.: Canine Orthopedics. Philadelphia, Lea & Febiger, 1974.

42. Withrow, S. J.: Principles of IM pinning and cerclage wiring. *In* Scientific Proceedings of the 47th Annual Meeting of the American Animal Hospital Association. Los Angeles, 1980.

43. Withrow, S. J.: Use and misuse of full cerclage wires in fracture repair. Vet. Clin. North Am., *18*:201, 1978.

44. Withrow, S. J., and Holmberg, D. L.: Use of Full Cerclage Wires in the Fixation of 18 Consecutive Long-Bone Fractures in Small Animals. JAAHA 13 (Nov/Dec): 735, 1977.

45. Wolff, E. F.: Rush pins in veterinary orthopedics—a review. J. Am. Vet. Med. Assoc., *11*:756, 1975.

47 * Thoracic Limb

Fractures of the Humerus

by DENNIS A. JACKSON

The surgical management of humeral fractures may be influenced by several factors. Of utmost importance is providing necessary emergency care and performing a thorough physical examination to detect other injuries. Because of their close proximity to the humerus, the thorax and its contents should be carefully evaluated for multiple injuries such as pulmonary contusion, pulmonary collapse, hemothorax, pneumothorax, fractured ribs, diaphragmatic hernia, and cardiac trauma. Thoracic radiographs and an electrocardiogram should be obtained if these injuries are suspected. The presence of thoracic injuries may take priority over or may delay the treatment of an existing humeral fracture. Also important is careful evaluation of the nerve components to the injured limb. Injury to the brachial plexus, avulsion of spinal nerves from the cord, or peripheral nerve injury may occur. Midshaft humeral fractures can injure the radial nerve near the site at which the nerve courses from medial to lateral over the musculospiral groove. In these cases, a careful neurologic evaluation with electrodiagnostic testing and surgical exploration of the nerve helps to determine the extent of injury.

The treatment and prognosis for uncomplicated healing can be determined by accurate classification of humeral fractures. Many factors must be considered in arriving at this classification; for example, if the fracture is open, delayed healing or infection is possible. Fractures with associated skin wounds are considered open fractures. Full assessment of any fracture requires two diagnostic radiographic views. One method of fixation may be suggested over another by evaluating the radiographs for extent of damage to bone, the degree of displacement, and the direction, location, and type of fracture. Other factors to consider include the age, weight, activity, and function of the patient, as well as the client's economic limitations. If the use of a Kirschner splint is considered, the potential for proper postoperative care should be assessed on an individual basis.

My preferred methods of managing humeral fractures are outlined in the following discussion. Certainly, other methods of repair exist and prove equally effective in the hands of individuals familiar with their use. It is important to remember that the principles and limitations of each technique must be understood and adhered to no matter what method is chosen. In this discussion, the management of fractures is based on the anatomic region of the humerus in which they occur. Conservative management with closed reduction and external fixation is discussed when applicable; however, in most cases, open reduction with internal fixation is preferred. Emphasis should be placed on limited exposure to the bone, along with atraumatic dissection of muscle planes, except when more extensive exposure is required to facilitate repair. The discussion of surgical approaches to the bone is brief, and the reader is referred to Piermattei and Greeley for a more complete description.[7]

Proximal Fractures

These include fractures of the proximal epiphysis, proximal metaphysis, humeral head, and greater tubercle. As a group, they are seen infrequently.

EPIPHYSEAL

Epiphyseal fractures occur in young growing animals that have an open growth plate. These fractures are also seen in young animals in which the epiphysis appears closed on radiographs. Most of these fractures required open reduction and internal fixation, with the exception of selected Salter type I fractures. Salter type I fractures of less than 24 to 48 hours' duration in small dogs and cats can be managed by closed reduction.

The proximal segment is immobilized by grasping the acromion of the scapula, and the distal segment is reduced by gentle abduction and adduction of the elbow. Care must be taken to avoid splitting the proximal physis at the thin junction between the humeral head and greater tubercle. Fixation can be achieved with a Velpeau sling or by normograde pinning through the greater tubercle with Kirschner wires or Steinmann pins (Fig. 47-1). Healing is rapid, and the pins or Velpeau sling can usually be removed in 2 to 3 weeks following radiographic examination. Failure to obtain

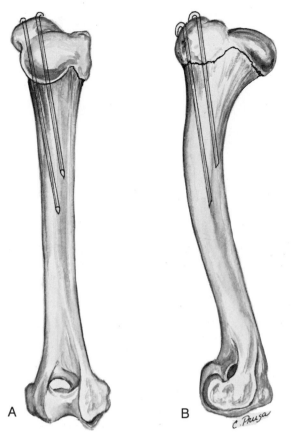

Fig. 47-1. *A Salter type I proximal epiphyseal fracture repaired with two pins or Kirschner wires passed in a normograde fashion from the greater tubercle into the metaphysis following closed or open reduction. A, Caudocranial view. B, Lateral view.*

satisfactory closed reduction or prolonged fracture duration necessitates an open approach to the proximal shaft through a craniolateral incision.

Double Rush pinning is the preferred method of internal fixation, with pin placement craniolateral and craniomedial through the greater tubercle (Fig. 47-2). Prebending the pins and using a Rush awl to create guide holes facilitate their insertion. Rush pins of appropriate size are driven at an angle of approximately 20° to the long axis of the bone. The lateral pin is directed toward the caudomedial cortex and the medial pin toward the caudolateral cortex of the shaft. The pins should cross distal to the fracture site and should seat firmly to provide rigid 3-point fixation. No additional fixation is required, and early restricted weight-bearing should be encouraged. For cats and small dogs, Kirschner wires can be substituted for Rush pins by a similar technique.

METAPHYSEAL

Proximal metaphyseal fractures of short duration can also be managed by closed reduction with normograde intramedullary pinning through the greater tubercle. Because many of these fractures are impacted, a single intramedullary pin usually provides adequate stabiliza-

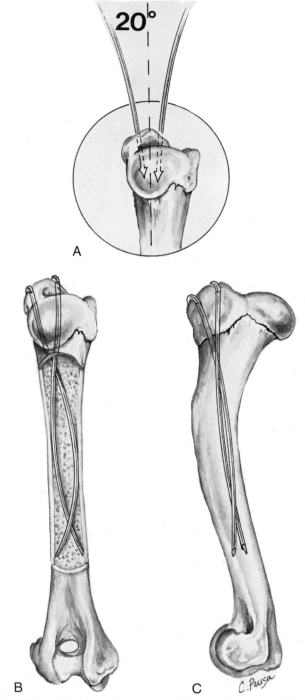

Fig. 47-2. *A Salter type I proximal epiphyseal fracture stabilized with double Rush pins. Prebent pins are placed craniolateral and craniomedial through the greater tubercle at an angle of approximately 20° to the long axis of the bone (A). B, Craniocaudal view. C, Lateral view.*

tion. For patients with rotational instability, a second pin or a half-Kirschner splint can be added. Open reduction is required if the fracture is of some duration or if soft tissue swelling is significant. The fracture is exposed through a craniolateral approach, and fixation is achieved with two Rush pins placed as described for a Salter I epiphyseal fracture (Fig. 47-3).

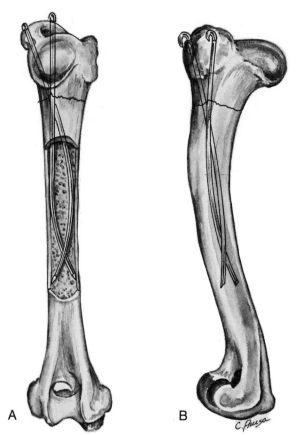

Fig. 47-3. *A proximal metaphyseal fracture repaired using double Rush pins. The pins cross distal to the fracture and provide rigid three-point fixation. A, Caudocranial view. B, Lateral view.*

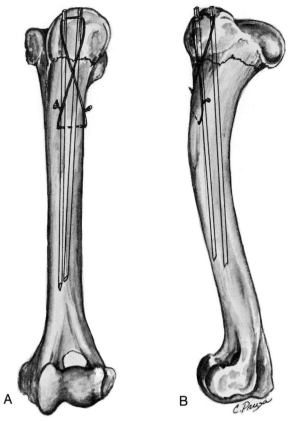

Fig. 47-4. *A proximal metaphyseal fracture stabilized with a tension-band wire and two Kirschner wires or small Steinmann pins passed normograde from the greater tubercle into the shaft. A, Craniocaudal view. B, Lateral view.*

Alternatively, a tension-band wire may be applied using appropriate size Kirschner wires or Steinmann pins and orthopedic wire (Fig. 47-4). With this technique, pins are placed parallel in the bone entering at the midpoint of the greater tubercle. The wire is positioned in figure-8 fashion over the pins and is anchored in the distal fragment through a hole drilled in the bone.

GREATER TUBERCLE AND HUMERAL HEAD

Fractures involving only the greater tubercle in young animals can be stabilized with two Kirschner wires or small Steinmann pins. In mature animals, a tension-band wire technique is recommended. In both cases, open reduction is required through a craniolateral approach to the proximal humerus.

Fractures involving the head of the humerus occur infrequently. Open reduction is required and should be performed as early as possible. The fracture is exposed through a craniolateral approach to the shoulder joint by osteotomy of the acromion process combined with an infraspinatous tenotomy for additional exposure. In young animals, fixation can be obtained with multiple Kirschner wires or Stille nails driven through the lateral humeral head into the neck and countersunk

below the articular cartilage. In the mature animal, fractures of the humeral head can be stabilized with a lag screw and Kirschner wire placed from the cranial surface of the proximal metaphysis into the humeral head. The osteotomized acromion process is replaced during closure using a tension-band wire.

The techniques described for fixation of greater tubercle or humeral head fractures may be combined when repairing injuries of the entire physis resulting in simultaneous fracture of these two structures. In young growing animals, this technique involves combined pinning of the greater tubercle and humeral head (Fig. 47-5). These techniques are used in young animals to avoid interfering with the future growth potential of the physis.

In mature animals, tension-band wire fixation of the greater tubercle with lag screw and Kirschner wire stabilization of the humeral head can be performed (Fig. 47-6). Adequate surgical exposure requires both a craniolateral approach to the proximal humerus and a craniolateral approach to the shoulder joint.

Postoperative care for humeral head and proximal epiphyseal fractures may require application of a Velpeau sling or a spica bandage for 1 to 2 weeks to provide additional support. After bandage removal, active range-of-motion exercises are recommended, followed by restricted activity until the bone is healed.

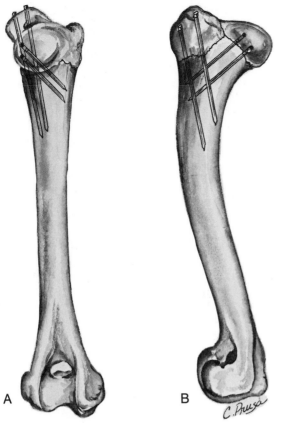

Fig. 47-5. *Capitus and greater tubercle fractures in a young animal. The greater tubercle is repaired with Kirschner wires. The capitus is stabilized with Kirschner wires or Stille nails driven through the lateral surface of the humeral head and countersunk below the articular cartilage. A, Caudocranial view. B, Lateral view.*

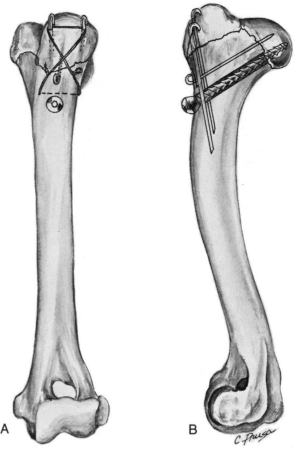

Fig. 47-6. *Capitus and greater tubercle fractures in a mature animal. The greater tubercle is repaired with tension-band wire. The capitus fracture is stabilized with a Kirschner wire, and a cortical lag screw is placed in the neck of the humerus. A, Caudocranial view. B, Lateral view.*

Shaft Fractures

Shaft fractures can occur at the proximal, middle, or distal diaphyseal regions of the bone. They may be classified as transverse, oblique, spiral, comminuted, or multiple. Types of fixation used to stabilize shaft fractures include intramedullary pins, Kirschner splints, and bone plates. Intramedullary pinning is most applicable to transverse and short oblique fractures in cats and in small to medium breed dogs. This type of pinning can also be used for long oblique, spiral, comminuted, or multiple fractures in combination with cerclage wiring, stack pinning, or Kirschner splintage. Kirschner splints alone are most commonly used for open, contaminated, multiple, or comminuted fractures. They may be placed during closed reduction, or they may be combined with a limited approach to the fracture site to facilitate reduction. These splints cause minimal disruption of blood supply to the bone and allow for free joint movement and treatment of open wounds during the healing period. Bone plating is usually reserved for shaft fractures in large and giant breed dogs. It is applicable to most types of shaft fractures and can be combined with lag screw fixation or cerclage wiring.

PROXIMAL DIAPHYSEAL

Proximal diaphyseal fractures usually occur at or just distal to the deltoid tuberosity. Contraction of the deltoideus and latissimus dorsi muscles results in caudal displacement of the proximal fragment. Closed reduction with normograde Steinmann pinning or application of a Kirschner splint may be considered, but can be difficult because of fragment distraction and soft tissue swelling. Open reduction is preferred, using a craniolateral approach to the proximal shaft with subperiosteal elevation of the deltoideus muscle. Fixation can be obtained by intramedullary pinning alone or in combination with a half-Kirschner splint.

MIDSHAFT AND DISTAL DIAPHYSEAL

INTRAMEDULLARY PIN FIXATION. Midshaft diaphyseal fractures are seen more frequently and typically occur where the radial nerve crosses the musculospiral groove as it passes from medial to lateral. These patients can have considerable overriding of the bone fragments, especially with oblique or spiral fractures. As mentioned earlier, radial nerve function should be carefully evaluated in these animals because of the close proximity of the nerve to the fracture site.

In medium to large breed dogs, closed reduction can be difficult because of the large muscle mass and fragment distraction. In small dogs and cats with recent transverse or short oblique fractures, closed reduction may be possible if the fracture site can be readily palpated. Normograde intramedullary pinning is performed by inserting the pin through the midpoint of the greater tubercle. An intramedullary pin that fills 70 to 75% of the medullary cavity at the fracture site is selected. The size of the medullary cavity can be estimated from the preoperative craniocaudal radiograph.

The pin is passed down the medullary cavity to the fracture site. The fracture is reduced, the pin is advanced into the distal fragment, and the pin is seated at a point just proximal to the supratrochlear foramen; one must take care to avoid penetrating the olecranon fossa (Fig. 47-7). Following pin placement, the joint is palpated to ensure a full range of crepitus-free motion. For closed or open pinning of fractures at the junction of the middle and distal third of the bone, a smaller pin is used to allow pin placement into the medial condyle. A pin is selected of sufficient size to fill the medial condyle on a preoperative craniocaudal radiograph. The pin is inserted at the midpoint of the greater tubercle, is passed in a normograde direction down the medullary cavity, and is seated in the medial condyle. The pin is advanced until the tip is felt to penetrate the distal surface of the condyle. To ensure that the pin has not penetrated the olecranon fossa, the joint should be palpated for crepitus and limited range of motion. Persistent rotational instability following insertion of an intramedullary pin for either middle or distal shaft fractures can be controlled by closed placement of a half-Kirschner splint (Fig. 47-8).

Open reduction of middle and distal diaphyseal fractures is preferred for medium to large breed dogs with fractures of greater than 24 to 48 hours' duration. A lateral approach to the bone allows exposure of the proximal three-fourths of the humeral shaft. The cephalic vein, as well as the radial nerve lying between the brachialis muscle and the lateral head of the triceps brachii muscle, should be identified and preserved. Proximal exposure of the shaft can be obtained by sub-

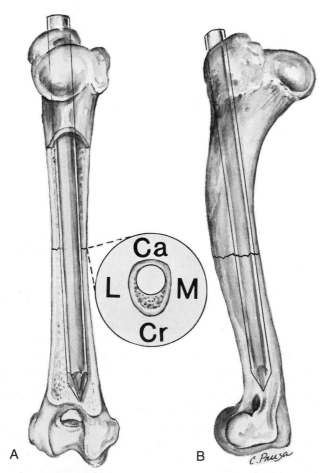

Fig. 47-7. *A transverse midshaft fracture demonstrating pin placement at the fracture site. The pin, which fills approximately 70 to 75% of the medullary cavity and contacts the caudal cortex of the bone at the fracture site, is inserted into the medullary cavity to a point just proximal to the supratrochlear foramen. A, Caudocranial view. (Ca, caudal cortex; L, lateral cortex; M, medial cortex; and Cr, cranial cortex). B, Lateral view.*

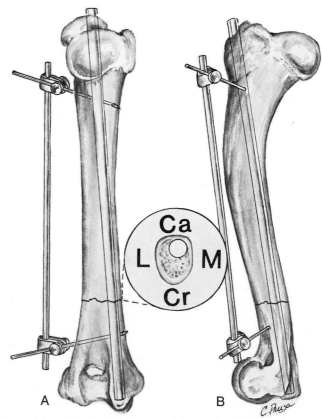

Fig. 47-8. *A distal transverse shaft fracture showing pin placement at the fracture site and application of a half-Kirschner splint. The intramedullary pin can be directed in a retrograde fashion against the caudomedial cortex of the proximal fragment to accentuate placement in the medial condyle. A, Caudocranial view. (Ca, caudal cortex; L, lateral cortex; M, medial cortex; and Cr, cranial cortex). B, Lateral view.*

periosteal elevation of the deltoideus muscle. Distal exposure can be gained by extending the incision to the lateral epicondyle and by dissecting the brachialis muscle to allow cranial and caudal retraction of the muscle and associated radial nerve.

Reduction of these fractures requires considerable traction with bone-holding forceps to correct overriding caused by spastic contraction of the muscles. In small dogs and in cats, fixation may be achieved with a single intramedullary Steinmann pin, as described for midshaft fractures handled by closed reduction. With open reduction, a pin of appropriate size is passed retrograde out the greater tubercle, the fracture is reduced, and the pin is seated in the distal fragment. To ensure proper pin placement in the distal fragment, the pin is directed in a retrograde fashion to accentuate placement either in the medullary cavity just proximal to the supratrochlear foramen or in the medial condyle.

For midshaft fractures requiring pin placement in the medullary cavity, the pin is started against the caudal cortex of the proximal fragment and is directed toward the greater tubercle (see Fig. 47-7).

For distal shaft fractures in which pin placement is desired in the medial condyle, the pin is started against the caudomedial cortex of the proximal fragment and is directed toward the midpoint of the greater tubercle (see Fig. 47-8). If the fracture remains unstable following single Steinmann pinning, additional fixation in the form of cerclage wires, stack pinning, or a half-Kirschner splint may be added. The intramedullary pin can be included within a hemicerclage wire if additional stability is achieved by pulling it against the cortex. Fractures most applicable to full-cerclage wiring include fissure fractures of the diaphysis and long oblique and spiral fractures. With both types of cerclage techniques, monofilament wire of sufficient size and strength should be used. A minimum of two cerclage wires is recommended to avoid the fulcrum effect associated with the use of one wire.

In large dogs with big medullary cavities, stack pinning provides more points of bone contact and improves rotational stability. Two pins of appropriate size are placed by directing the first pin in a retrograde fashion so that it seats in the medial condyle. The second pin is started at a point cranial and distal to the greater tubercle and is passed in a normograde direction down the medullary cavity to a point just proximal to the supratrochlear foramen (Fig. 47-9).

As mentioned earlier, half-Kirschner splints can also be used with intramedullary pinning to provide rotational stability. A single intramedullary pin is seated in the medial condyle to allow sufficient room between the pin and the cranial cortex of the shaft for placement of 2 Kirschner pins. Estimation of the Kirschner and intramedullary pin diameters can be obtained by studying the preoperative lateral radiograph. One Kirschner pin is placed in each fragment at 35 to 40° to the long axis of the bone and penetrates both cortices. Both pins should enter the bone through separate stab wounds away from the incision site. The pins are joined by a connecting bar and 2 single Kirschner

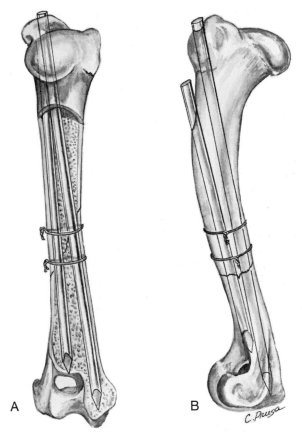

Fig. 47-9. *An oblique midshaft fracture repaired with stack pinning and full-cerlage wires. The first pin is passed in a retrograde direction from the caudomedial cortex of the fracture site and is placed in the medial condyle. The second pin is inserted in a normograde fashion from craniodistal to the greater tubercle to a point proximal to the supratrochlear foramen. A, Caudocranial view. B, Lateral view.*

clamps (see Fig. 47-8). In most cases, the half-Kirschner splint can be removed in 3 to 5 weeks following demonstration of a bridging callus on radiographic examination.

FULL KIRSCHNER SPLINT FIXATION. A full Kirschner splint can be used as the sole means of fixation for shaft fractures in cats and in small to medium breed dogs (Fig. 47-10). Before deciding on pin placement with the Kirschner splint, preoperative radiographs should be carefully evaluated for the presence and location of fissure fractures. The presence of fissure fractures may necessitate altering pin placement or may contraindicate the employment of the Kirschner splint.

When using a full Kirschner splint, 2 pins are placed craniolaterally in each major fragment. When possible, all pins are placed at 35 to 40° to the long axis of the bone and should penetrate both proximal and distal cortices. The proximal pin is placed just distal to the greater tubercle and the distal pin just proximal to the supratrochlear foramen or in transcondylar fashion using the epicondyles as landmarks. The 2 pins are joined with a connecting bar containing empty Kirschner clamps for placement of the 2 middle pins. The

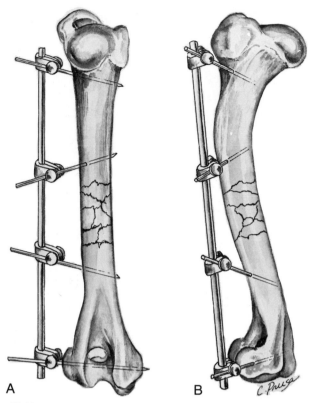

Fig. 47-10. *A comminuted midshaft fracture repaired with a full Kirschner splint. The splint is positioned on the craniolateral surface of the humerus, with the pins are driven through both cortices at approximately 35° to the long axis of the bone. A, Caudocranial view. B, Lateral view.*

deltoid tuberosity is used as a landmark for placement of the second pin in the proximal fragment. The second pin in the distal fragment is placed just proximal to the condylar ridges; one must take care to avoid the radial nerve. As mentioned earlier, the Kirschner splint can be placed during closed reduction, or a limited lateral approach may be used to facilitate fracture reduction. In both situations, a half Kirschner splint is initially positioned, and traction is applied to obtain axial alignment of the proximal and distal fragments. The two end clamps are tightened to maintain the reduction while the two middle pins are driven into the bone through clamps positioned on the connector bar. When inserting the middle pins, medial support should be given to the fragments to prevent distraction and loss of reduction. Lag screws or cerclage wires can be combined with the Kirschner splint as needed to provide additional fixation for oblique, spiral, multiple, or fissure fractures.

BONE PLATE FIXATION. Bone plates can be applied to most shaft fractures, but are especially useful for large and giant breed dogs and for multiple and comminuted fractures. A dynamic compression plate with three screws placed on each side of the fracture is recommended. In cases with oblique, spiral, or multiple fractures, lag screws or cerclage wires can be combined with plate fixation as required.

For fractures involving the proximal and midshaft regions, the plate is conformed to the bone and is placed on the cranial surface of the shaft (Fig. 47-11). Exposure is obtained using a craniolateral approach to the proximal shaft with subperiosteal elevation of the superficial pectoral and deltoideus muscles and caudal retraction of the brachialis and triceps brachii muscles.

For distal shaft fractures, the plate is positioned laterally along the musculospiral groove, the lateral condyle, and the lateral epicondylar crest (Fig. 47-12). The plate is conformed to the surface of the distal musculospiral groove and lateral condyle and is positioned under the brachialis muscle. Exposure is obtained using a lateral approach to the shaft, and the incision is extended proximally and distally as required.

For distal-third shaft fractures with a comminuted medial cortex, the plate can be applied to the caudal medial surface of the medial condyle (Fig. 47-13). Surgical exposure can be obtained using a medial approach to the distal shaft; one must take care to preserve the brachial and collateral ulnar vessels and the ulnar and median nerves. The nutrient artery located on the caudal surface of the bone should also be preserved. A transolecranon osteotomy can be performed when additional exposure is needed.

BONE GRAFTS. Autogenous cancellous bone grafts may be required to enhance healing of severely com-

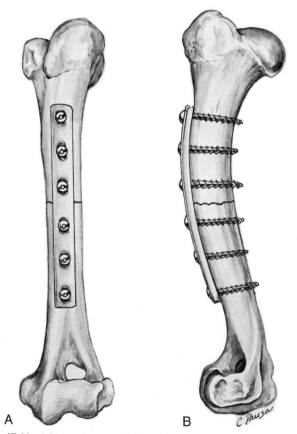

Fig. 47-11. *A bone plate applied to the cranial surface of the humerus for fixation of proximal or midshaft fractures. Three screws should be placed in the plate on each side of the fracture site. A, Craniocaudal view. B, Lateral view.*

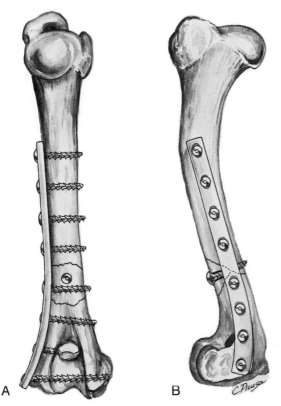

Fig. 47-12. *A bone plate placed on the lateral surface of the humerus for repair of a distal shaft fracture. The plate is conformed to the musculospiral groove, the lateral condyle, and the lateral epicondylar crest. Lag screw compression of a butterfly fragment is combined with plate fixation. A, Caudocranial view. B, Lateral view.*

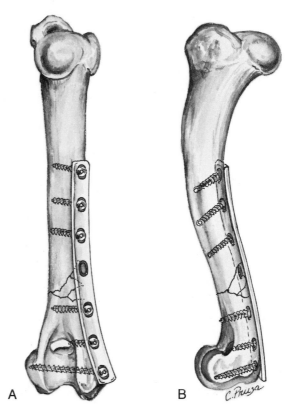

Fig. 47-13. *A bone plate positioned on the caudomedial surface of the shaft and the medial condyle for repair of distal shaft fractures with a comminuted medial cortex. A, Caudocranial view. B, Lateral view.*

minuted or multiple shaft fractures repaired with open reduction and internal fixation. Indications include middle-aged and older patients or patients with large bone defects at the fracture site. Cancellous bone is taken from surgically prepared sites at the greater tubercle, the tibial crest, or the wing of the ilium. The graft is harvested and is immediately placed in the fracture site prior to closure of the soft tissues.

Severely comminuted shaft fractures with large bone defects may require full cylinder cortical bone grafting. Suitably prepared cortical bone allografts can be used for this purpose. Bone grafts of this type are usually reserved for comminuted shaft fractures that cannot be repaired by normal reconstructive techniques.

Supracondylar Fractures

Most supracondylar fractures pass through the supratrochlear foramen. In young animals, an epiphyseal separation may occur with the supracondylar fracture. Metaphyseal fractures with no involvement of the supratrochlear foramen may be seen in other animals. Closed reduction is not advised with this type of fracture. Open reduction with internal fixation, to allow early joint motion with weight-bearing, produces the best results. Surgical exposure through a medial or lateral approach to the distal shaft may be used, or the

two approaches can be combined. When combing approaches, a lateral skin incision is made, and the skin and subcutaneous layers are reflected to expose both sides of the joint.

A transolecranon approach provides the best exposure in large dogs requiring double bone plating for multiple or comminuted supracondylar fractures. When approaching the supracondylar area in cats, one must realize that the median nerve passes through the supratrochlear foramen and that the ulnar nerve lies under the medial head of the triceps brachii muscle. Special care should be taken to preserve these structures.

TRANSVERSE

The preferred method of fixation of transverse supracondylar fractures involving the foramen is intramedullary pinning combined with Kirschner or Steinmann pinning of the lateral condyle. (Fig. 47-14). This technique provides rigid internal fixation for most transverse supracondylar fractures and is applicable to all sizes of dogs by appropriate alteration of the pin sizes. The fracture is reduced, and the proximal fragment is immobilized with bone-holding forceps. With the patient's elbow flexed, the veterinary surgeon passes a pin of sufficient size to fill the medial condyle

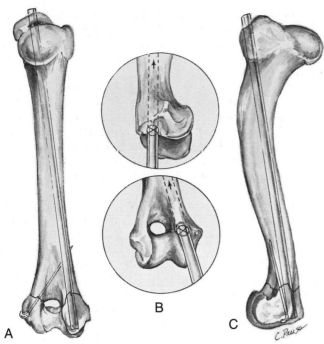

Fig. 47-14. *A transverse supracondylar fracture showing normograde placement of an intramedullary pin parallel to the caudal cortex of the medial condyle. A Kirschner wire or a small Steinmann pin is passed through the lateral condyle to penetrate the medial cortex and to provide rotational stability. A, Caudocranial view. B, Details of pin placement. C, Lateral view.*

normograde from the medial condyle to the greater tubercle. The pin is passed up the shaft parallel to the caudomedial cortex of the condyle to the greater tubercle. During pin placement, reduction is maintained by counterforce applied to the bone-holding forceps attached to the proximal fragment. Rotation of the distal fragment is controlled by bone-holding forceps placed over the fracture site of the lateral condyle. The fracture is checked repeatedly during pin advancement to ensure that reduction is maintained. When the pin penetrates the greater tubercle, the bone chuck is removed, and the distal point is cut off. The chuck is reapplied to the proximal portion, the distal part of the pin is drawn into the medial condyle, and the proximal pin is cut off as short as possible at the greater tubercle.

An alternate method of pin placement passes the pin retrograde up the caudomedial cortex of the proximal fragment. Following reduction, the pin is advanced into the distal fragment and is seated in the medial condyle. With both methods, a Kirschner wire or a small Steinmann pin is passed from distal and caudal to the lateral epicondyle to penetrate the medial cortex of the humeral shaft. The pin in the lateral condyle should pass between the intramedullary pin and cranial cortex of the shaft.

Postoperatively, a Robert Jones bandage is placed on the limb for 2 to 3 days to control postsurgical swelling and edema. Early physiotherapy and restricted exercise following weight-bearing is advised. Removal

of the intramedullary pin is recommended when the bone has healed.

Double Rush pinning offers an alternative for repair of transverse supracondylar fractures. Rush pins of appropriate size are prebent to facilitate their insertion and are placed slightly distal and caudal to the medial and lateral epicondyles. Guide holes are made with a Rush awl to allow introduction of the pins at approximately 20 to 30° to the long axis of the bone. The pins should be placed so that they cross above the fracture site and provide rigid 3-point fixation (Fig. 47-15). In small dogs and in cats, Kirschner wires or small Steinmann pins can be substituted for Rush pins and passed in similar fashion.

Oblique

Oblique supracondylar fractures can be repaired with intramedullary pinning and hemicerclage wiring. The intramedullary pin is directed in a retrograde fashion into the proximal fragment, the fracture is reduced and immobilized, and the pin is advanced and seated in the medial condyle. Hemicerclage wire, preplaced through the bone and around the pin, is tightened to provide additional stability and rotational control. A Robert Jones bandage is applied for 2 to 3 days, fol-

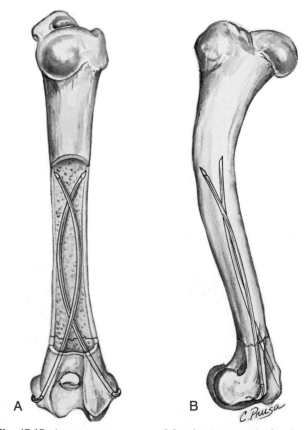

Fig. 47-15. *A transverse supracondylar fracture repaired using a double-Rush-pin technique. The pins are placed in the bone slightly distal and caudal to the epicondyles and at an angle of approximately 20 to 30° to the shaft of the humerus. A, Caudocranial view. B, Lateral view.*

lowed by physiotherapy and early, restricted weight-bearing.

MULTIPLE AND COMMINUTED

Fixation of multiple or comminuted supracondylar fractures in dogs of small to medium size can be achieved by intramedullary pinning of the medial condyle combined with cerclage wiring and a full Kirschner splint (Fig. 47-16). Surgical exposure for repair of these fractures usually requires a combined medial and lateral or transolecranon approach. A double-trocar-point Steinmann pin is passed in a retrograde fashion into the medial condyle, and the fracture site is reduced. The pin is then advanced in a normograde direction into the proximal fragment to exit at the greater tubercle. Next, a half-Kirschner splint is placed on the craniolateral aspect of the bone. The proximal pin is inserted below the greater tubercle and is passed between the intramedullary pin and the cortex of the bone. The distal pin is placed in transcondylar fashion by entering the bone at the lateral epicondyle and angling toward the medial epicondyle.

A connector bar containing empty Kirschner clamps for placement of two middle pins is positioned between the proximal and distal pins. Using traction, the major fragments are placed in axial alignment and are temporarily stabilized by tightening the proximal and distal clamps. Comminuted or multiple fragments are reduced and are stabilized with cerclage wires or lag screws. Kirschner wires can be placed across the bone, or the cortex may be grooved to prevent the cerclage wire from slipping down the metaphysis and becoming loose. The half-Kirschner splint is adjusted as required to allow manipulation to obtain reduction. The proximal and distal clamps are tightened after stabilizing the small bone fragments with wire or lag screws. The second pin in the proximal fragment is inserted into the bone between the intramedullary pin and the cranial cortex of the shaft. The second pin in the distal fragment is placed in transcondylar fashion in the distal fragment from the lateral to medial epicondyle. The two distal pins are placed within the condylar bone in cross-pin fashion. Care should be taken to support the fracture site during placement of the two middle pins to prevent distraction and loss of reduction.

In large dogs, double bone plating may be required to provide fixation of comminuted or multiple supracondylar fractures (Fig. 47-17). A transolecranon approach provides the best exposure for application of two

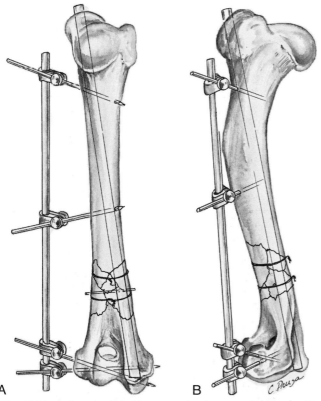

Fig. 47-16. *A comminuted supracondylar fracture stabilized with an intramedullary pin placed in the medial condyle, cerclage wiring, and a full Kirschner splint. The intramedullary pin is directed in a retrograde fashion into the medial condyle and then is advanced into the proximal fragment. Full cerclage wires are used to stabilize the multiple bone fragments. A, Caudocranial view. B, Lateral view.*

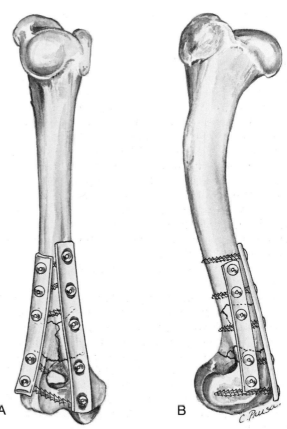

Fig. 47-17. *A double bone plate repair of a multiple supracondylar fracture. The plates are positioned on the caudomedial surface of the medial condyle and the caudal surface of the lateral condyle. A minimum of two screws should be placed distal to the fracture site in each plate. A, Caudocranial view. B, Lateral view.*

plates of appropriate size. To use the bone plating technique, the condylar fragment must be large enough to allow placement of at least two screws distal to the fracture. The larger plate is positioned on the caudomedial surface of the medial condyle. The second, smaller plate is conformed to the caudal surface of the lateral condyle and the lateral epicondylar crest. Consideration must be given to placement of all screws prior to drilling, and the plates should be positioned to allow interdigitation of the screws. Lag screw compression through the plate should be used whenever possible. Placement of screws into the joint or olecranon fossa must be avoided to ensure an unrestricted, crepitus-free range of motion.

Postoperative care includes the use of a Robert Jones bandage for 3 to 5 days, with early active physiotherapy and restricted weight-bearing. Removal of the bone plates may be necessary following healing of the fracture if the screws loosen or if the implant interferes with joint function.

CANCELLOUS BONE GRAFTS. Comminuted or multiple supracondylar fractures may require autogenous cancellous bone grafting, as described previously for comminuted shaft fractures. When bone grafting is anticipated, one or more donor sites are surgically prepared. Following reduction and fixation, the graft is harvested and is placed into the fracture site prior to closure of the wound.

Condylar Fractures

Fractures of the lateral condyle of the humerus are seen more frequently than medial condyle fractures. The presumed reason for difference is that the lateral condyle bears the major portion of the weight transferred through the joint and is biomechanically weaker than the medial condyle. Preoperative radiographs of lateral condyle fractures usually reveal a subluxated elbow joint with cranial and outward rotation of the fragment caused by contraction of the extensor muscles of the forearm. Fracture of the medial condyle causes caudal and inward displacement of the fragment.

Closed reduction of lateral condyle fractures is possible if swelling is minimal and if the fracture is not of greater than 24 to 36 hours' duration. The fragment is reduced by digital manipulation and is temporarily stabilized with a condyle clamp placed over the epicondyles. The clamp is positioned to allow access to the area slightly distal and cranial to the epicondyles. In small dogs and in cats, a Vulsellum clamp can be substituted for the larger condyle clamp. Reduction is checked prior to stabilizing the fracture by palpating the caudal surface of the lateral condyle, by moving the joint through a full range of motion, and by taking radiographs. Failure to obtain anatomic reduction is an indication for a limited open lateral approach to facilitate repair.

If closed reduction is achieved, a stab incision is made over the epicondyle and a guide hole created distal and cranial to the epicondyle with an intramedullary pin. A drill bit is placed in the guide hole and is advanced across the condyles parallel to the joint surface to a point distal and cranial to the opposite epicondyle. A depth gauge is used to determine the length of screw required, and the hole is threaded with a bone tap. A cancellous screw is inserted to create a lag effect and to provide compression at the fracture site. If rotational instability persists, a Kirschner wire can be placed from the epicondyle to the cortex of the shaft.

Lateral or medial condyle fractures of greater than 36 hours' duration or fractures that are nonreducible because of excessive swelling or early callus formation should be handled by open reduction. A transolecranon approach provides the best exposure, although a medial or lateral approach may be adequate in selected cases. Subperiosteal elevation of the extensor carpi radialis muscle allows better visualization and easier reduction for lateral condyle repairs. Accurate anatomic reduction of the articular surface is paramount to a successful repair. Gentle curettage of the fracture surface, to remove organizing fibrin clots and interposed soft tissue, facilitates reduction. The fracture is stabilized with a condyle clamp or Vulsellum forceps, and a hole is drilled across the condyles as described for closed reduction. In cats and in small dogs, the use of a C-clamp placed across the condyles ensures proper drilling of the condylar hole. The depth of the hole is measured and is tapped to receive a cortical bone screw. The fracture is separated, and the threaded hole in the condyle fragment is overdrilled to create a glide hole. The fracture is reduced, and a transcondylar cortical screw is inserted to provide lag screw compression at the fracture site.

An alternate technique is to drill the condyle fragment from the fracture site, reduce the fracture, and use the condylar hole as a guide to drill the opposite condyle. With both techniques, a Kirschner wire is placed caudal to the screw head and driven up the condyle to the cortex of the distal shaft to prevent rotation (Fig. 47-18). If the transolecranon approach is used, the olecranon is replaced and is stabilized using a tension-band wire. Postoperative care includes the use of a Robert Jones bandage for 3 to 5 days, followed by physiotherapy and restricted weight-bearing until the bone is healed. The implants are not removed unless they loosen or cause irritation to the soft tissues.

Intercondylar Fractures

Supracondylar fractures of the humerus occurring with a condyle fracture are referred to as "T" or "Y" fractures. They are usually seen in mature animals in which the epiphysis has fused. Because the fracture involves articular surface, closed reduction with external fixation is not an acceptable method of repair, and open reduction with internal fixation should be recommended as early as possible.

A transolecranon approach provides the best visualization and facilitates anatomic reduction of the fracture. The surface of the fracture is exposed and cleaned of organizing fibrin and interposed soft tissue.

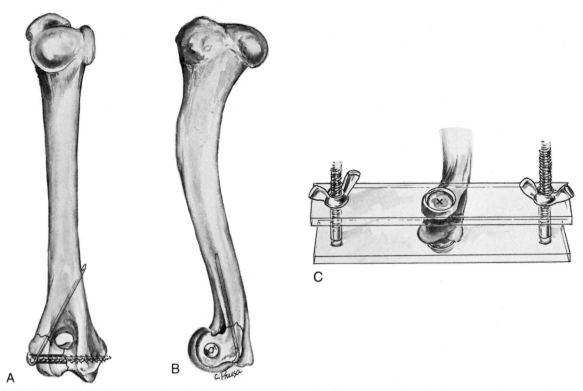

Fig. 47-18. *A lateral condylar fracture stabilized with a transcondylar cortical lag screw and a Kirschner wire. The lateral condyle can be temporarily reduced with a condyle clamp (C) during placement of the transcondylar screw. Overdrilling the lateral condyle provides lag screw compression at the fracture site. The Kirschner wire placed in the condyle prevents rotation of the fragment. A, Caudocranial view. B, Lateral view.*

Reduction is performed and is evaluated by visualizing the articular surface of the condyles and the alignment of the humeral shaft with the condylar ridges. The intercondylar fracture is repaired by first reducing the fracture to a single supracondylar fracture. The condyles are immobilized with a condyle clamp or Vulsellum forceps, and one or two small Kirschner wires are passed across the fracture to provide temporary fixation.

A guide hole for a drill bit is started distal and cranial to the lateral epicondyle using an intramedullary pin. The drill site is located on a line 45° cranial and distal to a line passing through the lateral epicondyle and the shaft of the humerus (Fig. 47-19). The drill is directed toward a similar point cranial and distal to the medial epicondyle. Placement of the screw should be in the center of both condyles and parallel to the joint surface. In small dogs and cats, a C-clamp is useful for immobilizing the condyles and for providing a guide for proper screw placement. A depth gauge is used to determine the screw's length, and the hole is threaded with a bone tap. The lateral condyle fragment is overdrilled to create a glide hole, and a cortical screw is inserted to provide lag screw compression at the fracture site. Care should be taken to avoid overcompression of the soft cancellous bone.

An alternate method for drilling is first to reduce the fracture, then to separate it to allow drilling from the fracture surface of the lateral condyle to a point cranial and distal to the lateral epicondyle. With this technique, the hole must be carefully centered in the lateral condyle. The fracture is again reduced and is immobilized with an appropriate clamp or a small Kirschner wire. The medial condyle fragment is drilled using the hole in the lateral condyle as a guide. The depth of the hole is measured, and the entire length is threaded with a bone tap. The lateral condyle is overdrilled as previously described, and a cortical screw is selected and is inserted to provide lag screw compression at the fracture site. The Kirschner wires are usually removed, except in large dogs in which additional fixation may be desirable. In tiny animals, threaded pins or Kirschner wires can be used to provide fixation if available bone screws are too large. Following stabilization, the joint should be flexed and extended to ensure a crepitus-free, nonrestricted range of motion.

The repaired condyles can now be attached to the shaft using the intramedullary pinning technique described for supracondylar fractures. Following reduction, a pin of sufficient size to fill the medial condyle is selected, based on an assessment of the craniocaudal preoperative radiograph. The pin is passed parallel to the caudal cortex of the medial epicondyle to penetrate the greater tubercle. The distal point is cut off, and the bone chuck is applied to the proximal portion of the pin. The distal end is drawn into the medial condyle, and the proximal portion is cut as close to the greater tubercle as possible. During placement of the

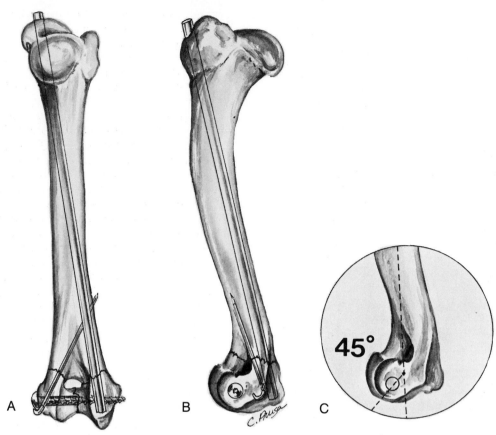

Fig. 47-19. *An intercondylar "T" fracture repaired with a transcondylar cortical lag screw, pinning of the medial condyle, and a Kirschner wire placed in the lateral condyle. The site for screw placement (C) is located on a line 45° cranial and distal to a line drawn through the shaft of the humerus and lateral epicondyle. A, Caudocranial view. B, Lateral view.*

intramedullary pin, the supracondylar fracture site should be checked repeatedly to ensure that reduction is maintained.

An alternate method of pin placement is to pass the intramedullary pin retrograde into the medial condyle. The fracture is reduced, and the pin is passed normograde up the humeral shaft to the greater tubercle. The pin is cut off as described for the previous technique. A Kirschner wire of appropriate size or a small Steinmann pin is passed up the lateral condyle to provide rotational stability. This pin enters the bone immediately caudal to the screw head and is directed between the intramedullary pin and the cranial cortex of the humeral shaft until it penetrates the medial cortex. This combination of transcondylar screw fixation of the condyles with pinning of the supracondylar fracture is applicable to all sizes of dogs and cats and provides an excellent method of fixation.

Another, but more difficult, technique uses lag-screw fixation for the condylar fracture, and double Rush pinning of the supracondylar fracture (Fig. 47-20).

Postoperative care with both types of fixation includes placement of a Robert Jones bandage for 3 to 5 days, followed by physiotherapy in the form of swimming or range-of-motion exercises and controlled weight-bearing. The intramedullary pin can be removed when the bone has healed. The transcondylar screw

and Kirschner wires or small Steinmann pin are usually not removed unless they loosen or cause irritation.

Comminuted "T" or "Y" fractures are unstable and usually require double bone plating for repair. A transolecranon approach provides the best exposure for stabilizing these fractures. A transcondylar screw is placed in the condyles, and bone plates are applied to the medial condyle and humeral shaft and to the lateral condyle and lateral epicondylar crest. For each plate, two screws are placed in the condylar fragment and three in the humeral shaft. An autogenous cancellous bone graft should be harvested and placed in the fracture site prior to closure.

Acknowledgement

I wish to thank Carol G. Prusa, Biomedical Communications Center, College of Veterinary Medicine, University of Illinois, for preparing the illustrations used in this article.

References and Suggested Readings

1. Archibald, J. (ed.): Canine Surgery. 2nd Ed. Santa Barbara, CA, American Veterinary Publications, 1974.
2. Braden, T. D.: The humerus. *In* Current Techniques in Small Animal Surgery. Edited by M. J. Bojrab. Philadelphia, Lea & Febiger, 1975.

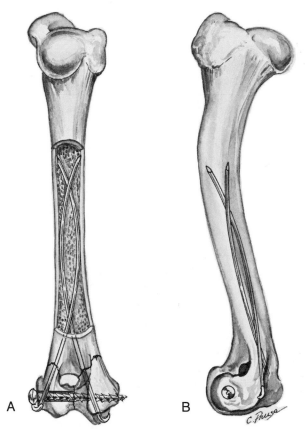

Fig. 47-20. *An intercondylar "T" fracture stabilized with a transcondylar cortical lag screw and double Rush pins. A, Caudocranial view. B, Lateral view.*

3. Brinker, W. O., and Flo, G. L.: Principles and application of external skeletal fixation. Vet. Clin. North Am., 5:197, 1975.

4. Evans, H. E., and Christensen, G. C.: Miller's Anatomy of the Dog. 2nd Ed. Philadelphia, W. B. Saunders, 1979.

5. Muller, M. E., Allgower, M., Schneider, R., and Willenegger, H.: Manual of Internal Fixation. 2nd Ed. New York, Springer-Verlag, 1979.

6. Piermattei, D. L.: Orthopedic conditions of the shoulder region. *In* Proceedings of the 47th Annual Meeting of the American Animal Hospital Association, 1980.

7. Piermattei, D. L., and Greeley, R. G.: An Atlas of Surgical Approaches to the Bones of the Dog and Cat. 2nd Ed. Philadelphia, W. B. Saunders, 1979.

8. Rush, L. V.: Atlas of Rush Pin Technics. Meridian, MS, Berivon, 1955.

9. Withrow S. J.: Principles of intramedullary pinning and cerclage wiring. *In* Proceedings of the 47th Annual Meeting of the American Animal Hospital Association, 1980.

Luxation of the Elbow

by Joseph M. Stoyak

The elbow joint is formed by articulation of the humerus with the radius and ulna. Approximately 80% of the weight is borne by the concave articular surface of the head of the radius. The remainder of the articular surface distally is comprised of the medial and lateral coronoid processes of the ulna. Dislocation of the elbow implies displacement of one or more bones that form this joint. As a result of the displacement, the articular surfaces are no longer in normal contact.

In the dog, elbow luxation is less common than hip luxation, which occurs ten times more frequently. This dislocation may be of either congenital or traumatic origin. The congenital type is least common and is associated with an anatomic deformity. Surgical correction is complicated and difficult. Owing to the deformity, such correction is rarely completely successful even when a series of operative procedures have been performed. The traumatic luxation requires great force and is often associated with other injuries. A local fracture may also be present. It is not possible to reduce a dislocation of the elbow complicated by a fracture unless the fracture segments are stabilized either before or concomitant with the reduction of the dislocation.

Traumatic dislocation is manifested by acute lameness. The limb is carried slightly abducted and rotated externally. Flexion and extension are restricted. The width of the joint is enlarged, and pain is present.

The possibility of the presence of other conditions must be considered. Distal humeral and condylar fractures are conditions most frequently confused with dislocation. When the joint is grossly swollen, differentiation is difficult.

It is imperative that the area be radiographed to confirm the diagnosis and to ascertain that no fractures are present. Because the lateral radiographic view may be deceiving, a craniocaudal view should also be obtained. Examination for extensor paralysis, which can accompany forelimb trauma, should be made.

Most commonly, the radius and ulna are luxated caudolaterally. The anconeal process is thus the main obstacle to reduction. Elbow dislocations are accompanied by severe damage to the soft tissues, especially the ligaments and joint capsule. The ligaments may be torn, or at least severely stretched, compromising their function as joint stabilizers.

Closed Reduction

If luxation alone is present, closed reduction is attempted before open procedures are considered. Closed reduction is effective in most patients.

General anesthesia is required. The use of deep anesthesia with analgesia, such as with inhalation anesthetics, affords a degree of relaxation that renders the procedure less traumatic to the already injured tissues. In the difficult case, the type of anesthesia used may mean the difference between open and closed reduction.

The patient is placed in the lateral recumbent position with the affected limb upward. Thomas splint traction for a few minutes with the elbow in flexion can be helpful. It is important to palpate carefully and to determine the exact location of the radial head, the tip of the anconeal process, and the lateral epicondylar ridge. The elbow is flexed sufficiently to allow the anconeal process to clear the impingement on the humeral con-

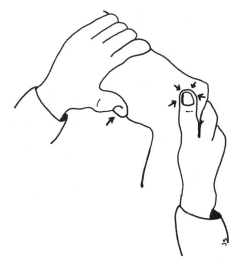

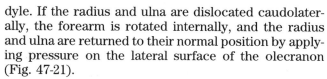

Fig. 47-21. *Application of pressure over the olecranon while the patient's elbow is severely flexed and the forearm is rotated outward. The veterinarian's left hand stabilizes the upper limb.*

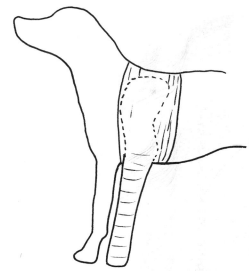

Fig. 47-22. *Full forelimb coaptation splint made of plywood and attached around the patient's chest.*

dyle. If the radius and ulna are dislocated caudolaterally, the forearm is rotated internally, and the radius and ulna are returned to their normal position by applying pressure on the lateral surface of the olecranon (Fig. 47-21).

In a stubborn dislocation, the anatomic peculiarities of the elbow joint may be used to accomplish the reduction. In this approach, the anconeal process is used as a fulcrum. If the anconeal process lies medial to the lateral condyle, only rotation of the radius and ulna, with extension of the joint by application of lateral pressure on the olecranon, is required to effect reduction. If the anconeal process lies lateral to the lateral condyle, however, it is first placed medially by flexing the elbow to 45° or less and working it to a medial position, usually in a stepwise fashion, by manipulating the leg while applying force on the olecranon medially.

Almost all luxated elbows treated shortly after the luxation has taken place can be reduced if adequate relaxation is obtained, provided the operator understands the anatomy of the region and performs the manipulation thoughtfully.

After reduction, a general impression of the resultant stability can be obtained by gently manipulating the joint. Examination of the elbow for evidence of rupture of the medial and collateral ligaments, as described by Campbell, is now performed.[1] This examination provides vital information for making the decision as to whether surgical repair of these ligaments is necessary. At this point, a decision is required regarding the next step in management.

CRITERIA FOR TREATMENT FOLLOWING CLOSED REDUCTION

1. If the joint is stable and the patient is not hyperactive, the leg is not immobilized, but the animal's activity is restricted for a week.

2. If instability persists and reluxation is threatened, the patient's leg is placed in a soft bandage to restrict elbow motion. Alternatively, it may be desirable to use a well-padded plywood coaptation splint or a plaster splint extending to the shoulder in spica fashion applied around the chest. Because this splint restricts elbow motion and cannot slip distally, it allows stretched tissues to rest and to regain their normal configuration (Fig. 47-22). This splint may be left in place 1 to 4 weeks as needed; however, joint ankylosis is possible if the splint is left in place for the full 4 weeks.

3. Should the elbow readily reluxate on manipulation, surgical repair of the damaged structures may be required. Usually all that is needed, however, is the application of a shoulder spica bandage for 3 to 4 weeks. If the collateral ligaments are ruptured, surgical treatment is preferable to prolonged splintage.

Open Reduction

Open reduction is usually required only when a delay occurs in presenting the patient for treatment, or when the condition has not been recognized in its early stages. In patients with severe dislocation, however, both open reduction and ligament repair can be expected to be necessary.

Open reduction is accomplished through an incision on the lateral aspect of the joint when the patient's leg has been aseptically prepared and draped. The incision is made by dissecting between the common and lateral digital extensor muscles just distal to their origin on the lateral epicondyle. Entry into the joint is made along the side of the lateral collateral ligament. Either a bone skid or blunt curved Mayo scissors may be used as a lever. The instrument selected is inserted with its convexity directed dorsally over the radial head, then medially and ventrally until it is under the lateral condyle (Fig. 47-23*A*). When placed, the instrument is then turned with its concavity directed dorsally. Downward

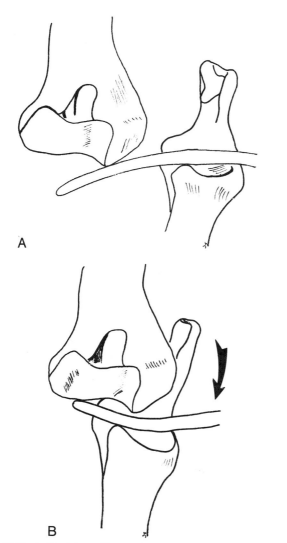

A

B

Fig. 47-23. A, *Position of lever after insertion, with its convexity directed dorsally. B, Position of lever when it has been turned, with its convexity directed ventrally and downward pressure exerted.*

pressure on the handle forces the lateral condyle up and allows it to slide laterally on the scissors while the elbow is flexed sufficiently to allow the anconeal process to clear the caudal border of the condyle (Fig. 47-23B). When the reduction is accomplished, the joint is examined for stability and the need for ligament repair. A splint is required following open reduction.

If the luxation has been of long duration, it may not be reducible by the leverage method just described. In such an instance, the veterinary surgeon should be prepared to provide extensive exposure of the joint to facilitate inspection and reduction. This exposure is best accomplished by either the transolecranon or the triceps brachii tenotomy approach. Again, a splint is usually applied following this approach. Its use is dependent on the status of the reduction. The olecranon osteotomy site is stabilized with a tension-band wire and requires no splintage. A judicious return to early weight-bearing may improve function in the joint, although degenerative changes frequently occur.

References and Suggested Readings

1. Campbell, J. R.: Nonfracture injuries to the canine elbow. J. Am. Vet. Med. Assoc., *155:*735, 1969.
2. Evans, H. E., and Christensen, G. C.: Miller's Anatomy of the Dog. 2nd Ed. Philadelphia, W. B. Saunders, 1979.
3. Leighton, R. L.: Surgical correction of complete luxation of the elbow in the dog. J. Am. Vet. Med. Assoc., *126:*17, 1955.
4. Leonard, E. P.: Orthopedic Surgery of the Dog and Cat. 2nd Ed. Philadelphia, W. B. Saunders, 1971.
5. Piermattei, D. L., and Greeley, R. G.: An Atlas of Surgical Approaches to the Bones of the Dog and Cat. 2nd Ed. Philadelphia, W. B. Saunders, 1979.
6. Smith, F. M.: Surgery of the Elbow. 2nd Ed. Philadelphia, W. B. Saunders, 1972.

Amputation of the Forelimb

by WILLIAM R. DALY

Amputation of the forelimb is occasionally indicated as a primary treatment for severe traumatic injuries resulting in irreparable fractures and soft tissue injuries. Other indications are severe neurologic injuries such as brachial plexus avulsion, irreparable vascular occlusion, and severe congenital or acquired deformities. Amputation may also be considered as an adjunct to the treatment of neoplasia or severe infections involving the limb. With the possible exception of neoplastic disease, amputation should be considered as a last-resort "salvage" procedure, indicated only when no alternative exists that would allow the retention of a useful limb.

Preoperative Considerations

Amputation performed at the shoulder joint or above is preferable because a stump below this level serves no useful function and is prone to abrasions and infection from frequent trauma. Small animals invariably adapt well to forelimb amputation; however, some giant breeds of dogs have difficulty. If the patient is able to ambulate while carrying the affected limb, it usually does well with a forelimb amputation.

The veterinary surgeon can choose to perform a forelimb amputation either through or directly below the scapulohumeral joint, or a forequarter amputation can be performed in which the scapula is removed with the limb. Forequarter amputation offers the advantages that major vessels and nerves are easily visualized, bone-cutting instruments are not required, and no prominent scapular spine remains behind. The procedure of choice, however, is the one that works best for each individual veterinary surgeon.

Forelimb amputation is a major procedure that should be performed only with a thorough knowledge of the patient's physical status. Because blood loss is likely to be greater than in most major operations, it is essential to evaluate both hematocrit and plasma proteins preoperatively. Anemic or hypoproteinemic patients should be treated medically, if time allows, or

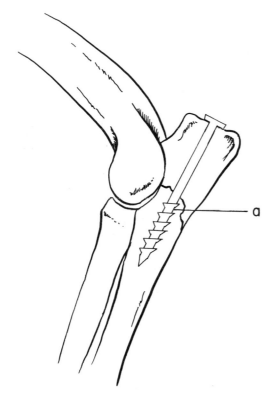

Fig. 47-27. *Cancellous screw in position with threaded portion completely across the fracture line (a).*

It is important to note carefully the conformation of the ulna prior to drilling of screw holes or driving the pins. The lateral curvature and narrow intramedullary canal make it difficult to drill the hole without exiting through the side of the ulna. The proximal ulnar fragment may be easily fragmented in the process of drilling and overdrilling. The use of screw fixation should be reserved for medium to large breed dogs. An additional drawback to this technique is the complication of breakage of the bone screw before the fracture has healed. The incidence of screw breakage can be decreased by the addition of a tension-band wire.

Another acceptable method of repair is the application of a bone plate on the caudal aspect, or tension-band side, of the ulna. This technique is especially useful in comminuted fractures of the proximal ulna and in large breed dogs in which at least two or three screws can be inserted in the proximal fragment (Fig. 47-29).

Surgical exposure of the fracture site, as described, avoids any vital structures. If reduction is difficult and tissue dissection is extensive, care must be taken to identify and to preserve the branch of the ulnar nerve that courses near the medial humeroulnar articulation.

Two methods of repair that may be fraught with complications are single intramedullary pin fixation and external coaptation. These types of fixation allow the pull of the triceps brachii muscle to distract the

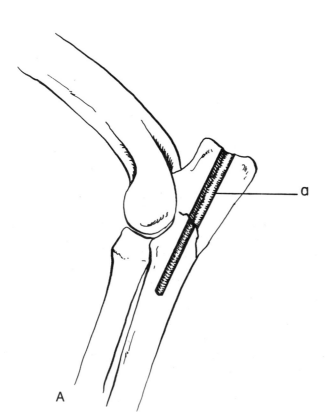

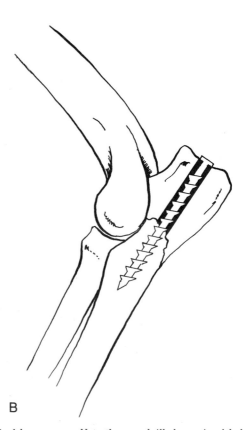

Fig. 47-28. A, *Fractured olecranon with holes drilled for placement of a cortical bone screw. Note the overdrilled proximal hole (a).* B, *Cortical screw in place, to reduce the fracture under compression.*

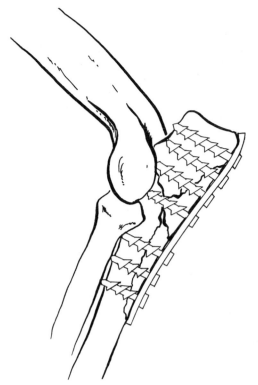

Fig. 47-29. *Fixation of a comminuted olecranon fracture with a bone plate and screws.*

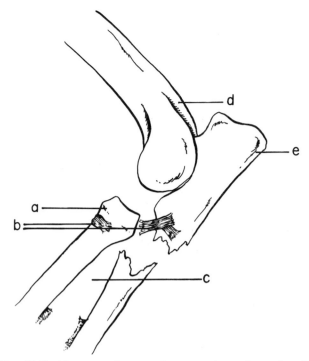

Fig. 47-30. *Monteggia fracture demonstrating a luxated radial head (a), torn anular ligaments (b), separation of interosseous attachment of the radius and ulna (c), and the relation of the humerus (d) and the olecranon (e) to each other.*

fracture fragments. The result may be prolonged lameness, malunion, delayed union, nonunion, and secondary degenerative joint disease.

Fractures of the Proximal Ulnar Shaft with Dislocation of the Head of the Radius

Monteggia described a fracture in man that involved the proximal ulna with concurrent dislocation of the radial head (Fig. 47-30). This type of fracture must be surgically reduced with the application of internal fixation. Surgical repair, however, is not without frequent complications. Repair of a Monteggia fracture can result in chronic luxation of the radial head, nonunion of the ulna, traumatic ossification around the radial head, osteoarthritis, and a decreased range of motion of the elbow joint.[5]

The fracture is approached surgically by a combination of a lateral approach to the elbow joint and a caudal approach to the proximal ulna. Reduction of the radial head luxation may be difficult because the extensor carpi radialis muscle is interposed between the radial head and the ulna. Primary emphasis must be placed on reducing the radial head luxation and restoring congruity of the elbow joint. These priorities are especially important in severely comminuted fractures of the ulna, in which loss of bone substrate may result in limb shortening and chronic radial head luxation.

After reduction of the radial head luxation, many alternatives for fixation exist. If possible, restoration of

the attachments of the anular ligament is preferred. The severed ends of the ligament are reattached with nonabsorbable sutures (Fig. 47-31). Identification of the ligamentous support to the elbow may be difficult in the face of severe soft tissues trauma. If the ends of the anular ligament cannot be reconstructed, other methods are available. The fascia lata from the rear leg can be used as a fascial strip for ligament reconstruction. Prosthetic ligaments can be made from suture material such as stainless steel, polyester, or nylon.

A more secure method of fixation of the radial head, and one that I prefer, is the use of a bone screw. This bone screw can be used in conjunction with a bone plate on the ulna or as one or two screws combined with or without external coaptation of the ulnar fracture (Figs. 47-32 and 47-33). The importance of accurate reduction of the radial head prior to insertion of the screws cannot be overemphasized. If difficulty is encountered in maintaining the radial head in place prior to fixation, self-centering bone holding forceps or reduction forceps* placed transversely over the lateral proximal radius and ulna provide solid reduction. The dislocated radial head is easier to reduce when the elbow is flexed and the radial head is slid medially over the humeral condyle.

The ulnar portion of the Monteggia fracture must also be reduced and internally fixed. If the fracture is above the joint, it may be repaired with a pin and a tension-band wire (see Fig. 47-26D). If the fracture is

*Both available from Synthes, Ltd., 983 Old Eagle School Road, Wayne, PA 19087

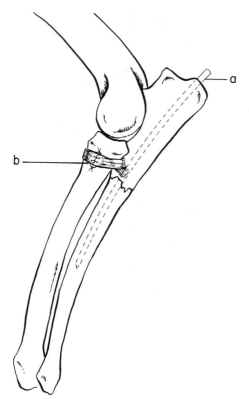

Fig. 47-31. *Reduction of ulnar portions of a Monteggia fracture with an intramedullary pin (a) and suture repair of torn ligaments (b).*

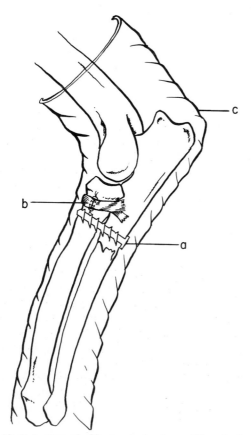

Fig. 47-32. *Reduction of a Monteggia fracture with a single cortical screw (a), ligament repair (b), and application of a plaster cast (c).*

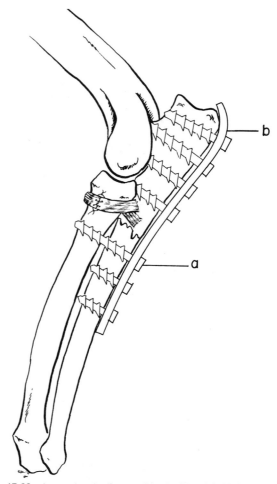

Fig. 47-33. *A repair similar to that in Fig. 47-32, but with the incorporation of a screw (a) into a bone plate (b).*

below the elbow, a single intramedullary pin is adequate (see Fig. 47-31). In small and medium breed dogs, a semitubular plate may be applied to the caudal aspect with incorporation of one or two screws through the ulna and into the repositioned radial head.

Postoperative radiographs should be taken to assess the degree of reduction of the radial head because this degree affects the prognosis. A soft, padded bandage, such as a modified Robert Jones bandage, should be used to support the affected limb for 5 to 7 days. The patient's exercise should be restricted for the next 4 to 6 weeks. Following radiographic and clinical evidence of healing, plates and pins should be removed. The prognosis for complete recovery with Monteggia fractures must be guarded because of the high incidence of postoperative complications.

Fracture of the Proximal Ulna and Dislocation of the Radius and Ulna

This type of fracture results in cranial displacement of the radius and distal ulnar fragment (Fig. 47-34A). If the injury is recent, closed reduction and closed normograde insertion of an intramedullary pin in the ulna may

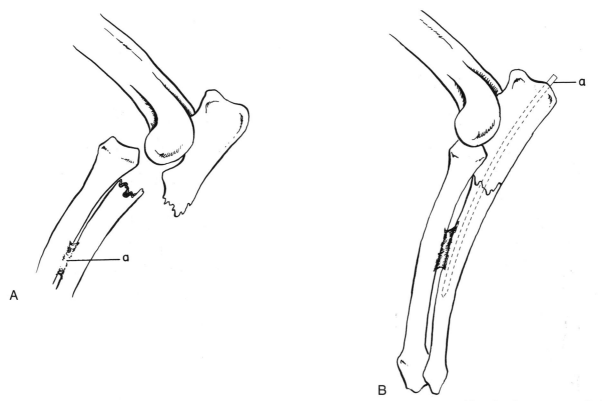

Fig. 47-34. A, *Fracture of the proximal ulna with displacement of distal ulna with the radial head. Note that interosseous attachments remain intact (a).* B, *Reduction of the fracture with an intramedullary pin (a).*

be attempted (Fig. 47-34*B*). More frequently, open reduction is necessary, in combination with traction and countertraction along with caudal pressure on the radius until anatomic alignment is reached. Another acceptable method of repair is reduction of the luxated radial head and ulnar fracture and then internal fixation with bone screws (see Fig. 47-32). If screw fixation is used alone, external support in the form of a plaster cast or a coaptation splint should be applied. Postoperative management is similar to that for the Monteggia fracture; however, the prognosis is better because of the retention of the interosseus attachments of the radius to the ulna.

Fracture and Fracture-Separation of the Radial Head

Fractures of the radial head may be classified as fracture-separations of the physis or intra-articular or metaphyseal fractures. Separation of the radial head at the physis (Salter I) is encountered infrequently (Fig. 47-35*A*). The radial physis closes at 5 to 8 months of age. The proximal radial physis contributes almost 40% of the longitudinal growth of the radius, and as a result, an injury of this type may disturb growth. Owners of the injured animal should be made fully aware of this possibility. Open surgical reduction of the separation is necessary if fracture displacement is significant. Soft tissue swelling makes digital manipulation difficult, and precise reduction and rigid fixation are required.

A lateral approach to the elbow joint is used to expose the radial head. Medial pressure on the radial epiphysis allows reduction. If this maneuver is unsuccessful, a combined medial approach may be undertaken. In addition, the radial physis may be gently levered onto the metaphysis with a small blunt instrument. Once accurate anatomic alignment is reached, a Kirschner wire is driven from the lateral side of the radial head at the edge of the articular surface across the fracture-separation to anchor in the medial cortex of the radius (Fig 47-35*B*). The wire is then bent at a sharp angle distally, is cut off near the sharpest bend, and then is seated slightly more deeply to avoid interference with the joint motion. A similar Kirschner wire is inserted from the medial side of the radial head to cross the lateral wire (Fig. 47-35*B*). If a medial surgical approach is not used, the wire may be inserted through a stab incision.

Postoperative craniocaudal and lateral radiographs must be taken to assess reduction. A light, padded bandage is placed on the patient's operated leg to extend from the distal third of the humerus to and including the digits. This bandage is kept in place for 3 to 5 days to help control swelling. Postoperative activity is restricted to leash exercise for 2 to 3 weeks. Following radiographic evidence of healing, the wires may be removed.

As with physeal separations, radial head fractures must be reduced open and internally fixed (Fig. 47-36*A*). The surgical approach is as described for physeal separations of the radial head. Preservation of as much

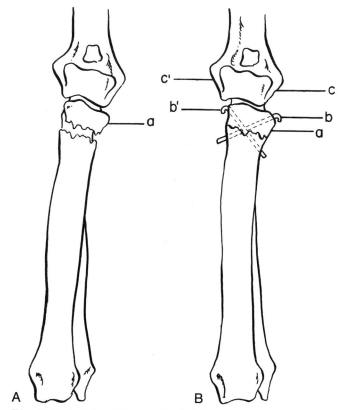

Fig. 47-35. A, *Salter I fracture through the proximal radial physis. Note the displacement of the radial head (a) from a cranial view.* B, *Reduction of the radial head (a) and placement of Kirschner wires (b and b¹) at the edge of the articular surface, bending away from humeral condyles (c and c¹).*

joint capsule as possible is important to stability at closure. The incision may be extended farther distally to allow reduction of the metaphyseal portion of the fracture. It must be emphasized that because of the articular nature of the fracture, accurate reduction is paramount. Temporary reduction may be maintained with bone clamps, cerclage wire, or Kirschner wires. Internal fixation with bone screws or Kirschner wires is the preferred method (Fig. 47-36*B* and *C*).

With the fracture reduced, a hole of appropriate size is drilled and then tapped. If the fracture fragments are large enough, use of a lag screw is desirable; this procedure requires overdrilling of the proximal hole (Fig. 47-36*B*). In addition, a small Kirschner wire or hemicerclage wire should be added to prevent rotation of the fracture fragments. Two Kirschner wires placed at angles to each other and anchored in both cortices of the radius also yield stable fixation (Fig. 47-36*C*).

Postoperatively, additional external support in the form of a modified Robert Jones bandage or a plaster cast is recommended for 2 to 3 weeks. Too early and vigorous weight-bearing may place excessive shearing forces on the radial head.

Severely comminuted radial head fractures require extensive tissue dissection and surgical skill to reduce anatomically (Fig. 47-37*A*). It is preferable to reconstruct the articular surface initially and then to reattach the aligned fragments to the radial metaphysis. Lag screw fixation or a combination of Kirschner wires and figure-8 stainless steel wire should be used to reconstruct the radial head. Attachment to the radial metaphysis is most difficult and is best accomplished by

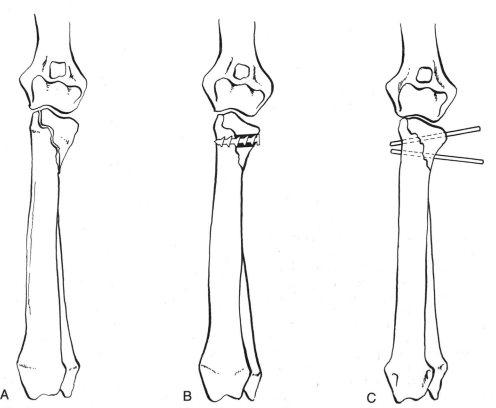

Fig. 47-36. A, *Radial head fracture. Note articular involvement.* B, *Radial head fracture repaired with a bone screw lagged into position by overdrilling.* C, *Radial head fracture repaired with two Kirschner wires.*

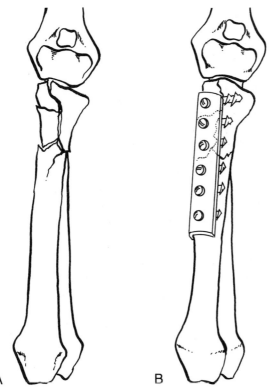

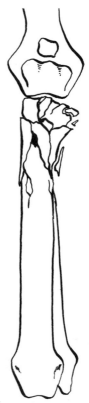

Fig. 47-37. A, *Comminuted fracture of the radial head with disruption of the articular surface. B, Fracture reduced with bone screws and a bone plate. Proximal screws are inserted as lag screws whenever possible to restore the articular surface.*

Fig. 47-38. *Severely comminuted radial head fracture necessitating excision of the radial head.*

incorporation of the lag screws into a bone plate (Fig. 47-37B).

Postoperative external support in the form of a plaster cast is necessary for 4 to 6 weeks unless the bone plate affords extremely rigid and accurate fixation.

If the radial head is too severely comminuted for primary reconstruction, then radial head excision is an alternative. Unfortunately, this procedure has much less satisfactory results in animals than in humans because of the necessity for weight-bearing on the radial head. This type of injury is often associated with a gunshot wound to the elbow joint (Fig. 47-38).

The approach for excision of the radial head is identical to that for internal fixation. Attempts should be made to preserve as much joint capsule as possible. The collateral ligaments are usually sacrificed. A length of the radial neck is removed, so that compression of the elbow during weight-bearing does not allow the humeral condyle to contact the remainder of the radial shaft (diaphysis). This salvage procedure is an alternative to joint fusion. The end result is a decreased range of motion of the elbow joint with accompanying foreleg lameness.

Fractures of the Diaphysis (Shaft) of the Radius or the Ulna

It is uncommon for a fracture to involve the radius and not the ulna. More frequently, a fractured ulna is encountered without subsequent radial fracture. Such isolated fractures may be greenstick or may demonstrate minimal displacement of the fracture fragments (Fig. 47-39A). The animal may actually be able to bear part of its weight on the affected limb. A closed reduction and external fixation procedure is the preferred method of repair. A plaster-of-Paris cast, a Schroeder-Thomas splint, or other types of casting materials may be applied. The application of the external coaptation device should be performed with the animal in a state of general surgical anesthesia, to provide adequate relaxation. Realignment of the fracture fragments is enhanced by placing traction on the limb during application of the external fixation. I prefer the application of a plaster-of-Paris cast or Fiberglass casting tape. The cast should extend from the distal third of the humerus over the entire length of the affected limb. Digits 3 and 4 should partially protrude from the distal end of the cast (Fig. 47-39B). Half-pin Kirschner-Ehmer splinting or intramedullary pin fixation should be used in patients that are extremely mobile or in which early ambulation is desired (Fig. 47-39C). In these patients, closed application of the fixation devices is desired.

Fractures of the Shafts of the Radius and the Ulna

More frequent are fractures involving the radius in combination with the ulna (Fig. 47-40). These fractures may occur at any point along the diaphysis, but are more commonly encountered in the middle and distal

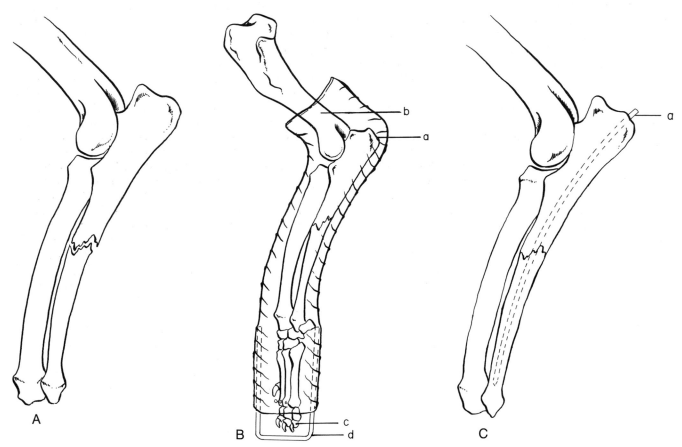

Fig. 47-39. A, *Fractured ulnar diaphysis with minimal displacement.* B, *Plaster-of-Paris cast (a) applied to the fracture. Note that the cast extends from the distal third of the humerus (b) to include all but the third and fourth digits (c). A walking bar has been applied (d).* C, *Intramedullary pin (a) fixation as the sole method of internal fixation.*

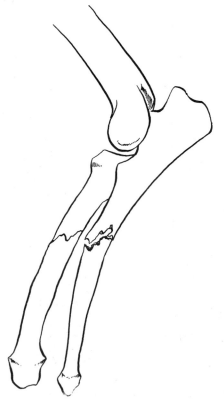

Fig. 47-40. *Typical shaft fracture of the radius and ulna.*

third. Radial and ulnar fractures may take any form and therefore must be handled individually by applying sound orthopedic principles. The ability to pronate and to supinate the forelimb in the dog and cat is much less important than in man, and successful repair is therefore possible even with resultant synostosis of the radius and ulna.

It is not unusual for attempts to repair fractures of the radius and ulna to result in delayed union, malunion, and nonunion, especially in fractures of the distal third of the radius and ulna in small and toy breeds of dogs. Complications can be caused by excessive tissue dissection, failure to prevent axial rotation, and premature ambulation. To minimize such disastrous results, the veterinary surgeon needs to provide accurate reduction, rigid fixation, early return to function, and the addition of cancellous autogenous bone grafts where indicated.

The fixation of diaphyseal fractures of the radius and ulna can be divided into external coaptation, external pin splintage, and internal fixation. Although the combination of internal and external fixation should be avoided, indications for such combinations exist.

CLOSED REDUCTION AND EXTERNAL FIXATION

Many fractures of the radius and ulna of the dog and cat are amenable to closed reduction and external fixation. Types of external coaptation include plaster-of-Paris or other casts, coaptive splints, and Schroeder-Thomas splints. The advantages of external fixation include decreases in tissue trauma, risk of infection, and cost of application. External fixation is more desirable for closed than for open fractures unless the veterinarian is willing to make frequent cast or splint changes. Fractures that respond well to external fixation include incomplete or greenstick fractures, transverse fractures of the shaft, and spiral or oblique fractures that are relatively stable. Comminuted fractures in which disturbances of the periosteal sleeve are minimal can be adequately immobilized with external fixation. Although younger animals under 25 kg are more favorable candidates for such fixation, I have placed plaster-of-Paris casts on dogs of the giant breeds with excellent results. In addition, a fracture may be so severely comminuted that it defies repair with internal fixation (Fig. 47-41). External fixation is more desirable in fractures of the proximal two-thirds of the diaphysis, but should be avoided in severely displaced or overriding fractures.

Of the different types of external fixation, I prefer plaster or Fiberglass casts because of their ease of application, adaptability, and tolerance by the patient. After closed manipulation of the fractured radius and ulna, care should be taken not to disturb the reduction during application of the cast. The cast should extend from the distal third of the humerus to and including all the digits, except for the distal portions of digits 3 and 4 (see Fig. 47-39B).

The cast is applied with the patient in a plane of general surgical anesthesia. The patient is positioned in dorsal recumbency with the affected limb suspended above the patient's body by means of adhesive stirrups taped to the cranial and caudal aspects of the limb. The leg is pulled slightly across the chest of the patient (Fig. 47-42). By positioning the limb in this fashion, it is much easier to apply the cast with the carpus in a slightly varus position to avoid external rotation. The elbow and the carpus are slightly flexed. Positioning of the limb in this manner counteracts the tendency for the carpus to dorsiflex, to develop a valgus deformity, and to rotate outward postoperatively. This abnormality is in part due to the loss of tone in the flexor muscle group and position of the foot when walking or standing. The olecranon and metacarpal pad are lightly cushioned with gauze sponges with center holes cut in them over the prominences. Small wisps of cotton are inserted between the toes. The dog is draped to prevent plaster from falling on the hair coat during application. A stockinette is slipped over the tape stirrups and is rolled over the entire limb. The stockinette should conform to the shape of the patient's leg.

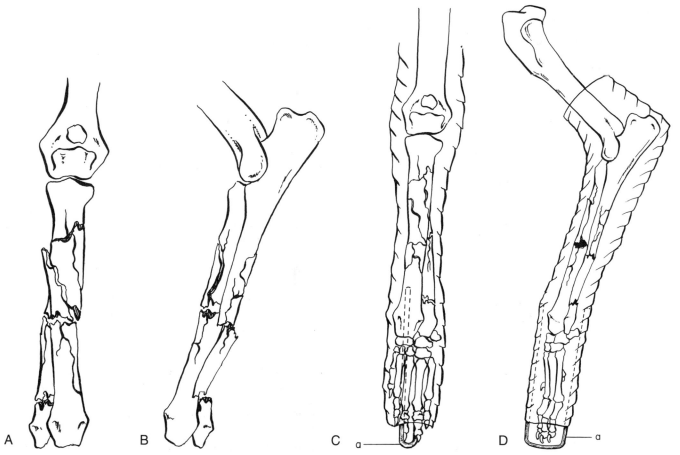

Fig. 47-41. *Cranial* (A) *and lateral* (B) *views of severely comminuted radius and ulnar shaft fracture. Note the minimal displacement and numerous fissure lines. Cranial* (C) *and lateral* (D) *views of reduction and external fixation with a plaster-of-Paris cast. A walking bar* (a) *has been added. The elbow and carpus are slightly flexed.*

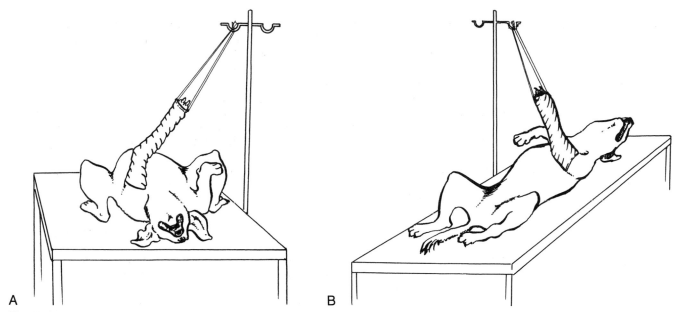

Fig. 47-42. A *and* B, *The patient is positioned on the table, and the foreleg secured in such a manner to avoid casting the limb with the carpus outwardly rotated or hyperextended.*

The cast padding is then applied, beginning from the patient's toes, and is continued proximally to extend 1 cm beyond the proposed cast. The cast padding is overlapped half of its width and is pulled firmly against the patient's leg. The padding is wrapped from outside to inside in an attempt to avoid outward rotation of the leg. Following conformation of correct reduction of the fracture fragments, the plaster of Paris is applied. A roll of plaster is submerged vertically in tepid water for 5 seconds, it is removed, and then it is gently squeezed. The rolls of plaster are applied in the same direction as the cast padding, starting with 2 wraps at the digits and then overlapping half the width to above the elbow. The plaster material must be applied firmly to conform to the shape of the limb. As at the digits, 2 wraps of plaster are applied per layer of plaster at the proximal end of the cast.

During application of the plaster, the layers are smoothed gently with the moistened palm of the hand. The layers of plaster should be smoothed with wet hands until the laminations disappear. One should avoid any digital pressure on the plaster. The number of layers of plaster depends upon the size of the dog. A rule of thumb is not to make the cast more than a quarter-inch in thickness or it will be too heavy and take too long to dry. Additional support can be added by applying vertical strips of plaster on the cranial and caudal aspect of the cast. Prior to application of the last layer of plaster, the stockinette is pulled down over the edges of the cast and is covered with plaster. A hot-air dryer decreases the setting time of the plaster. Although the setting time may be advertised as 5 to 8 minutes, the plaster-of-Paris cast may take 24 to 48 hours to dry completely. The cast may be firm in 5 to 8 minutes, but it is easily damaged. Therefore, following the casting procedure, the patient should be confined to a cage overnight and should be prevented from wetting the cast.

A walking bar, made from an aluminum splint rod, is attached 24 hours after casting (see Fig. 47-39). This bar protects the bottom of the cast and helps to keep debris from between the digits. A radiograph should be taken following application of the cast. The cast should be kept dry at all times and should be checked by the veterinarian at least every 2 weeks. The patient's owner should be counseled to look for signs of possible complications. Such signs include tissue swelling, of the toes especially, discharges, foul smells, or mutilation of the cast by the animal. The patient should be strictly confined and should only be allowed leash exercise while the cast is in place. In a young, growing animal, the cast may have to be changed every 2 weeks. Depending upon the age of the animal, the fractured radius and ulna should heal in 6 to 8 weeks, at which time the cast is removed. An oscillating cast cutter is used to remove the cast.

Other external coaptation devices such as Schroeder-Thomas splints, Mason metasplints, and yucca board have been advocated in the past. These methods do not allow proper positioning of the limb as does a plaster cast, nor do they immobilize the fracture fragments as well. For example, the Mason metasplint does not extend above the elbow. Improper application of these devices often leads to complications in fracture healing.

EXTERNAL PIN SPLINTAGE

External pin splintage can take the form of half- or full-pin splintage. Half-pin splintage involves the insertion of two pins in each of the proximal and distal bone segments, with the pins connected by an external bar or bars (Fig. 47-43). The device is commonly referred to as a Kirschner-Ehmer pin splint. Numerous other pin splints are available. Full-pin splintage differs from the half-pin technique in that the pins penetrate both sides of the leg and are connected by bars on both sides (see Fig. 47-46). The Kirschner-Ehmer device is available in small and medium sizes for small animals. This type of fixation allows movement of the joint above and below the fracture while stabilizing the fracture fragments and allowing weight-bearing by the patient.

Half-pin Kirschner-Ehmer splintage may be used to augment additional internal fixation devices such as intramedullary pins, wires, or screws. The Kirschner-Ehmer splint incorporates 2 pins in each fracture fragment that are placed at 35 to 45° angles to each other (Fig. 47-43D). The pins must penetrate both cortices of the radius or ulna. If the fracture is easily reduced, the splint may be applied during closed reduction. More commonly, the fractured radius and ulna are reduced by an open approach.

The surgical approach to the radius is a craniomedial exposure as described by Piermattei and Greeley.[9] In the majority of radial and ulnar fractures, the radial fracture is reduced and is held in position with bone-holding forceps. The ulnar fracture usually follows the radius in reduction. Two methods of application of the Kirschner-Ehmer device are described in the literature (Figs. 47-43 and 47-44). I prefer the method involving the single bar (see Fig. 47-43). The pins of the apparatus are inserted from a cranial or craniomedial direction, through the skin adjacent to the incision, and not through the incision. The anatomic features of the radius facilitate insertion of the pins from this direction. Because the radius is flattened in the lateral-to-medial plane, insertion of the pins in that direction is difficult. The Kirschner-Ehmer device is protected on the craniomedial edge of the leg. The pins are inserted in the same plane. First, the most proximal and distal pins are inserted on each side of the fracture. The connecting bar with four single clamps is attached. The clamps on the two inserted pins are tightened. This maneuver is followed by insertion of the two pins through the single clamp holes into the bone segments. All four clamps are then securely tightened.

The use of a single bar instead of multiple bars results in less manipulative flexibility, but the device is just as stable and burdens the patient with less weight and bulk. The pins of the Kirschner-Ehmer device should penetrate the fracture fragments at least 2 cm from the fracture site; if that is not possible, the pins

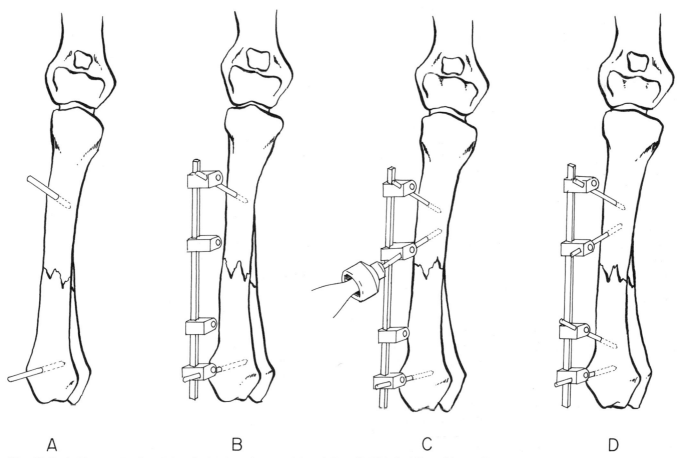

A   B   C   D

Fig. 47-43. A, *The proximal and distal pins have been positioned first.* B, *This is followed by application of the connecting bar and four single clamps. The proximal and distal clamps are tightened around the pins.* C and D, *The third and fourth pins are driven through the clamp holes in the same plane as the proximal and distal pins. All clamps are securely tightened. Although not visible in the diagrams because of the craniomedial direction of the splint placement, the pins must penetrate both cortices of the radius.*

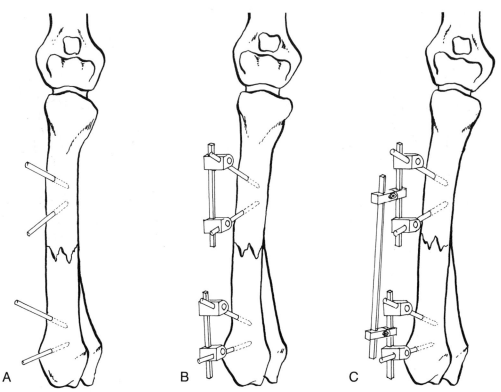

Fig. 47-44. *The application of multiple bars for the Kirschner-Ehmer splint proceeds as in Figure 47-43, except all four pins are driven before the clamps are applied (A). B, The two pins in each segment are connected by a connecting bar containing one double clamp. C, The proximal and distal bars are then connected by an additional bar through the double clamps.*

may be crossed (Fig. 47-45). The pins of the splint must penetrate both cortices of the radius. Except in young, growing dogs, it is not a problem if the pins also penetrate the cortex of the ulna. The pins of the Kirschner-Ehmer splint should be driven by hand with a Jacobs' pin chuck because it allows a tighter fit than a power tool. The clamps of the splint should be adjusted to lie roughly 1 cm above the skin's surface.

Postoperative radiographs should be taken following wound closure. If adjustments need to be made, the clamps are loosened, and the fracture is manipulated closed. A light support wrap is placed over the patient's leg and under the Kirschner-Ehmer splint for 24 to 48 hours to control swelling. The leg is checked closely following the surgical procedure, to ensure that pressure necrosis is not caused by the clamps against the skin. The splint is wrapped with gauze and tape to prevent it from becoming entangled with household objects.

The Kirschner-Ehmer splint is well accepted by most patients. The device should be followed closely and should be removed when the fracture has healed or replaced if the pins have loosened prior to fracture healing. In approximately 4 to 6 weeks, it is not unusual for the pins of the device to loosen.

The veterinary surgeon encounters certain radial and ulnar fractures that are open, possibly severely comminuted, with bony defects, accompanied by severe soft tissue wounds that are contaminated or infected. The attending veterinarian must respect the soft tissue and must treat it properly in order for the fracture to heal.

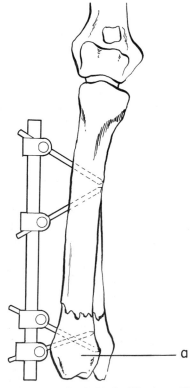

Fig. 47-45. *Application of a half-pin Kirschner-Ehmer splint to hold in reduction a distal radius and ulnar shaft fracture. The small size of the distal fragment of the radius (a) has dictated that the distal two splint apparatus pins be crossed in order to gain a purchase and to be far enough away from the fracture site.*

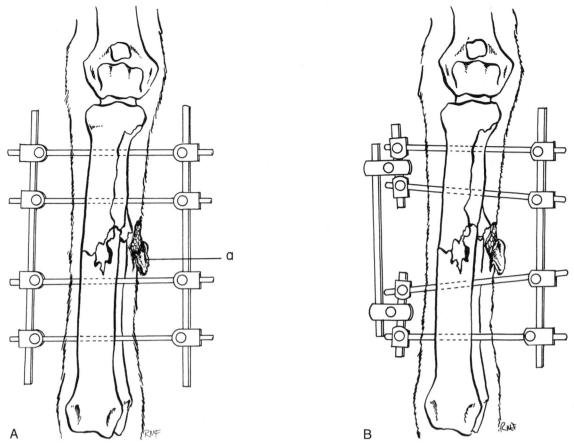

Fig. 47-46. A *and* B, *Application of full-pin splintage to a comminuted open fracture of the radius and ulna. Note the soft tissue wound (a). The parallel pins have been placed with minimal disturbance of bone fragments. The middle two pins in Figure 47-46B have been driven so as not to be parallel to the most proximal and distal pins. This may delay premature loosening of the splint and prevent it from sliding from side to side, resulting in pressure necrosis of the skin.*

Extensive surgical invasion into this type of fracture often leads to postoperative complications such as osteomyelitis, nonunion, sequestrum formation, or implant failure. This type of fracture is ideal for full-pin splintage, which allows for minimal invasion of the injured soft tissues and preserves the tenuous blood supply of fragmented bone. Full-pin splintage maintains the fracture fragments in distraction if large pieces of bone are missing or are severely comminuted. This technique allows the veterinary surgeon to debride and to cleanse the soft tissues so that a suitable environment for osteosynthesis can develop. Often, fracture healing takes place with the full-pin splint in place before a secondary orthopedic repair is attempted. This type of splint can be applied open or closed, preferably with a Jacobs' hand chuck, but a power tool may be used. The full-pin splint differs from the half-pin device in that the four pins pass through the skin on both sides of the radius or ulna (Fig. 47-46). The pins are connected on each side of the leg with a connecting bar. If one bar is used on each side, the pins must be driven as described for the half-pin splint (Fig. 47-46A). Multiple connecting bars may be used if the fracture cannot be realigned and the pins kept in the same plane (Fig. 47-46B). If the proximal portion of the fractured radius is too small to accommodate external pins, the proximal portion of the external pin splintage may be placed in the proximal ulna. The full Kirschner-Ehmer splint is managed postoperatively similarly to the half-splint apparatus. Care must be taken to cover the pin splintage on the lateral portion of the leg with a padded bandage, to keep it from catching on an object.

INTRAMEDULLARY PINNING

I use intramedullary pins infrequently for sole fixation of radial shaft fractures. The diaphysis of the radius anatomically is not as amenable to intramedullary pins as are the ulna and other long bones. An intramedullary pin may be used to maintain alignment in the radius in combination with a pin in the ulna. The oval configuration of the medullary cavity of the radius allows axial rotation even if the ulna is pinned. The small amount of rotation can lead to nonunion of the fracture fragments. Whether the intramedullary pin is positioned to fill the entire medullary cavity or is just inserted across the fracture line as a toggle pin, the main purpose is that of alignment. The rigid internal fixation of the radius is achieved with the addition of external pin splintage or, at least, with the application of a plaster cast. Insertion of an intramedullary pin in the radius is more difficult than in other long bones. The pin may be inserted in a retrograde fashion through the distal fragment and out, cranial to the radial carpal joint, and may then be driven into the proximal fragment. The pin may involve the joint in such a case. A better method is to direct the pin in an antegrade fashion (direct grade or normograde) from the distal end of the radius, proximal to the radial carpal joint. A detailed description of intramedullary pinning of the radius and ulna is available in the literature.[8]

BONE PLATING

Fractures of the radius and ulna may also be repaired with bone plates (Fig. 47-47). It is beyond the scope of this chapter to discuss the principles of bone plating in detail. Additional indications for plate fixation include nonunions, delayed unions, and correction of malunions. Plating should be used in any fracture of the radius and ulna in which extreme rotational stability and early weight-bearing are desired. Large or giant breeds of dogs may require plating of both the radius and ulna in order to provide adequate support for early ambulation. Small and toy breeds of dogs are notorious for developing nonunions following fractures of the distal third of the radius and ulna, and bone plating provides the extreme rotational stability needed for healing.

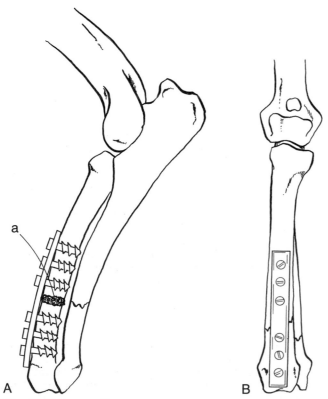

Fig. 47-47. *Lateral* (A) *and cranial* (B) *views of a shaft fracture of the radius and ulna reduced with a bone plate. Note six cortices of purchase on each side of fracture line and the application of a cancellous bone graft (a) to the fracture site following bone plate fixation.*

The craniomedial approach is used to expose a diaphyseal fracture of the radius. The extent of the incision is determined by the type of fracture and length of bone plate applied. If the ulna is to be plated or pinned, it can be approached through a separate caudal or lateral incision. Initial alignment and intramedullary pinning of the ulnar fracture may aid in alignment of the radial fracture. The radius is usually all that is necessary to repair. Plate application requires more extensive tissue dissection in an effort to place a minimum of three cortical bone screws on each side of the fracture.

Exposure of either the most proximal or most distal metaphysis of the radius is more difficult because of the attachments of ligamentous structures and muscle insertions proximally and the presence of tightly adhered extensor tendons distally. These structures must be carefully elevated, and the plate must be placed beneath them. The bone plate is placed on the cranial surface of the radius because it is the tension-band side of the bone. Semitubular plates may be used in smaller animals and may be placed on the craniomedial surface of the radius; these plates conform well to this area. A guideline for choosing the appropriate size and type of plate has been published.[3] Additionally, the veterinary surgeon should choose the appropriate method of application based on the goal of neutralization or compression bone plating. Closure of the surgical site after plating may be compounded by a lack of soft tissue, especially distally on the radius. Care should be taken to appose the antebrachial fascia and the subcutaneous tissues in an effort to cover the plate. If the plate lies directly under tightened skin edges, pressure necrosis may ensue. The idea of plate fixation should not be discarded if soft tissue trauma is severe and if it is anticipated that wound closure will not be possible. In the face of rigid immobilization and proper wound management, an exposed bone plane eventually is covered by granulation and epithelialization.

The addition of cancellous bone grafts is as important in plating as in other methods of internal fixation (Fig. 47-47). An excellent source is the proximal humerus, and it is easily incorporated into the surgical site. This technique is especially important in older patients, in cases nonunion of fractures, and in severely comminuted fractures.

Postoperatively, a light, padded bandage is applied to the entire limb from the distal humerus to and including the digits. The bandage is removed in 48 to 72 hours. Early ambulation in moderation is encouraged, and the progress in fracture healing is followed at monthly intervals, starting 8 weeks after the surgical procedure. Upon evidence of clinical and radiographic union, I recommend removal of the bone plate.

Fractures of the Distal Radius and Ulna

Named after an Irish surgeon, Abraham Colles, this type of injury consists of fracture of the distal 3 cm of the radius with or without fracture of the ulnar styloid

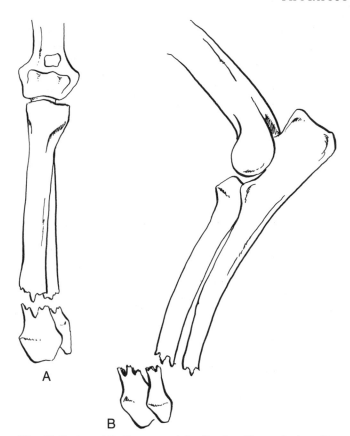

Fig. 47-48. A and B, *Fracture of the distal radius and ulna. The lateral view (B) demonstrates the cranial displacement of the distal fracture fragments. The minimal displacement (A) demonstrates the importance of two radiographic views.*

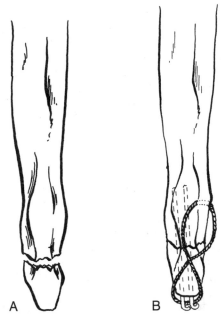

Fig. 47-49. A, *Ulnar styloid process fracture. B, Reduction of the fracture by means of pins and a tension-band wire.*

process (Fig. 47-48). Leaps from high places frequently cause this type of fracture, which results in cranial displacement of the distal segment of the radius. The fracture is commonly repaired by closed reduction and casting. Besides casting, any of the methods described for diaphyseal fractures may be used. Owing to the high incidence of nonunion of distal radial fractures, however, plating this type of fracture in small or toy breed dogs and adding a cancellous autogenous bone graft to the fracture site may be warranted (see Fig. 47-47A). Additional external support such as a plaster cast or coaptation splinting is recommended when a short plate has been placed on distal radial fractures, because of the extreme forces levered at the proximal plate edge. This external support may be removed in 2 to 3 weeks. Half-pin splintage may also be used, and the two distal Kirschner-Ehmer pins may be criss-crossed in the distal fragment (see Fig. 47-45).

Fractures of the Ulnar Styloid Process

Although unusual in occurrence, fractures of the ulnar styloid process should be repaired by internal fixation (Fig. 47-49A). The ulnar styloid process is important in maintaining lateral support to the carpus by means of the ulnar collateral ligament. The fracture is approached through a distal lateral incision and is held in reduction with either a tension-band wire, a bone screw, or a Rush pin (Fig. 47-49B). A small, padded bandage is used for postoperative support. If the distal fracture fragment of the styloid process is too small to accept internal fixation, the fracture is externally coapted in plaster of Paris, with the carpus in slight flexion.

References and Selected Readings

1. Brinker, W. O.: Small Animal Fractures. East Lansing, Michigan State University Continuing Education Service, 1978.
2. Brinker, W. O.: Types of fractures and their repair. *In* Canine Surgery, 2nd Ed. Edited by J Archibald. Santa Barbara, CA, American Veterinary Publications, 1974.
3. Brinker, W. O., et al.: Guidelines for selecting proper implant size for treatment of fractures in the dog and cat. J. Am. Anim. Hosp. Assoc., *13:*476, 1977.
4. Evans, H. E., and Christensen, G. C.: Miller's Anatomy of the Dog. 2nd Ed. Philadelphia, W. B. Saunders, 1979.
5. Hohn, R. B., et al.: Fractures of the radius and ulna. Scientific Presentations and Seminar Synopses of 38th Annual Meeting of the American Animal Hospital Association, April, 1971.
6. Knecht, C. D., et al.: Fundamental Techniques in Veterinary Surgery. Philadelphia, W. B. Saunders, 1975.
7. Leonard, E. P.: Orthopedic Surgery of the Dog and Cat. 2nd Ed. Philadelphia, W. B. Saunders, 1971.
8. Neal, T. M.: The radius and ulna. *In* Current Techniques in Small Animal Surgery. Edited by M. J. Bojrab. Philadelphia, Lea & Febiger, 1975.
9. Piermattei, D. L., and Greeley, R. G.: An Atlas of Surgical Approaches to the Bones of the Dog and Cat. Philadelphia, W. B. Saunders, 1979.
10. Putnam, R. W.: Excision of the canine radial head. Mod. Vet. Pract., *49:*32, 1968.
11. Rudy, R. L. (ed.): Symposium on management of limb fractures in small animals. Vet. Clin. North Am., *5:*145, 1975.

Fragmented Medial Coronoid Process of the Ulna

by JOSEPH M. STOYAK

Anatomic Features

The medial coronoid process of the ulna is a beak-like projection distal to the trochlear notch that articulates with the radius cranially and the humerus proximally. This process, along with a less-prominent lateral coronoid process, increases the surface area of the joint without contributing materially to its weight-bearing function (Fig. 47-50).

History

Fragmented medial coronoid process of the ulna disorder was first described in the mid-1970s. The disease probably existed prior to this time, but was undiagnosed because of the esoteric nature of the early changes in the bones. Frequently associated with osteochondritis dissecans of the medial condyle of the humerus, the rapid progression to changes of degenerative joint disease makes a more definitive diagnosis by radiographic means less likely as time passes.

The condition is more prevalent in large breed dogs, with Labrador and golden retrievers, Newfoundlands, and rottweilers among those breeds frequently affected, but few large breeds appear to have been spared. These dogs are usually 6 to 12 months of age, but older dogs are seen.

Clinical Signs and Diagnosis

Commonly associated with the lesion is a lameness that occurs after rest. This lameness may resolve shortly after moderate use of the limb. Some animals exhibit lameness only after heavy exercise. On physical examination, the lameness may be precipitated or intensified by severe flexion of the elbow joint. Palpation of the medial joint space may elicit tenderness. Crepitus may also be heard on manipulation of the joint. The joint capsule is often thickened and distended. The experienced clinician recognizes that these signs are also frequently seen with an ununited anconeal process and are also related to the age of the animal and stage of the disease.

The diagnosis of this condition is not easily confirmed. It frequently relies on the patient's medical history, physical examination, and radiographic studies that may either confirm the diagnosis or eliminate others and may thus increase the index of suspicion on the examiner's part. It should be emphasized that radiographic changes may be subtle, if detected at all. The veterinarian must be prepared to devote significant time and effort to positioning the patient and making the radiographs. Radiographic technique must be meticulous, and multiple views are usually necessary and desirable. The fragmented medial coronoid process may not be seen because it is superimposed on the radial head in most views. Trial and error has shown that slightly oblique views give the best delineation of this process. The most frequent changes seen on the lateral view are osteophyte formation on the dorsal aspect of the anconeal process with the elbow flexed. The caudal border of the medial condyle may also show osteophytosis on this view. On the craniocaudal view, osteophytosis of the medial coronoid process is often seen, along with the appearance of osteophytosis and erosion on the medial condylar margins.

Surgical Treatment

Surgical repair appears to be the definitive treatment for this condition. The use of corticosteroids, either intra-articularly or systemically, has no place in the primary management of this disorder. The use of these agents may only complicate an already complex situation. The decision to operate is not always easy, because it is without the benefit either of significant numbers of cases or of long-term studies on patients. Limited experience seems to indicate that most patients without advanced osteoarthrosis can be expected to benefit from surgical treatment. Certain patients with degenerative changes, however, may also show relief of pain and improvement in function. The veterinary surgeon's confidence in his diagnosis and his experience with similar patients aid in making the decision. Once this hurdle is crossed, the procedure presents little hazard to the patient if one adheres to proper surgical principles. The veterinary surgeon must be intimately familiar with the anatomic features of the area before attempting the procedure.

The aim of the surgical procedure is to remove any fragmented portions of the medial coronoid process from the joint space. It is critical to inspect the articular surface of the medial humeral condyle for evidence of osteochondritis dissecans. This disease is common and may not be visible radiographically.

The surgical approach must allow adequate access to the medial compartment of the elbow joint. The ap-

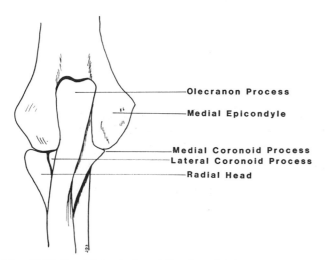

Olecranon Process

Medial Epicondyle

Medial Coronoid Process
Lateral Coronoid Process
Radial Head

Fig. 47-50. *Caudolateral view of the elbow joint.*

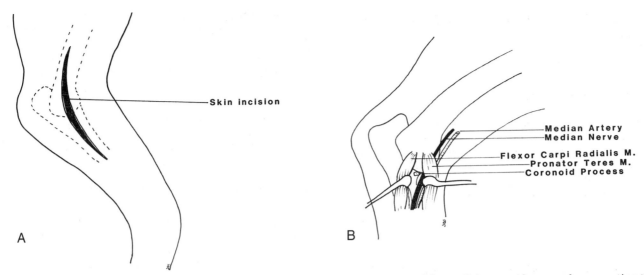

Fig. 47-51. A, *Site of the skin incision over the medial aspect of the elbow.* B, *Exposure of the medial coronoid process by separating the muscles.*

proach should be the least traumatic that allows the veterinary surgeon to accomplish his goal. I prefer a medial approach over the medial epicondyle (Fig. 47-51A). The flexor carpi radialis and pronator teres muscles are identified and are separated near their origins at the medial epicondyle (Fig. 47-51B). At this point, extreme care must be taken to identify and to protect the median artery and nerve, which lie directly under these muscles at the level of the joint. Separation of these muscles, along with adequate retraction, may allow adequate access to the joint after a vertical incision into the joint capsule.

More adequate exposure is attained by transection of the tendons of the pronator teres and flexor carpi radialis muscles near the epicondyle with reflection of both distally (Fig. 47-52). The medial collateral ligament may also be transected at this time. The joint capsule is incised in a horizontal plane. The joint may then

be further exposed by placing downward pressure on the radius and ulna and by thus "hinging" the joint open over the edge of the operating table or a pad placed under the patient's elbow. Lateral rotation of the radius also opens the joint for better exposure. An assistant, or a self-retaining retractor, is necessary for the maintenance of adequate exposure. The joint is then inspected thoroughly and all loose fragments are removed. The medial condylar articular surface is also inspected and any loose flaps of cartilage are removed, and curettage of subchondral bone in the area is performed. The joint is thoroughly flushed with saline solution. The joint is closed with absorbable suture material, whereas the ligaments and muscles are reattached with nonabsorbable suture material. The rest of the closure is routine.

A well-padded elbow bandage is used for 7 days, and the patient's exercise is restricted for 3 to 4 weeks.

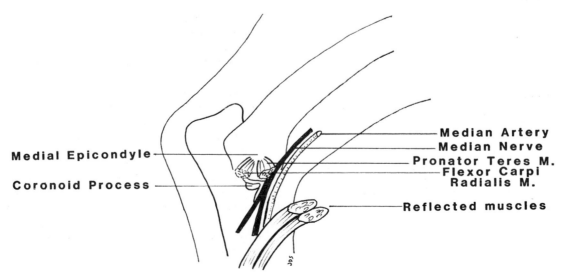

Fig. 47-52. *Exposure of the medial coronoid process by transecting the muscles at the medial epicondyle.*

References and Suggested Readings

Berzon, J. L., and Quick, C. B.: Fragmented coronoid process: anatomical, clinical, and radiographic considerations with case analyses. J. Am. Anim. Hosp. Assoc., *16*:241, 1980.

Denny, H. R., and Gibbs, C.: The surgical treatment of osteochondritis dissecans and ununited coronoid process of the canine elbow joint. J. Small Anim. Pract. *21*:323, 1980.

Evans, H. E., and Christensen, G. C.: Miller's Anatomy of the Dog. Philadelphia, W. B. Saunders, 1979.

McCurnin, D. M., Slusher, R., and Grier, R. L.: A medial approach to the canine elbow joint. J. Am. Anim. Hosp. Assoc., *12*:475, 1976.

Olsson, S. E.: Lameness in the dog. Proc. Am. Anim. Hosp. Assoc., *42*:363, 1975.

Tirgari, M.: Clinical, radiographical, and pathological aspects of arthritis of the elbow joint in dogs. J. Small Anim. Pract., *15*:671, 1974.

Growth Deformities of the Radius and Ulna

by JAMES W. WILSON

Deformities of the radius and ulna may appear clinically as a single entity, but in actuality they involve many distinct underlying pathophysiologic conditions. In order to correct the obvious deformity successfully, an understanding of radial and ulnar anatomy, growth rates, and physeal closure times is needed, as well as a knowledge of the varied methods of surgical repair. The following discussion outlines the present knowledge in these areas. For an in-depth understanding, the cited references should be examined.

Anatomic Features

The radius is the main weight-supporting bone of the forelimb. It is shorter than the accompanying ulna, and it articulates with the humerus at the elbow joint and with the radial carpal bone at the carpal joint. In both cases, the radius is the major weight-bearing antebrachial component of the joint.

The ulna parallels the radius and serves mainly for muscle attachment. It is longer than the radius and is, in fact, the longest bone in the canine body. The ulna articulates with the humerus at the trochlear notch and with the radius laterally at the elbow joint, and it stabilizes and restricts movement of the joint in a sagittal plane, but allows rotation of the antebrachium. Within the carpus, the ulna articulates with the ulnar and the accessory carpal bones and stabilizes the joint laterally.

Because of the close anatomic and functional relationship between the radius and ulna, their growth rates must be equal and coordinated.

Physeal Growth Rates and Closure Times

The 4 antebrachial physes grow at different rates and contribute different amounts to final adult forelimb length.[19] Although this growth rate may vary slightly among breeds of dogs, it is universally agreed that approximately 70% of radial growth occurs at the distal physis and 30% at the proximal. The olecranon physis contributes little to ulnar length, with at least 85% of ulnar growth occurring at the distal physis. Thus, any single change or combination of physeal growth changes can severely affect the shape and length of the forelimb.

Age at physeal closure varies among breeds of dogs and within individuals within the breeds.[3,9,25] In the smaller breeds, the physes may close earlier, and in the larger breeds, later. The proximal radial and distal ulnar physes close somewhere between 7.5 and 11 months of age. The distal radial physis closes slightly later, at 7.5 to 12 months, whereas the proximal ulnar physis closes slightly earlier, between 6 and 8 months of age.

As a physis approaches closure, its rate of growth and its contribution to adult bone length and shape decrease. Deformity resulting from physeal injury becomes less likely. The cited references document over 86 cases of forelimb deformity. The initiating cause occurred prior to 7 months of age in all the cases, prior to 6 months of age in 95% of the cases, and prior to 5 months of age in 86% of the cases. The likelihood of deformity is related to the remaining growth potential. Thus, an injury to a 5-month-old dog could possibly result in a forelimb deformity, whereas there would only be a 15% chance of deformity in the 5- to 6-month-old dog and a 5% chance in the 6- to 7-month-old dog, and minimal chance exists in the dog older than 7 months. Knowing these growth potentials and chances of deformity is also important in decisions regarding corrective procedures.

Pathologic Features

The problem with forelimb deformities lies not with the long bones themselves, but with the joints of which these bones are a part. Asynchronous growth of the antebrachial bones can result in abnormal joint stress, incongruence, increased joint laxity, joint impingement, subluxation, or decreased range of motion, depending on the particular deformity. These abnormalities can lead to pain, lameness, dysfunction, and ultimately, to degenerative joint disease. Detailed descriptions of the resulting pathologic manifestations can be found in the cited references.[1,2,12,13,16,17,19] The goal of surgical repair of forelimb deformities is to prevent, to arrest, or to minimize joint pathologic manifestations.

Initiating Causes

PREMATURE PHYSEAL CLOSURE

Because of the nutritional and structural oddities of the physis, trauma to the immature animal is more apt to cause physeal injury than diaphyseal fracture or ligamentous rupture. Accordingly, trauma is the most commonly reported cause of forelimb deformity related to premature physeal closure.[5,6,8,13,14,18,24] Because of this, physeal injuries have been divided into 5 types, based on appearance and clinical outcome.[4,11,21,23] Of these types, Salter types IV and V injuries are the most damaging to the physis and frequently cause the injured physis to close. If physeal closure occurs in a dog before 7 months of age, subsequent forelimb deformity is likely. Physes have also been reported to fuse prematurely following experimental x-irradiation[2,18] or hypergravity,[12] with hypertrophic osteodystrophy or nutritional secondary hyperparathyroidism,[13] as a recessive inherited genetic trait,[10] from retained enchondral cartilage cores,[13] and from unknown causes.[8,18,20,26]

DISTAL ULNA. In contrast to other animals, the dog has a uniquely shaped distal ulnar physis. It is conical in configuration with a pointed metaphysis projecting into an epiphyseal recess. This configuration makes the physis susceptible to Salter type V injuries. Any shearing force applied to the ulna could produce compression on the side of the cone. Retarded growth or premature closure is likely and is seen clinically. Distal ulnar physeal abnormalities account for the greatest incidence of forelimb deformities[17,24] and account for the bulk of veterinary publications.[2,5,8,10,12,13,17,24,26]

Growth deformities due to distal ulnar physeal abnormalities are particularly severe because this physis contributes approximately 85% to ulnar length. Once physeal growth ceases, ulnar length becomes fixed. As the radius continues to grow, the ulna acts as a retarding strap twisted around the radius causing the radius to bow outward. This abnormal growth results in a complex radial deformity of which three components are seen: cranial bowing (curvus); distal lateral deviation (valgus); and external rotation (supination) (Fig. 47-53). The effects of the radial deformity are most severe distally. The epiphysis of the radius is rapidly rotated craniolaterally off the carpal bones. This rotation invariably leads to caudolateral subluxation of the carpus and to degenerative joint disease. Proximally, the continued radial growth progressively forces the radial head into the elbow and pushes the humeral condyles out of the trochlear notch (Fig. 47-54). Last, the altered shape and position of the radius result in altered stress on the antebrachium transforming the cross-sectional configuration of the radius from oval to triangular while greatly increasing the diameter of the distal ulna.

Clinically, dogs with distal ulnar physeal growth disturbances are usually able to bear weight and have some degree of grossly visible valgus deformity. Limb pain and lameness may be minimal; if present, they are usually associated with the elbow or carpus. One may find pain, crepitation, or a limited range of motion on joint manipulation. If valgus is severe, an abnormal paw position during weight-bearing may result in abrasions and ulcerations to the surface of the paw.

Two approaches to surgical correction can be taken, depending on the growth potential of the animal. If the antebrachial physes are closed or if growth is nearly complete, a single-procedure total correction may be attempted. After ulnar osteotomy, an oblique or cuneiform radial osteotomy is performed at the point of greatest deformity. The forelimb is then straightened, and the radial osteotomy is stabilized with a bone plate and screws or an external fixation device. If the animal still has significant growth potential, then one of three dynamic corrections is preferred. In the first, a segmental ulnar ostectomy is performed, and an adjustable external fixation device* is applied to the ulna. This device is then adjusted periodically to spread the ostectomy, to lengthen the ulna, and to delay ostectomy

* Hoffman-type external fixation system, Zimmer, Warsaw, IN 46580, or, External compression clamp, Synthes Ltd., Wayne, PA 19087

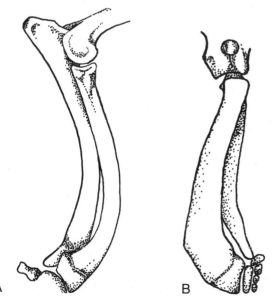

Fig. 47-53. *Lateral (A) and craniocaudal (B) views of complex radial deformity resulting from premature closure of the distal ulnar physis.*

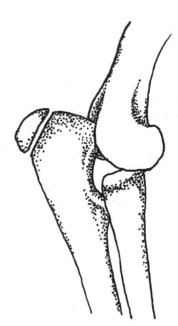

Fig. 47-54. *Elbow incongruence resulting from altered ulnar growth due to premature closure of the distal ulnar physis.*

re-union. The second procedure is ulnar transposition. A third option, ulnar osteotomy or ostectomy without fixation, has also been used as a method of releasing the retarding strap effect of the ulna. Because of continued radial growth and the rapid healing potential of immature bone, however, it is usually necessary to perform repetitive procedures.

DISTAL RADIUS. Unlike that of the distal ulna, this physis is not anatomically unusual.[4,8,14,17,20] All Salter types of injuries can occur. Thus, trauma to this physis may be less likely to result in forelimb deformity. Whether this reduced incidence actually occurs clinically is unclear, but fewer cases are reported in the veterinary literature.

Premature closure can be either symmetrical (closure of the entire physis) or asymmetrical (partial closure). Asymmetrical closures are the most common and usually involve retardation of growth or fusion of the lateral part of the physis. Radial growth then fails to keep pace with ulnar growth, resulting initially in distal subluxation of the radial head (Fig. 47-55). Because the humerus is anchored to the radial head by the collateral ligaments of the elbow, as the mismatch in growth progresses, the ulna subluxates proximally. This disorder may progress to complete proximal ulnar luxation (Fig. 47-56). Increased stress on the distal ulnar physis from the shortened radius may cause slower growth and thus a shorter ulnar length when compared to the contralateral leg. Depending on the degree of disparity between lateral and medial distal radial growth, a variable degree of carpal valgus, cranial carpal subluxation, and outward rotation of the paw will occur (Fig. 47-57).

Symmetrical closures of the entire distal radial physis are less common. When they do occur, the drastically shortened radius may act as a retarding strap on the ulna and may thereby cause the ulna to bow laterally. As this disorder progresses, carpal varus and inward rotation of the paw may occur. Abnormalities

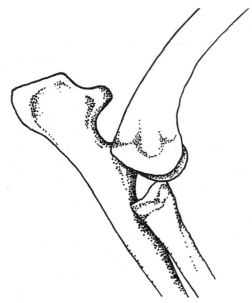

Fig. 47-56. *Elbow luxation in advanced deformity due to premature closure of the distal radial physis.*

within the elbow proceed as described for asymmetrical closures.

Dogs with premature closure of the distal radial physis are presented to the veterinarian with varying degrees of forelimb lameness. The leg may be noticeably shorter. Angular deformity may or may not be evident. The patient's elbow may be painful on passive manipulation, and the range of motion may be decreased. The elbow may crepitate. Carpal pain,

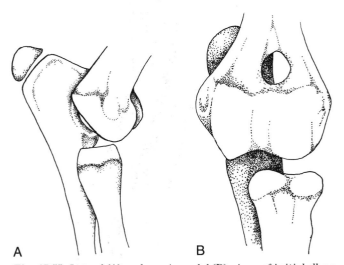

Fig. 47-55. *Lateral* (A) *and craniocaudal* (B) *views of initial elbow incongruence following premature closure of the distal radial physis.*

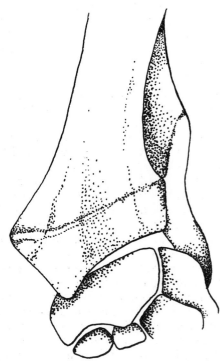

Fig. 47-57. *Carpal and distal radial deformity resulting from premature closure of the distal radial physis.*

joint distension, hyperextension, or crepitation may be present.

If the condition is recognized before the other antebrachial physes have closed, every attempt should be made to prevent the progression of limb deformity, to maintain normal joints, and to preserve the leg's length. These objectives necessitate radial osteotomy or ostectomy and progressive radial lengthening using one of the adjustable external fixation devices. If the antebrachial physes are all closed, surgical correction should be aimed at re-establishing elbow congruence and correcting any angular deformity. Osteotomy of the radius and subsequent spreading of the surgical site will allow one to shift the radial head proximally to correct elbow congruence. At the same time, the distal radius should be repositioned to correct any angular deformity. If the angulation is severe, ulnar osteotomy may facilitate positioning. The repositioned bones can then be stabilized using a bone plate and screws or an external fixation device. In severe cases requiring considerable radial shift, progressive spread using a dynamic fixator may be less traumatic and should be considered.

DISTAL RADIUS AND ULNA. Simultaneous premature closure of both distal antebrachial physes is rare.[6,17] Few cases have been documented. Minimal to marked leg shortening, depending on the growth potential remaining at the time of closure, is the most obvious sequela. Accompanying deformities are usually minimal. The radial head may overgrow and may impinge on the humeral condyles, or it may luxate laterally. On the other hand, one may see no elbow abnormalities at all. The diaphysis of the radius and ulna may bow laterally, and the paw may be slightly deviated laterally, or the leg may be relatively straight.

Presenting symptoms depend greatly on the degree of leg shortening and the presence of accompanying deformities. Amputation may be the only alternative when the degree of leg shortening is extreme. In less severe cases, leg lengthening procedures may be attempted, using osteotomy and progressive spreading or osteotomy, allogeneic cortical grafting, and rigid plate or external pin splint fixation. The osteotomy and fixation device can be positioned to correct any accompanying deviation. Radial head excision was used in the report of a patient with lateral radial head luxation.[6]

PROXIMAL RADIUS. This cause of forelimb deformity is the rarest.[17] Because this physis contributes only about 30% to adult radial length, premature closure results in minimal radial shortening. As the proximal radius ceases growth, the radiohumeral joint space increases. If the closure occurs when considerable growth potential still exists, this joint incongruence may progress to ulnar subluxation because of the downward pull of the elbow collateral ligaments on the humerus.

Correction should be aimed at establishing normal elbow congruence through proximal radial osteotomy and radial head shift. Because the proximal radial physis closes relatively early and contributes less than 30% to adult radial length, the veterinary surgeon may elect to delay correction of this condition until the dog is older than 7 months.

SYNOSTOSIS OF THE RADIUS AND ULNA

Because the distal ulnar physis must grow at a rate approximately equal to the combined growth of both the proximal and distal radial physes, a dynamic state of constant shifting between the bones of the forelimb exists.[1,15] If this normal shifting is altered by diaphyseal fusion (synostosis) of the radius and ulna (Fig. 47-58), abnormalities similar to those seen in premature physeal closure may occur. The olecranon is prevented from shifting proximally to keep pace with growth from the proximal radial physis. Consequently, luxation of the humeroulnar articulation takes place as radial growth pushes the humerus proximally out of the trochlear notch.

Dogs with this condition are lame from elbow pain. On physical examination, they usually have painful, stiff elbows with a decreased range of motion. Crepitation may be present. Surgical correction requires ulnar osteotomy with proximal ulnar shift. Following correct positioning, the proximal ulna may be secured to the radius with screws, or the ulnar osteotomy may be stabilized using an external fixation device or a bone plate and screws. In the growing animal, it may be advisable to provide continued spread using an adjustable external fixation device until all antebrachial physes close.

MALUNION OF FORELIMB FRACTURES

This last category of forelimb deformities is seen with less frequency now that rigid internal fixation of

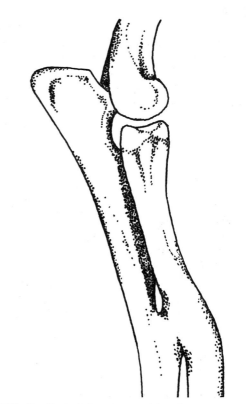

Fig. 47-58. *Forelimb deformity resulting from synostosis of the radius and ulna during growth.*

fractures is being used more and more in veterinary surgery. Malalignment is less likely to occur during fixation and is less likely to develop during healing. When malunion does occur, correction necessitates consideration of the degree of deformity, the growth potential of the animal, the original method of fixation, and the methods of fixation at hand. In the young, growing dog, malalignment and subsequent abnormal weight-bearing may cause secondary changes in one or more of the antebrachial physes and may require a more complex procedure or even staged surgical procedures. If all antebrachial physes have closed, then correction may be completed by transverse, oblique, or cuneiform osteotomy, realignment, and rigid fixation.

Surgical Techniques

The objective of any surgical correction should be to return the limb to functional use, to minimize pathologic joint manifestations, and to provide a pleasing cosmetic result. To accomplish these goals, the condition must be recognized early, and vigorous treatment must be instituted. When choosing a surgical repair, the etiopathologic features of the deformity, the age of the animal and its remaining growth potential, the skill of the veterinary surgeon, and the available methods of fixation must all be considered. Education of the patient's owners is of equal importance. The postoperative recovery period can be long and may require home nursing care, multiple recheck appointments, or close observation of external fixation devices. The most technically perfect surgical procedure can fail from negligent postoperative care.

Some veterinary surgeons prefer to postpone surgical correction in the young, growing animal until a complete correction can be attempted. I, on the other hand, consider it unwise to delay a surgical procedure until all antebrachial physes have fused. Associated joint disorders only worsen during this time and make the prognosis for eventual full recovery less likely.

CORRECTION OF ASYMMETRICAL

PHYSEAL CLOSURE

If the growth of only a part of a physis slows down or stops, the remaining physis continues to grow. This abnormal growth tilts the epiphyseal end of the bone toward the abnormal physeal area. This condition is asymmetrical physeal closure. It occurs in both the proximal and the distal radial physes, but has not been reported in the distal ulnar physis. The most effective treatment in the actively growing animal is conversion of the condition to a more symmetrical closure. The deformity can then be treated using the methods discussed later for the particular physis.

To convert an asymmetrical to a symmetrical closure, the remaining physeal growth needs to be slowed or arrested. The time-tested technique most commonly used is physeal stapling. The staple is positioned to straddle the physis opposite the abnormal physeal area. The veterinary surgeon may use either a commercially available driver and staple or may fashion a staple on his own. Screws, cross-pins, and wires have also been used.

TREATMENT PRIOR TO PHYSEAL CLOSURE

OSTEOTOMY AND OSTECTOMY. If growth of one of the antebrachial bones slows or stops, it may bow the other bone or may cause joint incongruence. Cutting the affected bone attempts to release this tension, allows the bones to orient normally, and provides length to the affected bone. Ideally, more than 1 cm should separate the cut ends at the end of the surgical procedure. Less of a gap causes a faster union of the ends and thus shortens the time for correct bone orientation and lengthening.

If an operation is performed to minimize the development of antebrachial deformity following premature closure of the distal ulnar physis, it is best done midshaft where it does not interfere with elbow or carpal stability. The interosseous membrane is cut to free the proximal end of the ulna from the radial shaft. If marked distal subluxation of the proximal ulna exists, it may move to a more normal position by itself or can be shifted intraoperatively. Ulnar osteotomies in the growing animal are not stabilized, so as to maximize future ulnar length and proximal shift within the elbow.

This procedure can be performed with radial physeal disorders, but because the radius is the major weight-bearing bone of the forelimb, continued compaction of the osteotomy site occurs if unstabilized. Because fixation would be mandatory, the cuts can be made adjacent to the affected physis, to allow a less traumatic and more precise realignment of the associated joint. The surgical site can then be stabilized by a bone plate and screws, an external fixation device, or by securing the jointward radial segment to the ulna with screws or pins.

Unfortunately, it is often necessary to repeat this type of correction. If the surgical site is rigidly fixed, the bone's position eventually becomes locked. Any additional growth in the other antebrachial bone results in reformation of the deformity. Leaving the surgical site unstabilized does not help. Most bone defects in immature animals heal readily. Once the cut ends of the operated bone unite, continued growth in the other antebrachial bone again results in reformation of the original deformity.

OSTEOTOMY, OSTECTOMY, AND PROGRESSIVE SPREAD. The drawback of osteotomy or ostectomy in the growing animal is that once the cut ends are united by rigid fixation or early bone union, the deformity is likely to reform and necessitate an additional surgical procedure. A method to provide needed stability, to lengthen the bone slowly, and also to delay early bone union is to span the surgical site with one of the dynamic external fixation devices.*[13,14] At the time of the surgical

*Hoffman-type external fixation system, Zimmer, Warsaw, IN 46580 or, External compression clamp, Synthes Ltd., Wayne, PA 19087

procedure, two pins are placed in both proximal and distal segments of the operated diaphysis. The device is attached and is manipulated to obtain appropriate diaphyseal lengthening, to correct the osteotomy gap size, and to provide proper joint alignment.

Postoperatively, the apparatus is progressively lengthened every fourth day. This maneuver delays rapid bone union at the osteotomy site and permits the affected bone to lengthen at approximately the same rate as the other antebrachial bone. The device can usually be adjusted when the dog is awake, with or without sedation. The limb should be radiographed routinely for positioning and length. Adjustment can be continued as long as necessary or until the osteotomy unites. The leg should then be supported in a Robert Jones dressing for a week after device removal. By forcing the affected bone to elongate as the other antebrachial bone grows, deformities can be minimized.

STYLOID TRANSPOSITION. The distal half of the ulna is approached through a lateral incision.[7] After adequate retraction of soft tissues, the periosteum of the exposed ulna is incised and is circumferentially elevated from midshaft to styloid. The distal quarter of the ulna is then excised, beginning with an oblique osteotomy at the midpoint of the distal ulna. The second osteotomy is made on the distal ulnar epiphysis, starting laterally at the level of the distal radial physis and angling dorsomedially toward the styloid tip. The lateral surface of the radial epiphysis is next cleared of overlying soft tissue to provide a site for styloid attachment, and the cut surface of the styloid is contoured to conform to this radial site. The styloid is then tilted into position against the radial epiphysis and is secured with small pins or a screw; one must be careful to avoid the physis and the radiocarpal joint (Fig. 47-59). The surgical site is closed routinely.

Postoperative care, recommended by the original authors, consists of a Robert Jones dressing on the patient's leg for the first 3 days, followed by 3 weeks of protection and support in a full-length cast. Ulnar styloid transposition permanently removes the retarding strap effect of the ulna, yet it maintains carpal stability and allows continued radial growth. This procedure is

of value in the treatment of premature distal ulnar physeal closure when significant radial growth remains.

TREATMENT AFTER PHYSEAL CLOSURE

OBLIQUE OR CUNEIFORM OSTEOTOMY. Correction by oblique osteotomies does not require preplanned, calculated cuts and has a theoretic advantage of ensuring or actually gaining limb length.[13,22] If this method is chosen, both the radius and ulna should be transected with 45° oblique cuts made in the region of maximal deformity. The proximal radial fragment is then bayoneted into the medullary cavity of the distal fragment. Using this reduction as a pivotal point, the realignment in all 3 planes can be accomplished simultaneously, then is held in position and is rigidly stabilized. If a bone plate and screws are used, they should be affixed first to the anatomic cranial surface of the distal fragment and then anchored to the proximal fragment, preferably with compression. If an external fixation device is used, one has the luxury of being able to make minor readjustments on limb alignment after surgical closure. In either case, rigid fixation and stability are of paramount importance inasmuch as only minimal bone contact exists between the cut ends.

Cuneiform osteotomy requires preoperative calculation of a radial wedge osteotomy. The shape and size of the wedge are determined by simple plane-geometric calculations on tracings of the lateral and craniocaudal radiographs of the affected limb (Fig. 47-60). Correction for valgus is calculated from the craniocaudal radiograph by determination of the angle at which the existing carpal and elbow joint planes are not parallel.

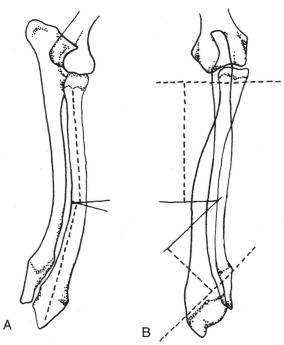

Fig. 47-60. A *and* B, *Method for calculation of wedge size and shape for cuneiform osteotomy.*

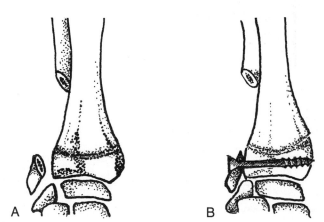

Fig. 47-59. A *and* B, *Diagrammatic representations of ulnar styloid transposition.*

Extension of lines drawn parallel to the two joint planes gives the size and shape of the wedge needed to be removed to return the plane of the carpal joint to parallel that of the elbow. From the lateral tracing, correction for cranial bowing is determined by calculation of the angle at which the axis of the radius has been shifted.

Surgical treatment is carried out in the patient by first making a transverse osteotomy of the radius proximal and adjacent to the region of maximal deformity together with an oblique osteotomy of the ulna. The calculated biplane wedge is then removed from the distal fragment with its base in a cranial-to-medial direction, tapering caudally and laterally. The cut surfaces of the radius can then be abutted to check the degree of limb straightening. If insufficient, the site can be further beveled, or the removed wedge can be reversed and inserted into the osteotomy for additional straightening. One last item needs to be corrected before the osteotomy is fixed. The calculation and cutting of the wedge cannot take into account rotational deformity. This adjustment can only be made visually after curvus and valgus have been corrected by the wedge.

Cuneiform osteotomy provides flat surfaces for bone union and thus potentially satisfactory stability. This technique is ideally suited for compression plate fixation. The plate should be kept straight and should not be contoured unless absolutely necessary. This technique helps ensure correction of cranial bowing. The plate is first secured to the distal fragment. The osteotomy site is then conformed to the straight plate, and the plate is anchored to the proximal fragment using compression. If external fixation is chosen, the pins should be placed as far proximally and distally as possible to gain maximal stability.

OSTEOTOMY AND SHIFT. Elbow subluxation is a prominent feature of many deformities. It is correctly treated by re-establishing joint congruence through lengthening and repositioning the epiphyseal end of the affected bone. To accomplish this end, the affected bone is transected transversely, and the osteotomy site is spread. Usually, a spreading instrument or a distractor is needed to force the epiphysis back into its normal anatomic position. The interosseous ligament often needs to be cut in order to ensure adequate bone movement. Once normal anatomic position is obtained, the bone needs to be held in place with rigid fixation, either by bridging the gap with a bone plate and screws or an external fixator or by anchoring the transected bone to the other antebrachial bone with multiple screws or pins (Fig. 47-61).

In some patients, it may be advisable to reposition the affected bone gradually. Gradual repositioning is less traumatic, it allows the interosseous membrane to stretch slowly, and it allows careful control and adjustment of repositioning. This procedure can be easily accomplished by spanning the osteotomy with a dynamic external fixation device. Associated deformities can be corrected simultaneously by proper pin placement and appropriate limb straightening. The apparatus is then progressively opened every fourth day until

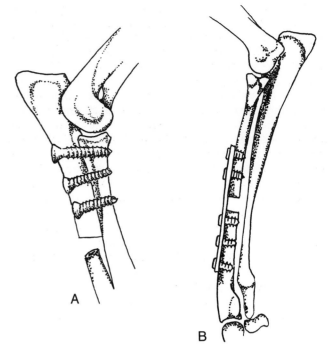

Fig. 47-61. A and B, *Methods of stabilization following osteotomy and repositioning.*

radiographs determine that the bone has been shifted sufficiently.

RADIAL HEAD EXCISION. In the human literature, radial head ostectomy is reported as a method of treatment for several defects at the radial-humeral articulation. Satisfactory postoperative results are generally reported. In the veterinary literature, radial head ostectomy has been reported as a method of treatment for lateral radial head luxation subsequent to premature distal ulnar physeal closure.[6] Satisfactory short-term results are also reported. It must be remembered, however, that man does not walk on his arms as dogs do on their front legs. Resection destroys the only possible normal antebrachial weight-bearing structure within the elbow. Joint instability and eventual loss of limb use appear probable. In addition, physiologic regrowth of the resected radial head with humeral condylar contact is a reported long-term complication in man. This regrowth has also been observed in the dog. For these reasons, radial head excision should not be an initial choice for treatment. Other methods of surgical management that attempt to restore joint congruence should be tried first.[8] If these procedures fail, then radial head ostectomy may be considered in an attempt to salvage a joint prior to elbow arthrodesis.

ARTHRODESIS. Often, degenerative changes within one or both of the antebrachial joints are so severe that, even if the forelimb deformity is corrected, the dog remains in severe pain, limps, or is unable to bear weight. In such a case, joint fusion is warranted. Whether performed as the initial treatment of choice or following attempts at correction, a straight forelimb is important; otherwise, problems may develop in the remaining joints.

The techniques for arthrodesis of the elbow or carpal joint are described in Chapter 48. Regardless of technique, certain principles always need to be followed. In order for bone union to occur, the cancellous bone of the epiphyses needs to be exposed and placed in close contact. This requirement necessitates thorough removal of all joint cartilage from the bones to be fused. To augment healing, additional fresh autogenous bone should be added to the surgical site. Commonly, this added bone is in the form of cancellous chips, obtained from a major metaphysis or from the wing of the ilium, which are packed in and around the fusion site. In the case of carpal arthrodesis, a variation of an unusual but excellent technique should be considered.[26] Because the function of the distal ulna is negated by arthrodesis, this structure becomes an excellent site for graft bone. It is already within the surgical field and is largely cancellous bone. The distal ulna may be used intact as an inlay graft, as reported, or it may be cut up and used as chip grafts.

Finally, the surgical site needs to be rigidly stabilized in the correct angle for the particular joint to be fused. This stability is best provided by placing the site to be fused under compression with a bone plate and screws or with one of the dynamic external fixation devices. A less rigid form of fixation increases the likelihood of nonunion.

References and Suggested Readings

1. Alexander, J. W., Walker, T. L., Roberts, R. E., and Dueland, R.: Malformation of canine forelimb due to synostosis between the radius and ulna. J. Am. Vet. Med. Assoc., *173*:1328, 1978.
2. Carrig, C. B., Morgan, J. P., and Pool, R. R.: Effects of asynchronous growth of the radius and ulna on the canine elbow joint following experimental retardation of longitudinal growth of the ulna. J. Am. An. Hosp. Assoc., *11*:560, 1975.
3. Chapman, W. L.: Appearance of ossification centers and epiphyseal closures as determined by radiographic techniques. J. Am. Vet. Med. Assoc., *147*:138, 1965.
4. Clayton-Jones, D. G., and Vaughan, L. C.: Disturbance in the growth of the radius in dogs. J. Small Anim. Pract., *11*:453, 1970.
5. Dieterich, H. F.: Repair of radius curvus in a two-stage surgical procedure: a case report. J. Am. Anim. Hosp. Assoc., *10*:48, 1974.
6. Dieterich, H. F.: Repair of a lateral radial head luxation by radial head ostectomy. VM SAC, *68*:671, 1973.
7. Egger, E. L., and Stoll, S. G.: Ulnar styloid transposition as an experimental treatment for premature closure of the distal ulnar physis. J. Am. Anim. Hosp. Assoc., *14*:690, 1978.
8. Gurevitch, R., and Hohn, R. B.: Surgical management of lateral luxation and subluxation of the canine radial head. Vet. Surg., *9*:49, 1980.
9. Hare, W. C. D.: The age at which epiphyseal union takes place in the limb bones of the dog. Wien. Tieraerztl. Monatsschr., *49*:210, 1961.
10. Lau, R. E.: Inherited premature closure of the distal ulnar physis. J. Am. Anim. Hosp. Assoc., *13*:609, 1977.
11. Llewellyn, H. R.: Growth plate injuries—diagnosis, prognosis, treatment. J. Am. Anim. Hosp. Assoc., *12*:77, 1976.
12. Morgan, J. P., Fisher, G. L., McNeill, K. L., and Oyama, J.: Abnormal canine bone development associated with hypergravity exposure. Am. J. Vet. Res., *40*:346, 1979.
13. Newton, C. D.: Surgical management of distal ulnar physeal growth disturbances in dogs. J. Am. Vet. Med. Assoc., *165*:479, 1974.
14. Newton, C. D., Nunamaker, D. M., and Dickinson, C. R.: Surgical management of radial physeal growth disturbance in dogs. J. Am. Vet. Med. Assoc., *167*:1011, 1975.
15. Noser, G. A., et al.: Asynchronous growth of the canine radius and ulna: effects of cross pinning the radius to the ulna. Am. J. Vet. Res., *38*:601, 1977.
16. O'Brien, T. R.: Development deformities due to arrested epiphyseal growth. Vet. Clin. North Am., *1*:441, 1971.
17. O'Brien, T. R., Morgan, J. P., and Suter, P. F.: Epiphyseal plate injury in the dog: a radiographic study of growth disturbance in the forelimb. J. Small Anim. Pract., *12*:19, 1971.
18. Olson, N. C., Brinker, W. O., and Carrig, C. B.: Premature closure of the distal radial physis in two dogs. J. Am. Vet. Med. Assoc., *176*:906, 1980.
19. Olson, N. C., Carrig, C. B., and Brinker, W. O.: Asynchronous growth of the canine radius and ulna: effects of retardation of longitudinal growth of the radius. Am. J. Vet. Res., *40*:351, 1979.
20. Passman, D., and Wolff, E. F.: Premature closure of the distal radial growth plate in a dog. J. Am. Vet. Med. Assoc., *167*:391, 1975.
21. Rudy, R. L.: Correction of growth deformity of the radius and ulna. *In* Current Techniques in Small Animal Surgery. Edited by M. J. Bojrab. Philadelphia, Lea & Febiger, 1975.
22. Rudy, R. L.: Corrective osteotomy for angular deformities. Vet. Clin. North Am., *1*:549, 1971.
23. Salter, R. B., and Harris, W. R.: Injuries involving the epiphyseal plate. J. Bone plate. Joint Surg. [Am.], *45*:587, 1963.
24. Skaggs, S., DeAngelis, M. P., and Rosen, H.: Deformities due to premature closure of the distal ulna in fourteen dogs: a radiographic evaluation. J. Am. Anim. Hosp. Assoc., *9*:496, 1973.
25. Smith, R. N., and Allcock, J.: Epiphyseal fusion in the greyhound. Vet. Rec., *72*:75, 1960.
26. Tadmor, A., and Herold, H. Z.: Central inlay bone graft for correction of radiocarpal deformity in a dog. J. Am. Vet. Med. Assoc., *162*:640, 1973.

Ununited Anconeal Process

by Kenneth R. Sinibaldi

Ununited anconeal process is a disease of young, rapidly growing dogs in which nonunion or partial union of the anconeal process to the olecranon of the ulna occurs. This disorder is more commonly seen in the German shepherd dog, although other breeds may be affected. Males are affected more commonly than females (2:1). This condition leads to front-leg lameness of varying degree and to secondary osteoarthritis. The term elbow dysplasia should not be used to describe the condition of ununited anconeal process. This term denotes a developmental anomaly, with or without ununited anconeal process, that progresses to osteoarthritis of the joint.

The pathogenesis of ununited anconeal process has not been definitely established, but strong evidence supports an inherited developmental anomaly in the fusion of the anconeal process to the ulna. A comparative study of the elbow development of young greyhounds and German shepherd dogs showed that the delayed union of the anconeal process in the German shepherd dogs was due to the presence of a large mass of cartilage in the process. The blood supply of the anconeal process was the same in both breeds, but the greyhound completed ossification and union of this process 1 to 5 weeks sooner.

Clinical Signs

Affected dogs are presented for examination between 6 and 9 months of age. The condition may be present for several months prior to presentation, but because of the varying degrees of lameness, which may be subtle, few cases are observed early by the owner. The condition may be unilateral or bilateral. The degree of lameness is subtle to severe. In bilateral cases, one leg may be affected more than the other, and lameness may vary from day to day, with severe involvement shifting from leg to leg. When the dog is at rest, it may stand with little weight on the affected limb and with the toes pointed laterally (external rotation). This stance has been described as the "wing out" stance. The patient should be examined while moving to determine which limb is involved. A shortened reach in the cranial stride is seen as the elbow is flexed and the limb is advanced. Palpation of the joint usually elicits pain. Crepitus, both soft tissue and bony, may also be present. Joint swelling is only seen early in the course of the disease and decreases with the chronicity of the condition. Muscle atrophy is present in advanced cases, owing to disuse.

This disease is a juvenile orthopedic disease in which age is important in establishing a diagnosis. Radiographically, in the normal dog, the ossification centers appear in the region of the anconeal process when the dogs are 11 to 12 weeks old. These centers are usually numerous, and they eventually merge to form a large center that gradually fuses with the diaphysis of the ulna adjacent to the articular cartilage of the trochlear notch. Complete fusion is seen at 16 to 20 weeks in the German shepherd dog. Therefore, a diagnosis of ununited anconeal process should not be made before a dog is 4½ months old.

Radiographic Examination

If ununited anconeal process is suspected, radiographs of the elbow joint should be taken to confirm the diagnosis. This procedure is best done with the patient anesthetized. Prior to the radiographic examination and while the animal is anesthetized, the limb should be taken through a range of motion, and the normal as well as affected joints should be palpated to rule out any possible coexisting diseases. Radiographs should be taken with the elbow flexed as much as possible. In this position, the anconeal process moves caudoventrally out of the supracondylar fossa and away from the condyles so it can be seen in its entirety. A craniocaudal view should also be taken to demonstrate early osteophyte changes and degree of osteoarthritis. Both elbows should be radiographed, so that a

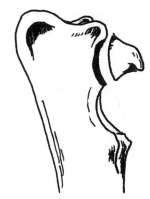

Fig. 47-62. *Diagrammatic illustration of an ununited anconeal process.*

comparison between the normal and the abnormal elbow can be made. This bilateral examination also reveals the presence of a bilateral lesion, even though one leg may not show obvious clinical signs.

Radiographic findings reveal that the anconeal process is not fused to the ulna (Fig. 47-62). Depending on the duration of the condition, various degrees of osteoarthritis are present. In some chronic cases, the process may be anchored high in the supracondylar fossa even in flexion. Some sclerotic change is usually present in the ulna at the site of normal attachment of the anconeal process. Osteolysis may be present in chronic cases.

Treatment

Basically, one has three choices of treatment for this condition: no treatment, removal of the anconeal process, or reattachment of the process. The first choice is rarely acceptable because this condition is progressive and usually leads to pain and advanced osteoarthritis. Few cases that are not surgically treated heal or become asymptomatic.

REMOVAL OF THE ANCONEAL PROCESS

Removal of the anconeal process has been the most accepted method of treatment. Much debate exists on the resultant instability of the elbow joint after surgical removal of the anconeal process. Some feel that although this instability is better than no treatment, the unstable joint is susceptible to lateral "wobbling" that ultimately leads to secondary osteoarthritis and future lameness. Others, however, have shown that the degree of osteoarthritis present at the time of surgical removal of the process remains stable and progresses little thereafter.

Surgical removal of the anconeal process, if performed before the development of severe osteoarthritis, can restore the animal to clinical soundness. Removal of the ununited anconeal process is a simple, safe, and feasible procedure. The patient is placed in lateral recumbency, with the affected leg uppermost.

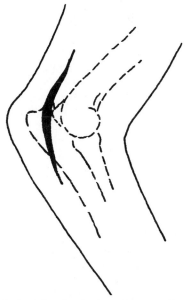

Fig. 47-63. *Skin incision for the lateral approach to the anconeal process. Directly under this incision are the fascia and muscle belly of the anconeal process.*

The limb is prepared for the surgical procedure and is draped in the usual aseptic manner. A lateral approach to the elbow joint is used.

The skin is incised caudal to the lateral humeral condyle, and the lateral head of the triceps muscle is retracted cranially, to expose the underlying anconeus muscle (Fig. 47-63). An incision is then made into the anconeus muscle by directing the surgical blade at a slightly cranial angle, incising across the muscle fibers. This incision penetrates the joint capsule and allows synovial fluid to escape. By lengthening this incision dorsally and ventrally, the anconeal process is exposed. The process is then grasped with suitable forceps, and gentle traction is applied. Sharp dissection with scissors or a scalpel is used to free the anconeal process. A fibrous attachment is usually seen at the caudal end of the process where the vascular supply to the process enters from the ulna. After incising this structure, the anconeal process can be removed. The joint should be inspected for free fragments and flushed well with saline solution, and the joint capsule, muscle, and subcutaneous tissue should be closed with an absorbable suture. The skin is closed with nonabsorbable sutures of the veterinary surgeon's choice.

Postoperative care consists of a padded cotton bandage for 7 to 10 days, and the patient's activity is limited to leash exercise only. After suture removal, swimming therapy can be beneficial and has worked well in limiting joint stiffness.

REATTACHMENT OF THE ANCONEAL PROCESS

Inasmuch as removal of the anconeal process may not leave the elbow joint as stable as if the process were intact, surgical reattachment of the process may be of benefit. This procedure can be accomplished with a cortical bone screw used in a lag fashion.

The preparation and positioning of the patient are the same as for removal of the anconeal process. The approach is also the same, except the incision length is greater, to allow for adequate exposure for screw implantation. After exposing the anconeal process, the nonfused surfaces of the process and its normal attachment on the ulna should be curetted to stimulate bleeding. The patient's elbow is placed in extreme flexion, and the radius and ulna are externally rotated to allow visualization of the anconeal process. The process is positioned, and a hole is drilled from just behind the tip of the process through the bone and into the ulna. The hole in the anconeal process must be large enough to allow for passage of the screw threads without contact (gliding hole). This goal is accomplished by overdrilling the original pilot hole (Fig. 47-64). The hole in the ulna is then tapped, and the screw is positioned so that the threads contact only the bone of the ulna and therefore compress the process to the ulna (Fig. 47-64*A* and *B*). This compression enhances stability and fusion of the anconeal process to the ulna. The head of the screw must be countersunk to eliminate contact with the cartilage of the condyles. It usually takes 6 to 8 weeks for fusion to occur. Postoperative care is the same as for surgical removal of the anconeal process.

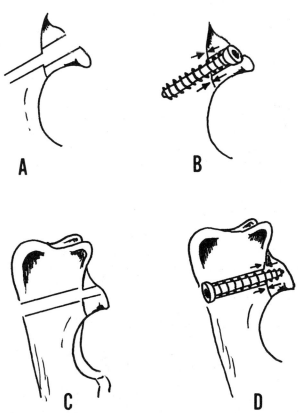

Fig. 47-64. *Reattachment of the anconeal process. A and B, The lag principle, with the gliding hole in the anconeal process. C and D, The procedure is reversed, with the gliding hole in the ulna.*

If this technique is used, it must be noted that if performed on young or rapidly growing puppies (5 to 7 months), the possibility exists that they will overgrow the attached anconeal process and will shear off the screw even if the process has healed. For this reason, it is recommended that lag screw fixation be postponed until the patient's growth rate slows (9 to 10 months).

This problem of overgrowing may be eliminated if the screw is placed in the opposite direction (Fig. 47-64C and D). The procedure is the same, except the anconeal process should be tapped to accept the screw threads, and the ulna should be overdrilled to serve as the gliding hole. This maneuver also allows for screw removal once radiographic healing has taken place.

In summary, ununited anconeal process is most common in male German shepherd dogs. The condition leads to front-leg lameness of varying degrees. If the disorder is untreated, secondary osteoarthritis and pain result. The diagnosis can be made by considering breed, age, and clinical findings. Conformation of the condition is best made by radiographic examination.

Surgical intervention is the treatment of choice, despite the controversy over removal or reattachment of the anconeal process. I currently feel, as do others, that the surgical removal of the anconeal process is a simple, safe, and feasible procedure that yields consistently rewarding results.

References and Suggested Readings

Archibald, J. (ed.): Canine Surgery. 2nd Ed. Santa Barbara, CA, American Veterinary Publications, 1974.

Bojrab, M. J. (ed.): Current Techniques in Small Animal Surgery. Bojrab, Philadelphia, Lea & Febiger, 1975.

Herron, M. R.: Ununited anconeal process—a new approach to surgical repair. Mod. Vet. Pract., 51:30, 1970.

Piermattei, D. L., and Greeley, R. G.: Atlas of Surgical Approaches to the Bones of the Dog and Cat. 2nd Ed. Philadelphia, W. B. Saunders, 1979.

Sinibaldi, K. R., and Arnoczky, S. P.: Surgical removal of the ununited anconeal process in the dog. J. Am. Anim. Hosp. Assoc., 2:192, 1975.

Van Sickle, D. C.: The relationship of ossification to canine elbow dysplasia. J. Am. Anim. Hosp. Assoc., 2:24, 1966.

Whittick, W. G.: Canine Orthopedics. Philadelphia, Lea & Febiger, 1974.

Fractures of the Scapula

by WILLIAM W. RYAN

Fractures of the scapula are uncommon because the bone is well protected from trauma by the thoracic cage and associated musculature. The three most common fractures sites are the scapular spine or acromion, the neck, including the supraglenoid tubercle and the articular surface of the glenoid cavity, and the scapular body.[1-3] Frequent complications are injury to the suprascapular nerve, especially with scapular neck fractures, rib fractures, thoracic trauma, and brachial plexus injury. Examination for these complications is essential.

Diagnosis

Diagnosis is based on physical and radiographic examinations. Animals with scapular fractures usually show both a swinging and a standing leg lameness. With fractures of the scapular neck, the shoulder may be dropped and the limb may be held in internal rotation. Crepitus is not a common finding, except with scapular neck fractures, and pain is more severe the closer the fracture is to the shoulder joint.[3] It is imperative to examine both craniocaudal and lateral radiographs to confirm the diagnosis of scapular fractures.

Conservative Treatment

Most scapular fractures are not severely displaced, owing to the protective nature of the surrounding muscles and the rib cage. These fractures can be managed successfully by simply limiting the animal's activity to a minimum for 3 or 4 weeks. A modified Velpeau sling or an over-the-shoulder spica splint may also be used and should be maintained for at least 3 weeks.

Surgical Treatment

Surgical intervention is required in patients with marked displacement of the fracture segments, fractures involving the articular surface of the shoulder joint, and avulsion fractures.

SURGICAL APPROACHES

The surgical approach for fractures of the body of the scapula, the spine of the scapula, or the acromion starts with an incision directly over the spine of the scapula. The skin and subcutaneous fascia are incised and are retracted. An incision is then made in the deep fascia along the spine of the scapula and is deepened to free the origins of the deltoideus and omotransversarius muscles and the insertion of the trapezius muscle. These muscles are retracted to expose the spine of the scapula and the deep infra- and supraspinatus muscles. The supra- and infraspinatus muscles are then elevated subperiosteally from their attachments on the spine of the scapula to expose the body of the scapula. Following surgical repair, closure consists of a single row of simple interrupted sutures including the deep fascia and the external sheath of the deep infra- and supraspinatus muscles. Closure of the skin and subcutaneous tissues is routine.[4]

When approaching fractures of the neck of the scapula, the supraglenoid tubercle, or the articular surface of the glenoid cavity, a more extensive approach is required. A skin incision is made beginning at the middle of the scapula, following the spine distally, crossing the joint and continuing over the lateral surface of the proximal humerus. The skin and subcutaneous fascia are retracted. An incision is then made in the deep fascia over the spine of the scapula and is deepened to free the origin of the scapular head of the deltoideus and omotransversarius muscles and the insertion of the trapezius muscle on the spine. The incision is continued distally through the deep fascia over the acromial head of the deltoideus muscle and is stopped before reaching the cephalic vein. This fascia is undermined and is retracted from the acromial head of the deltoideus muscle. The omotransversarius and trapezius muscles are then retracted cranially. The two parts of the deltoideus muscle are then divided by blunt dissection, and the scapular head of the deltoideus muscle is retracted caudally.

The acromion then undergoes osteotomy to include all the origin of the acromial head of the deltoideus muscle, which is then freed from the shaft of the humerus and is reflected distally, leaving its insertion on the deltoid tubercle undisturbed. The deep infra- and supraspinatus muscles are then bluntly elevated from the spine and body of the scapula and are retracted. During elevation and retraction of the infraspinatus muscle, care must be taken to avoid the suprascapular nerve as it crosses over the neck of the scapula. Exposure of the articular surface of the joint requires tenotomy of the infraspinatus muscle. This incision is made near the muscle's insertion on the humerus; one must leave enough of a stump to receive one or two sutures.

After reduction and surgical stabilization of the fracture, closure is accomplished by first joining the infraspinatus tendon with horizontal mattress sutures. The acromion is reattached to the spine by two monofilament stainless steel sutures placed through holes drilled in the bones (Fig. 47-65). A single row of simple interrupted sutures may be used to close the remaining muscles and fascia. Starting proximally, these sutures engage the deep fascia, the trapezius muscle, the external sheath of the infraspinatus and supraspinatus muscles, the spinous part of the deltoideus muscle, and the deep fascia. The pattern is continued distally, with the omotransversarius muscle replacing the trapezius muscle as the acromion is approached. Distal to the acromion, the deep fascia alone is closed. The skin and subcutaneous tissues are closed in a routine manner.[4]

ACROMION, SPINE, AND SCAPULAR BODY FRACTURES

Fixation of acromion fractures, just as with the previously described procedure for reattachment of an acromion that has undergone osteotomy, can usually be accomplished with two monofilament stainless steel sutures (Fig. 47-65).

In cats and small dogs, fractures of the spine and scapular body can also be stabilized with monofilament stainless steel wires placed through predrilled holes (Fig. 47-66). In larger dogs, it is often necessary to use small bone plates[2] (Fig. 47-67) or a combination of a small bone plate and stainless steel wires (Fig. 47-68).

It is difficult to hold the scapular fracture fragments in reduction prior to application of the bone plate. Instead, the bone plate should be first secured with screws to the proximal fragment. The distal fragment is then levered into reduction, and screws are then

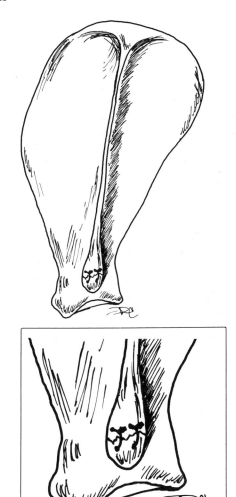

Fig. 47-65. *The acromion is reattached to the spine with stainless steel sutures.*

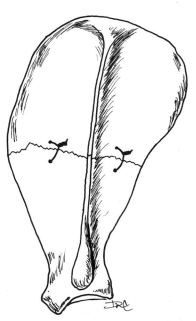

Fig. 47-66. *Stabilization of scapular spine and body fractures with stainless steel wires in cats and small dogs.*

a modified Velpeau sling is advisable following reduction of a medial dislocation because this immobilization directs the humeral head laterally. In animals with a lateral dislocation, a non-weight-bearing sling is used. In both instances, the external support should be maintained for 2 to 3 weeks.

Failure of closed reduction and external immobilization techniques results in recurrent dislocation of the shoulder and necessitates open reduction and internal stabilization. The principle of using an existing anatomic structure, the biceps brachii tendon, as a functional collateral ligament seems more physiologic than the use of synthetic materials for stabilization. When the biceps brachii tendon has torn free from its origin on the supraglenoid tubercle, a portion of the supraspinatus tendon may be substituted in the repair. Both techniques are further supported by plication of the joint capsule.

MEDIAL LUXATION

BICIPITAL TENDON TECHNIQUE. This technique is initiated with a craniomedial parahumeral incision over the shoulder (Fig. 47-78A, inset). The skin and subcutaneous tissues are reflected, and the medial border of the brachiocephalicus muscle is separated and retracted laterally, exposing the superficial and deep pectoral muscles, the supraspinatus muscle, and the distal communicating branch of the cephalic vein (Fig. 47-78A). The proximal half of the insertion of the superficial pectoral muscle is transected and is retracted medially to expose the deep pectoral muscle, which is incised in a similar fashion along the length of its insertion on the humerus (Fig. 47-78B). Incision of the fascial attachment between the supraspinatus muscle and the deep

pectoral muscles, with medial retraction of the latter, allows for a full medial exposure of the shoulder joint (Fig. 47-78C). The insertion of the subscapularis muscle is elevated, is detached from the lesser tubercle, and is reflected medially. The tissues over the bicipital groove and the transverse humeral ligament are transected, and the dorsal aspect of the joint capsule surrounding the bicipital tendon is incised to allow mobilization of the tendon from the bicipital groove (Fig. 47-78D).

At this point, the joint is inspected, and any torn portions of the capsule are identified. A crescent-shaped osteotomy is made in the lesser tubercle, with the bottom of the crescent following the curve of the humeral head. The bone flap is elevated, leaving it hinged cranially. A small amount of cancellous bone is curetted beneath the bone flap. The dislocation is reduced, and the bicipital tendon is transplanted beneath the bone flap, which is secured over the tendon with 2 0.045-inch Kirschner wires or a 2.7-mm screw and spiked Teflon washer (Fig. 47-78D). The medial joint capsule is closed in a plicating fashion. The tendinous insertion of the subscapularis muscle is advanced toward the crest of the greater tubercle of the humerus and is sutured near the insertion of the deep pectoral muscle. The remaining musculature, subcutaneous tissues, and skin are closed in layers (Fig. 47-78E). The limb is placed in the modified Velpeau sling for 2 weeks.

SUPRASPINATUS TENDON TECHNIQUE. This technique for medial luxation uses the same surgical approach as the bicipital tendon technique to the insertion of the deep pectoral muscle (Fig. 47-79A). The deep pectoral muscle is separated from the fascial attachment to the medial fleshy border of the supraspinatus muscle and

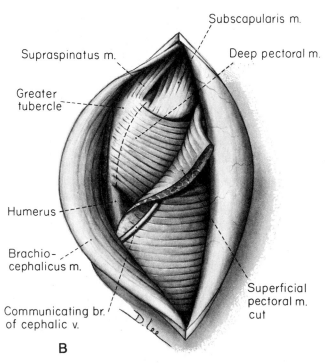

Fig. 47-78. *Legend on facing page.*

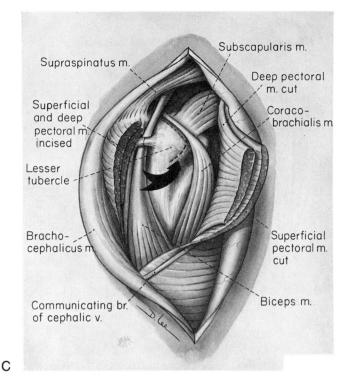

C

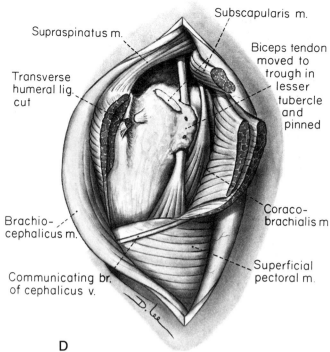

D

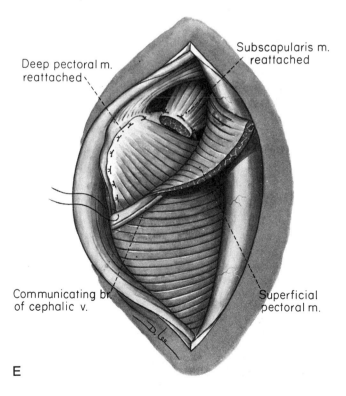

E

Fig. 47-78. A, *Cranial view of muscles of the canine shoulder and proximal humerus following the craniomedial parahumeral incision (inset) and retraction of the brachiocephalicus muscle laterally. B, Craniomedial view of the shoulder following incision and retraction of the superficial pectoral muscle. C, Craniomedial view of the shoulder with the pectoral muscles retracted medially exposing the lesser tubercle and the medial aspect of the joint. Note the line for the incision in the transverse humeral ligament. The osteotomy line on the lesser tubercle is identified (arrow). D, Craniomedial view of the shoulder showing the bicipital tendon fixed in place beneath the bone flap on the lesser tubercle. E, Craniomedial view of the shoulder showing reattachment of the subscapularis and deep pectoral muscles in a more cranial fashion. (A to E, From Hohn, R. B., Rosen, H., Bohning, R. H., Jr., and Brown, S. G.: Surgical stabilization of recurrent shoulder luxation. Vet. Clin. North Am. 1:537, 1971).*

from its insertion on the greater and lesser tubercles of the humerus (Fig. 47-79B). It is important to make an accurate separation between the tendinous fold of the supraspinatus muscle and the deep pectoral muscle (Fig. 47-79B). Distally, the strong muscular belly of the supraspinatus curves far around the neck of the scapula so that it appears on the medial surface of the shoulder. This portion of the muscle has a tendinous fold that inserts on the cranial surface of the greater tubercle. This fold should not be mistaken for the division between the deep pectoral muscle and the supraspinatus muscle. Retraction of the deep pectoral muscle exposes the medial aspect of the shoulder. A partial osteotomy of the greater tubercle is accomplished by positioning the osteotome on the crest of the greater tubercle of the humerus and directing it so that the

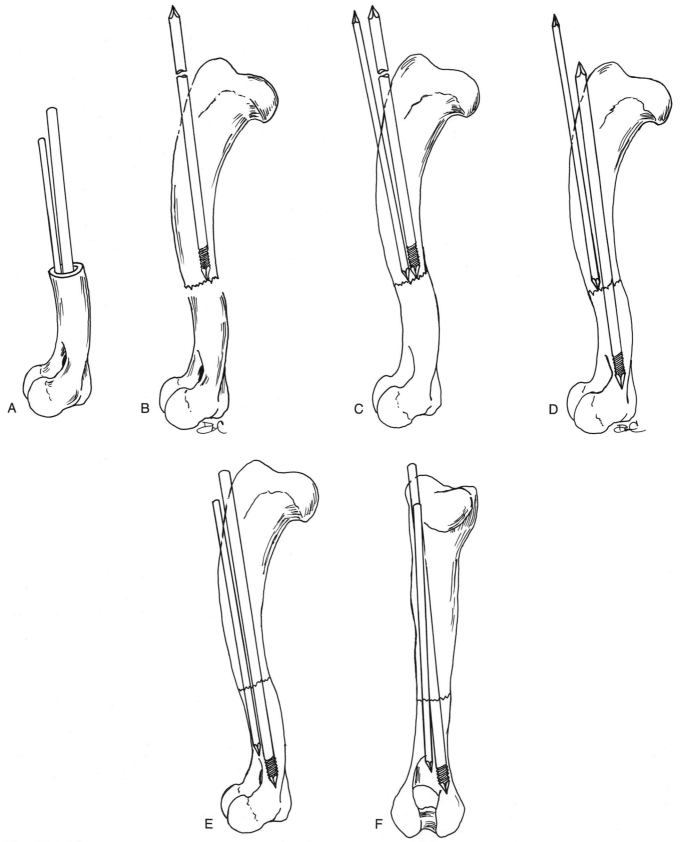

Fig. 48-3. A, *Determining the intramedullary pins needed to fill the canal of the humerus.* B, *A large pin is passed in a retrograde fashion first, following the cranial cortex of the intramedullary canal.* C, *Next, the smaller pin is inserted in a retrograde direction in the same manner and usually emerges cranial to the large one. The fracture is reduced.* D, *The large, threaded pin is driven deeply near the medial condyle.* E and F, *The smaller pin is driven to a point just proximal to the supratrochlear foramen.*

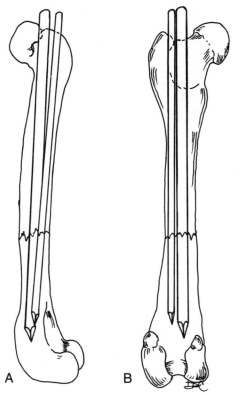

Fig. 48-4. *Stack pinning of the femur.* A, *Lateral view.* B, *Caudocranial view.*

nary surgeon can direct the intramedullary pins out the greater trochanter or the trochanteric fossa during the retrograde step. Placement of the pins in the greater trochanter may enhance the stability of a proximal fracture.[3] The placement of the intramedullary pins in both the trochanteric fossa and the greater trochanter can be accomplished from the proximal end of the proximal fragment for fixation of fractures in the middle or proximal third of the femur; however, proper placement of the intramedullary pins into the distal fragment is then unreliable, and I do not recommend it for the stack-pin technique.

Postoperative Considerations

Recovery time can be shortened with the postsurgical application of a leg wrap, which enhances venous return. This bandage must incorporate the entire foot to prevent strangulation of venous return. The bandage should be changed if wet and should be removed when soft tissue swelling is no longer significant. Cage rest is recommended for 5 to 10 days postoperatively with mild, leash exercise. The length of confinement depends upon the stability of the dog's personality. Appropriate bacteriocidal antibiotics should be administered prior to surgical preparation and should be continued during the recovery stage, as necessary. Restricted daily exercise (leash only) is advised for an additional 3 to 4 weeks in giant breed, obese, or hunting dogs. The intramedullary pins are removed when clinical union of the fracture is radiographically evident.

Acknowledgment

I wish to acknowledge the suggestions offered by Dr. Charles, Knecht in the preparation of the publication[2] that led to this discussion of the stack-pin technique.

References and Suggested Readings

1. Brinker, W. O.: Fractures. *In* Canine Surgery. 2nd Ed. Edited by J. Archibald. Santa Barbara, CA, American Veterinary Publications, 1974.
2. Chafffee, V. W.: Multiple (stacked) intramedullary pin fixation of humeral and femoral fractures. J. Am. Anim. Hosp. Assoc., *13*:599, 1977.
3. DeAngelis, M. P.: Fractures of the femur. *In* Current Techniques in Small Animal Surgery. Edited by M. J. Bojrab. Philadelphia, Lea & Febiger, 1975.
4. De Lahunta, A.: Veterinary Neuroanatomy and Clinical Neurology. Philadelphia, W. B. Saunders, 1977.
5. Piermattei, D. L., and Greeley, R. G.: An Atlas of Surgical Approaches to the Bones of the Dog and Cat. 2nd Ed. Philadelphia, W. B. Saunders, 1979.
6. Rudy, R. L.: Principles of intramedullary pinning. Vet. Clin. North Am., 5:209, 1975.

Bone Grafting in Small Animal Orthopedics

Cortical Allografts

by WILLIAM B. HENRY, JR.

The use of allograft bone to replace comminuted segments of diaphyseal bone was first reported in the veterinary literature in 1976.[17] This information, as well as the recent success of frozen allograft transplantation involving 45 allografts,[6] 11 of which were large, segmental tubular grafts rigidly fixed with bone plates, led my colleagues and me to apply similar techniques in the repair of severely comminuted long-bone fractures in dogs and cats.[1] Recent research on allograft acceptance in cats has helped to establish guidelines for the use of allograft bone in clinical veterinary medicine.[13]

Bone Banking Procedures

Donor selection is based on the animal's age and freedom from infectious and contagious disease. Young donors whose epiphyseal plates are radiographically closed are generally selected. An animal with an abnormal complete blood count, urinalysis, or physical examination is not used. If an animal has any evidence of infection (dental, otic, or skin) it is not considered to be an acceptable donor.

The bones are harvested under completely sterile conditions. Skin preparation consists of clipping with a No. 40 blade, followed by at least 3 surgical scrubs with cotton and an iodinated surgical soap.* This scrubbing is followed by an iodinated surgical spray, which is allowed to remain on the limb for 3 to 5 minutes before an alcohol† cleansing with cotton swabs is performed. This procedure is followed by an alcohol spray of the entire limb, which is allowed to dry before one applies a plastic adhesive drape.‡ Routine orthopedic operative draping and gowning procedures, using towels, stockinette, double muslin drapes, and double surgical gloving are used during all bone harvests. The bone is harvested either while the donor is under general surgical anesthesia or minutes after the donor's death. All muscle and most of the periosteum are removed from the bone using a No. 10 surgical blade. On occasion, an entire femur, tibia, or humerus, is harvested. If only diaphyseal segments are taken, an osteotomy is made at the metaphyseal ends of the bone. No attempt is made to remove the marrow from the medullary cavity.

The harvested bone is doubly wrapped in muslin towels and is placed either in gas-sterilized, heavy-gauge polyethylene bags or in autoclaved Nalgene§ bottles. The bottles are tightly sealed, are dated, and are labeled as to species of animal and bone type. Each graft is then radiographed, and the radiograph is filed for future matching before grafting. The bone grafts can be stored in a standard home refrigerator freezer. The average temperature in this type of freezer varies between −15 and −20° C. Although grafts have been used for up to 3 years after harvest,[11] I do not use bone grafts stored in this manner after 12 months. It is unknown whether long-term dehydration has adverse biomechanical effects.

Case Selection

The majority of fractures that my colleagues and I have allografted have had 10 or more comminuted pieces, not counting the proximal and distal segments of bone.[1] Allografts should only be used in highly comminuted fractures of the diaphysis of long bones that cannot be reconstructed. A comminuted fracture can seldom be repaired without compromise. When evaluating preoperative radiographs, the veterinary surgeon may not be able to foresee all possible compromises in the repair. When faced with this preoperative dilemma, the criteria for successful allografting must be reviewed, and a tentative plan must be prepared.

The two major criteria for successful allografting are as follows:

*Prepodyne scrub (contains polaxamer-iodine complex and titratable iodine 1%), West Chemical Products, Inc., New York, NY
†Lavacol (70% ethyl alcohol), Parke-Davis, 201 Tabor Road, Morris Plains, NJ 07950
‡Vidrape Parke-Davis, 201 Tabor Road, Morris Plains, NJ 07950
§Scientific Products Co., 20 Wiggins Avenue, Bedford, MA 01730

1. One must not allograft contaminated or infected fractures. All open or fresh contaminated fractures should be closed, immobilized, and determined to be sterile 7 to 14 days following closure before allografting. All fractures infected from previous surgical procedures should not be allografted until the infection is resolved. Infection in orthopedics is disastrous, especially when using allografts.[2,5]

2. Allografts must be rigidly fixed in order for primary bone healing to occur. The most rigid fixation for consistently successful allografts is provided by bone plates and Association for the Study of Internal Fixation (ASIF)‖ bone plating techniques.[2,6] The veterinary surgeon must understand the ASIF techniques well and must be equipped with the appropriate instruments to apply these techniques properly. Other methods or combinations of methods of fixation have been used in allograft repair of fractures or in tumor resection with unsatisfactory results.[7]

Primary bone healing can be obtained if the following four principles of graft fixation are not violated:

1. The number of cortices of screw purchase in the host bone is important. In the dog, at least 6 cortices and 3 screws are needed in the proximal and distal host bone. Use of a 4.5-mm bone plate requires at least 5.5 cm of proximal host bone and a similar amount of distal host bone. The correct method of measuring the proximal and distal host bone is demonstrated in Figures 48-5 and 48-6. This dog's proximal and distal segments of bone measure 8.5 cm and thus easily provide enough bone for 3 screws, proximally and distally, using a 4.5-mm ASIF bone plate (Fig. 48-7). If a 3.5-mm ASIF bone plate is used, 4.5 cm of bone must be present in the proximal and distal host bone segments for the insertion of 3 proximal and 3 distal screws. In the cat, 6 cortices of screw purchase are ideal; however, successful allografts with primary bone healing have been obtained with 4 cortices.[2] When using a 2.7-mm ASIF bone plate, at least 3.5 cm of proximal and distal host bone must be available for 6 cortices of screw purchase. Measurement of the cat's bone for allograft replacement of comminuted segments is the same as in the dog (see Figs. 48-5 and 48-6).

2. Dynamic compression plates should be used when interpositioning allografts between the two segments of host bone. This maneuver permits compression of the host-graft interfaces at both ends (Fig. 48-8). Because transverse osteotomies are used, the compression of both host-graft interfaces provides rigid bone fixation.

3. The degree of osteotomy contact at both host-graft interfaces is important. The veterinary surgeon must think of the cross-section of cortical bone and must attempt to gain contact of the allograft and host bone, both proximally and distally, throughout the entire 360°. In order to obtain this end, a bone of correct diameter must be selected from the bone bank. It is much more difficult to obtain this contact throughout 360° in dogs because of the curvature of their bones.

‖Synthes, Ltd., 983 Old Eagle School Road, Wayne, PA 19087

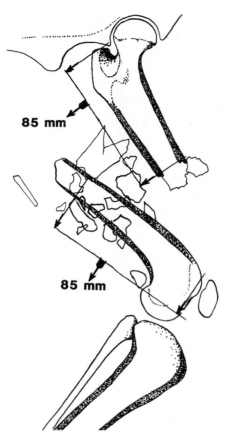

85 mm

85 mm

Fig. 48-5. *The lateral radiograph is more accurate when determining the length of the allograft and the presence of sufficient host bone to obtain six cortices of fixation both proximally and distally.*

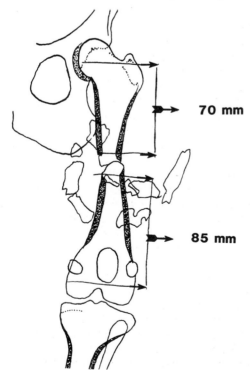

70 mm

85 mm

Fig. 48-6. *Preoperative measurements from craniocaudal radiographs to determine both the proposed length of the allograft and the presence of adequate host bone for rigid fixation result in error due to muscle contracture.*

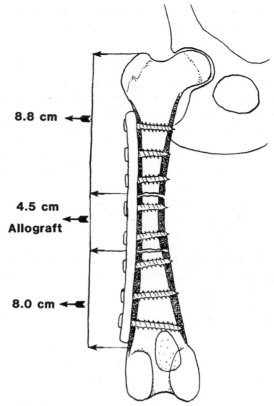

8.8 cm

4.5 cm Allograft

8.0 cm

Fig. 48-7. *Optimal allograft fixation in the dog with six cortices of screw purchase in the host bone above and below the allograft.*

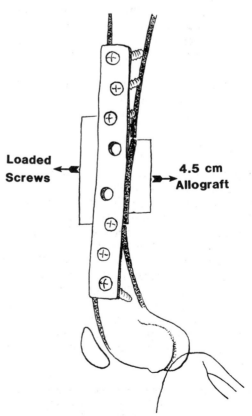

Loaded Screws

4.5 cm Allograft

Fig. 48-8. *Counting from the proximal end of the femur, the third and sixth screws have been loaded to compress the allograft segment of bone both proximally and distally.*

The straight bones of the cat make this objective much easier to attain. The 360° contact cannot be obtained in either species quickly and easily unless the veterinary surgeon has an air drill* with a wide assortment of sharp burs.

4. The last principle is that tubular allografts fail when interpositioned on interfragmentary reconstructed host bone. One should not rebuild the metaphyseal ends of the bone in order to obtain additional cortices of screw purchase in host bone. The cortices of screw purchase must be in intact host bone (see Fig. 48-7). When partially reconstructed metaphyseal host bone was used as a buttress for the allograft, the repairs uniformly failed in the dog,[2] although one success was reported in the cat.[1] Instability in the fracture repair results in failure.

If these four principles of rigid fixation can be adhered to when using large diaphyseal allografts, a high rate of success can be expected.

Technique of Allograft Repair

Preoperative radiographs of the fractured bone and the contralateral normal bone are used to determine the diameter and the approximate length of the allograft. The diameters of banked bone radiographs are compared with the diameter of the contralateral bone. The approximate length of the allograft can be determined preoperatively by measuring the proposed proximal and distal osteotomy sites of fractured bone, then by subtracting these segment lengths from the length of the contralateral bone; thus, the approximate length of the allograft is given (see Figs. 48-5 and 48-6).

The veterinary surgeon may, if possible, determine the exact length of the graft intraoperatively by reconstructing the comminuted pieces until the allograft length is found. The surgical preparation of the recipient is identical to that of the donors. Standard surgical approaches are used to the tension side of the bone. Often, because of the literal explosion of the bone when a comminuted fracture occurs, soft tissue damage is extensive. This damage frequently necessitates removal of large amounts of clot and debridement of lacerated, devitalized muscle. The allograft bone is removed from its sterile container and is placed in saline solution or in a 10% solution of povidone-iodine† to defrost while the veterinary surgeon makes his approach to the fracture.

The proximal and distal osteotomies are performed, following the preoperative length-measurement guidelines, using either a reciprocating or an oscillating saw.* One must be careful to make the osteotomies perpendicular to the long axis of the bone. The allograft is then measured and is cut to size; again, one must try to maintain a perpendicular cut. Bone plates of appropriate size and length are selected and are contoured to fit the contralateral bone using the preoperative radiographs. The allograft bone is then applied to

* Animal Care Products, 3M Center, St. Paul, MN 55101
† 100 ml diluted in 900 ml Ringer's lactated solution.

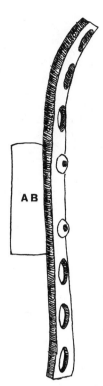

Fig. 48-9. *The plate is contoured to fit the contralateral bone using the preoperative radiographs, and the allograft is applied to the plate using at least two screws. This technique facilitates implantation of the allograft segment between the host bone segments. AB, Allograft bone.*

the contoured plate. At least two screws are used to fix the allograft to the plate (Fig. 48-9). The plate is now checked for contour on the distal and proximal segments of host bone.

The osteotomy interfaces are contoured to the shaft to obtain a perfect 360° host-graft interface and to maintain proper hip and knee alignment. Achievement of this objective is facilitated by applying the allograft to the contoured plate. Disparity in limb length caused by inappropriate allograft length should be kept to less than 1 cm in the cat and 2 cm in the dog. In large dogs with fractures, a distractor‡ must be used occasionally to overcome muscle contracture and to obtain limb length. Autogenous cancellous bone grafts can be used at the osteotomy sites; however, segmental allografts heal without such grafts when rigidly fixed.[1]

Following the grafting procedure, surgical wounds are liberally flushed with a 10% povidone iodine solution for 2 to 3 minutes before wound closure. The soaking solution is removed with suction. During wound closure, care is taken to approximate the adjacent musculature closely to the allograft bone. This maneuver is important because the primary portion of graft revascularization comes from the surrounding soft tissue. Close approximation of the musculature also diminishes dead space and prevents fluid sequestration and possible infection. I administer no preoperative, intraoperative, or postoperative antibiotics.

‡ Synthes, Ltd., 983 Old Eagle School Road, Wayne, PA 19087

Postoperative Care

Compressive and supportive Robert Jones bandages can be used in tibial fractures for 3 to 5 days. Humeral and femoral fractures are not immobilized postoperatively. If no preoperative or postoperative complications are seen, the hospitalization period can be as short as 5 days. On discharge from the hospital, the patient's owners are instructed to confine the animal to the house and to a leash when outside. Monthly physical and radiographic examinations are advisable for the first 3 to 6 months. If no complications exist, the animal is allowed unrestricted activity 6 months postoperatively.

Healing of Allograft Bone

In rigidly fixed allografts, the osteotomy sites at the host-graft interface fill with woven bone perpendicular to the long axis of the graft within 3 months of implantation. This woven bone rigidly cements together the interface between the host bone and the allograft bone. By 6 months, the host-graft interface of woven bone is replaced by lamellar bone.[13] The osteotomy line is barely visible at this time, and numerous osteons cross the graft-host interface directly.[13] Cutting cones (new osteons) are led by large osteoclasts that remove the dead allograft bone. The accompanying neocapillaries and osteoblasts follow the osteoclast into the dead allograft bone and lay down new host bone. This revascularization process of dead bone has been called "creeping substitution" or appositional new bone growth.[15]

The host medullary corticocancellous bone provides a ready source of vascular components that cross both distal and proximal host-graft interfaces and allow the rapid production of new bone on the dead corticocancellous bone of the allograft.[2] As revascularization occurs across the host-graft interface and through the endosteal canal, the surrounding soft tissue (musculature, for example) provides mesenchymal cells that differentiate into osteoclasts, neocapillaries, and osteoblasts. Creeping substitution occurs from the newly formed "periosteal sleeve" that forms over the dead allograft bone with new cutting cones (osteons) traversing the cortical bone from the periosteal side to the endosteal canal. At 12 months, the dead allograft bone is not completely replaced by living host bone.[13]

When an allograft fails, the allograft cortical bone is treated by the body in the same manner as avascular cortical autograft bone that is not rigidly fixed. The graft becomes a sequestrum that the body attempts to decalcify and to resorb. If the segment of dead bone, whether allograft or autograft, is large, wound drainage occurs during the attempted resorption process.

The drainage and infection that ensue are not primary, but are secondary to the presence of the dead bone that has not been rigidly fixed to permit revascularization. These failures all have similar radiographic appearance. The sequestrated allograft bone is surrounded by a periosteal cuff of new bone that attempts to bridge the transplant proximally and distally. The loosening of the bone plate and screws is depicted by the radiolucent zones that surround them and by their displacement from their original immediate postoperative location. Clinically, the animal is not weight-bearing, and draining fistulous tracts are seen in the soft tissue in 2 to 4 months postoperatively. One or more bacterial strains can be cultured from the draining tracts. Most often, these strains are staphylococci or coliform organisms. At this point, the veterinary surgeon's alternatives are limited to either amputation or removal of the allograft bone and autogenous cancellous bone grafts.[2]

Experience with plate removal on allograft fracture repair has been minimal. I have left bone plates in indefinitely without complications. One plate was removed from a patient 18 months after the allografting procedure without complications.[17] A biopsy had been performed on bone at 6 month intervals prior to removal of the bone plate.

In summary, the alternatives to allograft transplantation in severely comminuted fractures are attempted reconstruction, with autogenous cancellous bone grafting either alone or in combination with autogenous corticocancellous bone grafting, or amputation.

Allograft bone for transplantation can be obtained and frozen easily and inexpensively. It should be used only in selected patients in which the degree of diaphyseal comminution is so severe that the fracture cannot be reconstructed and fixed rigidly. It is a last-resort alternative to amputation in these fractured limbs. Allograft bone is immunogenic; however, this property does not compromise the fate of the transplant.[14]

References and Suggested Readings

1. Henry, W. B., Jr., and Wadsworth, P. L.: Diaphyseal allografts in the repair of severely comminuted long bone fractures. J. Am. Anim. Hosp. Assoc., *17*:525, 1981.
2. Henry, W. B., Jr., and Wadsworth, P. L.: Retrospective failure analysis of large diaphyseal allografts used in the repair of severely comminuted long bone fractures. J. Am. Anim. Hosp. Assoc., *17*:525, 1981.
3. Lexer, E.: Joint transplantations and arthroplasty. Surg. Gynecol. Obstet., *40*:782, 1925.
4. Lexer, E.: Die Verwendung der freien Knochenplastic nebst Bersuchen uber Gelenkversteifung und Gelenktransplantation. Arch. Klin. Chir., *86*:939, 1908.
5. Mankin, H. J.: Personal communication, 1973.
6. Mankin, H. J., Fogelson, F. S., Thrasher, A. Z., and Jaffer, R.: Massive resection and allograft transplantation in the treatment of malignant bone tumors. N. Engl. J. Med., *294*:1247, 1976.
7. Mankin, H. J., and Schachar, N. S.: The role of allograft transplantation in the treatment of malignant bone tumors. In Proceedings of the 1977 Annual Meeting of the American Association of Tissue Banks. Edited by K. W. Sell, V. P. Perry, and M. M. Vincent. Rockville, Md, 1978.
8. Ottolenghi, E. E.: Massive osteo and osteo-articular bone grafts: technic and results of 62 cases. Clin. Orthop. *87*:156, 1972.
9. Parrish, F. F.: Allograft replacement of all or part of the end of a long bone following excision of a tumor: report of twenty-one cases. J. Bone Joint Surg. (Am.), *55*:1, 1973.

10. Parrish, F. F.: Treatment of bone tumors by total excision and replacement with massive autologous and homologous grafts. J. Bone Joint Surg. (Am.), 48:968, 1966.
11. Parrish, F. F., et al.: Personal communication, 1977.
12. Ray, R. D.: Bone grafts and implants. Clin. Orthop., 87:2, 1972.
13. Schachar, N. S., Henry, W. B., Wadsworth, P. L., and Mankin, H. J.: A feline model for the study of osteo-articular joint transplantation: qualitative and quantitative assessment of bone healing and articular cartilage viability. Submitted for publication.
14. Schachar, N. S., et al.: A feline model for the study of frozen osteoarticular joint transplantation. II. Development of lymphocytotoxic antibodies in allograft recipients. Submitted for publication.
15. Turek, S. L.: Orthopaedics: Principles and Their Application. 3rd ed. Philadelphia, J. B. Lippincott, 1977.
16. Volkov, M.: Allotransplantation of joints. J. Bone Joint Surg. (Br.), 52:49, 1970.
17. Wadsworth, P. L., and Henry, W. B.: Entire segment cortical bone transplant. J. Am. Anim. Hosp. Assoc., 12:741, 1976.
18. Wilson, J. W.: Uses of bone grafts: the results of experiments with cancellous and cortical grafts. Third Annual Advanced Course on Internal Fixation of Fractures, Non-Unions and Reconstructive Surgery, Columbus, Ohio, March, 1980.

Autogenous Cancellous Bone Grafts

by WAYNE R. RENEGAR

The use of bone grafts can be a valuable adjunct to many orthopedic procedures and may be necessary for the successful outcome of a procedure. The successful management of (1) nonunion and delayed union of fractures, (2) defects following fracture repair, (3) defects caused by bone cysts, tumors, and infection, (4) arthrodesis of joints, and (5) fractures repaired with avascular pieces of bone can all depend on the proper use of fresh cancellous bone grafts. With the exception of the replacement of large bone defects, the fresh cancellous bone graft applies to all of these indications.

Cancellous bone grafts are most commonly used to stimulate or to complement osteogenesis in a variety of orthopedic procedures. Fresh cancellous bone grafts are used primarily to enhance osteogenesis by the transfer of viable osteogenic cells or by stimulating the induction of osteogenesis by the host. The autogenous cancellous bone graft is far superior to all other types of grafts with regard to acceptance of the graft, new bone production by the graft, and host induction of new bone.[2,4,7]

Vascularization is the most important factor in acceptance of the graft.[5] The blood supply to any long bone is derived from 3 afferent sources: (1) the nutrient artery, which provides most of the medullary and 70% of the cortical blood supply, (2) the metaphyseal vessels, which are numerous and freely anastamose with the medullary vessels, and (3) the periosteal blood supply, which provides blood to the remaining 30% of the cortex and also anastamoses with the medullary circulation.[6-8] When a complete fracture occurs, the medullary circulation is interrupted. Therefore, bone distal to a fracture separated from the nutrient artery must derive all its blood supply from the metaphyseal and periosteal vessels.

When a fracture does occur, a fourth important source of blood enters into the healing process. This source is the extraosseus blood supply and arises from the ingrowth of capillaries from the traumatized surrounding soft tissues.[7] Periosteal callus and bone grafts receive most of their blood supply from the invasion of capillaries from the extraosseus tissues.

Graft-particle size plays an important role in the rate of revascularization and the survival of transplanted osteogenic cells.[1] Grafts less than 0.3 mm by 0.7 mm in size not only are devoid of living osteogenic cells, but also may stimulate a foreign-body response by the host that delays healing. The greatest number of osteogenic cells survive in fresh autogenous cancellous grafts approximately 2.8 mm by 1 mm in size. Grafts of this particular size had the best revascularization rate when implanted into the anterior chamber of the eyes of rats.

Cancellous bone is present in the metaphyseal region of most long bones. It is also abundant in the wing and body of the ilium. In man, the wing of the ilium and the proximal tibia are popular donor sites for cancellous bone. These areas are chosen because of the abundance of cancellous bone and the ease with which it is obtained. Cancellous bone from the ilium is more osteogenic because of the amount of marrow it contains. Cancellous bone from the proximal tibia has less marrow and more fat. The proximal tibia and proximal humerus are better sources in animal patients, however, because most small animals do not have a large, thick ilial wing.

Indications for Fresh Cancellous Autogenic Grafts

The use of fresh autogenic cancellous bone grafts should be considered in the following conditions or procedures[3,9]:

1. To stimulate osteogenesis, especially in delayed union or nonunion of fractures.
2. To fill defects in a fracture repair (Fig. 48-10).
3. To fill defects caused by the curettage of bone cysts, bone tumors, and osteomyelitis (Fig. 48-11).
4. To fuse joints surgically (arthrodesis) (Fig. 48-12).
5. To stimulate osteogenesis in fresh complicated fractures, especially in open (compound) fractures.
6. To replace an avascular piece of bone (Fig. 48-13).
7. To assist in the correction of bone deformities.
8. To aid in plastic surgical procedures in which bone is required.
9. To stimulate osteogenesis in fractures of the distal extremities (radius, ulna, tibia) in toy dog breeds in which nonunion of fractures is common.

The advantages of fresh autogenic cancellous bone grafts in these procedures include the following: (1) the grafts are generally easily obtained through a small

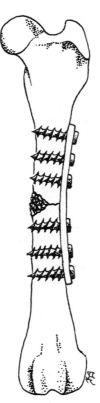

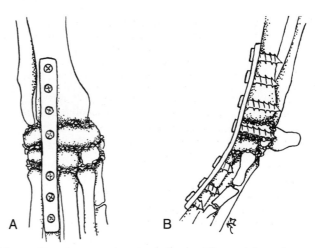

Fig. 48-12. *Fresh cancellous bone chips used to pack in and around a carpus during a carpal fusion. A, Craniocaudal view. B, Lateral view.*

Fig. 48-10. *Fresh cancellous bone chips used to pack a medial defect in the midshaft femur following fracture repair.*

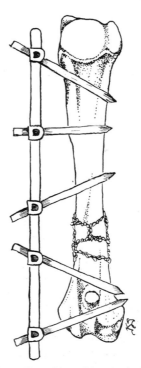

Fig. 48-13. *Fresh cancellous bone chips packed around avascular pieces of bone following fracture repair.*

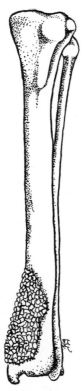

Fig. 48-11. *Fresh cancellous bone chips used to pack a large medial defect in the tibia following curettage of a localized destructive lesion.*

exposure, (2) minimal instrumentation is required, and (3) osteogenesis is enhanced. The disadvantages of fresh autogenic cancellous bone grafts are as follows: (1) an extra procedure must be performed, (2) it is often necessary to expose another bone, (3) it is possible to set up a dual infection if contaminated instruments are used, and (4) it is possible to create a second, iatrogenic fracture. It must be emphasized, however, that when a grafting procedure is anticipated and care is taken in obtaining the graft, the advantages far outweigh the disadvantages.

Collection Sites

Fresh autogenous cancellous bone can be obtained from a number of sites in the dog and cat. These sites include: (1) the proximal lateral or medial tibia, (2) the greater tubercle of the humerus, (3) the greater trochanter of the femur, (4) the iliac crest and wing of the ilium, and (5) the ribs, although rib grafts in small animal patients function more as corticocancellous grafts than as purely cancellous grafts.

PROXIMAL MEDIAL TIBIA

A 1- to 2-cm skin incision is made on the medial aspect of the tibia extending from the tibial tubercle distally. The subcutaneous tissues and the insertions of the sartorius and gracilis muscles are separated by sharp dissection to reveal the periosteal surface of the bone. The medial cortex of the tibia is perforated with a quarter-inch Steinmann pin or a drill bit. A bone curette is now inserted, and fresh cancellous bone is harvested. Because of the shape of the proximal tibia, care must be taken to avoid penetrating the cranial and lateral cortices with the bone curette. It is often helpful to direct the bone curette caudolaterally (Fig. 48-14). If more than one hole is needed to harvest the graft, the holes should be in a vertical rather than a horizontal plane. Numerous holes in a horizontal plane or overzealous use of the bone curette in toy breeds or in active dogs often results in iatrogenic fractures of the proximal tibia following autogenic graft harvests.

PROXIMAL LATERAL TIBIA

Harvesting fresh cancellous bone from the proximal lateral tibia is similar to the procedure for the proximal medial tibia, except the tibialis cranialis muscle is reflected distally to expose the proximal tibia. Care should be taken to avoid the tendon of the long digital extensor muscle.

GREATER TUBERCLE OF THE HUMERUS

A 1- to 2-cm skin incision is made over the craniolateral aspect of the greater tubercle of the humerus. The subcutaneous tissues are separated by sharp dissection to reveal the periosteal surface of the bone. A quarter-inch Steinmann pin or a drill bit is used to perforate the craniolateral cortex of the greater tubercle. The bone curette is directed caudomedially to obtain the greatest amount of cancellous bone (Fig. 48-15). If numerous holes are used to harvest the cancellous bone the holes should again be made in a vertical plane. In my experience, the greater tubercle of the humerus and proximal humerus provide easy access to large amounts of fresh cancellous bone.

GREATER TROCHANTER OF THE FEMUR

A 1- to 2-cm skin incision is made directly over the lateral aspect of the greater trochanter. The subcutaneous tissues and superficial gluteal muscle are sharply incised to reveal the periosteal surface of the bone. The

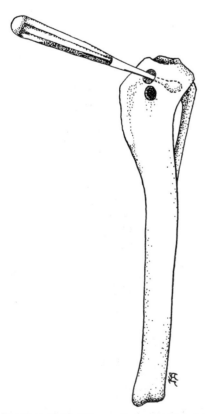

Fig. 48-14. *Proper method of harvesting cancellous bone from the proximal medial tibia. Additional holes for harvesting should be in a perpendicular plane, as opposed to a horizontal plane.*

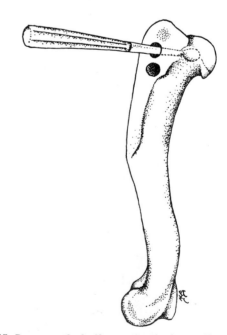

Fig. 48-15. *Proper method of harvesting fresh cancellous bone from the greater tubercle and proximal humerus. Again, additional holes for harvesting should be in a perpendicular plane, as opposed to a horizontal plane.*

procedure already described is used to harvest fresh cancellous bone from the proximal femur. Again, care should be taken to place several holes in a vertical plane because perforations of the cranial and caudal cortices of the greater trochanter can result in iatrogenic fractures. Of all sources of cancellous bone, the greater trochanter provides perhaps the least amount, and I have rarely used it.

ILIAC CREST AND WING AND BODY
OF THE ILIUM

The iliac crest is an excellent source of both cancellous and corticocancellous autogenous grafts. A 5- to 6-cm skin incision is made directly over the dorsal aspect of the iliac crest. The deep fascia is sharply incised for the entire length of the incision. The middle gluteal muscle is sharply incised from its attachment to the dorsal edge of the iliac crest and is subperiosteally elevated from the wing of the ilium. The lateral and dorsolateral cortex of the exposed iliac crest can now be removed with a rongeurs, an osteotome, or an oscillating saw (Fig. 48-16). The cancellous bone is then harvested with a bone curette. Large amounts of cancellous bone can be obtained from the ilium by directing the curette vertically and caudally and by actually removing bone from the entire wing and body of the ilium (Fig. 48-17).

The iliac crest and wing of the ilium also serve as excellent sources of fresh autogenic corticocancellous bone. The procedure is similar, except in addition to elevating the middle gluteal muscle laterally, the iliocostalis and longissimus lumborum muscles are elevated medially. The entire iliac crest and wing of the ilium are now free of muscle attachments cranial to the sacrum. Using a sharp osteotome or an oscillating saw, the iliac crest and the cranial wing of the ilium can now be removed. Care must always be taken to avoid the sacrum.

The iliac crest and the cranial wing of the ilium can be used in 2 different fashions. First, if a large number of corticocancellous bone chips are required, the entire

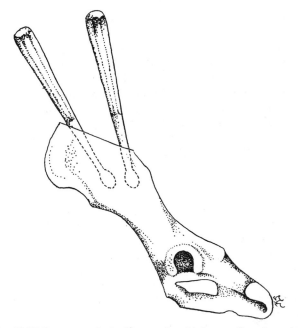

Fig. 48-17. *Proper method of harvesting fresh cancellous bone from the iliac crest and the wing and body of the ilium.*

segment can be rongeured into small, 2- to 3-mm by 1-mm pieces. These particles are used in a manner similar to fresh cancellous grafts in that they can be packed around a fracture or can be used to pack defects in a bone. The iliac crest and the cranial wing of the ilium can also be used as a large corticocancellous graft in large defects. The graft should be rongeured to fit a defect snugly and then should be rigidly fixed in place with lag screws or cerclage wires (Fig. 48-18).

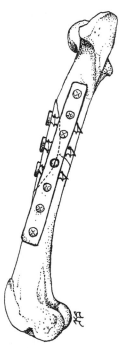

Fig. 48-18. *The iliac crest used as a large corticocancellous graft to fill a large cranial defect in the femur. The graft is rigidly fixed in place with three lag screws.*

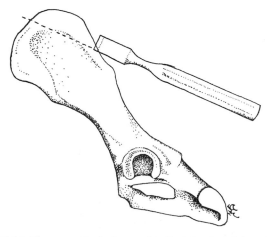

Fig. 48-16. *Proper method of removing the lateral and dorsolateral cortex of the iliac crest to obtain fresh cancellous bone.*

Large defects can be repaired by the use of fresh corticocancellous grafts taken from the wing of the ilium.

Storage of Fresh Cancellous Autogenic Grafts

Following the harvest of a fresh cancellous bone graft, the graft should be placed in a dry, sterile, stainless steel container until it is ready for use. It may be helpful to place a moistened gauze sponge over the top of the container, but not in direct contact with the graft, to keep the graft from becoming too dry. Timing the graft harvest just prior to closure is perhaps the easiest way of ensuring that the graft will not become too dry. Moreover, the fracture site should be thoroughly lavaged prior to graft placement, so that the fracture site can be closed immediately after graft placement.

References and Suggested Readings

1. Anderson, K. J.: The behavior of autogenous and homogenous bone transplants in the anterior chamber of the rats' eye. J. Bone Joint Surg. [Am.], *43*:980, 1961.
2. Burinell, R. G.: Recent Advances in Orthopedics. Edited by A. G. Apley. London, J. & A. Churchill, 1969.
3. Gambardella, P. C.: Bone grafts in small animal orthopedics: a review. Compend. Contin. Ed. Practicing Vet., *1*:596, 1979.
4. Ham, A. W., and Harris, R.: The Biochemistry and Physiology of Bone. 2nd Ed. Edited by G. Bourne. New York, Academic Press, 1971.
5. Ray, R. D.: Vascularization of bone grafts and implants. Clin. Orthop., *87*:43, 1972.
6. Rhinelander, F. W.: The normal circulation of bone and its response to surgical intervention. J. Biomed Mater. Res., *8*:87, 1974.
7. Rhinelander, F. W.: Tibial blood supply in relation to fracture healing. Clin. Orthop., *105*:34, 1974.
8. Rhinelander, F. W.: The normal microcirculation of diaphyseal cortex and its response to fracture. J. Bone Joint Surg. [Am.], *50*:784, 1974.
9. Whittick, W. G.: Bone transplantation. *In* Current Techniques in Small Animal Surgery. Edited by M. J. Bojrab, Philadelphia, Lea & Febiger, 1975.

Allogeneic and Autogenous Corticocancellous Bone Grafts

by JAMES W. WILSON

Corticocancellous grafting employs transplantation of a bone fragment containing a large percentage of both cortical and cancellous bone. Although zenografts can be used, only the fresh autograft and the frozen allograft are of clinical importance in veterinary surgery today. The two bones used are the ilium and the rib.

The fresh autogenous transplant combines the structural strength of cortical bone with the osteoconductive and osteogenic properties of cancellous bone. It is ideally suited for combined support and augmentation of deficits in long-bone fracture repair and in joint fusions.

The stored allogeneic transplant can be used in the same sites as the autogenic transplant. Although allografts lack osteogenic properties, the trabeculae of the cancellous bone provide an excellent trellis for host bone replacement. Depending on the method of storage, this transplanted bone can be minimally antigenic and may be included in the repair process.

Harvesting Iliac Bone

The procedure described in the preceding section of this chapter applies. In this case, the harvested ilium is split and is shaped to approximate the recipient site and is then used intact.

Harvesting Ribs

The skin incision is placed over the sixth or seventh rib, from the vertebral articulation to just below the costochondral junction. The subcutaneous tissue and the latissimus dorsi muscle are incised to expose the lateral surface of the selected rib. The periosteum is incised in the center of the rib and is stripped circumferentially with a scalpel blade or a periosteal elevator. The exposed rib is cut dorsally and ventrally with bone-cutting forceps and is removed from its periosteal envelope. Additional ribs may be harvested in a similar fashion. If the harvesting site is to be repaired, the incised periosteal envelope should be closed with absorbable suture followed by standard closure of the incised overlying tissues.

If the harvested rib is to be used as frozen allogeneic bone, it should be split in half longitudinally before storage. This maneuver facilitates preparation of the graft when used. It is also advisable to split longitudinally ribs used as fresh autogenous grafts, to expose the osteoprogenitor cells to an adequate nutrition and to increase the amount of participation they have in new bone formation. Autografts should be sized and used as soon as possible. If they need to be set aside for a short time, they are best placed in blood-soaked sponges or on a moist, bloody tissue bed.

Arthrodesis

by THOMAS M. TURNER

and ALAN J. LIPOWITZ

Arthrodesis is achieved by surgically stabilizing a joint to obtain a bony ankylosis or fusion. Because arthrodesis is a salvage procedure, it should be performed only when the possibility for return of a healthy, functional joint has been eliminated.

Several criteria are necessary for any arthrodesis to be successful.[1] The remainder of the limb must be functional and capable of compensating for the stresses that will be transmitted to it as a result of the arthrodesis. Second, the joint must be fused in the most functional position possible. This position is determined preoperatively by evaluating the normal as well as the abnormal limb and by using a goniometer to note the appropriate fusion angle of extension or flexion as well as varus or valgus. A sterile goniometer can then be provided at the time of operation to determine the precise angles required to maintain proper leg angulation and length. Third, a method of rigid fixation is necessary, using either external or internal devices. Although several techniques are available for performing an arthrodesis, our preferences in most cases are internal plate fixation, use of compression screws and tension-band wires, or use of an external fixation device. The principle of compression is applied whenever possible.[8] Fourth, all cartilage, adjacent synovium, and soft tissue must be removed, to expose healthy subchondral bone while preserving the contour of the articular surface where possible. This objective may be achieved by using a power-driven bur, an osteotome, curettes, or rongeurs. Any areas of cartilage or soft tissue not excised can lead to delayed fusion. The joint should be liberally packed with autogenous cancellous bone to fill all defects at the fusion site. The limb is then placed in the proper degree of angulation and axial alignment, and the fixation device is applied.

Strict asepsis and proper surgical technique are mandatory when performing an arthrodesis, particularly one involving joints with minimal soft tissue coverage, such as the carpus and hock.

Postoperatively, the patient's limb is supported in a splint for 4 to 8 weeks, and only minimal activity is allowed. The fusion site is radiographed at intervals of 4 to 6 weeks until the arthrodesis is complete.

Indications

An arthrodesis is especially justified for particular conditions. The main neurologic indication is an irreparable peripheral nerve injury resulting in loss of function of an extremity joint, such as the carpus or hock, that is not amenable to tendon transfer. The proximal aspect of the limb must be completely functional, however. Function can be determined by a neurologic examination of the limb and evaluation of the animal's use of the limb with the affected joint in a temporary splint.

Orthopedic indications for an arthrodesis include chronic instability or subluxation not amenable to reconstructive procedures and painful arthritis not responsive to medical therapy, such as septic arthritis, immune-mediated arthritis, or degenerative joint disease.[3,4,9,13] A painful intra-articular nonunion, failure of a previous joint reconstruction, and severe growth deformities may also require arthrodesis. A primary arthrodesis may be necessary in cases of severe joint derangement or luxation, irreparable articular fractures, or a severe open avulsion injury of a joint with extensive loss of soft tissue and bone.

Complications

An arthrodesis failure can generally be attributed to lack of adherence to proper surgical and grafting techniques, development of a postsurgical infection, or recurrence of a previous disease process. Moreover, a failure can result from lack of obtaining functional angulation and alignment of the joint. The inability of the implant to maintain apposition and position can also cause failure, as well as the use of an implant of inadequate size or strength. Neglect of the biomechanics in arthrodesis predisposes the procedure to failure. Frequent postoperative physical and radiographic examinations ensure the detection of these failures.

Carpus

Arthrodesis of the carpus may be performed as either a partial or a total joint fusion (panarthrodesis), depending on the area of instability.[9,13] Preoperative stress radiographs of the involved joint should reveal the area of instability. The intraoperative use of an Esmarch bandage or a tourniquet reduces hemorrhage and thus facilitates the surgical procedure. Moreover, the use of plastic adherent drapes allows the entire limb to be seen during the operation and aids in maintenance of aseptic technique. A cranial approach is preferable; however, the skin incision should be placed so that closure is not directly over the implant.

PARTIAL CARPAL ARTHRODESIS

Partial carpal arthrodesis involves only the carpometacarpal, middle carpal, and intercarpal joints. This procedure requires that the antebrachiocarpal joint be functional, stable, and pain free. A cranial approach is used to expose these joints.[10] The angular relation of the metacarpal bones to the radial carpal and ulnar carpal bones is neutral. A Kirschner wire or a small Steinmann pin is inserted into the distal aspect of the medullary canal of each of the second, third, and fourth metacarpal bones, emerges at the base of the metacarpal bones, and is then imbedded into the radial carpal and ulnar carpal bones (Fig. 48-19). Cancellous bone graft is then liberally packed into all defects. In some patients with ligamentous injury, additional stability may be desirable. If so, an appropriate bone screw is inserted into the medial aspect of the radial carpal bone, and another is placed in the second metacarpal base. A figure-8 heavy-gauge wire is then passed around the screws and is tightened to achieve compression and stability. Postoperatively, the limb is protected for 6 weeks in a caudal splint. When the arthrodesis has healed, the pins are removed, and the animal should have approximately a 90° range of motion of the radial carpal joint.

An alternate method of fixation is the use of a cranial finger "T" or "L" plate. The plate is applied to either the third or fourth proximal metacarpal bone, with the "T"

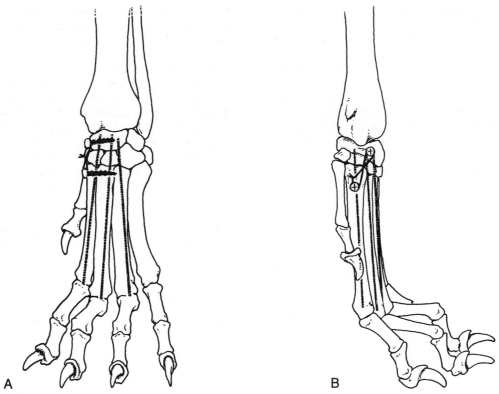

Fig. 48-19. *Partial carpal arthrodesis using intramedullary pins in the second, third, and fourth metacarpal bones. Additional stability is gained by figure-8 wire around screws placed in the radial carpal bone and the second metacarpal bone. A cancellous bone graft is packed in the fusion site. A, Craniocaudal view. B, Lateral view.*

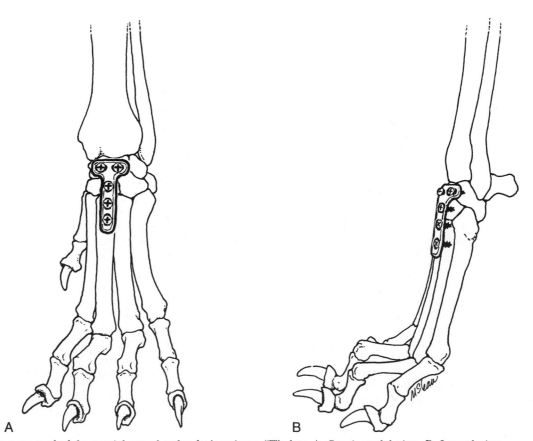

Fig. 48-20. *Alternate method for partial carpal arthrodesis using a "T" plate. A, Craniocaudal view. B, Lateral view.*

or "L" portion attached to the radial carpal bone (Fig. 48-20).

A fusion of the antebrachial joint only is not advocated because it places excessive stress on the remaining joints and may lead to further degenerative joint disease and subluxation.[3]

If the accessory carpal-ulnar carpal joint is unstable or subluxated, an arthrodesis may be performed. The joint is approached laterally[10] and is prepared for arthrodesis. A lag screw is inserted through the accessory carpal bone and into the ulnar carpal bone. In addition, a tension-band wire of heavy gauge is passed around the screw and through the proximal aspect of the fourth and fifth metacarpal bones.

CARPAL PANTHRODESIS

Panarthrodesis is necessary when the entire carpus is involved in the disease process or is unstable. The fixation device of choice is a bone plate to achieve compression and stability. An external fixation device is reserved for cases of extensive bone and soft tissue damage. All carpal joints are prepared for arthrodesis through a cranial approach. Three locations are possible for plate application: cranial, medial, and caudomedial. Each of these has advantages and disadvantages. The joint is normally in about 10° of hyperextension; however, the most desirable angle

must be determined prior to the surgical procedure. In addition, when applying a bone plate, strict attention must be given to maintain proper valgus angulation and axial alignment.

In most cases, medial application of a plate is the method of choice and has the advantage of using one narrow plate while allowing excellent purchase for the distal screws, which are inserted transversely into the proximal metacarpal bones and the radial carpal bone[6] (Fig. 48-21). When applying a bone plate to the carpus, it is preferable for at least three screws to obtain purchase distally in the metacarpal bones and three screws proximally in the radius. A craniomedial approach to the carpus is performed. Excision of the first phalanx may be necessary for placement of the bone plate. The degree of hyperextension is obtained by adjusting the position and the contour of the proximal aspect of the bone plate along the medial aspect of the distal radius.

A plate applied to the cranial surface of the joint is easily contoured; however, it is applied to the compression rather than the tension side of the joint. A straight bone plate may be applied along the cranial surface of the radius to the third or fourth metacarpal and radial carpal bones[4,9,13] (Fig. 48-22). The disadvantage of this method is the necessity of relying on purchase in only one metacarpal bone. Therefore, in larger breed dogs, two plates applied cranially are advantageous. One

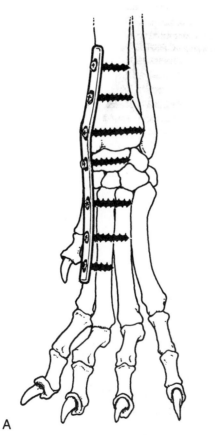
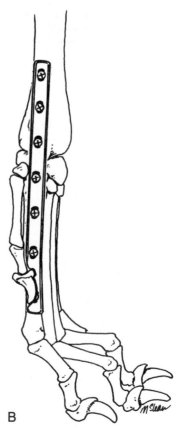

Fig. 48-21. *Pancarpal arthrodesis using a medially applied plate. The plate is contoured to the desired fusion angle, and cancellous bone is packed within the fusion site.* A, *Craniocaudal view.* B, *Lateral view.*

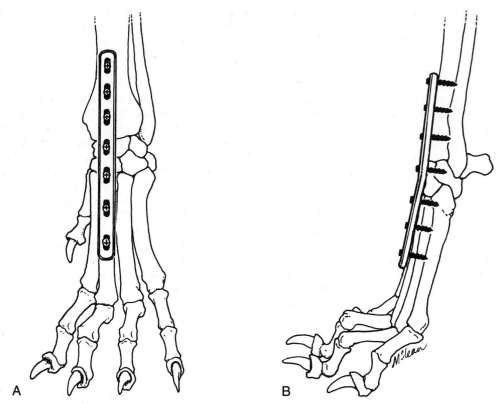

Fig. 48-22. *Pancarpal arthrodesis using a cranially applied compression plate secured to the radius, radial carpal bone, and third metacarpal bone. The plate is contoured for desired angulation. A cancellous bone graft is applied to the fusion site. A, Craniocaudal view. B, Lateral view.*

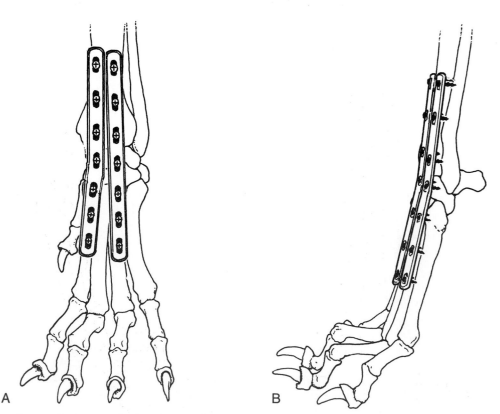

Fig. 48-23. *Pancarpal arthrodesis using double plates applied cranially to the radius, radial carpal bone, and the second and fourth metacarpal bone. The plates are contoured for desired angulation, and a cancellous bone graft is applied to the fusion site. A, Craniocaudal view. B, Lateral view.*

plate is applied along the cranial aspect of the radius to the cranial surface of the second metacarpal bone, and the other is placed along the cranial surface of the radius to the cranial aspect of the fourth metacarpal bone (Fig. 48-23). Special bone plates such as the "T" plate may be applied cranially to allow purchase in more than one metacarpal bone (Fig. 48-24).

Biomechanically, a caudomedially positioned plate is the most desirable; however, it may be technically difficult to contour and apply the plate to obtain the necessary angulation and alignment (Fig. 48-25).

Postoperatively, all carpal arthrodeses are protected by a padded bandage with a caudal splint for 6 weeks. Because carpal arthrodesis can cause moderate postoperative swelling of the limb, frequent examinations of the limb and bandage are necessary in the early postoperative period.

The successful use of bone plates in open fractures is well known. The use of an external fixation device may be even more advantageous, however, particularly in the carpus and hock that have sustained severe trauma and bone loss. It has been found that an external fixation device may be beneficial for performing arthrodesis of the carpus and the hock. The joint is properly prepared for arthrodesis, and a graft is applied. Kirschner wires are then used to obtain purchase in the bone above, below, and in the joint. These wires are then connected medially and laterally in cement bars (methyl methacrylate). The precise angle of arthrodesis is rigidly held while the cement cures (Fig. 48-26). This device allows treatment of the wound while providing rigid external fixation with minimal metal implantation. (See also the section of this chapter by Earley, "Carpus and Tarsus.")

Elbow

Arthrodesis of the elbow creates a long lever from the shoulder to the carpus. The result is an altered, awkward gait; however, the limb is functional. An elbow fusion can also predispose the limb to fracture. Regardless of these disadvantages, some conditions, as indicated previously, may necessitate elbow arthrodesis. Conditions that in particular may require arthrodesis are severe growth abnormalities of the radius and ulna, painful intra-articular nonunions, and severe degenerative joint disease.[9]

A transolecranon approach is used to expose the caudal surfaces of the humerus and ulna and to prepare the joints for arthrodesis.[9,10] The radial and ulnar nerves are isolated and are retracted. Additional exposure of the joint may be gained by using the craniolateral approach to the elbow[12] or by incising the ulnarcollateral ligament. The joint is prepared for arthrodesis as previously described. The plate is contoured to the predetermined angle and is secured to the caudal aspect of the humerus and ulna, to achieve compression of the humeroulnar joint. The plate should have a minimum of 8 holes, 4 proximally and 4 distally (Fig. 48-27). When feasible, a lag screw should be inserted through the lateral humeral condyle into the radial head. In cases of severe deformity, the radial

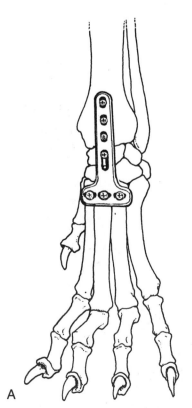 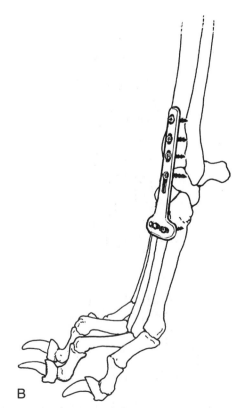

A   B

Fig. 48-24. *Pancarpal arthrodesis using a cranially applied "T" plate. The plate is secured to the radius, radial carpal bone, and the second, third, and fourth metacarpal bones.* A, *Craniocaudal view.* B, *Lateral view.*

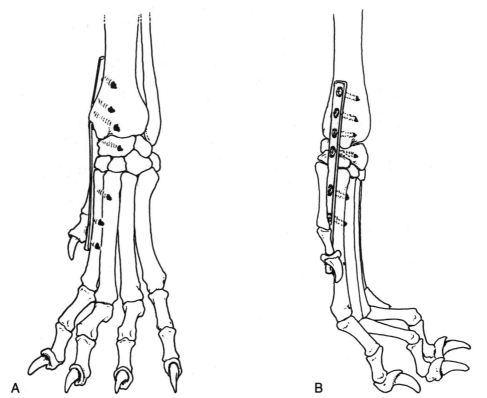

Fig. 48-25. *Pancarpal arthrodesis using a plate applied to the caudomedial aspect of the carpus. A, Craniocaudal view. B, Lateral view.*

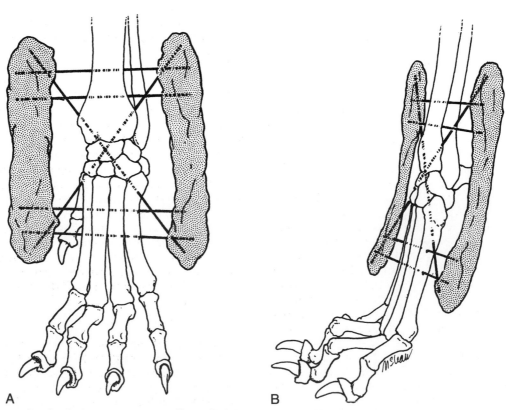

Fig. 48-26. *Pancarpal arthrodesis using an externally applied fixation device. Methyl methacrylate bars connect the pins medially and laterally. A cancellous bone graft is applied to the fusion site. A, Craniocaudal view. B, Lateral view.*

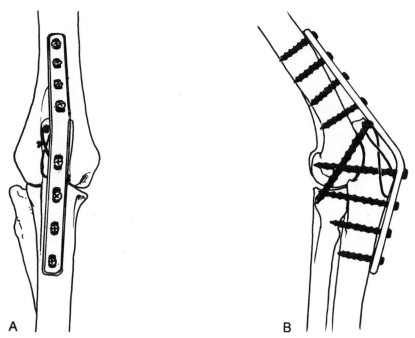

Fig. 48-27. *Elbow joint arthrodesis using a plate applied to the caudal aspect of the humerus and ulna. A cancellous bone graft is applied to the fusion site. The olecranon is reattached lateral to the plate with a screw and a figure-8 wire. A, Craniocaudal view. B, Lateral view.*

head may be excised, and the radius may be fixed to the ulna. The olecranon is reattached lateral to the plate with a lag screw and a figure-8 tension-band wire. Following the surgical procedure, the limb is maintained in a padded bandage for 2 weeks, and the animal is then allowed limited activity for 4 weeks until it has adapted to the limb.

Stifle

Stifle arthrodesis has been advocated for those patients in which the knee is severely internally deranged.[9] Indications for fusion may include concomitant loss of the cruciate and collateral ligaments and severely comminuted fractures of the distal femur or proximal tibia that are irreparable. Arthrodesis is also advocated in cases of severely painful joint disease. Fusion of the stifle affected by osteoarthritis or immune-mediated articular disease in many cases restores nearly normal function to the limb that otherwise cannot be used because of pain or instability.

Fusion of the stifle requires removal of the cruciate ligaments, menisci, and the opposing articular surfaces of the femoral condyles and the tibial plateau. Stabilization can be achieved by the use of two Steinmann pins or two compression screws placed in cruciate fashion across the fusion site.[9] Application of a compression plate to the cranial surfaces of the distal femur and proximal tibia, to cross the fusion site, is the method of choice, however. This technique provides greater stability and compression at the fusion site than cross-pins or compression screws.

Preoperative considerations include the usual evaluation procedures. Prior to the surgical procedure, the

patient's owners must be made aware of the expected change in limb function resulting from the fusion. A successful result, that is, fusion and weight-bearing, still leaves the patient with an abnormal gait. Dogs with a stifle arthrodesis abduct the limb slightly when it is brought forward during walking and running.

Because articular cartilage and subchondral bone are removed in creating the fusion site, some leg length is lost. Leg length discrepancies accentuate gait abnormalities following fusion. To minimize these gait abnormalities and to overcome the loss of leg length, the fusion site should be placed in a few more degrees of extension than the opposite, normal stifle. Prior to the surgical procedure, the joint angle of the normal stifle should be measured with a goniometer when the patient is standing in a normal weight-bearing position. A sterile goniometer is then used during the operation to align the fusion site properly prior to fixation. The bone plate to be used for the fusion should be selected before the surgical procedure. The plate's length is dictated by the patient's size; however, the plate should cover at least half the length of the femur and tibia. The bone plate may be contoured prior to the operation according to measurements of the normal stifle.

SURGICAL TECHNIQUE

The patient is placed in lateral recumbency with the affected leg uppermost, and the entire limb from above the hip to below the tarsus is surgically prepared. A curved, lateral parapatellar skin incision is made from the midshaft of the femur to the distal third of the tibia. The subcutaneous tissues are incised in the same line. Another curved incision is made through the fascia lata between the vastus lateralis and the biceps femoris muscles. The incision continues distally through the lateral fascia of the stifle and parallel to the patellar ligament. As the incision crosses the joint, it is slightly lateral and parallel to the tibial crest. The crural fascia overlying the cranial tibial muscle is then incised to approximately the midshaft region of the tibia.

A parapatellar incision is now made through the joint capsule to expose the lateral femoral condyle. The incision is lengthened proximally by separation between the vastus lateralis and biceps femoris muscles. Subperiosteal dissection is necessary to elevate the musculature from the cranial surface of the femur. Extending the joint and luxating the patella and vastus lateralis muscle medially aid in dissection. Distally, subperiosteal dissection is needed to elevate the cranial tibial and long digital extensor muscles from the surface of the proximal tibia.

The joint is then flexed to better expose the cruciate ligaments and menisci, which are removed, as is the infrapatellar fat pad. An oscillating saw, an osteotome or a Gigli wire is used to remove the articular cartilage carefully from the distal femur and proximal tibia (Fig. 48-28). The properly contoured plate is used as a template to determine the fusion angle and the line of transection through the femoral condyles and articular surface of the proximal tibia. The resulting apposing surfaces of the distal femur and proximal tibia must be parallel and must have maximum contact.

To achieve better plate-to-bone contact, the trochlear groove of the distal femur and the most cranial surface of the tibial tubercle are removed. The patella is also removed, or it may be preserved for reattachment later. The compression plate is then fitted to the cranial surfaces of the femur and the tibia. Compression across the fusion site increases stability and enhances healing. At least three screws should be placed above and below the fusion site (Fig. 48-29). Gaps in and about the fusion site should be packed with cancellous bone. Closure is in layers in a routine manner.

Postoperative radiographs are taken to ensure proper plate placement and fusion site alignment. A padded bandage is then applied to the entire limb, to help reduce postoperative swelling and to lend some temporary support to the fusion site. Assuming the bandage does not become soiled or wet and thereby necessitates earlier removal, it is removed on the fourth or fifth postoperative day. Continued external support for several weeks in a bandage or cast may be warranted in larger animals. Exercise is restricted to walking on a leash; running and jumping should be discouraged for 4 to 6 weeks following the surgical procedure. The bone plate and screws are removed when radiographic evidence of bony union is seen. The surgical approach for plate removal is similar to that for plate application. Following plate removal, the patient's limb should be supported in a bandage for 2 to 4 weeks.

COMPLICATIONS

Complications of stifle arthrodesis include nonunion, loosening of the orthopedic appliance, fractures of the bone plate or screws, and fractures of the femur or tibia at the proximal or distal ends of the plate.

Maximum contact between the cancellous bone of the femur and proximal tibia, rigid stability of the fusion site, and packing of the fusion site with cancellous

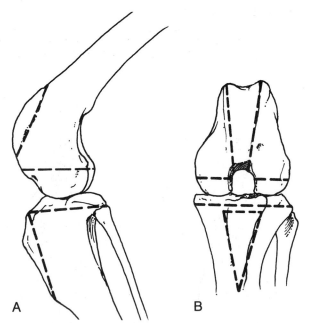

Fig. 48-28. *Lateral (A) and craniocaudal (B) views of the stifle; dashed lines indicate the approximate line for removal of the articular surfaces of the distal femur, proximal tibia, femoral trochlea, and tibial tuberosity in preparing joint for arthrodesis.*

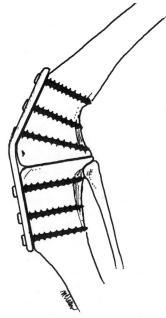

Fig. 48-29. *Lateral view of the stifle illustrating plate application to cranial surfaces of the femur and tibia for arthrodesis. A cancellous bone graft is packed in the fusion site to fill any gaps between bony surfaces.*

bone produce a successful bony union. Failure of arthrodesis is usually the result of inadequate support and stabilization, which allows motion at the fusion site.

Loosening of the screws and plate soon after their application is usually due to technical oversight and can be avoided by the proper use of a drill and tap and by selecting screws of appropriate length. A minimum of three screws above and below the fusion site is recommended. In some cases, cancellous rather than cortical screws hold better in the distal femur and proximal tibia. Appliance failure, breaking of the screws or plates, is also due to technical errors. Plates should not be bent over screw holes, nor should they be bent at severe angles. Correct bending procedures and the use of a plate of appropriate length should help to avoid implant failure.

Bone fractures at the proximal or distal ends of well-applied plates may be due to a combination of factors. Although rigidly applied, the plate may be just long enough that the plate's end acts as a fulcrum for the oscillating forces applied to the bone during weight-bearing. Because the plate is more rigid than the bone, excessive bone oscillation occurs at the plate's ends, and fractures may result. Bone plates applied across the stifle should cover at least half the length of the femur and tibia. Excessive stress protection or osteoporosis beneath a rigidly applied plate can also result in loosening of the device, fractures adjacent to the plate, or both.

Hock

Ligamentous injuries of the hock resulting in joint instability are uncommon.[7] Similarly, degenerative joint disease and severe articular fractures of this joint are not often seen. In many cases of tibiotarsal instability, ligament reconstruction with wire or nylon suture may suffice,[4,7] but the rare patient with severe joint derangement may indeed require arthrodesis.[4,9,11]

Like the carpus, the tarsal joints are composite articulations.[5] The tibiotarsal articulation occurs between the talus or tibiotarsal bone and the distal end of the tibia. This joint has the greatest degree of motion of all the tarsal articulations. The proximal intertarsal articulations occur between the talus and the calcaneus or fibular tarsal bone, between the talus and central tarsal bone, and between the calcaneus and the fourth tarsal bone. The distal intertarsal articulations are between the central tarsal bone and the second and third tarsal bones. Between the numbered tarsal bones and the metatarsal bones are the tarsal-metatarsal joints. Between the individual bones of the tarsus are the rigid, vertical intratarsal articulations.

Methods of tibiotarsal arthrodesis include crossed Steinmann pins or compression screws, or the use of a large compression screw across the joint with a tension-band wire placed through the caudal cortex of the distal tibia and the calcaneus.[9,11] This second method is the one of choice.

TIBIOTARSAL ARTHRODESIS

The patient is placed in lateral recumbency with the affected limb uppermost and surgically prepared from the midthigh to and including the toes. The patient's foot and toes should be thoroughly scrubbed and then exposed during the surgical procedure.

The tibiotarsal joint is approached through a curved incision, which is begun several centimeters above the medial malleolus, crosses the cranial surface of the joint, and ends several centimeters below the fifth metatarsal head. The subcutaneous tissues are incised in a similar line, and the long digital extensor tendon, on the cranial aspect of the joint, is identified. An arthrotomy is made medial to the tendon, and the joint capsule is sufficiently reflected to expose the articular surfaces. The articular cartilage of both the distal tibia and that of the tibial tarsal bone is removed, exposing bleeding subchondral bone.

The joint is placed in the previously determined fusion angle (approximately 125 to 135° for dogs, 115 to 125° for cats[11]), and a small incision is made on the caudal aspect of the tibiotarsal bone. A guide pin inserted through the incision traverses the tibiotarsal bone and penetrates the medullary cavity of the tibia (Fig. 48-30A). With the guide pin in place, the joint angle should be measured with a sterile goniometer, and the foot should be examined for proper alignment with the leg. A screw hole is then drilled parallel to the guide pin; the size of the drill bit should correspond to the desired screw size. The hole depth is measured and is then tapped for screw threads, and a cancellous or a large cortical bone screw is inserted. All screw threads must be on the tibial side of the fusion site, well seated in the tibia, to achieve maximum compression (Fig. 48-30B). In larger animals, two or more screws may be inserted at different angles.

A tension-band orthopedic wire is then placed through both the fibular tarsal bone and the caudal cortex of the distal tibia (Fig. 48-31). This wire helps to

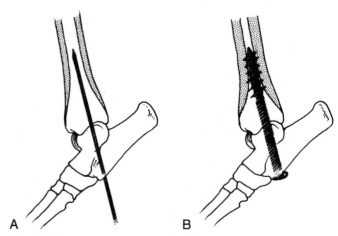

Fig. 48-30. A, *Guide pin placement, traversing the tibiotarsal bone and penetrating the medullary cavity of the tibia, prior to placement of a compression screw for tibiotarsal arthrodesis.* B, *Placement of a cancellous bone screw for tibiotarsal arthrodesis.*

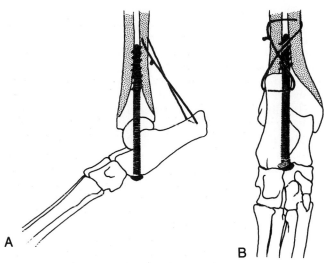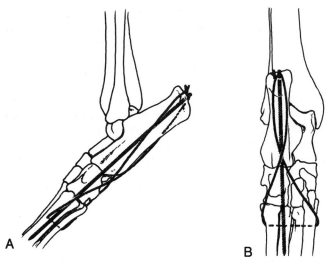

Fig. 48-31. *Lateral (A) and caudocranial (B) views showing placement of a tension-band wire through the fibular tarsal bone and the caudal cortex of the distal tibia.*

Fig. 48-32. *Lateral (A) and caudocranial (B) views showing placement of a Steinmann pin and tension-band wire for intertarsal arthrodesis.*

neutralize the bending forces placed on the screw during weight-bearing. Cancellous bone, taken from a previously prepared site, is then packed into any gaps or defects between the apposing surfaces of the fusion site, and the compression screw is tightened.

The incision is closed in a routine manner, postoperative radiographs are taken, and the limb then placed in a padded bandage. When the soft tissue swelling has subsided, usually within 48 to 72 hours postoperatively, a splint is applied to the patient's leg. The cast extends from the toes to the midthigh. Radiographic evaluation is done periodically, and the splint is removed when evidence of fusion is seen. Following the surgical procedure, the animal is allowed only minimal activity for 4 to 6 weeks. The compression screw should be removed when radiographic evidence of fusion is present. The limb should be protected in a reinforced bandage for 2 to 4 weeks following removal of the compression screw.

INTERTARSAL ARTHRODESIS

Arthrodesis of the intertarsal joints is indicated when injury has caused extensive ligamentous damage resulting in gross joint instability.[2,4,9] These articulations are approached from the cranial surface of the joint, as previously described.[10] All articular cartilage is removed from the intertarsal bones and proximal joint surfaces of the metatarsal bones. Stabilization is achieved by either a large Steinmann pin or a compression screw placed through the fibular tarsal bone, through the central tarsal bone, and into the third metatarsal bone. A tension-band wire is placed through the base of the metatarsal bones and around the screw head or proximal end of the pin at the tuber calcanei[2,4,9] (Fig. 48-32).

If a Steinmann pin is used, power equipment may be necessary for pin placement because of the difficulty in hand drilling a pin through the compact bone of the

calcaneus. The pin's diameter should be gauged by the size of the medullary canal of the third metatarsal bone and by the width of the central tarsal bone. Too large a pin may fracture these bones.

A cortical bone screw placed in lag screw fashion across the intertarsal joints gives excellent stability to the fusion site. The size of the screw is dictated by the size of the patient. A gliding hole must be drilled through the calcaneus and central tarsal bone so that the screw threads only engage bone in the third metatarsal bone. If the threads engage bone elsewhere, distraction rather than compression of the fusion site will occur.

The orthopedic wire for the tension band is placed in the usual manner and is passed beneath the Achilles (calcanean) tendon around the screw head or pin. Cancellous bone taken from a previously prepared site should be packed in any gaps or defects at the fusion site.

Postoperatively, the limb is placed in a padded bandage until soft tissue swelling subsides, and a cast is then applied. Periodic radiographic examination determines the time of fusion, usually 4 to 6 weeks. The cast is then removed. The pin or screw should be removed once bony union is achieved.

In cases of severe open joint injury with loss of bone and soft tissue and the potential for wound infection, an external fixation device may be more beneficial than implants in achieving arthrodesis (See also the section of this chapter by Earley, "Carpus and Tarsus.")

COMPLICATIONS

Complications of the foregoing method of tibiotarsal arthrodesis include delayed or nonunion, loosening of the compression screw, fracture of the screw, and malalignment.[11] Nonunion of the fusion site, without screw fracture, may be due to technical errors such as removal of an insufficient amount of articular cartilage, poor contact of the fusion site surfaces, and failure to achieve sufficient stability at the fusion site. Loosening of the compression screw may be due to poor placement originally or to excessive motion at the fusion site following the surgical procedure. All screw threads must be on the tibial side of the fusion to achieve maximum compression. Drilling and tapping of the screw holes must be done carefully to ensure maximum purchase of the screw threads in the distal tibia. Protection of the fusion site with the tension-band wire and external support decreases the forces to which the screw is subjected and aids in preventing its loosening.

A screw that is too large for the medullary cavity of the tibia may cause fissure fractures of the distal tibial cortices leading to screw loosening and overall instability of the fusion site.[11] Should this complication occur, the limb must be immobilized in a cast until radiographic evidence of union is seen. The screw may break if it is continually subjected to the oscillating forces generated by weight-bearing. Protection of the screw with external support and a tension-band wire has already been mentioned. Moreover, the screw must be removed when bony union has occurred; otherwise, screw fracture may result, and a sound patient with a successful arthrodesis may once again be lame.[11]

Malalignment of the fusion site is a technical error that can easily be avoided by proper planning and technique. The patient's entire foot should be visible during the operation, and a sterile goniometer should be available. Prior to placement of the guide pin, the apposing surfaces of the fusion site should be brought together, and the fusion angle and orientation of the foot with the limb should be assessed. Once the guide pin is in place, these parameters should be re-evaluated.

The proper fusion angle should be obtained from the opposite limb prior to the surgical procedure, with the patient standing in a normal, relaxed position. Consideration must also be given to the loss of limb length incurred by the removal of articular cartilage. This loss may be overcome by placing the fusion site in extension several degrees greater than normal.

Complications of intertarsal arthrodesis are similar to those described for tibiotarsal fusion.

In summary, arthrodesis of a painful or unstable joint can preserve a functional limb with nearly normal usage. The remaining functional joints compensate for the loss of joint motion, provided proper techniques of arthrodesis are observed.

References and Suggested Readings

1. Crenshaw, A. H. (ed.): Campbell's Operative Orthopedics. 5th Ed. St. Louis, C. V. Mosby, 1971.
2. Dieterich, H. F.: Arthrodesis of the proximal intertarsal joint for repair of rupture of proximal plantar intertarsal ligaments. VM SAC, 69:995, 1974.
3. Early, T. D.: Canine carpal ligament injuries. Vet. Clin. North Am., 8:183, 1978.
4. Early, T. D., and Dee, J. F.: Trauma to the carpus, tarsus, and phalanges of dogs and cats. Vet. Clin. North Am., 10:717, 1980.
5. Evans, H. E., and Christensen, G. C.: Miller's Anatomy of the Dog. 2nd Ed. Philadelphia, W. B. Saunders, 1979.
6. Hohn, R. B.: Personal communication.
7. Holt, P. E.: Treatment of tibio-tarsal instability in small animals. J. Small Anim. Pract., 18:415, 1977.
8. Müller, M. E., Allgöwer, M., and Willenegger, H.: Manual of Internal Fixation. New York, Springer-Verlag, 1970.
9. Olds, R. B.: Arthrodesis of elbow, carpus, stifle and hock. In Current Techniques in Small Animal Surgery. Edited by M. J. Bojrab. Philadelphia, Lea & Febiger, 1975.
10. Piermattei, D. L., and Greeley, R. C.: An Atlas of Surgical Approaches to the Bones of the Dog and Cat. 2nd Ed. Philadelphia, W. B. Saunders, 1979.
11. Stoll, S. G., Sinibaldi, K. R., De Angelis, M. P., and Rosen, H.: A technique for tibiotarsal arthrodesis utilizing cancellous bone screws in small animals. J. Am. Anim. Hosp. Assoc., 11:185, 1975.
12. Turner. T. M., and Hohn, R. B.: Craniolateral approach to the canine elbow for repair of condylar fractures or joint exploration. J. Am. Vet. Med. Assoc., 176:1264, 1980.
13. Wind, A.: Surgical diseases of the carpal joint and methods of treatment. In Current Techniques in Small Animal Surgery. Edited by M. J. Bojrab. Philadelphia, Lea & Febiger, 1975.

Principles and Application of Cerclage Wires

by STEPHEN J. WITHROW

The use of wire to hold pieces of bone together during fracture healing is an important aspect of small animal orthopedic surgery. Attention to details of equipment, case selection, and actual application of the wires aids in successful healing of bone. The details of bone vascularity as it relates to encircling wire loops is adequately covered elsewhere.[2] Suffice it that properly applied cerclage wire neither deleteriously influences blood supply to bone nor suppresses fracture healing.

Equipment

Only monofilament stainless steel wire should be used for cerclage wiring. The size may vary from 18-gauge wire (animals over 15 kg) to 20-gauge (animals 2 to 15 kg) or 22- to 26-gauge (for animals and birds 2 kg or less) wire.

The 2 most common means of securing a tight wire are with a lariat-like loop or with standard twists (Fig. 48-33). Both methods have their proponents. The loop

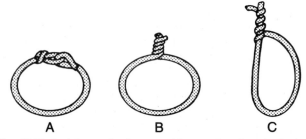

Fig. 48-33. A, *A loop wire is secured by turning the wire back on itself.* B, *Standard twists should have each arm equally twisted.* C, *Slip knots should be avoided because they easily loosen and also put excessive stress on the twisted arm.*

may be slightly less secure against an expansile loading (shearing) force than the standard twist,[3] but this difference is probably not significant in fractures in dogs and cats. Recent work has shown greater compression is attainable with loops than with twisted wire.[7] In over 600 loop-wire applications in dogs and cats, followed to radiographic union, only 1 wire has been seen to straighten out. I prefer a loop wire because of speed and convenience of application.

Many wire tighteners are on the market today (Fig. 48-34). A special point of concern for the prospective buyer of a wire tightener, apart from the loop versus standard twist decision, is whether to purchase one with a strain gauge. Strain gauges should theoretically allow more exacting and uniform wire tightening. Interestingly, uniform tension with loops was attainable without the use of strain gauges.[7]

Indications

FULL CERCLAGE

The simplest indication for full-cerclage wires is stabilization of nondisplaced fissures in a fractured bone. Once the fracture is visualized and fissures are seen, full-cerclage wires should be applied. These wires prevent the fissure from widening when the veterinary surgeon reduces the fracture or places an intramedullary pin.

Long oblique or spiral two-piece fractures are also ideal for full-cerclage wiring. Biomechanically, the longer the obliquity or the more parallel the fracture to the long axis of the bone, the better it responds to full-cerclage wiring. Another rule of thumb is that the fracture line should be two or three times as long as the cross-sectional diameter of the bone because more interfragmentary compression is achieved with long oblique or spiral fractures than with short oblique fractures. When a wire is tightened on a short oblique fracture, it potentiates shearing forces (Fig. 48-35).

The last indication is the comminuted fracture that can be anatomically reconstructed. Several large pieces of bone can usually be reduced anatomically with full-cerclage wires. If the pieces of bone are small or are missing, solid and permanent stabilization is less likely. This idea has been equated to the old-fashioned, wood-slatted water barrel,[6] which is stable as long as all pieces of wood (bone) are present and the metal bands (cerclage wires) are tight. Once a piece of wood is gone (missing bone, small unstable pieces), however, the stability is poor, and the barrel collapses.

HEMICERCLAGE

The use of wire patterns that do not fully encircle the bone, or hemicerclage, is indicated for short oblique or transverse fractures. The main goal is to prevent rotational instability.

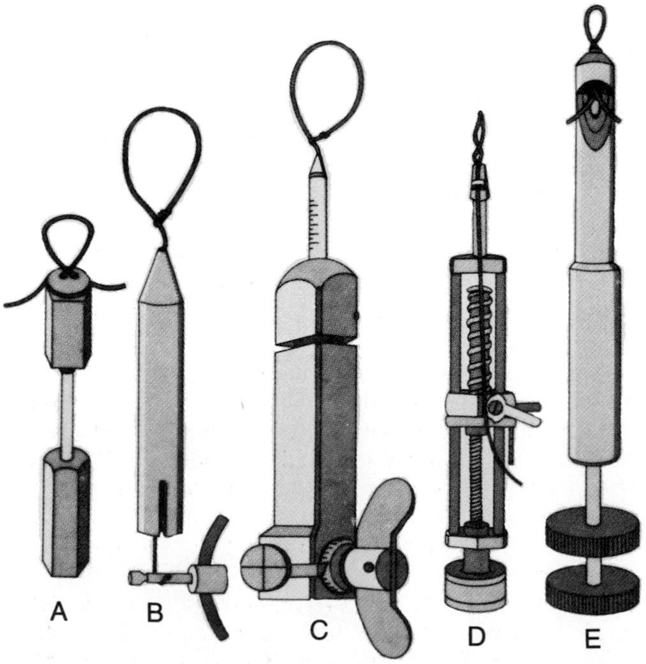

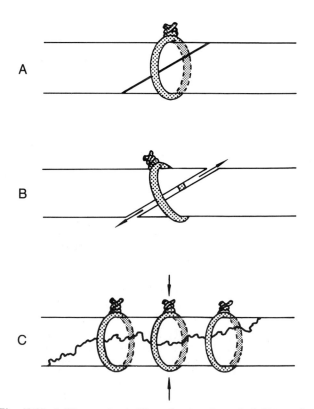

Fig. 48-34. *The more commonly used wire twisters are shown. A, Richards standard wire twister. B, Richards loop wire tightener. C, Osteo Systems through Richards wire tightener. D, Rhinelander wire tightener-twister. E, Bowen wire twister-cutter. A and B use loops, whereas C and D feature strain gauges. Tightener E is designed to both twist and cut the wire off in the same motion. Standard hardware pliers are not shown because they do not produce consistent results.*

Fig. 48-35. *A, When a short oblique fracture is encircled by a wire, compression of the wire potentiates gliding and distraction of the bone (B). C, Fractures with longer obliquity allow direct compression perpendicular (arrows) to the fracture line.*

Cerclage Techniques

Once the proper patient is selected for cerclage wiring, the following technical points apply.

When wires must be placed in an area that has muscle attachments, care should be taken not to remove or destroy these tissues, if possible. The wire should travel through and not over these muscle attachments. The wire should be passed as close to the bone as possible. This objective may be accomplished by pushing the wire, by pulling it with curved hemostats, or by means of various commercially available wire passers (Fig. 48-36). If muscle or fascia is trapped between the wire and the bone, significant problems can result, the most important of which is eventual loosening of the wire. If muscle is trapped under the wire, the wire may feel tight on the operating table, but the wire loosens as this muscle necroses. Another consideration is transient loss of blood supply to the bone when muscle and its associated blood supply are lost (Fig. 48-37).

Wires can and should be placed *over* loose fitting periosteum, for example, the cranial femur. This periosteum, without associated muscle attachments, contributes little or nothing to osseous vascularity. In fact, elevation of this periosteum for cerclage placement may induce unnecessary callus formation, especially in the growing animal.[4]

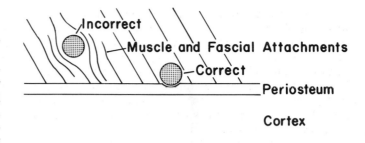

Fig. 48-37. *Wires should lie directly on the bone, over the periosteum, rather than away from the bone and in soft tissues.*

Wires must be placed *tightly* in order to be of benefit. A loose wire allows fracture movement, may impede external callus formation, and can prevent early revascularization of cortex by muscle and fascia. Each wire tightener requires a special technique and practice before it can be used effectively. No matter which tightener is chosen, veterinary surgeons should practice on cadaver bones until they feel confident that consistent and reproducible wire tightness is achieved. Without the help of strain gauges, wire tension is more of an art than a science, and practice is mandatory. Twisted wires should be bent over perpendicular to the long axis of the wire, twisting slightly as they are bent. This maneuver helps prevent loosening by putting equal strain on each arm of the twist. If the wire is bent over parallel to the long axis, one arm may be loosened. Even when the wire is "properly" bent over, up to 50% of the attained tension may be lost.[7] Wires should also be bent over away from major gliding muscle bellies or nerves. Some veterinary surgeons prefer to leave the twists (4 to 6) sticking straight up in hope of maintaining tension.[1]

Wires should rarely be used without an intramedullary pin in fractures of long bones. If a fracture heals without infection, wires need not be removed because they induce little or no stress protection.

FULL CERCLAGE

Full-cerclage wires should be placed perpendicular to the long axis of the bone for maximal long-term stability. If a wire is placed obliquely to the shaft, it often moves to the perpendicular plane and becomes loose (Fig. 48-38).

Wires are generally placed 5 mm from each end of the fracture and roughly 1 cm apart between the end wires. A special problem with full-cerclage wires is the placement of wire around bone of changing diameter, such as in metaphyseal regions. The wire slips to the area of least resistance, the narrowest area, and becomes loose. This problem can be prevented by (1) placing a hemicerclage wire, (2) slightly notching the bone in 1 or 2 places to seat the wire in the outer 10% of the cortex, or (3) driving a transcortical Kirschner wire and laying the wire on top of the pin (Fig. 48-39).

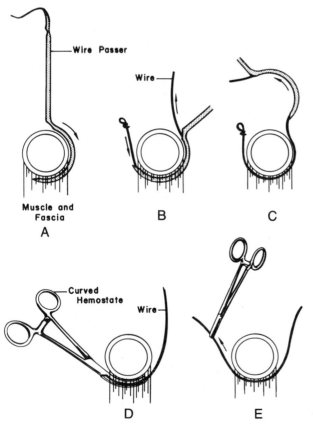

Fig. 48-36. A, *A wire passer is inserted adjacent to and around the bone.* B, *The wire is then partially pushed through the passer.* C, *Then the passer removed, leaving the wire.* D and E, *Hemostats may also be used to pull the wire around the bone.*

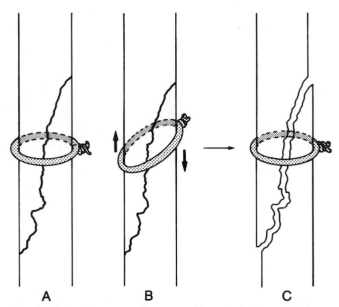

Fig. 48-38. A, *The correct placement of the wire is perpendicular to the diaphysis.* B, *If a wire is placed obliquely to the diaphysis, even though it may feel tight on the operating table, it will often shift, with resultant fracture instability* (C).

In a two-bone system, such as radius and ulna and tibia and fibula, it is preferable to encircle just one bone, although in the distal tibia it may be difficult to avoid encircling the fibula with the tibia.

HEMICERCLAGE

Hemicerclage wires are inserted partially through the cortex rather than completely around it. These wires are usually indicated for short oblique or transverse fractures and are principally used to counteract rotation. Many wire patterns have been described, but little objective biomechanical work exists to evaluate their relative efficacy. It can probably be said that the simple "suture" hemicerclage is the least stable design because the bone can pivot around the one point of fixation. Similarly, figure-8 wires that cross at the fracture line can rotate. Figure-8 cerclage that does not cross at the fracture line or a horizontal mattress pattern seems to afford the best stability (Fig. 48-40).

Holes are usually drilled in the bone about 1 or 2 cm away from the fracture ends. Care should be taken to avoid placing a wire in a fissure line or less than 3 mm

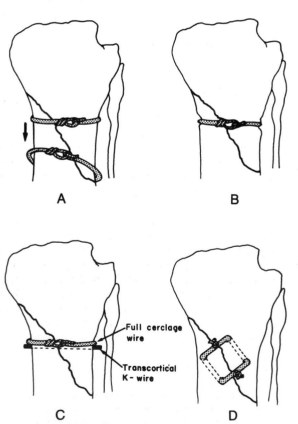

Fig. 48-39. A, *Placing a full-cerclage wire on conical bone often causes slippage of the wire to a narrower area. This problem can be avoided by notching the bone slightly* (B), *by passing a Kirschner wire (K-wire) below it* (C), *or by using hemicerclage techniques* (D).

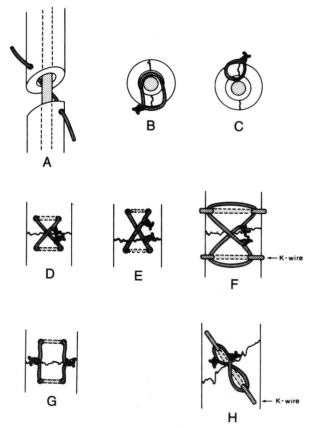

Fig. 48-40. A, B, *and* C, *Simple suture hemicerclage entails drilling one hole in each side of the fracture. The wire may or may not encircle the pin.* D, E, *and* F, *Figure-8 cerclage patterns can be used. Pattern E is preferable to D.* G, *Horizontal mattress cerclage seems to be more stable than the figure-8 patterns.* H, *Another variation includes a Kirschner wire (K-wire) across the fracture with a figure-8 over the top.*

from the main fracture line. Holes are usually drilled with an appropriate sized Kirschner wire in a Jacobs' hand chuck or with a power drill. When drilling 2 holes in one segment, such as for a figure-8 or a mattress pattern, it is best to drill both holes on the same plane with the same Kirschner wire (Fig. 48-41). This maneuver facilitates wire passage. In general, wires should be passed through these holes before the fracture is fully reduced or the pin is driven. The wire may or may not encircle the pin. Probably, encircling the pin is advantageous only when the pin is small and therefore deformable and can be "pulled up" to the cortex for another potential point of fixation. Once the fracture is reduced and the pin is driven, the excess wire is pulled up, and tightening can begin.

When using the figure-8 or mattress patterns, it is best to tighten each arm of the pattern separately. This technique affords more uniform tension on all aspects of the wire. If only one arm is tightened, the opposite arm will usually be loose because tension cannot be transferred around the areas where the wire is sharply bent (Fig. 48-41). Uniformly tight twists are mandatory, and twisting is performed as for full-cerclage wires.

Special Considerations

Special care must be exercised when applying cerclage wires, especially full-cerclage wires, to young dogs and cats. Excessive tension, which is generally impossible to attain in the mature animal, can crush the soft bone. Another common question concerns the fate of the bone and wire in an animal that is still growing. In most cases, the "knot" stays on the periosteal sur-

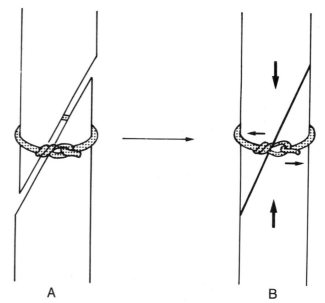

Fig. 48-42. A, *Accentuation of "proposed" unstable fracture when wire has been applied.* B, *With weight bearing, however, this shearing force is converted to a compressive force as the bones are forced into an ungiving wire.*

face, and the wire is slowly pulled into the cortex and is overgrown. Slight thinning of the diaphyseal diameter occurs, but this change is usually transitory, and the bone re-establishes normal or near-normal thickness. When wires are buried in cortical bone, no effect on the vascularity of the bone has been observed. I have seen no refracture through these areas in all my patients followed to date.

It has been stated that tension cannot be sustained by full-cerclage wires and that they loosen when the tightener is removed or when the wires are bent over. If the patient has been chosen correctly, however, a form of dynamic compression can theoretically take place. As the apposing obliquely fractured bone ends attempt to shear or to override, they work to expand the wire, and the result is a tight wire (Fig. 48-42). From a clinical viewpoint, primary bone healing is seen radiographically in over half the patients I have treated. If primary bone healing implies stability, then wires apparently can be made tight and appear to hold this tension. Loose wires seen clinically have almost invariably been applied improperly. When applied properly in the correct fracture, cerclage wire can and does afford an economical, simple, fast, and stable means of fixation. If poorly applied, as with any other means of fracture repair, only the expected poor result can occur.[5]

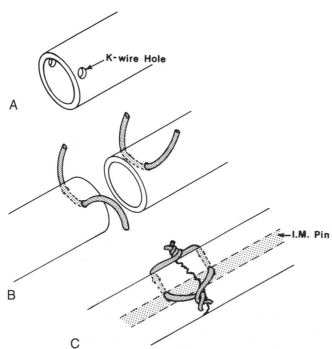

Fig. 48-41. A, *A Kirschner wire (K-wire) hole is usually drilled before bone reduction or pin placement.* B, *Wires are then passed.* C, *The fracture is reduced, and the wires are tightened.*

References and Suggested Readings

1. Griffiths, R. C: Presented at the American Animal Hospital Association annual meeting, Los Angeles, April, 1980.
2. Rhinelander, F. W.: Tibial blood supply in relation to fracture healing. Clin. Orthop., *105:*34, 1974.
3. Rhinelander, F. W.: Personal communication, 1980.
4. Wilson, J. W.: Tenth Annual Course on Internal Fixation of Fractures and Nonunions. Columbus, Ohio, March, 1980.

5. Withrow, S. J.: Use and misuse of full cerclage wires in fracture repair. Vet. Clin. North Am., *8*:201, 1980.

6. Withrow, S. J., and Holmberg, D. L.: Use of full cerclage wires in the fixation of 18 consecutive long-bone fractures in small animals. J. Am. Anim. Hosp. Assoc., *13*:735, 1977.

7. Rooks, R. L., et al.: In vitro carclage wiring analysis. Vet. Surg., *11*:31, 1982.

Open Fractures

by PAUL C. GAMBARDELLA

An open fracture is one that communicates with the outside environment through a break in the skin. Open fractures were previously called "compound" fractures. This term should no longer be used, however, because "open" more accurately describes the condition and can be easily compared to "closed" fractures. Open fractures are always contaminated and are threatened by infection. It is for this reason that treatment is considered an emergency and should be carried out in an aggressive manner.

Fracture Wound Mechanism

Fractures are made open by two mechanisms. The first is an externally applied force that penetrates the skin and underlying soft tissues and directly fractures the bone. An example is a fracture created by the penetration of a bullet. The second is the internally applied force of a fracture fragment penetrating through the soft tissues and skin. An example is the open wound created by the pointed edge of an oblique or spiral fracture as the fragments are distracted.[2] Some of the more severe open fractures are created by a combination of the two mechanisms. Examples are the fractures and wounds of the distal limbs that occur as an animal is twisting under a moving automobile. The medial or lateral aspect of the tarsus and the cranial surface of the carpus may be dragged along the pavement; skin, ligaments, and bone are lost, and the surface of the road is deeply embedded into the exposed tissues.

Physical Examination

Before undertaking the management of an open fracture, one must be aware that a traumatized patient with a fracture may also have other more life-threatening injuries. Even severe open fractures must be temporarily neglected while the animal is evaluated for airway obstruction, blood loss, and shock. Life-threatening conditions such as a diaphragmatic hernia, active internal bleeding, or a rupture in the urinary tract must be treated before definitive fracture repair is undertaken. Cursory cleansing and covering of the wound and temporary immobilization of the fracture should be performed as part of the initial treatment of the patient, but more definitive management of the wound and fracture should begin once life-threatening problems are successfully treated.

A proper and complete examination of the musculoskeletal system is essential. The open fracture is usually obvious and therefore should be examined last. Closed fractures, ligament injuries, and luxations may simultaneously exist in other limbs or in the limb with the open fracture. It is important to establish the extent of the soft tissue injury and the viability of the limb. Some injuries are so severe that a decision to amputate the leg can be made after initial examination. In other cases, 2 to 4 days may pass before the limb's viability can be determined. The viability of the soft tissues surrounding the fracture may be more easily determined during the debridement phase of treatment. The color of the tissue, the presence of pulsating arteries, and the occurrence of bleeding edges after debridement all indicate living tissue. The prognosis associated with the soft tissue injury may influence the owner's willingness to proceed with treatment. Wounds with large areas of skin loss that require grafting may add considerable expense to the total cost of treatment.

Bone fragments protruding through the skin or otherwise exposed should not be replaced or reduced before radiographic examination is made. A sterile moistened dressing is placed over the wound and fragments, and a thorough radiographic examination of the limb is made before surgical treatment. Two radiographic views of the entire bone are made, including the joints above and below the fracture.

Classification of Open Fractures

It is helpful to classify open fractures according to severity in order to establish more easily a treatment regimen and prognosis for each patient. The following classification, based on the one by Gustilo and Anderson for open fractures in man,[1] has been modified to reflect the needs of the small animal patient and the veterinary surgeon.

Type I: Open fractures with wounds less than 1 cm long, no exposed bone, no appreciable skin loss, no bone loss, and no obvious gross contamination; low-velocity bullet wounds are included in this type.

Type II: Open fractures with wounds greater than 1 cm long, exposed bone with or without bone loss, obvious gross contamination to the wound and bone, and no major skin loss.

Type III: Open fractures with large-to-massive wounds, obvious skin loss, and gross contamination of bone and soft tissues; bone loss is usually associated with these injuries; high-velocity bullet wounds are included in this type.

In my experience, the majority of open fractures encountered in small animals are Type I injuries of the tibia and radius. Open fractures of the femur, humerus, and bones distal to the carpal and tarsal joints are less frequently seen. Unfortunately, Type III injuries are seen next in order of frequency. More specifically, common Type III injuries are of the medial or lateral aspect of the hock joint. These injuries result from automobile accidents and usually fulfill all the criteria for Type III injuries.

Treatment

Once the patient's condition is stable, and thorough physical and radiographic examinations have been made, definitive treatment of the open fracture should begin. Three goals should be met in the treatment of open fractures in small animals: (1) prevention of infection, (2) stabilization of the fracture, and (3) promotion of wound healing. The third goal is of major importance in Type III open fractures with severe soft tissue wounds.

Before any major cleansing of the wound, a culture of the open soft tissues should be taken for future reference. Next, a broad-spectrum antibiotic is administered. Studies in man have shown that a cephalosporin is the antibiotic of choice.[1,5] I suggest the use of cephaloridine (10 mg/kg bid), to be administered immediately following culture and continued for 5 days postoperatively unless the culture results dictate differently. All open fractures are contaminated and contain some devitalized tissue in the wound. It is important to remember that antibiotics are not a substitute for proper cleansing, irrigation, and debridement of the wound.

The patient should be given a general anesthetic for cleansing, debridement, and irrigation of the wound. Once the limb has been properly clipped of hair and the skin cleansed with an appropriate surgical soap*, the remainder of the procedure is performed in the operating room under aseptic conditions. The veterinary surgeon should be properly scrubbed and dressed, and a routine sterile draping procedure is used on the injured limb. The wound should be irrigated extensively with normal saline solution or lactated Ringer's solution.

Agents of gross contamination, such as pebbles and other foreign matter, should be picked out of the wound with forceps. In Type I and II injuries, it may be necessary to extend the wound or surgically to approach the bone before proper debridement can be completed. Osseus fragments that protrude from the wound are cleansed with Betadine solution before they are replaced. Bone that is grossly impregnated with dirt should be thoroughly cleansed, but it should not be discarded unless it is a small and insignificant fragment. I prefer to save all butterfly fragments, even those freed from the soft tissues, because stabilization of the fracture may depend on them. The remainder of the wound, that is, skin and other soft tissues, must be thoroughly debrided of all gross contamination and devitalized tissue. The most useful criteria for the determination of viable muscle are contractibility and the capacity to bleed.

*Betadine, Purdue Frederick Co., 50 Washington Street, Norwalk, CT 06856

FRACTURE FIXATION

The accepted practice in the management of open fractures in human medicine is to avoid internal fixation of the fracture. External fixation and traction are the methods of choice. Neither method involves metal implantation, and both are satisfactory for human patients. Internal fixation is used routinely for the treatment of open fractures in small animals. Bed rest and traction are impossible in small animal patients. It is imperative that stable, lasting fixation be applied to the fracture because healing may be delayed either by infection or by the large amount of surrounding soft tissue damage. Controversy surrounds the use of intramedullary pins, because they have the potential to carry bacteria throughout the medullary canal.[4]

Lasting stability is the most important factor in choosing the method of fixation, whether it be bone plates and screws or pins and wires. The method of internal fixation should reflect the stabilization requirements of the fracture. I have successfully used bone plates and screws, intramedullary pins and wires, and the Kirschner-Ehmer apparatus for fixation of open fractures. Fractures of Type III injuries with significant damage to soft tissues and skin are best stabilized with the Kirschner-Ehmer apparatus. This device provides adequate fixation and also allows for easier management of the open wound. Fractures distal to the carpus and tarsus are usually immobilized by external means because small animal patients tolerate casts and splints in these areas well. Frequent splint changes are necessary until the wound is healed, however. Moreover, internal fixation of the bones distal to the carpus and tarsus is generally not necessary. No thorough retrospective or prospective studies of the treatment of open fractures in small animals have been conducted, but in my experience, open fractures, regardless of type, treated within 12 hours of injury and in the manner described rarely become infected.

Autogenous cancellous bone grafts should be used to fill defects in the bone and to promote healing of the fracture. Cancellous bone is plentiful in the wing of the ilium and in the proximal metaphyseal regions of the tibia and humerus. The graft is harvested and is transplanted to the fracture site just before closure of the wound. The wound should not be further irrigated after transfer of the graft. Allogenic cortical bone grafts should not be used in open fractures because of the high risk of infection and subsequent sequestration of the graft.

CLOSURE OF THE SKIN WOUND

In most cases in which skin loss is minimal, the wound should be closed primarily. Penrose drains are placed within the wound adjacent to the bone and are made to emerge distal to the primary incision. The drains are generally removed on the third postoperative day, if no infection is evident. Type III injuries can seldom be closed primarily because of skin loss. Wounds of this type should be allowed to remain open and to heal by second intention. Once the process of wound contraction is complete, a skin graft is used to cover the remaining defect.

In Type III injuries that leave the veterinary surgeon in doubt as to the amount of viable soft tissue, a delayed primary closure may be used. The wound is irrigated and debrided, and the fracture is repaired in the usual manner. The wound is packed with sponges soaked in Betadine solution, and the leg is bandaged. On the third postoperative day, the patient is anesthetized, and the packing is removed. The remainder of the nonviable tissue is recognizable at this time and is debrided. The wound is closed primarily with Penrose drains. The drains are removed on the third postoperative day, if no infection is evident.

BULLET WOUNDS

The majority of bullet wounds with associated fractures in small animals are caused by low-velocity (under 1000 feet per second) bullets. These injuries may be treated much differently from the bullet wounds created by the high-velocity bullets of war weapons. The fractured bone should be approached in the manner used for closed fractures of the same region. Any devitalized tissue is excised. An extensive debridement of the bullet tract is not necessary, and only those bullet fragments that are easily located during the exposure are removed. The exceptions to this rule are bullet fragments lodged in joints. All bullet fragments and other osteochondral fragments should be removed from the joint. The presence of lead within the synovium may cause severe periarticular fibrosis.[3] The fracture is repaired in the usual manner, and the surgical wound is closed primarily with a Penrose drain emerging through the skin distal to the incision. The drain is removed on the third postoperative day. The wound should be cultured at the time of operation, and the patient should be treated with cephaloridine as for other open fractures. High-velocity (greater than 2000 feet per second) bullets create much soft tissue trauma and may fracture the bone without even striking it. These bullet pathways must be thoroughly flushed and debrided, and the entire wound is treated as a severe Type III injury. Limbs traumatized with high-velocity bullets often require amputation.

References and Suggested Readings

1. Gustilo, R. B., and Anderson, J. T.: Prevention of infection in the treatment of 1025 open fractures of long bones. Retrospective and prospective analyses. J. Bone Joint Surg. [Am.], 58:453, 1976.

2. Heppenstall, R. B. (ed.): Fracture Treatment and Healing. Philadelphia, W. B. Saunders, 1980.

3. Leonard, M. H.: Solution of lead by synovial fluid. Clin. Orthop., 64:255, 1969.

4. Nunamaker, D.: Treatment of open fractures in small animals. Compend. Contin. Ed. Practicing Vet., 1:66, 1979.

5. Patzakis, M. J., Harvey, J. P., and Ivler, D.: The role of antibiotics in the management of open fractures. J. Bone Joint Surg. [Am.], 56:532, 1974.

Carpus and Tarsus

by THOMAS D. EARLEY

Because so many carpal and tarsal injuries are seen, I have chosen to present only the most common. Owing to the many bones and joints in these regions, at least two radiographic views are necessary to establish a diagnosis. In some instances, oblique and stress radiographic positions are needed. Because of the complex nature of the anatomic structures in these joints, it is tempting to regard the injuries as minor and to use splints as the sole treatment, often with fair-to-poor results. Many of the injuries to the carpus and tarsus have articular considerations, and principles of joint repair should be followed strictly for the best results.

Preoperative Considerations

Most carpal and tarsal injuries are painful, and a moderate amount of swelling may occur. A temporary coaptation splint with several layers of cast padding is recommended to aid in reduction of the swelling and to minimize the discomfort to the patient. Often, the most diagnostic radiographs are obtained when the patient is heavily sedated, especially when stressed views are needed. Reviewing the pertinent anatomy of the surgical area is helpful and usually reduces the surgical time. Some veterinary surgeons prefer to apply an exsanguinating tourniquet during the procedure. Care should be taken not to leave the tourniquet on for more than 90 minutes.

Fractures of the Carpus

Fractures of the carpus are infrequent; however, most of these fractures involve articular surfaces or compromise joint stability.

Fractures of the ulnar styloid process result in instability of the lateral aspect of the antebrachiocarpal joint. Although this instability is not severe, many animals are partially weight-bearing when presented to the veterinarian. Anatomic realignment using a tension-band wire is recommended (Fig. 48-43). A lateral approach with retraction of the ulnaris lateralis tendon gives adequate surgical exposure.

Fractures of the radial styloid process are infrequent, but may also be repaired using a tension-band wire (Fig. 48-44). The medial approach involves knowledge of the tendon of the abductor pollicis longus muscle and the radial collateral ligament.

Fractures of the radial carpal bone generally involve either the body, which constitutes the articular surface and should be repaired striving for anatomic reduction using a compression screw (Fig. 48-45), or the palmar medial process, which represents an avulsion fracture of the attachment of the palmar radial carpal-metacarpal ligament and should be repaired using a tension-band wire (Fig. 48-46).

Fractures of the accessory carpal bone, generally seen in racing greyhounds, involve the free end as an

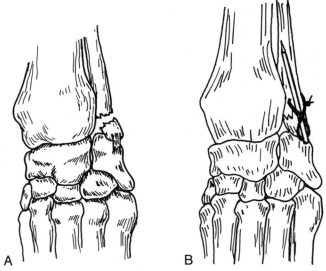

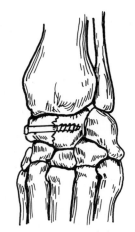

Fig. 48-45. *Intra-articular fracture of the radial carpal bone repaired with a compression screw.*

Fig. 48-43. *Fracture (A) of the lateral styloid process repaired with a tension-band wire (B).*

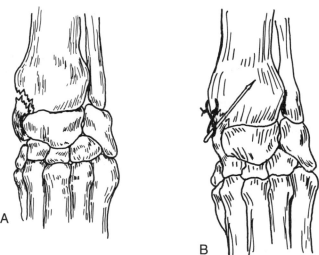

Fig. 48-44. *Fracture (A) of the medial styloid process repaired with a tension-band wire (B).*

avulsion fracture that may be repaired with a compression screw or Kirschner wires and tension band (Fig. 48-47) or the base as an avulsion fracture caused by the pull of the ligament between the ulnar carpal bone and the accessory carpal bone. This fracture may also be repaired with a screw or Kirschner wires (Fig. 48-48).

A unique avulsion fracture of the base of the fifth metacarpal bone is seen in hyperextension injuries and is the result of the pull of the lateral palmar accessory carpal-metacarpal ligament. This fracture can be repaired with either a compression screw or a tension-band wire (Fig. 48-49).

Fractures of the metacarpal and metatarsal bones, if simple and well aligned, can be successfully treated using coaptation splinting until radiographic healing has occurred. When simple fractures are displaced, intramedullary pinning is recommended, especially for the major weight-bearing (third and fourth) digits, in

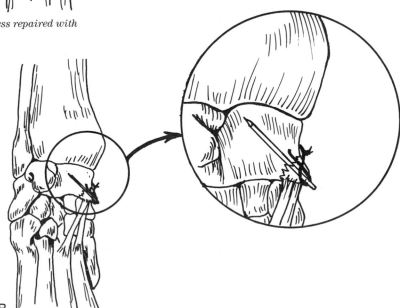

Fig. 48-46. *Avulsion fracture (A) of the palmar prominence of the radial carpal bone repaired with a tension-band wire (B, inset).*

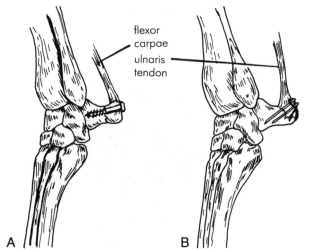

Fig. 48-47. *Fracture of the free end of the accessory carpal bone repaired with a compression screw (A) or Kirschner wires and tension band (B).*

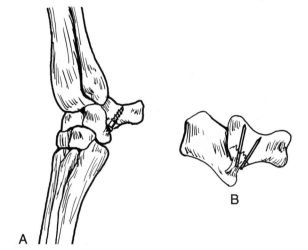

Fig. 48-48. *Avulsion fracture of the base of the accessory carpal bone repaired with a compression screw (A) or Kirschner wires (B).*

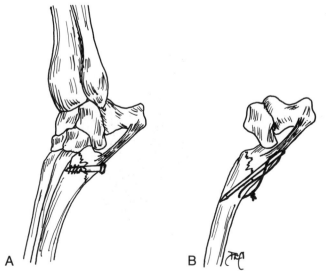

Fig. 48-49. *Avulsion fracture of the base of the fifth metacarpal repaired with a compression screw (A) or a tension-band wire (B).*

conjunction with external support (Fig. 48-50). The pins may be introduced through a dorsal approach driven in Rush-pin fashion and countersunk if desired. If the bones are comminuted, bone plates are useful (Fig. 48-51).

Fractures of the Tarsus

Malleolar fractures result in instability of the tarsocrural joint. Fractures of both malleoli should be anatomically reduced and stabilized with tension-band wires (Fig. 48-52). Accurate Kirschner wire placement can be ensured by directing the wire in a retrograde fashion through the distal fragment. In small dogs and cats, the Kirschner wire should penetrate the tibia when stabilizing the lateral malleolus.

Calcaneus fractures, if simple, are best stabilized with small pins or tension-band wires. If the tension-band wire is used, the orthopedic wire should pass underneath the superficial digital flexor tendon to guarantee adequate tightening (Fig. 48-53). The wires should be removed after the fracture has healed. Comminuted calcaneus fractures that do not lend themselves to pinning can be repaired with small bone plates secured to the lateral surface (Fig. 48-54).

Fractures of the talus are rare; however, because this bone bears much of the patient's weight, secure fixation is important. Fractures of the condyles represent articular surfaces and must be replaced anatomically. To approach condyle fractures of the talus, an osteotomy of the appropriate malleolus must be accomplished. Countersinking Kirschner wires below the articular surfaces is mandatory (Fig. 48-55). Oblique fractures of the body and head of the talus may be repaired using a compression screw (Fig. 48-56). If these fractures are transverse, small bone plates may be applied to the medial surface (Fig. 48-57).

Fractures of the central tarsal bone occur mainly in racing greyhounds and range in severity from simple vertical transverse fractures to comminuted fractures that cannot be reconstructed. Fractures that can be repaired should be stabilized with either one or two screws. The medial-to-lateral bone screw may be anchored in the fourth tarsal bone if the lateral fragment is narrow (Fig. 48-58).

Acute Luxations and Subluxations of the Carpus

Hyperextension injuries result in loss of palmar support to any of the 3 carpal joints. Often, this injury is misdiagnosed because abnormalities are not always seen in the 2 normal radiographic positions. The mild-to-moderate swelling in the carpal region is often regarded as "just a sprain," and either no treatment or short-term support is offered. The dog invariably walks on the palmar aspect of its metacarpal bones if proper surgical treatment is not accomplished. Most of these injuries occur when the dog jumps or falls off a high place, and the owner often sees the injury take place. A

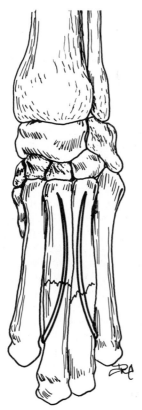

Fig. 48-50. *Simple metacarpal shaft fracture repaired with intramedullary Kirschner wires.*

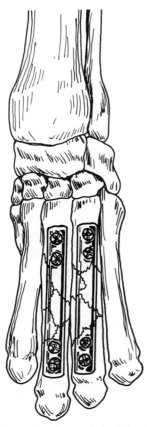

Fig. 48-51. *Comminuted metacarpal shaft fracture repaired with bone plates.*

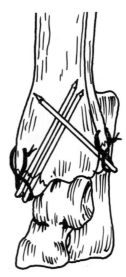

Fig. 48-52. *Bilateral malleolar fracture repaired with tension-band wires.*

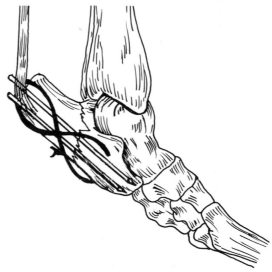

Fig. 48-53. *Simple fracture of the calcaneus repaired using a tension-band wire.*

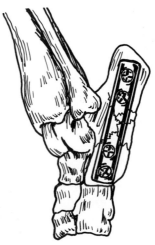

Fig. 48-54. *Comminuted fracture of the calcaneus repaired using a bone plate.*

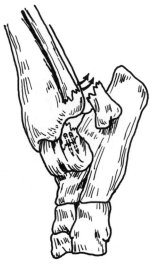

Fig. 48-55. *Fracture of the lateral condyle of the talus (arrows) using a lateral malleolus osteotomy approach and Kirschner wires for fixation.*

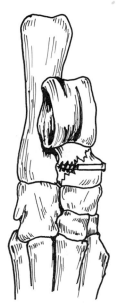

Fig. 48-56. *Fracture of the body and head of the talus repaired using a compression screw.*

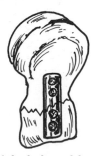

Fig. 48-57. *Fracture of the body and head of the talus repaired using a bone plate.*

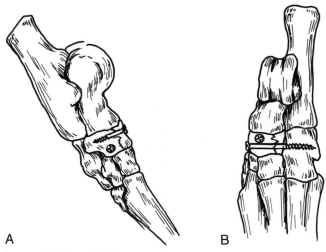

Fig. 48-58. A *and* B, *A common fracture of the central tarsal bone repaired using compression screws.*

lateral-to-medial hyperextension radiograph, with the dog under heavy sedation, demonstrates which joint is subluxated or luxated. In my experience, the percentage of joint involvement is as follows: antebrachiocarpal 5 to 10%, middle carpal 65 to 70%, and carpometacarpal 15 to 20%.

The surgical correction of these injuries demands a thorough anatomic knowledge of the palmar region of the carpus. To date, treatment of hyperextension of the antebrachiocarpal joint has only occasionally been successful using long-term coaptation splints. Recently, reconstruction of the oblique part of the short radial collateral ligament using the tendon of the abductor pollicis longus muscle or the tendon of the flexor carpi radialis muscle, in addition to coaptation, has been advocated (Fig. 48-59).

Surgical treatment of hyperextension injury of the middle carpal joint has been more successful using orthopedic wire and screws to maintain a proper bone and joint relationship during the ligament healing process (Fig. 48-60). The ruptured ligaments, which normally attach the free end of the accessory carpal bone to the fourth and fifth metacarpal bones, should be sutured once the orthopedic wire is secured.

Coaptation support for 6 to 8 weeks is recommended. The phalanges should be left free for the last 3 to 4 weeks. The wire that attaches the free end of the accessory carpal bone to the metacarpal bones should be removed at approximately 4 months. The wire from the ulnar carpal bone to the base of the fifth metacarpal bone is not removed.

Carpometacarpal hyperextension generally ruptures the palmar carpal fibrocartilage's attachment to the base of the metacarpal bones.

Often, the ligaments that support the middle carpal joint are also ruptured. The middle carpal joint reconstruction technique is recommended, in addition to wiring of the fibrocartilage to the metacarpal bones (Fig. 48-61). Occasionally, carpometacarpal luxation

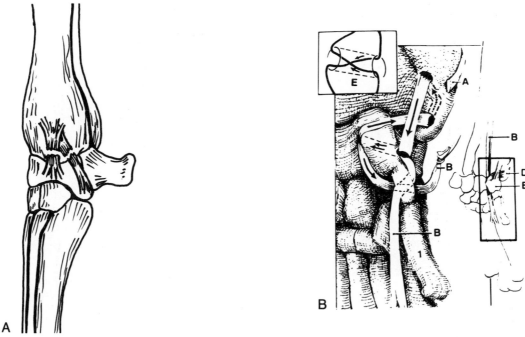

Fig. 48-59. *Loss of radial collateral ligament support (A) and reconstruction using the tendon of the flexor carpi radialis (B). B, End of excised abductor pollicis longus tendon (A); tendon of the flexor carpus radialis (B); medial styloid process (D); and radial carpal bone (E). 1, First metacarpal bone. Inset, Direction of the tendon of the flexor carpi radialis as it passes through the radial carpal bone twice. (B, From Earley, T.: Canine carpal ligament injuries. Vet. Clin. North Am., 8:183, 1978.)*

occurs unrelated to hyperextension. Closed reduction results in a stable realignment that, in addition to coaptation splint support for 6 weeks, is satisfactory. If stability is not satisfactory after closed reduction, 2 or 3 Kirschner wires are driven in a Rush-pin fashion, from the third and fourth metacarpal bones into the distal row of carpal bones (Fig. 48-62). These pins are removed in 6 to 8 weeks.

Luxation of the radial carpal bone is a rare injury that results in the detachment of the radial carpal bone from the ulnar carpal bone, from the palmar ulnar carpal ligament, the palmar radial carpal ligament, and the short radial collateral ligament (Fig. 48-63). Open reduction, with ligament reconstruction of the short radial collateral ligament, and splinting for 6 weeks are curative.

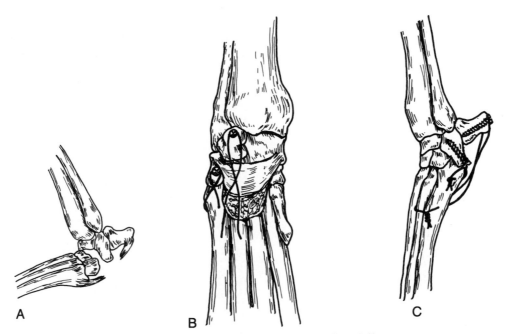

Fig. 48-60. *Hyperextension of the middle carpal joint (A) with wire stabilization (B and C).*

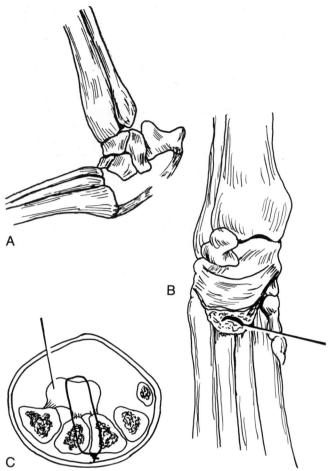

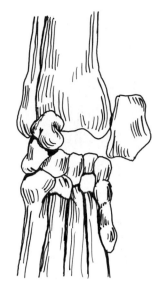

Fig. 48-63. *Palmar medial luxation of the radial carpal bone. See Figure 48-59B for radial collateral ligament reconstruction.*

Medial shearing injuries to the carpus destroy the medial styloid process and the short radial collateral ligament and its attachment on the radial carpal bone. The result is subluxation of the medial antebrachiocarpal joint. Using the tendon of the flexor carpi radialis muscle, the straight and oblique parts of the ligament can be reconstructed. Splinting for 6 to 8 weeks with periodic changes for wound management is indicated (see Fig. 48-59B).

Acute Tarsal Luxations and Subluxations

Tarsocrural luxations may be the result of bilateral malleolar fractures (Fig. 48-64). In the past, an intramedullary pin through the joint was advocated. At present, repair of each malleolar fracture with tension-band wires is advocated (see Fig. 48-52). Restricted activity and external support for 4 to 5 weeks are recommended for the tissues to heal.

Tarsocrural subluxation often occurs when one of the malleoli and its attached collateral ligament are sheared off (Fig. 48-65A). Debridement and wire reconstruction can be accomplished during the same operation.

A screw is placed in the imaginary center of an arc made by the outline of the appropriate condyle of the talus (Fig. 48-65B). Another screw is then placed in the distal tibia, and orthopedic wire connects these screws in a figure-8 pattern (Fig. 48-65B and C). It is important not to tighten this wire too much. Additional stabilization may be required, as shown in Figure 48-65D. One of the main advantages of this repair is the convenience of changing the soft dressing on the wound without fear of altering the stability. The wire eventually breaks, but is not generally removed.

Luxation of the talus is a unique injury that separates the head from the central tarsal bone and the body from the calcaneus. A medial approach and positional screw fixation to the calcaneus comprise the surgical

Fig. 48-61. *Hyperextension of the carpometacarpal joint (A) repaired using wire (B, leader line) to secure the palmar carpal fibrocartilage (C, leader line) to the third and fourth metacarpal bones.*

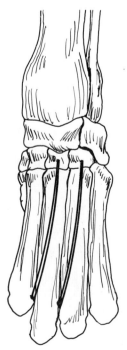

Fig. 48-62. *Carpometacarpal stabilization using Kirschner wires.*

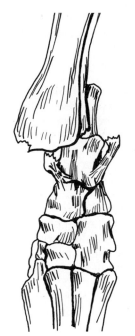

Fig. 48-64. *Bilateral malleolar fractures resulting in luxation of the tarsocrural joint.*

treatment of choice (Fig. 48-66). Placement of an additional screw in the central tarsal bone with a figure-8 wire secured to the proximal screw is recommended.

Proximal intertarsal luxations usually represent a rupture of the plantar ligaments and result in a loss of support on the plantar side. Two surgical techniques are commonly employed to stabilize this joint. Either a screw or a pin is inserted through the long axis of the calcaneus and into the fourth tarsal bone. A tension-band wire that passes through the plantar process of the fourth or central tarsal bone and over the tuber calcanei can be added (Fig. 48-67). The second technique requires a bone plate to be applied to the lateral surface, the calcaneus, the fourth tarsal bone, and the fifth metatarsal bone. (Fig. 48-68).

Both techniques usually result in a functional arthrodesis of the intertarsal and tarsometatarsal joints unless the metal is removed soon after the joints have become stable, as a result of the healing ligaments and joint capsule.

Luxation of the central tarsal bone is occasionally seen in the pet animal. Through a medial approach, the bone is easily reduced and should be secured to the fourth tarsal bone using a bone screw (Fig. 48-69).

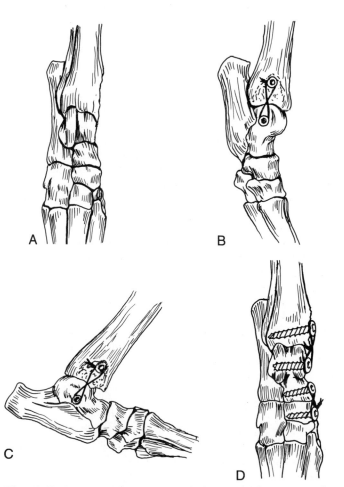

Fig. 48-65. *Shearing injury to the medial aspect of the tarsocrural joint (A) with collateral ligament reconstruction using screws and orthopedic wires (B to D).*

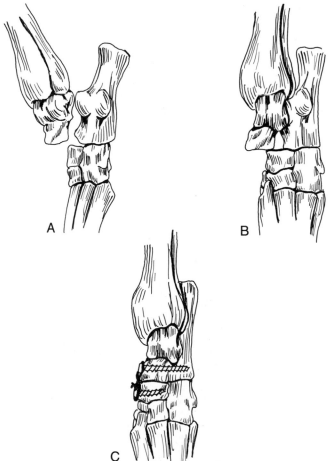

Fig. 48-66. *Talus-calcaneus luxation (A and B) with positional screw fixation. C, A screw in the central tarsal bone with a figure-8 wire to the proximal screw provides additional support.*

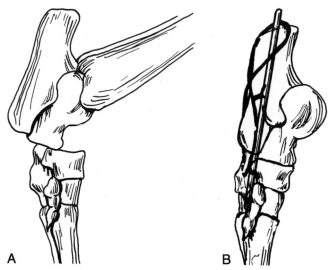

Fig. 48-67. *Proximal intertarsal luxation* (A) *using a tension-band wire for stabilization* (B).

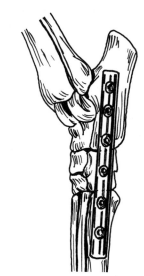

Fig. 48-68. *Proximal intertarsal luxation using a bone plate for stabilization.*

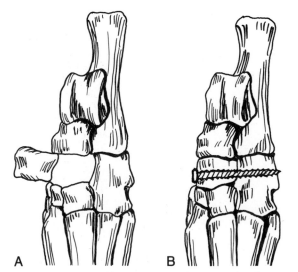

Fig. 48-69. *Central tarsal bone luxation* (A) *repaired using a positional screw* (B).

Acute tarsometatarsal luxations are handled in the manner described for carpometacarpal luxations.

Carpal Arthrodesis

If the antebrachiocarpal joint is irreparably damaged or diseased and arthrodesis is indicated, a total carpal arthrodesis of all three carpal joints should be performed. The most effective technique is to secure a compression bone plate to the dorsum of the carpus (radius to third metacarpal bone) when the articular cartilage has been excised and a cancellous bone graft has been applied. If possible, the veterinary surgeon should ensure that one screw enters the radial carpal bone and that compression of all joints is achieved. A 5° flexion contour should be placed in the bone plate (Fig. 48-70). The plate should be removed in 6 to 9 months as long as radiographic evidence of arthrodesis is complete.

If either the middle carpal or the carpometacarpal joint is severely damaged or diseased, a partial arthrodesis of both distal joints is indicated. Two surgical techniques are generally offered, both accomplished through a dorsal approach separating the tendons of the common digital extensor and the extensor carpi radialis muscles. The first technique employs a small, "T"-shaped bone plate with 2 screws, which should not exit the opposite side of the radial carpal bone. One should secure the plate to the dorsum of the radial carpal bone. One screw should be inserted into the third carpal bone and 2 screws into the third metacarpal (Fig. 48-71). The plate is generally removed once radiographic evidence of arthrodesis is observed, in 6 to 9 months. The second technique uses 3 small pins or Kirschner wires introduced into the second, third, and fourth metacarpal bones, driven proximally through the second, third, and fourth carpal bones, and seated into the radial and ulnar carpal bones, respectively (Fig. 48-72). These pins are generally not removed. Whichever technique is used, external support is recommended for 4 to 6 weeks. (See the section of this chapter, Turner and Lipowitz, "Arthrodesis.")

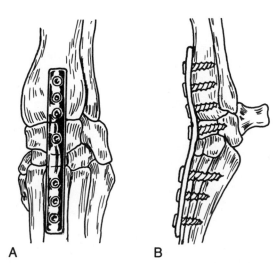

Fig. 48-70. A *and* B, *Total arthrodesis of the carpus using a bone plate.*

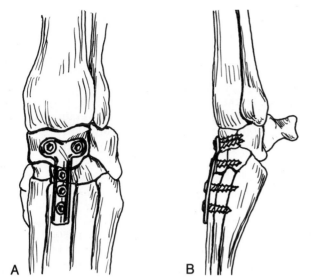

Fig. 48-71. A *and* B, *Partial arthrodesis of the carpus using a bone plate.*

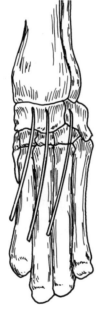

Fig. 48-72. *Partial arthrodesis of the carpus using small pins.*

Tarsal Arthrodesis

Tarsocrural arthrodesis is advocated when a joint is severely injured or diseased. The cochlea of the tibia tends to ride over the condyles of the talus, and this motion often causes failure of arthrodesis techniques. To prevent this movement, I advise surgically flattening the tibial cochlea and talar condyles prior to applying the internal fixation device. This flattening can be accomplished with a rongeur or an osteotome. The correct joint angle can be determined by using a goniometer to measure the standing angle of the normal tarsus. A compression screw is directed from the medial distal tibia, proximal to the medial malleolus, and emerges at the base of the calcaneus where the plantar ligament attaches. An intramedullary pin is inserted between the

tuber calcanei and the distal tibia for added stability (Fig. 48-73).

It is important to use external support, such as a coaptation splint, until the arthrodesis is complete. The pin should be removed at this time; however, the screw is left in place. The eventual increase in stress transferred to the distal tarsal joints may cause degenerative joint disease and may warrant arthrodesis of these distal joints.

Distal tarsal arthrodesis generally refers to arthrodesis of the proximal and distal intertarsal joints, in addition to the tarsometatarsal joint or just the distal intertarsal and tarsometatarsal joint. This arthrodesis is generally accomplished with bone plates (Fig. 48-74) or partially threaded screws (Fig. 48-75A). Coaptation splinting is recommended until the arthrodesis is complete. (See the section of this chapter by Turner and Lipowitz, "Arthrodesis.")

Total arthrodesis of the tarsus in one surgical procedure is effectively accomplished by applying a bone plate on the dorsal surface of the distal tibia, tarsus, and third metatarsal bone (Fig. 48-75B). Splint support is applied for 6 weeks. The plate is removed in 6 to 9 months, once radiographic arthrodesis is complete.

Luxations of the Phalanges

These injuries, which occur as a result of collateral ligament and joint capsule ruptures, are best handled by suturing the joint capsule and collateral ligament with a slowly degrading suture material. Coaptation splinting is used for 4 weeks, with leash restraint for 2 additional weeks. If reconstruction of the joint is not possible, amputation of the luxated part is recommended. If the amputation is to be performed at the metatarsal(carpal)-phalangeal level, the sesamoid bones should be excised.

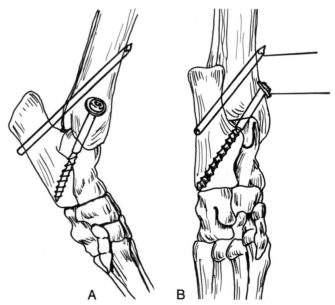

Fig. 48-73. A *and* B, *Tarsocrural arthrodesis using a permanent compression screw and a temporary Steinmann pin (B, leader lines).*

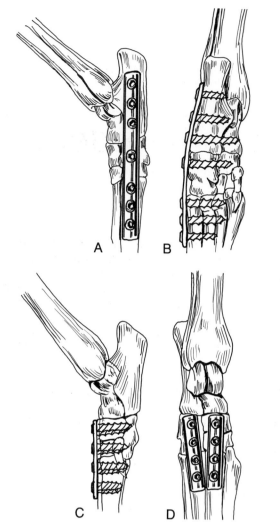

Fig. 48-74. A *to* D, *Proximal intertarsal joint arthrodesis using bone plates.*

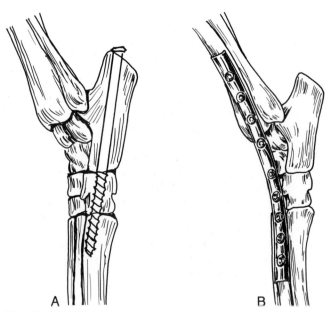

Fig. 48-75. A, *Distal intertarsal joint arthrodesis using threaded screws.* B, *Total arthrodesis using a bone plate.*

Flexor Tendon Injuries

Severing of the deep and superficial flexor tendons should be handled aggressively initially because subsequent attempts at reconstruction are not rewarding. Fortunately, injuries generally occur at the proximal metacarpal and metatarsal levels, where surgical exposure is easy and the tendons have not yet divided. Each tendon should be sutured individually with nonabsorbable suture material, and the patient's paw should be placed in a coaptation splint for 4 weeks. This splint should be constructed to maintain the phalanges in a neutral position. A minimal walking bar can be secured to the end of the splint to protect the tendons from stress. This bar should be removed at 4 weeks, and the patient's paw should start experiencing some stress, but only in the neutral position for the next 4 weeks. The paw should then be placed in a support wrap to allow more stress to be applied, but the dog should not be allowed other than leash activity during the next 2 weeks. This gradual return of stress ensures longitudinal orientation of collagen fibers and enhances the strength and healing of the tendons.

When the flexor tendons are severed below the point of division, the stress protection is even more critical. Sudden weight-bearing breaks down the repair, with little chance of reconstruction. The consequence of a loss of flexor tendon support is a flat foot and severe abrasion of the carpal or tarsal pad.

Postoperative Considerations

Most surgical procedures demand a coaptation splint for several weeks to reduce the stress on the healing area until adequate strength is achieved at the surgical site. I generally use a coaptation splint made of plastic or plaster. The splint is applied to the palmar surface of the carpus and to the dorsal surface of the tarsus.

References and Suggested Readings

Campbell, J. R., Bennett, D., and Lee, R.: Intertarsal and tarso-metatarsal subluxations in the dog. J. Small Anim. Pract., *17*:427, 1976.

Dee, J. F.: Fractures in the racing greyhound. *In* Pathophysiology in Small Animal Surgery. Edited by M. J. Bojrab. Philadelphia, Lea & Febiger, 1981.

Dee, J. F., and Earley, T. D.: Fractures of the carpus and tarsus and paw. *In* Veterinary Manual of Internal Fixation. In press.

Dietrich, H. F.: Arthrodesis of the proximal intertarsal joint for repair of rupture of proximal plantar intertarsal ligaments, VM SAC, 995, 1974.

Earley, T. D.: Canine carpal ligament injuries. Vet. Clin. North Am., *8*: 183, 1978.

Earley, T. D.: Hyperextension injuries of the canine carpal joint. Georgia Vet., *29*, 1976.

Earley, T. D., and Dee, J. F.: Trauma to the carpus, tarsus and phalanges of dogs and cats. Vet. Clin. North Am., *10*:717, 1980.

Farrow, C. S.: Carpal sprain injury in the dog. J. Am. Vet. Radiol. Soc., *18*:38, 1977.

Punzet, G.: Fixation of the os carpi radialis in the dog: pathogenesis, symptoms and treatment. J. Small Anim. Pract., *15*:751, 1974.

49 * Miscellaneous Disorders

Delayed Union and Nonunion of Fractures

by Dennis N. Aron

Delayed union and nonunion of fractures in small animals are occasionally encountered as an orthopedic complication. These problems can become crippling to the patient, annoying to the client, and frustrating to the veterinary surgeon. If the cause for the delayed union or nonunion can be identified, then a method of management becomes more evident. Furthermore, by understanding the cause and management of these problems, the chance of preventing them is improved.

Delayed Union

Delayed union can be defined as the condition that exists in a fracture that is not healed, or is not healing, in the time normally required for that particular bone and that type of fracture. Although this definition is explicit, in clinical practice it is frequently difficult to differentiate among normal healing, delayed union, and nonunion because no absolute criteria define them.

CAUSES

The causes of delayed union of fractures can be many and, as is later pointed out, are the same as the causes for nonunion of fractures. First, fractures can be subjected to multiple forces such as bending, shearing, and rotation and conditions such as distraction and overriding. If immobilization and reduction of the fracture are not sufficient to overcome these conditions and forces, motion will result and healing will be delayed or interrupted. Rotational forces are particularly difficult to overcome and are probably the primary cause of delayed healing. As a consequence to any form of instability, fine capillary buds, which initially attempt to bridge the fracture gap, are easily destroyed. Bone healing is delayed without an adequate blood supply to provide mesenchymal cells and nutrients. Second, a gap between fracture fragments may predispose the fracture to delayed union. This gap can be caused by soft tissue interposition, malposition, over-riding, displacement, or distraction. It is difficult for the blood supply to bridge the fracture gap, and the gap predisposes the fracture site to further instability.

A third cause of delayed union involves the nutrient artery. The blood supply to the diaphyseal cortical bone is provided by the nutrient and metaphyseal arteries to the medullary canal and a network of periosteal arteries. Damage to this blood supply by the trauma of a complete fracture and the compromise of remaining blood supply through various fracture fixation techniques can result in delayed healing. Fourth, infection caused by contamination from the original trauma or iatrogenically at the time of fracture repair may interfere with healing. Infection can lead to bone death and sequestra formation.

Finally, some less common causes for delayed unions are osteopenic bones of old age, poor nutrition and resulting negative nitrogen balance, metabolic defects, usage of corticosteroids or anticoagulants, and radiation.

DIAGNOSIS

The diagnosis of delayed union is determined by the patient's medical history, physical examination, and radiographic evaluation. The patient's history provides a "time factor." Delayed union is present when a fracture has not healed in the time normally required for that particular bone and type of fracture. Usually, in a mature dog, over 1 year of age, a fracture takes at least 8 weeks to heal, whereas in young dogs, it may heal twice as rapidly.

Obviously, many variables exist. For example, cancellous bone, as in a metaphyseal fracture, heals faster than cortical bone, as in diaphyseal fractures. Further, small bones usually heal faster than large bones such as the femur. Various types of fractures heal at different rates; for example, oblique and interlocking fractures heal more rapidly than transverse fractures.

Physical examination may demonstrate that the patient is reluctant to bear weight on the affected limb. On palpation, muscle atrophy, persistence of pain, and instability at the fracture site are present. Radiographs of the fracture may reveal an absence of bone healing, as evidenced by the lack of a bony callus or callus formation bridging the fracture gap. Most important, sclerosis of the bone ends is not seen; this condition is more indicative of a nonunion than a delayed union. It becomes obvious that a diagnosis of a delayed union can be subjective, and no definitive way exists to prove that healing is not progressing as expected. Because a fine line often separates the diagnosis of delayed union from that of nonunion, nonunion of a fracture is said to exist when all healing has ceased.

TREATMENT

Once delayed union of a fracture has been established, but bone healing is still progressing, a conservative approach to hasten healing should be considered. In most situations, the means of fixation of the fracture is assessed and is found to be inadequate. External devices may have to be improved, the animal may have to be restrained physically or by drugs, or an internal device may have to inserted or replaced.

Delayed union due to infection should be treated with immobilization, warm compresses, and antibiotics based on results of culture and sensitivity tests.

Nonunion

Nonunion of a fracture can be defined as the condition that exists in a fracture in which signs of repair have ceased. Causes of nonunion are the same as those of delayed union. The difference between the two conditions is that with nonunion, the condition has proceeded to a point that further healing does not occur without assistance.

DIAGNOSIS

The diagnosis of nonunion, as that of delayed union, is provided by a combination of medical history, physical examination, and radiographic evaluation. Progressive muscle atrophy, deformity, pain, and failure to use the limb are evidenced. In a nonunion of long duration, gross instability may be present, but the animal may indicate no pain on palpation of the limb. Further, with a nonunion of long duration, the animal may bear weight on the distorted limb.

Radiographically, the nonunion can show two distinct appearances: it can be vascular (hypertrophic) or avascular (atrophic), depending on the integrity of the blood supply to the fractures. Mesenchymal cells and nutrients are provided from the blood, and with existing periosteal osteoblasts, provide visible callus formation. Conversely, without blood supply, the precursors of bone, mesenchymal cells and nutrients, are not provided, and no bony callus is visible. Radiographic features common to both vascular and avascular nonunions are sclerotic fracture ends, a gap between fragments, a sealed marrow cavity, and fracture surfaces that are usually smooth and well defined (Figs. 49-1 and 49-3A).

Vascular nonunions are classically characterized by a nonbridging, "elephant's foot" type of callus. In other

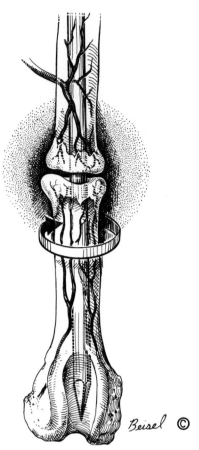

Fig. 49-1. *This schematic drawing of a vascular nonunion reveals the rotational instability (arrow) causing the problem. Note the well-established blood supply, sclerotic fracture ends, and "elephant's foot" callus production.*

words, plenty of callus is present, both proximal and distal to the fracture, but none bridges the fragments. An avascular nonunion shows little, if any, callus formation and bone atrophy above and below the fracture site. Pseudoarthrosis (false joint) is a term commonly used for the radiographic and clinical appearance of the fracture gap present with a nonunion. Histologically, this gap contains fibrous tissue and cartilage. A pseudoarthrosis may contain a synovial membrane and synovial fluid as well as cartilage (Figs. 49-1 and 49-3 A).

TREATMENT

The treatment of a nonunion depends upon the basic principle of recognizing the reason for the nonunion and correcting its cause. Principles of nonunion treatment include the following:

1. If the nonunion is due to instability, one must improve stability.
2. If due to infection, one must debride the wound and provide stability.
3. If due to inadequate blood supply and, therefore, osteoblasts, one must provide a cancellous bone graft.

4. Fibrous tissue and cartilage within a nonunion are pluripotential; they can convert to bone, given the proper environment.

The amount of blood supply and stability of the fracture appear to determine whether fibrous or cartilaginous tissue is laid down at the nonunion site. If the blood supply is adequate, fibrous tissue is laid down, whereas cartilaginous tissue is present if the blood supply is compromised. With an adequate blood supply, the fibrous tissue converts to bone when stability is provided. In the presence of cartilage, if stability is provided, a blood supply develops, and the cartilage converts to bone. In clinical situations, the nonunion is usually due to a combination of factors, all of which must be considered.

Considerations for treatment of vascular nonunions (Fig. 49-2) include the following:

1. A compression technique is preferred for fixation.
2. Debridement of tissue between bone ends is not necessary with compression techniques.
3. Bone grafting is usually not necessary.

Advantages of using a compression technique to treat vascular nonunions are the reduced fracture gap and rigid fixation afforded by the technique. The rigid fixation facilitates early exercise function, increases

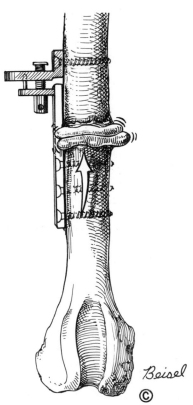

Fig. 49-2. *This illustration shows axial compression (arrow) being applied to the fracture to cause the pseudoarthrosis tissue to be "squeezed out" of the fracture site. (The compression jig is then removed from the plate, and the proximal screws are inserted). This method helps to speed the conversion of nonunion tissue to bone and to initiate primary bone healing.*

circulation, and prevents muscle atrophy. Moreover, as a direct stimulus, compression speeds the conversion of pseudoarthrosis tissue to bone. Therefore, the nonunion is simply managed by aligning and compressing the fracture ends, using any of a variety of compression plating systems.* Bone grafting is not necessary because the blood supply to the bone ends is already established, and plenty of osteoblasts are probably present. Bone healing occurs by direct ossification from the haversian canal, as evidenced by the lack of radiographic periosteal callus.

Considerations for treatment of avascular nonunions due to lack of stabilization and vascularity (Fig. 49-3) include:

1. Debridement of bone ends and opening up of the medullary canal.
2. Provision of stability under compression for rigid fixation, with a bone plate.
3. Decortication or fish scaling (Fig. 49-3 *D*), a process that involves chiseling a flap in the outer quarter to third of the cortex.
4. Provision of a cancellous bone graft.

INFECTED NONUNION

Infection is a common cause of nonunion and is often associated with fracture instability. The patient's medical history provides information as to the source of an infection, such as an open wound due to trauma or iatrogenic contamination due to surgical repair of the fracture. The patient's history and the physical examination may reveal draining tracts, not necessarily in the vicinity of the original fracture, with systemic and local signs of inflammation. The patient is not usually bearing normal weight on the limb, which may be painful to palpation. Radiographs typically show a combination of osteoproliferative and osteodestructive lesions.

Considerations for treatment of nonunions due to infection (Fig. 49-4) include:

1. Debridement of all infected tissue including sequestra, abscess cavities, dead bone ends, and scar tissue.
2. Intraoperative culture with sensitivity testing.
3. Provision of a bone plate under compression, if possible.
4. Maintenance of existing fixation devices if they contribute to stability.
5. Provision of a primary or delayed autogenous cancellous bone graft.
6. Wound drainage.
7. Intraoperative antibiotic or antiseptic flush with a 10% Betadine† solution (100 ml Betadine in 1000 ml normal saline solution) and postoperative parenteral or oral antibiotics.

* Supplied by the following, for example: Synthes, Ltd., 983 Old Eagle School Road, Wayne, PA 19087; Zimmer-Shaffner, Warsaw, IN 46580; Richards Manufacturing Co., Inc., 1450 Brooks Road, Memphis, TN 38116; and Kirschner-Collision, P.O. Box 459, Aberdeen, MD 21001.
† Purdue Frederick Co., 50 Washington Street, Norwalk, CT 06856

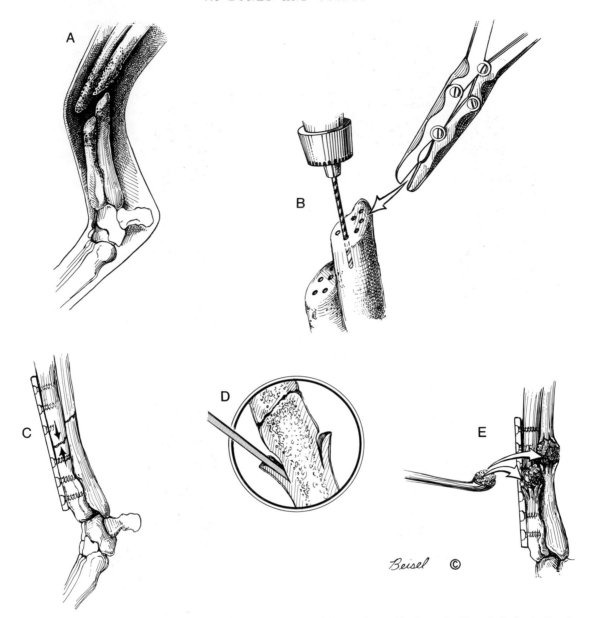

Fig. 49-3. A, *Avascular nonunion of the radius and ulna due to chronic instability and poor blood supply. Note the lack of callus formation, sealed marrow cavities, and bone atrophy above and below the fracture. B, Initially, the fracture ends are debrided (arrow), and the medullary cavities, both proximal and distal, are opened up by drilling small holes in the bone ends. C, Reduction and stabilization of the avascular nonunion are achieved using a six-hole dynamic compression plate. D, The cortical bone in the vicinity of the fracture is "fish-scaled" (decorticated) in order to expose osteogenic cells and to provide a greater surface area on which to pack a cancellous graft. E, An autogenous cancellous bone graft is harvested and is packed (arrow) around the fracture site.*

It is important to realize that infected nonunions of fractures heal in the presence of infection *if the nonunion is stable;* therefore, existing devices should not be removed if they are contributing to the stability of a fracture. Conversely, instability plays a large role in perpetuating an infected nonunion; thus, all loose fixation devices should be removed and replaced. An autogenous cancellous bone graft can be used, either primarily or as a delayed graft (when infection is under control) to hasten bone healing. Cancellous bone grafts are preferred to cortical grafts because cancellous bone, if infected, is resorbed, whereas cortical grafts can sequestrate. Wound drainage is necessary postoperatively to control dead space and to allow instillation of antibiotics or antiseptics.

It should not be assumed that a nonunion of a fracture can be treated only by means of a bone plate and compression. On the contrary, a nonunion can heal if compression is not used, but the nonunion site should be opened, and fibrous tissue or cartilage should be debrided down to bleeding bone (Fig. 49-5). A cancellous bone graft is then necessary for either vascular or

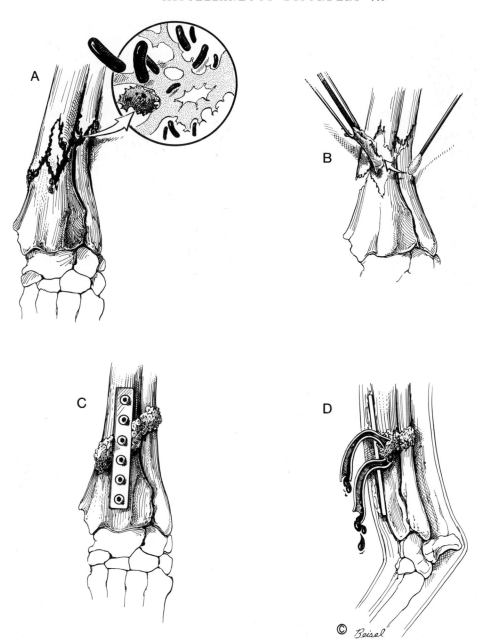

Fig. 49-4. A, *Nonunion of the radius and ulna due to infection and fracture instability. Inset, note the dead bone (sequestrum) surrounded by "pus." B, Initially, a bone culture is obtained, then all nonviable and infected tissues are debrided. (Vigorous flushing of the infection site, with an antiseptic solution or a lavage solution, is necessary with debridement of tissues). C, The fracture is reduced, and rigid stabilization is provided. Bone defects can be filled with an autogenous bone graft to eliminate dead space and to hasten bone healing. D, Drains are placed to prevent the buildup of fluid and to control dead space.*

avascular nonunions. All forms of fixation devices can be used, such as bone plates and screws, pins, Kirschner-Ehmer apparatus, transfixation pins, and tension-band wire. The result must, of course, be to achieve stabilization of the fracture.

Acknowledgment

I would like to express a special thanks to Dan Beisel for his incredible talent in putting my words into pictures.

References and Suggested Readings

Aron, D. N.: Management of delayed union and nonunion fractures in small animals. Compend. Contin. Ed. Practicing Vet., *1*:697, 1979.

Aron, D. N.: Pathogenesis, diagnosis, and management of osteomyelitis in small animals. Compend. Contin. Ed. Practicing Vet., *1*:824, 1979.

DeAngelis, M. P.: Causes of delayed union and nonunion of fractures. Vet. Clin. North Am., *5*:251, 1975.

Meyer, S., Weiland, A. J., and Willenegger, H.: The treatment of infected nonunion of fractures of long bones. J. Bone Joint Surg. [Am.], *57*:836, 1975.

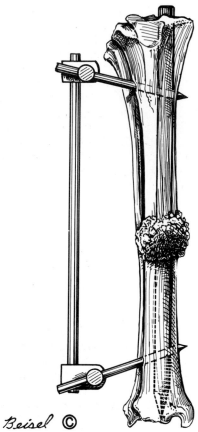

Beisel ©

Fig. 49-5. *This avascular nonunion of the tibia was treated by debridement of bone ends, opening of the medullary canals, placement of a Steinmann pin with a half-Kirschner splint for rigid stability, decortication, and placement of an autogenous cancellous bone graft.*

Müller, M. E., Allgöwer, M., Schneider, R., and Willenegger, H.: Manual of Internal Fixation. 2nd Ed. New York, Springer-Verlag, 1977.

Müller, M. E., and Thomas, R. J.: Treatment of nonunion in fractures of long bones. Clin. Orthop., *138*:141, 1979.

Piermattei, D. L.: Treatment of nonunion of fractures in the dog. *In* Proceedings of the 33rd Annual Meeting of the American Animal Hospital Association, San Francisco, 1966.

Rosen, H.: Compression treatment of long bone pseudoarthroses. Clin. Orthop., *138*:154, 1979.

Sumner-Smith, G.: Bone in Clinical Orthopaedics: A Study in Comparative Osteology. Philadelphia, W. B. Saunders, 1982.

Sumner-Smith, G., and Cawley, A. J.: Nonunion of fractures of the dog. J. Small Anim. Pract., *11*:311, 1970.

Osteochondritis Dissecans

by Joseph W. Alexander

Osteochondritis dissecans is a syndrome of the immature joint characterized by localized separation of articular cartilage and subchondral bone that may lead to the formation of a cartilage flap or ossicle. The cause

of this lesion in the dog is unknown. Several theories as to the etiology of osteochondritis dissecans have been proposed, including hypercalcitonism associated with overnutrition,[3] trauma to immature cartilage,[2] hormonal disturbances,[8] and osteonecrosis.[12] In a study of the development of the microcirculation of the humeral head in the dog, it was demonstrated that the bony epiphysis and its vasculature develop last on the medial aspect.[1] Because this region is the most common location for osteochondritis dissecans of the shoulder, it was suggested that the developing ossification front would be exposed to the effects of trauma for an extended period of time. It was postulated that this delay in ossification could be a factor in the development of the lesion.

Although this syndrome has been seen most frequently in the proximal end of the humerus, it has also been reported to occur in the distal humerus, distal femur, femoral head, distal radius, cervical spine, and recently, the tibial tarsal bone.

The natural course of the disease, which is intimately related to the history of the lesion itself, is variable. Free-floating "joint mice," partially detached chondroosseous fragments, and intact, essentially asymptomatic defects are all seen. It is not uncommon for the lesion to be bilateral; however, the clinical signs, radiographic findings, and course of the syndrome in one limb may differ from those in contralateral limbs.

Shoulder Joint

Osteochondritis dissecans of the shoulder is a lesion of the proximal humeral epiphysis. It has been reported to affect primarily young dogs, 4 to 12 months old, belonging to the large and giant breeds. The syndrome has rarely been reported in smaller breeds. Males are 2 to 5 times more likely to be affected than females.[11]

The most common presenting sign is a variable degree of lameness of one or both front limbs. Physical examination should localize the lesion because affected animals usually show pain or crepitation on extension or flexion of the shoulder joint(s).

A tentative diagnosis of osteochondritis dissecans can be confirmed by demonstration of the characteristic lesion on accurate mediolateral radiographs. Heavy sedation or general anesthesia is necessary to obtain diagnostic films. Pulling the affected shoulder forward, rotating the chest out of the radiographic field, and pulling the opposite shoulder caudally help to ensure satisfactory radiographs. The osteochondral defect is usually evident on the central portion of the caudal third of the articular surface of the humeral head. Both shoulders should be radiographed because a significant number of dogs have bilateral lesions.

Although it is possible that the loose cartilage flap may become partially reattached or may break off completely and subsequently lead to a resolution of the lameness, this phenomenon is the exception rather than the rule. In dogs showing pain and lameness, surgical intervention is indicated to relieve the immediate clinical signs and to prevent the development of degenerative joint disease.

SURGICAL TREATMENT

Several surgical approaches to the shoulder joint have been advocated. The following technique was originally described by Hohn.[5] The dog is positioned in lateral recumbency, and a craniolateral curved skin incision is made from the midpoint of the scapular spine to the midhumeral shaft (Fig. 49-6A). The subcutaneous fat is incised in the same line as the initial skin incision. The skin margins are undermined and are retracted. The underlying branches of the cephalic vein, the two bellies of the deltoideus muscle, and the omotransversarius muscle can now be identified (Fig. 49-6B). Using a periosteal elevator, the insertion of the acromial head of the deltoideus muscle is elevated subperiosteally off the humerus and is retracted in a caudal direction. This retraction exposes the underlying tendons of insertion of the infraspinatus muscle proximally and the teres minor muscle distally (Fig. 49-6C). The distal portion of the omotransversarius muscle is sharply dissected off the acromion and is retracted in a cranial direction along with a distal portion of the supraspinatus muscle. The infraspinatus tendon is then transected close to its insertion on the humerus.

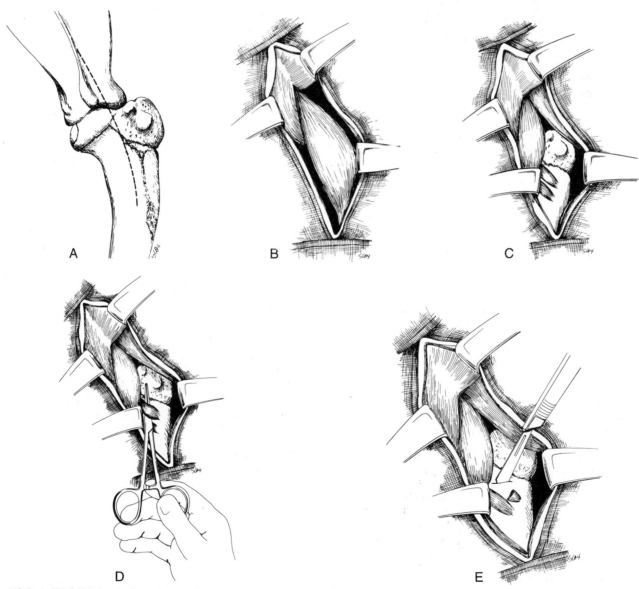

Fig. 49-6. A, *With the dog in lateral recumbency, a craniolateral curved incision is made from the midpoint of the scapular spine to the midhumeral shaft. B, The skin and subcutaneous tissues are reflected to expose the underlying acromial head of the deltoideus muscle and the supraspinatus muscle. C, The acromial head of the deltoideus muscle is retracted caudally to expose the underlying tendons of insertion of the infraspinatus muscle proximally and the teres minor muscle distally. D, The infraspinatus tendon is isolated and is transected close to its insertion on the humerus. E, The joint capsule is incised along the line of curvature of the humeral head.*

Special care must be taken to leave sufficient infraspinatus tendon on the humerus to allow reattachment at the time of closure (Fig. 49-6D). In order to make retrieval of the severed infraspinatus muscle easier at the time of closure, the muscle and its associated tendon can be "tagged" with a suture prior to severing the tendinous insertion. The capsule of the shoulder joint should now be exposed and is incised along the line of curvature of the humeral head so as to allow adequate capsular tissue on both sides of the incision for closure (Fig. 49-6E). Once the joint is opened, the lesion on the humeral head can be visualized by internally rotating the humerus and by dislocating the humeral head laterally.*

In the majority of patients, the loose cartilage flap is removed, and the flap bed is curetted down to bleeding subchondral bone. Initially, granulation tissue and, ultimately, fibrocartilage fill in the curetted defect in the articular surface. The joint is thoroughly irrigated, and any floating "joint mice" or bony ossicles attached to the joint capsule are removed.

In selected cases, I have attempted to bring about a primary repair, by gently lifting up the cartilage flap, taking care not to break it off, and curetting the underlying subchondral bed. At least three cortical "matchstick" grafts are then collected from the proximolateral humeral shaft with an oscillating saw or an osteotome and mallet. (Fig. 49-7A). A small Steinmann pin is used to drill guide holes through the dorsal surface of the

*Editor's Note: An alternate approach to the shoulder joint involves dissecting between the acromial and scapular heads of the deltoideus muscle to expose the teres minor muscle. Unless the patient is unusually heavily muscled in this area, the teres minor muscle can then be "rolled" craniodorsally to expose the joint capsule without muscle transection.

cartilage flap into the underlying subchondral bed. The matchstick grafts are then driven into the guide holes. These grafts fix the cartilage flap to the prepared subchondral bed and allow primary healing to take place (Fig. 49-7B).

Closure is accomplished by suturing the joint capsule with an absorbable suture in a simple continuous pattern. The tendon of the infraspinatus muscle is reattached to its insertion on the humerus with a nonabsorbable suture using a horizontal mattress pattern. The subcutaneous tissue and skin are closed in a routine manner. Postoperatively, the patient's activity is restricted to leash exercise for 2 weeks.

Elbow

Osteochondritis dissecans of the canine elbow develops on the medial humeral condyle. Although the condition is uncommon, it is one of several disorders that must be included in the differential diagnosis of osteoarthritis of the elbow joint. The syndrome has been reported to occur as an isolated lesion and in combination with an ununited coronoid process.[13] Osteochondritis dissecans of the elbow joint is seen most often in growing large and giant breeds of dogs. Unlike in man, in whom osteochondritis dissecans of the elbow occurs almost exclusively in males, both canine sexes have been reported to be affected.

Dogs with this syndrome are presented to the veterinarian because of a lameness of the involved limb(s). Pain upon manipulation of the elbow, reduced range of motion in the joint, and crepitation are the most common clinical findings. Craniocaudal radiographs of the elbow reveal a saucer-shaped defect surrounded by a

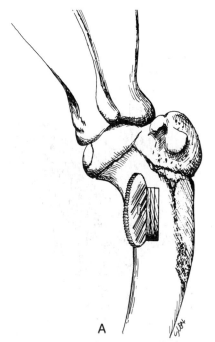

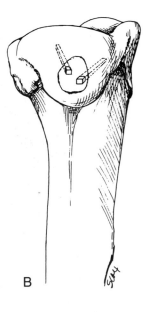

Fig. 49-7. A, *Cortical "matchstick" grafts are collected from the proximolateral humeral shaft with an oscillating saw.* B, *Two of the three cortical "matchstick" grafts have been placed in the osteochondral flap.*

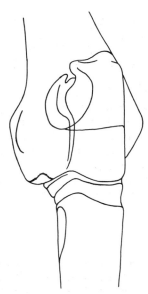

Fig. 49-8. *Diagrammatic representation of radiographic findings in osteochondritis dissecans of the elbow.*

sclerotic zone in the articular cartilage of the medial condyle of the humerus (Fig. 49-8).

SURGICAL TREATMENT

The treatment for osteochondritis dissecans of the elbow is the same as that of the shoulder, that is, osteochondroplasty by removal of the cartilage flap and curettage of the remaining cartilage defect. Two approaches to the medial side of the elbow have been described in the veterinary literature.[4,7] The technique outlined in this discussion involves a flexor muscle tenotomy.

In this approach, a medial skin incision is made from midhumerus to midradius and ulna, with the medial humeral epicondyle as the midpoint (Fig. 49-9A). Following dissection of the subcutaneous tissue, the pronator teres muscle and the flexor carpi radialis muscle are identified at their tendons of origin on the medial humeral epicondyle. Both muscles are isolated by blunt dissection and are individually transected close to their origin. Care should be taken to leave sufficient tendon on both the epicondyle and the muscle bellies to allow a strong closure. The median artery and nerve lie deep to the pronator teres muscle and should be identified at the time of this muscle's transection (Fig. 49-9B). An incision is then made through the medial collateral ligament and the underlying joint capsule parallel to the joint space. To expose the articular surface of the medial condyle of the humerus, the forearm is rotated laterally and pulled distally. The loose cartilage flap is removed and the cartilage crater is curetted down to bleeding subchondral bone. Prior to closure the joint should be lavaged with a saline solution. Closure is accomplished by suturing the flexor carpi radialis muscle and the pronator teres muscle back to their respective tendons of origin. The remainder of the closure is routine.

Postoperatively, the limb is placed in a Robert Jones dressing for 5 days. Early weight-bearing is encouraged, but the patient's activity is restricted to leash exercise for 2 weeks.

Stifle

Although osteochondritis dissecans of the stifle has been reported to occur in both the lateral and medial femoral condyles, the most common site for this lesion is the medial aspect of the weight-bearing surface of

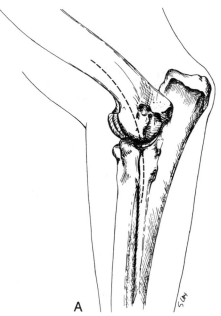

A

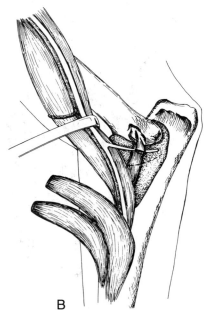

B

Fig. 49-9. A, *A medial skin incision is made from the midhumerus to the midradius and ulna with the medial humeral epicondyle as the midpoint.* B, *The pronator teres muscle and the flexor carpi radialis muscle are both transected at their respective tendons of origin.*

the lateral femoral condyle. The disease is usually seen in large or giant breeds of dogs between the ages of 3 and 9 months. This disorder has been reported to occur in littermates and in conjunction with osteochondritis dissecans of the shoulder.[6]

The dog is usually presented to the veterinarian because of a weight-bearing lameness of the involved limb. Physical examination usually reveals discomfort and, in long-standing cases, crepitation upon flexion and extension of the stifle joint. The diagnosis can be confirmed by an arthroscopic examination of the stifle joint and by radiographic studies. A craniocaudal radiograph demonstrates the characteristic radiolucent area on the distal end of the affected condyle. An osteochondral flap may be partially detached from the articular surface or may even be free-floating within the joint space (Fig. 49-10).

SURGICAL TREATMENT

Surgical intervention through a standard arthrotomy, with removal of the offending osteochondral flap and any free floating "joint mice," usually is successful in resolving the lameness if osteoarthritic changes within the joint are not already advanced.

Hock

Osteochondritis dissecans of the canine hock joint affects the tibial tarsal bone, primarily the medial ridge of the trochlea. Most dogs are presented to the clinician because of a sudden onset of a weight-bearing lameness. The clinical signs usually develop between the ages of 4 and 8 months, affect primarily large or giant breeds, and although both sexes have been reported to have the syndrome, it is seen most frequently in males. The disease commonly occurs bilaterally; however, the clinical signs and course in one limb may differ from those in the opposite limb.

Physical examination usually reveals joint distension, especially on the medial aspect of the tarsus, and pain upon flexion of the tibiotarsal joint. In advanced

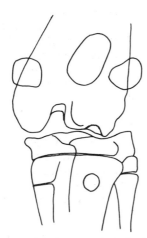

Fig. 49-10. *Diagrammatic representation of radiographic findings in osteochondritis dissecans of the stifle joint.*

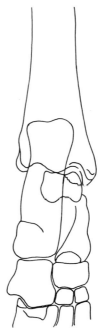

Fig. 49-11. *Diagrammatic drawing of radiographic findings in osteochondritis dissecans of the hock joint.*

cases, crepitation and a reduced range of motion may be a feature of this syndrome. Marked hyperextension of the hock is a common conformational fault associated with osteochondritis dissecans of this joint.

Radiographic findings include joint distension, a radiolucent bony defect on the medial ridge of the talus, the presence of variably sized mineralized joint bodies, and evidence of remodeling of the distal tibia and lateral medial malleolus (Fig. 49-11).

SURGICAL TREATMENT

The surgical goal in treating osteochondritis dissecans of the hock is the same as for other joints: removal of the cartilaginous flap and any free-floating "joint mice." A caudomedial approach to the tibiotarsal joint is used to accomplish these objectives. For this approach, the dog is placed in lateral recumbency with the affected leg down. An incision is made, following the angle of the hock, just caudal to the medial malleolus of the tibia (Fig. 49-12A). The superficial branch of the tibial nerve, the plantar branch of the saphenous artery, the superficial plantar metatarsal vein, and the deep digital flexor tendon should be identified and should be retracted caudally toward the tuber calcanei (Fig. 49-12B). The joint capsule is then incised in a longitudinal direction, and the hock is flexed to expose the affected trochlear ridge. When increased exposure is required, a technique has been described that involves a medial malleolar osteotomy.[10]

Surgical treatment of osteochondritis dissecans of the hock differs from that of other joints in that curettage of the cartilage flap bed is contraindicated. A follow-up study on dogs with this hock disorder that had undergone flap removal and curettage down to sub-

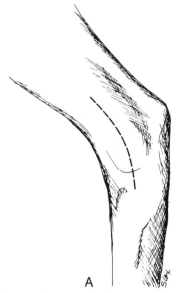
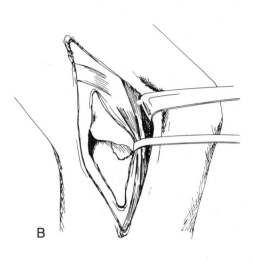

Fig. 49-12. A, *An incision is made, following the angle of the hock, just caudal to the medial malleolus of the tibia.* B, *Incising the joint capsule in a longitudinal direction and flexing the hock joint expose the lesion of the trochlear ridge (talus).*

chondral bone revealed that osteoarthritic changes had become progressive after surgical treatment.[9] This investigator concluded that this complication was due to increased joint instability caused by a flattening of the medial ridge of the trochlea of the tibial tarsal bone secondary to curettage of the flap bed.

The joint space is irrigated with a saline solution, and closure of the surgical site is routine. The tarsal joint is supported with a soft bandage for the first 7 to 10 postoperative days, after which controlled exercise is encouraged. The progress in patients with osteochondritis dissecans of the hock is generally good if surgical therapy is initiated prior to the development of advanced degenerative joint disease.

References and Suggested Readings

1. Carrig, C. B., and Morgan, J. P.: Microcirculation of the humeral head in the immature dog. J. Am. Vet. Radiol. Soc., *25*:28, 1974.
2. Craig, P. H., and Riser, W. H.: Osteochondritis dissecans in the proximal humerus of the dog. J. Am. Vet. Radiol. Soc., *6*:40, 1965.
3. Hedhammer, A., et al.: Overnutrition and skeletal disease. an experimental study in growing Great Dane dogs. Cornell Vet., *64*:1, 1974.
4. Henry, W. B., Wadsworth, P. L., and Mehlhoff, C. J.: Medial approach to elbow joint with osteotomy of medial epicondyle. J. Am. Coll. Vet. Surg., *8*:46, 1979.
5. Hohn, R. B.: Osteochondritis dissecans of the humeral head. J. Am. Vet. Med. Assoc., *163*:69, 1973.
6. Knecht, C. D., et al.: Osteochondritis of the shoulder and stifle in 3 of 5 border collie littermates. J. Am. Vet. Med. Assoc., *170*:58, 1977.
7. McCurnin, D. M., Slusher, R., and Grier, R. L.: A medial approach to the canine elbow joint. J. Am. Anim. Hosp. Assoc., *12*:475, 1976.
8. Paatsama, S., et al.: Somatotropin, thyrotropin and corticotropin hormone—induced changes in the cartilage and bones of the shoulder and knee joints in young dogs. J. Small Anim. Pract., *12*:595, 1971.
9. Rosenblum, G., Rogins, G. M., and Carlisle, C. H.: Osteochondritis dissecans of the tibiotarsal joint in the dog. J. Small Anim. Pract., *19*:759, 1978.
10. Sinibaldi, K. R.: Medial approach to the tarsus. J. Am. Anim. Hosp. Assoc., *15*:77, 1979.
11. Smith, C. W., and Stavater, J. L.: Osteochondritis of the canine shoulder joint. A review of 35 cases. J. Am. Anim. Hosp. Assoc., *11*:658, 1978.
12. Vaughn, L. C., and Jones, D. G. C.: Osteochondritis dissecans of the head of the humerus in dogs. J. Small Anim. Pract., *9*:283, 1968.
13. Wolfe, D. A.: Surgical correction of osteochondritis dissecans of the medial humeral condyle and ununited coronoid process in a dog. VM SAC, *71*:1554, 1976.

Osteomyelitis

by Dennis D. Caywood

Osteomyelitis is an inflammation of the bone marrow and adjacent bone. Although generally a result of infection, osteomyelitis may occur following local radiation therapy, implant corrosion, or trauma. In spite of recent developments, refinements in surgical techniques, and continued developments in antibiotic therapy, the treatment of osteomyelitis still presents a significant challenge to the veterinary clinician.

Etiopathogenesis

Bacteria can reach bone by a number of pathways; however, the presence of bacteria in bone alone is not enough to cause disease. It appears that bacteria, vascular occlusion secondary to septic thrombosis, and the resulting bone necrosis are equally important in establishing infection.

As osteomyelitis develops, the acute inflammatory response results in the production of exudate-containing bacteria. Enzymes from disintegrating polymorphonuclear leukocytes cause further necrosis. Destruction of cancellous bone, thinning of cortical bone, and erosion of the periosteum lead to soft tissue abscess. In addition, necrotic cortical bone, from inflammation, fracture, or surgical procedures, in the presence of bacteria allows the infection to persist. Inflammatory cells isolate the necrotic bone from viable granulation tissue and prevent demineralization and subsequent resorption. Later, fibrous tissue and newly formed bone further isolate bone from the body's defense mechanisms in an attempt to heal the lesion. This repair is the maximum that the body can ordinarily accomplish. Unfortunately, infection may become reactivated at any time following necrosis of the involucrum.

The majority of bone infections are associated with fractures. In most cases, bacteria gain access to bone during open reduction procedures. Open fractures with initial direct contamination account for a smaller percentage of infections. Many cases of osteomyelitis involving the feet result from an extension of soft tissue infections. Unlike osteomyelitis in humans, hematogenous infections are not commonly observed in the dog and cat.

Diagnosis

The patient's medical history and the physical examination generally enable the clinician to localize the disease process. Local pyrexia, swelling, draining abscesses, pain, and lameness are common clinical signs. Leukocytosis is not a consistent finding, particularly in chronic osteomyelitis. The diagnosis must be based on radiographic studies and positive culture results.

The bony changes associated with infection are limited primarily to local destruction and new bone formation. These changes are observed radiographically as lytic lesions, periosteal new bone, and areas of increased bone density. Typical lytic and periosteal bone changes do not appear until 10 to 14 days following the onset of infection. Soft tissue changes are occasionally observed within 24 hours, however. Such changes are characterized by local swelling and loss of demarcation between fascia and muscle planes.

The majority of the organisms isolated from cases of canine and feline osteomyelitis are gram-positive. Staphylococcus is isolated in 45 to 50% of patients and is the most frequent isolate, regardless of the source of infection. Although staphylococcus is identified in a high percentage of infections, gram-negative bacteria are often present when more than one species is involved. The high percentage of mixed infections in the dog and cat commonly results from exposed traumatic or operative wounds and extension of soft tissue infections. Mixed infections generally involve 2 or 3 species of organisms.

Treatment

A combination of surgical and antibiotic therapy is usually essential in the treatment of bone infections. Early infections without extensive vascular fibrous tissue and necrotic bone involvement may respond to antibiotic therapy alone. Selection of the appropriate antibiotic depends on the proper identification and antibiotic sensitivity of the causative organism(s). Fine-needle aspiration and a culture of the affected bone may avoid many surface bacterial contaminates encountered in a draining wound. A bone biopsy and culture are necessary when other culture techniques do not isolate an organism.

It is often necessary to begin parenteral antibiotic therapy while awaiting positive culture and sensitivity test results. It is advisable to begin with a combination of bacteriocidal antibiotics. I prefer the combination of gentamicin and ampicillin until a specific organism(s) and sensitivity pattern are identified.

Treatment of osteomyelitis of the digits presents unique problems. Early infections may respond to antibiotic therapy and wound management, but patients with extensive soft tissue involvement associated with chronic osteomyelitis of the phalanges, metacarpals, and metatarsals are best managed by amputation.

ACUTE OSTEOMYELITIS

Although antibiotics are of great benefit, they are usually not curative. The mainstay of therapy is surgical intervention. Decompression and drainage of the affected bone are recommended in acute osteomyelitis to prevent further cortical and medullary bone necrosis.

SURGICAL TECHNIQUE. The surgical approach is generally directly over the lesion of the affected bone. When possible, the incision should be placed to allow dependent drainage. The skin and subcutaneous incision is limited to a length of 2 to 4 cm. The deeper muscle and fascial layers are separated by a combination of sharp and blunt dissection. Knowledge of the regional anatomic structures is important to prevent damage to nerve and blood supply. If the infection is confined to the medullary cavity, surgical decompression can be accomplished by trephinization (Fig. 49-13A and B). Culture and biopsy samples may be obtained at this time. The medullary cavity and surrounding areas are flushed with either a saline-antibiotic or a saline-povidone-iodine solution. All visible exudates and fluids are aspirated from the wound. The wound is then packed open using antibiotic dressings or umbilical tape impregnated with povidone-iodine solution (Fig. 49-13C). The area should be protected against contamination of its surroundings, and the limb should be immobilized. A Robert Jones bandage accomplishes both objectives. The bandage and dressings need to be changed daily until wound exudation diminishes. Wound dressings are removed 10 to 14 days following decompression, and the wound is allowed to heal by granulation. Parenteral antibiotics should be continued for 30 to 60 days, and the bone should be evaluated radiographically every 10 to 14 days.

Subsequent draining abscesses mark the onset of chronic osteomyelitis and the need for a more vigorous surgical approach.

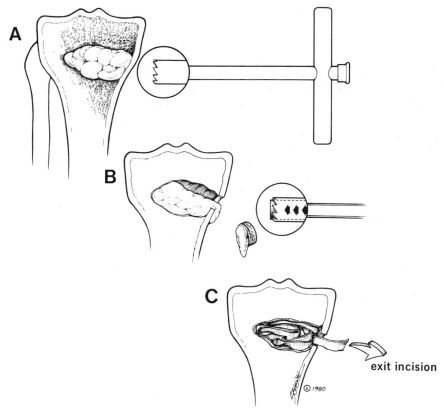

Fig. 49-13. *Treatment of acute osteomyelitis. A, Infection confined to the medullary cavity. B, Surgical decompression by trephinization. C, Wound packed open using umbilical tape impregnated with povidone-iodine solution.*

CHRONIC OSTEOMYELITIS

Because the majority of bone infections result from open reduction of fractures, the veterinary surgeon often encounters chronic osteomyelitis associated with metallic implants. Implants should not be removed if they maintain bone stability and if radiographic evidence of healing exists. The infection often is not eliminated until the implant is removed following fracture union, however. If the implant does not provide stability, it should be removed, and stability should be achieved by other means. The use of full-pin and half-pin splintage is preferred to intramedullary pins, bone plates, and screws for two reasons: (1) chronic osteomyelitis persists as long as a metallic implant is located at the site of infection, and (2) intramedullary pins spread infection through the medullary canal. In addition, full- or half-pin splintage devices can be positioned without disruption of the blood supply to the soft tissues near the fracture site.

In chronic infection, vascular fibrosis tissue, inflammatory cells, and newly formed bone isolate necrotic bone and organisms from the body's defense mechanisms and systemically administered antibiotics. Therefore, the treatment of chronic osteomyelitis necessitates meticulous debridement of all infected tissues.

Although closed irrigation-suction techniques have gained considerable popularity in human medicine, semiclosed packing techniques are advocated in the management of chronic osteomyelitis in the dog and cat. A semiclosed packing technique has been shown to have a success rate similar to that with closed irrigation-suction procedures. In addition, three disadvantages encountered with closed irrigation-suction systems make them inconvenient in veterinary practice: (1) constant monitoring of the patient is required to ensure fluid infusion and suction; drain obstruction disrupts the blood supply to the limbs; (2) large volumes of fluids and antibiotics are needed; and (3) it may be difficult to prevent the animal from pulling out the tubing and associated devices needed for irrigation-suction techniques.

Bone debridement commonly leaves large bony deficits associated with either the initial fracture or the remaining weakened bone. For this reason, autogenous cancellous and cortical cancellous bone grafts are used in the surgical management of osteomyelitis.

A two-step surgical approach allows initial elimination of the infection from the wound and subsequent grafting and fixation of the bone. This approach eliminates the possibility of interfering with the graft when treating the infected wound and decreases reinfection at the graft site.

SURGICAL TECHNIQUE: STEP 1. The surgical approach should give wide exposure to the bone and should allow complete visualization of all infected tissues. The sequestra are removed individually, and ostectomy is performed on infected bone with rongeurs, to create a "saucer" in the remaining viable bone (Fig. 49-14*A* to *C*). Infected and vascular fibrous soft tissues are also removed. The area is flushed with a saline-antibiotic or a saline-povidone-iodine solution, and all fluids and exudates are aspirated. The bone is often severely weakened following partial ostectomy and creation of the saucer-shaped defect. A half- or a full-pin splint may be applied to provide stabilization or to prevent fracture (Fig. 49-14*D*). The bony deficit is then packed with umbilical tape impregnated with povidone-iodine solution, with one end of the tape exiting the wound through a stab incision away from the approach incision (Fig. 49-14*E* and *F*). The approach is closed routinely, and the limb is immobilized in a Robert Jones bandage. The bandage may need to be changed daily until exudation diminishes. The umbilical tape is removed from the wound 10 to 14 days following the operation, and the patient is given antibiotics for a 30- to 60-day period. The bone is evaluated radiographically every 2 to 3 weeks.

In approximately 30 to 60 days, when the infection is eliminated from the wound, bone grafting and other forms of fracture fixation may be used. Success rates are lower if fixation and grafting are attempted before wound sterilization is ensured.

SURGICAL TECHNIQUE: STEP 2. The skin over the proximal humerus, ribs, and wing of the ilium is prepared for an aseptic surgical procedure. Preparation of several potential autogenous cancellous and corticocancellous bone graft sites ensures adequate graft to fill large

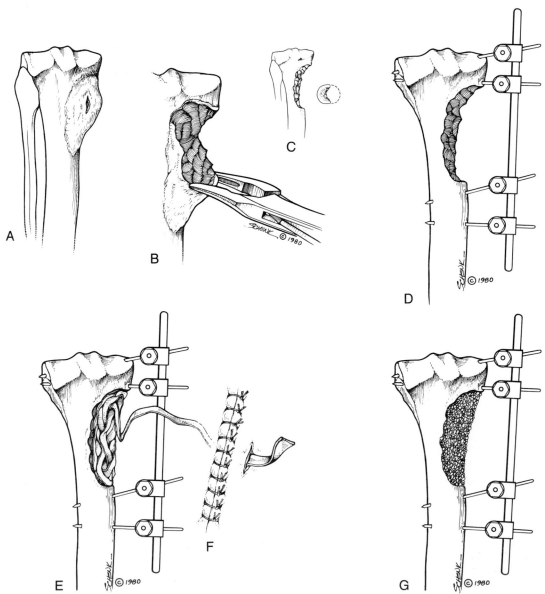

Fig. 49-14. A *to* C, *Partial ostectomy of infected bone using rongeurs.* D, *A full Kirschner apparatus is applied to stabilize the weakened bone following partial ostectomy.* E, *The bone deficit is packed with umbilical tape impregnated with povidone-iodine solution.* F, *One end of the tape exits through a stab incision away from the approach incision.* G, *The entire bone deficit is filled with a cancellous bone graft. (The proximal pin should ideally remain distal to the joint.)*

bone deficits. Each area is draped separately, and strict asepsis is maintained. The area of the previous infection is approached as in Step 1 of this technique. A separate veterinary surgeon, or a single surgeon regloving and regowning, approaches the graft sites using separate instruments. Cancellous or corticocancellous bone is obtained and is passed in sponges moistened with saline solution to the site to be grafted. The donor sites are closed to prevent their possible contamination.

If the medullary cavities have sealed, they may be re-established by drilling with an intramedullary pin. Sclerotic bone ends may be removed with rongeurs. The entire deficit is filled with bone graft (Fig. 49-14G). Previous half- or full-pin splintage is maintained, or alternate fixation may be applied. The wound is closed primarily.

Prognosis

The prognosis of this disorder depends on the location, duration, and severity of bone involvement as well as on the development of clinical complications, if any. Acute infections with limited bone involvement, particularly those involving the feet, have a good prognosis. Chronic infections with extensive bone necrosis and soft tissue abscessation warrant a guarded prognosis. If clinical complications develop in a patient with osteomyelitis, the prognosis depends on the systems affected, the severity of the complications, and the surgical accessibility of the lesion.

References and Suggested Readings

Caywood, D. D., Wallace, L. J., and Braden, T. D.: Osteomyelitis in the dog: a review of 67 cases. J. Am. Vet. Med. Assoc., *172*:943, 1978.

Nunamaker, D. M.: Management of infected fractures: osteomyelitis. Vet. Clin. North Am., *5*:259, 1975.

Smith, C. W., Schiller, A. G., Smith, A. R., and Dorner, J. L.: Osteomyelitis in the dog: a retrospective study. J. Am. Anim. Hosp. Assoc., *14*:589, 1978.

Walker, M. A., et al.: Radiographic signs of bone infections in small animals. J. Am. Vet. Med. Assoc., *166*:908, 1975.

Wingfield, W. E.: Surgical treatment of chronic osteomyelitis in dogs. J. Am. Anim. Hosp. Assoc., *11*:568, 1975.

Index

Numbers followed by a "t" indicate tables.